# Head and Neck Imaging

# Head and Neck Imaging

## —— FOURTH EDITION ——

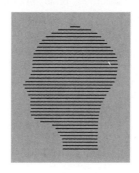

*EDITED BY*

### Peter M. Som, M.D.

Professor of Radiology and Otolaryngology
Mount Sinai School of Medicine of New York University;
Chief of Head and Neck Radiology
Mount Sinai Hospital
New York, New York

### Hugh D. Curtin, M.D.

Professor of Radiology
Harvard Medical School;
Chief of Radiology
Department of Radiology
Massachusetts Eye and Ear Infirmary
Boston, Massachusetts

Mosby

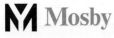

*An Affiliate of Elsevier Science*

11830 Westline Industrial Drive
St. Louis, Missouri 63146

HEAD AND NECK IMAGING

Set ISBN:0-323-00942-5
Volume 1: 9997626044

FOURTH EDITION

**Library of Congress Cataloging-in-Publication Data**

Head and neck imaging/[edited by] Peter M. Som, Hugh D. Curtin—4th ed.
     p. ; cm.
   Includes bibliographical references and index.
   ISBN 0-323-00942-5
     1. Head—Imaging. 2. Neck—Imaging. I. Som, Peter M. II. Curtin, Hugh D.
   [DNLM: 1. Head—radiography. 2. Magnetic Resonance Imaging. 3.
Neck—radiography. 4. Tomography, X-Ray Computed. WE 705 H43031 2003]
   RC936 .H43 2003
   617.5′10754—dc21

          2002075146

*Acquisitions Editor:* Janice Gaillard
*Developmental Editor:* Hazel Hacker, Heather Krehling

GW/MVY

Printed in the United States of America

Last digit is the print number:  9  8  7  6  5  4  3  2  1

*To Judy and Carole,*

*As we worked the long hours on this edition, the two of you gave us encouragement, support, love, and showed exceptional tolerance. We truly appreciate all that you did for us and the time that you allowed us to have in order to make this fourth edition possible. It is with our love and thanks that we dedicate* Head and Neck Imaging *to you.*

**P.M.S. and H.D.C.**

# Preface

When we embarked on the fourth edition of *Head and Neck Imaging,* every attempt was made to address the constructive comments we received from readers and reviewers of the third edition. Thus, the organization of this book has been modified and because many readers wanted *Head and Neck Imaging* to serve as a single definitive reference, the fourth edition has been expanded. *Head and Neck Imaging* is now more encyclopedic and detailed, presents more pathology, contains more images, and covers new imaging technologies. Although space limitations and a publishing date never allow a text to be truly all-encompassing, we have attempted to comply as thoroughly as possible with these requests.

The table of contents reflects a re-organization of the book. Compared to the third edition, this edition not only contains several new atlases of normal anatomy, but in many areas there are more detailed discussions of the anatomy. Pertinent physiology is now more thoroughly discussed to allow a better understanding of the function of the specific anatomic units. The pathology sections throughout the book have been enlarged to not only be more inclusive, but also to provide updated and more complete nomenclature and references for each disease. These enlarged sections also discuss pertinent statistics, new genetic concepts relating to a disease, epidemiological data, and contain a more detailed description of the pathology. As pathology is ever more becoming the final arbiter of disease, we believe that *Head and Neck Imaging* should serve, as much as possible, as a resource for this information.

Toward the pursuit of a more complete understanding of the field of head and neck imaging, a chapter discussing the current concepts of the genetics of tumor development and metastasis has been included. This chapter was added because we believe that in the near future, genetic-based imaging, a field now in its infancy, will become a considerably more important technology.

Being an imaging book, many new images have been included and unique older images have been upgraded. In addition, there is now a long overdue new chapter on ultrasound. The inclusion of this chapter fills a deficiency in the prior editions of *Head and Neck Imaging.* There is also a chapter dealing with the use of newer imaging modalities such as PET, MR-spectroscopy, and Thallium-201 imaging. The inclusion of these new sections better rounds out the scope of modalities that are currently being utilized in the field. There are also new chapters on swallowing studies, the trachea, skin and soft tissue lesions, and neural tumor spread. The paranasal sinus plain film section of the third edition was retained, as the growth of emergency room medicine has resulted in a resurgence of the use of these films.

The quality of any book is dependent on the excellence of the contributors' chapters. We were especially fortunate that our contributors submitted thorough, current, and detailed chapters accompanied by high quality images. As editors, it is always a pleasure to work with such wonderful material. In addition to asking some contributors from previous editions to again help us, there are many new contributors to the fourth edition. We are especially pleased with the enthusiastic contributions made by these new contributors, as these radiologists represent the future of the field.

Last, but far from least, the editors want to thank all of the editorial people at Saunders/Mosby, without whose guidance, patience, and knowledgeable advice this edition could not have been made. It was through their efforts that a new fresh format for the book was created. This includes more reference charts and tables, and a ''new look'' that we believe will make the fourth edition more accessible to our readers.

It is our hope that our readers will utilize the fourth edition of *Head and Neck Imaging* to not only help them in the diagnosis of head and neck imaging cases, but as a resource for the knowledge that is necessary to attain a well informed understanding of this fascinating and rewarding field.

Sincerely,

P.M.S.
H.D.C.

# Contributors

**Nadir G. Abdelrahman, M.D.**
Post-Doctoral Fellow,
Massachusetts General Hospital,
Boston, Massachusetts

**James J. Abrahams, M.D.**
Professor of Diagnostic Radiology (Neuroradiology)
  and Surgery (Otolaryngology),
Director of Medical Studies,
Yale University School of Medicine,
New Haven, Connecticut

**Yoshiaki Akimoto, D.D.S., Ph.D.**
Department of Oral Surgery,
Nihon University School of Dentistry at Matsudo,
Chiba, Japan

**Sait Albayram, M.D.**
Assistant Professor, Radiology,
Cerrahpasa Medical School,
Department of Radiology,
Kocamustafapasa Istanbul, Turkey

**Suzanne Aquino, M.D.**
Associate Radiologist,
Massachusetts General Hospital,
Assistant Professor of Radiology,
Harvard Medical School,
Boston, Massachusetts

**Derek C. Armstrong**
Staff, Division of Neuroradiology,
The Hospital for Sick Children,
Assistant Professor,
University of Toronto,
Toronto, Canada

**Armand Balboni, M.Phil**
Center for Anatomy and Functional Morphology,
The Lillian and Henry M. Stratton-Hans Popper
  Department of Pathology,
Mount Sinai School of Medicine,
New York University,
New York, New York

**Mark A. Augustyn, M.D.**
Ohio State University,
Columbus, Ohio

**Shahid Aziz, D.M.D., M.D.**
Assistant Professor,
University of Medicine and Dentistry of New Jersey,
New Jersey Dental School,
Newark, New Jersey

**Bruce S. Bauer, M.D., F.A.C.S.**
Chief, Division of Plastic Surgery,
The Children's Memorial Hospital,
Associate Professor of Surgery,
The Feinberg School of Medicine,
Northwestern University,
Chicago, Illinois

**Mark L. Benson, M.D.**
President, Radiology Associates, Inc.
Wheeling Hospital,
Wheeling, West Virginia

**Jorge Bianchi, D.M.D., M.M.Sc.**
Clinical Fellow in Head and Neck Radiology,
Massachusetts Eye and Ear Infirmary,
Boston, Massachusetts

**Larissa T. Bilaniuk, M.D.**
Staff Neuroradiologist,
Children's Hospital of Philadelphia,
Professor of Radiology,
University of Pennsylvania School of Medicine,
Philadelphia, Pennsylvania

**Susan I. Blaser, M.D.**
Staff Neuroradiologist,
Division of Neuroradiology,
The Hospital for Sick Children
Associate Professor,
Medical Imaging,
University of Toronto,
Toronto, Canada

**Margaret S. Brandwein, M.D.**
Associate Professor of Pathology and Otolaryngology,
Mount Sinai School of Medicine,
New York, New York

**Jan W. Casselman, M.D., Ph.D.**
Director of MRI and Head and Neck Radiology,
Department of Medical Imaging—MRI
A.Z. Sint-Jan Brugge A.V., Bruges
A.Z. Sint-Augustinus, Antwerp, Belgium

**J.A. Castelijns**
Professor Doctor,
VU Medical Centre,
Amsterdam, The Netherlands

**Donald W. Chakeres, M.D.**
Professor of Radiology,
Department of Radiology,
Head of Neuroradiology and MRI Research,
Ohio State University,
Columbus, Ohio

**Hugh D. Curtin, M.D.**
Chief of Radiology,
Massachusetts Eye and Ear Infirmary,
Professor of Radiology,
Harvard Medical School,
Boston, Massachusetts

**Bradley N. Delman, M.D.**
Assistant Attending Radiologist,
Mount Sinai Medical Center,
Assistant Professor of Radiology,
Mount Sinai School of Medicine of New York
    University,
New York, New York

**Nancy J. Fischbein, M.D.**
Assistant Professor of Radiology,
University of California at San Francisco,
San Francisco, California

**Lawrence E. Ginsberg, M.D.**
Associate Professor, Radiology and Head
    and Neck Surgery,
University of Texas,
M.D. Anderson Cancer Center,
Houston, Texas

**Tessa Goldsmith, M.A., C.C.C./S.L.P**
Clinical Specialist-Speech Language Pathologist,
Massachusetts General Hospital,
Boston, Massachusetts

**Anton N. Hasso, M.D.**
Professor, Department of Radiological Sciences,
Director, Neuroimaging Research and Development,
College of Medicine,
Professor of Radiological Science,
Professor of Otolaryngology,
Head and Neck Surgery,
University of California at Irvine,
Orange, California

**Roy A. Holliday, M.D.**
Director of Radiology,
The New York Eye and Ear Infirmary,
Professor of Clinical Radiology,
Albert Einstein College of Medicine,
New York, New York

**Michael W. Hayt, M.D., D.M.D.**
Director of Neuroradiology,
Center for Diagnostic Radiology,
Winter Park, Florida

**Patricia A. Hudgins, M.D.**
Professor of Radiology/Neuroradiology,
Director of Neuroradiology Fellowship Program,
Emory University School of Medicine/Hospital,
Atlanta, Georgia

**Edward M. Johnson, Ph.D.**
Vice-Chairman for Research,
Department of Pathology,
Associate Director for Shared Resources,
D.H. Ruttenberg Cancer Center,
Professor,
Pathology, Molecular Biology, and Cancer Biology,
Mount Sinai School of Medicine,
New York, New York

**Takashi Kaneda, D.D.S., Ph.D.**
Chief and Professor of Radiology,
Department of Radiology,
Nihon University School of Dentistry at Matsudo,
Japan

**Edward E. Kassel, D.D.S., M.D., F.R.C.P.C.,
F.A.C.R**
Neuroradiologist,
Mount Sinai Hospital and University Health Network,
Associate Professor,
Departments of Medical Imaging, Otolaryngology,
    and Ophthalmology,
University of Toronto,
Toronto, Canada

**Todd T. Kingdom, M.D.**
Director, Rhinology and Sinus Surgery,
Associate Professor,
Department of Otolaryngology,
University of Colorado Health Sciences Center,
Denver, Colorado

**Ilhami Kovanlikaya, M.D.**
Research Director,
Cedars-Sinai Medical Center,
Los Angeles, California

**Jeffrey T. Laitman, Ph.D.**
Distinguished Professor,
Professor and Director of Anatomy and Functional
  Morphology,
Professor of Otolaryngology,
Director of Gross Anatomy,
Mount Sinai School of Medicine,
New York, New York

**J.S. Lameris, M.D., Ph.D.**
Professor of Radiology,
University of Amsterdam,
Academic Medical Center,
Amsterdam, The Netherlands

**William Lawson, M.D.**
Professor, Vice-Chairman,
Department of Otolaryngology,
Mount Sinai Medical Center,
New York, New York

**Michael H. Lev, M.D.**
Director, Emergency Neuroradiology
  and Neurovascular Laboratory,
Massachessetts General Hospital,
Staff Radiologist,
Massachessetts Eye and Ear Infirmary,
Assistant Professor of Radiology,
Harvard Medical School,
Boston, Massachusetts

**William W.M. Lo, M.D.**
Section Chief, Neurology,
St. Vincent Medical Center,
Clinical Professor of Radiology,
University of Southern California,
Los Angeles, California

**Laurie A. Loevner, M.D.**
Associate Professor of Radiology and
  Otorhinolaryngology: Head and Neck Surgery,
University of Pennsylvania Medical System,
University of Pennsylvania School of Medicine,
Philadelphia, Pennsylvania

**Mahmood F. Mafee, M.D.**
Head, Department of Radiology,
Professor of Radiology,
University of Illinois at Chicago

**M. Marcel Maya, M.D.**
Neuroradiologist,
Department of Imaging,
Cedars Sinai Medical Center,
Los Angeles, California

**David G. McLone**
Surgeon-in-Chief,
Childrens Memorial Hospital,
Professor of Neurosurgery,
Northwestern University's Feinberg School of Medicine,
Chicago, Illinois

**Manabu Minami, M.D.**
Department of Radiology,
Faculty of Medicine,
University of Tokyo,
Tokyo, Japan

**Suresh K. Mukherji, M.D.**
Chief of Neuroradiology and Head and Neck Radiology,
University of Michigan,
Department of Radiology,
Ann Arbor, Michigan

**Thomas P. Naidich, M.D., F.A.C.R.**
Vice Chairman for Academic Affairs,
Professor of Radiology,
Professor of Neurosurgery,
Professor of Anatomy and Functional Pathology,
Mount Sinai Medical Center,
New York, New York

**William R. Nemzek, M.D.**
Medford Radiological Group,
Medford, Oregon

**Kuni Ohtomo, M.D., Ph.D.**
Department of Radiology,
Faculty of Medicine,
University of Tokyo,
Tokyo, Japan

**Hiroyuki Okada, D.D.S., Ph.D.**
Department of Pathology,
Nihon University School of Dentistry at Matsudo,
Chiba, Japan

**Tomohiro Okano, D.D.S., Ph.D.**
Professor,
Department of Radiology,
Showa University School of Dentistry,
Tokyo, Japan

**Patrick J. Oliverio, M.D.**
Neuroradiologist,
Fairfax Radiological Consultants,
Inova Fairfax Hospital,
Fairfax, Virginia

**James Rabinov, M.D.**
Interventional Neuroradiology,
Massachusetts General Hospital,
Instructor in Radiology,
Harvard University,
Boston, Massachusetts

**Deborah L. Reede, M.D.**
Associate Professor,
New York University,
New York, New York

**Joy S. Reidenberg, Ph.D.**
Associate Professor,
Mount Sinai School of Medicine,
New York, New York

**Caroline D. Robson, M.D.**
Assistant Professor, Division of Radiology,
Children's Hospital,
Assistant Professor of Radiology,
Harvard Medical School,
Boston, Massachusetts

**Reuben Rock, D.D.S., M.D.**
Staff Radiologist,
Hartford Hospital,
Hartford, Connecticut

**Laura V. Romo, M.D.**
Assistant in Radiology,
Harvard Medical School,
Massachusetts Eye and Ear Infirmary,
Boston, Massachusetts

**Osamu Sakai, M.D., Ph.D.**
Research Fellow,
Department of Radiology,
Massachusetts Eye and Ear Infirmary,
Harvard Medical School,
Boston, Massachusetts
Assistant Professor,
Department of Radiology,
Jichi Medical School,
Tochigi, Japan

**Pina C. Sanelli, M.D.**
Clinical Assistant Attending,
New York Presbyterian Hospital,
Cornell Campus,
Assistant Professor of Radiology,
Weill Medical College of Cornell University,
New York, New York

**Tsukasa Sano, D.D.S., Ph.D.**
Assistant Professor,
Department of Radiology,
Showa University School of Dentistry,
Tokyo, Japan

**J. Pierre Sasson, M.D.**
Director of MRI Services,
Associate Director of Radiology Residency,
Mount Auburn Hospital,
Cambridge, Massachusetts
Clinical Instructor,
Harvard Medical School,
Boston, Massachusetts

**Peter J. Savino, M.D.**
Director, The Neuro-Ophthalmology Service,
Wills Eye Hospital,
Chairman, Department of Ophthalmology,
The Graduate Hospital,
Philadelphia, Pennsylvania

**Charles J. Schatz, M.D., F.A.C.R.**
Director of Head and Neck Imaging,
Tower Radiology,
Beverly Hills, California
Clinical Professor of Radiology,
Clinical Professor of Otolaryngology,
University of Southern California School of Medicine,
Los Angeles, California

**Steven J. Scrivani, M.D., D.D.S., D.S.C.**
Director,
The Center for Oral, Facial, and Head Pain,
The Pain Management Center,
New York Presbyterian Hospital,
Columbia Presbyterian Medical Center,
Edward V. Zegarelli Assistant Professor,
Oral and Maxillofacial Surgery,
Columbia University,
Columbia-Presbyterian Medical Center,
New York, New York

**Joel M.A. Shugar, M.D.**
Attending Physician,
Mount Sinai Hospital,
Associate Clinical Professor of Otolaryngology
Mount Sinai School of Medicine,
New York, New York

**Peter M. Som, M.D.**
Chief of Head and Neck Imaging,
Mount Sinai Hospital and Medical Center,
Professor of Radiology, Otolaryngology, and Anatomy
    and Functional Morphology,
Mount Sinai Medical School,
New York University,
New York, New York

**Wendy R.K. Smoker, M.D.**
Professor of Radiology,
Director of Neuroradiology,
Department of Radiology,
University of Iowa Hospitals and Clinicals,
Iowa City, Iowa

**Joel D. Swartz, M.D.**
President,
Germantown Imaging Associates,
Gladwyne, Pennsylvania,
Medical Director,
National Medical Imaging,
Philadelphia, Pennsylvania

**Mark L. Urken, M.D.**
Professor and Chairman,
Department of Otolaryngology,
Mount Sinai School of Medicine of New York
    University,
New York, New York

**Michiel W.M. van den Brekel, M.D., Ph.D.**
Head and Neck Surgeon,
Netherlands Cancer Institute,
Antoni van Leenwenhoek Hospital,
Assistant Professor,
Department of Otolaryngology,
Academic Medical Center,
University of Amsterdam,
Amsterdam, The Netherlands

**Alfred L. Weber, M.D.**
Chief of Radiology (Emeritus),
Department of Radiology,
Massachusetts Eye and Ear Infirmary,
Boston, Massachusetts
Professor of Radiology,
Harvard Medical School,
Cambridge, Massachusetts

**Jane L. Weissman, M.D., F.A.C.R.**
Director of Head and Neck Imaging,
Professor of Radiology and Otolaryngology,
Oregon Health and Science University.
Portland, Oregon

**P.L. Westesson, M.D., Ph.D., D.D.S.**
Chief of Diagnostic and Interventional Neuroradiology,
University of Rochester Medical Center,
Professor of Radiology and Professor
    of Clinical Dentistry,
University of Rochester,
Rochester, New York,
Professor of Oral Diagnostic Science,
State University of New York at Buffalo,
Buffalo, New York,
Associate Professor of Oral Radiology,
University of Lund,
Lund, Sweden

**Hirotsugu Yamamoto, D.D.S., Ph.D.**
Department of Pathology,
Nihon University School of Dentistry at Matsudo,
Chiba, Japan

**Mika Yamamoto, D.D.S.**
Research Fellow,
Department of Radiology,
Massachusetts Eye and Ear Infirmary,
Boston, Masssachusetts,
Instructor,
Department of Radiology,
Showa University School of Dentistry,
Tokyo, Japan

**Mitsuaki Yamashiro, D.D.S.**
Department of Radiology,
Nihon University School of Dentistry at Matsudo,
Chiba, Japan

**Robert A. Zimmerman, M.D.**
Vice-Chairman of Radiology,
Chief, Division of Radiology,
Children's Hospital of Philadelphia,
Professor of Radiology and Professor of Radiology
    in Neurosurgery,
University of Pennsylvania School of Medicine,
Philadelphia, Pennsylvania

**S. James Zinreich, M.D.**
Department of Neuroradiology,
Johns Hopkins Hospital,
Baltimore, Maryland

# Contents

# Volume 2

# Sinonasal Cavities

# 1

# Embryology and Congenital Lesions of the Midface

*Thomas P. Naidich, Susan I. Blaser, Bruce S. Bauer, Derek C. Armstrong, David G. McLone, and Robert A. Zimmerman*

# INTRODUCTION

Traditionally, congenital malformations have been defined by their effect on gross anatomy and classified by phenotypic similarities.[1] Clinically valid constellations of pathology have been called syndromes and named for the authors who reported them. Recent work has begun to elucidate the molecular bases for the phenotypes observed to provide an improved method for defining disease entities.[2–25] This chapter reviews selected congenital malformations of the midface, both classically and as examples of the evolving classification by molecular genetics. Limitations in the information available make this approach uneven, but still useful.

Craniofacial malformations result from misregulation of normal tissue patterning.[2] In utero, signal transduction pathways normally relay information from outside the cell, through the plasma membrane and cytoplasm, into the nucleus in order to regulate and coordinate the expression of target genes (Fig. 1-1). From the nucleus, related information then passes outward to alter cytoplasmic structures, to modulate the cell response to incoming signals, and to coordinate activities of other cells, nearby or distant.[2] The signals employed often take the form of *ligands*, which may be diffusable (e.g., growth factors) or stationary (e.g., extracellular matrix–associated proteins). The ligands bind to molecules designated transmembrane receptors.[2] These transmembrane receptors present an extracellular domain, which can interact with external signals; a transmembrane domain, which spans the cell membrane; and an intracellular domain, which effects changes within the cell.[2] Binding of the ligand to the extracellular domain of the receptor alters receptor conformation and initiates changes that propagate along the molecule to alter enzymatic activity or regulatory properties within the intracellular domain. Receptors such as fibroblast growth factor receptors (FGFRs) and bone mophogenic protein (BMP) receptor are often kinases that catalyze the transfer of a phosphate group from adenosine triphosphate (ATP) to the side chains of amino acids within other proteins (the substrates).[2] The substrates may themselves be kinases. Therefore, binding of ligand to the extracellular domain of the receptor may cause phosphorylation of the intracellular domain of the receptor, leading to phosphorylation of intracellular substrates and altered

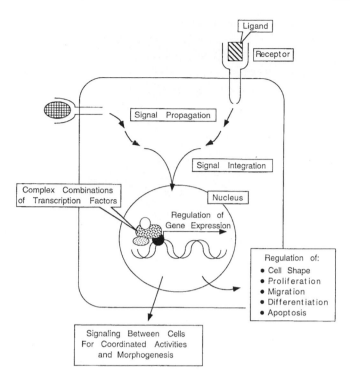

FIGURE 1-1 Cell signaling and signal transduction. Diagramatic representation. The outer square represents the cell surface. Ligand binding to the extracellular domain of the transmembrane receptor conveys information to the nucleus, where it affects gene regulation and transcription, alterations in cell shape, proliferation, migration, differentiation, apoptosis, and coordination of cell populations for further embryogenesis. (From Nuckolls GH, Shum L, Slavkin HC. Progress toward understanding craniofacial malformations. Cleft Palate-Craniofac J 1999;36:12–26.)

activity of other intracellular proteins. In like fashion, interactions among proteins to form a complex can alter their conformation and activity, either subtly or substantially.[2] Complexes of proteins designated transcription factors associate with DNA to increase or decrease transcription of specific genes and to modify protein synthesis qualitatively and/or quantitatively. Through these changes in protein activity, signals are propagated and integrated into circuits or networks that regulate gene expression and control cell proliferation, migration, differentiation, bilateral symmetry, and even death (apoptosis).[2] The coordinated control of cell populations is fundamental to the formation of complex structures such as the human face during embryonic development.[1–25] Derangements in this coordinated signaling lead to the malformations observed. Figures 1-2 and 1-3 depict the developing forebrain and its relationships to the developing face.[5–7]

# EMBRYOLOGY OF THE FACE AND SKULL

## Development of the Face and Jaws

The tissue that gives rise to the face and jaws derives from three major sources (Figs. 1-2 and 1-3):

1. The *ectoderm* provides the surface cover, and by ectodermal–mesenchymal interactions helps to pattern the developing structures.[3, 4, 20, 21]

2. *Neural crest cells* provide most of the facial mesenchyme.[3, 4, 7, 17, 23]

3. The *paraxial and prechordal mesoderm* contribute tissue that evolves into the myoblasts of the voluntary craniofacial muscles.[4]

The first sign of the future face is a surface depression, the stomodeum, situated just below the developing brain (Fig. 1-4). The ectoderm that overlies the early forebrain extends into the stomodeum, where it lies adjacent to the developing foregut. The junction between the surface ectoderm and the subjacent endoderm is called the oropharyngeal membrane. The line of attachment of the oropharyngeal membrane corresponds to Waldeyer's ring. Dissolution of the oropharyngeal membrane by the end of

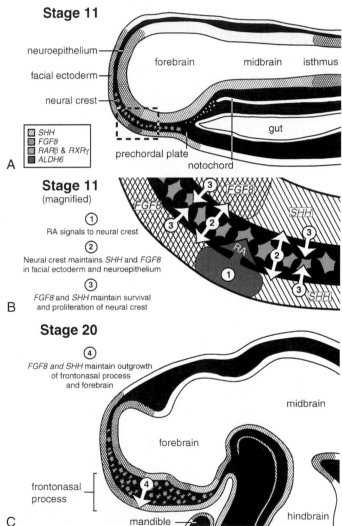

FIGURE 1-2 Establishing the forebrain. **A** to **C**, Patterning the forebrain and the frontonasal process in relation to the prechordal plate, anterior to the notochord. Roles of Sonic Hedgehog (*SHH*), fibroblast growth factor 8 (*FGF8*), retinoic acid (RA), retinoic acid receptor beta (RARβ), retinoic acid "X" receptor gamma (RXRγ), and aldehyde dehydrogenase 6 (ALDH6) in maintaining the outgrowth of the forebrain and the neural crest to establish the frontonasal process. In this and all future sagittal (lateral) images, anterior is displayed to the reader's left. (From Schneider RA et al. Local retinoid signaling coordinates forebrain and facial morphogenesis by maintaining *FGF8* and *SHH*. Development 2001;128:2755–2767.)

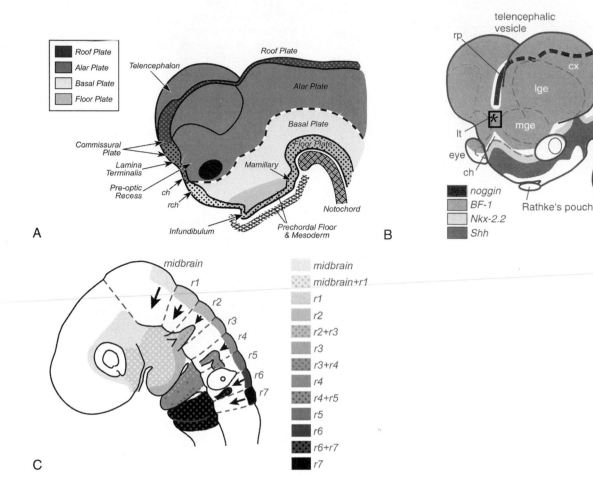

**FIGURE 1-3** **A,** Schematic representation of the longitudinal organization of the forebrain. The optic stalk appears as a black oval. Black lines indicate the boundary of the telencephalic vesicle and the contours of the medial and lateral ganglionic eminences within it. Note the relationships among the alar-basal junction, the optic stalk, the chiasmatic plate anlage (*ch*), and the retrochiasmatic (rch) (anterobasal region) of the basal plate, and the relationships among the notochord, floor plate, prechordal floor, and infundibulum. **B,** Molecular designation of topography. Compare the topographc distribution of Sonic Hedgehog (*Shh*), *Nkx-2.2*, *BF-1*, and *noggin* with the anatomic locations shown in **A.** *Shh* is a gene that encodes a diffusable protein implicated in specifying the notochord and floor plate of the neural tube. It helps to regulate *Nkx-2.2*. *Nkx-2.2* is a homeobox gene first detectable at the 1-somite stage in a median rostral region of the neural plate just anterior to the rostral tip of the notochoral plate. *Shh* and *Nkx-2.2* define adjacent and nonoverlapping longitudinal neuroepithelial zones that extend along the entire central nervous system (CNS) and end anteriorly, where they cross the midline in the optochiasmatic region. Brain factor 1 (BF-1) may be regarded as an alar plate marker of the prosencephalon. It is expressed in most of the telencephalon, the preoptic region, the adjoining one half of the optic stalk, and one half of the optic cup. It is reciprocal to the expression of BF-2 in the other halves of the optic stalk and cup. *noggin* is a gene that encodes a secreted polypeptide with neural-inducing properties. It is expresssed in the roof plate along the entire neural axis. Its anterior end approximates the anterior extent of the prosencephalic vesicle and does not enter the lamina terminalis. *Rh*, rhombencephalon; *me*, mesencephalon; *cx*, embryonic cerebral cortex; *lge*, lateral ganglionic eminence; *mge*, medial ganglionic eminence. The anterior-medial alar region of the neural plate maps to the lamina terminalis of the brain (square with asterisk). *Shh* present in the mge is not shown for simplicity. **C,** Neural crest migration. Chick embryo model. The facial mesenchyme derives from cohorts of neural crest cells that migrate to specified regions within the developing face and branchial arches from defined segments of the forebrain, midbrain, and hindbrain rhombomeres r1 to r7. Note the relationships of the pathways of migration to the optic vesicle, the otic placode, and the developing cranial nerves 5, 7/8, and 9/10. Clonal variations and mutations in specific cohorts of neural crest cells can lead to malformations restricted to subsets of cells in specific topographies. In mammals, r2, r4, and r6 send streams of neural crest cells into branchial arches 1, 2, and 3, respectively. The streams of neural crest cells that arise in r3 and r5 turn sharply to join the streams from adjacent rhombomeres. (**A** and **B** from Shimamura K et al. Longitudinal organization of the anterior neural plate and neural tube. Development 1995;121:3923–3933. **C** from Köntges G, Lumsden A. Rhombencephalic neural crest segmentation is preserved throughout craniofacial ontogeny. Development 1996;122:3229–3242.)

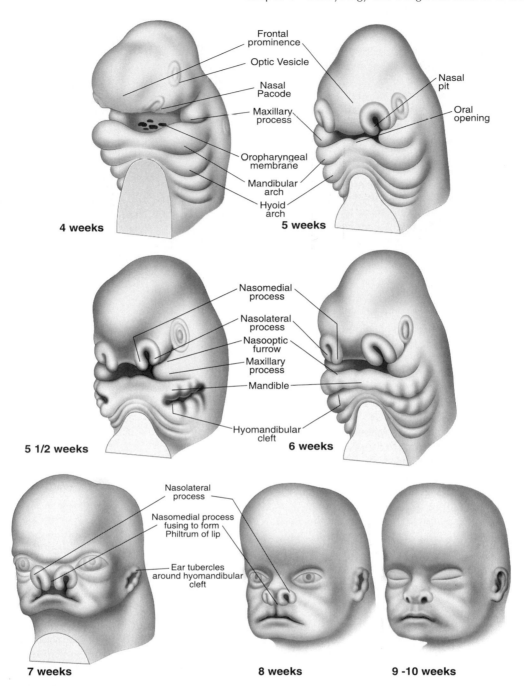

**FIGURE 1-4**   Embryogenesis of the face from 4 to 10 wg. See text. (Modified from Carlson BM. Human Embryology and Developmental Biology, 2nd ed. St. Louis: CV Mosby, 1999.)

the fourth week of gestation (wg) permits communication between the mouth and the foregut.[3] Waldeyer's ring connects the nasopharyngeal adenoids, the palatine tonsils, and the lingual tonsils.[14] The depth of Waldeyer's ring within the mouth of the newborn indicates the extent to which facial development results from thickening of the surface tissue external to the original ectodermal level.[14]

During the fourth week of gestation (wg), neural crest cells migrate to the developing face from the lower forebrain, the midbrain, and rhombomeres 1 and 2 of the upper hindbrain (Fig. 1-3C). Neural crest cells also migrate to other pharyngeal arches from the lower rhom-

bomeres.[3, 6, 7] These migratory neural crest cells are the predominant source of facial connective tissue, including cartilage, bone, and ligaments. Since the neural crest cells migrate to the face as cohorts of cells from different portions of the brain, they carry with them different developmental programs. Mutations arising in the premigratory or early migratory neural crest cells may affect one specific clone of cells, which then carries that mutation to a predestined site in the face.

At 4 wg, five identifiable primordia surround the stomodeum (Fig. 1-4). The single, unpaired frontonasal prominence lies in the midline just superior to the stomodeum. Embryologically, this prominence is related to the forebrain. Paired maxillary prominences lie on each side of the stomodeum superiorly, and paired mandibular prominences lie on each side of the stomodeum inferiorly. These processes originate from the first branchial (pharyngeal) arch.[3, 11] During the fourth to eighth wg, the frontonasal prominence gives rise to the median facial structures, and the paired maxillary and mandibular prominences give rise to the lateral facial structures.[3] Since the medial and lateral structures derive from different tissues, malformations of the face tend to affect either the median or the lateral structures separately, or their lines of junction.

By the end of the fourth wg, even before the neural folds close, paired thickenings of ectoderm appear on the surface of the frontonasal prominence just superolateral to the stomodeum.[3] These oval nasal placodes, located at 1 and 11 o'clock, give rise to the future nose and nasal cavities. Development of the nasal placodes (and the lens placodes) requires the paired box gene *Pax 6*.[3] In the absence of *Pax 6*, neither the nasal nor the lens placode develops.[3] During the fifth wg, mesenchyme in the margins of the nasal placodes proliferates to form horseshoe-shaped elevations (Fig. 1-4). The medial limbs of the horseshoes are designated the nasomedial processes. The lateral limbs of the horseshoes are designated the nasolateral processes. The nasomedial processes are longer than the nasolateral processes.[4] The tissue surrounding the placodes thickens and elevates, so the nasal placodes appear to become recessed within depressions in the surrounding tissue. The depressions are then designated nasal pits. The nasal pits are the primordia of the anterior nares (the future nostrils) and the nasal cavities.[4]

From 4 to 5 wg, the mandibular processes enlarge on both sides. From 5½ to 8 wg, their medial components merge in the midline, forming the point of the lower jaw (mentum) (Fig. 1-4).[3] Incomplete fusion at the mentum leaves the common midline chin dimple.[4] From 4 to 6 wg, the paired maxillary processes grow toward each other and toward the paired nasomedial processes.[3] The maxillary processes will ultimately give rise to the lateral two thirds of the upper jaw, the upper teeth (except for the incisors), and the palatal shelves that contribute to the hard palate. By the end of the sixth wg, the nasolateral processes begin to merge with the maxillary processes to form the ala nasi and the lateral border of the nostril on both sides (Fig. 1-4).[3] Along the junctions between the maxillary and nasolateral processes on both sides, nasolacrimal grooves still extend between the developing nose and eyes. The ectoderm along the floor of these grooves thickens to form solid epithelial cords, which detach from the grooves and then canalize to form the nasolacrimal ducts and lacrimal sacs. By the late fetal period, the nasolacrimal ducts extend from the medial corners of the eyes to the inferior meatuses in the lateral walls of the nasal cavity.[4] These ducts usually become completely patent only after birth. The nasomedial processes on both sides remain unfused.

From the sixth to the eighth wg, the cheeks and the corners of the mouth form by the merging of the maxillary and mandibular processes. The upper lip is completed during the seventh and eighth wg (Fig. 1-4).[3] The expanding nasomedial processes merge with the superficial regions of the maxillary processes on both sides along epithelial seams (fusion lines) designated nasal fins.[3] Mesenchyme pen-

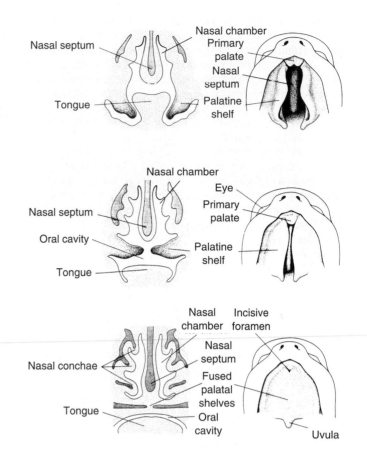

**FIGURE 1-5**   Embryogenesis of the palate from 6½ to 10 wg. (From Langman J. Medical Embryology: Human Development, Normal and Abnormal, 2nd ed. Baltimore: Williams & Wilkins, 1969.)

etrates the nasal fins, forms a continuous union between the nasomedial and the maxillary processes, and completes much of the upper lip and upper jaw on both sides. The two nasomedial processes then merge with each other across the midline to form the intermaxillary segment. The fusion of the two nasomedial processes displaces the frontonasal prominence posteriorly. Therefore, the frontonasal prominence does not contribute significantly to the definitive upper lip, jaw, or nasal tip, even though it formed a prominent portion of the stomodeal border at 4 to 5 wg.[3] The intermaxillary segment formed by the nasomedial processes is the precursor for the medial portion of the upper lip (the prolabium), the premaxillary component of the upper jaw containing the four upper incisors (the gnathogingival segment), and a triangular midline anterior wedge of palate (the primary palate) (Fig. 1-5).[3] The primary palate will later become continuous with the most rostral portion of the nasal septum. Fusion of the paired nasomedial processes also forms the tip and the crest of the nose and a portion of the nasal septum.[3]

From the sixth wg, the primordia of the auricles of the external ear begin to develop (Fig. 1-4). By the seventh wg, six mesenchymal swellings designated auricular hillocks form around the first pharyngeal groove on each side: three from the first branchial arch and three from the second branchial arch[3] (see the section on Hemifacial Microsomia). The auricular hillocks will merge with each other to form the auricle. The groove between them will form the external auditory meatus.[3] Initially, the external ears are located inferomedially in the neck. As the mandible develops, the ears ascend laterally to the sides of the head at the level of the eyes.[4] During this time, descent of the nose and medial migration of the orbits above the nose are also observed.

Until the end of the sixth wg, the primitive jaws are composed of masses of mesenchyme.[4] A linear thickening of ectoderm, designated the labiogingival lamina, then begins to grow into the underlying mesenchyme. This lamina "carves out" a labiogingival groove, creating the separate lips and gingiva. It then degenerates, except in the midline, leaving the labiogingival groove between the lips and the gingivae, and a midline frenulum for the upper lip.[3, 4] Separation of the lips from the gingivae occurs only after the mesenchyme within the individual facial processes merge to form the upper lip, and is not found in regions where the facial processes fail to merge successfully (e.g., such a sulcus is deficient in patients with complete cleft lips).

Once the basic facial structures take shape, they are invaded by mesodermal cells associated with the first and second pharyngeal arches. These cells form (1) the muscles of mastication (first arch derivatives innervated by cranial nerve 5) and (2) the muscles of facial expression (second arch derivatives innervated by cranial nerve 7).[3] The relative proportions of the facial structures change during life. The midface remains underdeveloped during embryogenesis and early postnatal life and grows to full size later.[3] The mandible is initially small and shows later "catch-up" growth.

## Molecular Signaling and Tissue Patterning in the Face

The facial primordia are analogous to limb buds and depend on highly similar molecular signaling for patterning and elongation. In both the face and limbs, for example, (1) mesenchymal–ectodermal interactions pattern the tissue, (2) sonic hedgehog, fibroblast growth factor (FGF), and retinoic acid signaling are critical for growth, (3) aristaless-like homeobox genes (*Prx1, Prx2, Alx3, Alx4*) serve as upstream regulators of sonic hedgehog, and (4) the homeobox gene *Msx1* is expressed in the rapidly proliferating mesenchyme near to the leading edge of the process.[3, 5, 11, 12] In the face, sonic hedgehog may be the morphogenic organizer, while fibroblast growth factors may serve as the stimuli for mesenchymal outgrowth.[3]

Facial and limb malformations are known to result from deficiency or excess of molecular signaling. Similar phenotypes, such as clefting, may result from either deficiency of the appropriate midline tissue or such excess of other midline tissue that the appropriate processes cannot meet to fuse in the midline. In experimental animals, *reduced* retinoic acid signaling diminishes expression of sonic hedgehog and fibroblast growth factor 8 (FGF8) in the mesenchyme, increases apoptosis (programmed cell death) locally, and decreases proliferation of tissue in the forebrain and frontonasal processes. These animals show holoprosencephalic phenotypes with hypoplastic forebrain, fused eyes, and absence of structures derived from the frontonasal

process. Timely replacement of retinoic acid prevents this malformation.[5] Conversely, excess sonic hedgehog stimulates frontonasal growth and widens the frontonasal process (an average of 48%), so that (1) the developing palatal shelves fail to abut, leaving a cleft palate, and (2) more severe phenotypes show ectopic midfacial structures with duplication of the nasal bone.[12, 15]

## Development of the Palate

The palate is formed from the seventh to the tenth wg from three primordia: an unpaired median palatine process and paired lateral palatine processes (Fig. 1-5).[6, 8, 9] The newly merged nasomedial processes form the median palatine process. This grows posteriorly to form a triangular bony structure designated the primary palate. In adult life, this portion is called the premaxillary component of the maxilla and gives origin to the four upper incisors.[3] The incisive foramen marks the posterior midline extent of the premaxilla. The lateral palatine processes first appear during the sixth wg and grow vertically downward on both sides of the tongue.[3] The growth of the palatal shelves also resembles the growth of the limb bud. It involves both ectodermal–mesenchymal interaction and growth factors like epidermal growth factor (EGF) and transforming growth factor alpha (TGF-alpha). The growing palatal processes may even display an apical ectodermal thickening similar to the apical ectodermal ridge of the limb bud.[3] During the seventh wg, hydration of hyaluronic acid within the palatal processes generates an intrinsic shelf-elevating force that elevates the palatal shelves from their early vertical position alongside the tongue into a definitive horizontal position above the dorsum of the tongue.[11] The epithelial cells along the medial edge of each palatal shelf contact each other and fuse together along an epithelial seam.[11] The two palatal shelves also fuse with the triangular primary palate anteromedially to form the Y-shaped fusion line (Fig 1-5). The success or failure of palatal fusion is strongly influenced by genetics and by physical constraints of the space available within the dividing nasooral cavity.

Following fusion of the palatal shelves, the seam cells migrate, orally and nasally, into epithelial triangles and subsequently into the oral and nasal epithelia.[23] Developmental programs for epithelial–mesenchymal interactions promote regionally specific palatal epithelial differentiation into nasal pseudostratified ciliated columnar cells and oral stratified squamous cells.[11] Growth factors localized within the developing palate appear to underlie the epithelial–mesenchymal interactions. Fibroblast growth factor 7 (FGF7), for example, is synthesized by the mesenchymal cells, while its receptor is synthesized in the overlying epithelia, establishing an integrated signaling system.[2]

## Development of the Nasal Cavities and Septum

From 5 wg, the nasal pits deepen toward the oral cavity, forming substantial depressions. By 6½ wg, only a thin oronasal membrane separates the oral cavity from the nasal cavities.[3] This oronasal membrane then breaks down, so that the oral cavity can communicate with the nasal cavities through openings posterior to the primary palate.[3] These openings are designated the nasal choanae. Fusion of the two palatal shelves then lengthens the nasal cavity and carries the communication posteriorly to the upper pharynx.[3] The nasal septum grows down from the frontonasal prominence to reach the level of the palatal shelves when the shelves fuse to form the definitive secondary palate. Anteriorly, the septum is continuous with the primary palate.[11] The actual fusion of the palate begins posterior to (not at) the incisive foramen and extends from there, both anteriorly and posteriorly, to complete the formation of the palate. The point of fusion of the secondary palatal shelves with the primary palate is marked by the incisive foramen.[11]

## The Facial Skeleton

The cartilage of the nasal capsule is the foundation of the upper part of the face (Figs. 1-6 and 1-7).[24] The bony elements of the facial skeleton appear around it and replace it in part. The lateral masses of the ethmoid form by enchondral ossification of the nasal capsule. The frontal processes of the maxillary bones, the premaxillary bone, the nasal bones, the lacrimal bones, and the palatine bones all form in membrane in close relationship with the roof and lateral walls of the cartilaginous nasal capsule.[24] The vomer develops in membrane in relation to the perichondrium of the septal process.[24] Eventually, nearly all of the nasal capsule becomes ossified or atrophied. All that remains of the cartilage of the nasal capsule in adults is the anterior part of the nasal septum and the alar cartilages that surround the nostrils.

Specifically, the midline septal cartilage is directly continuous with the cartilaginous skull base. At birth, the skull base has three major ossification centers: the *basioc-*

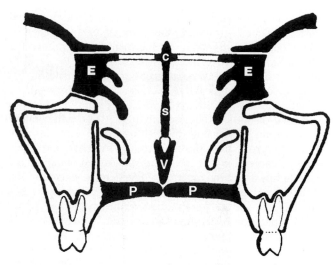

**FIGURE 1-7** Diagram of the pattern of ossification around the nasal cavity. The ossified crista (*C*) and septal cartilage (*S*) form a "cristal" cross that is isolated from the lateral ethmoid centers (*E*) by the unossified cribriform plates and from the vomer (*V*) by the sphenoidal tail. Although the maxillae are ossified, only the palatal shelves (*P*) have been inked in to emphasize their relationships to the vomer. (Modified from Scott JH. The cartilage of the nasal septum (a contribution to the study of facial growth). Br Dent J 1953;95:37.)

*cipital* center, the *basisphenoidal* center, and the *presphenoidal* center. The septal cartilage has not yet ossified. The lateral masses of the ethmoid have ossified, forming paired paramedian bones, but the cribriform plate is still cartilaginous or fibrous.[24] At birth, therefore, the entire midline of the face may be a lucent strip of cartilage situated between the paired ossifications in the lateral masses of the ethmoids. This lucent midline can simulate a midline cleft on imaging studies. The septal cartilage extends along the midline from the nares to the presphenoid bone.[24] Anteriorly and inferiorly, the septal cartilage attaches to the premaxillary bone by fibrous tissue.[24] Posteriorly, the septal cartilage is continuous with the cartilage of the cranial base. Inferiorly, the lower edge of the septal cartilage is slotted into a U- or V-shaped groove that runs along the entire upper edge of the vomer (Figs. 1-7 to 1-9).[24] This groove is designated the vomerine groove. It should not be mistaken for a midline cleft in the septum.

At about the time of birth or during the first year of life, a fourth center, the *mesethmoidal* center, appears in the septal cartilage anterior to the cranial base. This center will form the perpendicular plate of the ethmoid.[24] The residual portion of still unossified septal cartilage that extends posterosuperiorly toward the cranial base between the perpendicular plate of the ethmoid and the vomer is designated the sphenoidal tail of the septal cartilage.[24] Initially, the ossifying perpendicular plate is separated from the rest of the facial skeleton by (1) the unossified cartilage or fibrous tissue of the cribriform plates and (2) the sphenoidal tail (Figs. 1-7 to 1-9). At about the third to sixth year, the lateral masses of the ethmoid and the perpendicular plate of the ethmoid become united across the roof of the nasal cavity by ossification of the cribriform plate.[24, 25]

Somewhat later, the perpendicular plate unites with the vomer below.[24] As the two bones approach, the vomerine

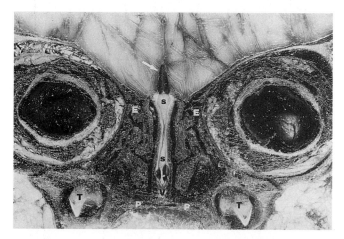

**FIGURE 1-6** Coronal cryomicrotome section through the nasal cavity of a full-term stillborn infant at the level of the optic globes. The lateral ethmoid centers (*E*), the midline vomer (*V*), and the palatal shelves (*P*) of the maxillae are well ossified. The unossified septal cartilage (*S*) slots into the vomerine groove in the upper surface of the Y-shaped vomer. The crista galli (*arrow*) is beginning to ossify, forming a pointed "cap." The cribriform plates have not ossified. Note the normal position of the floor of the anterior fossa with respect to the two orbits and optic globes. *T*, Unerupted teeth.

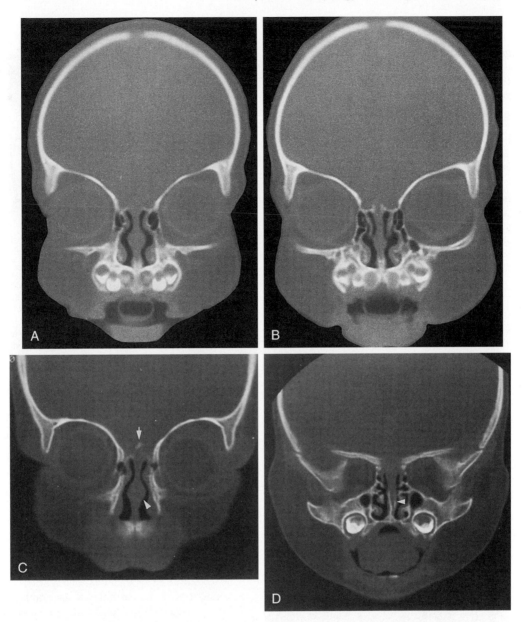

**FIGURE 1-8**  Normal patterns of ossification of the nasal capsule, as shown by direct coronal CT in progressively older patients. **A** and **B**, Four-month-old girl. The lateral ethmoid centers and a small segment of vomer are ossified. The midline septal cartilage is entirely unossified. **C** and **D**, Five-month-old boy. The lateral ethmoid centers, the palatal shelves, the vomer, and the tip (*white arrow*) of the crista galli are ossified. The widened midportion of the septum (*white arrowhead* in **C**) is designated the septal diamond. The two sides of the vomerine groove give the posterior septum a bilaminar appearance (*white arrowhead* in **D**).

*Illustration continued on following page*

groove may become converted into a vomerine tunnel. This should not be mistaken for a bony canal around a dermal sinus or cephalocele. Growth of the septal cartilage continues for a short period after craniofacial union is complete. This may explain the common deflection of the nasal septum away from the midline.[24]

Because the appearance of the nasal septum varies with the patient's age, one must interpret imaging "evidence" of midline defects and sinus tracts carefully. Review of the CT appearance of the midline anterior fossa and nasal septum in 100 children aged 2 days to 18 years revealed the following normal patterns (Figs. 1-7 to 1-9):[1, 26]

1. The lateral ethmoid centers are ossified in all patients.
2. No *midline* ossifications of the anterior fossa or septum are present in 14% of patients less than 1 year of age.
3. The cribriform plate is not ossified in patients less than 2 months of age. It can be ossified from 2 to 8 months of age. It is fused across the midline from 8 months on.
4. The tip of the crista can be ossified from 2 days on. It is invariably ossified from 2½ years on.
5. The crista plus the cribriform plate forms a _/\\_ os-

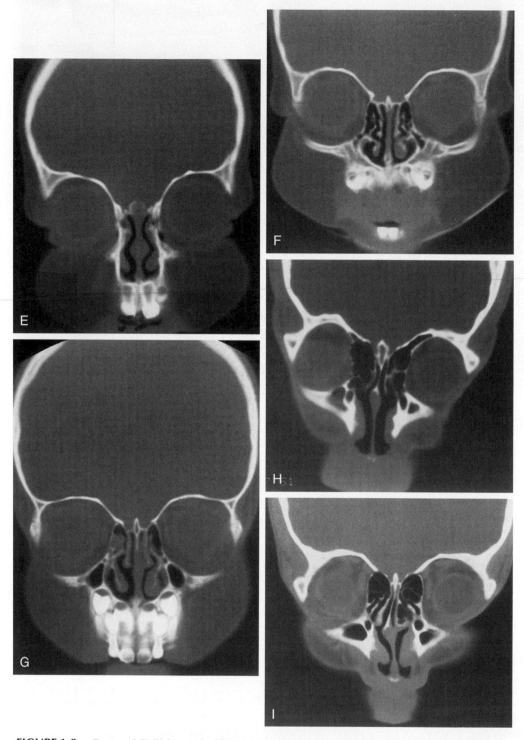

**FIGURE 1-8** *Continued.* **E,** Eight-month-old boy. Anteriorly, the crista galli is incompletely ossified, forming a hollow cap. **F,** Further posteriorly, the crista and the cribriform plates have ossified together, roofing over the nasal cavity. The perpendicular plate of ethmoid is beginning to ossify as a bilaminar plate. The Y-shaped vomer is larger. **G,** Nine-month-old girl. The ossified perpendicular plate has enlarged and extended inferiorly toward the septal diamond. The ossified crista resembles a hollow diamond. **H,** Seventeen-year-old boy. The ossified perpendicular plate reaches the top of the septal diamond, where it may widen into a knob or fork. **I,** Eleven-month-old boy. The nasal septum frequently buckles at the septal diamond.

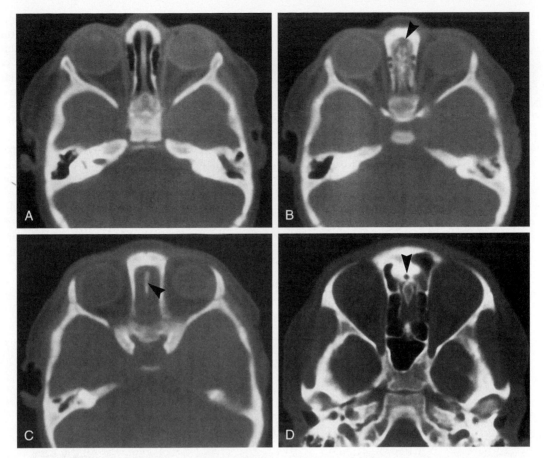

**FIGURE 1-9** Normal pattern of ossification as shown on axial noncontrast CT. In the 11-month-old girl shown in **A** to **C**, serial axial images display the following: (**A**) The normal, thin nasal septum with faint parallel ossifications representing the vomer, (**B**) the normal midline defect (*black arrowhead*) anterior to the normal parallel ossification within the closing cribriform plates and crista, and (**C**) the upper portion of the crista (*arrowhead*) with a small fossa anterior to it. Comparing these images with the coronal sections in Figures 1-6 through 1-8 aids understanding of how the parallel ossifications arise. **D**, Twelve-year-old boy. The foramen cecum (*black arrowhead*) is a well-defined ostium situated just anterior to the diamond shaped ossified crista galli.

sification, with *no* ossification of the perpendicular plate, in patients 2 months to 5 months of age.

6. The ossified crista, cribriform plate, and perpendicular plate can form a bony "cristal cross" from 4 months on. These ossifications invariably form a cross from 11 months on.

7. A zone of *un*ossified tissue is seen within the crista in 60% of patients with a cristal cross. Such ostia can be present at any age from 4 months on.

8. The perpendicular plate of the ethmoid can be ossified as a single plate in patients aged 11 months to 18 years. It is ossified in the vast majority of patients older than 2 years.

9. The perpendicular plate is ossified as two parallel laminae in 15% of patients.

10. The nasal septum is widest at the midpoint of its vertical height in nearly all patients of all ages. This widening is designated the septal diamond.

11. The perpendicular plate widens inferiorly or splits to form an inverted Y at the septal diamond in 30% of patients, all older than 6 years of age.

12. The perpendicular plate reaches as far inferiorly as the septal diamond in 32% of all patients, 92% after age 6 years and 100% after age 13 years.

The ossified vomer exhibits a V- or Y-shaped superior border in 80% of patients at any age. The vomerine ossification appears as a single point anteriorly and as a V or Y posteriorly in 21% of patients. In 8% it is seen only as a single point.

In the *normal* patient then, one may expect to see no ossification in the midline of children under 1 year of age, an unossified zone within 60% of the cristal crosses, a "bilaminar" perpendicular plate of ethmoid in 15%, and a V- or Y-shaped upper surface of the vomer in at least 80% of patients (Figs. 1-6 and 1-7). These should not be overinterpreted as pathology.

The development of the ethmoid labyrinth is often asymmetric in contour and position.[27] As a consequence, 48% of normal patients show contour asymmetry of the fovea ethmoidalis with flattening of the ethmoid roof on one side, and 9.5% show an asymmetric position of the fovea ethmoidalis.[27] Of those with positional asymmetry, the fovea is lower on the right in 63% and lower on the left in 37%.[27] This normal variation must not be misinterpreted as pathology.

## TORI PALATINUS, MAXILLARIS, AND MANDIBULARIS

Torus palatinus is a benign thickening of normal cortical and medullary bone on the oral surface of the hard palate (Fig. 1-10).[28–35] It is covered by a thin, pale mucosa. The torus typically aligns along the median intermaxillary-interpalatine suture, protrudes downward from the apex of the palatal arch, and extends to both sides, approximately symmetrically. The regions of the palatal rugae and the greater palatine foramina are usually spared, so the tori have a ''faceted,'' triangular/diamond configuration.[32] The nasal aspect of the hard palate is never affected by simple torus palatinus.[31] *Torus maxillaris* signifies one or multiple unilateral or bilateral hyperostoses arising from the alveolar portion of the maxilla, usually in the molar region. Torus maxillaris internus arises along the lingual surface of the dental arch opposite the roots of the molars and may coalesce into lobular or irregular masses. Torus maxillaris externus appears as broader, sausage-shaped, or alate expansion(s) of the buccal aspect of the superior alveolar ridge.[28–32] *Torus mandibularis* signifies unilateral or bilateral hyperostoses arising along the lingual surface of the mandible between the alveolar border and the mylohyoid line (Fig. 1-11). They usually are found in relation to the apex of the second premolar[33] opposite the mental foramen.[29–32] *Multiple tori* may occur together. Tori maxillaris and mandibularis are found more commonly in skulls with torus palatinus (Figs. 1-10 and 1-11). Buccal hyperostoses of the maxilla and mandible commonly occur together in both sexes.[22] Torus palatinus and torus mandibularis may both be associated with a thick posterior wall of the glenoid fossa (tympanic plate).[37]

Torus palatinus is found in 19% to 60% of diverse ethnic

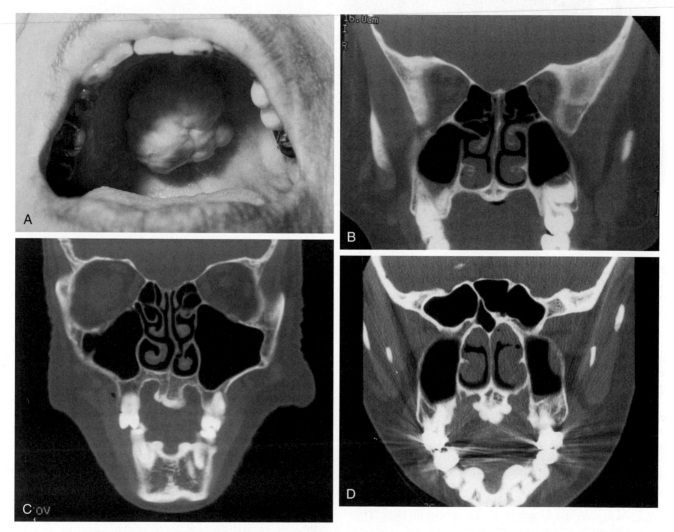

**FIGURE 1-10** Torus palatinus. **A,** Open-mouth view. Large lobular torus palatinus in a 78-year-old woman. **B** to **D,** Coronal CT. **B,** Small, symmetric torus palatinus in a 30-year-old man. **C,** Large lobular asymmetric, pedunculated torus palatinus with bilateral tori mandibulares. **D,** Lobular pedunculated torus palatinus in a 45-year-old woman. (**A** and **D** from Naidich TP, Valente M, Abrams K, Spreitzer JJ, Doundoulakis SH. Torus palatinus. Int J Neuroradiol 1997;3:229–243.)

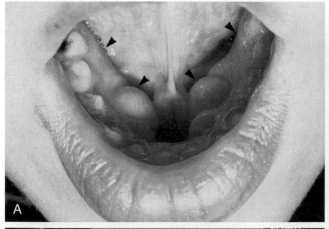

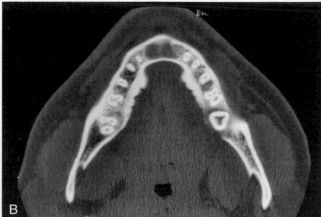

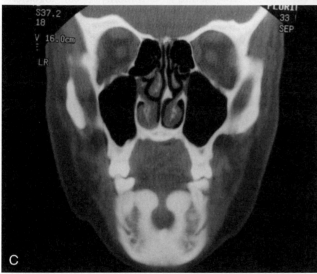

**FIGURE 1-11**   Torus mandibularis. **A,** Open-mouth view. A 30-year-old woman with bilateral tori mandibulares (*arrowheads*). **B,** A 39-year-old man. On axial CT, the tori manifest as marked denticulate cortical thickenings along the inner aspects of the mandibular arch. **C,** A 33-year-old woman. On coronal CT the tori manifest as marked cortical exostoses with minimal encroachment on the medullary cavity. (From Naidich TP. Pits, patches and protuberances. Hyperostosis mandibularis. Int J Neurol 1997;3:224–228.)

populations and in 20.9% of 2478 dental subjects of mixed heritage in the United States.[35, 37, 38] Tori have a distinct tendency toward heritability, with Oriental and Amerindian populations showing a particularly high incidence (44% to 60%).[30] In one study of approximately 150 Japanese families, Suzuki and Sakai showed that the incidence of torus palatinus in parents of Japanese children was 87.7% if the child had a torus but only 23.8% if the child had no torus.[33] Further, the larger the torus in the parent, the greater the incidence of tori in the children, the earlier their appearance, and the larger their size in the offspring.[19]

Tori are found in approximately 2% of newborns and increase in incidence with age.[34, 39, 40] After the newborn period, torus palatinus is approximately twice as common in females as in males.[35, 38–42] Tori grow as the patients grow, until maturity at 20 to 30 years of age, and then stabilize.[30, 33, 42] Unusual tori continue to increase in size in later decades of life.[30] Woo found no sex difference in the size or shape of the tori palatini in 2348 skulls.[30]

Torus palatinus is classified by shape into four major categories[34, 35]:

1. *Flat torus* is a smooth, bilaterally symmetric, broad-based exostosis that is mildly elevated, slightly convex, and oriented along the midline intermaxillary-interpalatine suture of the palate.

2. *Spindle torus* is a midline palatine ridge (the cresta palatina), which may contain a prominent median groove, signifying bilateral origin.

3. *Nodular torus* is a more bulbous hyperostosis formed from close juxtaposition of paired bilateral hemitori or from multiple smooth, discrete, bony protuberances.

4. *Lobular torus* is a large, pedunculated, mushroom-like mass that typically arises from a single base to form multiple secondary lobules separated by variably deep grooves.

Overall, flat and spindle-shaped tori palatini are the most common (86% combined). The larger nodular and lobular forms are seen in only 6% to 8% of patients.[21]

Most tori palatini are small, clinically insignificant, incidental findings on imaging studies. Only 22% are more than 2 cm in length.[42] Very rarely, large tori may restrict motion of the tongue, distort the oral air cavity, and cause speech disturbance. Substantial tori may have to be resected before a patient can be fitted with dental prostheses.

## FACIAL CLEFTS

Deranged development of the frontonasal process and/or failure of adjacent processes to merge successfully results in

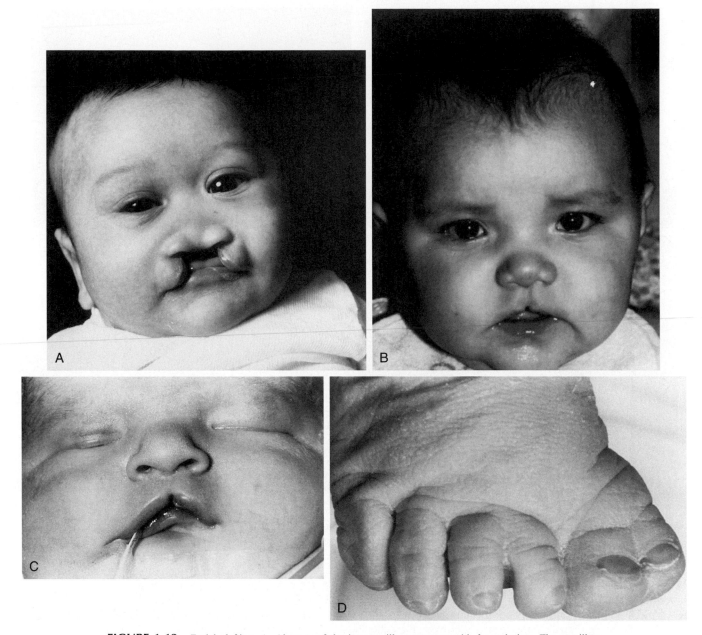

**FIGURE 1-12**   Facial clefting. **A**, Absence of the intermaxillary segment with *hypo*telorism. The maxillary processes form the normal lateral thirds of the upper lips. The midline rectangular defect indicates the site of the deficient intermaxillary segment with absent prolabium, incisors, and primary palate. There was consequent clefting of the secondary palate. Absent intermaxillary segment with hypotelorism signifies a high likelihood of holoprosencephaly. **B**, True midline cleft of the upper lip and philtrum with *hyper*telorism. The nose is normal. A 7-month-old girl with transethmoidal cephalocele and left optic nerve dysplasia (morning glory syndrome). True midline cleft lip signifies the high likelikhood of midline craniofaciocerebral and optic dysraphysm. **C** and **D**, Midline cleft lip is also found in association with Mohr syndrome (orofacial digital syndrome II [OFD II]). The presence of reduplicated great toes bilaterally helps to identify OFD II and to distinguish it from OFD I.

a coherent series of malformations. Insufficiency of the frontonasal and nasomedial processes may result in hypoplasia or absence of the nose and intermaxillary segment, with a roughly rectangular defect in the middle one third of the upper lip, absence of the incisors, absence of the primary palate with a cleft in the secondary palate, and *hypo*telorism. This is one common manifestation of holoprosencephaly[1, 6, 43, 44] (Fig. 1-12A). Failure of the two nasomedial processes to merge in the midline produces the rarer, true midline cleft lip and palate with *hyper*telorism.

This is typically associated with cleft primary palate, diastasis of the medial incisors, double frenulum of the upper lip, dehiscence of the skull base, and basal encephaloceles (Fig. 1-12B). True midline cleft is also a feature of Mohr syndrome (Fig. 1-12D). Failure of the nasomedial processes to merge with the maxillary processes on one or both sides produces the typical unilateral or bilateral common cleft lip and/or cleft palate (Fig. 1-13). Discordant growth of the two divided processes may then result in offset of the premaxillary segment from the maxillary segment, a

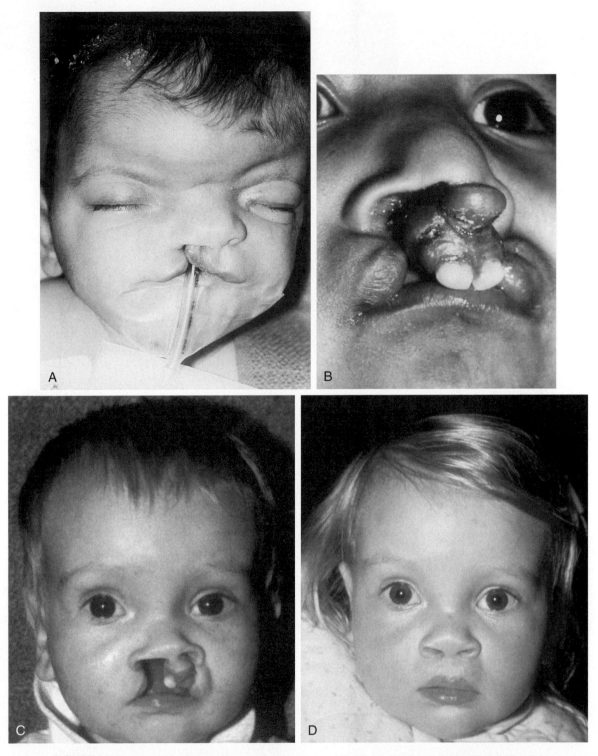

**FIGURE 1-13**   Facial clefting. **A,** Right unilateral common cleft lip and palate in a 4-day-old girl. The cleft extends into the base of a widened nostril. The intermaxillary segment is distorted. **B,** Bilateral common cleft lip and cleft palate with discordant forward growth of the intermaxillary segment in a 4-year-old boy. The normal canthi, alae nasi, and lateral thirds of the lip and jaw indicate normal formation and merging of the maxillary and nasolateral processes. The abortive prolabium, premaxillary segment, and central incisors attach to the vomer and project well anterior to their expected position, because failure to merge the facial processes led to discordant growth of the maxillary and intermaxillary segments. **C** and **D,** Bilateral common cleft lip and palate prior to (**C**) and following (**D**) surgical repair. There is near-symmetric restoration of the nose and upper lip, with some residual distortion caused by scar.

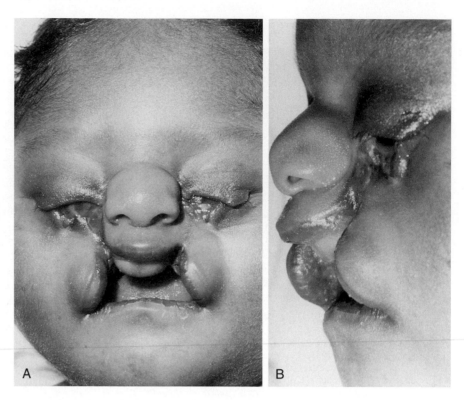

**FIGURE 1-14** Facial clefting. Bilateral oblique orooocular clefts with bilateral common cleft lip. **A,** Frontal view. **B,** Lateral view.

widened nostril, a depressed ala nasi, and an anomalous nasal septum.[4] Failure to merge the nasolateral process with the maxillary process results in an oblique facial cleft extending from the inner canthus of the eye into the nose (Fig. 1-14). This cleft may occur in association with bilateral common cleft lip and/or palate. Failure to merge the maxillary with the mandibular process, unilaterally or

bilaterally, results in a transverse facial cleft, also designated "wolf mouth" or macrostomia[45] (Fig. 1-15). The transverse cleft may occur in isolation or as part of syndromes such as hemifacial microsomia (see the section on Hemifacial Microsomia). Clefts that do not align along known lines of embryonic fusion likely represent the syndrome of amniotic bands (see the section on Syndrome of Amniotic Bands) (Fig. 1-16). The relative incidences of the facial clefts are given in Table 1-1.[30]

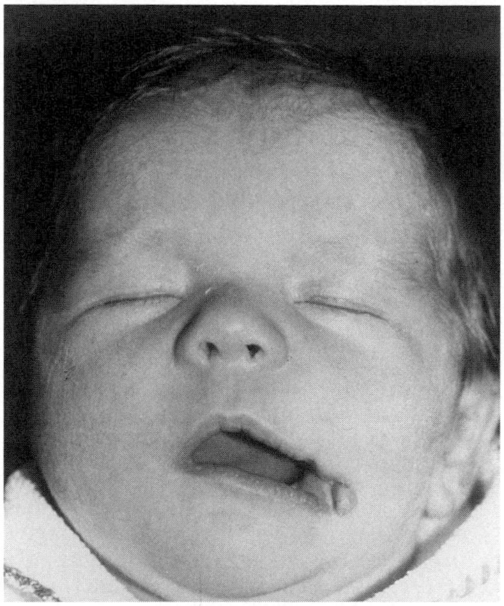

## Common Cleft Lip and/or Cleft Palate

Common clefts of the lip and/or palate account for 98.8% of all facial clefts.[46] They may involve the lip only, the lip and palate, or the palate only, unilaterally or bilaterally. Approximately 50% to 70% of all cases of cleft lip/palate are nonsyndromic.[13] The rest are divided among more than 300 presently recognized entities.[13] Cleft lip (with or without cleft palate) should be recognized as an entity distinct from cleft palate only, but the two conditions are usually considered together in series of facial clefting.[47]

The nature and incidence of clefting vary among populations. Caucasians show nonsyndromic clefting of the lip and/or palate in 1 per 700 to 1000 live births.[48] Clefting of the palate alone (cleft palate only) occurs less fequently: 6.5 per 10,000 births.[48] In 460 patients with oral clefts in France, the lesion was an isolated cleft lip in 19.1%, combined cleft lip plus cleft palate in 37.2%, and cleft palate only in 43.7%.[49] Of the 171 infants with complete cleft lip and palate, the clefts were unilateral in 58.5% and bilateral in 41.5%.[49] Study of 1669 consecutive *surgically treated* cleft lips and cleft palates in Iran found that, in that group, isolated cleft lips were slightly more common in women

**FIGURE 1-15** Facial clefting. Unilateral transverse facial cleft and macrostomia in an infant girl. (From Bauer BS, Wilkes GH, Kernahan DA. Incorporation of the W-plasty in repair of macrostomia. Plast Reconstr Surg 1982;70:752–757.)

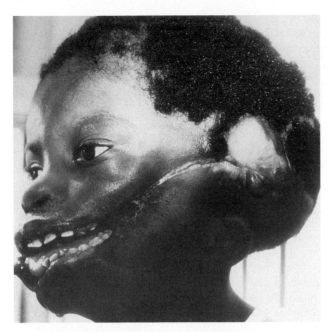

**FIGURE 1-16** Facial clefting. Nonanatomic clefts in a 12-year-old mentally retarded girl with the syndrome of amnionic bands. Lateral view. A long, thin band-like scar extends across the scalp and face from the temporoparietal region through the cheek and the corner of the mouth to the lower lip. The large posterior zone of atrophic skin, absent hair, tissue bulging, and inferior displacement of the ear indicate the site of an associated temporoparietal encephalocele. Imaging studies showed notching and separation of teeth where the band crossed the alveolar ridge.

(1.16:1) and that combined cleft lip/cleft palate was significantly more common in men (2.2:1).[50] Cleft palate only was very slightly more common in women (1.1:1).[50] The combination of cleft lip plus cleft palate is more common than either isolated cleft lip or isolated cleft palate.[50] Both isolated cleft lip and combined cleft lip/cleft palate are more often unilateral than bilateral and affect the left side more than the right (Table 1-2).[50] Unilateral left-sided clefting, unilateral right-sided clefting, and bilat-

### Table 1-1
### INCIDENCE OF FACIAL CLEFTS (N = 3988)

| Cleft Type | Number | Percent |
| --- | --- | --- |
| Common cleft lip/cleft palate | 3940 | 98.8 |
| True midline cleft lip | 8 | 0.20 |
| True midline cleft lip (part of the oro-facial-digital syndrome) | 3 | 0.08 |
| Pseudo-median cleft lip (holoprosencephaly) | 7 | 0.18 |
| Midline cleft nose | 8 | 0.20 |
| True bifid cleft nose | 4 | — |
| Unilateral and bilateral cleft ala nasi | 4 | — |
| Transverse facial cleft (macrostomia) | 12 | 0.30 |
| Oblique oro-orbital clefts | 3 | 0.08 |
| Cleft scalp | 7 | 0.18 |
| Total | 3988 | 100 |

From Fogh-Andersen P. Rare clefts of the face. Acta Chir Scand 1965;129:275–281.

eral clefting occur in a ratio of 6:2:3 (Table 1-2).[50] Table 1-3 summarizes a 50-year experience with 2297 clefting patients in Denmark.[47]

### Pathogenesis of Cleft Lip/Cleft Palate and of Cleft Palate

Both genetics and environment have been implicated in facial clefting. The risk of a child's being born with a cleft lip and palate is 4% if one parent *or* one sibling is affected but 17% if both one parent *and* one sibling are affected.[51] This indicates a heritable component. Dietary supplementation with vitamins $B_6$ and folic acid during the first trimester markedly decreases the risk of recurrence in women who had previously borne children with cleft lip and palate.[48] This indicates a potential role for teratogens (or deficiencies). Teratogens linked to facial clefting include cortisone, anticonvulsants such as phenytoin, salicylates, aminopterin, organic solvents, maternal alcohol ingestion, maternal diabetes mellitus, maternal rubella, and the season of gestation. Increased maternal and paternal age may also play a role.[48] Maternal smoking during early pregnancy is a clear risk factor for cleft lip/palate. Study of 2207 pregnancies leading to cleft lip/palate showed a definite increase in the incidence of cleft lip/palate in children of mothers who smoked during pregnancy and an increasing risk of cleft lip/palate with increasing amounts of smoking.[52] The odds ratio for clefting increases from 1.32 for women who smoke 1 to 10 cigarettes daily to 1.69 for those who smoke 21 or more cigarettes daily.[52] Smoking seems to synergize with uncommon polymorphisms in the TGF-alpha gene at chromosome 2p13 to increase the risk of cleft palate sixfold.[2] Statistically significant elevations in lactate dehydrogenase and creatine phosphokinase have been reported in the amnionic fluid of human fetuses with cleft lip/cleft palate (vs. control normal fetuses).[53]

### Genes and Heritability

Families of patients with cleft lip (with or without cleft palate) rarely include individuals with isolated cleft palate, and vice versa, probably because the primary and secondary palates form independently.[48] Nonsyndromic orofacial clefting (OFC) (cleft lip with or without cleft palate) has been mapped to genes designated *OFC1* at chromosome 6p23, *OFC2* at 2p13, interactions between *OFC1* and *OFC2*, and *OFC3* at 19q13.2.[48] Patients with OFC constitute a heterogeneous group, with some clefts inherited by autosomal dominance, others as a multifactorial threshold trait, and still others by oligogenic inheritance.[48]

The gene products related to cleft lip and cleft palate have been characterized as TGF-alpha (2p13), retinoic acid receptor alpha (RARA) (17q21.1), MSX1 (4p16.1), and BCL3 (19q13.2).[48] In animals the gene *endothelin-1* lies in the OFC1 region at chromosome 6p23-24.[48] "Knockout" mice deficient in OFC1 show craniofacial malformations including cleft palate.[48] Mice deficient in endothelin converting enzyme-1 or in endothelin-A receptor show nearly identical malformations. END1, the transcription factor dHAND, and the gene *MSX1* (*Hox 7*) may form a signal cascade that regulates the development of neural crest–derived branchial arch mesenchyme.[48, 54, 55]

Nonsyndromic cleft palate only (CPO) has uncertain inheritance but may arise as a recessive single major locus

**Table 1-2**
**CLASSIFICATION OF CLEFTS BY TYPE AND SIDE (N = 1669 CONSECUTIVE SURGICALLY TREATED CLEFTS IN IRAN)**

| Type of Cleft | Unilateral Right | Unilateral Left | Bilateral | Total |
|---|---|---|---|---|
| Cleft lip | 121 (24.1%) | 297 (59.3%) | 83 (16.6%) | 501 (30%) |
| Cleft lip and palate | 128 (16.5%) | 373 (48%) | 276 (35.5%) | 777 (46.5%) |
| Cleft lip (not classified) | | | | 42 (2.6%) |
| Cleft lip and palate (not classified) | | | | 60 (3.6%) |
| Cleft palate | | | | 289 (17.3%) |
| Total | 249 (14.9%) | 670 (40.1%) | 359 (21.5%) | 1669 (100%) |

From Rajabian MH, Sherkat M. An epidemiological study of oral clefts in Iran: analysis of 1669 cases. Cleft Palate-Craniofac J 2000;37:191–196.

with low penetrance.[48] *TGF-β3* is a major candidate gene for mutation in human isolated cleft palate.[22] It is localized in a temporally and spatially restricted fashion in the medial edge epithelia of the fusing palate. Culture of palatal shelves in the presence of neutralizing antibody to *TGF-β3* or anti-sense oligonucleotides to *TGF-β3* prevents fusion of the palatal shelves.[56] *TGF-β3* knockout mice show isolated cleft palates extending from the posterior soft palate into the hard palate for a variable distance.[11] Cleft secondary palates are seen in knockout mice with deficiency of the GABA-producing enzyme glutamic acid decarboxylase and deficiency of the β-3 subunit of the $GABA_A$ receptor genes.[48] A different lesion would appear to explain the rare human X-linked cleft palate.[11]

### Clinical Features

Children with cleft lip and palate face aesthetic and functional problems (Fig. 1-13). The extent of these difficulties depends on the type of cleft and its severity. Functionally, the cleft in the *palate* is most significant, because the palate is critical to achieving adequate intraoral suction for early feeding and to closing the nasopharynx (velopharyngeal valve) for later speech. Aesthetically, children with cleft lip with or without cleft primary palate face potential postoperative asymmetries of the lip and nose, visible scars, and either tissue deficiencies or excess. Functionally, they face potential dental and orthodontic problems related to the effect of the cleft on the alveolar-maxillary position and on dental development. Those with complete cleft lip and palate and those with isolated clefts of the secondary palate face problems with speech and language, including limitation of the phonemic repertoire, poor intelligibility, and delayed development of expressive

and receptive language skills. The degree of delay is directly related to the adequacy and timing of palate repair.

Further problems relate to the growth of the midface, dental occlusion, and the effect of the clefting on eustachian tube function. The degree of later midface deformity depends on the initial distortion in facial development, the timing and type of surgical repair, and the integration of cleft care for all aspects of cleft palate management. Clefting causes concurrent abnormalities in development and orientation of the palatal muscles (particularly the levator palatini and tensor veli palatini). Abnormality in these muscles directly affects the function of the eustachian tube, the child's ability to aerate the middle ear, and the incidence of otitis media. Special attention must be directed to the potential for loss of hearing secondary to infection and to any additional impact that this complication would have on speech development.

### Facial Deformities

Physical examination and imaging reveal structural changes in most areas of the face.

#### Lip

The clefts of the lip may be complete, incomplete, unilateral, or bilateral. Incomplete clefting, whether unilateral or bilateral, can occur in isolation or in combination with a complete clefting of the opposite side of the lip. The distortions in the soft tissues of the lip vary with the cleft and its severity. *Complete unilateral clefts* of the lip extend from the floor of the nostril, through the lip, to a point below the nostril (Fig. 1-17). The lip is shortened on both sides of the cleft, usually asymmetrically, with greater shortening on the medial side. The normal landmarks of the vermillion-

**Table 1-3**
**POINT PREVALENCE OF CLEFT PALATE AT BIRTH IN DENMARK (1936–1987) (N = 2297 PATIENTS)**

| Datum | Total Number of Live Births | Type of Cleft and Number with That Type of Cleft | | | | | | Total |
|---|---|---|---|---|---|---|---|---|
| | | CPH | CPS | CPSM | $CPSM_C$ | CP (?) | CPAA | |
| Cleft type | | | | | | | | |
| Males | 1,951,353 | 362 | 244 | 231 | 152 | 38 | 177 | 1052 |
| Females | 1,841,710 | 563 | 268 | 198 | 149 | 44 | 172 | 1245 |
| Gender ratio (M:F) | 1.06 | 0.64 | 0.91 | 1.17 | 1.02 | 0.86 | 1.03 | 0.84 |
| Totals | 3,793,063 | 925 | 512 | 429 | 301 | 82 | 349 | 2297 |
| Incidence per 10,000 live births | | 2.44 | 1.35 | 1.13 | 0.79 | 0.22 | 0.92 | 6.06 |

Abbreviations: *CPH*, Overt, isolated cleft palate involving the hard and soft palates; *CPS*, Overt isolated cleft of the soft palate only; *CPSM*, submucous isolated cleft palate; *$CPSM_C$*, the subgroup of CPSM that fulfills the Calnan criteria and were operated on for *CPSM* (this is a subgroup of the prior column); *CP (?)*, isolated cleft palate, type unknown; *CPAA*, syndromic isolated cleft palate; isolated cleft palate and clefts associated with anomalies, syndromes, and mental disabilities. All cleft types are included.
Christensen K, Fogh-Andersen P. Etiological subgroups in non-syndromic isolated cleft palate. A genetic-epidemiological study of 52 Danish cohorts. Clin Genet 1994;46:329–335.

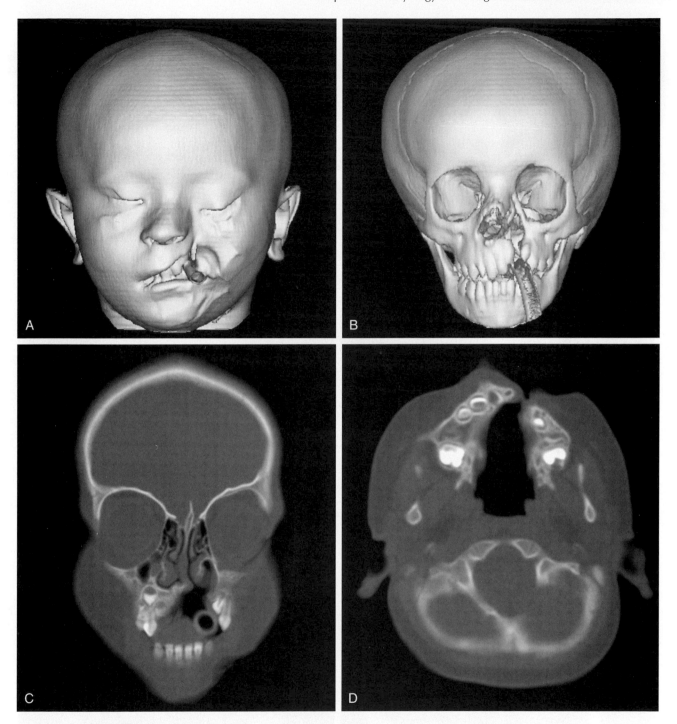

**FIGURE 1-17**   Unilateral cleft lip and palate in a 2-year-old boy. **A**, Three-dimensional CT of the skin surface. **B**, Three-dimensional CT of bone surface. **C**, Coronal CT. **D**, Axial CT. The unilateral cleft extends through the lip, the alveolar ridge, and the palate on the left. In this patient, the soft-tissue cleft lies lateral to the deformed ala nasi and extends toward the lacrimal sac fossa.

cutaneous junction and the vermillion-mucosal junction are distorted. The vermillion tapers upward along the cleft toward the nostril sill. There is a deficiency of vermillion on the medial side. The underlying muscle of the upper lip does not decussate in the midline of the lip, but streams parallel to the border of the cleft and inserts at the alar base. This altered course, failure of decussation, and concurrent distortion of the levator labii superioris create a "fullness" in the segment of the lip lateral to the cleft termed the orbicularis bulge. Patients with *incomplete unilateral cleft lips* show lesser degrees of vertical lip deficiency and muscle distortion proportional to the completeness of the cleft. There may be a small coloboma in the *lower* portion of the lip, a groove in the skin overlying the cleft, and absence of hair and sweat glands in the skin overlying the cleft.[57] Patients with *complete bilateral cleft lip* show similar disorganization of structure on both sides (Fig. 1-18). The central lip segment (prolabium) develops no underlying

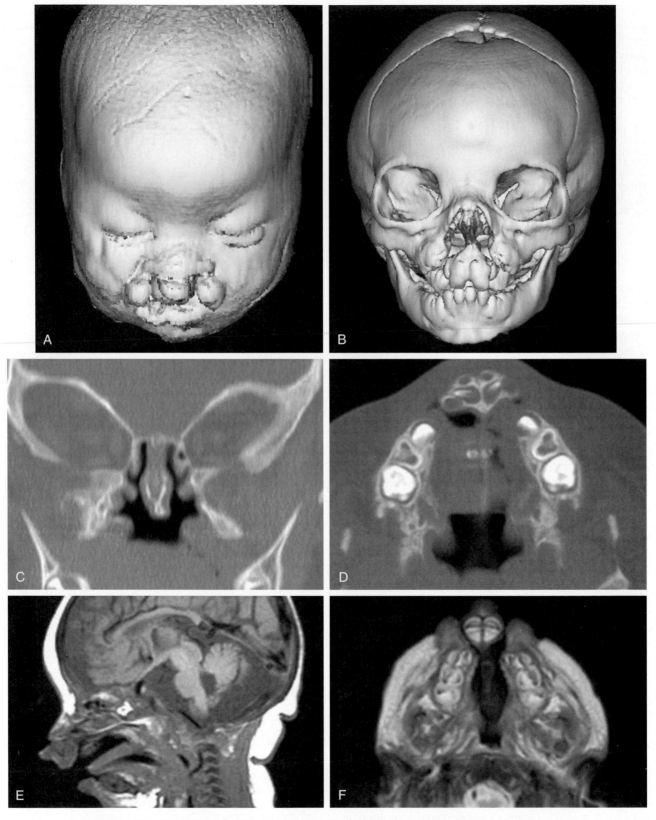

**FIGURE 1-18**   Bilateral cleft lip and palate in a 2-month-old boy. **A**, Three-dimensional CT of the skin surface. **B**, Three-dimensional CT of bone surface. **C**, Coronal CT. **D**, Axial CT. **E**, Saggital T1 MRI. **F**, Axial T2 MRI. The symmetric clefts extend through the lips, the bases of the nostrils, the alveolar ridges, and the palate, leaving a distorted premaxillary segment with the central prolabium isolated from the paired maxillary processes. The prominent central incisors and smaller lateral incisors are positioned far anterior to the maxillary arches. The clefts course obliquely from anterolateral to posteromedial between the primary and secondary palates (cf. Fig. 1-5) before continuing directly posteriorly between the two maxillary palatal shelves to either side of the ununited septum.

muscle, only connective tissue. The degree of deficiency of prolabial tissue varies in width and vertical extent. Minimal vermillion is present. The labial sulcus is absent. The underlying premaxilla varies in position and may project forward or remain in reasonable alignment. The position of the premaxilla significantly affects the appearance and position of the prolabial segment of the lip.

### Maxilla

In comparison to persons with normal palates, those with cleft palates show consistent but variable degrees of midfacial hypoplasia. The anterior hemimaxilla shows a narrowed curvature on the side of the cleft ("arch collapse") and upward tilting of the premaxillary segment.[58, 59] The palatal (inferior) end of the nasal septum nearly always lies on the side of the cleft, while the anterior nasal spine of the maxilla nearly always lies on the noncleft side.[58, 59] This asymmetry probably arises as the tongue pushes into the cleft, and the divided lip and cheek muscles pull asymmetrically on the anterior nasal spine. The posterior maxillary arch is widened in patients with unilateral cleft lip and palate, but the vertical development of the posterior maxilla is normal.[58–62]

### Nose

**Unilateral Cleft** On the cleft side, the angle between the medial and lateral crura is obtuse, the ala is caudally displaced, the alar-facial groove is absent, and the alar-facial attachment is at an obtuse angle. There is real or apparent bony deficiency of the maxilla. The circumference of the naris is greater. The naris is retrodisplaced. The columella is shorter in the anteroposterior dimension, and the medial crus is displaced. The nasal septum is typically deflected toward the cleft side, both superiorly and posteriorly, then deflects back toward the noncleft side, with the caudal septum presenting in the normal nostril. The bony pyramid is also deflected toward the cleft side, with varying deficiencies of the skeletal support for the nose due to the deficiency of the maxillary segment on the side of the cleft.

**Bilateral Cleft** The most visible feature of the bilateral cleft nose is shortening and deficiency of the columella centrally, with splaying and caudal displacement of the alar cartilages to both sides. These distortions create the typical blunted flat nose, widened nostrils, and displaced alar bases. The nasal septum may be midline or variably deflected, depending on whether the cleft is incomplete or asymmetric. Similarly, variations in the position of the smaller segments of the lips and the underlying hemimaxillae affect the degree of nasal widening and flattening.[57]

### Concurrent Malformations

Malformations of other body parts occur in 7.73% (Iranian series) to 36.8% (French series) of patients with cleft lip and/or cleft palate.[49, 50, 63] Malformations are more common with isolated cleft palate (46.7%) than with combined cleft lip plus cleft palate (36.8%) or isolated cleft lip (13.6%).[49] An American series of 3804 cases confirmed that concurrent malformations were more common with isolated cleft palate (51.7%) than with cleft lip plus cleft palate (26.2%).[63] In the French series, infants with clefting showed concurrent chromosomal syndromes (7.8%), recognized nonchromosomal syndromes (3.3%), facial anoma-

lies (11.1%), eye anomalies (2.6%), ear anomalies (1.1%), and diverse malformations of the central nervous system (8.5%), skeletal system (7.8%), urogenital system (6.3%), cardiovascular system (4.6%), digestive system (3.3%), abdominal wall (1.3%), skin (0.43%), and other regions (2.6%).[49]

### Subtle Deformities in Parents of Patients with Common Clefts

Parents of children with cleft lip and palate show an increased incidence of facial asymmetry, wider bizygomatic distance and wider tragus-subnasal distance than do controls, and an increased incidence of nasal deformity and microform cleft lip.[51] However, parents of children with clefts show no divergence from the normal population in their occlusion or dentition.[57] Compared to parents of normal children, parents of children with unilateral clefts show no asymmetry in tooth size and no difference in the incisor relationship, overjet, overbite, and intercanine widths.[57] Parents of children with unilateral and bilateral clefts display equal tooth number, tooth width, and intercanine widths.[57]

## Midline Cleft Lip and Median Cleft Face Syndromes

Median cleft lip is a rare anomaly related to midline craniofacial-cerebral dysraphism.[46] In Fogh-Andersen's series of 3988 craniofacial clefts collected over 30 years (Table 1-1), median clefts of the upper lip were observed in only 15 cases (0.38).[46] Five (0.13%) were true median cleft lips (as considered here) (Fig. 1-12B), three more (0.08%) were true medial cleft lips occurring as part of the orofacial digital syndrome (Fig. 1-12C,D), and seven (0.17%) were pseudomedian cleft lips. An additional four (0.10%) were cases of median cleft nose. Nearly all cases of median cleft face syndrome occur sporadically.[64, 65] Only a few familial cases have been reported.[44, 66–68] An unexpectedly high 12% to 18% of patients with median cleft face syndrome are the products of twin gestation,[44, 66, 67] but the other twin is usually normal. Focal neurologic deficits are not reported with median cleft face syndrome[66, 67, 69–78] and do not appear to form part of the disease. These patients have variable intellectual development. Patient IQ does not appear to be related to the severity of facial clefting.

The midline craniofacial dysraphisms fall naturally into two groups: (A) an inferior group in which the clefting primarily involves the upper lip (with or without the nose) and (B) a superior group in which the clefting primarily affects the nose (with or without the forehead and upper lip). Group A is associated with basal encephaloceles, callosal agenesis (rarely lipoma), and optic nerve dysplasias such as optic pits, colobomas, megalopapilla, persistent hyperplastic primary vitreous with hyaloid artery, and morning glory syndrome (Figs. 1-19 and 1-20). Group B consists of patients with the median cleft face syndrome. This group is characterized by hypertelorism, a broad nasal root, and a median cleft nose (with or without median cleft upper lip, median cleft premaxilla, and cranium bifidum occultum frontalis).[66, 69] Group B patients manifest an increased incidence of

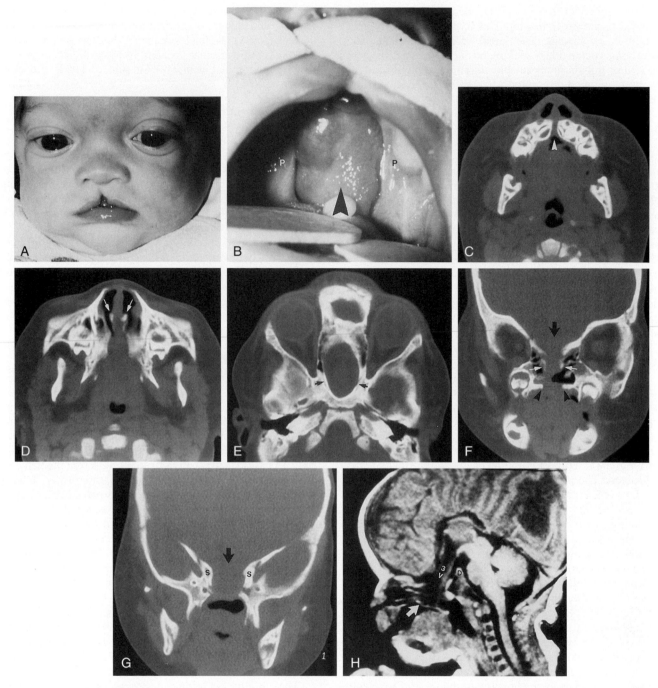

**FIGURE 1-19** Craniofacial cerebral dysraphism. True midline cleft vermillion and philtrum with *hyper*telorism in a 4-month-old boy with progressive compromise of the airway. **A**, Facial clefting. **B**, View through the open mouth toward the palate demonstrates cleft palate with wide separation of the palatal shelves (*P*) and downward protrusion of a soft-tissue mass (*arrowhead*) into the oral cavity. CT in the axial (**C** to **E**) and coronal (**F** and **G**) planes demonstrates midline clefting in the superior alveolar ridge (*arrowhead* in **C**), abnormally wide nasal septum with cleft ethmoids (*white arrows* in **D** and **F**), cleft palate (*black arrowheads* in **F**), and a soft-tissue mass (*black arrow* in **F** and **G**) that bulges inferiorly through the sharply marginated ovoid canal (*black arrows* in **E**) in the cleft sphenoid (*S*) and ethmoid bones. **H**, Sagittal T1-weighted MR image demonstrates callosal agenesis and a transsphenoidal-ethmoidal cephalocele (*white arrows*) containing the third ventricle (*3V*), hypothalamus, and portions of the frontal lobes. The cephalocele extends downward into the oral cavity through the cleft sphenoid just anterior to the dorsum sellae (*D*). (Courtesy of Dr. Sharon Byrd, Chicago.)

frontonasal and intraorbital encephaloceles, anophthalmos/microphthalmos, and callosal lipomas (less frequently, callosal agenesis). Group B has only a weak association with basal encephaloceles or with optic nerve dysplasia (Fig. 1-21).[44]

## Group A

True clefting of the *upper* lip is typically associated with *hyper*telorism and is a clear stigma of the likely concurrence of basal encephalocele, callosal agenesis or lipoma, and any of the diverse forms of optic nerve

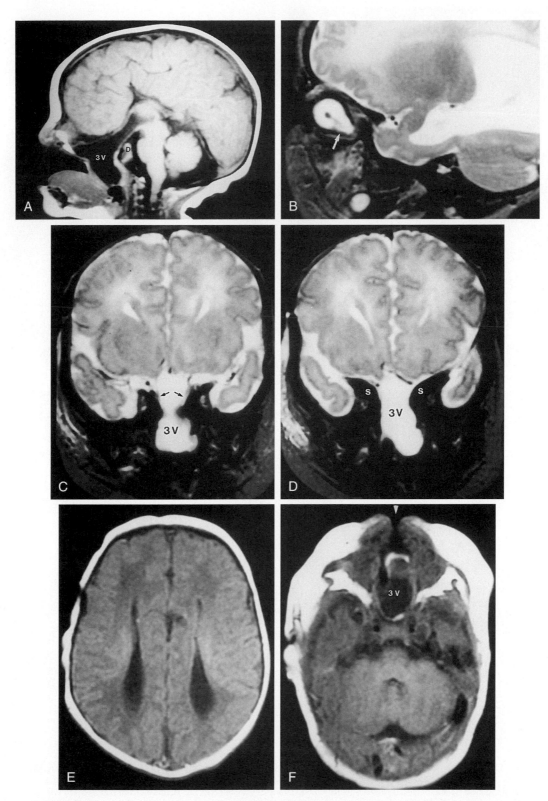

**FIGURE 1-20**    Craniofacial-cerebral dysraphism. True midline cleft upper lip. **A,** Midsagittal T1-weighted MR image shows a transsphenoidal-ethmoidal cephalocele, with the third ventricle (*3V*) and optic apparatus protruding downward through the defect in the sphenoid bone immediately anterior to the dorsum sellae (*D*) to rest on the tongue. The corpus callosum is absent. **B,** Sagittal T2-weighted MR image through the ocular globe demonstrates microphthalmia with coloboma (*arrow*). **C** and **D,** Coronal T2-weighted images through the cleft in the sphenoid (*S*). The cavernous sinuses (*arrows*) form the lateral walls of the hernia ostium. **E** and **F,** Axial T1-weighted images display the callosal agenesis (**E**), the ovoid contour of the third ventricle (*3V*) within the midline defect in the sphenoid, and the midline cleft upper lip (*arrowhead*) (**F**).

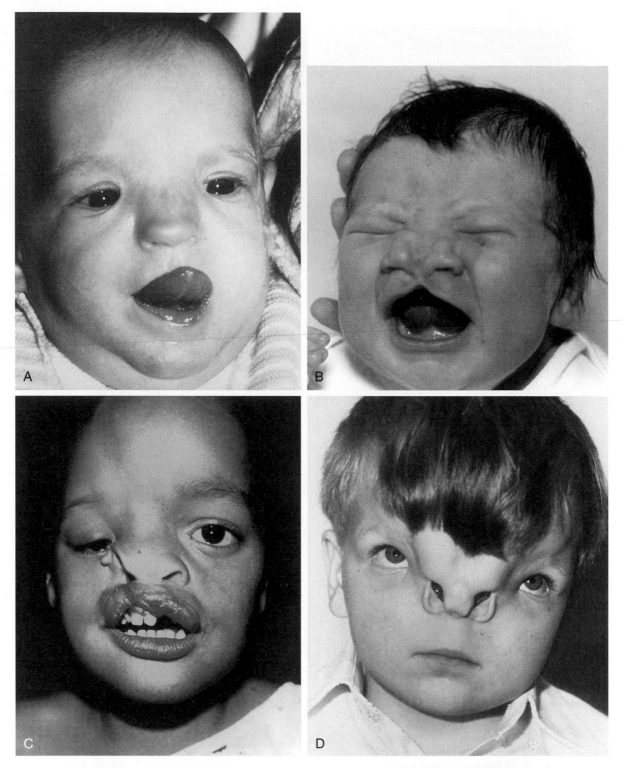

**FIGURE 1-21**    Median cleft face syndrome, typical facies. **A,** Sedano facies type A in 3-month-old boy. **B,** Sedano facies type B in 4-day-old boy. **C,** Sedano facies type C in a young boy after repair of concurrent bilateral common cleft lip and palate. **D,** Sedano facies type D in a 3½- year-old boy. (**A, B,** and **D** from Naidich TP, Osborn RE, Bauer B, et al. Median cleft face syndrome: MR and CT data from 11 children. J Comput Assist Tomogr 1988;12:57.)

dysplasia (Figs. 1-12B, 1-19, and 1-20). The labial defect observed varies from a small notch, to a vertical linear cleft, to a small triangular deficiency of the midline upper lip vermillion (with or without philtrum), with absence of the labial tubercle. This defect is designated *true midline cleft*

*upper lip*. Rarely, this defect may also occur as an isolated finding or as part of the orofacial digital syndromes I and II (Fig. 1-12C,D).[79–81]

Patients with median cleft upper lip may show basal encephaloceles, rare anomalies estimated to constitute

1.2% of all encephaloceles (Figs. 1-12B, 1-19, and 1-20).[82, 101–104] Table 1-4 summarizes the findings in a total of 30 cases collected from the literature and personal material.[43, 66, 83–100] In this series, 50% manifested midline cleft lip (but not nose), an additional 13% manifested midline cleft lip plus nose, 40% to 43% manifested callosal agenesis, and 40% manifested optic nerve dysplasia (i.e., any of the spectrum of optic pit, optic/periopticcoloboma, morning glory disc, and/or megalopapilla). Since the reports are incomplete in many cases, the true concurrence of these anomalies is likely to be even higher.

To date, no report details the true incidence of encephalocele, callosal agenesis, and facial clefting in patients with optic nerve dysplasias.[90–93, 105–109] However, Beyer et al.[110] found one sphenoidal encephalocele in eight patients with 10 morning glory discs, a single-series incidence of 10% to 15%. Lipoma of the corpus callosum is observed in approximately 0.06% of all patients in both in vivo and necropsy studies.[111] Agenesis of the corpus callosum is present in 35% to 50% of such cases.[111] Midline interhemispheric lipoma may be associated with midline subcutaneous lipomas, cranium bifidum, and frontonasal encephaloceles.[66, 112, 113]

### Group B

Median cleft face syndrome (frontonasal dysplasia) is a rare form of dysraphism that affects the midface (Figs. 1-21 and 1-22). The characteristic physical findings in median cleft face syndrome include hypertelorism, cranium bifidum occultum frontalis, widow's peak hairline, and midline clefting of the nose (with or without cleft upper lip, premaxilla, and palate).[44, 66, 69, 114–116] There may also be common clefts of the upper lip and palate, primary telecanthus, ocular colobomas, microphthalmia, and notch-

ing of the alae nasae. Hypertelorism is present in all cases of median cleft face syndrome and is the one *obligatory* finding.[69] The next most constant finding is true midline bony clefting of the nose. The other facial deformities may be present or absent in varying degree.

The types of facial clefting seen in this syndrome have been classified differently by different authors.[64, 66, 69] DeMyer classified the median cleft face syndrome into four classical facies, which represent the most frequently encountered combinations of the major and minor defects of median cleft face syndrome (Table 1-5).[64, 66] Sedano et al.[69] proposed an alternative classification of median cleft face syndrome (Table 1-6). These systems differ, in part, in the importance attributed to notching of the alae nasae (Table 1-7). In our opinion, the Sedano et al. classification appears to correlate best with the intracranial pathology and is the most useful system.

### Molecular Genetics

In mice, severe nasal clefting results from defects in the aristaless-related genes (*Alx3* and *Alx4*), which are upstream regulators of *sonic hedgehog*.[117] Mice with the compound null mutation *Alx3/Alx4* show severe midline clefts of the nose with malformation, truncation, or absence of most of the facial bones, skull base, and other elements derived from neural crest.[117] There is significantly increased apoptosis localized to the outgrowing frontonasal process at (mouse) embryonic day (ED) 10.0, leading to an abnormal position of the nasal processes when they appear at ED 10.5.[117] Thereafter, failure of the medial nasal processes to fuse in the midline leaves defects ranging in severity from partial splitting of the nasal tip to wide separation and anterior truncation of the lateral halves of the nose.[117] The nasal capsule may form as two separate halves, each closed by a

**Table 1-4**
**ANOMALIES ASSOCIATED WITH 30 BASAL ENCEPHALOCELES***

| Anomaly | Manifestation | Number | % |
|---|---|---|---|
| Encephalocele site† | Sphenoidal | 18 | 60.0 |
| | Sphenoethmoidal | 10 | 33.3 |
| | Ethmoidal | 2 | 0.7 |
| | Hypothalamus, third ventricle or pituitary in cephalocele | 15 | 50.0 |
| Endocrine dysfunction | Hypothalmic/pituitary | 6 | 20.0 |
| | Diabetes insipdus with normal anterior pituitary | 1 | 0.3 |
| Corpus callosum | Agenesis | 12 (+1?) | 40.0 (43.0?) |
| | Median cleft lip but not nose | 15 | 50.0 |
| | Median cleft lip and median cleft nose | 4 | 13.3 |
| | ''Fissure lip''‡ | 1 | 0.3 |
| | ''Harelip''‡ | 1 | 0.3 |
| | Cleft palate‡ (of any type) | 14 | 47.0 |
| Eye anomalies | Hypertelorism | 22 | 73.0 |
| | Optic nerve dysplasia§ | 12 | 40.0 |
| | Persistent fetal ocular vasculature | 1 | 0.3 |
| | Microphthalmos | 2 | 0.7 |
| Other pathology | Absent optic chiasm | 1 | 0.3 |
| | Absent chiasm and tracts | 1 | 0.3 |
| | Polymicrogyria | 1 | 0.3 |
| | Preauricular skin tags | 1 | 0.3 |
| | Hypospadias, chordee, lumbar dimple plus hemangioma | 1 | 0.3 |

*Includes data from references 67 (patient 13), 123, 24 (case 1), 25, 26 (case 3), 131, 133 (cases 1 and 2), 134, 135 (cases 1 and 2), 132 (case 7), 136, 138, 141, 142, 143, 145, 146, 152, 149 (cases 1 through 5), 153, 154, 155, and 345.
†In many cases this is the best guess from the limited data available.
‡In these cases the exact nature of the cleft is uncertain.
§Any of the spectrum: optic pit, optic coloboma, megalopapilla, morning glory disc.

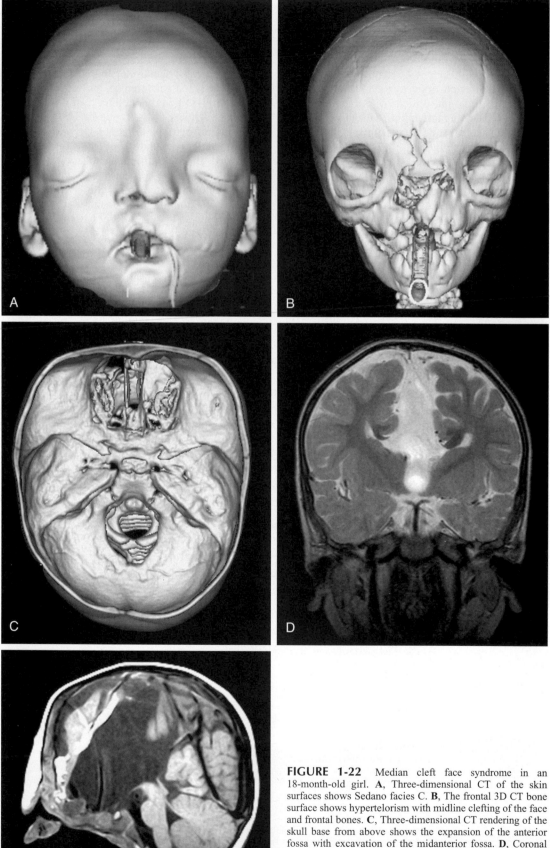

**FIGURE 1-22** Median cleft face syndrome in an 18-month-old girl. **A**, Three-dimensional CT of the skin surfaces shows Sedano facies C. **B**, The frontal 3D CT bone surface shows hypertelorism with midline clefting of the face and frontal bones. **C**, Three-dimensional CT rendering of the skull base from above shows the expansion of the anterior fossa with excavation of the midanterior fossa. **D**, Coronal T2-weighted MR image of the brain shows callosal agenesis, interhemispheric fissure, and wide third ventricle. **E**, Sagittal T1-weighted MR image shows the typical flat frontal contour, callosal agenesis with high third ventricle, and interhemispheric lipoma.

**Table 1-5**
**DeMYER CLASSIFICATION OF MEDIAN CLEFT FACE SYNDROME**

| Facies | Characteristics |
|---|---|
| I | Hypertelorism<br>Median complete cleft nose<br>Absence, hypoplasia, or median clefting of upper lip and premaxilla<br>Cranium bifidum |
| II | Hypertelorism<br>Median cleft nose<br>A. Nose completely cleft<br>B. Cleft nose with divided nasal septum<br>C. Slight hypertelorism<br>No median cleft of upper lip, premaxilla or palate<br>Cranium bifidum present or not |
| III | Hypertelorism<br>Median cleft nose and upper lip with or without median cleft premaxilla<br>No median cleft palate<br>No cranium bifidum |
| IV | Hypertelorism<br>Median cleft nose<br>No median cleft of upper lip, premaxilla or palate<br>No cranium bifidum |

From DeMyer W. The median cleft face syndrome: differential diagnosis of cranium bifidum occultum, hypertelorism, and median cleft nose, lip and palate. Neurology 1967;17:961–971.

remnant of the nasal septum, while a median nasal septum is absent.[117] The nasal labyrinth and anterior part of the nasal capsule are severely malformed and curved.[117] The premaxilla and maxilla are strongly affected and positioned laterally.[117] The palatine bones are cleft.[117] Portions of the skull base that derive from neural crest (the basipresphenoid and pterygoid processes) are severely malformed and broadened, whereas posterior elements of the skull base, derived from cephalic and somitic mesoderm, are normal.[117]

**Table 1-6**
**SEDANO CLASSIFICATION OF FRONTONASAL DYSPLASIA***

| Facies | Characteristics |
|---|---|
| A | Hypertelorism<br>Broad nasal root<br>Median nasal groove with absence of nasal tip<br>No true clefting of the facial midline<br>Anterior cranium bifidum present or not |
| B | Hypertelorism<br>Broad nasal root<br>Deep medial facial groove or true cleft of the nose or nose and the upper lip<br>Cleft palate present or not<br>Anterior cranium bifidum present or not |
| C | Hypertelorism<br>Broad nasal root<br>Nasal alar notching (unilateral or bilateral)<br>Anterior cranium bifidum present or not |
| D | B and C |

*Anterior cranium bifidum may be present or not in all four facies, A through D. Sedano HO, Cohen MM Jr, Jirasek J, et al. Frontonasal dysplasia. J Pediatr 1970;76:906–913.

**Table 1-7**
**CORRELATION OF SEDANO AND DeMYER CLASSIFICATIONS**

| Sedano Classification | Corresponding DeMyer Classification (Per Sedano) | Corresponding DeMyer Classification (Observed in this Series) |
|---|---|---|
| Type A | IV | IIB, IV |
| Type B | IA,* IIB, III | I, IIA, IIB |
| Type C | IIC | — |
| Type D | IA,* IB, IIA | I, IIA, IIC |

*Patients who would be classified into DeMyer's Group IA may be classified as either Sedano facies type B or Sedano facies type D.
Modified from Sedano HO, Cohen MM Jr, Jirasek J, et al. Frontonasal dysplasia. J Pediatr 1970;76:906–913.

Compound null *Alx3/Alx4* mice also show severe reduction in the frontal and parietal bones, with widened fontanelles.[117]

### Concurrent Malformations

Median cleft face syndrome has been found to coexist with many other syndromes.[44, 67, 68, 70–78, 113, 114, 118–125] One review of 11 cases of median cleft face syndrome found 3 type A facies, 4 type B, 4 type D, and no type C. Hypertelorism and a broad nasal root were found in 100% (by definition), true midline bony cleft of the nose in 8 of 11 (all cases except type A facies), median cleft upper lip in 3 of 11, common cleft lip in 3 of 11, common cleft palate in 3 of 11, cranium bifidum in 6 of 11, calcified falx in 6 of 11, interhemispheric lipoma in 5 of 11, Gorlin-Goldenhar syndrome in 2 of 11, and twinning in 2 of 11 patients.[44] We have also seen one patient with concurrent Kallmann syndrome, midline facial cleft, and hypotelorism.[126, 127]

The imaging features of median cleft face syndrome include hypertelorism, cranium bifidum, facial clefting, and intracranial calcifications related to interhemispheric lipoma and/or calcification of the anterior aspect of the falx (Fig. 1-22).[44, 123, 126, 127] The calcification of the falx produces a thick frontal crest that is most commonly found when a lipoma is present, but may be present without associated lipoma.[114]

## Transverse Facial Clefts

Transverse facial clefts represent failure of the maxillary and mandibular processes to form the corner of the mouth and the cheek (Fig. 1–15).[45] (These are discussed in greater detail in the section on Hemifacial Microsomia.)

## Clefts of the Lower Lip and Mandible

Median clefts of the lower lip and the mandible are rare in humans. They vary widely from a simple notch of the vermillion to a complete cleft of the lower lip involving the tongue, the chin, the mandible, the supporting structures of the median of the neck, the hyoid, and the manubrium sterni.[128] The anterior tongue is often bifid (rarely absent). It may be bound to the divided mandible (ankyloglossia).[128, 129] The hyoid bone may be cleft or absent.[128] The clefting of the neck may be accompanied by cysts, chords, contractures, and even midline dermoids of the neck.[128, 129] These lower midline clefts may also be associated with midline clefting of the upper lip and nose.[129]

Cleft lower lip, mandible, and neck may result from mutations in upstream regulators of *sonic hedgehog* (e.g., the aristless-like homeobox genes *Prx1* and *Prx2*) that control cell proliferation during morphogenesis. *Prx1* and *Prx2* mutant mice show reduced size or absence of the midline mandible, an absent or single mandibular incisor, and reduction in their limbs. The mandibular features are consistent with reduced lateral expansion of the medial elements of the jaw. Treatment with the plant alkaloid jervine inhibits end organ response to sonic hedgehog and produces very similar phenotypes in the treated mice.[15, 117]

## Syndrome of Amniotic Bands

Rupture of the amnion can precipitate a cascade of secondary events collectively designated the *amniotic band disruption complex*.[130] In this complex, bands of amnion may interrupt normal morphogenesis, crowd fetal parts, or actually disrupt previously formed parts.[130] Facial clefts may then result from a strand of amnion situated between and preventing the expected fusion of two facial processes, or from a strand of amnion that cleaves through a region not normally formed by fusion, leading to nonanatomic facial clefts and encephaloceles (Fig. 1-16).[130] The frequency and extent of such malformations are greater when the disruption occurs earlier in pregnancy.[130] In 33 cases of this syndrome wherein the timing of the amniotic rupture could be estimated, facial clefts were found in 96% of cases when the rupture occurred prior to 45 days' gestation but in no case in which the rupture occurred after 45 days.[130] Severe defects in the central nervous system and the calvarium such as anencephaly, cephalocele, and hydrocephalus were also common (88%) when the amnion ruptured before 45 days' gestation and were not seen thereafter.[130]

## NASAL DERMAL SINUSES, CYSTS, HETEROTOPIAS, AND CEPHALOCELES

In the early embryo, the developing frontal bones are separated from the developing nasal bones by a small fontanelle called the fonticulus frontonasalis.[131–133] The nasal bones are separated from the subjacent cartilaginous nasal capsule by the prenasal space (Figs. 1-23 and 1-24). This space extends from the base of the brain to the nasal tip.[132] Midline diverticula of dura normally project *anteriorly* into the fonticulus frontonasalis and *anteroinferiorly* into the prenasal space. These diverticula touch the ectoderm. Normally, the diverticula regress prior to the closure of the bone plates of the anterior skull base. Normally, the fonticulus frontonasalis is closed by union of the nasal bones with the nasal processes of the frontal bone to make the frontonasal suture.[134] The prenasal space becomes obliterated as the cartilaginous nasal capsule develops into the upper lateral nasal cartilages and the

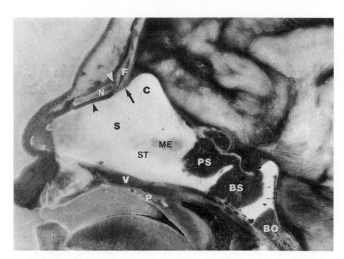

**FIGURE 1-23**   Midsagittal cryomicrotome section of a full-term newborn demonstrates the normal relationships at birth among the ossified frontal bone (*F*), the ossified nasal bone (*N*), the frontonasal suture (*white arrowhead*), and the cartilaginous nasal capsule (*large white structure*) that forms the still-unossified nasal septum (*S*) and crista galli (*C*). The ossified hard palate (*P*) and ossified vomer (*V*) lie below the septal cartilage. Note the direct line from the prenasal space (*black arrowhead*) through the foramen cecum (*black arrow*) to the normal depression or "fossa" just anterior to the crista galli. The midline septal cartilage is directly continuous with the cartilaginous skull base. The basioccipital (*BO*), basisphenoidal (*BS*), and presphenoidal (*PS*) ossification centers are well formed. The mesethmoidal (*ME*) ossification center is just beginning to form. When the vomer and mesethmoid enlarge, the residual cartilage between them is designated the sphenoidal tail (*ST*).

ethmoid bone including the crista galli, cribriform plates, and perpendicular plate of the septum.[132] The two leaves of the falx normally insert into the crista galli, one leaf passing to each side of the crista. At the skull base, the frontal and ethmoid bones close together around a strand of dura, leaving a small ostium designated the foramen cecum. Normally, this transmits a small vein. This foramen is easily

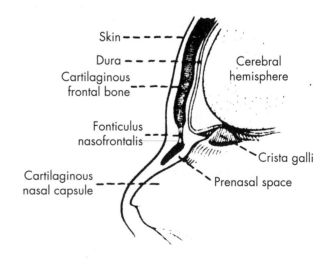

**FIGURE 1-24**   Diagram of the normal embryonic relationships among the dura, fonticulus frontonasalis, prenasal space, and surrounding structures. (From Gorenstein A, Kern EB, Facer GW, et al. Nasal gliomas. Arch Otolaryngol 1980;106:536.)

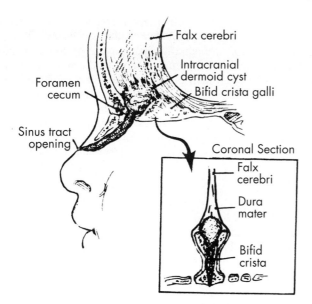

**FIGURE 1-25** Diagram of a typical nasal dermal sinus and cyst traversing the prenasal space and the enlarged foramen cecum to form a mass anterior to and within a groove in the anterior concavity of the crista galli. *Inset*: The anatomic relationships of the leaves of the falx to the sides of the crista galli direct upward extension of the mass into the interdural space between the leaves of the falx. (From Gorenstein A, Kern EB, Facer GW, et al. Nasal gliomas. Arch Otolaryngol 1980;106:536.)

seen at the bottom of a small depression that lies just in front of the crista galli. It is not certain whether the foramen is situated exactly at the frontoethmoidal junction or between the nasal processes of the frontal bones.[132]

If the embryonic diverticula of dura become adherent to the superficial ectoderm, they may not regress normally. Instead, they may pull ectoderm with them as they retreat, creating an (ecto)dermal tract that extends from the glabella through a canal at the frontonasal suture to the crista galli or beyond the crista to the interdural space between the two leaves of the falx.[131, 132, 135] A similar persistent tract may pass from the external surface of the nose, under or through the nasal bones, and ascend through the prenasal space to enter the cranial cavity at the foramen cecum just anterior to the crista galli (Fig. 1-25). Such a tract would be associated with a widened foramen cecum, distortion and grooving of the crista galli, and extension into the interdural space between the two leaves of the falx. Depending on the precise histology of the portions of the tract that persist, these tracts could develop into superficial glabellar and nasal pits, fully patent glabellar and nasal dermal sinuses, and/or one or several (epi)dermoid cysts and/or fibrous cords. Rarely, the sinus tracts, cysts, and cords may extend into or become adherent to the brain itself.[136] Nasal cephaloceles and gliomas may arise by an analogous mechanism. Indeed, there are no valid *histologic* criteria to differentiate between the two entities.[137] If the dural diverticulum persists as a patent communication that contains leptomeninges, CSF and neural tissue, that state would constitute a glabellar or nasal meningoencephalocele (Fig. 1-26). If the developing structure becomes "pinched off" and (nearly) isolated from the cranial cavity by subsequent constriction of the dura and bone, it constitutes a heterotopic focus of meninges and neural tissue at the glabella and nose. Such a benign,

nonneoplastic glial heterotopia is given the dreadful misnomer glabellar and nasal glioma (Fig. 1-27).

## Dermoids and Dermal Sinuses

### Dermoids of the Skull

Dermoids of the skull occur at sites related to the closure of the neural tube, the diverticulation of the cerebral hemispheres, and the lines of closure of the cranial sutures (Fig. 1-28). Pannell et al.[138] classified 94 dermoids of the skull into three groups: A. *Midline dermoids* (43%) affect the anterior fontanelle (25), glabella (1), nasion (2), vertex (1), and the occipital/suboccipital region (11). B. *Frontotemporal dermoids* (45%) affect the sphenofrontal (15), frontozygomatic (16), and sphenosquamosal (11) sutures. C. *Parietal dermoids* (13%) affect the squamosal (8), coronal (1), lambdoid (1), and parietomastoid (2) sutures. Bartlett et al.[139] categorized 84 orbitofacial dermoids into three slightly different groups. In this classification: A. *Frontotemporal dermoids* (64%) are single, slowly growing, asymptomatic lesions ranging from a few millimeters to several centimeters in size. They cluster about the eyebrows, are equally frequent on the left and right sides,

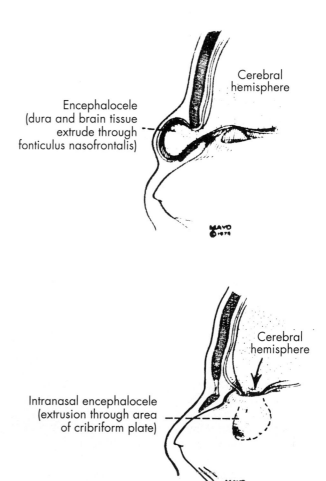

**FIGURE 1-26** Schematic representation of the origin of (**A**) extranasal (glabellar) cephaloceles and (**B**) intranasal transethmoidal cephaloceles. (From Gorenstein A, Kern EB, Facer GW, et al. Nasal gliomas. Arch Otolaryngol 1980;106:536.)

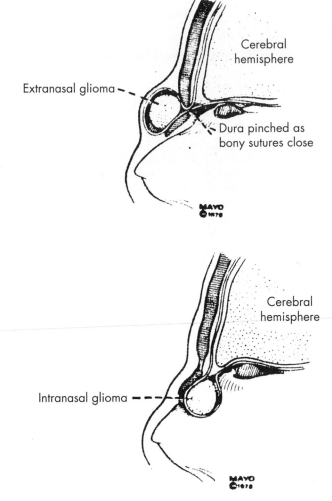

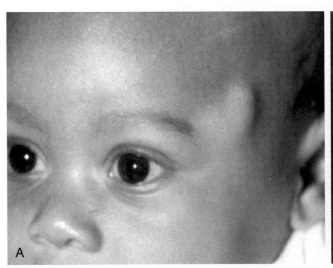

**FIGURE 1-27** Schematic representation of the origin of (**A**) extranasal gliomas and (**B**) nasal gliomas. (From Gorenstein A, Kern EB, Facer GW, et al. Nasal gliomas. Arch Otolaryngol 1980;106:536.)

and show a slight female preponderance. None extends intracranially. B. *Orbital dermoids* (25%) are single lesions of variable size, are equally frequent on the left and right sides, and are more common lateral to the midaxis of the globe (two thirds) than medial to the midaxis of the globe (one third). Thirty percent of the orbital dermoids adhere to the orbital wall: 20% at the frontozygomatic suture laterally or the confluence of the sutures medially, and 10% away from the sutures. Females predominate in this group (2:1). C. *Nasoglabellar dermoids* (11%) are equally frequent on the left and right sides and equally frequent in males and females.[139]

### Nasal Dermal Sinuses

Nasal dermal sinuses are thin (1-3 mm) epithelium-lined tubes[140] that (1) arise at external ostia situated along the midline of the nose and (2) extend deeply for a variable distance, sometimes reaching the intradural intracranial space. *Nasal dermoid and epidermoid cysts* are midline epithelium-lined cysts that arise along the expected course of the dermal sinus. They may coexist with dermal sinuses or present as isolated masses (Table 1-8[142]; Figs. 1-29 and 1-30). Nasal dermal cysts and sinuses constitute 3.7% to 12.6% of all dermal cysts of the head and neck and 1.1% of all such cysts throughout the body.[131, 140] There is no sex predilection.[131, 141–143] They may occur in isolation, as one of a small number of concurrent malformations, or as part of well-known syndromes, including hemifacial microsomia, frontonasal dysplasia, oro-facial-digital syndrome type I, and the *v*ertebral defects, imperforate *a*nus, *t*racheoesophageal fistula, and *r*adial and *r*enal dysplasia (VATER) association.[144] Familial cases are known but rare.[144–146]

### Nasal Dermoids and Epidermoids

Nasal dermoids and epidermoids cluster in three areas: the midline just superior to the nasal tip, the junction of the upper and lower lateral cartilages, and near the medial canthus. Glabellar cysts external to the frontal bone

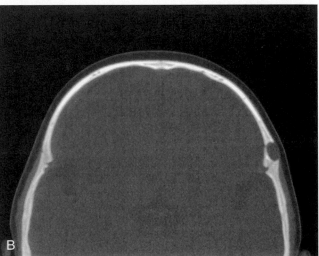

**FIGURE 1-28** Left frontotemporal dermoid. Two patients. **A**, Infant boy with a soft-tissue "bump" close to the pterion. **B**, Noncontrast axial bone algorithm CT displays a sharply marginated, slightly expansile dermoid abutting onto the coronal suture.

**Table 1-8**
**PRESENTING FEATURES OF NASAL DERMAL SINUS/CYST (N = 32)**

| Patient Presentation | Number of Patients | Superficial Infection | Behavior Change from Frontal Abscess | Recurrent Meningitis | Osteomyelitis |
|---|---|---|---|---|---|
| Sinus ostia | 14 | 2 | 2 | 1 | — |
| Midline cyst | 18 | 1 | 1 | 1 | 1 |
| Combined | 32 | 3 (9%) | 3 (9%) | 2 (6%) | 1 (3%) |

From Pensler JM, Bauer BS, Naidich TP. Craniofacial dermoids. Plast Reconstr Surg 1988;82:953–958.

are less common (Figs. 1-31 and 1-32). True epidermoids occur as often as true dermoids, but epidermoids are more common at the glabella-nasion, whereas dermoids are more common along the bridge of the nose (Figs. 1-33 and 1-34).[141] On occasion, multiple sinus ostia are present or sinuses and cysts coexist at both the glabella and the nasal bridge.[131, 147]

Nasal dermal sinuses and cysts are usually detected early in life (mean age, 3 years) as midline nasal cysts (56%) or midline pits (44%), which may contain sparse wiry hairs (Table 1-8) (Figs. 1-35 and 1-36).[142, 148, 149] There may be intermittent discharge of sebaceous material and/or pus; intermittent inflammation; increasing size of the mass with variable degrees of broadening of the nasal root and bridge; intermittent episodes of meningitis; or behavioral change

secondary to a frontal lobe abscess (Table 1-8).[142] The sinus ostium may be "pinpoint" and undetectable until pressure is applied against the nose to express cheesy material.[131] Nasal dermal cysts may be soft and discrete or indurated. They may erode through the overlying skin to form secondary sinus pits. True epidermoids are seven times more likely than dermoids to become infected.[141] Together, nasal dermal sinuses and cysts account for approximately 5% of the intracranial abscesses found in relation to all types of nasal, sinus, and orbital infections.[150]

Nasal dermal sinuses open at any site from the glabella downward along the bridge (dorsum) of the nose to the base of the columella.[151] In one family of identical triplets, each child had a nasal dermal sinus, but the ostia lay at three different sites (nasion, bridge, and tip).[144] Overall, the

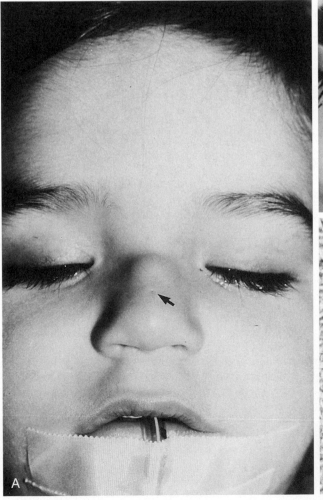

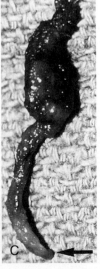

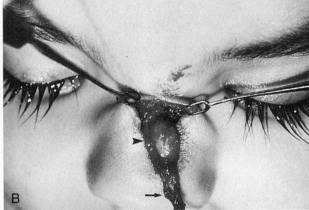

**FIGURE 1-29** Nasal dermal sinus in a 10-month-old boy with increasing swelling of the nose. **A,** Swelling and a pinpoint ostium (*arrow*) on the dorsum of the nose. **B,** Surgical dissection traces the sinus tract (*black arrow*) inward from the ostium to a well-defined ovoid dermoid cyst (*black arrowhead*) within the septum. The cyst reached just to the cribriform plate. **C,** Operative specimen demonstrates the proportions and contours of the dermal sinus and cyst. The arrow indicates the superficial cutaneous end of the tract.

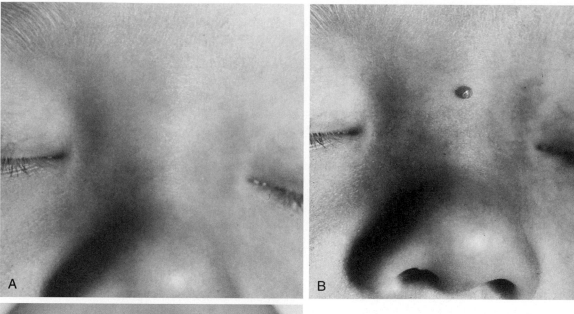

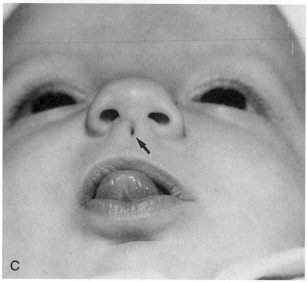

FIGURE 1-30   **A** and **B**, Infected dermal sinus in a 16-month-old boy with intermittent painful swelling, redness, and discharge at the glabella. **A**, Frontal view of the glabella shows swelling of the nasal root but no ostium or discharge. **B**, Immediately thereafter, pressure applied at both sides of the nasal root expressed pus. **C**, Nasal dermal sinus in a 3-month-old girl. When the sinus ostium (*arrow*) lies at the base of the columella, extension to the intracranial space is rare.

external ostium of the sinus is found at the glabella-nasion in 25%, the bridge of the nose in 31%, the nasal tip in 19%, and the base of the columella in 25% (Table 1-9).[148]

The depth to which nasal dermal sinuses and cysts extend is highly variable. The lesions can be shallow pits that end blindly in the superficial tissue (Fig. 1-30C) or long tubes that wander extensively extra- and intracranially (Figs. 1-36 and 1-37).[131] In Bradley's review of 67 children with nasal dermoids, the lesion was confined to the skin in 61% and extended deeply to invade the nasal bones in 10%. The lesion extended into the septal cartilage in 10%, the nasal bones and cartilage in 6%, and the cribriform plate in 12%.[141] Rare sinuses may traverse the entire anteroposterior extent of the nasal septum to end at the basisphenoid, where they attach to the dura just anterior to the sella.[131] Intracranial extension of the dermal sinus is more frequent in patients with multiple anomaly syndromes (67%) than in those with isolated nasal dermal sinuses (31%).[144] The location of the sinus ostium does *not* predict whether there is any intracranial extension. Intracranial extension can be

associated with cysts and sinuses at *nearly* any site, but the frequency of such extension does change with sinus location (Table 1-9).[142] In Pensler et al.'s series,[142] each of four sinuses situated at the base of the columella passed directly to the nasal spine of the maxilla, with no intracranial extension. However, Muhlbauer and Dittmar[145] report a similar sinus that ascended to end in the ethmoid air cells; it did not enter the cranial cavity.

The intracranial end of (epi)dermoids usually affects the anterior epidural space near the crista galli, and from there may pass deeper, between the two leaves of the falx, as an *inter*dural mass.[142, 144] Rare lesions also extend into the brain.[136] In approximately 31% of cases with intracranial extension, the tissue extending inward is a fibrous cord devoid of (epi)dermal elements. At present, intracranial extension of a fibrous cord is not considered significant and has not been associated with sequelae on follow-up examination.[142]

Nasal dermal sinuses are resected for three major reasons: for cosmesis, to avoid/treat complications of local infection, and to avoid/treat secondary meningitis and cerebral abscess (Fig. 1-38).[151] Late development of squamous cell carcinoma has not been observed with *nasal* dermal sinuses to date.

Imaging studies successfully display the course of sinus tracts and any sequelae of infection. The ostium and tract usually appear as isodense fibrous channels or as lucent dermoid channels that extend inward for a variable distance. Bony canals indicate the course of the sinus through the nasal bones, ossified nasal septum, and skull base (Fig.

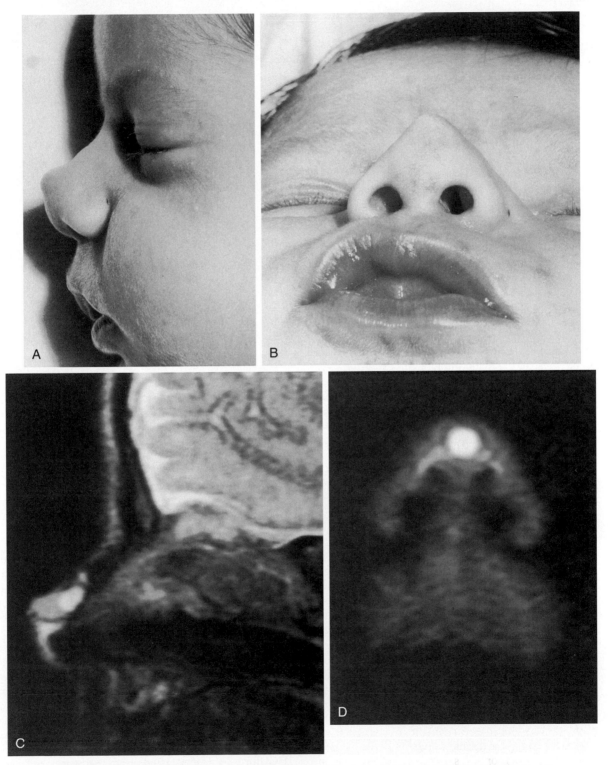

**FIGURE 1-31**   Dermal cyst at the nasal tip in an 11-month-old boy. **A** and **B**, Lateral (**A**) and inferior (**B**) view of the nose shows a focal "elfin" expansion and upturning of the cartilaginous nose. **C** and **D**, Corresponding T2-weighted MR images in the sagittal (**C**) and coronal (**D**) planes show a focal mass and a signal change corresponding to the dermal cyst.

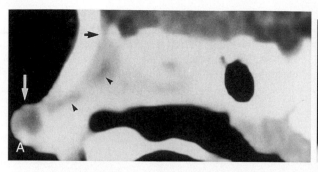

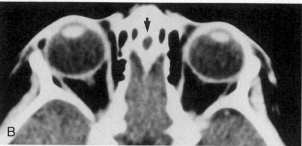

**FIGURE 1-32**   Dermal cyst the nasal tip. **A,** Sagittal reformatted CT. The lucent dermoid cyst (*white arrow*) at the nasal tip connects via a lucent track (*black arrowheads*) to an expanded foramen cecum (*black arrow*). **B,** Axial CT confirms the expansion of the foramen cecum (*arrowhead*).

1-32). An uncomplicated dermoid cyst appears as a well-defined lucency/signal with a sharply marginated capsule (Figs. 1-31 to 1-33). Swelling and edema around the cyst suggest secondary inflammation (Fig. 1-34).[152] The intracranial ends of dermoid cysts typically lie in a hollowed-out gully along the anterior surface of a thickened, enlarged crista.[131] This hollow gives a false impression of a *bifid* crista.[131] The intracranial portion of the dermoid may be lucent or dense. Unfortunately, the only proof of intracranial extension is actual demonstration of an intracranial mass. Imaging demonstration of an enlarged foramen cecum and distorted crista galli only *suggests* such extension; it does not prove it. Foraminal enlargement and distortion of the crista seem to form part of the malformation and may be present (1) with intracranial extension, (2) without intracranial extension, or (3) with intracranial extension of a *fibrous* cord rather than a dermoid.[142] In our own series of 32 cases,[142] the foramen cecum was wide and the crista was grooved anteriorly (bifid) in 6 of 6 cases (100%) with intracranial extension. However, the foramen

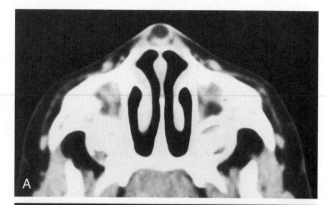

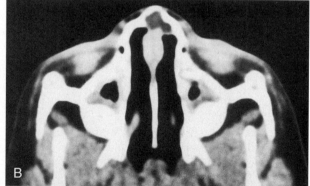

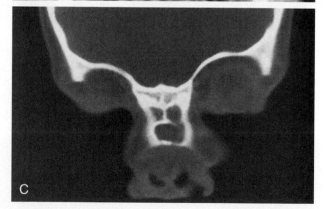

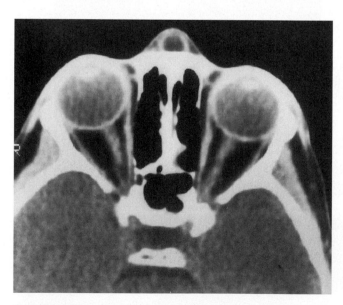

**FIGURE 1-33**   Extranasal epidermoid cyst with no infection. Axial noncontrast CT in a 4-year-old boy. The well-defined isodense cyst wall and lucent center are clearly separable from the adjoining soft tissues. The nasal bones are flattened. No intracranial component was present.

**FIGURE 1-34**   Mixed extranasal-intranasal dermoid with infection. **A** and **B,** Axial noncontrast CT demonstrates an extranasal (**A**) and an intranasal (**B**) mass, scalloped erosion of the nasal bones, and edema of the fat planes surrounding the cyst. **C,** Direct coronal CT shows the broadening and erosion of the nasal bridge.

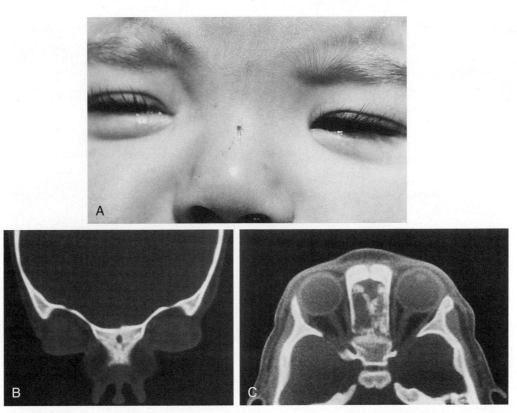

**FIGURE 1-35**   Nasal dermal sinus with intracranial extension. **A,** Frontal view of a 1-year-old girl shows a small tuft of hairs protruding from a midline dermal sinus on the dorsum of the nose. **B,** Direct coronal CT. A well-marginated canal penetrates between the nasal processes of the frontal bones. **C,** Axial CT scan reveals a large foramen cecum with anterior grooving of the crista galli. At surgery the dermal sinus tract and extranasal dermoid were traced upward through the foramen cecum into a 2 to 3 cm intracranial dermoid. This extended intradurally but did not attach to brain. A second ''arm'' of the intranasal dermoid passed posteriorly toward the sphenoid bone.

cecum was also wide in 10 of 26 cases (38%) with no intracranial extension, and the crista was grooved anteriorly in 7 of those 10 cases. To avoid unnecessary craniotomies, therefore, surgical studies suggest that the best approach is to dissect the extracranial portion of the tract along its entire length from the superficial ostium to the *extra*cranial surface of the enlarged foramen cecum, to sever the tract at the extracranial end of the foramen cecum, and then to send the severed end for pathologic examination. If the specimen shows (epi)dermal elements at the foramen cecum, the dissection is extended intracranially. If no (epi)dermal elements are found at the foramen cecum and if no mass is shown by imaging studies, the procedure is concluded without intracranial exploration.[131, 142]

## Heterotopic Brain Tissue

### Nasal Heterotopias (Gliomas)

Nasal gliomas are congenital masses of glial tissue that occur intranasally and/or extranasally at or near the root of the nose. They may or may not be connected to the brain by a pedicle of glial tissue. By definition, they do not contain any CSF-filled space that is connected with either the ventricles or the subarachnoid space of the head.[153]

Nasal gliomas and cephaloceles form a spectrum of related diseases (Figs. 1-23 to 1-27). Characteristic encephaloceles contain ependyma-lined ventricles filled with CSF. Prototypical nasal gliomas consist of solid masses of glial tissue that are entirely separate from the brain.[153] Transitional forms include solid lesions with *microscopic* ependyma-lined canals, solid lesions intimately attached to the brain by glial pedicles with no ependyma-lined spaces, and solid lesions attached to the dura by fibrous bands with no glial pedicles.[153] Analysis of cases reveals that the presence or absence of a pedicle and the presence or absence of *thin* ependyma-lined channels are not helpful in making surgically and radiologically useful distinctions among these lesions. Thus the medically significant differential diagnosis between nasal gliomas and encephaloceles depends on the presence (encephalocele) or absence (nasal glioma) of communication between the intracranial CSF and any fluid spaces within or surrounding the mass.[154, 155] Indeed, nasal gliomas remain connected with intracranial structures in 15% of cases, usually through a defect in or near the cribriform plate.[132]

Nasal gliomas are uncommon, accounting for only 4.5% of congenital nasal masses.[131, 156] They occur sporadically, with no familial tendency.[132] They usually affect both genders equally,[132] although a 3:1 male preponderance has been reported.[156] Up to 15% of patients with nasal heterotopias also manifest multiple cerebral heterotopias.[137] Other congenital malformations of the brain or body are

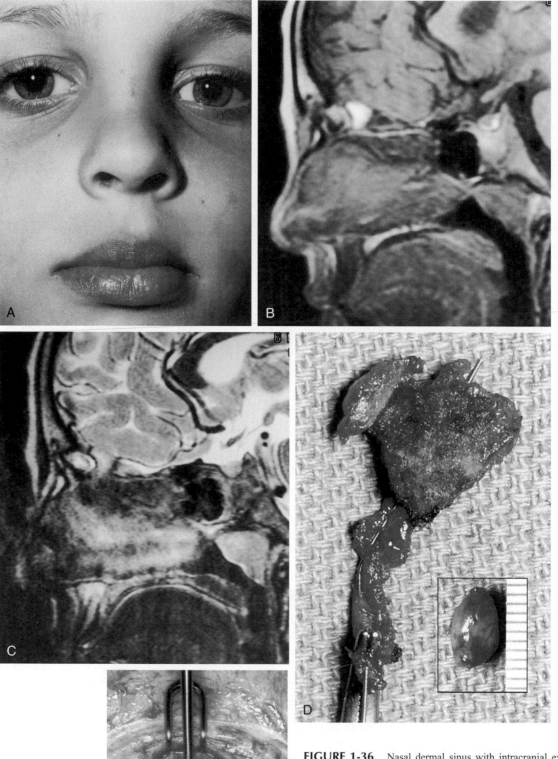

**FIGURE 1-36** Nasal dermal sinus with intracranial extension. **A,** Frontal view of a 7-year-old boy shows a single hair protruding from a midline raised ostium at the dorsum of the nose and subtle fullness at the glabella. **B** and **C,** Sagittal T1-weighted (**B**) and T2-weighted (**C**) MR images show an extranasal tract leading to a glabellar soft-tissue mass that continues intracranially to a well-defned dermoid cyst seated anterior to a concave crista galli. **D,** The probe demonstrates the course of the excised tract in relation to the mass and the dermoid. *Inset in* **D,** Close-up of the dermoid that nested in the anterior concavity of the crista galli. **E,** Intraoperative photograph, from above, shows the probe passing from the surgical defect in the nasal bones, through the tract, to the intracranial space anterior to the crista, between the two layers of dura that constitute the falx (see Fig. 1-25 inset).

**Table 1-9**
**NASAL DERMAL SINUSES: LOCATION OF OSTIUM VERSUS INTRACRANIAL EXTENSION (N = 16)**

| Location of Sinus Ostium | Number of Patients | Number (%) with Intracranial Extension |
|---|---|---|
| Glabella | 4 | 2 (50%) |
| Nasal bridge | 5 | 4 (80%) |
| Nasal tip | 3 | 1 (33%) |
| Base of columella | 4 | 0 (rare) |

From Paller AS, Pensler JM, Tadinori T. Nasal midline masses in infants and children: dermoids, encephaloceles, and gliomas. Arch Derm 1991;127:362–366.

rare. Nasal gliomas are subclassified into extranasal, intranasal, and mixed forms (Fig. 1-27).[132, 157]

Extranasal gliomas (60%) lie external to the nasal bones and nasal cavities.[137, 157] They typically occur at the bridge of the nose, to the left or right of the midline, but, curiously, not in the midline itself. Extranasal gliomas may also be found close to the inner canthus, at the junction of the bony and cartilaginous portions of the nose, or between the frontal, nasal, ethmoid, and lacrimal bones. They may extend into the maxillary antrum between the lateral edge of the nasal bone and the nasal cartilage.[158] Clinically, extranasal gliomas present in early infancy or childhood as

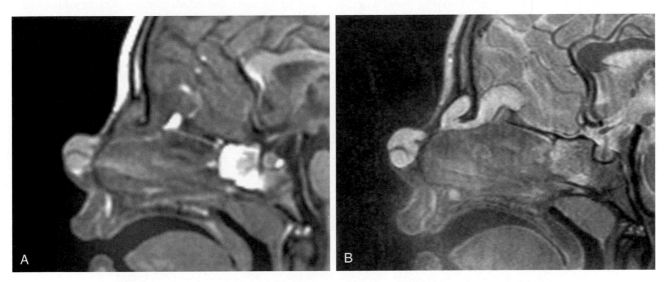

**FIGURE 1-37**  Nasal dermoid with intracranial extension. **A** and **B**, Sagittal T1-weighted (**A**) and T2-weighted (**B**) MR images in a 2-year-old girl with a bulbous nasal tip. The lesion expands the nasal tip and continues via a narrow tract to the glabella, where it forms a confluent transcranial mass at the glabella, the expanded prenasal space, the expanded foramen cecum, and the midline interdural space between the two leaves of the falx.

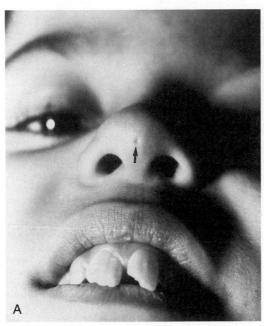

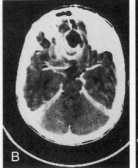

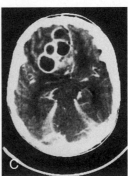

**FIGURE 1-38**  Nasal dermal sinus, intranasal dermoid, intracranial dermoid, and multilocular cerebral abscesses in 10-year-old boy. **A**, Frontal view shows the dermal sinus ostium (*arrow*) at the nasal tip. **B** and **C**, Contrast-enhanced axial CT scans demonstrate the multilocular right frontal abscesses extending upward from the skull base. The very lucent right paramedian cyst (*arrow*) is the intracranial dermoid itself.

firm, slightly elastic, reddish to bluish, skin-covered masses. Capillary telangiectasias may cover the lesion. They are typically unilateral, most frequently on the right, and are rarely bilateral.[156] Nasal gliomas exhibit no pulsations, do not increase in size with the Valsalva maneuver (crying), and do not pulsate or swell following compression of the ipsilateral jugular vein (negative Fürstenburg sign).[132, 149, 155, 159–161] These lesions usually grow slowly in proportion to adjacent tissue but may grow more or less rapidly.[132] They can cause severe deformity by displacing the nasal skeleton, the adjoining maxilla, and the orbital walls, potentially causing hypertelorism.[132]

Intranasal gliomas (14% to 30%) lie within the nasal or nasopharyngeal cavities (Figs. 1-29, 1-39).[137, 157] Intranasal gliomas usually present as large, firm, polypoid, submucosal masses that may extend inferiorly toward or nearly to the nostril.[132, 160] They may protrude through the nostril

secondarily.[159] They usually attach to the turbinates and come to lie medial to the middle turbinate, between the middle turbinate and the nasal septum.[132] Rarely, they attach to the septum itself. They expand the nasal fossa, widen the nasal bridge, and deviate the septum contralaterally. Obstruction of the nasal passage may lead to respiratory distress, especially in infants. Blockage of the nasolacrimal duct may cause epiphora on the affected side. CSF rhinorrhea, meningitis, and epistaxis may be the presenting complaints. Intranasal gliomas are commonly confused with inflammatory polyps. However, nasal gliomas usually have a firmer consistency and appear less translucent than inflammatory polyps.[127, 153] Intranasal gliomas typically lie medial to the middle turbinate, whereas inflammatory polyps typically lie inferolateral to the middle turbinate. Only posterior ethmoid polyps project into the same space as the nasal glioma. As an additional criterion, nasal gliomas

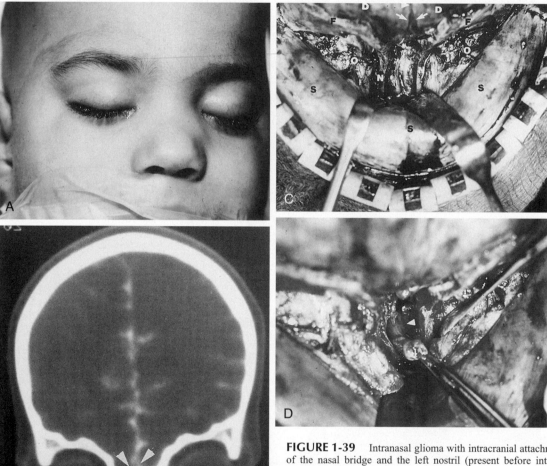

**FIGURE 1-39**    Intranasal glioma with intracranial attachments. **A**, Facies. Widening of the nasal bridge and the left nostril (present before intubation). **B**, Water-soluble positive-contrast cisternography. Direct coronal CT demonstrates a large left unilateral intranasal mass (*arrows*) that deviates the nasal septum rightward, bows the left nasal bone outward, and extends superiorly through a widened foramen cecum into the interdural space between the leaves (*white arrowheads*) of the falx. Opacified CSF outlines the intracranial portion of the mass but does not extend extracranially into or around the intranasal portion of the mass. **C** and **D**, Frontal intraoperative photographs oriented like **A** and **B**. **C**, The scalp (*S*) has been reflected over the orbits (*O*). Keyhole resection of the frontonasal junction exposes the frontal dura (*D*) and nasal cavity, bounded by a remnant of frontal bone (*F*) at the supraorbital ridges and a remnant of nasal bone (*N*) laterally. The frontal dura of either side is reflected inward in the midline (*white arrowhead*) to form the falx. The interdural space (*white arrows*) is widened inferiorly. **D**, Further dissection frees the interdural portion (between the forceps) of the nasal glioma and proves that it is directly continuous with the intranasal portion (*white arrowhead*) of the mass.

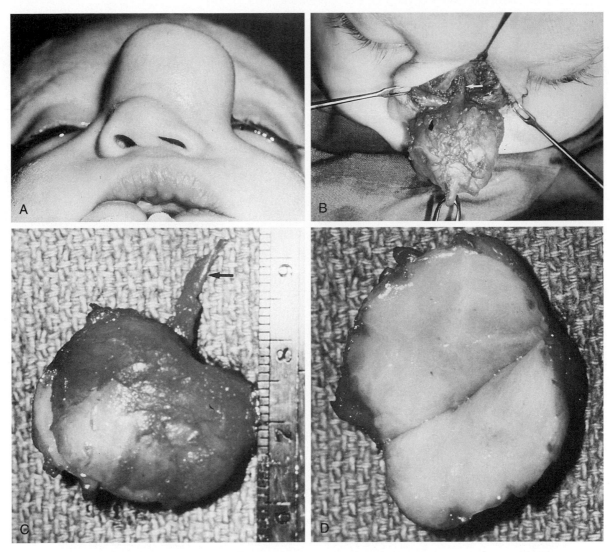

**FIGURE 1-40**   Mixed extranasal-intranasal glioma in an 8-month-old boy with a nasal mass that was present at birth and grew in proportion to the child. **A,** View of the face demonstrates a 3 by 3 by 3 cm firm left paramedian subcutaneous mass that displaces the septal and alar cartilage, narrowing the nostril. The mass did not pulsate or change size with crying. **B and C,** At surgery the mass was not bound to the subcutaneous tissue. It lay almost entirely external to the nasal bones, to the left of midline. A narrow stalk (*arrows*) passed directly through the left nasal bone and extended upward to the left cribriform plate. **D,** Bisecting the specimen revealed a homogeneous mass of smooth grayish-white shiny tissue. Histologic examination revealed brain and fibrous tissue consistent with nasal glioma.

typically present in infancy, whereas ordinary nasal polyps are exceptionally rare under 5 years of age.[161]

Mixed nasal gliomas (10% to 14%) consist of extranasal and intranasal components that communicate via a defect in the nasal bones or around the lateral edges of the nasal bones (Figs. 1-40 to 1-42).[137, 157] Rarely, these two portions communicate through defects in the orbital plate of the frontal bone or the frontal sinus. When *extra*nasal gliomas lie on *both* sides of the nasal bridge, the two components communicate with each other via a defect in the nasal bones, constituting a mixed nasal glioma.[155]

Histologically, nasal gliomas resemble reactive gliosis rather than neoplasia.[161] They consist of large aggregates or small islands of glial tissue with evenly spaced fibrous or gemistocytic astrocytes within vascularized fibrous tissue.[137, 158] The astrocytes may be multinuclear, but they

exhibit no mitotic figures and no bizarre nuclear forms.[160] Fibrous connective tissue enwraps the blood vessels and extends outward to form collagenous septa that partially subdivide the mass.[160] Prominent zones of granulation tissue may be present.[160] The lesion is usually not encapsulated, but astrocytic processes, fibroblasts, and collagen may form a loose or dense connective tissue capsule.[132, 160, 162] *Extra*nasal gliomas are surrounded by dermis with dermal appendages.[132] *Intra*nasal gliomas are surrounded by minor salivary glands, fibrovascular tissue, and nasal mucosa.[132] Only 10% of reported nasal gliomas contain neurons.[160] Occasional lesions show distinct laminated "cortical" architecture, with an external acellular zone resembling the molecular layer of the cortex and an inner, more cellular zone.[137] Still other lesions have zones suggesting a pial layer around the glial tissue.[137] Calcification is rare.[153] Invasion

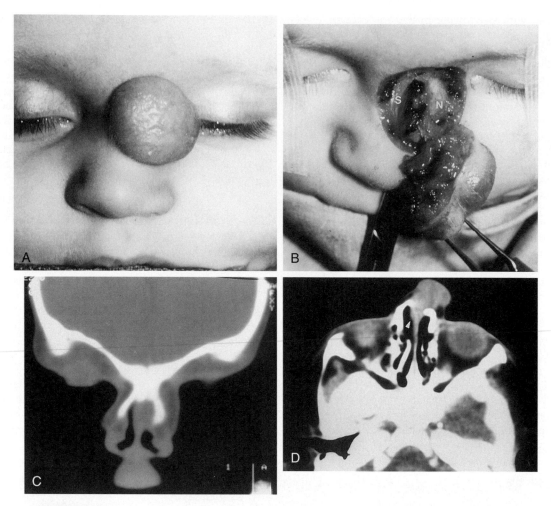

**FIGURE 1-41**   Mixed extranasal-intranasal glioma in a 6-month-old boy. **A,** Facies. The globular mass overlies the dorsum of the nose on the left. **B,** At surgery the lesion was found to have extended through the left nasal bones, bowed the septum (*S*) rightward, and bowed the residual left nasal bones (*N*) leftward. It was attached by a pedicle to the foramen cecum. **C** and **D,** Coronal and axial CT scans show that the mass extends through the resultant defect into the thickened nasal septum (*white arrowhead* in **D**). The crista galli and brain were normal. (Courtesy of Dr. Sharon Byrd, Chicago.)

of surrounding tissue has never been observed, and no metastases have been reported.[162] Thus, these lesions are classified as glial heterotopias, not neoplasias.[161, 163]

### Nonnasal Heterotopias

Heterotopic brain tissue has also been identified at numerous nonnasal sites, including the orbit, hard palate, soft palate, nasopharynx, pterygopalatine fossa, tongue, upper lip, neck, and even lung.[164–170] These heterotopias may be grouped with the nasal gliomas but are probably better considered separately. Both nasal gliomas and nonnasal heterotopias contain glial cells within a fibrous matrix, but the nonnasal brain heterotopias typically show more advanced maturation and differentiation into neural components such as choroid plexus, ependyma-like epithelium, Nissl substance, and rare ganglion cells.[170] Nonnasal heterotopias are usually benign lesions. Solid lesions typically grow in proportion to the body. Cystic lesions may enlarge disproportionately rapidly, especially if they contain functioning choroid plexus.[170–172] Rarely, tumors have been reported in association with nonnasal heterotopias. Bossen

and Hudson[173] reported a small oligodendroglioma arising within heterotopic brain tissue in the soft palate and nasopharynx. Lee et al.[174] reported a melanotic neuroectodermal tumor (melanotic progonoma) within an oropharyngeal mass of brain tissue.

Cleft palates have been reported in 6 of 17 patients (35%) with nasopharyngeal brain heterotopias.[175] Other nasopharyngeal lesions such as teratoid tumors, epignathi, dermoids, hairy polyps, and lipomas have also been associated with clefting of the soft palate.[176] It is unclear whether these concurrences reflect mechanical impediments to the formation of the palate or a midline "clefting/twinning" derangement of molecular signaling.

### Epignathus Teratoma

Epignathus teratomas are congenital teratomas of the oropharynx found in 1 per 35,000 (up to 1 per 800,000) live births.[177] They occur sporadically, are more frequent in girls (female : male ratio = 3 : 1), and are more frequent in children of younger mothers.[177] Fetal history may disclose an elevated alpha-fetoprotein level and polyhydramnios due to fetal difficulty with swallowing in utero.[177] These tumors are typically single masses attached to the skull base in the midline of the posterior nasopharynx, close to Rathke's pouch and the craniopharyngeal canal.[177] Infrequently, they may be multiple and/or may arise laterally.[177] Small epignathus teratomas are frequently pediculated and vary in position. Large tumors may extend intracranially via the craniopharyngeal canal, extend inferiorly to involve the hard palate, fill the oral cavity, deform the maxilla, and even protrude from the oral cavity.[177] Epignathus lesions are regarded as mature teratomas that do not recur after complete resection.[177] Malignant degeneration has not been described, but intracranial extension is often fatal.[177] Six percent of epignathus teratomas are associated with other malformations, most frequently cleft palate of mechanical origin.[177] Other concurrent malformations include duplicate pituitary glands, bifid noses, bifid tongues, and glossoptosis.[177] In the literature, five of seven patients with duplicate pituitary glands (71%) had concurrent epignathus teratomas, with or without callosal agenesis.[177]

### Epulis

Congenital epulis is a rare tumor that affects the gingiva of infants.[178] The lesions may be single or multiple, are eight times more common in girls than in boys, and are three times more common in the maxilla than in the mandible.[178, 179] Epulides are usually not associated with malformations of the teeth, but hypoplasia or absence of the underlying tooth is seen occasionally.[178] Pathologically,

the lesion is composed of large cells with eosinophilic granular cytoplasm within a vascular fibrous connective tissue.[178, 180] Electron microscopy shows that the tumor cells are filled with autophagosomes containing collagen precursors. Immunohistochemical stains are positive for vimentin and neuron specific enolase. These features suggest that epulis may arise from early mesodermal cells that express pericytic and myofibroblastic features, and which undergo cytoplasmic autophagocytosis.[180] Epulis may resolve spontaneously or require resection.[181] The lesions do not recur after resection and show no malignant potential.[178, 182]

## Cephaloceles

Cephaloceles are congenital herniations of intracranial contents through a cranial defect.[183] When the herniation contains only meninges, it is designated a *cranial meningocele*. If the herniation also contains brain, it is called a *meningoencephalocele*. Cephaloceles are classified by the site of the cranial defect through which the brain and meninges protrude.[183, 190]

### Sincipital Cephaloceles

Sincipital cephaloceles are cephaloceles situated in the anterior part of the skull.[161, 184–191] These include both interfrontal cephaloceles (Fig. 1-43) and frontoethmoidal cephaloceles (Figs. 1-44 to 1-49).[161] Sincipital cephaloceles

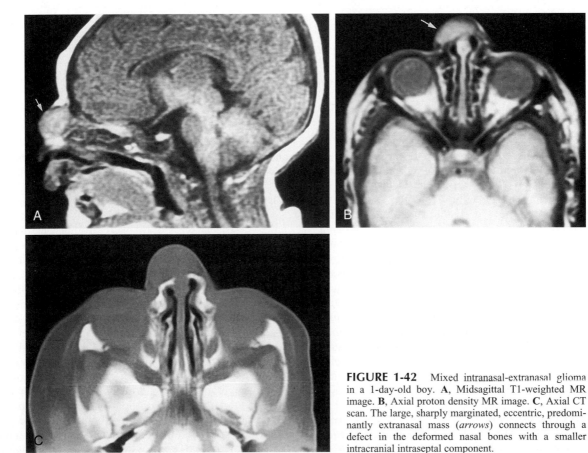

**FIGURE 1-42**  Mixed intranasal-extranasal glioma in a 1-day-old boy. **A**, Midsagittal T1-weighted MR image. **B**, Axial proton density MR image. **C**, Axial CT scan. The large, sharply marginated, eccentric, predominantly extranasal mass (*arrows*) connects through a defect in the deformed nasal bones with a smaller intracranial intraseptal component.

always present as external masses along the nose, orbital margin, or forehead.

Cephaloceles are common lesions, occurring in 1 per 4000 live births.[192, 193] The specific cephaloceles observed vary widely in different populations (Table 1-10). Sincipital cephaloceles are found in 1 in 35,000 live births in North America and Europe but in 1 per 5000 to 6000 live births in Southeast Asia.[194–196] Among Caucasians, occipital cephaloceles are most frequent (67% to 80%), while sincipital cephaloceles (2% to 15%) and basal cephaloceles (10%) are infrequent.[183, 190] Among Australian aborigines, Malaysians, and select Southeast Asian groups, sincipital cephaloceles are the most frequent form encountered. Occipital cephaloceles are closely linked with neural tube defects such as myelomeningocele and show a female preponderance (female : male ratio = 2.4 : 1).[197] Sincipital cephaloceles show no linkage to neural tube defects and no gender predominance.[190, 197]

### Interfrontal Cephalocele

The interfrontal cephalocele presents anteriorly as a midline mass situated above the frontonasal suture. In this form, the cranial defect lies between the two frontal bones (Fig. 1-43).

### Frontoethmoidal Cephaloceles

Frontoethmoidal cephaloceles are defined as cephaloceles that pass outward from the skull through a defect at the junction of the frontal and ethmoid bones, immediately anterior to the crista galli.[161, 185, 198, 199] Frontoethmoidal cephaloceles are then subclassified into nasofrontal, nasoethmoidal, and nasoorbital subtypes by the point at which the skull defect and hernia emerge *externally* (Fig. 1-44).[185, 196] In 120 Thai patients with frontoethmoidal cephalocele seen from 1992 to 1996, Boonvisut et al.[200] found that the internal ostium was a single opening centered at the foramen cecum anterior to the crista galli in 117 cases (97.5%), and paired, bilateral openings occurred at either side of the crista galli in 3 cases (2.5%). The external ostia of the frontoethmoidal cephaloceles were single or multiple and variable in position.[200] In all cases, the crista galli was intact, and the edge of the defect flared outward like a funnel.

Boonvisut et al.[200] classified the external ostia into type I (a single external opening between two adjacent bones) and type II (multiple external openings clustered in the same region). They then used the term *limited* to mean restricted to the territories within or between two adjacent bones and *extended* to signify extension of the bone defect to adjacent bones beyond the confines of the two bones affected primarily. For simplicity, they considered the narrow frontal processes of the maxilla to be nasal bones when classifying lesion ostia into limited or extended types.[200] In their system, type IA signifies a single ostium situated between or within a single pair of bones (e.g., limited to the frontonasal suture). Type IIA signifies multiple external ostia, each of which is limited to two adjacent bones, and type IIB signifies multiple external ostia, at least one of which is of the extended type. In their 120 cases, 106 (88.3%) of the external ostia were type I (85 type IA and 21 type IB). Fourteen (11.7%) of the external ostia were type II (10 type IIA and 4 type IIB).[200] The individual variations are tabulated in their paper.[200]

The relative frequencies of the individual subtypes of frontoethmoidal cephaloceles may vary with the population. In 120 cases of frontoethmoidal cephalocele from Southeast Asia, 39% were frontonasal, 42% were nasoethmoidal, and 18% were nasoorbital (Table 1-11).[196] In 30 cases from India, however, only 6.7% were frontonasal, 87% were nasoethmoidal, and 6.7% were nasoorbital.[195]

**Frontonasal subtype** In the frontonasal form of frontoethmoidal cephalocele, the cephalocele emerges from the bony canal between the frontal and nasal bones. The frontal bones are displaced superiorly. The nasal bones, frontal processes of maxillae, and nasal cartilage are all displaced inferiorly, away from the frontal bone, but retain their normal relationship to each other. The ethmoid bone is displaced inferiorly, so that the anterior end of the cribriform plate is depressed, the midline portion of the anterior fossa is very deep, and the crista projects into the defect from its inferior rim. The anterior portions of the medial orbital walls are displaced laterally. In this subtype, the bone canal is short, because the intracranial (frontoethmoidal) and extracranial (frontonasal) ends of the defect lie close together.[185]

In patients with the frontonasal subtype, the associated soft-tissue mass usually lies at the glabella or nasal root, between deformed orbits (Fig. 1-45).[184, 185] The mass may be small (1 to 2 cm) or larger than the infant's head. Large masses stretch and thin the skin (partially), obscure vision, and may block the airway.[201, 202] Large masses may also cause pressure deformities of the adjacent soft tissue and bone at the forehead, nose, and orbits and thereby cause telecanthus or true bony hypertelorism. Inferior displacement or lengthening on the medial orbital wall may cause an

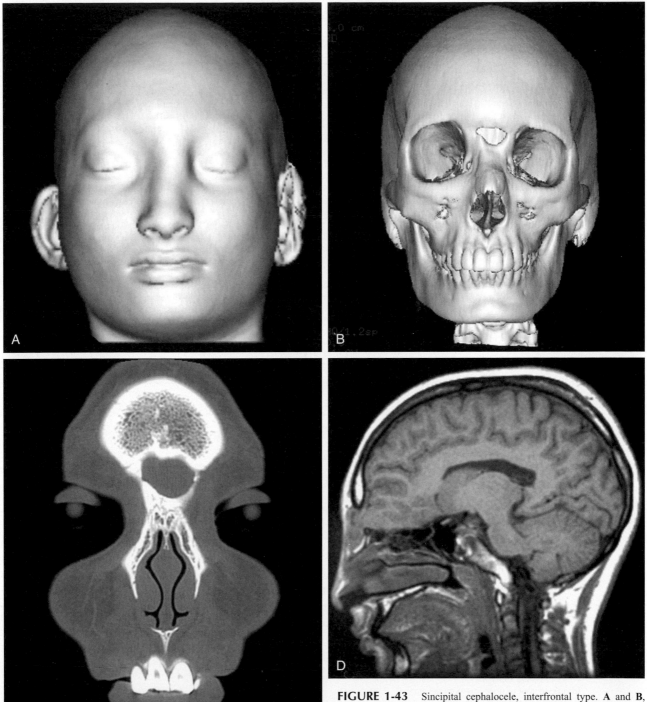

**FIGURE 1-43**  Sincipital cephalocele, interfrontal type. **A** and **B**, Three-dimensional CT of the skin surface (**A**) and the bone (**B**) in a 9-year-old girl shows minimal swelling above the glabella with midline cranium bifidum and concavity of the external surface of the frontonasal suture. **C**, Direct coronal CT documents that the sharply marginated defect lies superior to the nasofrontal suture, between the two frontal bones. **D**, Sagittal T1-weighted MR image shows fullness at the glabella and herniation of intracranial content through the cranial defect above and external to the nasal bones and nasal capsule.

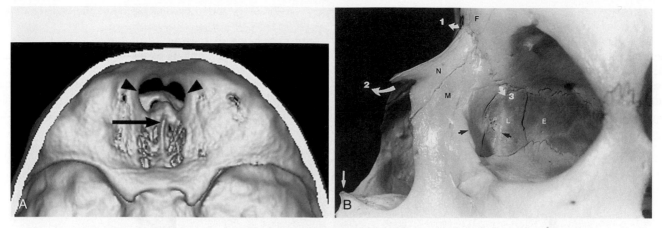

**FIGURE 1-44**　**A,** Three-dimensional bone CT of the internal aspect of the skull base shows the internal ostium of a frontoethmoidal cephalocele. All frontoethmoidal cephaloceles exit the skull via a single defect (97.5%) (*arrowheads*) or paired paramedian defects (2.5%) in the anterior fossa just anterior to the crista galli (*arrow*). **B,** Sites of the anterior ostia of frontoethmoidal cephaloceles. Dried adult skull displays the contours and relationships of the individual bones of the skull and face and the intervening sutures. Ethmoid bone or lamina papyracea (*E*), frontal bone (*F*), lacrimal bone (*L*), frontal process of the maxilla (*M*), and nasal bones (*N*). Note the interfrontal, internasal, frontonasal, and frontomaxillary sutures; the nasal spines (*arrow*) of the maxillae; and the lacrimal sac fossa (between the *black arrows*). The anterior crest of the lacrimal sac fossa is formed by the frontal process of the maxilla. The posterior crest is formed by the lacrimal bone. Cartilaginous structures are not displayed. The sites through which the three subtypes of the frontoethmoidal cephaloceles protrude are indicated by the numbered arrows. *1,* Frontonasal cephalocele. The frontonasal forms emerge at the frontonasal junction. The frontal bones form the superior margin of the defect. The nasal bones, frontal processes of the maxillae, and nasal cartilage form the inferior margin of the defect. *2,* Nasoethmoidal cephalocele. The nasoethmoidal forms emerge beneath the nasal bones superior to the cartilaginous nasal capsule. The nasal bones and the frontal processes of the maxillae form the superior margin of the defect. The nasal cartilage and nasal septum form the inferior margin of the defect. *3,* Nasoorbital cephalocele. The nasoorbital forms emerge along the medial wall of the orbit between the frontal processes of the maxilla and the lacrimal-ethmoid bones. The frontal process of the maxilla forms the anterior margin of the defect. The lacrimal bone and lamina papyracea of the ethmoid form the posterior wall of the defect.

### Table 1-10
### GEOGRAPHIC INCIDENCE OF CEPHALOCELE TYPES

| Cephalocele Location | Boston[186] N = 265 (%) | Indiana[187] N = 67 (%) | Europe[188] N = 68 (%) | Japan[189] N = 40 (%) | Australia[190] N = 74 (%) |
|---|---|---|---|---|---|
| Cervico-occipital | | | 11 (16%) | | 2 (3%) |
| Occipital | 196 (74%) | 55 (82%) | 34 (50%) | 14 (35%) | 34 (46%) |
| Parieto-occipital | | | | 4 (10%) | |
| Parietal | 34 (13%) | 3 (4%) | 6 (9%) | 15 (38%) | 13 (18%) |
| Lateral | | | 1 (1%) | | |
| Sicipital | 31 (12%) | 8 (12%) | 16 (24%) | 3 (7%) | 25 (34%) |
| Nasopharyngeal | 4 (2%) | 1 (1%) | | 4 (10%) | |

Modified from Naidich TP, Altman NR, Braffman BH, et al. Cephaloceles and related malformations. AJNR 1992;13:655–690.

### Table 1-11
### SITE OF MASS OR MASSES IN FRONTOETHMOIDAL CEPHALOCELES (*N* = 120)

| Subtype of Frontoethmoidal Cephalocele | Total Number (Percent) | Number Presenting at Each Site |
|---|---|---|
| I. Frontonasal subype | 47 (39%) | |
| Glabella | | 30 |
| Middle of root of nose (between the eyes) | | 17 |
| II. Nasoethmoidal subtype | 50 (42%) | |
| Middle of root of nose (between the eyes) | | 29 |
| Both sides of the base of the nose | | 9 |
| Lower bridge of the nose | | 7 |
| Widened bridge of the nose | | 5 |
| III. Nasoorbital subtype | 22 (18%) | |
| Inner canthus on one side | | 14 |
| Both sides of the nose | | 6 |
| Widened base of nose with one eye absent | | 2 |
| IV. Multiple sites | 1 (0.8%) | |

From Charoonsmith T, Suwanwela C. Frontoethmoidal encephalomeningocele with special reference to plastic reconstruction. Clin Plast Surg 1974;1:27-47.

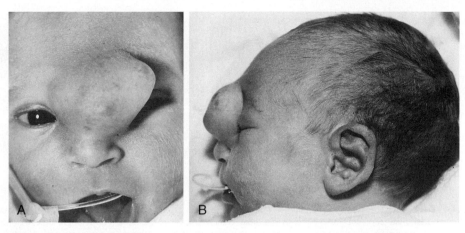

**FIGURE 1-45**  **A** and **B**, Facies. Frontonasal form of a frontoethmoidal cephalocele in 1-week-old girl. The lobulated 3 by 3 by 3 cm skin-covered mass protrudes between the orbits to overlie the nasal bones and nasal cartilage.

antimongoloid slant of the eyes.[202] The size of the soft-tissue mass tends to be proportional to the intracranial pressure, not the size of the internal ostium.[200]

Most frontonasal cephaloceles are firm, solid masses that exhibit no transmitted pulsations. Some are cystic, compressible, and pulsatile and increase in size with the Valsalva maneuver (crying). The mass usually grows as the child grows. Cystic masses may increase in size disproportionately rapidly as CSF pools within the sac. The cephalocele may be covered by intact skin, thin skin that ruptures to leak CSF, or no skin at all, exposing the meninges and brain to the environment. The falx frequently extends into the sac, partially subdividing it. The herniated brain may be well preserved, with recognizable gyri and sulci that converge toward the hernia ostium, or the herniated brain may be reduced to a mass of distorted gliotic tissue. Typically, the brain is not adherent to the base of the sac at the ostium but may be adherent to the meninges at the dome of the sac (60%).[201] The tips of the frontal lobes usually protrude into the defect symmetrically or asymmetrically (Figs. 1-46 and 1-47). The olfactory bulbs may herniate with the brain. The olfactory tracts are stretched. The optic nerves enter the skull normally, but may then recurve sharply anteriorly toward the hernia orifice. The internal carotid arteries course with the optic nerves. The anterior communicating artery may lie near the ostium. Concurrent anomalies such as holoprosencephaly and hydrocephalus may be present.[201]

**Nasoethmoidal subtype**  In the nasoethmoidal form of frontoethmoidal cephalocele, the cephalocele emerges from the bony canal between the nasal bones and the nasal cartilage.The nasal bones and the frontal processes of the maxillae remain attached to the frontal bones above the sac, forming the anterosuperior wall of the canal. The nasal cartilage, nasal septum, and ethmoid bone are displaced posteroinferiorly, forming the posterior-inferior wall of the canal. The crista projects upward into the canal from the depths of the floor. The medial walls of the orbit form the lateral borders of the defect. These can be bony or membranous. In this group, the canal is long, because the intracranial (frontoethmoid) and extracranial (nasoethmoid) ends of the defect lie far apart. In the nasoethmoidal form, the bone defect is usually circular and is situated between the

orbits, increasing the interorbital distance. The nasal bones remain attached to the frontal bones along the upper margins of the ostium. The cribriform plate lies at a normal height with respect to the orbits. The soft-tissue mass lies to one side of the midline, beside the nasal cartilage. It may be bilateral.[203] In patients with nasoethmoidal cephaloceles, the soft-tissue mass usually presents below the glabella, along a widened dorsum of the nose.[184, 185] Cystic swellings may be present on both sides of the nose and may extend to the inner canthus. Hydrocephalus is common. In Suwanwela's series, one of three patients had concurrent agenesis of the corpus callosum with an interhemispheric cyst.[185]

**Nasoorbital subtype**  In the nasoorbital form of frontoethmoidal cephalocele, the cephalocele emerges from the bony canal at the medial wall of the orbit between the maxilla and the lacrimal/ethmoid bones (Figs. 1-48 and 1-49). The abnormal frontal process of the maxilla is displaced anteromedially to form the anterior margin of the defect. The lacrimal bone and lamina papyracea of the ethmoid are displaced posterolaterally to form the posterior edge of the defect.[161] The frontal bones, nasal bones, and nasal cartilage retain their normal relationship to each other. In this subtype, the canal is very long, because the intracranial (frontoethmoidal) and extracranial (medial orbital) ends of the defect are widely separated. Patients with nasoorbital cephaloceles commonly present with cystic soft-tissue masses at the nasolabial folds between the nose and the lower eyelid. These contain nubbins of brain.[185]

Frontoethmoidal cephaloceles induce secondary deformities in the facial skeleton. They impede development of the frontal sinuses, and increase the interorbital and intercanthal distances in most cases. The bitemporal widths and the angles between the lateral orbital walls are usually normal (97.5%), except in cases with microphthalmia or anopia (in which they are slightly decreased).[200] Displacement of the crista galli, the cribriform plate, and the perpendicular plate of the ethmoid bone may lead to maxillary hypoplasia.[204] In all cases, the faces of the patients appear longer than normal and the nasal cartilages are misshapen. The pyriform aperture is shorter and broader than normal and is displaced inferiorly.

Concurrent malformations found in 25 patients with

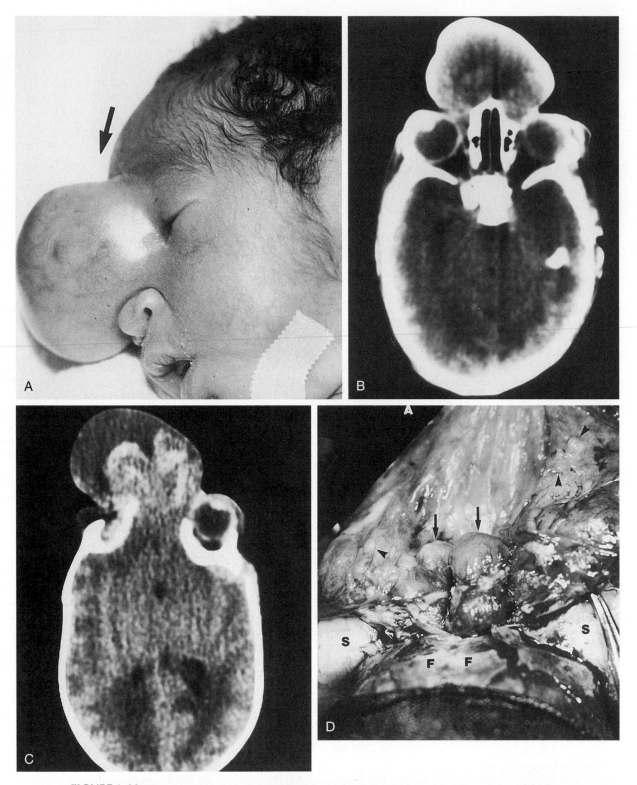

**FIGURE 1-46**    Frontonasal form of a frontoethmoidal cephalocele in a newborn girl. **A**, Lateral view of the face. A large skin-covered midline mass protrudes between the two orbits, overlies the nasal bones and nasal cartilage, and compresses the nostrils. The arrow indicates the angle of observation for the surgical photograph. Noncontrast CT (**B**) and contrast-enhanced CT (**C**) on 2 different days, oriented as in **D**, the surgical specimen. The ostium of the cephalocele lies above the ethmoid and nasal bones but below the frontal bones, so the lesion is a frontonasal type of frontoethmoidal cephalocele. The mass is predominantly cystic. The inferior portions of both frontal lobes protrude directly into the sac to different degrees, greater on the left. **D**, Surgical photograph. Anterior (*A*) view of the frontal bone (*F*) after reflection of the scalp (*S*) anteriorly and opening of the upper wall of the cephalocele to expose its contents. Most of the sac was filled by CSF. Portions of both frontal lobes (*arrows*) protrude into the sac, separated by the interhemispheric fissure. Multiple glial nodules (*black arrowheads*) stud the meninges that form the inner lining of the sac.

frontoethmoidal cephaloceles include microcephaly (24%), unilateral or bilateral microphthalmos (16%), hydrocephalus (12%), and seizures (4%).[161] Mental retardation was present in 43% of those old enough to test. CSF leakage and continuous bleeding from the exposed brain were major problems in those cephaloceles that lacked a skin cover or in which the thin skin cover ruptured. Rappoport et al.[201] found significant associated congenital anomalies such as microphthalmos, mental retardation, and syndactyly with appendicular constriction bands in 33% of these patients. In one patient with a large frontoethmoidal cephalocele, an arachnoid cyst overlying the right frontal lobe communicated with the external sac. Mahapatra et al.'s 30 cases of frontoethmoidal cephalocele from India showed hypertelorism (83%), enlarged head (from hydrocephalus) (16%), and microcephaly.[195]

The etiologies of frontoethmoidal cephaloceles have not been established satisfactorily. Clear variations in cephalocle incidence with geographic location and population suggest the possibility of a genetic basis for the lesions. David et al.[204] corrrelated advanced paternal age with frontoethmoidal cephaloceles and suggested an autosomal dominant inheritance pattern. Alternatively, Richards[205] noted an increased incidence of frontoethmoidal cephaloceles in impoverished rice farmers of Cambodia but a reduced incidence of encephaloceles in infants conceived in winter months, leading him to propose that aflatoxins, notably ochratoxin A, may represent a teratogenic cause of frontoethmoidal cephaloceles. Approximately 60% to 85% of frontoethmoidal cephaloceles have a good outcome unless there are concurrent severe anomalies.[191] In Brown and Sheridan-Pereira's series,[206] severe mental, motor, and/or visual handicaps were seen in only 30% and mild motor/visual handicaps in another 10%. The size of the fluid spaces does not determine the patient's prognosis. Imaging of these cephaloceles displays the bony defect, the nature of the herniating tissue, the effect on the adjacent tissue, and any concurrent intracranial ear, nose, and throat malformations.[126, 127, 207, 208]

### Basal Cephaloceles

Basal cephaloceles are cephaloceles that protrude through the skull base. They include the sphenoorbital, sphenomaxillary, and sphenopharyngeal cephaloceles.[154, 191]

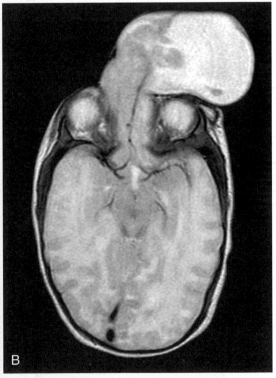

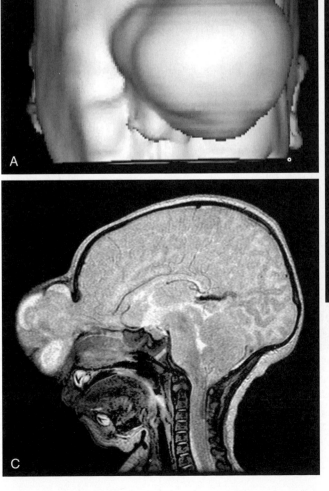

**FIGURE 1-47** Frontonasal form of frontoethmoidal cephalocele. **A,** Three-dimensional CT of the skin surface. The asymmetric glabellar mass obscures the left orbit and projects over the bony and cartilaginous nose. **B** and **C,** T2-weighted MR images in the axial (**B**) and sagittal (**C**) planes demonstrate hypertelorism, anterior herniation of both frontal lobes into the cephalocele through a defect between the frontal bones and the nasal bones, and asymmetric distention of the sac by CSF. The medial frontal anatomy is distorted by the herniation.

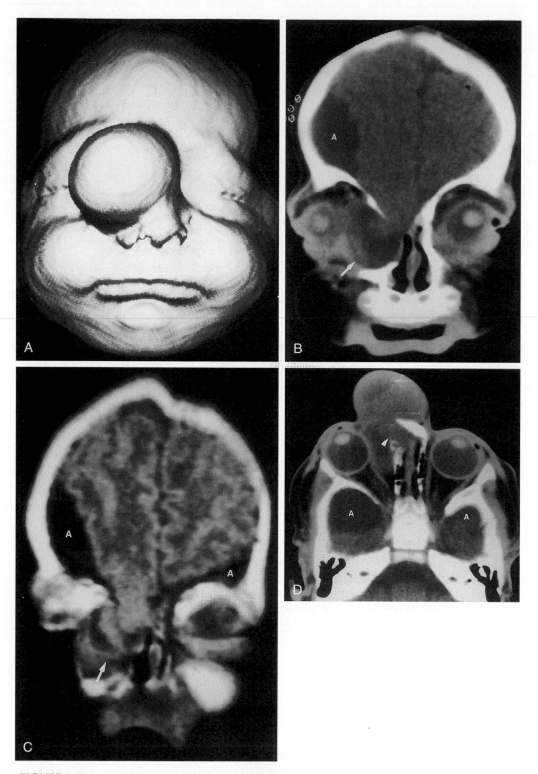

**FIGURE 1-48**    Unilateral nasoorbital cephalocele. **A,** Three-dimensional CT of the skin surface shows a large, eccentric, skin-covered mass at the medial right canthus. The cartilaginous nose is deviated inferiorly and leftward. Coronal CT (**B**) and coronal T1-weighted MR image (**C**) show lateral deviation of the right globe and muscle cone by inferior protrusion of a unilateral cephalocele (*white arrows*) containing brain and meninges. The cephalocele displaces the nasal mucosa medially and the orbital contents laterally. Bilateral anterior temporal fossa CSF spaces suggest concurrent arachnoid cysts (*A*). **D,** Axial CT demonstrates the defect (*arrowhead*) in the medial wall of the right orbit, the characteristic displacement of the muscle cone, and the narrowing of the ipsilateral nasal passage.

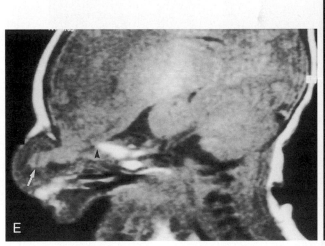
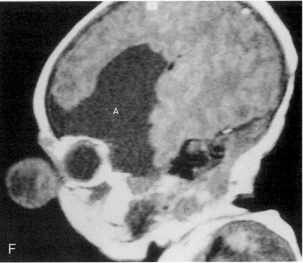

**FIGURE 1-48** *Continued.* **E** and **F**, Sagittal T1-weighted MR images. The paramedian section (**E**) demonstrates the intracranial end (*black arrowhead*) of the osseous canal and direct extension of brain tissue (*white arrow*) into the medial orbit. The lateral section (**F**) demonstrates the prominent arachnoid cyst commonly found in these lesions.

Basal cephaloceles are not visible externally unless they grow large enough to protrude secondarily through the nostril or mouth.[25] They are classified by their point of exit from the skull as sphenoorbital, sphenomaxillary, and sphenopharyngeal.[154] In combined data on 20 basal cephaloceles, 1 (5%) was sphenoorbital, none was sphenomaxillary, and 19 (95%) were sphenopharyngeal.[197, 209]

### Sphenoorbital Cephaloceles

Sphenoorbital cephaloceles exit the skull via the superior orbital fissure and come to lie in the orbit posterior to the globe.

### Sphenomaxillary Cephaloceles

Sphenomaxillary cephaloceles exit the skull via the superior orbital fissure to enter the orbit, but then pass further inferiorly via the inferior orbital fissure to reach the pterygopalatine space. From there they may extend further into the infratemporal fossa.[210]

### Sphenopharyngeal Cephaloceles

Sphenopharyngeal cephaloceles exit from the skull through or between the sphenoid and ethmoid bones. This group is then subclassified (from anterior to posterior) as purely transethmoidal, sphenoethmoidal, or purely transsphenoidal. In the same combined series of 20 cephaloceles, the subtypes of the 19 sphenopharyngeal cephaloceles were transsphenoidal (5 of 19, 26%), sphenoethmoidal (2 of 19, 11%), and transethmoidal (12 of 19, 63%).[158, 197]

*Transethmoidal cephaloceles* (63%) extend downward anteriorly, through a defect in the midline or along the cribriform plate, and do not involve the sella turcica.[197, 204, 209, 210] The hernia sac extends inferiorly into the sinuses or the nasal cavity[211] and typically contains portions of the frontal lobes and olfactory apparatus. *Transsphenoidal cephaloceles* (26%) extend downward posteriorly, through a defect in the floor of the sella turcica, to reach the

nasal cavity (Figs. 1-19 and 1-20).[197, 209] If the palate is cleft, they may also extend further inferiorly into the oral cavity. The posterior margin of these defects is always the dorsum sellae. The lateral walls are the cavernous sinuses and the widely separated halves of the sphenoid bone. The anterior extent is very variable. The defect may involve the sella only or the sella plus the planum sphenoidale. *Sphenoethmoidal cephaloceles* (11%) extend downward through a combined sphenoidal and ethmoidal defect.[197, 204] In our experience, these are nearly always especially large transsphenoidal cephaloceles that extend unusually far anteriorly to involve the ethmoid bone.

As a group, the transethmoidal, transsphenoidal, and sphenoethmoidal cephaloceles are associated with hypertelorism, midline facial clefting, ocular clefting/colobomas, optic nerve dysplasia, and midline cerebral defects. They may be considered together as a craniofacial-cerebral dysraphic complex (Table 1-4). Blustajn et al.[217] noted dysgenesis of the internal carotid artery in two patients with transsphenoidal cephaloceles, hypopituitarism, hypertelorism, and optic nerve coloboma and suggested that all aspects of the syndrome might represent a disorder of neural crest migration. The transethmoidal group tends to have minor facial anomalies (two of three hypertelorism, two of three cleft lip/cleft palate), so they present later in life.[209] The transsphenoidal cephaloceles typically show more severe hypertelorism and facial clefting. The cephalocele sac contains the pituitary gland and the hypothalamus, the anterior recesses of the third ventricle, and the optic apparatus. Symptoms vary. In neonates and infants, the intranasal/pharyngeal soft-tissue mass usually causes a runny nose, nasal obstruction, mouth breathing, or snoring. Frequently, these symptoms are ignored.[218] If they are noted, the intranasal lesions then discovered may be mistaken for nasal polyps, as is true of nasal gliomas.[134] If the early signs are not appreciated, the basal cephaloceles may not be detected until adulthood, when they tend to

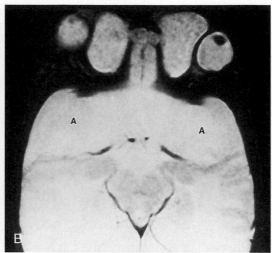

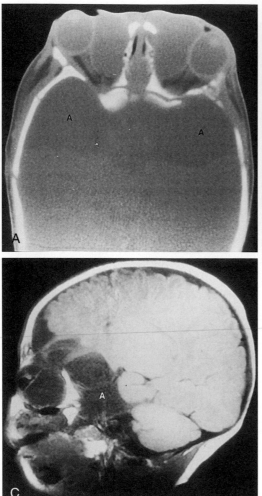

**FIGURE 1-49**   Bilateral nasoorbital cephaloceles in a 5-week-old boy. **A** and **B**, CT and T2-weighted MR image in the axial plane demonstrate lateral displacement of the globes and muscle cones by large, predominantly cystic cephaloceles that extend into the orbit via bilateral defects in the medial walls of the orbits. There are prominent bilateral temporal fossa arachnoid cysts. **C**, Paramedian sagittal T1-weighted MR image shows a direct connection between the brain and the intraorbital sac, indicating cephalocele. (Courtesy of Dr. Robert Dorwart, Indianapolis.)

present with visual disturbance, pituitary-hypothalamic dysfunction, or CSF rhinorrhea.[218] Basal cephaloceles, particularly transsphenoidal cephaloceles, carry a high operative mortality rate (50%) and a high risk of chronic severe neuroendocrine handicaps (70%).[191]

### Rarer Basal Cephaloceles

Other forms of basal cephalocele are seen very infrequently. Losken et al.[210] identified a group of cephaloceles that entered the orbit directly by downward extension between the ethmoid bone medially and the orbital plate of the frontal bone laterally, *not* via the cribriform plate and *not* via the superior orbital fissure.[210] These authors designated this new group anterior ethmoidal cephaloceles (if the ostium lay close to the anterior ethmiodal foramen) and posterior ethmoidal cephaloceles (if the ostium lay close to the posterior ethmoidal foramen). Elster and Branch[219] and Soyer et al.[220] each reported a transalar form of sphenoidal cephalocele that extended downward through the greater wing of the sphenoid into the pterygoid fossa. Raftopoulos et al.[221] described a variation in which the cephalocele appears to have extended inferiorly through the sphenopetral fissure via the anterior foramen lacerum, displacing the foramen ovale anterolaterally.

## DACRYOCYSTOCELES

Dacryocystoceles are the distended nasolacrimal ducts/sacs that result from imperforation of the lacrimal system in the newborn period and shortly thereafter.[222, 223] They are the second most common cause of neonatal nasal obstruction, after choanal atresia, and may require prompt therapy.[208] Dacryocystoceles commonly present as 5 to 12 mm round, tense blue to blue-gray masses situated just inferior to the medial canthi (Fig. 1-50).[222] In the newborn, therefore, dacryocystoceles may be confused with cephaloceles, especially the nasoorbital form of frontoethmoidal cephalocele.

Dacryocystoceles are usually unilateral, in either eye, but may be bilateral in 13% to 65% of cases.[223–226] Males and females are affected equally.[225–228] Nearly all cases are sporadic. The lacrimal *production* system is mature at birth, so full-term infants make tears from the first day of life on.[229] The volume of tears does not correlate with birth weight, placental weight, Apgar score, or maturity of the placenta.[229] However, the distal end of the nasolacrimal duct remains imperforate in many full-term newborns, estimated variably at 6% to 84%.[230–232] The incidence is known to be higher in premature and stillborn infants, perhaps because stretching of the mucosa by breathing and crying helps to open the inferior end of the nasolacrimal duct.[233] Most neonatal dacryostenoses resolve spontaneously. In two series of uncomplicated congenital dacryostenoses, 90% of obstructed tear ducts opened spontaneously at 1 to 13 months of age.[227] Eleven percent required probing to open the duct.[223] Some of those with spontaneous opening of the obstruction re-present in adulthood with renewed stenosis and/or infection.

In 2% of patients with imperforate *distal* nasolacrimal ducts, concurrent obstruction of the *proximal* ducts creates a distended lacrimal sac cyst designated a lacrimal sac mucocele, amniocele, or dacryocystocele.[233, 234] Dacryocystoceles are sterile at birth and asymptomatic. They manifest as excessively large tear menisci along the lower lid margins, crusting of dried mucoid material along the lashes, and epiphora. Secondary dacryocystitis occurs in 0.5% to 6% of these patients and infrequently (2%) leads to a dacryopyocele (lacrimal sac abscess).[225] Periorbital cellulitis and septicemia may ensue.[232]

In approximately 11% to 24% of patients with dacryocystoceles, the distal intranasal end of the nasolacrimal duct distends to form an endonasal cyst (the nasolacrimal mucocele), which may cause partial or complete airway obstruction (Fig. 1-51).[231, 235, 236] These cysts are bilateral in about half of the patients (43% to 48%). Unilateral or partial bilateral obstruction presents as noisy breathing, increased inspiratory effort, restless sleep, and poor sucking. Because 80% of neonates show normal cyclic vasocongestion of the nasal mucosa on alternating sides, patients with unilateral endonasal cysts or partial bilateral obstruction may suffer cycles of respiratory distress when normal nasal engorgement reduces the residual airway. Because neonates breathe predominantly through the nose and will not open

their mouths spontaneously to breathe, significant bilateral endonasal obstruction becomes an acute airway emergency, relieved suddenly when crying or mechanical devices open the mouth. Patients with an endonasal component of the dacryocystocele suffer dacryocystitis more frequently.[237, 238]

## HOLOPROSENCEPHALY

The term *holoprosencephaly* was coined by DeMyer and Zeman[239] to include a group of cerebral malformations characterized by "the tendency for the prosencephalon to remain as a whole, as a simple vesicle incompletely transformed into a complex di- and telencephalon with lobes and hemispheres" (Fig. 1-52). It is characterized by hypoplasia or aplasia of the rostral brain and of the premaxillary segment of the face. Holoprosencephaly is the most common congenital brain malformation in humans.[240] It is found in 1 per 250 concepti but shows very high intrauterine lethality.[240–242] For that reason, the *clinical* incidence of holoprosencephaly is estimated to be 1 in 13,000 to 18,000 live births.[243] There is a female predominance.[244] Surviving patients with severe holoprosencephaly suffer developmental delay, failure to thrive, seizures, poor temperature control, and spastic quadriparesis.[245] Individuals with less severe forms of holoprosencephaly may survive past infancy, with developmental delay. They may even appear to be normal, only to be discovered later to have holoprosencephaly. Those with the least severe forms may show only mental retardation.

Approximately 50% of patients with holoprosencephaly show alteration in the number or structure of their chromosomes,[232] especially chromosomes 13 and 18.

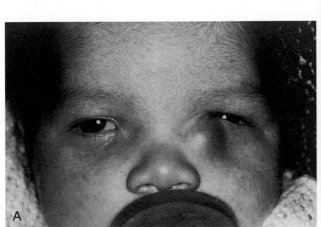

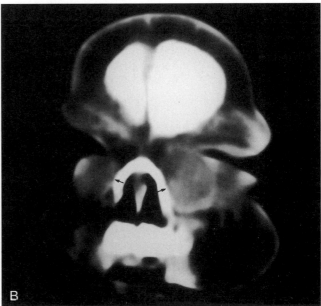

**FIGURE 1-50**  Dacryocystocele. **A**, Frontal view of a 13-day-old girl with a tense bluish mass inferior to the medial canthus on the left. A far smaller lesion of the same type on the right had just subsided. **B**, Direct coronal CT demonstrates the large, tense left cyst (*arrow*) and a smaller right cyst (*arrow*). (**A** from Naidich TP, Heier LA, Osborn RE, Castillo M, Bozorgmanesh A, Altman N. Facies to remember number 6. Congenital dacryocystocele. Int J Neurol 1996;2:389–396.)

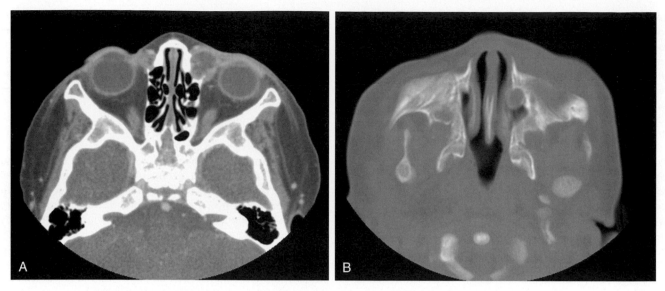

**FIGURE 1-51** Dacryocystocele. **A** and **B**, Axial CT images of a 2-day-old girl with complex cardiac anomalies and asymmetric periorbital edema show asymmetric widening of the left nasolacrimal sac fossa by a tense dacryocystocele. The distended inferior end of the dacryocystocele protrudes into the nasal cavity, causing partial obstruction.

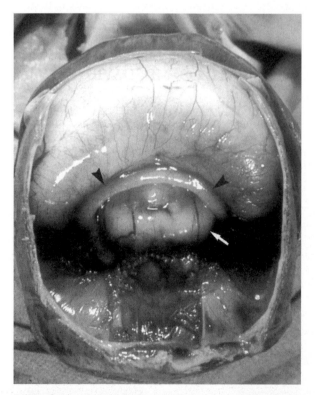

**FIGURE 1-52** Alobar holoprosencephaly with dorsal cyst in a 1-month-old patient with cebocephaly. Gross pathology in situ. View from above at postmortem examination discloses the lissencephalic shield-shaped holoprosencephalon displaced anteriorly against the frontal bones by the large dorsal cyst. The cyst leads directly into the monoventricle deep to an everted hippocampal ridge (*arrowheads*). The holoprosencephalon shows no division into lobes. The diencephalon (*white arrow*) is similarly undivided. There is no falx cerebri. (From Smith MM, Thompson JE, Naidich TP, Castillo M, Thomas D, Mukherji SK. Facies to remember. Cebocephaly with single midline proboscis. Alobar prosencephaly. Int J Neuroradiol 1996;2:251–263.)

Approximately 70% of patients with trisomy 13 have holoprosencephaly.[243] Only 2.1% of patients with trisomy 18 have holoprosencephaly (but holoprosencephalic patients often show trisomy 18).[246] There is a definite association with the Meckel, Kallman, and hydrolethalis syndromes.[247] Recently, holoprosencephaly has been related to deletions and translocations in at least 12 chromosomal regions[248] (Table 1-12).

*SIX3* is a transcription factor related to the *Drosophila* sine oculis/optix family of master regulatory genes that can lead to ectopic eye formation. The gene *Sonic Hedgehog* produces an extremely powerful secreted signaling protein (sonic hedgehog) that organizes adjacent tissues, including the notochord, the floor plate of the neural tube, the zone of polarizing activity of the limb bud, the ectodermal tips of the facial processes, and the apical ectoderm of the second pharyngeal arch.[3] To act, hedgehog protein normally undergoes autoproteolytic cleavage and interacts with cholesterol to create an active, cholesterol-modified amino-terminal segment that remains associated with the membrane and initiates signal transduction.[2, 3, 10, 249] *TGIF* is transforming growth-interacting factor, a modulator of transforming growth factor-alpha. *ZIC2* is a zinc-finger transcription factor gene. The *PATCHED* gene (ptc) codes for a transmembrane receptor that downregulates expression of certain growth factors. *PATCHED* functions in a regulatory feedback pathway with sonic hedgehog, GLI, and Wnt1 (see also the section on Syndromic Craniosynostosis). The hedgehog proteins upregulate several genes, including *PATCHED*. Patched protein then builds up until it interrupts transmission of the hedgehog signal from the cell membrane to the nucleus. Mutations in the *PATCHED* gene cause Gorlin's basal cell nevus syndrome and some sporadic basal cell carcinomas.[250]

Other groups of genes may also play a role in at least some forms of holoprosencephaly. The genes *Otx1* (chromosome 2p13), *Otx2* (chromosome 14q21-q22), *Emx1* (chromosome 2p14-p13), and *Emx2* (chromosome 10q26.1) are intimately involved with patterning large portions of the cerebrum, including the medial cerebral wall.[251–254] Recent work on the role of fibroblast growth factor 8 (fgf8) in modulating the expression of *Otx2* and *Emx2* suggest that this factor could also be related to holoprosencephaly.[255]

In humans, holoprosencephaly may be inherited as an autosomal dominant trait that causes haploinsufficiency for sonic hedgehog. At least 27 different mutations of the *Sonic Hedgehog* gene are known to cause a wide range of holoprosencephalic phenotypes.[240, 248, 256, 257] Translocations that mutate upstream regulators of *Sonic Hedgehog* are associated with mild phenotypes of holoprosencephaly.[258]

Classically, holoprosencephaly has been related to maternal diabetes and in utero exposure to radiation, alcohol, cocaine, *Toxoplasma gondii*, and syphilis.[259] Many teratogens that cause holoprosencephaly are now known to affect *Sonic Hedgehog*. The plant alkaloid jervine, for example, causes holoprosencephaly by inhibiting the tissue response to Sonic Hedgehog.[12] Severe cholesterol deficiency prevents formation of the active signaling moiety of *Sonic Hedgehog* and is the basis for the holoprosencephaly seen in 5% of the RSH/Smith-Lemli-Opitz syndrome.[2] Cleft palate and postaxial polydactyly are also part of this syndrome.[2, 10]

## Holoprosencephaly Facies

Patients with severe forms of holoprosencephaly manifest a spectrum of orbital, ocular, nasal, and aural anomalies, including an elongated tube-like nasal analog termed the *proboscis*.[260] As a group, the facies of holoprosencephaly are characterized by hypotelorism (Fig. 1-12A). These facies must be carefully differentiated from the facies of the midline craniofacial-cerebral dysraphisms, in which *hyper*telorism is associated with true midline clefting of the nose and/or lip, cranium bifidum occultum, anophthalmos-microphthalmos, colobomas of the peripapillary retina, basal cephaloceles, dysgenesis of the corpus callosum, and intracranial lipomas. The holoprosencephalic facies are grouped into five major categories (Fig. 1-53).

### Cyclopia

Cyclopia (Fig. 1-53A) is characterized by a single median bony orbit, which usually contains a variably well-formed eye. The "eye" may consist only of rudiments, may be a single globe with partial formation of one or two cornea(s), or may have partial or complete doubling of the globe(s) within the single orbit. The eyebrows may be absent, present only laterally, or united across the midline (synophrys). The nose may be absent or may consist of an elongated, fleshy, tube-like proboscis that arises from the glabella above the orbit and projects anteriorly. The proboscis has a single external ostium that leads to a blind-ending, mucous membrane–lined canal. No midline septum exists, but other septa, reminiscent of turbinates, may partition the channel. The mouth may be small or absent. The upper lip is present and uncleft, but the philtrum and labial tubercle are usually absent.

### Ethmocephaly

Ethmocephaly (Fig. 1-53B) is characterized by two separate hypotelorotic orbits, two separate eyes, and a median (or, rarely, a double) proboscis that projects anteriorly from a narrow attachment *between* the two eyes. There is no cleft lip or cleft palate. This facies is transitional between cyclopia and cebocephaly and is exceptionally rare.[261]

### Cebocephaly

Cebocephaly (Fig. 1-53C) is characterized by two separate hypotelorotic orbits, two separate eyes, and a single tubular proboscis that attaches along the expected course of the nose and "reclines on its side" rather than projecting outward, as in cyclopia or ethmocephaly. The proboscis has a single midline ostium and a single blind-ending, mucous membrane–lined canal. There are no nasal bones or nasal septum; the presence of a nasal septum rules out cebocephaly. No olfactory epithelium or ganglia are present. The upper lip is typically present but may be hypoplastic. The philtrum may be partially formed, but there is usually no well-developed labial tubercle.

### Absent Intermaxillary Segment with Central Defect and Hypotelorism

Absence of the intermaxillary segment (Fig. 1-53D) is characterized by two hypotelorotic orbits with two eyes, a flat or absent nasal bridge with hypoplastic alae nasi but no nasal septum, and a pseudomedian cleft of the upper lip (absent intermaxillary segment). The missing intermaxillary segment includes (1) the entire thickness of the middle third of the upper lip (prolabium) that normally forms the philtrum and the labial tubercle, (2) the premaxillary bone with the upper incisors, and (3) the primary palate. The secondary palate may be cleft or not.

### Intermaxillary Rudiment with Hypotelorism

This facies (Fig. 1-53E) is characterized by bilateral lateral (common) cleft lip and a hypoplastic intermaxillary segment. The nasal bridge is flat or incompletely elevated but is better developed than in Facies 4 above. The nasal septum is present, but incomplete. The residual intermaxillary segment may be highly rudimentary or moderately well developed. These facies form a continuous spectrum with facies 4 (see above).

Major anomalies of the lower face may also be present in patients with alobar holoprosencephaly, including agnathia, microstomia, anostomia, and otocephaly (ear head).[262]

**Table 1-12**
**GENES RELATED TO HOLOPROSENCEPHALY**

| Gene Name | Gene Product | Chromosome Location |
|---|---|---|
| *HPE1* | Product unknown | 21q22.3 |
| *HPE2* | SIX3 | 2p21 |
| *HPE3* | Sonic hedgehog | 7q36 |
| *HPE4* | TGIF | 18p11.3 |
| *HPE5* | ZIC2 | 13q32 |
| *PATCHED* | Patched protein | 9q22.3 |

Data from Odent S. Attie-Bitach T, Blayau M, et al. Expression of the Sonic Hedgehog (*SHH*) gene during early human development and phenotypic expression of new mutations causing holoprosencephaly. Hum Mol Genet 1999;8:1683–1689.

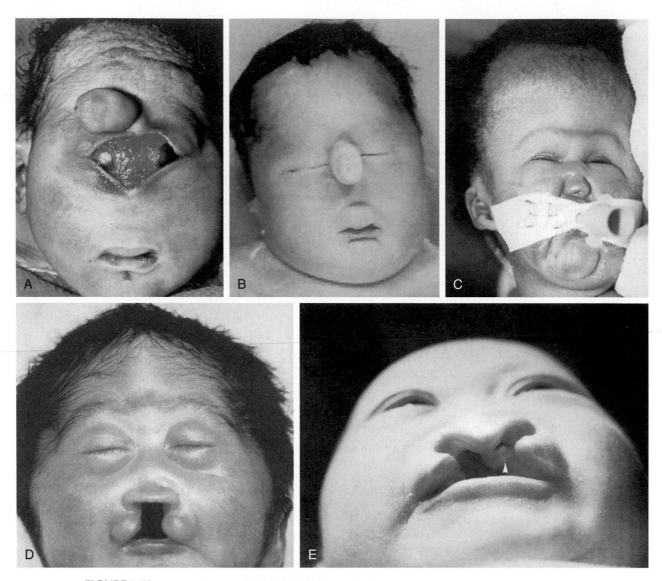

**FIGURE 1-53**    Typical facies associated with holoprosencephaly. Five types. **A,** Facies 1: cyclopia. (Courtesy of Dr. Fred Epstein, New York.) The complete upper lip, with a hint of a labial tubercle in the midline, could represent either fusion of the nasomedial processes independent of the frontonasal process or fusion of the two maxillary processes across the midline. **B,** Facies 2: ethmocephaly. (Courtesy of Dr. Michael Cohen, Halifax, Nova Scotia, Canada.) **C,** Facies 3: cebocephaly with synophrys (fusion of the two eyebrows across the midline). **D,** Facies 4: absent intermaxillary segment, flat nasal bridge, and rudimentary alae nasi (cf. Fig. 12A). Imaging disclosed alobar holoprosencephaly with dorsal cyst. **E,** Facies 5: hypotelorism with an intermaxillary rudiment (*white arrowhead*). Imaging disclosed lobar holoprosencephaly. (From Smith MM, Thompson JE, Naidich TP, Castillo M, Thomas D, Mukherji SK. Facies to remember. Cebocephaly with single midline proboscis. Alobar prosencephaly. Int J Neuroradiol 1996;2:251–263.)

## Brain Malformations

Holoprosencephaly is regarded as a generalized reduction in the forebrain and the frontonasal prominence. As a consequence, the brain is typically microencephalic, weighing only 100 to 150 g at birth (vs. the normal 200 to 300 g).[263] The head is usually microcephalic but may manifest macrocrania when marked expansion of a dorsal cyst distends the intracranial space. Classically, the spectrum of brain anomalies seen with holoprosencephaly is divided into three groups: alobar, semilobar, and lobar forms. In the most severe *alobar form*, the supratentorial brain shows no differentiation into hemispheres or lobes (Fig. 1-52). There is no falx, no interhemispheric fissure, and no superior or inferior sagittal sinus. The deep gray nuclei including the thalami form a single deep gray mass with no (or a rudimentary) third ventricle. The holoprosencephalon contains an undivided monoventricle with no septum pellucidum and no differentiation into lateral ventricles or horns. This monoventricle frequently continues posteriorly into a large dorsal cyst, which displaces the holoprosencephalon anteriorly, close to the frontal bones (Fig. 1-52). The intermediate *semilobar form* is the one most frequently seen in clinical practice. Semilobar holoprosencephaly shows partial development of the interhemispheric fissure, falx, and sagittal sinuses, especially posteriorly. The monoventricle shows partial differentiation into posterior and temporal horns in a ''batwing'' configuration, but no septum pellucidum. A small, partly formed third ventricle partially subdivides the deep gray matter into paired, partially united thalami. A dorsal cyst may be present or absent. The least severe form, *lobar holoprosencephaly*, is characterized by variably complete formation of the interhemispheric fissure, falx, and dural sinuses and at least partial formation of the lobes of the prosencephalon, the horns of the lateral ventricles, and the third ventricle. The development of the brain is most nearly normal posteriorly and substantially less advanced anteriorly. By definition, however, all forms of holoprosencephaly exhibit continuity of the frontal cortex across the midline, where normally the two frontal lobes would be separate.

## Correlations Between Facies and Holoprosencephaly

Patients with *alobar* holoprosencephaly show facial abnormalities in 83% to 90% of cases.[239, 264] These abnormalities may be any of the five major categories of facies but often are facies 1 to 3. Therefore, detection of cyclopia, ethmocephaly, or cebocephaly strongly suggests the presence of alobar holoprosencephaly. However, 10% to 17% of patients with alobar holoprosencephaly have milder atypical facial changes or normal facies.[265] Patients with *semilobar* holoprosencephaly show facial anomalies less often, in 30% of cases in some series.[265] These usually are the milder facies 4 and 5 (Fig. 1-54). Facies 3—cebocephaly—can be seen with semilobar holoprosencephaly. Patients with *lobar* holoprosencephaly usually have normal facies but may also show facies 4 or 5 or subtle findings such as a single central incisor.[244]

Osaka and Matsumoto[265] correlated the presence of facial anomalies with the type of holoprosencephaly. In this review, facial anomalies were considered to be clefting of the lip and palate, not milder forms. These authors found an imperfect correlation: facial anomalies were seen in 47 of the 100 cases (47%). In these cases the holoprosencephaly was alobar in 80%, semilobar in 10%, lobar in 0%, ''abortive'' in 0%, and unclassified in 9%. Facial anomalies

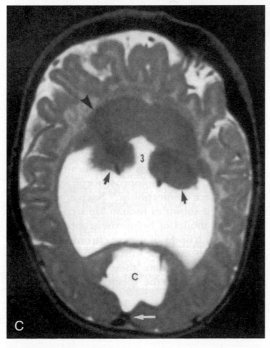
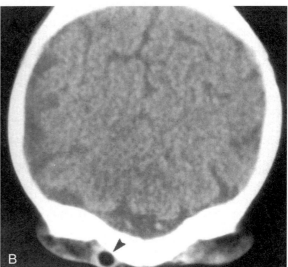
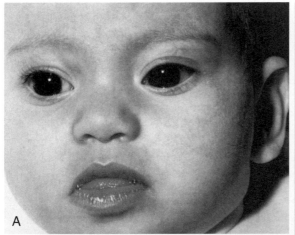

**FIGURE 1-54** Normal facies with semilobar holoprosencephaly. **A,** Frontal view. This normal-appearing child was evaluated for the small bulge at the upper medial right orbit. **B,** Direct coronal noncontrast CT documents that the orbital lesion (*arrowhead*) is a small dermoid. Absence of the interhemispheric fissure led to MR imaging. **C,** Axial T2-weighted MR image shows semilobar holoprosencephaly with absence of the interhemispheric fissure and falx anteriorly, partial subdivision of a monoventricle into temporal and occipital horns posteriorly (batwing configuration), incomplete third ventricle (*3*), partial separation of the thalami (*arrows*) with union of the deep gray matter (*arrowhead*) anteriorly, and a dorsal cyst (*C*). (From Smith MM, Thompson JE, Naidich TP, Castillo M, Thomas D, Mukherji SK. Facies to remember. Cebocephaly with single midline proboscis. Alobar prosencephaly. Int J Neuroradiol 1996;2:251–263.)

were absent in 53 of the 100 cases (53%). In those patients with no facial anomalies, the holoprosencephaly was alobar in 8%, semilobar in 20%, lobar in 50%, "abortive" in 20%, and unclassified in 0%. In at least one study, four patients with concurrent Dandy-Walker cyst and holoprosencephaly had normal facies.[264]

## FACIAL AND BRANCHIAL ARCH SYNDROMES

The syndromes of the first and second branchial arches manifest as deficiencies of tissue and as hypoplasias of the maxillary and mandibular arches.

### Pathogenesis

Differences among the dysplasias of the first and second branchial arch derivatives may reflect differences in the time of insult with respect to neural crest cell migration and differences in the cells targeted.[266] In mice, neural crest cells destined for the first and second visceral arches begin to migrate out of the neural folds when the embryo has five to nine somites.[266] Exposure to retinoic acid at and just prior to this time causes malformations of the visceral arches that appear to constitute the Goldenhar oculoauriculovertebral (OAV) spectrum (see the section on Hemifacial Microsomia).[266] Exposure to retinoic acid later, after the migration of neural crest cells into the first and second visceral arches is nearly complete, affects the formation of cells from the ectodermal placodes associated with the first and second visceral arches.[266] Excessive cell death initially involving placode-derived cells appears to underlie mandibulofacial dysostosis (MFD) (see the section on Mandibulofacial Dysostosis [Treacher Collins Syndrome]).[266] The normal ganglia are composed entirely of neural crest cells.

Placodal cells then migrate into the distal part of the ganglia, where they differentiate rapidly into neuroblasts, while the crest cells contribute to later-differentiating neurons, and supporting Schwann sheath cells and satellite cells.[266] MFD appears to be directly related to excessive and/or premature cell death in the cell populations derived from the first and second ectodermal placodes.[266] Subsequent deficiencies in the tissues that form the dorsal aspects of the maxillary and mandibular prominences of the first visceral arch and the dorsal aspect of the second visceral arch may result directly from localized tissue damage or secondarily from inadequate promotion of growth and/or cytodifferentiation.[266]

## Hemifacial Microsomia (Goldenhar Syndrome, OAV Complex)

Concurrent auricular, ocular, and facial anomalies are found in a heterogeneous group of overlapping conditions. Goldenhar described the triad of (1) epibulbar choristomas, (2) preauricular skin appendages and pretragal blind-ending fistulae in association with (3) mandibular facial dysostosis, now called Goldenhar syndrome.[267–269] To these, Gorlin and colleagues added concurrent vertebral anomalies and renamed the complex oculo-auriculovertebral (OAV) *dysplasia*.[270] Rollnick and Kaye then added microtia and called the condition the OAV *complex*.[271] In similar fashion, unilateral hypoplasia of the face and transverse facial clefts, previously termed hemifacial microsomia (HFM), and bilateral, more nearly symmetrical bifacial microsomia (BFM), have also been incorporated into the expanded OAV complex.[272] Further work has linked the OAV complex with the VATER sequence.[272, 273]

HFM is the second most common facial birth defect after cleft lip and palate (Fig. 1-55).[274] Males are affected more frequently than females: (1.2 to 1.8) to 1. The OAV complex

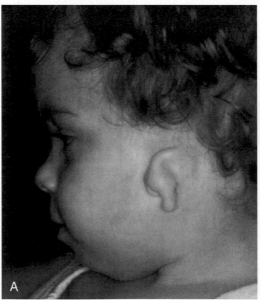
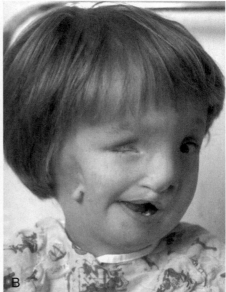

**FIGURE 1-55** Microtia and hemifacial microsomia in two patients. **A,** Microtia. The pinna is deformed. The face appears normal. **B,** Hemifacial microsomia. The line formed by the two palpebral fissures and the line formed by the mouth converge to the region of the deformed, hypoplastic pinna. The right orbit, right eye, and entire right side of the face are asymmetrically smaller. The skin tag falls along the line between the pinna and the mouth.

usually arises sporadically but may be familial in up to 21% of cases.[275] About 45% of patients have affected relatives, and 5% to 10% have affected sibs.[271] The specific mode of inheritance and the effect of environmental factors are hotly debated but may be autosomal or X-linked dominant in at least some cases.[276] Among 204 patients with malformations of the external ear (microtia), HFM constitutes 70.5%, isolated microtia 23.5%, Goldenhar syndrome alone 3%, and Goldenhar syndrome within the OAV complex 3% of cases.[275] Goldenhar syndrome accounts for approximately 19% of cases of HFM and 4% to 8% of all cases of OAV complex.[274, 277] The specific incidences of the OAV conditions are estimated at 1 per 3500 to 5600 births for Goldenhar syndrome and 1 per 45,000 live births for the OAV complex.[267]

The OAV spectrum is believed to develop during the first 4 wg, during the period of blastogenesis.[278] Its pathogenesis is unknown. Three theories have been offered[280]: 1. OAV could result from interference with the vascular supply to the region, notably the primordial stapedial artery, leading to local hemorrhage in the developing first and second branchial arches.[276, 279] 2. OAV could reflect impaired interaction between neural crest cells and the branchial arch mesenchyme.[276] 3. OAV could reflect mutations in the *Msx* genes. These genes are a class of homeobox genes expressed in cephalic neural crest cells prior to their migration to form the craniofacial mesenchyme and are critical for differentiation of first branchial arch ectoderm-mesenchyme.[276] Manipulation of the *Msx* genes in mice leads to major abnormalities in first branchial arch derivatives.[281, 282] Similar genes function throughout the body. At present, therefore, the *Msx* genes are candidate genes for the OAV complex and other craniofacial malformations.[276] Some similarity exists between bilateral OAV syndrome and hypoglycemia associated with diabetic embryopathy, but the children with hypoglycemia do not manifest the facial asymmetry typical of HFM-OAV complex.[283]

The stigmata of the OAV complex include anomalies of the face, ears, and eyes, with numerous concurrent malformations of the central nervous system (CNS) (15%), skeleton (41%), heart (26%), gut (12%), and lungs (9%).[284]

### Face

Facial asymmetry is seen in about 65% of patients, is severe in 20%,[272] and progresses during childhood.[272] The asymmetry may *not* be appreciable in the infant, but it becomes evident by age 4 years in most cases.[285] The hypoplasia may be predominantly vertical or predominantly transverse, but most patients show mixed vertical-transverse hypoplasia, with the greatest hypoplasia along the oblique line from the (residual) ear to the corner of the mouth (Fig. 1-55). Most HFM is unilateral (up to 94% in some series), but the microsomia may be bilateral in 16% to 35%.[286] The right side of the face is affected far more often than the left. In the *upper face*, the zygoma and the lateral maxilla are most affected.[287–289] The orbits are approximately equal in size in 96%, but differ in their vertical position in two thirds and in their horizontal position in 15% of HFM patients.[290] The

interorbital distance remains normal. The nose and columella deviate toward the hypoplastic side. In the *lower face*, the mandible is affected most severely, so *mandibular* hypoplasia accounts for most of the asymmetry seen in HFM (Fig. 1-56). The ramus of the mandible is more severely hypoplastic than the body, so the mandible acquires a steeper slope. These changes cause anteroinferomedial displacement of the temporomandibular joint, lateral rotation of the lower jaw, and posterior displacement of the mandibular angle.[287–289]

The muscles of mastication show reduced volume that is ipsilateral to the side of HFM and roughly proportional to the degree of mandibular hypoplasia. Muscle mass is reduced about 50% in each of the masseter, temporalis, medial pterygoid, and lateral pterygoid muscles in grade 3 mandibular hypoplasia, but muscle mass is symmetrical and nearly normal in patients with only minimal manidibular hypoplasia.[291]

Sessile or pedunculated preauricular skin tags are found between the ear and the corner of the mouth in 20% to 88% of cases.[267] The skin tags are unilateral in 37% and bilateral in 25% of Goldenhar patients (Fig. 1-55). Skin tags may also arise at aberrant sites: retroauricular, nostril, nasal tip, and eyelids. They occasionally are seen in patients with apparently normal ears (4%). Preauricular and facial pits occur in 7% and preauricular sinuses in 6% to 29% of patients, with or without associated skin tags.

### Mouth

The mouth may have a short transverse dimension (microstomia) or show marked elongation by unilateral or bilateral transverse facial clefts (Tessier No. 7) (macrostomia) (Figs. 1-15, 1-57). These clefts may appear as open clefts extending well lateral to the vermilion or as thickened fibrous bands on the buccal mucosa, Macrostomia is present in 17% to 62% of HFM patients. Cleft lip and/or cleft palate is common in the Goldenhar group (20%) and those with the full OAV complex (15% cleft palate, 7% cleft lip with or without cleft palate). The upper lip may have a shortened vertical height.[267] The palatal and tongue muscles may be hypoplastic, paralyzed, or both. The palate deviates to the affected side in 39% of HFM patients. Bifid tongue, bifid uvula, and double lingual frenulum have also been reported. About 35% of patients suffer velopharyngeal insufficiency secondary to asymmetric movement of the palate and the lateral pharyngeal wall. The ipsilateral parotid and other salivary glands may be normal, agenetic, or displaced. Ectopic salivary gland tissue may be present as a nasal mass in Goldenhar syndrome. There may be salivary fistulae.[267]

HFM often includes malocclusion and buccal crossbite on the affected side.[292] Dental maturation is asymmetric in half of these patients; however, the side of greater maturation may be either the affected or the unaffected side with equal frequency.[292] The teeth show defects in the primary enamel.[292] The distribution of these defects is concordant with the laterality of the craniofacial anomalies and is most pronounced on the maxillary incisors.[292]

### Ears

#### External Ear

*Microtia* signifies an ear that is too small and/or malformed (Figs. 1-55 and 1-56).[286] Isolated nonsyndromal microtia is found in 0.016% of all newborns. Approximately 3.1% of microtia patients have Goldenhar syndrome, but microtia is found in up to 68% of Goldenhar patients. The microtia is typically unilateral (66%). Where it is bilateral, it is asymmetric in 65% to 90% of cases. The severity of the malformatiom in the external auditory canal parallels the change in the auricle. The external auditory canal is normal in 98% of those with a normal auricle and abnormal in 58% of grade 1, 100% of grade 2, and 86% of grade 3 microtia.[267]

#### Middle Ear

The severity of ossicular chain malformation parallels the severity of microtia and of mandibular hypoplasia. The ossicular chain is normal in 96% of those with normal auricles and abnormal in 52% of grade 1, 89% of grade 2, and 95% of grade 3 microtia. Radiologically, middle ear structures are abnormal in 70% of cases. Approximately one third of HFM patients have normal hearing. The rest show sensorineural hearing loss (6% to 16%), mixed conductive-

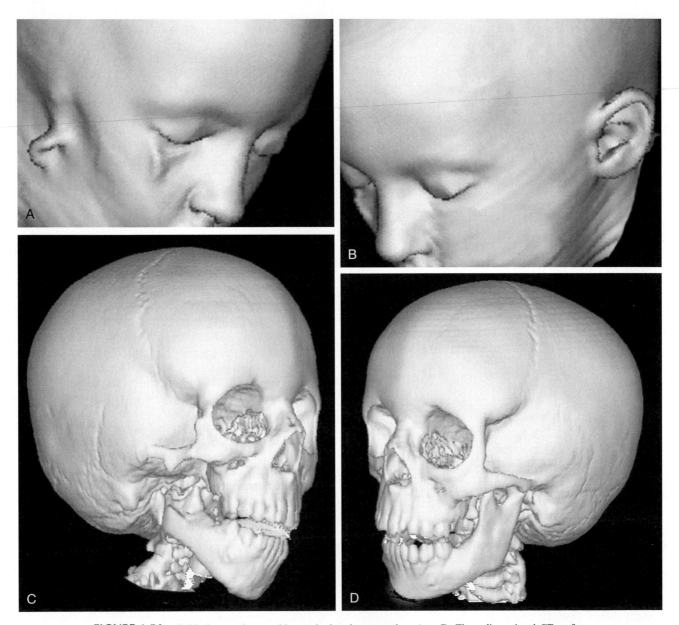

**FIGURE 1-56** Goldenhar syndrome with vertebral malsegmentation. **A** to **D**, Three-dimensional CT surface renderings of the skin (**A** and **B**) and bone (**C** and **D**) of the two sides show right hemifacial microsomia with right microtia and hypoplasia of the right zygomatic arch, right maxilla, and right mandible, especially the angle and condylar process of the mandible. The lower right eyelid shows depression of the skin surface that corresponded to a coloboma.

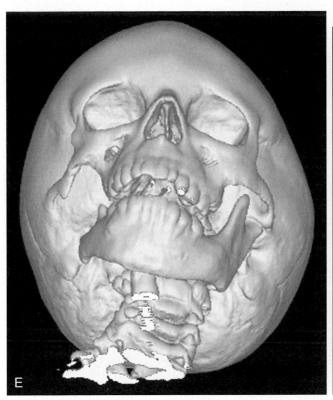
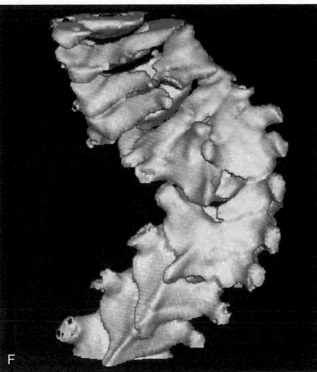

**FIGURE 1-56**   *Continued.* **E,** Frontal bone surface shows the marked deficiency of the right facial skeleton. **F,** The thoracolumbar spine shows malsegmentation and sharp-angle scoliosis.

sensorineural hearing loss (6%), or purely conductive hearing loss.[293]

*Inner Ear*

Inner ear anomalies are present in at least 6% of patients with Goldenhar and HFM syndromes (Fig. 1-57).[294, 295] Seventh nerve palsy is seen in 45% of HFM patients and correlates with the severity of the microtia. Radiologically, the facial nerve canal is abnormal in 83% of patients: 7% of grade 1 microtia, 38% of grade 2 microtia, and 63% of grade 3 microtia. The vestibules and semicircular canals may be dilated or small. The common crus may be absent.[296] The internal auditory canal can be asymmetrically smaller, shorter, and inclined upward. The cochlea and vestibule may be abnormal or absent.

*Eyes*

Characteristic ocular features of Goldenhar syndrome include epibulbar choristomas, colobomas of the upper lid, impaired ocular motility, and dacryostenosis (Fig. 1-58). Epibulbar choristomas are congenital, benign, nonproliferative masses of normal epidermal and connective tissue structures that are situated at abnormal sites. Their etiology is unknown. Choristomas are the most common epibulbar tumor in children.[269, 275, 297, 298] They are found in 4% to 32% of Goldenhar cases, 21% of HFM cases,[290]

and 88% of OAV complex cases. Of 50 children with ocular "dermoids," 46% had HFM. Half of these (22%) had signs of Goldenhar syndrome. Among 127 personal and published cases of Goldenhar, Feingold and Baum[269] found that 76% had dermoids (53% unilateral, 23% bilateral) and 47% had lipodermoids (28% unilateral, 19% bilateral). Most choristomas are subconjunctival (59%), often encroaching on the corneo-scleral limbus. A smaller number are limbal (41%). None are corneal.[275] A few arise on the eyelids.

Unilateral or bilateral colobomas of the *upper* lid are seen in 11% to 71% of Goldenhar cases, usually in the medial third or at the junction of the medial and middle thirds (Fig. 1-58).[275] *Lower*-lid colobomas may be seen in 6% of Goldenhar patients' eyes without concurrent upper-lid colobomas, but specific involvement of the lower lid suggests a diagnosis of MFD (Treacher Collins syndrome) rather than the Goldenhar-OAV complex.[293, 299] Other ocular features include ectropion (eversion of the lid margin) (25%), unilateral blepharostenosis (11%), blepharoptosis (2%), anophthalmia/cryptophthalmia/microphthalmia (2% to 12%), impaired ocular motility including esotropia, exotropia, and Duane's retraction syndrome (presumably secondary to hypoplasia of the oculomotor nerve or brain stem nuclei) (10% to 19%), and dacryostenosis (with or without lacrimal fistulae secondary to obstruction at the nasolacrimal duct or lower canaliculus) (11%).[275]

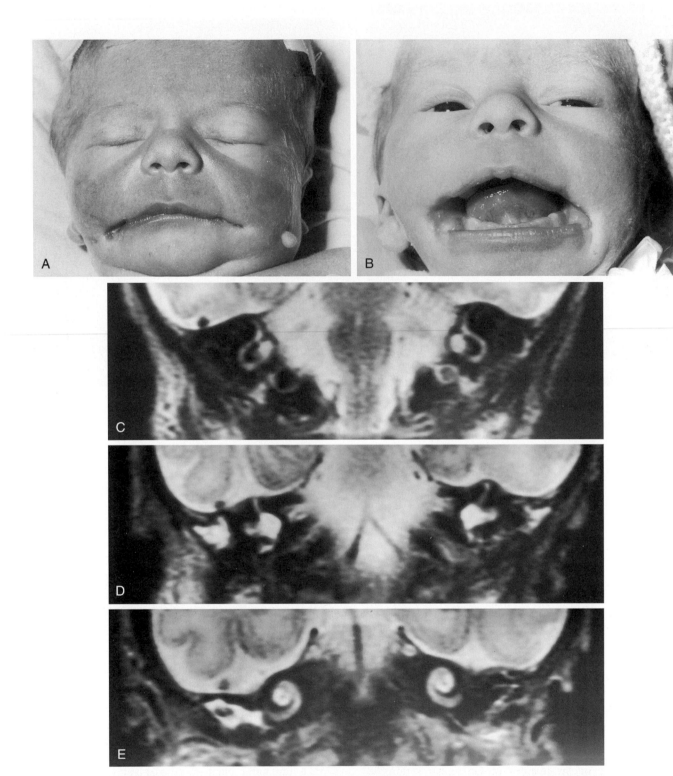

**FIGURE 1-57** Hemifacial microsomia with some bilateral elements. **A** and **B**, This newborn girl shows bilateral preauricular skin tags (removed in **B**) and bilateral transverse facial clefts with macrostomia. She had malformed pinnae bilaterally, more severe on the right, and decreased hearing bilaterally, with an absent response on brainstem auditory-evoked potentials at 90 and 105 dB bilaterally. **C** to **E**, Serial coronal T2-weighted MR images, displayed from posterior to anterior, show hypoplasia of the external auditory canals bilaterally, large vestibules, and malformed lateal semicircular canals bilaterally. (**A** and **B** from Naidich TP, Smith MS, Castillo M, Thompson JE, Sloan GM, Jayakar P, Mukherji SK. Facies to remember. Number 7. Hemifacial microsomia. Goldenhar syndrome. OAV complex. Int J Neuroradiol 1996;2:437–449.)

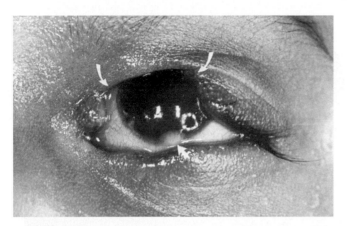

**FIGURE 1-58** Hemifacial microsomia. Goldenhar syndrome. This 4-month-old girl shows a large coloboma of the medial portion of the left upper lid (*between the curved white arrows*) and a whitish choristoma (*straight white arrow*) that straddles the corneoscleral limbus inferotemporally. There is a second, small coloboma of the lower lid medial to the choristoma. The caruncle is unusually prominent. (Case courtesy of Dr. Myron Tannenbaum, Miami, Florida.) (From Naidich TP, Smith MS, Castillo M, Thompson JE, Sloan GM, Jayakar P, Mukherji SK. Facies to remember. Number 7. Hemifacial microsomia. Goldenhar syndrome. OAV complex. Int J Neuroradiol 1996;2:437–449.)

### Central Nervous System

Total or partial peripheral seventh nerve palsies have been seen in 12% of microtia patients and 22% to 45% of patients with HFM.[290] Seventh nerve palsies correlate well with both the severity of mandibular hypoplasia and the presence of sensorineural hearing loss. Facial paralysis is found in about 50% of grades 1 and 2 mandibular hypoplasia, increasing to almost 70% in grade 3. The trigeminal nuclei and nerve and other cranial nerves may also be deficient. Other CNS malformations, found in 5% to 15% of patients with the OAV complex, include hydrocephalus, absent septum pellucidum, absent corpus callosum, Arnold-Chiari and Dandy Walker malformations, microcephaly with partial anencephaly, anterior cephaloceles, posterior cervicooccipital cerebellocele with vermian agenesis, lipoma of the corpus callosum and vermis, frontal lobe hypoplasia, and unilateral arrhinencephaly ipsilateral to the side of the Goldenhar microtia and HFM.[267]

### Plagiocephaly

Approximately 10% of patients with HFM show deformation of the frontal bone on the side of the predominant HFM.[300] The resultant HFM plagiocephaly phenotype mimics coronal synostosis, except that the affected ear is displaced anteroinferiorly, as expected for HFM, rather than posteroinferiorly, as expected for coronal synostosis. These plagiocephalic patients have orbital dystopia (86%), more severe microtia (57%), and a 43% incidence of parenchymal CNS anomalies such as callosal agenesis, encephalocele, and hydrocephalus. Goldenhar syndrome may be found in association with frontonasal dysplasia.[272]

## Mandibulofacial Dysostosis (Treacher Collins Syndrome, Franceschetti-Zwalen-Klein Syndrome)

MFD is an autosomal dominant syndrome found in 1 per 50,000 live births. It is now linked to the *TCS* (*TCOF1*) gene at chromosome 5q31.3-q32 and shows variable expression within families.[10, 301] Approximately 60% of cases arise as new mutations. The mutation is thought to interfere with coding for a protein designated *treacle*, leading to haploinsufficiency for this protein.[301] Multiple different mutations within this gene may give rise to the Treacher Collins syndrome.[10] Allelic mutations in the *TCS* gene could explain the partial clinical overlap of the Treacher Collins syndrome with Goldenhar syndrome and Nager acrofacial dysostosis (see the section on Nager Acrofacial Dysostosis Syndrome), but this mechanism has not been proved.[301]

The obligatory features of MFD are marked hypoplasia of the malar bone, with or without malar clefts, hypoplasia of the mandibular ramus and condyle, marked antimongoloid slant of the palpebral fissures, obliteration of the frontonasal angle, colobomas of the lateral third of the *lower* lid with or without those of the upper lid, and/or malformations of the eyelashes (Fig. 1-59).[266, 293, 299, 302] Other stigmata include inferior extension of the hairline onto the cheeks, malformed auricles, deformity or absence of the external auditory canal, malformed middle ear and ossicles with conductive hearing loss, blind fistulae and/or skin tags situated between the auricle and the corner of the mouth, microstomia or macrostomia, abnormal dentition with malocclusion, and antegonial notching of the mandible.[266, 293, 299, 300] Orbital hypoplasia, microphthalmos, lacrimal duct atresia, craniosynostoses, and skeletal malformations have also been reported. Miscarriage or early death is common.[302] One tries to differentiate MFD from the Goldenhar-HFM-OAV complex by observing that MFD mandibles are symmetric bilaterally, with little variation among patients. Patients with MFD show far greater frequency of *lower*-lid colobomas, *marked* antimongoloid slant of the palpebral fissures, and infrequent choristomas, skin tags, and upper-lid colobomas. Facial asymmetry, phenotypic characteristics, and lack of inheritance patterns distinguish bifacial microsomia from MFD.[267]

## Branchio-Oto-Renal Syndrome (Ear Pits-Deafness Syndrome)

Branchio-oto-renal syndrome (BORS) is characterized clinically by ear anomalies, hearing loss, preauricular pits, branchial fistulae, lacrimal duct stenoses, and renal dysplasia. There is variable expression within families; first-degree relatives may show varying features of HFM or BORS, but hemifacial microsomia is not a component of BORS itself. The syndrome is inherited as an autosomal dominant trait with high penetrance and variable expressivity. Patients with BORS show multiple different mutations and deletions in the *EYA1* gene at 8q13.3.[10] The gene affected is analogous to the *Drosophila eyes absent* gene.[10]

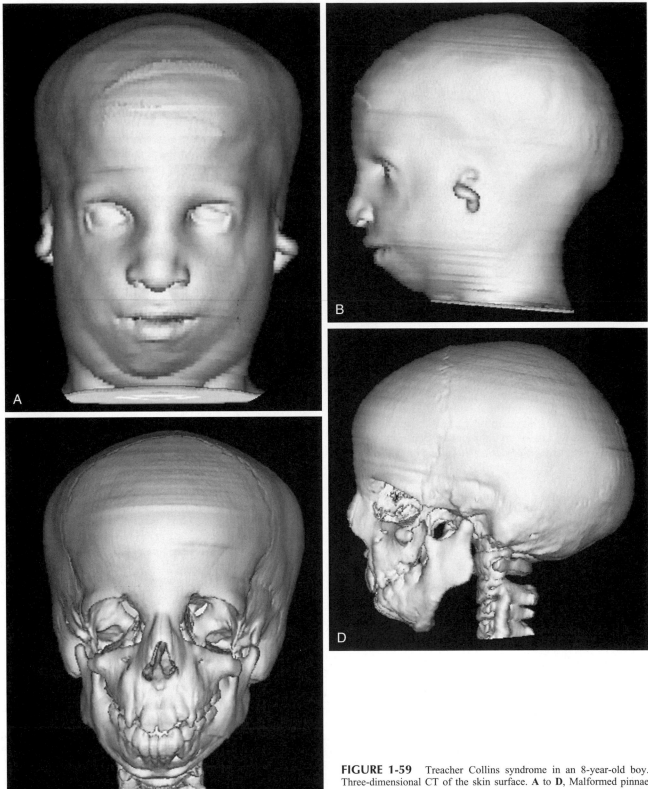

**FIGURE 1-59** Treacher Collins syndrome in an 8-year-old boy. Three-dimensional CT of the skin surface. **A** to **D**, Malformed pinnae bilaterally, an antimongoloid slant of the transverse orbital axis, malar hypoplasia with deficient lateral orbital walls bilaterally, hypoplastic mandible with prominent antegonial notch, narrow anterior vault, and overprojection of the central face.

## Nager Acrofacial Dysostosis Syndrome (AFD Nager)

AFD Nager is a form of MFD associated with radial defects. The condition may be sporadic or familial.[303] Craniofacial features include mandibular and malar hypoplasia, dysplastic ears with defects of the external auditory canal, conductive deafness, downward slanting of the palpebral fissures, absent eyelashes in the medial one third of the lower lids, microstomia, cleft palate, and a tongue-shaped extension of hair onto the upper cheek. The radial defects range from thumb hypoplasia to absent radial ray.

Some patients with Goldenhar syndrome and radial defects appear to overlap with those with AFD Nager.[303]

## Pierre Robin Sequence

The Pierre Robin sequence is characterized by micrognathia, glossoptosis, and cleft palate (Fig. 1-60). Girls are affected more than boys (female : male ratio = 3 : 2).[304] The sequence presents clinically as difficulty breathing, difficulty swallowing, and recurrent attacks of cyanosis.[304] Pierre Robin patients typically have palatal cleft-

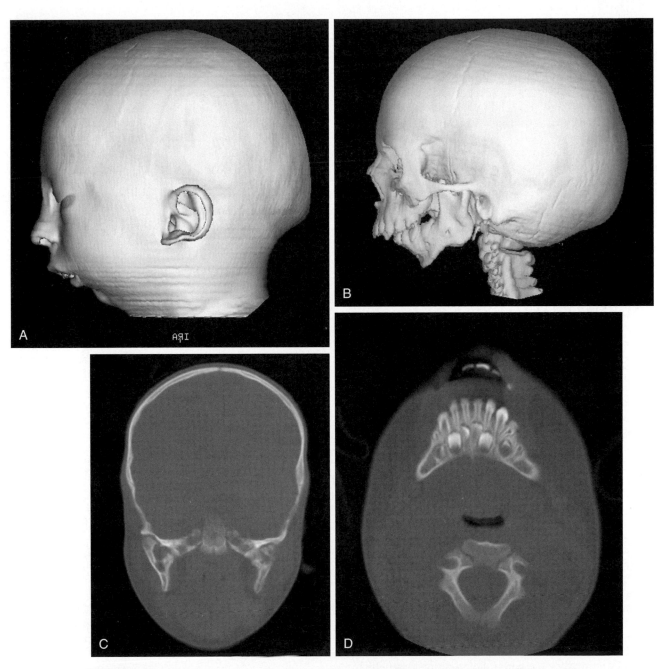

**FIGURE 1-60**   Pierre Robin sequence in a 2½-year-old boy with no catch-up growth of the mandible. **A** and **B**, Lateral 3D CT of the skin surface (**A**) and facial skeleton (**B**) show severe retrognathia and micrognathia. **C**, Coronal bone CT shows marked butressing of the mandibular condyle. **D**, Axial CT section shows a vertical orientation of the maxillary incisors but a horizontal course of the mandibular dentition.

**Table 1-13**
**RELATIVE FREQUENCIES OF SYNDROMIC AND NONSYNDROMIC**
**PRIMARY CRANIOSYNOSTOSES (1976–1999) (N = 2137)**

| Nonsyndromic Synostoses | Number | Percent | Syndromic Synostoses | Number | Percent |
|---|---|---|---|---|---|
| Scaphocephaly | 870 | 40.7 | Apert syndrome | 88 | 4.1 |
| Trigonocephaly | 334 | 15.6 | Crouzon syndrome | 98 | 4.6 |
| Lambdoid synostosis | 18 | 0.8 | Pfeiffer syndrome | 30 | 1.4 |
| Plagiocephaly | 252 | 11.8 | Saethre-Chotzen syndrome | 54 | 2.5 |
| Brachycephaly | 107 | 5.0 | Craniofrontonasal syndrome | 22 | 10 |
| Oxycephaly | 147 | 6.9 | Other syndromes | 36 | 1.7 |
| Complex | 81 | 3.8 | — | | |
| Subtotal | 1809 | 84.7% | Subtotal | 328 | 15.3% |

From Renier D et al. Management of craniosynostosis. Childs Nerv Syst 2000;16:645–658.

ing that may involve both the hard and soft palates or the soft palate only.[304] In 36 Brazilian children with isolated Pierre Robin sequence, all patients showed palatal clefting. The clefts were U-shaped in 27 (75%) (26 complete, 1 incomplete), and V-shaped in 9 (25%). The family history was positive for cleft lip/cleft palate in 27.7% of cases.[304] Thus, "the primary event occurring in isolated Robin sequence may be cleft palate and not micrognathia. . . ."[304] The Pierre Robin sequence may be observed as an isolated sequence, as one of multiple nonsyndromal defects, or as one component of Stickler syndrome, velo-cardio-facial syndrome (22q11 deficiency), or other named syndromes.[304] Marques et al.[304] suggest that a multifactorial polygenic inheritance best accounts for the features of the Pierre Robin sequence.

## PREMATURE CRANIAL SYNOSTOSES

Premature cranial suture synostosis signifies premature closure of one or more of the cranial sutures from any cause.[305, 306] Primary cranial synostoses occur in the absence of underlying brain or metabolic disease. Secondary cranial synostoses occur as the indirect consequence of reduced intracranial volume, often after shunting of hydrocephalus or a cerebral insult. Metabolic cranial synostoses arise from underlying disorders such as vitamin D–related rickets, familial hypophosphatasia, hyperthyroidism, and idiopathic hypercalcemia.[306, 307] Primary synostoses may occur as isolated phenomena (nonsyndromic synostosis, 85%) or as one part of multimalformation syndromes (syndromic synostosis, 15%).[308] Table 1-13 summarizes the distribution of 2137 primary craniosynostoses.[308]

Normally, the sutures become narrower and the fontanelles become smaller as the skull matures (Fig. 1-61). Closure of the suture does not occur along the whole length simultaneously, nor does it necessarily involve the entire depth.[309] The inner endosteal aspect of a suture appears to fuse in a more orderly fashion, whereas the outer ectocranial serrated surface shows greater variation.[309] The fontanelles normally close early: the posterior fontanelle by 8 weeks, the anterolateral fontanelle by 3 months, the anterior fontanelle by 15 to 18 months, and the posterolateral fontanelle by 2 years.[310] The mendosal suture

closes first, at several weeks after birth. The metopic suture begins to close during the second year and is completely closed during the third year.[310] The sagittal, coronal, and lambdoid sutures normally close much later, in early to midadulthood.[309] The sagittal suture begins to close at 22 years, the coronal suture at 24 years, and the lambdoid suture at 26 years.[309] These sutures may become fully closed only at 35, 41, and 47 years, respectively.[309] On plain X-rays, the sagittal suture is frequently closed after 35 to 40 years and is usually closed after 50 years.[309] The coronal and lambdoid sutures are frequently closed, at least in part, after 50 years.[309] The sutures bordering the squamous portion of temporal bone never close completely, even in the elderly.[309] However, in analyzing cases of craniosynostosis, it is important to bear in mind that functional closure of the sutures usually occurs at about the time the fontanelles close, well before true bony synostosis develops.

Early descriptions of premature craniosynostosis were based on the physical appearance of the patient.[305, 311–314] Such descriptions of head shape and patient appearance, however, are not specific and do not necessarily predict whether specific sutures will be fused on imaging studies. Terms in common use will now be discussed.

## Skull Shape

### Scaphocephaly (Dolichocephaly, Canoe Head)
This signifies elongation of the calvarium in the anteroposterior (AP) direction, with narrowing in the transverse dimension (Fig. 1-62A). It usually results from premature closure of the sagittal suture but may reflect, instead, prior deformation of the head due to prematurity, soft bones, poor head control, and prolonged decubitus position of the premature infant's head in the intensive care unit.[311]

### Trigonocephaly (Ax Head, Keel-Shaped Deformity)
This signifies sharp, anteriorly directed ridging of the midline frontal contour, usually from metopic synostosis (Fig. 1-62B).[314]

### Brachycephaly (Broad Head)
This signifies abnormal widening of the transverse diameter of the calvarium, with a shortened AP dimension.

It typically results from coronal or lambdoidal synostoses that limit growth in the AP direction (Fig. 1-62C).

### Oxycephaly (Turricephaly, Tower Head)

This signifies superior elongation of the calvarium. It is usually associated with bilateral coronal or bilateral lambdoid synostoses, which redirect brain growth anteriorly toward the anterior fontanelle-metopic suture complex or posteriorly toward the posterior fontanelle and lambdoid sutures.

### Plagiocephaly (Skew Head, Asymmetric Head)

This signifies asymmetric contour of the calvarium from (1) positional deformation of the skull, (2) unilateral suture synostosis (usually unilateral coronal synostosis), or (3) asynchronous asymmetric synostoses of multiple sutures

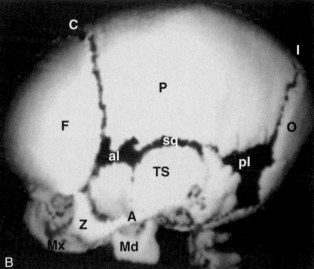

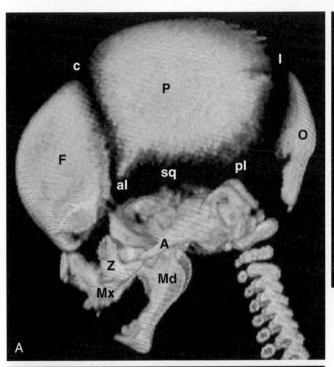

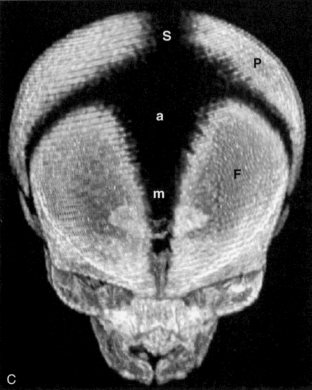

**FIGURE 1-61** Developing calvarium and sutures. Three-dimensional CT. **A**, Lateral fetal skull. **B**, Lateral newborn skull. **C**, Superior frontal view of **A**. The sutures and fontanelles narrow as the cranium matures. Uppercase black letters designate the bones: *F*, frontal bone, *P*, parietal bone, *O*, occipital bone, *TS*, temporal squama, *M*, maxilla, *Md*, mandible, *Z*, zygoma, *A*, zygomatic arch. Lowercase white letters designate the sutures and fontanelles: *c*, coronal suture, *l*, lambdoid suture, *sq*, squamosal suture, *al*, anterolateral fontanelle, *pl*, posterolateral fontanelle, *a*, anterior fontanelle, *m*, metopic suture, *s*, sagittal suture.

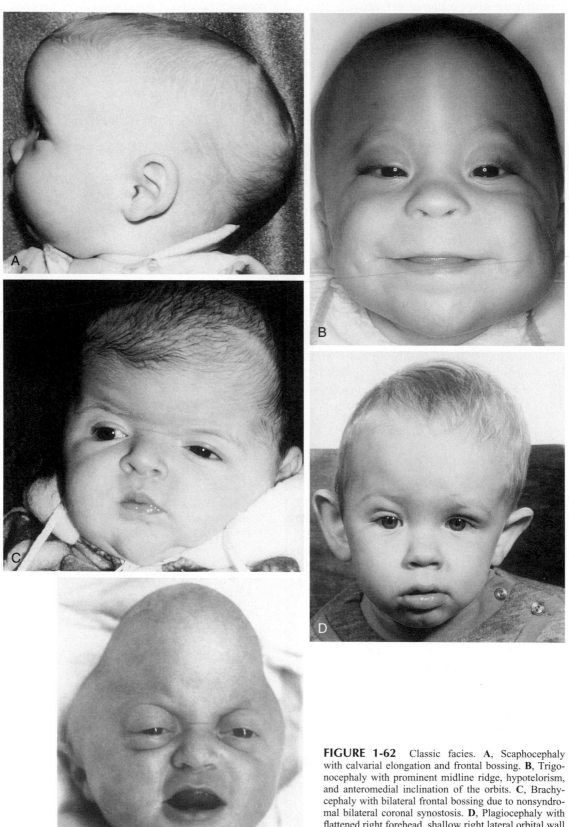

**FIGURE 1-62** Classic facies. **A,** Scaphocephaly with calvarial elongation and frontal bossing. **B,** Trigonocephaly with prominent midline ridge, hypotelorism, and anteromedial inclination of the orbits. **C,** Brachycephaly with bilateral frontal bossing due to nonsyndromal bilateral coronal synostosis. **D,** Plagiocephaly with flattened right forehead, shallow right lateral orbital wall (right harlequin eye), and compensatory left frontal bossing due to nonsyndromal unilateral right coronal synostosis. **E,** Kleeblattschädel (cloverleaf skull).

bilaterally (Fig. 1-62D). At present, the most common cause of cranial asymmetry is a positional deformation of the posterior aspect of the head designated posterior positional plagiocephaly. At present, therefore, the most common referral for possible synostosis is a benign, remediable positional deformation of the skull, not a true premature suture synostosis.[307–313]

### Kleeblattschädel (Cloverleaf Skull)

This signifies a trefoil deformity of the calvarium related to severe constriction of calvarial growth at the coronal, lambdoid, and/or squamosal sutures bilaterally. In this condition, remarkable expansion of the temporal fossae inferolateral to the orbits creates the lateral lobes of the cloverleaf, while redirection of growth toward the sagittal suture and fontanelles raises the midline superior lobe (Fig. 1-62E). Exorbitism is often marked. Kleeblattschädel is found most frequently in the syndromal forms of craniosynostosis.

## Nonsyndromic Primary Craniosynostoses

Nonsyndromic synostoses constitute 85% of all primary craniosynostoses (Table 1-13). Premature sagittal, coronal, and metopic synostoses are the most frequent forms. Lambdoid synostosis is least common (1% to 3%), affects the midface only incidentally, and will not be discussed specifically.

### Premature Sagittal Synostosis

Premature sagittal synostosis is found in 2 to 10 per 10,000 live births and accounts for 40% to 70% of all nonsyndromal craniosynostoses.[306, 313] From 6% to 10% of cases are familial, with autosomal dominant inheritance and 38% penetrance. There is a male predominance (70% to 85% of cases).[313] The abnormal suture is often closed at birth. This restricts transverse growth of the skull, so the patients show scaphocephaly. A palpable ridge or indentation may mark the site of closure. Compensatory growth at the adjacent coronal and lambdoid sutures may lead to frontal bossing, occipital bossing, or both.[313] The anterior fontanelle is often closed. The sphenoid wings and orbits are not affected. As a result, these patients show very prominent foreheads that project far anterior to the orbits but remarkably little facial asymmetry. In contrast to other synostoses, concurrent intracranial abnormalities are exceptionally rare.

### Premature Unilateral Coronal Synostosis

Premature unilateral coronal synostosis occurs in 0.7 to 4.8 per 10,000 births and accounts for 14% to 55% of synostoses.[313] Most cases are sporadic. Only 6.6% to 14.4% of cases are familial, with 60% penetrance. There is a slight female predominance (57% to 68%). The curvature of the coronal suture normally extends into the skull base along the adjoining sphenozygomatic, sphenofrontal, and sphenoethmoidal sutures. Unilateral coronal synostosis typically causes growth restriction along much of this arc unilaterally, leading to flattening of the forehead, zygoma, and orbit on the affected side (Figs. 1-62D and 1-63).[313] The eye and eyebrow appear to be

displaced up and back (harlequin eye). Compensatory contralateral frontal bossing displaces the contralateral eye inferolaterally. These patients commonly show mild exorbitism, vertical strabismus, horizontal strabismus, and amblyopia.[313] Bone thickening at and surrounding the closed suture may cause a palpable coronal ridge and temporal prominence, but such thickening is far less apparent than is the midsagittal ridging associated with scaphocephaly. The ipsilateral anterior fossa is small. The ipsilateral temporal fossa is rotated toward the midline. The root of the nose is drawn ipsilaterally unless concurrent involvement of the frontosphenoid suture deviates the nose to the opposite side. The ipsilateral maxilla may show vertical hypoplasia. The ipsilateral ear (tragus) is pulled antroinferiorly. The anterior fontanelle deviates to the opposite side. Torticollis is found in about one quarter of these cases.[313]

### Premature Metopic Synostosis

Premature metopic synostosis occurs in 1 to 10 per 70,000 births and accounts for 5% to 20% of all cranial synostoses. It is characteristically sporadic, with only 2% to 6% of cases showing familial inheritance, either as an autosomal recessive trait or as an autosomal dominant trait, with very low penetrance.[313] Closure of the metopic suture restricts expansion of the frontal midline, so these patients manifest symmetric lateral sloping of the forehead, short anterior fossa, forward bowing of the coronal sutures, orbital hypotelorism, and ethmoid hypoplasia (Figs. 1-62B and 1-64). The crista galli remains intact. The nasal septum and facial midline are usually straight. The medial walls of the orbits are thickened and rise unusually high. Therefore, the superomedial corners form the highest points of the orbital roofs, and the lateral orbits fall away inferiorly. The degree of orbital deformity correlates with the wedging of the forehead. The frontal lobes, frontal sulci, and ventricles are usually compressed. There may be callosal dysgenesis, hydrocephalus, or other intracranial anomalies.

## Syndromic Craniosynostosis (Craniofacial Dysostosis)

The term *craniofacial dysostosis*[2, 10, 307, 315–344] identifies a group of syndromes that exhibit premature synostoses of cranial sutures as one prominent feature. More than 100 such syndromes are recognized.[3] Together they account for 15% of all primary craniosynostoses.[308] Traditionally, craniofacial dysostoses have been classified by their characteristic phenotypes and named by author or place as Crouzon, Apert, Saethre-Chotzen, Pfeiffer, Jackson-Weiss, Boston, and Muenke (Adelaide) syndromes (Fig. 1-65).[321] Recent work shows that such phenotypic classification is imprecise. Mutations of different genes involved in the same pathway create similar phenotypes. Identical mutations in fibroblast growth factor receptor 2 (FGFR2) have been found in patients classified phenotypically as having Pfeiffer and Crouzon syndromes, and in patients classified phenotypically as having Jackson-Weiss and Crouzon syndromes.[10] Therefore, the eponymous craniosynostotic syndromes should now be regarded as phenotypic extremes of FGFR and other mutations, not as nosologic entities. With the

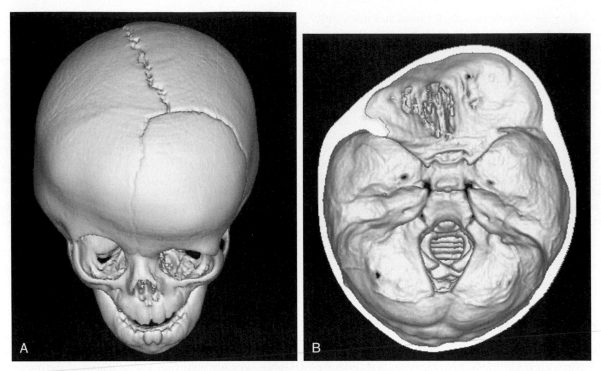

**FIGURE 1-63**   Nonsyndromal unilateral right coronal synostosis in a 7-month-old girl. **A** and **B**, Three-dimensional CT of the cranial surface (**A**) and a view of the skull base from within (**B**). The right coronal suture and anterior fontanelle are closed. The sagittal and left coronal sutures are patent. The metopic suture is faintly visualized. Asymmetric closure of the right coronal suture restricts growth of the ipsilateral anterior fossa and orbit, causing plagiocephaly, harlequin right eye, short right anterior fossa, high position of the right sphenoid wing-pterion, compensatory bossing of the left frontal contour, and inferior displacement of the left orbit.

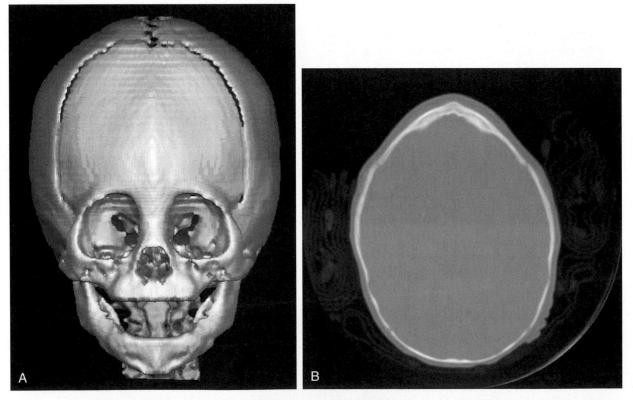

**FIGURE 1-64**   Trigonocephaly in a 3-month-old girl. **A**, Three-dimensional CT of the facial skeleton. **B**, Axial bone CT through the metopic suture. Premature closure of the metopic suture leads to hypotelorism, upward medial pointing of the orbital contours (''quizzical orbits'') and a keel-shaped brow.

exception of Apert syndrome (which does show consistent genetics), the clinical phenotypic classifications should be abandoned and replaced with molecular classifications of these syndromes.[326]

### Molecular Genetics

Understanding the craniofacial dysostoses requires a background in the cell signaling mechanisms that control suture maturation. The next sections review these mechanisms preparatory to adressing the eponymous craniosynostosis syndromes.

### Fibroblast Growth Factor Receptors

Four unlinked genes, *FGFR1* to *FGFR4*, constitute a family of genes that produce high-affinity receptors for the fibroblast growth factors (FGFs 1 to 9).[2] Of these, FGFR1, FGFR2, and FGFR3 are related to suture closure. The chromosomal locations of the FGF genes are: FGF1, 5q31-q33; FGF2, 4q26-q27; and FGF3, 11q13. FGFR genes 1 to 3 are located as follows: FGFR1, 8p11.2-11.1; FGFR2, 10q26; FGFR3, 4p16[326] (Table 1-14).

The FGFR genes encode a group of structurally related tyrosine kinase receptors of the subclass IV type. These FGFRs are situated at the cell membrane and share a three-part structure (Fig. 1-66; see also Fig. 1-1): (1) an *extracellular domain* composed of a variable number of immunoglobulin-like domains (Ig loops), (2) a *transmembrane domain* that bridges the cell wall, and (3) an *intracellular cytoplasmic domain* containing both a tyrosine kinase region responsible for tyrosine kinase activity and an

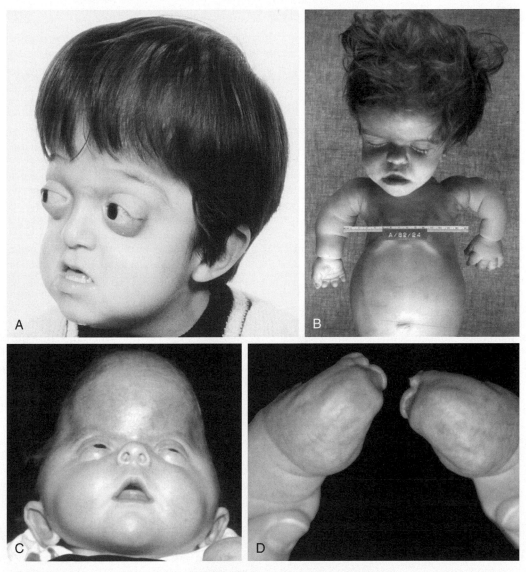

**FIGURE 1-65**   Facies of craniofacial dysostoses and achondroplasia. Four patients. **A**, Crouzon syndrome. Oblique view shows turricephaly, midface hypoplasia, hypertelorism, shallow bony orbits, marked bilateral exorbitism, and partial surgical closure of the eyelids to protect the globe. **B**, Homozygous achondroplasia in a 33-month-old girl with defective cartilage formation leading to a narrow skull base, secondary enlargement of the vault by hydrocephalus, and rhizomelic dwarfism. **C** and **D**, Apert syndrome (acrocephalosyndactylism type I). **C**, Frontal view shows brachycephaly, orbital hypertelorism, shallow orbits with bilateral exorbitism, maxillary hypoplasia and down-turned mouth. **D**, The hands show bilateral syndactylism involving all digits (type 3).

*Illustration continued on following page*

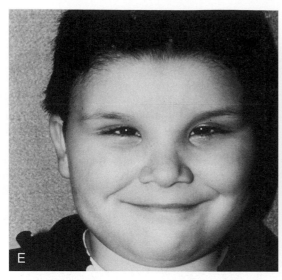

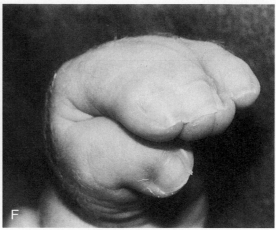

**FIGURE 1-65** *Continued.* **E** and **F**, Saethre-Chotzen syndrome (acrocephalosyndactylism type III). **E**, Frontal view shows relatively mild facial asymmetry, mild midface hypoplasia, and ptosis of the eyelids. **F**, The hand shows cutaneous syndactyly of the central fingers with broadening of the other digits. (**B**, From Pauli RM, Conroy MM, Langer LO Jr, et al. Homozygous achondroplasia with survival beyond infancy. Am J Med Genet 1983;16:459–473.)

interkinase region.[10] The immunoglobulin-like domains Ig II and Ig III are necessary for ligand binding.[326] The FGFRs are normally activated (and controlled) by the presence of ligands, which serve as "on" signals to initiate phosphorylation. The binding of a ligand to the receptor in the *extracellular* domain normally promotes receptor dimerization. This initiates a sequence of cross-phosphorylation of the *cytoplasmic* domains, provision of binding sites for downstream signaling molecules, conformational changes, and increased kinase activity.[2]

In the craniofacial dysostoses, mutations in the FGFR genes create mutant proteins that allow the receptors to function independently of their normal ligand signals. The mutant receptor proteins form constitutive dimers, which activate the kinase domain and downstream signaling events, even in the absence of ligand.[2] That is, the

mutated genes are always "on," a "gain-of-function" mutation. Since FGFRs and FGF signaling guide development of multiple different organ systems, including the cranio-facial-oral-dental complex, the group of FGFR malformations exhibits a coherent set of multisystem anomalies affecting the skeleton, the central nervous system, the skin, and the auditory system.[2] The mutations that cause the craniofacial dysostoses cluster in the third Ig loop and in the linker region between Ig loops II and III. FGFRs 1, 2, and 3 each contain an analogous proline in the linker region between Ig loops II and III. Replacement of this proline with an arginine in any of these receptors causes craniosynostosis, with or without other skeletal malformations.[2] In FGFR1, this substitution causes the Pfeiffer syndrome. In *FGFR2*, the equivalent substitution causes Apert syndrome, and in *FGFR3* it causes Muenke nonsyndromic coronal craniosynostosis.[2] By receptor:

**FGFR1** In FGFR1, replacement of the proline with an arginine at codon 252 (Pro252Arg) causes Pfeiffer syndrome.[2] Other proline substitutions at position 252 (Pro252) are seen with other nonspecific craniosynostoses.[10]

**FGFR2** The FGFR2 gene is involved in most craniofacial dysostoses. Nearly all cases of Apert syndrome show one of two specific missense mutations at codons 252 and 253, which encode the linker region between the Ig II and Ig III domains of the extracellular domain.[10] These Apert-specific mutations consist of substitutions of tryptophan for serine at nucleotide 252 (Ser252Trp) or of arginine for proline at nucleotide 253 (Pro253Arg).[10] The Ser252Trp mutation accounts for 65% of Apert cases and, more commonly, causes concurrent cleft palate. The Pro253Arg mutation accounts for 35% of Apert cases and has a greater association with syndactyly.[327] A mild form of Apert syndrome has also been related to a different FGFR2 mutation, predicted to substitute phenylalanine for serine at position 252 (Ser252Phen-predicted). A study of 57 Apert

**Table 1-14**
**CHROMOSOMAL LOCATIONS OF THE GENES FOR FIBROBLAST GROWTH FACTORS AND THEIR RECEPTORS**

| Fibroblast Growth Factors (FGF) | Chromosomal Location |
| --- | --- |
| FGF1 | 5q31-q33 |
| FGF2 | 4q26-q27 |
| FGF3 | 11q13 |
| FGF8 | 10q25-q26 |

| Fibroblast Growth Factor Receptors (FGFR) | Chromosomal Location |
| --- | --- |
| FGFR1 | 8p11.2-11.1 |
| FGFR2 | 10q26 |
| FGFR3 | 4p16 |

Data from Cohen MM Jr. Fibroblast growth factor receptor mechanisms. In: Cohen MM Jr, MacLean RE, eds. Craniosynostosis. Diagnosis, Evaluation and Management, 2nd ed. New York: Oxford University Press, 2000;77-94; Müller U et al. Molecular genetics of craniosynostotic syndromes. Arch Clin Exp Ophthalmol 1997;235:545–550.

patients has shown an exclusively paternal origin of the mutation, which is thought to be related to advanced paternal age.[328]

Other FGFR2 mutations also cause craniofacial dysostoses. Substitution of leucine for serine at position 252 (Ser252Leu) or of serine for proline at position 253 (Pro253Ser) causes Crouzon-like and Pfeiffer-like phenotypes with only mild craniosynostosis.[10, 326] Mutation in the Ig IIIc portion of the extracellular domain of FGFR2 may produce the Jackson-Weiss syndrome.[329]

**FGFR3** FGFR3 is the site of a spectrum of mutations that cause disorders of the axial and appendicular

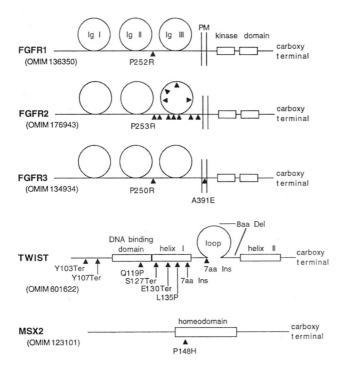

**FIGURE 1-66** Molecular genetics of craniosynostoses. The craniofacial dysostoses reflect underlying derangements in signal transduction (see also Fig. 1-1). Diagrammatic representations of FGFRs 1 to 3, the basic helix-loop-helix transcription factor TWIST, and the homeodomain transcription factor *MSX2*. Each molecule is oriented horizontally, with the amino terminal to the left and the carboxy terminal to the right. FGFR 1 to 3. These receptor tyrosine kinases show a similar structure with (1) an extracellular domain composed of three Ig-like loops (Ig I to Ig III) and interposed linker regions between the loops, (2) a transmembrane domain that spans the plasma membrane (PM), and (3) an intracellular kinase domain. By convention, amino acid substitutions are designated by citing from left to right: the normal amino acid, the position at which that amino acid normally resides (counting from the amino terminal of the protein), and last, the new amino acid that has replaced the normal original. Each FGFR has a highly conserved proline at a slightly different position within the linker region between Ig II and Ig III. Amino acid substitutions at that site lead to craniofacial dysostoses. Illustrated here are substitutions of arginine (R) for proline (P) in FGFR1 (P252R), in FGFR2 (P253R), and in FGFR3 (P250R). Numerous other mutations in FGFR2 (*arrowheads*) also produce craniosynostoses. **TWIST.** Multiple mutations along the *TWIST* gene cause Saethre-Chotzen syndrome. *MSX2.* A single point mutation in the homeodomain of *MSX2* can cause Boston-type craniosynostosis. *S,* serine; *P,* proline; *R,* arginine; *Y,* tyrosine; *L,* leucine; *Q,* glutamine; *H,* histidine; *A,* alanine; *E,* glutamic acid; *aa,* amino acid; *T,* termination, stop codon; *Del,* deletion; *Ins,* insertion. Additional mutations are discussed in the text. (From Nuckolls GH, Shum L, Slavkin HC. Progress toward understanding craniofacial malformations. Cleft Palate-Craniofac J 1999;36:12–26.)

skeleton. These include achondroplasia, hypochondroplasia, and thanatophoric dysplasia II, as well as skin disorders. Achondroplasia is associated with a point mutation in the transmembrane domain of FGFR3 (Fig. 1-65B). A study of 10 achondroplasia patients showed an exclusively paternal origin of the mutation, which is thought to be related to advanced paternal age.[317] Hypochondroplasia is associated with a mutation in the intracellular tyrosine kinase domain of FGFR3. The form of thanatophoric dysplasia with cloverleaf skull is associated with mutation of the *extra*cellular domain of FGFR3, whereas the form of thanatophoric dysplasia without cloverleaf skull is associated with a mutation of the *intra*cellular domain of FGFR3.[10] Crouzon patients with concurrent acanthosis nigricans and Chiari I malformation show a specific mutation in the transmembrane domain of FGFR3 (Ala391Glu) at 4p16.3, just 11 amino acids away from the mutation site of achondroplasia.[10] In FGFR3, substitution of arginine for proline at codon 250 (Pro250Arg) is associated with Pfeiffer syndrome. Other proline substitutions at this site have been observed with nonspecific craniosynostoses.

### Other Signaling Systems

Derangements of other genes and transcription factors may also be responsible for craniosynostoses.

**GLI3** GLI3 is one of three members of a vertebrate family of zinc finger transcription factor proteins designated GLI (because they may be found in gliomas).[2] GLI interacts with hedgehog to affect expression of hedgehog responsive genes. In the absence of hedgehog, GLI is cleaved to a short form that represses hedgehog target genes. The presence of hedgehog preserves the full-length, active form of GLI and thereby allows hedgehog-responsive genes to be expressed.[18, 325] Known homology to the cubitus interruptus (*Ci*) gene in *Drosophila* predicts several functional domains for *GLI3*, including a DNA-binding zinc finger domain and a microtubule-binding domain.[2] Mutations in *GLI3* causes three distinct clinical disorders, two of which result in craniofacial dysmorphogenesis:

1. *Greig cephalopolysyndactyly* (GCPS) is an autosomal disorder defined predominantly by postaxial polydactyly of the hands and preaxial polydactyly of the feet with syndactyly. The craniofacial features of this disorder include macrocephaly with broad forehead, hypertelorism, broad nasal root, and occasional craniosynostosis. Mutations in *GLI3* associated with GCPS cause truncation of the molecule within the centrally located zinc finger domain and probably result in functional haploinsufficiency.[2]

2. *Pallister-Hall syndrome* (PHS) is caused by a frameshift in the *GLI3* sequence just downstream of the zinc finger domains, resulting in a differently truncated protein, which potentially retains partial function and DNA binding. PHS patients exhibit hypothalamic hamartomas, craniofacial anomalies, and polydactyly of the hands, usually central or preaxial. They do not display the hypertelorism or broad forehead seen with GCPS. Imperforate anus and laryngeal clefts have been reported in PHS.[2, 10]

3. *Postaxial polydactyly A* (PAP-A). The third *GLI3* mutation causes PAP-A. This mutation lies further

downstream in the gene and causes truncation of the molecule after the microtubule-binding domain but before several hundred carboxy-terminal amino acids.[2]

**TWIST** TWIST is a basic helix-loop-helix type of nuclear transcription factor that is homologous to the *Drosophila* gene *twist*. In *Drosophila*, *twist* is involved with dorsoventral patterning and muscle differentiation. Both *twist* and FGFR are coexpressed in early mesoderm in *Drosophila*. TWIST appears to regulate the expression and activity of the FGFRs.[2] The Saethre-Chotzen syndrome is caused by missense, nonsense, and insertion-type mutations in the human TWIST gene. It may also arise, less often, by mutations in FGFR2 and FGFR3.[2] Mice with TWIST defects show the same craniofacial features as humans, plus reduplication of the first digit, an infrequent feature of Saethre-Chotzen syndrome in humans.[10]

**MSX2** *MSX2* (muscle segment homeobox gene 2) is a homeotic gene situated at chromosome 5q34-q35. *MSX2* normally interacts with a transcription factor, TFIIF, which acts on DNA to promote transcription of other genes. In the normal person, this binding occurs over a limited period of time, leading to a finite amount of "product."[326] In patients with Boston (type II) craniosynostosis and limb malformations, an autosomal dominant mutation substitutes histidine for a highly conserved proline (Pro148His) within the homeodomain of *MSX2* (Fig. 1-66). This substitution impedes proteolysis of the *MSX2* protein and affects the dissociation of (transcription-promoting) *MSX2* from DNA.[326] Reduced dissociation of *MSX2* from DNA leads to increased time of binding, increased production of the gene product, and the clinical syndrome. In mice, *MSX2* is expressed in the embryo, both in the calvarial sutures and in the distal portion of the limb bud during skeletal patterning. Transgenic mice that overexpress the wild-type molecule exhibit the same craniosynostosis as mice expressing the mutant form of *MSX2*.[2]

### Relationship of Cranial Suture Morphogenesis and Craniosynostosis

In humans, cranial neural crest cells differentiate into primary and secondary cartilage, enchondral bone, and membranous bone and give rise to most of the skeletal tissues of the skull.[330] In the vault, mineralization proceeds outward from several ossification centers from about 13 wg on. At about 18 wg the mineralizing bone fronts meet, and sutures are induced along the lines of approximation. The skull subsequently enlarges by appositional growth at the suture, with deposition of unmineralized bone matrix (osteoid) along the suture margins.[328]

The suture is anatomically simple. Two plates of bone are separated by a narrow space that contains immature, rapidly dividing osteogenic stem cells. One portion of these stem cells is recruited to differentiate into osteoblasts and make new bone. The remainder resist differentiation into osteoblasts, continue to proliferate, and maintain the suture.[328] These events are partially controlled by *Fgfr1*, *Fgfr2*, *Fgfr3*, *MSX2*, and TGF-beta, which are expressed in the sutures. Premature fusion at one suture prevents further growth at that suture. Excessive growth at other sutures then leads to skull distortion.[328]

### FGF 1, 2, and 3

FGF2 is a known survival factor for neural crest cells. Low concentrations of FGF2 cause concentration-dependent *proliferation* of osteogenic stem cells. High concentrations of FGF2 induce *osteoblastic skeletogenic differentiation* of these cells. Through an autoregulatory loop, high concentrations of FGF2 normally downregulate fgf2 to modulate the FGF2 concentration. FGF1 and FGF3 also play a role.[328, 330–332] The normal suture is maintained by a gradient of FGF2 that balances these signals, allowing osteogenic stem cells to proliferate in the center of the suture (where the concentrations of FGF2 are low) and to differentiate into osteoblasts at the margins of the sutures (i.e., at the edges of the growing calvarial plates), where the concentrations of FGF2 are higher (Fig. 1-67).

In mice, *Fgfr2* is expressed only in proliferating osteoprogenitor cells. Downregulation of *Fgfr2* and upregulation of *Fgfr1* signal the onset of differentiation into osteoblasts. Osteopontin, a marker of osteoblast differentiation, then appears, following which *Fgfr1* (plus osteonectin and alkaline phosphatase) become downregulated. *Fgfr3* is expressed both in osteogenic cells and in cranial cartilage, including a plate of cartilage that underlies the coronal suture.[331]

In mice, implantation of FGF2-soaked beads in the subcutaneous tissue over the coronal suture disrupts the normal suture and leads to synostosis. The local increase in the concentration of FGF2 causes three effects: (3) ectopic expression of *Fgfr1* and osteopontin (i.e., osteoblastic differentiation) in the sutural mesenchyme beneath the bead, (2) downregulation of *Fgfr2* locally (where the concentration of FGF2 is high), and (3) ectopic upregulation of *Fgfr2* in a ring surrounding the bead (where the concentration of FGF2 has fallen to a critical level around the circumference of the bead).[331] Since *low* levels of FGF2 maintain the proliferating population of osteogenic stem cells at the suture, and *high* levels of FGF2 stimulate osteoblastic differentiation, the *excessive* (constitutive "on") FGFR2 signaling due to FGF mutations causes osteogenic differentiation and premature cranial synostosis.[328, 332]

The role of *MSX2* and TWIST, and their interaction with the FGFRs, is poorly understood. *MSX2* expression is associated with apoptosis in several cell types during development. Therefore, the craniosynostosis seen in *MSX2* patients could be due to abnormalities in the programmed death of connective tissue cells at the suture site. *MSX2* may participate in the FGFR signaling pathway, since it is coexpressed with FGFRs at the apical epidermal ridge of developing limbs and at the periphery of membranous calvarial bones. BMP signaling also regulates MSX expression, suggesting that this transcription factor may serve as a focal point for integrating multiple pathways that regulate skeletal development.[2]

In other species, *twist* is known to be a critical gene for mesoderm induction and to function later as a myogenic switch. Expression of specific fibroblast growth receptors depends on *twist*. Null mutants for such receptors show abnormal directions of cell migration and defective muscle formation.[328] Mesodermal expression of the *msh* gene is turned on later in myogenesis and is abolished in *twist* mutants. Similar effects could contribute to the abnormal suture development seen in TWIST mutants.[328]

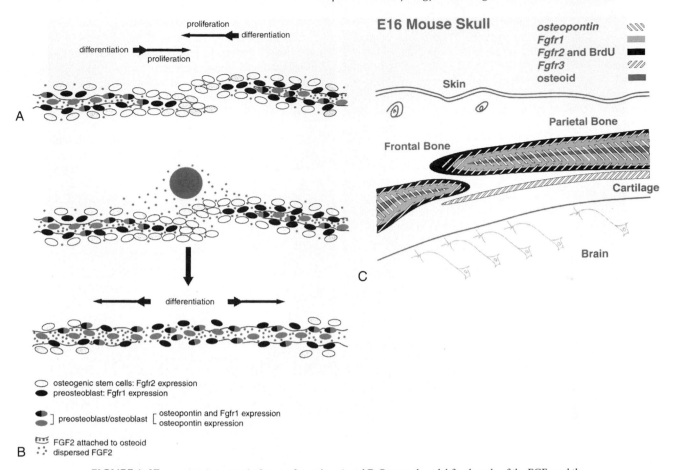

**FIGURE 1-67**    Molecular control of suture formation. **A** and **B**, Proposed model for the role of the FGFs and the FGFRs in balancing the proliferation and differentiation of osteogenic stem cells in the early fetal coronal suture of the mouse. **A**, Normal sutural growth. FGF2 is secreted by the osteoblasts. It is absorbed onto the unmineralized bone matrix. Lower levels of FGF2 diffuse into the extracellular environment of the sutural stem cells. These low levels of FGF2 stimulate the osteogenic stem cells to proliferate. These proliferating stem cells express *Fgfr2*. As new matrix is secreted by the differentiating cells, FGF2 levels rise in the environment of those osteogenic stem cells closest to the new matrix. The high levels of FGF2 stimulate these cells to differentiate into preosteoblasts. The process of differentiation involves downregulation of *Fgfr2*, exit from the cell cycle of proliferation, and subsequent upregulation of *Fgfr1*. Slightly later, there is upregulation of osteogenesis-related genes, including *osteopontin*. The preosteoblasts begin to secrete matrix and are then designated osteoblasts. *Fgfr1* is downregulated when differentiation is complete. **B**, Addition of ectopic FGF2 (*black circle* representing an FGF2-soaked bead) to the environment of the osteogenic stem cells raises the concentration of FGF2 locally and accelerates the process of differentiation, so the proliferating cell population is lost for the duration of the increased signal. This local increase in FGF2 mimics the effect of the gain-of-function, "constitutively on" mutations of FGFR1, FGFR2, and FGFR3 associated with the craniofacial dysostoses. **C**, Diagrammatic representation of the coronal suture of the fetal mouse. Summary of the expression patterns of the FGFR genes (*Fgfr 1, Fgfr2, and Fgfr3*) and of the osteogenesis-related gene *osteopontin*, a marker of osteoblast differentiation. *Fgfr2* is expressed only in proliferating osteogenic stem cells (osteoprogenitor cells). *Fgfr1* expression is associated with cell differentiation into osteoblasts. *Fgfr3* is expressed in both the osteogenic and chondrogenic portions of the skeletogenic membrane. The onset of differentiation toward osteoblasts is preceded by downregulation of *Fgfr2*, upregulation of *Fgrf1*, and upregulation of osteopontin. (From Iseki S, Wilkie AOM, Morriss-Kay GM. *Fgfr1* and *Fgfr2* have distinct differentiation- and proliferation-related roles in the developing mouse skull vault. Development 1999;126:5611–5620.)

## Eponymous Craniosynostoses

### Crouzon Syndrome

Crouzon syndrome (acrocephalosyndactyly type II) is the most frequent craniofacial dysostosis (1 per 25,000 births) (Figs. 1-65A, 1-68, and 1-69). It results from an autosomal dominant trait with variable expressivity. About 45% to 65% of cases are familial; the rest are sporadic.[308, 333] Clinically, Crouzon syndrome is characterized by bilateral coronal synostosis with a brachycephalic or oxycephalic vault. The sagittal and lambdoid sutures may also be affected. Typically, the sutures are not fused at birth but show progressive synostosis from about 1 year on.[308] Crouzon patients show maxillary hypoplasia with shallow orbits, bilateral exorbitism, and orbital hypertelorism. The nasal passages are partially obstructed, causing mouth breathing. *The hands and feet are spared.* Concurrent intracranial anomalies are common, including jugular venous obstruction with anomalous venous drainage (63%) and hydrocephalus. The hydrocephalus is more frequently progressive in Crouzon syndrome than in Apert syn-

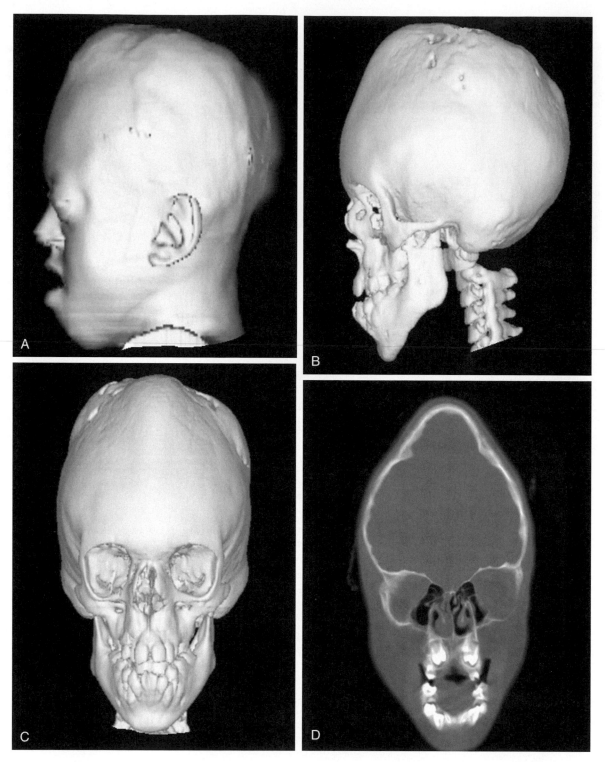

**FIGURE 1-68**  Crouzon syndrome in a 9-year-old girl. **A** to **C**, Three-dimensional CT of the lateral skin surface (**A**), the lateral facial skeleton (**B**), and the frontal facial skeleton (**C**). **D**, Direct coronal CT. The patient shows oxycephaly, shallow orbits with exorbitism, hypoplasia of the midface with narrow, partially obstructed nasal passages, relative prognathism, and an everted lower lip.

drome.[208, 334] Chiari I malformation is seen in 71.4% of Cruzon patients.[208] Other features reported in Crouzon patients include calcification of the stylohyoid ligament (50% of patients older than 4 years), cervical spine anomalies, especially fusions of C2-C5 (up to 40%), elbow malformations (18%), minor hand deformities (10%), and visceral anomalies (7%).[208] Of all craniofacial dysostoses, the Cruzon patients with the FGFR3 mutation have the highest incidence of jugular venous stenosis or atresia and enlarged emissary veins. This phenomenon could reflect a relationship to the FGFR3 achondroplasia spectrum, which classically displays such venous stenoses and hydrocephalus.[335]

*Apert Syndrome*

Apert syndrome (acrocephalosyndactyly type I) is an autosomal dominant craniofacial dysostosis. Most cases arise sporadically as new mutations, but the disorder may be transmitted through families with complete penetrance. Apert syndrome occurs in 1 per 50,000 to 100,000 births, so it is less common than Crouzon syndrome. Clinically, Apert syndrome is characterized by severe symmetric syndactylism of the hands and feet. This is subclassified by the digits affected as type I (affecting digits 2, 3, and 4), type II (affecting digits 2, 3, 4, and 5), and type III (affecting all five digits).[308] Apert patients show bilateral coronal synostoses with brachycephaly, a midline defect due to widened metopic and sagittal sutures, orbital hypertelorism, shallow orbits with bilateral exorbitism, exotropia, maxillary hypoplasia with downturned mouth, high-arched palate, class III malocclusion, and anterior open bite (Figs. 1-65C,D and 1-70).[333] In Apert syndrome, the cranial changes appear to be more severe than those in Crouzon syndrome. The midface hypoplasia is present from birth. There is more severe redirection of the ante-rior cranial base and orbits, with greater brain compression and more prominent bulging of the eyes.

Cleft palate is present in 30% to 42% of Apert patients.[308] Choanal stenosis is common, but atresia is rare. Hypoplasia of the posterior choanae may compromise the nasopharyngeal and oropharyngeal airways, increasing the risk of respiratory distress, sleep apnea, cor pulmonale, and sudden death.[208] Eustachian tube dysfunction, otitis media, and conductive hearing loss are common. Sensorineural hearing loss is rare.[208] Apert patients show an increased incidence of callosal agenesis, megalencephaly, and gyral anomalies. Hydrocephalus may require shunt decompression before craniofacial surgery is performed. Most patients have normal intelligence but display specific learning difficulties. Up to one third suffer mental retardation. Approximately 70% show fusion of the cervical vertebrae, usually C5 and C6.[333] Rhizomelic shortening of the lower limbs reduces the stature by 5% to 50%.[307] There may be ankylosis of the elbows, hips, and shoulders. Concurrent problems with the cardiovascular (10%), genitourinary (9.6%), gastrointes-

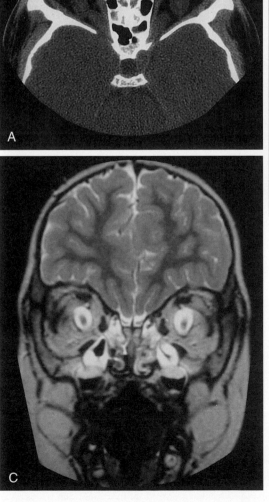

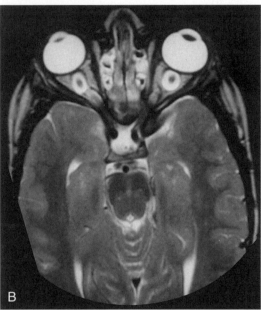

**FIGURE 1-69**  Untreated Crouzon syndrome in a 3-year-old. **A**, Axial CT demonstrates orbital hypertelorism, bilateral shallow orbits, and ocular exorbitism. Increased thickness along the optic sheaths could indicate enlarged optic nerves, sheaths, or neoplasm. **B** and **C**, Axial and coronal T2-weighted MR images demonstrate a bilateral prominent perineural subarachnoid space bilaterally and normal optic nerves. The optic canals appear small. There is a mild harlequin shape to the orbit.

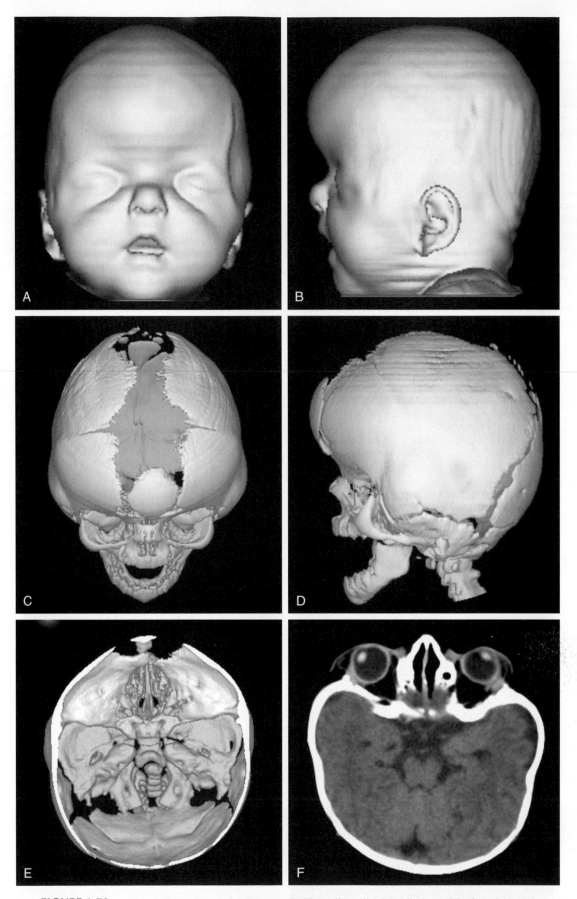

**FIGURE 1-70** Apert syndrome in an infant boy. **A** to **D**, Three-dimensional CT displays of the frontal (**A**) and lateral (**B**) skin surfaces, and the corresponding frontal (**C**) and lateral (**D**) facial skeletons. **E** and **F**, Three-dimensional CT of the skull base (**E**) and an axial CT section through the orbits (**F**). The patient shows brachycephaly with fused coronal sutures bilaterally, wide patency of the sagittal suture, metopic suture and anterior fontanelle with an intrasutural bone, consequent hypertelorism, shallow symmetric anterior fossa, and midface hypoplasia with marked exorbitism.

tinal (1.5%), and respiratory (1.5%) systems contribute to patient morbidity.[208] The stylohyoid ligament may calcify in 38% to 88% of Apert patients.[208]

### Saethre-Chotzen Syndrome

Saethre-Chotzen syndrome (acrocephalosyndactyly type III) is one of the more common craniofacial dysostoses, with an incidence of 1 per 50,000 to 1 per 100,000.[336] It is an autosomal dominant trait with complete penetrance (but variable phenotype) caused by mutations in TWIST, FGFR2, and FGFR3.[2] Saethre-Chotzen syndrome is characterized clinically by multiple suture synostoses with brachycephaly, hypertelorism with shallow orbits, maxillary hypoplasia, facial asymmetry, blepharoptosis, ear anomalies with prominent antihelical crura (crux cymbae), brachydactyly, and cutaneous syndactyly involving the second and third fingers (Fig. 1-65D,E).[326] Antimongoloid slant of the palpebral fissures, beaked nose, and a low-set frontal hairline are frequent. Increased intracranial pressure and mental retardation are infrequent.[326] The corresponding homozygous mutation causes cephalic neural tube defects and fetal lethality.

### Pfeiffer Syndrome

Pfeiffer syndrome (acrocephalosyndactyly type V) is an autosomal dominant craniosynostosis with complete penetrance. It occurs in about 1 per 200,000 live births.[336] About 40% of the cases are familial, and 60% are sporadic.[308] Pfeiffer patients present clinically with soft-tissue syndactyly, broad great toes, broad thumbs, and radial deviation of the phalanges of the fingers (varus deformity). The head displays brachycephaly, short anterior fossa, receding lower forehead, supraorbital bar, hypertelorism, antimongoloid slant of the eyes, and flat nasal bridge.[307] The jaw is prognathic.[288, 326, 337] The clinical outcome of Pfeiffer patients varies widely, leading Cohen[338] to subclassify the disorder into three types. Type I is classic Pfeiffer syndrome, with a good clinical outcome. Type II shows severe concurrent CNS malformations with Kleeblattschädel and a poor prognosis. Type III shows severe CNS malformations without Kleeblattschädel, but still with a poor prognosis. Pfeiffer cases with Kleeblattschädel appear to map to FGFR2, while those with milder phenotypes generally map to FGFR1.[339]

### Jackson-Weiss Syndrome

Jackson-Weiss syndrome is a clinically distinct autosomal dominant condition with craniosynostoses and concurrent foot anomalies.[333, 340, 341] The skull shape varies widely from brachycephaly to acrocephaly. Frontal prominence, hypertelorism, and strabismus have been noted. Intelligence is usually normal. The most consistent and distinctive feature of Jackson-Weiss syndrome is abnormality of the feet, with broad great toes, medial deviation of the toes, and tarsal-metatarsal coalitions. Hand anomalies are rare. There is great variability within families but high penetrance, so that some members have only foot deformities with no craniosynostosis.

### Boston (Type 2) Craniosynostosis

Boston syndrome is an autosomal dominant condition localized to chromosome 5qter. It has a variable phenotype, including forehead retrusion, frontal bossing, turricephaly, and Kleeblattschädel. All affected individuals have recession in the supraorbital region in relation to the superior surface of the cornea. Most exhibit myopia or hyperopia.[326]

### Muenke Syndrome

Muenke syndrome (Adelaide craniosynostosis) is an autosomal condition. Patients may show bicoronal synostosis (70%), unilateral coronal synostosis (30%), or simple macrocephaly.[333, 341] Muenke patients show midface hypoplasia (60%), downward slanting of the palpebral fissures (50%), strabismus and facial asymmetry (frequent), and sensorineural hearing loss (30%).[339] Broad halluces are seen clinically in 25%. Radiographs show short, broad middle phalanges in the hands but hypoplastic to absent middle phalanges in the toes.[339] Cone epiphyses are frequent in both hands and feet. Carpal and/or tarsal fusions are present in about 50%. Syndactyly and deviation of the great toes are not part of the syndrome.[339] A minority of Muenke patients show developmental delay.

### Baere-Stevenson Cutis Gyrata Syndrome

The Baere-Stevenson syndrome is an extremely rare autosomal dominant form of craniosynostosis that leads to early death. Patients show Kleeblattschädel and severe dermatologic anomalies including corrugated skin furrows (cutis gyrata), extensive acanthosis nigricans, cutaneous or mucosal tags, and small nails. Other features include choanal atresia, bifid scrotum, and an enlarged umbilical stump. The mutation affects FGFR2, either in the transmembrane domain or in the extracellular domain at the linker region between the third Ig-like loop and the transmembrane domain.[339]

## CONCLUSION

The broad spectrum of craniofacial malformations illustrates the differing ways in which basic embryologic mechanisms may deviate from the expected program.[342–344] Analysis of those malformations by molecular genetics is now providing increased understanding of the nature of those programs. Ultimately, it may be hoped that knowledge of the underlying mechanisms will allow us to tailor diets to meet the specific needs of each expectant mother to prevent these malformations and, at need, to call on the armamentarium of the body to effect scarless, seamless repair of any malformations that do occur.

## REFERENCES

1. Naidich TP, Zimmerman RA, Bauer BS, Altman NR, Bilaniuk LT. Midface: embryology and congenital lesions. In: Som PS, Curtin HD, eds. Head and Neck Imaging, Vol. 1. St. Louis: CV Mosby, 1996;3–60.
2. Nuckolls GH, Shum L, Slavkin HC. Progress toward understanding craniofacial malformations. Cleft Palate-Craniofac J 1999;36:12–26.
3. Carlson BM. Human Embryology and Developmental Biology, 2nd ed. St. Louis: CV Mosby, 1999.
4. Moore KL, Persaud TVN. The Developing Human. Clinically Oriented Embryology, 6th ed. Philadelphia: WB Saunders, 1998.

5. Schneider RA et al. Local retinoid signaling coordinates forebrain and facial morphogenesis by maintaining *FGF8* and *SHH*. Development 2001;128:2755–2767.

6. Shimamura K, Hartigan DJ, Martinez S, et al. Longitudinal organization of the anterior neural plate and neural tube. Development 1995;121:3923–3933.

7. Köntges G, Lumsden A. Rhombencephalic neural crest segmentation is preserved throughout craniofacial ontogeny. Development 1996; 122:3229–3242.

8. Patten BM. The normal development of the facial region. In: Pruzansky S, ed. Congenital Anomalies of the Face and Associated Structures. Springfield, Ill: Thomas, 1985.

9. Langman J. Medical Embryology: Human Development, Normal and Abnormal, 2nd ed. Baltimore: Williams & Wilkins, 1969.

10. Elmslie FV, Reardon W. Craniofacial developmental abnormalities. Curr Opin Neurol 1998;11:103–108.

11. Ferguson MWJ. Development of the face and palate. Cleft Palate-Craniofac J 1995;32:522–524.

12. Hu D, Helms JA. The role of Sonic hedgehog in normal and abnormal craniofacial morphogenesis. Development 1999;126: 4873–4884.

13. Murray JC. Invited editorial. Face facts: Genes, environment, and clefts. Am J Hum Genet 1995;57:227–232.

14. Davies J. Embryology and anatomy of the head, neck, face, palate, nose and paranasal sinuses. In: Paparella MM, Shumrick DA, eds. Otolaryngology, Vol. 1. Philadelphia: WB Saunders, 1980;63–123.

15. ten Berge D, Brouwer A, Korving J, et al. *Prx1* and *Prx2* are upstream regulators of sonic hedgehog and control proliferation during mandibular arch morphogenesis. Development 2001;128: 2929–2938.

16. Lu M-F, Cheng H-T, Kern MJ, et al. *Prx-1* functions cooperatively with another paired-related homeobox gene, *prx-2*, to maintain cell fates within the craniofacial mesenchyme. Development 1999;126: 495–504.

17. Borchers A, David R, Wedlich D. *Xenopus cadeherin-11* restrains cranial neural crest migration and influences neural crest specification. Development 2001;128:3049–3060.

18. Brivanlou AH, Darnell JE Jr. Signal transduction and the control of gene expression. Science 2002;295:813–818.

19. Schilling TF. Genetic analysis of craniofacial development in the vertebrate embryo. BioEssays 1997;19:459–468.

20. Wedden SE. Epithelial–mesenchymal interactions in the development of chick facial primordia and the target of retinoid action. Development 1987;90:341–351.

21. Richman JM, Tickle C. Epithelial–mesenchymal interactions in the outgrowth of limb buds and facial primordia in chick embryos. Dev Biol 1992;154:299–308.

22. Proetzel G, Paulowski S, Wiles MV, et al. Transforming growth factor β3 is required for secondary palate fusion. Nat Genet 1995;11:409–414.

23. Carette MJM, Ferguson MWJ. The fate of medial edge epithelial cells during palatal fusion in vitro: an analysis by DiI labelling and confocal microscopy. Development 1992;114:379–388.

24. Scott JH. The cartilage of the nasal septum (a contribution to the study of facial growth). Br Dent J 1953;95:37–43.

25. Mood GF. Congenital anterior herniations of brain. Ann Otol Rhinol Laryngol 1938;47:391–401.

26. Naidich TP, Takahashi S, Towbin RB. Normal patterns of ossification of the skull base: ages 0-16 years. Paper presented at the 71st scientific assembly and annual meeting of the Radiological Society of North America, Chicago, November 19, 1985.

27. Lebowitz RA, Terk A, Jacobs JB, Holliday RA, et al. Asymmetry of the ethmoid roof: analysis using coronal computed tomography. Laryngoscope 2001;111:2122–2124.

28. Naidich TP, Valente M, Abrams K, Spreitzer JJ, Doundoulakis SH. Torus palatinus. Int J Neuroradiol 1997;3:229–243.

29. Naidich TP. Pits, patches and protuberances. Hyperostosis mandibularis interna. Int J Neurol 1997;3:224–228.

30. Woo J-K. Torus palatinus. Am J Phys Anthropol 1950;8:81–112.

31. van den Broek AJP. On exostoses in the human skull. Acta Neirland Morph 1943;5:95–118.

32. Thoma KH. Tumors of the Jaw. Oral Pathology, 3rd ed. St. Louis: CV Mosby, 1950;1336–1344.

33. Suzuki M, Sakai T. A familial study of torus palatinus and torus mandibularis. Am Phys Anthropol 1960;18:264–272.

34. Thoma KH. Torus palatinus. Int J Orthodont Oral Surg 1937;23: 194–202.

35. Kolas S, Halperin V, Jefferis K, Huddleston S, Robinson HBG. The occurrence of torus palatinus and torus mandibularis in 2,478 dental patients. Oral Surg Oral Med Oral Pathol 1953;6:1134–1141.

36. Lasker GW. Penetrance estimated by the frequency of unilateral occurrences and by discordance in monozygotic twins. Hum Biol 1957;19:217–230.

37. Hooton EA. On certain Eskimoid characters in Icelandic skulls. Am J Phys Anthropol 1918;1:53–76.

38. Lasker GW. Genetic analysis of racial traits of the teeth. Cold Spring Harbor Symp Quant Biol 1950;15:191–203.

39. Miller SC, Roth H. Torus palatinus: a statistical study. J Am Dent Assoc 1940;27:1950–1957.

40. Koemer O. Der torus palatinus. Z Ohrenh Krankh Luft 1910;61: 24–27.

41. Lachmann H. Torus palatinus bei Degenerieten, f. d. ges. Neurol Psychiatr 1927;111:616.

42. King DR, Moore GE. An analysis of torus palatinus in a transatlantic study. J Oral Med 1976;31:44–46.

43. Naidich TP, et al. Midline craniofacial dysraphism: midline cleft upper lip, basal encephalocele, callosal agenesis, and optic nerve dysplasia. Concepts Pediatr Neurosurg 1977;4:186.

44. Naidich TP, Osborn RE, Bauer B, et al. Median cleft face syndrome: MR and CT data from 11 children. J Comput Assist Tomogr 1988;12:57–64.

45. Bauer BS, Wilkes GH, Kernahan DA. Incorporation of the W-plasty in repair of macrostomia. Plast Reconstr Surg 1982;70:752–757.

46. Fogh-Andersen P. Rare clefts of the face. Acta Chir Scand 1965;129:275–281.

47. Christensen K, Fogh-Andersen P. Etiological subgroups in nonsyndromic isolated cleft palate. A genetic-epidemiological study of 52 Danish birth cohorts. Clin Genet 1994;46:329–335.

48. Carinci F, Pezzetti F, Scapoli L, Martinelli M, Carinci P, Tognon M. Genetics of nonsyndromic cleft lip and palate: a review of international studies and data regarding the Italian population. Cleft Lip-Craniofac J 2000;37:33–40.

49. Stoll C, Alembik Y, Dott B, Roth MP. Associated malformations in cases with oral clefts. Cleft Palate-Craniofac J 2000;37:41–47.

50. Rajabian MH, Sherkat M. An epidemiological study of oral clefts in Iran: analysis of 1669 cases. Cleft Palate-Craniofac J 2000;37:191–196.

51. Sigler A, Ontiveros DS. Nasal deformity and microform cleft lip in parents of patients with cleft lip. Cleft Palate-Craniofac J 1999;36:139–143.

52. Raposio E, Panarese P, Santi P-L. Fetal unilateral cleft lip and palate: detection of enzymatic anomalies in the amniotic fluid. Plastic Reconstr Surg 1999;103:391–394.

53. Chung KC, Kowalski CP, Kim HM, Buchman SR. Maternal cigarette smoking during pregnancy and the risk of having a child with cleft lip/palate. Plast Reconstr Surg 2000;105:485–491.

54. Thomas T, Kurihara H, Yamagishi H, Kurihara Y, Yazaki Y, Olson EN, Srivastava D. A signaling cascade involving *endothelin-1*, dHAND and *Msx 1* regulates development of neural-crest-derived branchial arch mesenchyme. Development 1998;125:3005–3014.

55. Robert B, Sassoon D, Jacq B, Gehring W, Buckingham M, et al. *Hox-7*, a mouse homeobox gene with a novel pattern of expression during embryogenesis. EMBO J 1989;8(1):91–100.

56. Brunet CL, Sharpe PM, Ferguson MWJ. Inhibition of TGFβ 3, but not TGFβ 1 or TGFβ 2 activity, prevents normal mouse embryonic palate fusion. Int J Dev Biol 1995;39:345–355.

57. Haria S, Noar JH, Sanders R. An investigation of the dentition of parents of children with cleft lip and palate. Cleft Palate-Craniofac J 2000;37:395–405.

58. Laspos CP, Kyrkanides S, Tallents RH, Moss ME, Subtelny JD. Mandibular and maxillary asymmetry in individuals with unilateral cleft lip and palate. Cleft Palate-Craniofac J 1997;34:232–239.

59. Laspos CP, Kyrkanides S, Tallents RH, Moss ME, Subtelny JD. Mandibular asymmetry in noncleft and unilateral cleft lip and palate individuals. Cleft Palate-Craniofac J 1997;34:410–416.

60. Ross RB. Commentary on Laspos et al. Cleft Palate-Craniofac J 1997;34:232–239.

61. Kyrkanides S, Bellohusen R, Subtelny JD. Skeletal asymmetries of the nasomaxillary complex in noncleft and postsurgical unilateral cleft lip and palate individuals. Cleft Palate-Craniofac J 1995;32: 428–433.

62. Kyrkanides S, Klambani M, Subtelny JD. Cranial base and facial skeleton asymmetries in individuals with unilateral cleft lip and palate. Cleft Palate-Craniofac J 2000;37:556–561.

63. Croen LA, Shaw GM, Wasserman CR, Tolarova MM. Racial and ethnic variations in the prevalence of orofacial clefts in California, 1983-1992. Am J Med Genet 1998;79:42–47.

64. DeMyer W. Median facial malformations and their implications for brain malformations. Birth Defects (Orig Article Ser) 1975;11:155.

65. Johnston MC, Hassell JR, Brown KS. The embryology of cleft lip and cleft palate. Clin Plast Surg 1975;2:195–203.

66. DeMyer W. The median cleft face syndrome: differential diagnosis of cranium bifidum occultum, hypertelorism, and median cleft nose, lip and palate. Neurology 1967;17:961–971.

67. Cohen MM et al. Frontonasal dysplasia (median cleft face syndrome): comments on etiology and pathogenesis. Birth Defects 1971;7:117.

68. Warkany J, Bofinger MK, Benton C. Median facial cleft syndrome in half-sisters: dilemmas in genetic counseling. Teratology 1973;8:273–285.

69. Sedano HO, Cohen MM Jr, Jirasek J, et al. Frontonasal dysplasia. J Pediatr 1970;76:906–913.

70. Bakken AF, Aabyholm G. Frontonasal dysplasia: possible hereditary connection with other congenital defects. Clin Genet 1976;10:214–217.

71. Fontaine G, Walbaum R, Poupard B, et al. La dysplasie frontonasale. J Genet Hum 1983;31:351–365.

72. Fragoso R, Cid-Garcia A, Hernandez A, et al. Frontonasal dysplasia in the Klippel-Feil syndrome: a new associated malformation. Clin Genet 1982;22:270–273.

73. Francois J, Eggermont E, Evens L, et al. Agenesis of the corpus callosum in the median facial cleft syndrome and associated ocular malformations. Am J Ophthalmol 1973;76:241–245.

74. Fuenmayor HM. The spectrum of frontonasal dysplasia in an inbred pedigree. Clin Genet 1980;17:137.

75. Hori A. A brain with two hypophyses in median cleft face syndrome. Acta Neuropathol 1983;59:150–154.

76. Ide CH, Holt JE. Median cleft face syndrome associated with orbital hypertelorism and polysyndactyly. Eye Ear Nose Throat Monthly 1975;54:150–151.

77. Kinsey JA, Streeten BW. Ocular abnormalities in the median cleft face syndrome. Am J Ophthalmol 1977;83:261–266.

78. Roizenblatt J, Wajntal A, Diament AJ. Median cleft face syndrome or frontonasal dysplasia: a case report with associated kidney malformation. J Pediatr Ophthalmol Strabis 1979;16:16.

79. Gorlin RJ, Anderson VE, Scott CR. Hypertrophied frenuli, oligophrenia, familial trembling and anomalies of the hand: report of four cases in one family and a forme fruste in another. N Engl J Med 1961;264:486–489.

80. Townes PL, Wood BP, McDonald JV. Further heterogeneity of the oral-facial-digital syndromes. Am J Dis Child 1976;130:548–554.

81. Starck WJ, Epker BN. Surgical repair of a median cleft of the upper lip. J Oral Maxillofac Surg 1994;52:1217–1219.

82. Ingraham RD, Matson DD. Spina bifida and cranium bifidum. IV. An unusual nasopharyngeal encephalocele. N Engl J Med 1943;228:815–820.

83. Avanzini G, Crivelli G. A case of sphenopharyngeal encephalocele. Acta Neurochir 1970;22:205–212.

84. Baraton J, Ernest C, Poree C, et al. The neuroradiological examination of endocrine disorders of central origin in the child (precocious puberty, hypopituitarism). Pediatr Radiol 1976;4:69–78.

85. Byrd SE, Harwood-Nash DC, Fitz CR, et al. Computed tomography in the evaluation of encephaloceles in infants and children. J Comput Assist Tomogr 1978;2:81–87.

86. Corbett JJ, Savino PJ, Schatz NJ, et al. Cavitary developmental defects of the optic disc: visual loss associated with optic pits and colobomas. Arch Neurol 1980;37:210–213.

87. Danoff D, Serbu J, French LA. Encephalocele extending into the sphenoid sinus. J Neurosurg 1966;24:684–686.

88. Ellyin F, Khatir AH, Singh SP. Hypothalamic-pituitary functions in patients with transsphenoidal encephalocele and midfacial anomalies. J Clin Endocrinol Metab 1980;51:854–856.

89. Exner A. Uber basale Cephalocelen. Dt Z Chir 1907;908:23–41.

90. Goldhammer Y, Smith JL. Optic nerve anomalies in basal encephalocele. Arch Ophthalmol 1975;93:115–118.

91. Jacob JB. Les Meningoencephaloceles anterieures de la base du crane. Maroc Med 1961;40:73–104.

92. Koenig SB, Naidich TP, Lissner G. The morning glory syndrome associated with sphenoidal encephalocele. Ophthalmology 1982;89:1368–1373.

93. Larsen JL, Bassoe HH. Transsphenoidal meningocele with hypothalamic insufficiency. Neuroradiology 1979;18:205–209.

94. Lewin ML, Shuster MM. Transpalatal correction of basilar meningocele with cleft palate. Arch Surg 1965;90:687–693.

95. Lichtenberg G. Congenital tumour of the mouth involving the brain and connected with other malformations. Trans Lond Soc Pathol 1867;18:250.

96. Manelfe C, Starling-Jardin D, Toubi S, et al. Transsphenoidal encephalocele associated with agenesis of corpus callosum: value of metrizamide computed cisternography. J Comput Assist Tomogr 1978;2:356.

97. Modesti LM, Glasauer FE, Terplan KL. Sphenoethmoidal encephalocele: a case report with review of the literature. Childs Brain 1977;3:140–153.

98. Oldfield MC. An encephalocele associated with hypertelorism and cleft palate. Br J Surg 1938;25:757–764.

99. Pinto RS, George AE, Koslow M, et al. Neuroradiology basal anterior fossa (transethmoidal) encephaloceles. Radiology 1975;117:79–85.

100. Pollock JA, Newton TH, Hoyt WF. Transsphenoidal and transethmoidal encephaloceles: a review of clinical and roentgen features in 8 cases. Radiology 1968;90:442–453.

101. Sadeh M, Goldhammer Y, Shacked I, et al. Basal encephalocele associated with suprasellar epidermoid cyst. Arch Neurol 1982;39:250–252.

102. Sakoda K, Ishikawa S, Uozumil T, et al. Sphenoethmoidal meningoencephalocele associated with agenesis of corpus callosum and median cleft lip and palate: case report. J Neurosurg 1979;51:397–401.

103. Van Nouhuys JM, Bruyn GW. Nasopharyngeal transsphenoidal encephalocele, crater-like hole in the optic disc and agenesis of the corpus callosum: pneumoencephalographic visualization in a case. Psychiatr Neurol Neurochir 1964;67:243–258.

104. Weise GM, Kempe LG, Hammon WM. Transsphenoidal meningohydroencephalocele: case report. J Neurosurg 1972;37:475.

105. Kindler P. Morning glory syndrome: unusual congenital optic disk anomaly. Am J Ophthalmol 1970;69:376–384.

106. Krause U. Three cases of the morning glory syndrome. Acta Ophthalmol 1972;50:188.

107. Malbran JL, Maria-Roveda J. Megalopapila. Archos Oftal B Aires 1951;26:331–335.

108. Itakura T, Miyamoto K, Uematsu Y, et al. Bilateral morning glory syndrome associated with sphenoid encephalocele: case report. J Neurosurg 1992;77:949–951.

109. Wexler MR, Benmeir P, Umansky F, et al. Midline cleft syndrome with sphenoethmoidal encephalocele: a case report. J Craniofac Surg 1991;2:38–41.

110. Beyer WB, Quencer RM, Osher RH. Morning glory syndrome: a functional analysis including fluorescein angiography, ultrasonography, and computerized tomography. Ophthalmology 1982;89:1362–1367.

111. Yock DH Jr. Choroid plexus lipomas associated with lipoma of the corpus callosum. J Comput Assist Tomogr 1980;4:678–682.

112. Suemitsu T, Nakajima SI, Kuwajimak, et al. Lipoma of the corpus callosum: report of a case and review of the literature. Childs Brain 1979;5:476–483.

113. Zee CS, McComb JG, Segall HD, et al. Lipomas of the corpus callosum associated with frontal dysraphism. J Comput Assist Tomogr 1981;5:201–205.

114. Pascual-Castroviejo I, Pascual-Pascual SI, Perez-Higueras A. Frontonasal dysplasia and lipoma of the corpus callosum. Eur J Pediatr 1985;144:66–71.

115. Tessier P. Anatomical classification of facial, craniofacial, and lateral facial clefts. J Maxillofac Surg 1976;4:69–92.

116. Roarty JD, Pron GE, Siegel-Bartelt J, et al. Ocular manifestations of frontonasal dysplasia. Plast Reconstr Surg 1994;93:25–30.

117. Beverdam A, Brouwer A, Reijnen M, Korving J, Meijlink F. Severe nasal clefting and abnormal embryonic apoptosis in *Alx3/Alx4* double mutant mice. Development 2001;128:3975–3986.

118. Aleksic S, et al. Intracranial lipomas, hydrocephalus, and other CNS anomalies in oculoaricularvertebral dysplasia (Goldenhar-Gorlin syndrome). Childs Brain 1984;11:285–297.

119. Shokeir MHK. The Goldenhar syndrome: a natural history. Birth Defects 1977;13:67–83.

120. Ryals BD, Brown DC, Levin SW. Duplication of the pituitary gland as shown by MR. AJNR 1993;14:137–139.

121. Chapman S, Goldin JH, Hendel RG, et al. The median cleft face syndrome with associated cleft mandible, bifid odontoid peg and agenesis of the anterior arch of atlas. Br J Oral Maxillofac Surg 1991;29:279–281.

122. Kurlander GJ, DeMyer W, Campbell JA. Roentgenology of the median cleft face syndrome. Radiology 1967;88:473–478.

123. de Villiers JC, Cluver PF, Peter JC. Lipoma of the corpus callosum associated with frontal and facial anomalies. Acta Neurochir Suppl (Wien) 1991;53:1–6.

124. Aleksic S, Budzilovich G, Reuben R, et al. Unilateral arhinencephaly in Goldenhar-Gorlin syndrome. Dev Med Child Neurol 1975;17:498–504.

125. Aleksic S, Budzilovich G, Greco MA, Epstein F, Feigin I, Pearson J. Encephalocele (cerebellocele) in the Goldenhar-Gorlin syndrome. Eur J Pediatr 1983;40:137–138.

126. Castillo M, Mukherji SK. Facies to remember. Number 2. Median cleft face syndrome with Sedano facies type D, callosal agenesis, interhemispheric lipoma, and dermoid. Int J Neuroradiol 1995;2:154–160.

127. Castillo M. Congenital abnormalities of the nose: CT and MR findings. Am J Roentgenol I994;162:1211–1217.

128. Oostrom CAM, Vermeij-Keers C, Gilbert PM, van der Meulen JC. Median cleft of the lower lip and mandible: case reports, a new embryological hypothesis and subdivision. Plast Reconstr Surg 1996;97:313–320.

129. Surendran N, Varghese B. Midline cleft of the lower lip with cleft of the mandible and midline dermoid in the neck. J Pediatr Surg 1991;26:1387–1388.

130. Higginbottom MC, Jones KL, Hall BD, Smith DW. The amniotic band disruption complex: timing of amniotic rupture and variable spectra of consequent defects. J Pediatr 1979;95:544–549.

131. Sessions RB. Nasal dermal sinuses—new concepts and explanations. II. Laryngoscope 1982;92 (suppl 29):1–28.

132. Gorenstein A, Kern EB, Facer GW, et al. Nasal gliomas. Arch Otolaryngol 1980;106:536–540.

133. McQuown SA, Smith JD, Gallo AE Jr. Intracranial extension of nasal dermoids. Neurosurgery 1983;12:531–535.

134. Choudhury AR, Ladapo F, Mordi VP, et al. Congenital inclusion cyst of the subgaleal space. J Neurosurg 1982;56:540–544.

135. Choudhury AR, Taylor JC. Primary intranasal encephalocele: report of four cases. J Neurosurg 1982;57:552–555.

136. Card GG. Dermoid cyst of nose with intracranial extension. Arch Otolaryngol 1978;104:301–302.

137. Yeoh GPS, Bale PM, de Silva M. Nasal cerebral heterotopia: the so-called nasal glioma or sequestered encephalocele and its variants. Pediatr Pathol 1989;9:531–549.

138. Pannell BW, Hendrick EG, Hoffman JH, et al. Dermoid cysts of the anterior fontanelle. Neurosurgery 1982;10:317–323.

139. Bartlett SP, Lin KY, Grossmank R, Katowitz J. The surgical management of orbitofacial dermoids in the pediatric patient. Plast Reconstr Surg 1993;91:1208–1215.

140. Nocini PF, Barbaglio A, Dolci M, Salgarelli A. Dermoid cyst of the nose: a case report and review of the literature. J Oral Maxillofac Surg 1996;54:357–362.

141. Bradley PK. Nasal dermoids in children. Int J Pediatr Otorhinolaryngol 1981;3:63.

142. Pensler JM, Bauer BS, Naidich TP. Craniofacial dermoids. Plast Reconstr Surg 1988;82:953–958.

143. Griffith BH. Frontonasal tumors: their diagnosis and management. Plast Reconstr Surg 1976;57:692–699.

144. Wardinski TD, Pagon RA, Kropp RJ, Hayden PW, Clarren SK. Nasal dermoid sinus cysts: association with intracranial extension and multiple malformations. Cleft Palatal-Craniofac J 1991;28:87–95.

145. Muhlbauer WD, Dittmar W. Hereditary median dermoid cysts of the nose. Br J Plast Surg 1976;29:334–340.

146. Plewes JL, Jacobson I. Familial frontonasal dermoid cysts: report of four cases. J Neurosurg 1971;34:683–686.

147. Hacker DC, Freeman JL. Intracranial extension of a nasal dermoid sinus cyst in a 56-year-old man. Head Neck 1994;16:366–371.

148. Paller AS, Pensler JM, Tadinori T. Nasal midline masses in infants and children: dermoids, encephaloceles, and gliomas Arch Dermatol 1991;127:362–366.

149. Barkovich AJ, Vandermarck P, Edwards MSB, et al. Congenital nasal masses: CT and MR imaging features in 16 cases. AJNR 1991;12:105–116.

150. Maniglia AJ, Goodwin J, Arnold JE, Ganz E. Intracranial abscesses secondary to nasal, sinus, and orbital infections in adults and children. Arch Otolaryngol 1989;115:1424–1429.

151. Rohrich RJ, Lowe JB, Schwartz MR. The role of open rhinoplasty in the management of nasal dermoid cysts. Plast Reconstr Surg 1999;104:1459–1471.

152. Johnson GF, Weisman PA. Radiological features of dermoid cysts of the nose. Radiology 1964;82:1016–1021.

153. Black BK, Smith DE. Nasal glioma: two cases with recurrence. Arch Neurol Psychiatr 1950;64:614–630.

154. Harley EH. Pediatric congenital nasal masses. Ear Nose Throat J 1991;70:28–32.

155. Walker EA Jr, Resler DR. Nasal glioma. Laryngoscope 1963;73:93–107.

156. Puppala B, Mangurten HH, McFadden J, Lygizos N, Taxy J, Pellettiere E. Nasal glioma presenting as neonatal respiratory distress. Clin Pediatr 1990;29:49–52.

157. Morgan DW, Evans JNG. Developmental nasal anomalies. J Laryngol Otol 1990;104:394–403.

158. Choudhury AR, Bandey SA, Haleem A, Sharif H. Glial heterotopias of the nose. A report of two cases. Childs Nerv Syst 1996;12:43–47.

159. Braun M, Boman F, Hascoet JM, et al. Brain tissue heterotopia in the nasopharynx: contribution of MRI to assessment of extension. J Neuroradiol 1992;19:68–74.

160. Smith KR Jr, Schwartz HG, Luse SA, et al. Nasal gliomas: a report of five cases with electron microscopy of one. J Neurosurg 1963;20:968–982.

161. Suwanwela C, Hongsaprabhas C. Frontoethmoidal encephalomeningocele. J Neurosurg 1966;25:172–182.

162. Heacock GL, Taqi F, Biedlingmaler J. Pathology quiz case 1. Nasal glioma. Arch Otolaryngol 1992;118:548–550.

163. Kurzer A, Arbelaez N, Cassiano G. Gliomas of the face: case report. Plast Reconstr Surg 1982;69:678–682.

164. Scheiner AJ, Frayer WC, Rorke LB, Heher K. Ectopic brain tissue in the orbit. Eye 1999;13:251–254.

165. Ibekwe AO, Ikerionwu SE. Heterotopic brain tissue in the palate. J Laryngol Otol 1982;96:1155–1158.

166. Leclerc JE. Cerebral tissue heterotopia in the soft palate. J Otolaryngol 1997;26:327–329.

167. Anand VK, Melvin FM, Reed JM, Parent AD. Nasopharyngeal gliomas: diagnostic and treatment considerations. Otolaryngol Head Neck Surg 1993;109:534–539.

168. Kallman JE, Loevner LA, Yousem DM, et al. Heterotopic brain in the pterygopalatine fossa. Am J Neuroradiol 1997;18:176–179.

169. Pasyk KA, Argenta LC, Marks MW, Friedman RJ. Heterotopic brain presenting as a lip lesion. Cleft Palate J 1988;25:48–52.

170. Hendrickson M, Faye-Peterson O, Johnson DG. Cystic and solid heterotopic brain in the face and neck: a review and report of an unusual case. J Pediatr Surg 1990;25:766–768.

171. Lasjaunias P, Ginisty D, Comoy J, Landrieu P. Ectopic secreting choroid plexus in the oropharynx. Pediatr Neurosci 1985–1986;12:205–207.

172. Wismer GL, Wilkinson AH, Goldstein JD, et al. Cystic temporofacial brain heterotopia. AJNR 1989;10:S32–S33.

173. Bossen EH, Hudson WR. Oligodendroglioma arising in heterotopic brain tissue of the soft palate and nasopharynx. Am J Surg Pathol 1987;11:571–574.

174. Lee SC, Henry MM, Gonzalez-Crussi F. Simultaneous occurrence of melanotic neuroectodermal tumor and brain heterotopia in the oropharynx. Cancer 1976;38:249–253.

175. Uemura T, Yoshikawa A, Onizuka T, Hayashi T. Heterotopic nasopharyngeal brain tissue associated with cleft palate. Cleft Palate-Craniofac J 1999;36:248–251.

176. Mahabir RC, Mohammad JA, Courtemanche DJ. Lipoma on the cleft soft palate: a case report of a rare congenital anomaly. Cleft Palate-Craniofac J 2000;37:503–505.

177. Vandenhaute B, Leteurtre E, Lecomte-Houcke M, et al. Epignathus teratoma: report of three cases with a review of the literature. Cleft Palate-Craniofac J 2000;37:83–91.

178. Koch BL, Myer C III, Egelhoff JC. Congenital epulis. AJNR 1997;18:739–741.

179. Fuhr AH, Krogh PHJ. Congenital epulis of the newborn: centennial review of the literature and a report of a case. Oral Surg 1972;30:30–35.

180. Damm DD, Cibull ML, Geissler RH, et al. Investigation into the histogenesis of congenital epulis of the newborn. Oral Surg Oral Med Oral Pathol 1993;76:205–212.

181. Jenkins HR, Hill CM. Spontaneous regression of congenital epulis of the newborn. Arch Dis Child 1989;64:145–147.

182. Brito JA, Ragoowansi RH, Sommoerlad BC. Double tongue, intraoral anomalies, and cleft palate—case reports and a discussion of developmental pathology. Cleft Palate-Craniofac J 2000;37:410–415.

183. Naidich TP, Altman NR, Braffman BH, et al. Cephaloceles and related malformations. AJNR 1992;13:655–690.

184. Finerman WB, Pick EI. Intranasal encephalomeningocele. Ann Otol Rhinol Laryngol 1953;62:114–120.

185. Suwanwela C, Suwanwela N. A morphological classification of sincipital encephalomeningoceles. J Neurosurg 1972;36:201–211.

186. Matson DD. Neurosurgery in Infancy and Childhood, 2nd ed. Springfield, Ill: Thomas, 1969;61–75.

187. Mealey J Jr, Dzenitis AJ, Hockey AA. The prognosis of cephaloceles. J Neurosurg 1970;32:209–218.

188. Fisher RG, Uiklein A, Kaith HM. Spina bifida and cranium bifidum: study of 530 cases. Mayo Clin Proc 1952;27:33–38.

189. Yokota A, Kajiwara H, Kochi M, Fuwa I, Wada H. Parietal cephalocele: clinical importance of its atretic form and associated malformations. J Neurosurg 1988;69:545–551.

190. Simpson DA, David DJ, White J. Cephaloceles: treatment, outcome and antenatal diagnosis. Neurosurgery 1984;15:14–21.

191. Peter JC, Fieggen G. Congenital malformations of the brain—a neurosurgical perspective at the close of the twentieth century. Childs Nerv Syst 1999;15:635–645.

192. Blumenfeld R, Skolnik EM. Intranasal encephaloceles. Arch Otolaryngol 1965;82:527–531.

193. Kennedy EM, Gruber DP, Billmire DA, Crone KR. Transpalatal approach for the extracranial surgical repair of transsphenoidal cephaloceles in children. J Neurosurg 1997;87:677–681.

194. Hoving EW. Nasal encephaloceles. Childs Nerv Syst 2000;16:702–706.

195. Mahapatra AK, Tandon PN, Dhawan IK, Khazanchi RK. Anterior encephaloceles: a report of 30 cases. Childs Nerv Syst 1994;10:501–504.

196. Charoonsmith T, Suwanwela C. Frontoethmoidal encephalomeningocele with special reference to plastic reconstruction. Clin Plast Surg 1974;1:27–47.

197. Czech T, Reinprecht A, Matula CH, Svoboda H, Vorkapic P. Cephaloceles—experience with 42 patients. Acta Neurochir (Wien) 1995;134:125–129.

198. Jacob OJ, Rosenfeld JV, Watters DA. The repair of frontal encephaloceles in Papua New Guinea. Aust N Z J Surg 1994;64:8568–8600.

199. Smit CS, Zeeman BJ, Smith RM, et al. Frontoethmoidal meningoencephaloceles: a review of 14 consecutive patients. J Craniofac Surg 1993;4:210–214.

200. Boonvisut S, Ladpli S, Sujatanond M, et al. Morphologic study of 120 skull base defects in frontoethmoidal encephalomeningoceles. Plast Reconstr Surg 1998;101:1784–1795.

201. Rappoport RL II, Dunn RC, Alhady F. Anterior encephalocele. J Neurosurg 1981;54:213.

202. Sargent LA, Seyfer AE, Gunby EN. Nasal encephaloceles: definitive one-stage reconstruction. J Neurosurg 1988;68:571–575.

203. Blumenfeld R, Skolnick EM. Intranasal encephaloceles. Arch Otolaryngol 1965;82:527–531.

204. David DJ, Sheffield L, Simpson D, White J. Frontoethmoidal meningoencephaloceles: morphology and treatment. Br J Plast Surg 1984;37:271–284.

205. Richards CGM. Frontoethmoidal meningoencephalocele: a common and severe congenital abnormality in South East Asia. Arch Dis Child 1992;67:717–719.

206. Brown MS, Sheridan-Pereira M. Outlook for the child with a cephalocele. Pediatrics 1992;90:914–919.

207. Zinreich SJ, Borders JC, Eisele DW, Mattox DE, Long DM, Kennedy DW. The utility of magnetic resonance imaging in the diagnosis of intranasal meningoencephaloceles. Arch Otolaryngol Head Neck Surg 1992;118:1253–1256.

208. Lowe LH, Booth TN, Joglar JM, Rollins NK. Midface anomalies in children. RadioGraphics 2000;20:907–922.

209. Moore MH, Lodge ML, David DJ. Basal cephalocele: imaging and exposing the hernia. Br J Plast Surg 1993;46:497–502.

210. Losken HW, Morris WMM, Earle JW. Unilateral exophthalmos caused by an anterior ethmoidal meningoencephalocele. Plast Reconstr Surg 1992;89:742–745.

211. Hao S-P, Wang H-S, Lui T-N. Transnasal endoscopic management of basal encephalocele-craniotomy is no longer mandatory. Am J Otolaryngol 1995;16:196–199.

212. Pollock JA, Newton TH, Hoyt WF. Transsphenoidal and transethmoidal encephaloceles: a review of clinical and roentgen features in 8 cases. Radiology 1968;90:442–453.

213. Sadeh M, Goldhammer Y, Shacked I, et al. Basal encephalocele associated with suprasellar epidermoid cyst. Arch Neurol 1982;39:250–252.

214. Sakoda K, Ishikawa S, Uozumil T, et al. Sphenoethmoidal meningoencephalocele associated with agenesis of corpus callosum and median cleft lip and palate: case report. J Neurosurg 1979;51:397–401.

215. Van Nouhuys JM, Bruyn GW. Nasopharyngeal transsphenoidal encephalocele, crater-like hole in the optic disc and agenesis of the corpus callosum: pneumoencephalographic visualization in a case. Psychiatr Neurol Neurochir 1964;67:243–258.

216. Weise GM, Kempe LG, Hammon WM. Transsphenoidal meningohydroencephalocele: case report. J Neurosurg 1972;37:475.

217. Blustajn J, Netchine I, Fredy D, et al. Dysgenesis of the internal carotid artery associated with transsphenoidal encephalocele: a neural crest syndrome? AJNR 1999;20:1154–1157.

218. Yokota A, Matsukado Y, Fuwa I, et al. Anterior basal encephalocele of the neonatal and infantile period. Neurosurgery 1986;19:468–478.

219. Elster AD, Branch CL. Transalar sphenoidal encephaloceles: clinical and radiologic findings. Radiology 1989;170:245–247.

220. Soyer PH, Dobbelaere P, Benoit S. Case report: transalar sphenoidal encephalocele. Uncommon clinical and radiological findings. Clin Radiol 1991;43:65–67.

221. Raftopoulos C, David P, Allard S, Ickx B, Baleriaux D. Endoscopic treatment of an oral cephalocele. J Neurosurg 1994;81:308–312.

222. Naidich TP, Heier LA, Osborn RE, Castillo M, Bozorgmanesh A, Altman N. Facies to remember number 6. Congenital dacryocystocele. Int J Neurol 1996;2:389–396.

223. Mansour A, Cheng K, Mumma J, et al. Congenital dacryocele: a collaborative review. Ophthalmology 1991;98:1744–1751.

224. Broggi R. The treatment of congenital dacryostenosis. Arch Ophthalmol 1959;61:30–36.

225. Ffooks O. Dacryocystitis in infancy. Br J Ophthalmol 1962;46:422–434.

226. Noda S, Hayasaka S, Setogawa T. Congenital nasolacrimal duct obstruction in Japanese infants: its incidence and treatment with massage. J Pediatr Ophthalmol Strabismus 1991;28:20–22.

227. Petersen R, Robb R. The natural course of congenital obstruction of the nasolacrimal duct. J Pediatr Ophthalmol Strabismus 1978;15:246–250.

228. Nordlow W, Vennerholm I. Congenital atresiae of the lacrimal passages: their occurrence and treatment. Acta Ophthalmol 1953;31:367–371.

229. Patrick R. Lacrimal secretion in full-term and premature babies. Trans Ophthalmol Soc UK 1974;94:283–290.

230. Cibis G, Spurney R, Waeltermann J. Radiographic visualization of congenital lacrimal sac mucoceles. Ann Ophthalmol 1986;18:68–69.

231. Menestrina L, Osborn R. Congenital dacryocystocele with intranasal extension: correlation of computed tomography and magnetic resonance imaging. J Am Osteopathol Assoc 1990;90:264–268.

232. Meyer J, Quint D, Holmes J, Witrak B. Infected congenital mucocele of the nasolacrimal duct. AJNR 1993;14:1008–1010.

233. Rand P, Ball WJ, Kulwin D. Congenital nasolacrimal mucoceles: CT evaluation. Radiology 1989;173:691–694.

234. Divine R, Anderson R, Bumsted R. Bilateral congenital lacrimal sac mucoceles with nasal extension and drainage. Arch Ophthalmol 1983;10:246–248.

235. Edmond J, Keech RV. Congenital nasolacrimal sac mucocele associated with respiratory distress. J Pediatr Ophthalmol Strabismus 1991;28:287–289.

236. Castillo M, Merten D, Weissler M. Bilateral nasolacrimal duct mucocele, a rare cause of respiratory distress: CT findings in two newborns. AJNR 1993;14:1011–1013.

237. Yee S, Siebert RW, Bower C, Glasier C. Congenital nasolacrimal duct mucocele: a cause of respiratory distress. Int J Pediatr Otorhinolaryngol 1994;29:151–158.

238. Peloquin L, Arcand P, Abela A. Endonasal dacryocystocele of the newborn. J Otolaryngol 1995;24:84–86.

239. DeMyer W. Holoprosencephaly. In: Vinken PJ, Bruyn GW, eds. Handbook of Clinical Neurology. Amsterdam: North Holland, 1977; 431–478.

240. Roessler E, Muenke M. The molecular genetics of holoprosencephaly: a model of brain development for the next century. Childs Nerv Syst 1999;15:646–651.

241. Nishimura H, Tanimura T, Semba R, Uwabe C. Normal development of early embryos: observation of 90 specimens at Carnegie stages 7 to 13. Teratology 1974;10:1–5.

242. Matsunaga E, Shiota K. Holoprosencephaly in human embryos: epidemiologic studies of 150 cases. Teratology 1977;16:261–272.

243. Urioste M, Valcarcel E, Gomez MA, Pinel I, Garcia de Leon R, Diaz de Bustamante A, Tebar R, Martinez-Frias ML. Holoprosencephaly and trisomy 21 in a child born to a nondiabetic mother. Am J Med Genet 1988;30:925–928.

244. Manelfe C, Sevely A. Etude neuroradiologique des holoprosencephalies (Neuroradiological study of holoprosencephalies). J Neuroradiol 1982;9:15–45.

245. Pauli RM, Pettersen JC, Arya S, Gilbert EF. Familial agnathiaholoprosencephaly. Am J Med Genet 1983;14:677–698.

246. Cohen MM Jr. Perspectives on holoprosencephaly: part I. Epidemiology, genetics, and syndromology. Teratology 1989;40:211–235.

247. Bachman H, Clark RD, Salahi W. Holoprosencephaly and polydactyly: a possible expression of the hydrolethalus syndrome. J Med Genet 1990;27:50–52.

248. Odent S, Attie-Bitach T, Blayau M, et al. Expression of the *Sonic Hedgehog* (*SHH*) gene during early human development and phenotypic expression of new mutations causing holoprosencephaly. Hum Mol Genet 1999;8:1683–1689.

249. Porter JA, Young KE, Beachy PA. Cholesterol modification of *Hedgehog* signaling proteins in animal development. Science 1996;274:255–259.

250. Pennisi E. Gene linkd to commonest cancer. Science 1996;272:1583–1584.

251. Kastury K, Druck T, Huebner K, et al. Chromosome locations of human *EMX* and *OTX* genes. Genomics 1994;22:41–45.

252. Simeone A, Acampora D, Gulisano M, Stornaiuolo A, Boncinelli E. Nested expression domains of four homeobox genes in developing rostral brain. Nature 1992;358:687–690.

253. Simeone A, Gulisano M, Acampora D, Stornaiuolo A, Rambaldi M, Boncinelli E. Two vertebrate homeobox genes related to the *Drosophila* empty spiracles genes are expressed in the embryonic cerebral cortex. EMBO J 1992;11:2541–2550.

254. Yoshida M, Suda Y, Matsuo I, Miyamoto N, Takeda N, Kuratani S, Aizawa S. *Emx 1* and *Emx 2* functions in development of dorsal telencephalon. Development 1997;124:101–111.

255. Rakic P. Neurocreationism—making new cortical maps. Science 2001;294:1011–1012.

256. Oliver G, Mailhos A, Wehr R, et al. *Six3*, a murine homologue of the sine oculis gene, demarcates the most anterior border of the developing neural plate and is expressed during eye development. Development 1995;121:4045–4055.

257. Roessler E, Belloni E, Gaudenz K, et al. Mutations in the human *Sonic Hedgehog* gene cause holoprosencephaly. Nature Genet 1996;14:357–360.

258. Meisler M. Mutation watch. Mammalian Genome 1997;8:305–306.

259. Castillo M, Mukherji SK. Disorders of ventral induction: holoprosencephalies. In: Castillo M, Mukherji SK, eds. Imaging of the Pediatric Head, Neck, and Spine. Philadelphia: Lippincott-Raven, 1996;33–36.

260. Smith MM, Thompson JE, Naidich TP, Castillo M, Thomas D, Mukherji SK. Facies to remember. Cebocephaly with single midline proboscis. Alobar holoprosencephaly. Int J Neurol 1996;3: 251–263.

261. Probst FP, Brun A. Structural organization of holospheric brains. In: Probst FP, ed. The Prosencephalies. Berlin: Springer-Verlag, 1979; 35–43.

262. Porteous ME, Wright C, Smith D, Burn J. Agnathia-holoprosencephaly: a new recessive syndrome? Clin Dysmorphol 1993;2:161–164.

263. Friede RL. Developmental Neuropathology, 2nd ed. Berlin: Springer-Verlag, 1989.

264. Kurokawa Y, Tsuchita H, Sohma T, Kitami K, Takeda T, Hattori S. Holoprosencephaly with Dandy-Walker cyst: rare coexistence of two major malformations. Childs Nerv Syst 1990;6:51–53.

265. Osaka K, Matsumoto S. Holoprosencephaly in neurosurgical practice. Neurosurgery 1978;48:787–803.

266. Sulik KK, Johnston MC, Smiley SJ, Speight HS, Jarvis BE. Mandibulofacial dysostosis (Treacher Collins syndrome): a new proposal for its pathogenesis. Am J Med Genet 1987;27:359–372.

267. Naidich TP, Smith MS, Castillo M, Thompson JE, Sloan GM, Jayakar P, Mukherji SK. Facies to remember. Number 7. Hemifacial microsomia. Goldenhar syndrome. OAV complex. Int J Neuroradiol 1996;2:437–449.

268. Goldenhar M. Associations malformatives de l'oeil et de l'oreille, en particulier le syndrome dermoide epibulbaire-appendices auriculares-fistula auris congenita et ses relations avec la dysostose mandibulofaciale. J Genet Hum 1952;1:243–282.

269. Feingold M, Baum J. Goldenhar's syndrome. Am J Dis Child 1978;132:136–138.

270. Gorlin RJ, Jue KL, Jacobsen U, Goldschmidt E. Oculoauriculovertebral dysplasia. J Pediatr 1963;63:991–999.

271. Rollnick BR, Kaye CI. Hemifacial microsomia and variants: pedigree data. Am J Med Genet 1983;15:233–253.

272. Cohen MM Jr, Rollnick BR, Kaye CI. Oculoauriculovertebral spectrum: an updated critique. Cleft Palate J 1989;26:276–286.

273. Beals RK, Robbins JR, Rolfe B. Anomalies associated with vertebral malformations. Spine 1993;18:1329–1332.

274. David DJ, Mahatumarat C, Cooter RD. Hemifacial microsomia: a multisystem classification. Plast Reconstr Surg 1987;80:525–535.

275. Mansour AM, Wang F, Henkind P, Goldberg R, Shprintzen R. Ocular findings in the facioauriculovertebral sequence (Goldenhar-Gorlin syndrome). Am J Ophthalmol 1985;100:555–559.

276. Stoll C, Viville B, Treisser A, et al. A family with dominant oculoauriculovertebral spectrum. Am J Med Genet 1998;78: 345–349.

277. Gosain AK, McCarthy JG, Pinto RS. Cervicovertebral anomalies and basilar impression in Goldenhar syndrome. Plast Reconstr Surg 1994;93:498–506.

278. Zelante L, Gasparini P, Scanderbeg AC, et al. Goldenhar complex: a further case with uncommon associated anomalies. Am J Med Genet 1997;69:418–421.

279. Figueroa AA, Friede H. Craniovertebral malformations in hemifacial microsomia. J Craniofac Genet Dev Biol Suppl 1985;l:167–178.

280. Cousley RRJ, Wilson DJ. Hemifacial micosomia: developmental consequence of perturbation of the auriculofacial cartilage model? Am J Med Genet 1992;42:461–466.

281. Foerst-Potts L, Sadler TW. Disruption of *Msx-1* and *Msx-2* reveals roles for these genes in craniofacial, eye, and axial development. Dev Dyn 1997;209:70–84.

282. Satokata I, Maas R. *Msx1* deficient mice exhibit cleft palate and abnormalities of craniofacial and tooth development. Nat Genet 1994;6:348–356.

283. Sadler LS, Robinson LK, Msall ME. Diabetic embryopathy: possible pathogenesis. Am J Med Genet 1995;55:363–366.

284. Horgan JE, Padwa BL, LaBrie RA, Mulliken JB. OMENS-plus: analysis of craniofacial and extracraniofacial anomalies in hemifacial microsomia. Cleft Palate-Craniofac J 1995;32:405–412.

285. Kearns GJ, Dent B, Padwa BL, et al. Progression of facial asymmetry in hemifacial microsomia. Plast Reconstr Surg 2000;105: 492–498.

286. Rollnick BR, Kaye CI, Nagatoshi K, Hauck W, Martin AO. Oculoauriculovertebral dysplasia and variants: phenotypic characteristics of 294 patients. Am J Med Genet 1987;26:361–375.

287. Smahel Z, Horak I. Craniofacial changes in unilateral microtia: I. An anthropometric study. J Craniofac Genet Dev Biol 1984;4: 7–16.

288. Smahel Z. Craniofacial changes in unilateral microtia: II. An x-ray study. J Craniofac Genet Dev Biol 1984;4:17–31.

289. Smahel Z. Craniofacial changes in hemifacial microsomia. J Craniofac Genet Dev Biol 1986;6:151–170.

290. Vento AR, LaBrie RA, Mulliken JB. The O.M.E.N.S. classification of hemifacial microsomia. Cleft Palate-Craniofac J 1991;28: 68–77.

291. Marsh JL, Baca D, Vannier MW. Facial musculoskeletal asymmetry in hemifacial microsomia. Cleft Palate J 1989;26:292–302.

292. Johnsen DC, Weissman BM, Murray GS, et al. Enamel defects: a developmental marker for hemifacial microsomia. Am J Med Genet 1990;36:444–448.

293. Caldarelli DD, Hutchinson JG Jr, Pruzansky S, Valvassori GE. A comparison of microtia and temporal bone anomalies in hemifacial microsomia and mandibulofacial dysostosis. Cleft Palate J 1980;17: 103–110.

294. Bassila MK, Goldberg R. The association of facial palsy and/or sensorineural hearing loss in patients with hemifacial microsomia. Cleft Palate J 1989;26:287–291.

295. Kirkham TH. Goldenhar's syndrome with inner ear defects. J Laryngol Otol 1970;84:855–856.

296. Manfré L, Genuardi P, Tortorici M, Legalla R. Absence of the common crus in Goldenhar syndrome. AJNR 1997;18:773–775.

297. Baum JL, Feingold M. Ocular aspects of Goldenhar's syndrome. Am J Ophthalmol 1973;75:250–257.

298. Elsas FJ, Green WR. Epibulbar tumors in childhood. Am J Ophthalmol 1975;79:1001–1007.

299. Caldarelli DD, Hutchinson JC Jr, Gould HJ. Hemifacial microsomia: priorities and sequence of comprehensive otologic management. Cleft Palate J 1980;17:111–115.

300. Padwa BL, Bruneteau RJ, Mulliken JB. Association between ''plagiocephaly'' and hemifacial microsomia. Am J Med Genet 1993;47:1202–1207.

301. Edwards SJ et al. Am J Hum Genet 1997;60:515–524.

302. Rune B, Sarnas KV, Aberg M, et al. Mandibulofacial dysostosis— variability in facial morphology and growth: a long-term profile roentgenographic and roentgen stereometric analysis of three patients. Cleft Palate-Craniofac J 1999;36:110–122.

303. Halal F, Herrmann J, Pallister PD, Opitz JM, Desgranges M-F, Grenier G. Differential diagnosis of Nager acrofacial dysostosis syndrome: report of four patients with Nager syndrome and discussion of related syndromes. Am J Med Genet 1983;14: 209–224.

304. Marques IL, Barbieri MA, Bettiol H. Etiopathogenesis of isolated Robin sequence. Cleft Palate-Craniofac J 1998;35:517–525.

305. Fernbach SK, Naidich TP. Radiological evaluation of craniosynostosis. In: Cohen MM Jr, ed. Craniosynostosis. Diagnosis, Evaluation and Management. New York: Raven Press, 1986;191–214.

306. Cohen MM Jr, MacLean RE. Craniosynostosis. Diagnosis, Evaluation, and Management, 2nd ed. New York: Oxford University Press, 2000.

307. Zimmerman RA. Skull development and abnormalities. In: Zimmerman RA, Gibby WA, Carmody RF, eds. Neuroimaging. Clinical and Physical Principles. New York: Springer, 2000;457–489.

308. Renier D, Lajeunie E, Arnaud E, Marchac D, et al. Management of craniosynostosis. Childs Nerv Syst 2000;16:645–658.

309. Hodges FJ III. Alterations in the skull with aging. In: Newton TH, Potts DG, eds. Radiology of the Skull and Brain, Vol. One, Book One, The Skull. St. Louis: CV Mosby, 1971;132–153.

310. Gooding CA. Cranial sutures and fontanelles. In: Newton TH, Potts DG, eds. Radiology of the Skull and Brain, Vol. One, Book One, The Skull. St. Louis: CV Mosby, 1971;216–237.

311. Huang MH, Mouradian WE, Cohen SR, Gruss JS, et al. The differential diagnosis of abnormal head shapes: separating craniosynostosis from positional deformities and normal variants. Cleft Palate-Craniofac J 1998;35:204–211.

312. Smits M, Wilmink JT. Synostotic and positional plagiocephaly. Two types of skull deformity studied with three-dimensional computed tomography. Int J Neurol 1998;4:405–411.

313. Park TS, Robinson S. Nonsyndromic craniosynostosis. In: McLone DG, ed-in-chief. Pediatric Neurosurgery: Surgery of the Develop-

ing Nervous System, 4th ed. Philadelphia: WB Saunders, 2001;345–361.

314. Posnick JC, Lin KY, Chen P, et al. Metopic synostosis: quantitative assessment of presenting deformity and surgical results based on CT scans. Plast Reconstr Surg 1994;93:16–24.

315. Reardon W, Winter RM, Rutland P, et al. Mutations in the fibroblast growth receptor 2 gene cause Crouzon syndrome. Nature Genet 1994;8:98–103.

316. Muenke M, Schell U, Hehr A, et al. A common mutation in the fibroblast growth factor receptor 1 gene in Pfeiffer syndrome. Nature Genet 1994;8:269–274.

317. Wilkie AOM, Slaney SF, Oldridge M, et al. Apert syndrome results from localized mutations of *FGFR2* and is allelic with Crouzon syndrome. Nature Genet 1995;9:165–172.

318. Preston RA, Post JC, Keats BJ, et al: A gene for Crouzon craniofacial dysostosis maps to the long arm of chromosome 10. Nature Genet 1994;7:149–153.

319. Shiang R, Thompson LM, Zhu YZ, et al. Mutations in the transmembrane domain of *FGFR3* cause the most common genetic form of dwarfism, achondroplasia. Cell 1994;78:335–342.

320. Rousseau F, Bonaventure J, Legeai-Mallet L, et al. Mutations in the gene encoding fibroblast growth factor receptor-3 in achondroplasia. Nature 1994;371:252–254.

321. Pauli RM, Conroy MM, Langer LO Jr, et al. Homozygous achondroplasia with survival beyond infancy. Am J Med Genet 1983;16:459–473.

322. Brueton LA, van Herwerden L, Chotai KA, et al. The mapping of a gene for craniosynostosis: evidence for linkage of the Saethre-Chotzen syndrome to distal chromosome 7p. J Med Genet 1992;29:681–685.

323. Vortkamp A, Gessler M, Grzeschik KH. *GLI3* zinc-finger gene interrupted by translocations in Greig syndrome families. Nature 1991;352:539–540.

324. Hui CC, Joyner AL. A mouse model of Greig cephalopolysyndactyly syndrome: the extra-toes mutation contains an intragenic deletion of the *Gli3* gene. Nature Genet 1993;3:241–246.

325. Mo R, Freer AM, Zinyk DL, et al. Specific and redundant functions of *Gli2* and *Gli3* zinc finger genes in skeletal patterning and development. Development 1997;124:113–123.

326. Müller U et al. Molecular genetics of craniosynostotic syndromes Arch Clin Exp Ophthalmol 1997;235:545–550.

327. Gorlin RJ. Fibroblast growth factors, their receptors and receptor disorders. Am J Cranio-Maxillofac Surg 1997;25:69–79.

328. Wilkie AOM. Craniosynostosis: genes and mechanisms. Human Mol Genet 1997;6:1647–1656.

329. Lejeunie E et al. Craniosynostosis: from a clinical description to an understanding of bone formation of the skull. Childs Nerv Syst 1999;15:676–680.

330. Sarkar S et al. FGF2 promotes skeletogenic differentiation of cranial neural crest cells. Development 2001;128:2143–2152.

331. Iseki S, Wilkie AOM, Morriss-Kay GM. *Fgfr1* and *Fgfr2* have distinct differentiation- and proliferation-related roles in the developing mouse skull vault. Development 1999;126:5611–5620.

332. Iseki S, Wilkie AOM, Heath JK, et al. *Fgfr2* and *osteopontin* domains in the developing skull vault are mutually exclusive and can be altered by locally applied FGF2. Development 1997;124:3375–3384.

333. Ackerman A et al. Skeletal malformations linked to fibroblast growth factor receptors. Int J Neuroradiol 1999;5:252–260.

334. Rollins N et al. MR venography in children with complex craniosynostosis. Pediatr Neurosurg 2000;32:308–315.

335. Robson et al. Prominent basal emissary foramina in syndromic craniosynostosis: correlation with phenotypic and molecular diagnoses. AJNR 2000;21:1707–1717.

336. Di Rocco C, Velardi F. Syndromic craniofacial malformations. In: McLone DG, ed.-in-chief. Pediatric Neurosurgery: Surgery of the Developing Nervous System, 4th ed. Philadelphia: WB Saunders, 2001;378–395.

337. Pfeiffer RA et al. Further delineation and review of the literature. Am J Med Genet 1964;90:301–320.

338. Cohen MM Jr. Pfeiffer syndrome update: clinical subtypes and guidelines for differential diagnosis. Am J Med Genet 1993;45:300–307.

339. Gorlin RJ. Fibroblast growth factors, their receptors and receptor disorders. Am J Cranio-Maxillofac Surg 1997;25:69–79.

340. Jackson CE, Weiss L, Reynolds WA, et al. Craniosynostosis, midface hypoplasia, and foot abnormalities: an autosomal dominant phenotype in a large Amish kindred. J Pediatr 1976;88:963–968.

341. Muenke M, Gripp KW, McDonald-McGinn D, et al. A unique point mutation in the *FGFR3* gene defines a new craniosynostosis syndrome. Am J Hum Genet 1997;60:555–564.

342. Couly GF, Coltey PM, Le Douarin NM. The triple origin of skull in higher vertebrates: a study in quail-chick chimeras. Development 1993;117:409–429.

343. Kawamoto HK Jr. The kaleidoscopic world of rare craniofacial clefts: order out of chaos (Tessier classification). Clin Plast Surg 1976;3:529.

344. Goodman RM, Gorlin RJ. Atlas of the Face in Genetic Disorders, 2nd ed. St. Louis: CV Mosby, 1977.

345. Derkay CS, Tunnessen WW Jr. Pictures of the month case 1 nasal glioma. Arch Pediatr Adolesc Med 1994;148:953–954.

## 2

# Anatomy and Physiology

*Peter M. Som, Joel M.A. Shugar,*
*and Margaret S. Brandwein*

## INTRODUCTION TO THE SINONASAL CAVITIES

For most physicians, the ubiquitous nature of the allergic and infectious diseases that affect the paranasal sinuses and nasal cavities (sinonasal cavities) renders them the most often imaged and therefore the best known areas of the head and neck. In addition, facial fractures are common and range from the broken nose to the more severe complex fractures. Lastly, the disfiguring tumors of the sinonasal cavities have earned their fearsome reputation because of their poor prognosis and the facial carnage they wreak. It thus seems reasonable to start the discussion of head and neck imaging with the sinonasal region.

# ANATOMY AND PHYSIOLOGY

## The Nose and Nasal Fossae

The term *nose* usually refers to the external nose that projects ventral to the rest of the face, while the terms *nasal fossae* or *nasal cavities* refer to the internal nasal airways. Topographically the nose can be divided into subunits that have practical importance in reconstructive surgery.[1-6] These subunits consist of the nasal dorsum, nasal sidewalls, nasal tip and columella, alar lobule, and supraalar facets. The nasion is the junction of the root of the nose with the forehead, while the lower or caudal free margin of the nose is formed by the alar rim, columella, and tip. On either side, the lateral lower margin of the nose has an expanded, rounded area referred to as the alar lobule, which consists of skin and soft tissue posterior and inferior to the lateral crus of the lower lateral cartilage. The dorsum of the nose consists of the dorsum of the nasal bones superiorly and the dorsal border of the quadrangular cartilage with the medial attachments of the upper lateral cartilages inferiorly (Fig. 2-1). The bony-cartilaginous junction is called the rhinion. The junction of the alae with the face is known as the alar-facial junction.

The nose has an overall pyramidal shape. Superiorly on either side of the nose, the sidewall of the pyramid consists of the nasal bone and the ascending process of the maxilla with which it articulates. The nasal bones are narrower and thicker cranially where they articulate with the nasal process of the frontal bones. The posterior surface of the nasal bones in the midline articulates with the perpendicular plate of the ethmoid bone superiorly and the quadrangular cartilage of the nasal septum inferiorly. Caudally the nasal bones become wider and thinner. Inferiorly the nasal bones attach to and overlap the cephalic portion of the upper lateral cartilages. The bony pyramid thus stabilizes the upper lateral car-

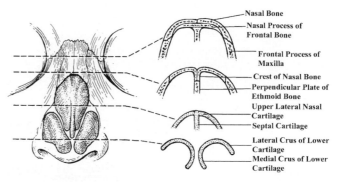

**FIGURE 2-2** Frontal view of the nose with cross-sectional diagrams at various levels illustrating the support structure of the nasal pyramid. (Modified from Hollinshead H. Anatomy for Surgeons. The Head and Neck. Vol 1. New York, NY: Hoeber-Harper, 1954.)

tilages that form the inferior sidewall of the nasal cartilaginous pyramid.[1] Rarely, the nasal bones are fused in the midline or are absent and replaced by an elongated frontal process of the maxilla. The nasal bones are very infrequently multiple.

The medial borders of the upper lateral cartilages are attached to the dorsum of the quadrangular cartilage of the septum and to each other. Laterally the upper lateral cartilages attach to the margin of the pyriform aperture (the osseous opening of the nasal cavity in the facial skeleton) by dense fibroareolar tissue. It is not uncommon to find accessory sesamoid cartilages in this area. The inferior border of the upper lateral cartilages are not attached and thus are mobile (Figs. 2-2 and 2-3).[2-5, 7]

On entering the nasal cavity, inspired air traverses the nasal valve. This is a circular area encompassed by the nasal septum, upper lateral cartilage, tip of the inferior turbinate, and floor of the nose. The total area encompassed by this valve provides the most important resistance to air flow in the nasal cavity.[8] Of slightly lesser importance is the angle formed by the meeting of the quadrangular cartilage of the nasal septum and the inferior border of the upper lateral cartilages, which is known as the nasal valve angle. Due to

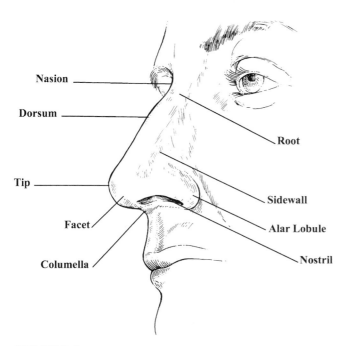

**FIGURE 2-1** The surface anatomy of the nose illustrated in a left anterior oblique view.

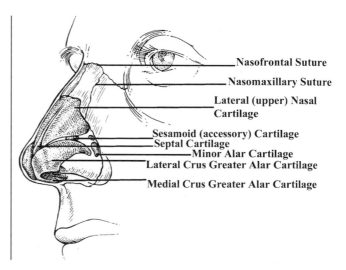

**FIGURE 2-3** Left anterior oblique view of the nasal skeleton indicating the osseous and cartilagenous anatomy.

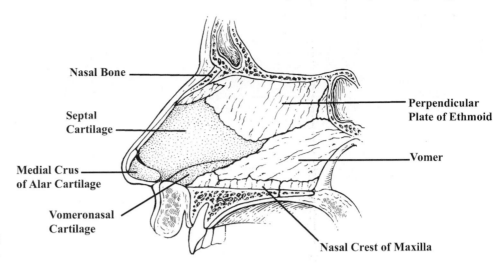

**FIGURE 2-4**  Diagram of a sagittal view of the nasal septum and hard palate.

Nasal Bone

Septal Cartilage

Medial Crus of Alar Cartilage

Vomeronasal Cartilage

Perpendicular Plate of Ethmoid

Vomer

Nasal Crest of Maxilla

its mobile nature, it is a dynamic structure that narrows and widens with the phases of respiration. It is thus a critical factor in determining airflow through the nasal cavity, and surgery in this area must preserve its integrity.

The lower paired lateral cartilages give the shape to the tip of the nose and base of the pyramid. Each lower lateral cartilage consists of medial crura and lateral crura. The point at which they meet dorsally is called the dome. The medial crura lie adjacent to the caudal end of the septum and attach to each other by loose connective tissue. At the dome, the lateral crura on either side extend superiorly and obliquely posteriorly toward the pyriform aperture, where they are attached by fibrous tissue. Sesamoid cartilages are also frequently found in this area of attachment. As each lateral crus extends superiorly, so does its lower border. The lower border thus does not parallel the alar rim. The soft tissue of the nose immediately below this area is devoid of cartilaginous support and is known as the alar lobule. The superior border of the lateral crus overlaps the distal ends of the upper lateral cartilages for a variable distance and is attached only by connective tissue. The skin covering the nose drapes across the angle formed at the junction of the medial and lateral crura, forming a triangular area called the facet (Figs. 2-2 and 2-3).

The nasal cavity on either side is separated by the nasal septum. The septum also helps support the bony and cartilaginous vault and the nasal tip. The main components of the nasal septum are the vomer, the perpendicular plate of the ethmoid, the quadrangular cartilage, the membranous septum, and the columella. Nasal bony crests from the upper surfaces of the palatine processes of the maxillae and the horizontal plates of the palatine bones also contribute to the inferior nasal septum (Fig. 2-4). The vomer may be bilaminar, due to its embryologic origin, and it and the perpendicular plate of the ethmoid bone are at times pneumatized. The perpendicular plate of the ethmoid fuses with the cribriform plate superiorly, and nasal septal surgery can cause a fracture of the cribriform plate, with a resultant cerebrospinal fluid leak. The vomer articulates superiorly with the perpendicular plate of the ethmoid and the crest of the sphenoid, anteriorly with the quadrangular cartilage, and inferiorly with the palatine bone and nasal crest of the maxilla. The vomer and quadrangular cartilage have a

tongue-in-groove relationship with the thin edge of the cartilage, fitting into a groove of the vomer. The posterior border of the vomer is free and divides the posterior choanae (Fig. 2-4).

The quadrangular cartilage is the most important surgical component of the septum due to its supportive function, and it is that portion of the septum anterior to the pyriform aperture that is the most significant in this role.[1] Thus the portion of the septum that provides the principal support to the nose lies anterior to a line drawn from the rhinion to the nasal spine, and injury to this region can result in a saddle nose deformity. The septal cartilage has an unusually mobile articulation with the surrounding bones, with only connective tissue stabilizing this junction. This relationship allows mobility that minimizes the chance of fracture or dislocation.

The membranous septum is that portion of the septum that lies between the caudal end of the cartilaginous septum and the columella. It is comprised only of a core of subcutaneous tissue lined on either side by vestibular skin. The columella is the most inferior part of the septum, and it has as its central support the medial crus of the right and left lower lateral cartilages. The inferior border of the columella and the lower margin of the nasal alae form the boundaries of the nostrils or nares, which are the external openings of the nose and which provide entrance into the nasal fossae.

The nasal muscles are the procerus, nasalis (compressor naris including both transverse and alar parts), levator labii superioris alaeque nasi (part of the quadratus labii), depressor septi, and the anterior and posterior dilator naris. The procerus and the forehead muscles elevate the skin over the dorsum of the nose. The nasalis (both the transverse and the alar portions) compresses the nares, and the dilators and the levator superioris alaeque nasi dilate the nostrils (Fig. 2-5). The depressor septi draws the nasal tip downward. The importance of the nasal muscles can be demonstrated in seventh nerve paralysis, in which the resultant alar collapse leads to nasal obstruction (Table 2-1).

The nasal cavities, or nasal fossae, are separated in the midline by the nasal septum. Each cavity is roughly pear-shaped, being narrow above (cranially) and wide below (caudally). The roof is formed by the thin cribriform plate of the ethmoid, which is only 5 mm across at its widest

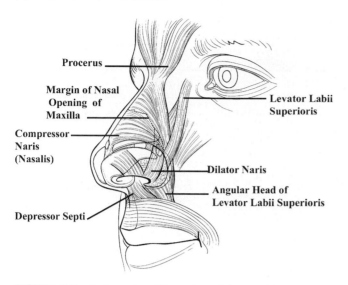

**FIGURE 2-5**    Left anterior oblique view of the nose illustrating the nasal musculature.

posterior margin. The floor of the nasal cavity is formed by the hard palate. The anterior two thirds of the hard palate is formed by the palatine processes of the maxillae, while the posterior one third is formed by the horizontal portions of the palatine bones.

The anterior portion of the nasal fossa that corresponds to the alar region of the nose is called the *vestibule*. It is lined with hair-bearing skin and sebaceous glands. Along the nasal septum there is no demarcation between the vestibule and the remaining nasal fossa. However, along the lateral wall there is a ridge, the limen vestibuli, that corresponds to the lower margin of the lateral crus of the cartilage, which marks the line of change from the skin of the vestibule into the mucous membrane of the remaining nasal fossa (Fig. 2-6).

The lateral wall of the nose is more intricate than the medial septal wall. Projecting from the lateral wall are three or four turbinates or conchae (Figs. 2-6 and 2-7). These conchae are scroll-like projections of bone that become smaller as they ascend the nasal cavity and that

**Table 2-1**
**MUSCLES OF THE FACE**

| Muscle | Origin | Insertion | Innervation | Action |
|---|---|---|---|---|
| Procerus (pyramidalis nasi) | Fascia over lower nasal bone and upper lateral nasal cartilages | Skin between and above eyebrow | Facial nerve (VII) [T, lower Z, B] | Draws down medial angle of eyebrows Produces transverse wrinkles over bridge of nose |
| Compressor naris (nasalis) | Canine eminence near maxillary incisive fossa | Aponeurosis on nasal cartilages | Facial nerve (VII) [lower Z, B] | Draws ala of nose toward septum Compressor of nostrils |
| Depressor septi (depressor alae nasi) | Incisive fossa of maxilla | Septum and back of ala of nose | Facial nerve (VII) [Lower Z, B] | Narrows nostril, draws septum down |
| Dilator naris (anterior and posterior) | Margin of nasal notch of maxilla and lesser alar cartilage | Skin near margin of nostril | Facial nerve (VII) [Z, B] | Enlarges nasal aperture |
| Levator labii superioris (infraorbital head) and levator labii superioris alaeque nasi (angular head) zygomaticus minor (zygomatic head) | *Angular head* from upper frontal process of maxilla *Infra-orbital head* from margin of orbit near infraorbital foramen *Zygomatic head* from alar surface of zygoma | *Angular head* to greater alar cartilage, skin of nose, and lateral upper lip *Infraorbital head* into muscles of upper lip between angular head and caninus *Zygomatic head* into skin of nasolabial groove and upper lip | Facial nerve (VII) [Z, B] | *Angular head* elevates upper lip and dilates nostril *Infraorbital head* raises angle of mouth *Zygomatic head* elevates upper lip laterally |
| Zygomaticus (major) | Zygomatic portion of zygomatic arch | Angle of mouth and orbicularis oris, depressor anguli oris, and caninus | Facial nerve (VII) [Z, B] | Draws angle of mouth upward and backward (laughing) |
| Levator anguli oris (caninus) | Canine fossa of maxilla below infraorbital foramen | Into angle of mouth and muscles of orbicularis oris, depressor anguli oris, and zygomaticus | Facial nerve (VII) [Z, B] | Elevates angle of mouth |
| Risorius | Fascia over masseter superficial to platysma | Skin at angle of mandible | Facial nerve (VII) [Z, B] | Retracts angle of mouth (grinning) |
| Depressor labii inferioris (quadratus labii inferioris) | Lateral surface of mandible between symphysis and mental foramen | Skin of lower lip and orbicularis oris | Facial nerve (VII) [M, B] | Depresses lower lip and draws it laterally (irony) |
| Depressor anguli oris (triangularis) (in 50% of people) transverse menti part of triangularis | Continuous with platysma on oblique line of mandible | Angle of mouth into orbicularis oris and skin | Facial nerve (VII) [M, B] | Depresses angle of mouth, associated with grief |

*Table continued on following page*

**Table 2-1**
**MUSCLES OF THE FACE** *Continued*

| Muscle | Origin | Insertion | Innervation | Action |
| --- | --- | --- | --- | --- |
| Mentalis | Incisive fossa of mandible | Skin of chin | Facial nerve (VII) [M] | Raises and protrudes lower lip, wrinkles skin, expresses doubt or disdain |
| Buccinator | Alveolar process of mandible opposite molar teeth and anterior border of the pterygomandibular raphe | Fibers converge toward angle of mouth where they blend with fibers of orbicularis oris muscle | Facial nerve (VII) [B] | Compresses cheeks, expels air from mouth, aids in chewing |
| Orbicularis oris | Sphincter muscle formed by contributions from various muscles and its own fibers Fibers from buccinator, levator anguli oris, depressor anguli oris, levator labii superioris, zygomaticus, depressor labii inferioris | Attaches to upper lip and lower lip, intermingles with fibers of origin, muscles, nasal septum | Facial nerve (VII) [lower Z, B, M] | Compression, contraction, and protrusion of lips. Involved in facial expression |
| Levator palpebrae superioris | Roof of orbit in front of optic foramen | Deep surface of upper eyelid, upper margin of superior tarsus, and superior fornix of conjunctiva | Cranial nerve III | Elevates eyelid voluntarily; attachment to superior tarsus acts involuntarily |
| Corrugater (supercilii) | Medial supraorbital | Skin of medial half of eyebrow | Facial nerve (VII) [Z, T] | Draws eyebrows downward and medially, produces wrinkles in frowning. Principal muscle in expression of suffering |
| Platysma | Fascia and skin over the upper part of the pectoralis and deltoid muscles | Lower border of the mandible and muscles of the lip | Facial nerve (VII) [C] | Produces a slight wrinkling of the skin surface of the neck, in an oblique direction, when entire muscle is brought into action. Anterior portion depresses the lower jaw and draws the lower lip and angles of the mouth down on each side |
| Oricularis oculi | *Orbital part* from medial orbital margin *Palpebral part* from palpebral ligament *Lacrimal part* from lacrimal bone | *Orbital fiber* arch around upper lid to lower lid and return to palpebral ligament *Palpebral fibers* go to *lacrimal fibers* to medial portion of upper and lower eyelids | Facial nerve (VII) [T, Z] | Sphincter of eyelids. The palpebral part is involuntary |
| Epicranius (occipitofrontalis) | Occipital bellies from lateral two thirds of superior nuchal line and mastoid process. Frontal bellies from epicranial aponeurosis at coronal suture | Skin of occipital region, skin of frontal region, and galea aponeurotica | Facial nerve (VII) [T, PA] | Moves scalp backward and forward, raises eyebrows (surprise) |
| Temporoparietalis | Temporal fascia above and anterior to the ear | Lateral border of the galea aponeurotica | Facial nerve (VII) [T] | Tightens scalp, draws back skin of temples |
| Auriculares (anterior, superior, posterior) | *Anterior:* temporal fascia and epicranial aponeurosis. *Superior:* epicranial aponeurosis and temporal fascia *Posterior:* mastoid process | *Anterior:* anterior and medial helix *Superior:* upper medial surface of auricle *Posterior:* Lower cranial surface of auricle | Facial nerve (VII) [T, PA] | Retracts and elevates ear |

Branches of the facial nerve: B = buccal, C = cervical, M = mandibular, PA = posterior auricular, T = temporal, Z = zygomatic, lower Z = lower zygomatic.

are named respectively from inferiorly as the inferior, middle, superior, and supreme turbinates. The supreme turbinate is present in only 60% of cases. The air space beneath and lateral to each concha is called the meatus. The paranasal sinuses drain into the nose via these meati. The anatomy of the lateral nasal wall is discussed further in Chapter 3.

## Physiology

There are three main physiologic functions of the nose: respiration, defense, and olfaction. In addition, a discussion of the physiology of the nose would not be complete without mention of the nasosystemic reflexes.

The nose plays an important role in respiration by

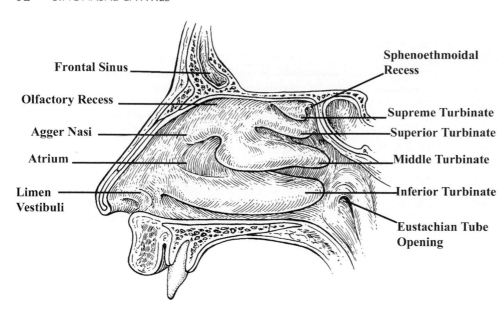

Frontal Sinus

Olfactory Recess

Agger Nasi

Atrium

Limen Vestibuli

Sphenoethmoidal Recess

Supreme Turbinate

Superior Turbinate

Middle Turbinate

Inferior Turbinate

Eustachian Tube Opening

**FIGURE 2-6** Diagram of a sagittal view of the lateral nasal fossa wall. The midline nasal septum has been removed.

effecting the nasal resistance and hence the airflow. The other effects of the nose on respiration are the humidification and warming of the inspired air.[8] In normal individuals with a tidal volume of <35 L/min, most respiratory airflow is nasal. Oral respiration is not physiologic and is a learned act that occurs during times of increased ventilatory demand.[9] This is well demonstrated in the case of newborns with bilateral choanal atresia, who, if not treated, would suffocate because they have not yet learned to breathe through their mouths.

Air enters the nares at an angle of 60° from the horizontal to reach the nasal valve, which has an area of only 0.32 cm². This is the most important factor contributing to nasal resistance and the resulting average airflow of 6.5 m/sec.[10] Once this point of resistance is passed, the nasal cross-sectional area increases with a decrease in airflow that results in turbulence. This turbulence is an important feature, as it allows increased contact of the air with the nasal mucosa. Once past the nasal valve area, the major airflow

passes through the middle meatus. A lesser amount passes along the floor of the nose, and the least airflow is superiorly in the olfactory area.

Another modifier of nasal resistance is the dilator nasis muscle. This muscle dilates the nares, with a resultant decrease in resistance.[8] This becomes an important factor when increased ventilatory demand results in flaring of the nostrils.

Maintaining nasal resistance within certain limits is required for efficient pulmonary ventilation and gas exchange.[9] It should not be surprising that among the different factors affecting nasal resistance, two of the most important are hypoxia and hypercarbia, which decrease nasal resistance.[8]

The effect of gravity on the pooling of blood in the excessively vascular tissues over the turbinates leads to increased nasal resistance. This is commonly demonstrated by the observation in many patients that when they lie on one side, the dependent nasal chamber becomes progres-

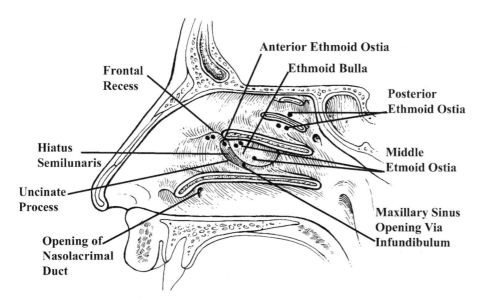

Frontal Recess

Hiatus Semilunaris

Uncinate Process

Opening of Nasolacrimal Duct

Anterior Ethmoid Ostia

Ethmoid Bulla

Posterior Ethmoid Ostia

Middle Etmoid Ostia

Maxillary Sinus Opening Via Infundibulum

**FIGURE 2-7** Diagram of a sagittal view of the lateral nasal fossa wall with the turbinates removed. The most common locations of the sinus ostia are indicated.

sively obstructed over a 15- to 20-minute period. When these patients turn to the opposite side, the clogged nasal fossa opens, and the dependent chamber becomes congested within 10 to 15 minutes.[7]

There are many other internal and external stimuli that affect nasal resistance by affecting the congestion of the nasal mucosa.[8] Some examples are vasomotor and allergic rhinitis, hormonal changes in pregnancy, thyroid dysfunction, and various medications. One phenomenon that affects nasal resistance is the nasal cycle. This occurs in 80% of individuals and results in one side of the nasal cavity being congested, with a decrease in serous and mucinous secretions, while the other side is decongested, with an increase in secretions.[8] The airflow through the nose is thus almost entirely through the patent side, and this alternates between the sides in a cyclical fashion every 1–4 hours. The function of the cycle is unclear; however, it can be documented on sectional imaging.[7] The appearance of the nasal cycle on imaging should not be confused with pathologic conditions.

Nasal resistance must be within certain limits; otherwise, the individual will have a subjective feeling of obstruction.[10] Thus the individual with a wide patent airway due to atrophic rhinitis or aggressive surgery will complain of nasal obstruction. When evaluating the cause of the patient's complaint, the clinician and radiologist should also be aware of the entity called paradoxical nasal obstruction. This situation occurs in patients who have learned to adapt to a long standing unilateral nasal obstruction.[8] The paradox exists because the patient complains of obstruction on the normal side when it becomes obstructed by congestion for various reasons, the most common being positional (with the normal side dependent), the nasal cycle, allergic rhinitis, or vasomotor rhinitis. The problem is corrected by directing treatment at the initially obstructed side.

Modification of the inspired air by humidification and warming are the other two main respiratory functions of the nose. The turbulent flow mentioned earlier allows the inspired air to interact over a large surface area.[10] Between 1 and 2 L of serous, watery secretions are produced daily by the serous glands of the nasal fossae, half of which is used to humidify inspired air.[11] The resultant nasal humidity is raised to 85%, which prevents drying of the lower airway and also enhances alveolar gas exchange.[8] Air entering the nose is efficiently warmed before reaching the lungs, and the average air temperature before entering the pharynx is 31 to 37° C . To perform this function, the average nose has about 160 $cm^2$ of mucous membrane, and the rich submucosal vasculature of the sidewalls of the nose makes an ideal surface for the conduction of heat to the air.[12]

The regulation of resistance, humidification, and temperature is performed by the specialized submucosal vascular network supplied by the autonomic nervous system.[13] There is a superficial capillary network that effects temperature change on the surface. At a deeper level there are venous lakes and sinuses that can produce changes in the thickness of the mucosa. Stimulation of the sympathetic nerves causes vasoconstriction, while stimulation of the parasympathetic system causes vasodilatation and nasal engorgement, with increased glandular secretions. The superficial mucosal vascular plexus works independently of the deep erectile vascular zone so that the surface temperature can vary

independently of the patency or resistance of the airway. There are thus four major responses that the nasal tissue can give, depending on the nature of the inspired air: (1) hyperemia of surface vessels and filling of the erectile cavernous tissue in response to cold, dry air, (2) ischemia of the surface vessels and shrinkage of the erectile cavernous tissue in response to warm, moist air, (3) ischemia of the surface vessels and filling of the erectile cavernous tissue in response to warm air of average relative humidity, and (4) hyperemia of the surface vessels and shrinkage of the erectile cavernous tissue in response to superficial irritation.[3]

The second main function of the nose is one of defense. The mucosa of the nasal fossa is a vascular, pseudostratified columnar ciliated epithelium that contains both serous and mucinous glands. The term *Schneiderian membrane* is given to this mucosa, which is derived embryologically from the invaginating ectodermal nasal placodes. The mucosa lining the paranasal sinuses is very similar to that of the nasal mucosa except that it is less vascular, thinner, and more loosely attached to the bone. The mucosal surface is covered with a mucoid blanket that is serous around the cilia and mucoid on the remaining surface. This sticky layer is ideal for trapping particulate matter.[8] This surface film of mucus traps more than 95% of particulate matter larger than 4.5 μm. Thus the cilia beat in the lower viscosity layer, while the upper layer is transported by the motion of the tips of the cilia.[10] The coordinated ciliary action of the nasal mucosa prevents infection by propelling the mucus backward and downward into the nasopharynx at the rate of about 6.7 to 10 mm/min. The cilia beat at a rate of 160 to 1500 beats/min. The cilia function normally under most circumstances unless the mucous blanket is removed and drying occurs. Other factors can interfere with ciliary function, such as viral infection and topical decongestants. In these circumstances, cilial function is impaired.[12] The absence of ciliary movement leads to a stagnation of mucus, with the resultant necessity to frequently blow the nose and achieve postnasal clearing.[14] This movement of mucus is also affected by gravity and the traction that results from swallowing. It has been estimated that three fourths of the bacteria entering the nose are trapped by the mucus and that this nasal mucous blanket is renewed about every 10 to 20 minutes.[11] The normal nasal mucosa resists infection because the mucous blanket removes bacteria and some viruses before they can penetrate the mucosa. The mucus also contains antibacterial and antiviral substances such as lysozyme, interferon, and immunoglobulins (IgA, IgE, IgG) that are important defense mechanisms.

Olfaction occurs in the upper recesses of the nasal fossa. This region is bounded laterally by the superior nasal concha and the lateral nasal wall above this level, superiorly by the cribriform plate, and medially by a portion of the nasal septum. This olfactory epithelium is thicker (60 to 70 μm) than the surrounding respiratory epithelium (20 to 30 μm), and it covers an area approximately 1 $cm^2$ on each side. The epithelium is pseudostratified columnar and rests on a vascular lamina propria with no submucosa. There are four cell types in the olfactory mucosa.[2–5, 8] The first is the olfactory bipolar neuron which detects odors. The peripheral processes of these cells extend to the surface of the epithelium forming a tuft of olfactory hairs. The central processes extend through the basal lamella to form a submucosal plexus that unites to form the 20 olfactory filia that pass through the cribriform plate. The bipolar neurons are replenished over a 7-week cycle. This is believed to be the only place in the body where special sensory cells are replaced after they die.[12] The remaining cells are microvillar cells whose function is still uncertain, supporting sustentacular cells, and basal cells that serve to replenish the bipolar cells. This mucosa has no ciliary action, and it is covered by a ''mucus'' that is derived from serous Bowman's glands deep in the lamina propria and from adjacent respiratory mucosal goblet cells. This mucous material spreads evenly over the surface of the olfactory epithelium, keeping it moist.

Although diffusion of odorants can provide access to the olfactory mucosa, the transport is facilitated by normal inhalation, and the most efficient transport of an odorant to the olfactory recess is accomplished by sniffing. Flavor, which is a combination of taste and smell, is thus affected if expired air does not reach the olfactory area.[14] The olfactory mucosa presents odorant molecules with certain constraints of absorption, solubility, and chemical reactivity.[12] Thus molecules may be perceived as being odorless for at least three reasons: (1) Their absorption by the mucus-lined respiratory nasal mucosal passages may be so high that all of the odorant is absorbed before it reaches the olfactory mucosa. (2) The molecules are not absorbed by the olfactory mucous secretions covering the olfactory mucosa and receptor cells. (3) A dried olfactory mucosa does not allow absorption, and thus there is no perception of smell.[3]

Once the odorant molecule reaches the receptor cell membrane, this molecule must alter the membrane potential of the olfactory receptor cell. The exact manner in which this is accomplished is not fully understood.[12] There are a number of theories of olfaction.[8] The molecular theory suggests that there are stereospecific receptors on the bipolar neurons. The temporal spatial theory suggests that the odor molecules are separated out in a manner that stimulates a specific area. Another theory claims that the odor molecules undergo some chemical reaction that depolarizes the bipolar cell. Regardless of which theory is correct, the ultimate event is depolarization of the bipolar cell, which results in a generator potential that leads to an action potential that travels along the first cranial nerve.

From the neuroepithelial receptor cells, fibers pass through the cribriform plate to terminate in the glomeruli of the olfactory bulb synapsing with the mitral and tufted cells that send their axons into the olfactory tract. The microcircuitry of these bulbs serves to narrow the spatial pattern of the glomerular inputs elicited by an odorant or a mixture of odorants.[12] From these bulbs, fibers then pass via the olfactory stria to medial and lateral septal nuclei situated just anterior and inferior to the rostrum of the corpus callosum. Then, from these septal nuclei, fibers pass into the limbic system, the uncus, the hippocampus, the parahippocampal region, the septum pellucidum, the fornices, the amygdala, and the gyrus rectus areas.[15] It has been noted that with orbitofrontal or medial thalamic lesions, odor discrimination and recognition are usually affected. However, in some cases, damage to these regions results in either no effect or an increased sensitivity to odor. It has also been noted that the recognition, interpretation, and memory of odors are located in the uncus and hippocampus, whereas the emotional response to odors is related to the entire limbic system.[15]

The maxillary division of the trigeminal nerve also plays a role in olfaction.[8] These nerve endings are sensitive to noxious stimuli such as ammonia. This can be used as a test for the malingering patient who feigns anosmia. The truly anosmic patient will respond to stimulation with ammonia, whereas the malingerer will deny it.

Olfaction is affected by the central processing of the messages from the olfactory area.[8] Clinically, olfactory cognition appears to develop between the ages of 3 and 5 years. Somewhere between the ages of 2 and 7 years, odor preferences are identified, and these are similar to those of adults living in the same area. That is, odors appear to be appreciated based upon individual experience and cultural restraints. It also appears that once an odor association is established, it is very difficult to erase it from memory and such an association may last for at least 1 year.[12] In humans, tests have shown that females have a better olfactory ability than males, both in threshold and in identification tasks.[12] In addition, olfaction is influenced by the menstrual cycle, being best at ovulation and poorest during menstruation. However, this effect is not simply hormonally related. Adaptation to odor also occurs so that the perception of an odor will fade if one is constantly exposed to it. This adaptation usually occurs within 5 minutes for chemical stimuli.

Abnormalities of the sense of smell include anosmia, which is the loss of the sense of smell; parosmia, which is a distortion or alteration of odors; and phantosmia, which is the usually constant perception of foul-smelling odors. Over 200 conditions have been associated with changes in olfaction, and these have been grouped into several categories.[12] The major categories associated with anosmia and the various percentages of occurrence from four major series are: (20% to 33%) obstructive nasal and sinus diseases (primarily nasal polyposis and chronic rhinitis), (15% to 32%) upper respiratory infection (URI) (persistent anosmia after the symptoms of the URI have resolved), and (9% to 32%) after head trauma (overall in adults, anosmia occurs in 5% to 10% of trauma cases, while in children transient anosmia occurs in 3.2% and permanent anosmia in 1.2%). Although frontal trauma most frequently causes anosmia, total anosmia is five times more likely after occipital trauma that results in a contra-coup shearing of the olfactory fibers) (0% to 8%) and with aging (More than half of the people 65 to 80 years old have a major decline in olfaction. This is also associated with Alzheimer's and Parkinson's diseases.), (0% to 8%) congenital (primarily familial anosmia and Kallmann's syndrome), (0% to 11%) toxic exposure (most toxins are either gases or aerosols), (8% to 16%) neoplasms (both sinonasal and intracranial tumors [25% of temporal lobe tumors are associated with olfactory disturbances]), (8% to 16%) psychiatric disorders (olfactory reference syndrome, Marcel Proust syndrome, etc.), parosmia and phantosmia (due to many causes, often associated with temporal lobe tumors or seizures), (0% to 26%) medications, (0% to 26%) surgery, and (0% to 26%) idiopathic causes (Table 2-2).[12]

The nasopulmonary and nasocardiac reflexes deserve mention.[8] The afferent pathway is via the maxillary division

**Table 2-2**
**MAJOR CATEGORIES OF ABNORMALITIES**
**ASSOCIATED WITH ANOSMIA**

Obstructive nasal and sinus diseases
Upper respiratory infection
Head trauma
Aging
Congenital
Toxic exposure
Neoplasms
Psychiatric disorders
Medications
Surgery
Idiopathic

of the trigeminal nerve. After central processing, the efferent pathway is via the vagus nerve to the various end organs including the heart, lungs, and vascular system. The effects include apnea, hyponea, bradycardia, cardiac arrhythmias, and a decrease in peripheral vascular resistance. These reflexes are responsible for those cases of hypoxia that can occur with posterior nasal packing. The high-risk patient should thus be closely monitored. Sneezing is also a reflex mediated via the trigeminal nerve. The resultant forceful expulsion of air is believed to be a basic protective mechanism.

## Vascular Supply

The vascular supply of the nasal fossa involves both external and internal carotid arterial supplies. Of the five arteries that supply the nasal cavity, the sphenopalatine artery is the most important.[16] This artery originates from the third segment of the internal maxillary artery. It then exits the superomedial aspect of the pterygopalatine fossa by way of the sphenopalatine foramen. The sphenopalatine artery then enters the nasal fossa behind and slightly above the posterior end of the middle concha.

The sphenopalatine artery has two major branches, the posterior lateral nasal branches and the posterior septal branches. The posterior lateral nasal arteries ramify over the nasal conchae, first giving off branches that supply the inferior turbinate and then giving rise to superior branches that supply the middle and superior turbinates. These lateral nasal branches also assist in supplying the maxillary, ethmoid, and sphenoid sinuses.

After giving origin to the posterolateral nasal branches, the main trunk of the sphenopalatine artery continues medially across the face of the sphenoid sinus. When it reaches the nasal septum, the sphenopalatine artery gives off its medial branches, the posterior septal arteries. These branches course anteriorly along the nasal septum. The most inferior of these branches becomes the nasopalatine artery. This vessel runs through the incisive canal to anastomose with the greater palatine artery (Fig. 2-8).

The anterior and posterior ethmoidal arteries originate from the ophthalmic artery, which is a branch of the internal carotid. They enter the nasal cavity at the level of the cribriform plate (frontoethmoidal suture line via the anterior and posterior ethmoidal canals) to anastomose with nasal branches of the sphenopalatine artery. They are the only arteries in the body that run lateral to medial. This rich anastomotic network provides an important potential collateral pathway between the internal and external carotid circulations.

There are two other arteries that also provide some blood supply to the nasal fossa. The terminal branch of the greater palatine artery enters the incisive foramen, where it anastomoses with the nasopalatine artery (a septal branch of the sphenopalatine artery). The final artery supplying the nasal fossa is the septal branch of the superior labial artery. It originates from the facial artery and supplies the medial wall of the nasal vestibule (Table 2-3).

Little's, or Kiesselbach's, area is a localized region of the anteroinferior nasal septum (Fig. 2-8). It is supplied by branches of the facial, sphenopalatine, and greater palatine arteries. This is often referred to as Kiesselbach's plexus and is the site of 90% of the cases of epistaxis (Table 2-4).[4]

The venous drainage of the nose is via the anterior facial vein, the sphenopalatine vein, and the ethmoid veins. The anterior facial vein and ethmoid veins communicate with the ophthalmic veins, which drain directly into the cavernous sinus. The sphenopalatine vein enters the pterygoid plexus, which ultimately drains into the cavernous sinus. Thus intracranial complications such as meningitis, abscess, and cavernous sinus thrombosis can result from nasal and sinus infections.[13]

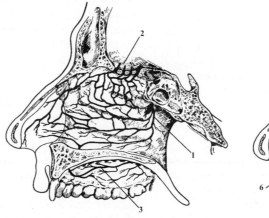 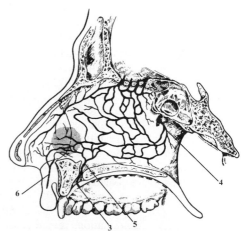

**FIGURE 2-8**   Diagrams of a sagittal view of the vascular supply of the (**A**) lateral nasal wall and (**B**) the nasal septum. 1, The posterior lateral nasal branches of the sphenopalatine artery; 2, the anterior and posterior ethmoidal arteries; 3, the greater palatine artery; 4, the posterior septal branches of the sphenopalatine artery; 5, the nasopalatine artery; and 6, the septal branch of the superior labial artery. The area of Kiesselbach's plexus is in dots on B. (From Osborn AG. The nasal arteries. AJR 1978; 130:89-97. Copyright 1978, American Roentgen Ray Society.)

**Table 2-3**
**ARTERIAL SUPPLY OF THE SINONASAL CAVITIES**

External carotid artery ↓
Internal maxillary artery ↓
Sphenopalatine artery ↓
Posterior lateral nasal branches
Posterior septal branches (anastomose with ethmoidal arteries) ↓
Nasopalatine artery (anastomoses with the greater palatine artery via incisive foramen)

Internal carotid artery ↓
Ophthalmic artery ↓
Anterior and posterior ethmoidal arteries (anastomose with nasal branches of the sphenopalatine artery)

External carotid artery ↓
Greater palatine artery enters the incisive foramen (anastomoses with the nasopalatine artery)

External carotid artery ↓
Facial artery ↓
Septal branch of the superior labial artery facial artery

↓ = artery gives off the following branch

The lymphatic drainage follows the veins rather than the arteries. The lymphatics of the anterior half of the nose drain across the face to enter the level IB nodes. The lymphatics of the posterior half of the nose and nasopharynx drain into the retropharyngeal nodes and levels II, III, IV, and V nodes.

## Nerve Supply

The motor supply to the nasal respiratory muscles (the procerus, the nasalis, and the depressor septi nasi) is mediated through the seventh cranial nerve. The integration of their contraction with the respiratory cycle is with the tenth cranial nerve. The physiologically important control of the circulation and secretomotor function to the normal airway is mediated by the autonomic system, primarily via the sphenopalatine ganglion. Sympathetic stimulation results in a pale, dry, shrunken mucosa, and parasympathetic stimulation causes a hypersecreting, hyperemic, swollen mucosa. Pain, temperature, and touch are mediated by branches of the first and second divisions of the fifth cranial nerve.[11, 12, 17]

The sensory innervation of the nasal mucosa is by branches of the maxillary and ophthalmic division of the trigeminal nerve. In the pterygopalatine fossa, the maxillary nerve gives branches to the sphenopalatine ganglion. These sensory nerves traverse the ganglion without synapsing. The nasal branch of the sphenopalatine ganglion enters the nasal cavity through the sphenopalatine foramen and then divides into the lateral posterior superior and medial posterior superior branches. The lateral posterior superior branch supplies the superior and middle turbinates. The medial

**Table 2-4**
**ARTERIAL SUPPLY TO KISSELBACH'S PLEXUS**

Kisselbach's plexus is supplied by branches of:
The Facial artery
The Sphenopalatine artery
The Greater palatine artery

posterior superior branch crosses the face of the sphenoid to reach the nasal septum as the nasopalatine nerve. Anteriorly, this nerve extends through the incisive canal to supply the gingiva and mucosa posterior to the incisor teeth.[12] The lower part of the nasal cavity is supplied by the greater palatine branch of the sphenopalatine ganglion. In the greater palatine canal this nerve gives off branches that pass through the perpendicular plate of the palatine bone to reach the nasal wall and supply the inferior turbinate and adjacent inferior and middle meatus. The anterior portion of the nasal cavity is supplied by the ophthalmic division of $V_2$. After the ophthalmic division of the trigeminal nerve ($V_1$) enters the orbit, it gives off branches, among which is the nasociliary nerve. This nerve runs in the medial orbit and gives off the anterior and posterior ethmoidal nerves, which then exit the orbit through the anterior and posterior ethmoidal canals, where they innervate the ethmoid mucosa, the dura in the anterior cranial fossa, and the roof of the nasal cavity. The posterior ethmoidal nerve supplies a small area of mucosa near the superior concha on both the medial and lateral nasal walls. The anterior ethmoidal nerve supplies both the medial and lateral nasal fossa walls via its lateral and medial internal nasal branches.

The autonomic innervation of the nasal fossa comes via the pterygopalatine (sphenopalatine) ganglion. Secretomotor (parasympathetic and motor) neural fibers originate in the brainstem at the nervous intermedius. These fibers run with the facial nerve to the geniculate ganglion, where they leave the facial nerve as the greater superficial petrosal nerve. This nerve runs along the anterior face of the petrous portion of the temporal bone to the cavernous sinus, where it receives sympathetic fibers from the deep petrosal nerve (originating from the cavernous portion of the internal carotid artery). The combined nerve then enters the vidian (pterygoid) canal as the vidian nerve, which goes to the pterygopalatine ganglion. The parasympathetic fibers synapse with postganglionic fibers in this ganglion and follow the branches of the trigeminal nerve to supply the nasal fossae and palatal region. The sympathetic fibers are already postganglionic, and thus they do not have synaptic connections in the sphenopalatine ganglion. They follow the blood vessels to supply the nasal fossae and palatal areas.[4, 6]

## THE PARANASAL SINUSES

All of the paranasal sinuses originate as evaginations from the nasal fossae.[18] As such, they are lined by a mucosa that is similar to that found in the nasal cavity, which is a pseudostratified columnar ciliated epithelium that contains both mucinous (goblet cells) and serous glands. The nasal septum, by contrast, is lined by squamous mucosa with a paucity of minor salivary glands and a thinner, tightly tethered lamina propria. Because the mucosa of the paranasal sinuses is attached directly to the bone, it is frequently referred to as mucoperiosteum.[19] Although the mucoperiosteum of the sinuses is slightly thinner than the nasal mucosa, it is continuous with the nasal mucosa at the various sinus ostia.

The functional reason for the presence of the paranasal sinuses has been debated since the sinuses were first described in 1800. The paranasal sinuses have been thought to contribute resonance to the voice, humidify and warm the inspired air, increase the olfactory membrane area, absorb shock to the face and head, provide thermal insulation for the brain, contribute to facial growth, represent vestigial structures, and lighten the skull and facial bones. Of these, the only documented reason appears to be that the paranasal sinuses form a collapsible framework that helps protect the brain from blunt trauma.[19] Also not understood are the reasons that cause some sinuses to be well developed, while others are hypoplastic. A question related to sinus growth is why some sinuses are routinely asymmetric.

## Ethmoid Sinus

The ethmoid sinuses are divided into groups of cells by bony basal lamellae that extend laterally to the laminae papyracea and superiorly to the fovea ethmoidalis.[20] These lamellae serve as attachments for the turbinates. There are thus five lamellae, one for each of the primary turbinates (middle, superior, and occasionally the supreme) and one for each of the secondary turbinates (bullae ethmoidalis and uncinate process). In the adult, the lamella is not a straight bony partition. Instead, it is almost inseparable from the other ethmoid septa due to the lamella's being pushed and distorted from its original straight configuration in the fetal ethmoid bone by the other ethmoid air cells.[21] The basal lamella of the middle turbinate is the most important, as it divides the ethmoid into anterior and posterior groups of cells that drain into the middle and superior meati, respectively. In addition, the basal lamella only extends from the posterior portion of the middle turbinate, where it is attached to the lateral nasal wall. No basal lamella is present along the anterior portion of the middle turbinate.[22] Instead, it is replaced by a medial lamella that attaches to the lateral cribriform plate. The anterior ethmoid cells are more numerous and smaller, whereas the posterior cells are larger and fewer.[21] The adult ethmoid has 3 to 18 cells. The lamellae of the remaining turbinates further subdivide the anterior and posterior groups of cells.[20] Each group of cells drains into grooves that appear at intervals running diagonally posteriorly to inferiorly and parallel to the lamella. The classification of the cells is therefore based on the drainage site of their ostium. Thus the anterior ethmoid is subdivided into frontal recess cells draining into the frontal recess, infundibular cells draining into the infundibulum and hiatus semilunaris, and bullar cells draining into a groove on the bullae ethmoidalis called the *superior hiatus*. The posterior ethmoid is subdivided into posterior and postreme cells draining into the posterior and postreme meati, respectively. This drainage pattern is of clinical significance because one would expect all cells draining into one groove to be similarly infected. The ostia of the ethmoid sinuses are the smallest of all of the paranasal sinuses, measuring only 1 to 2 mm in diameter. Of these ostia, those of the anterior ethmoid cells are smaller than those of the posterior cells, a factor probably contributing to the higher incidence of anterior ethmoid mucoceles.[21]

The ethmoid sinuses begin to form in the third to fifth fetal months, when numerous separate evaginations arise from the nasal cavity. The anterior cells are the first to so form as evaginations in the lateral nasal wall in the region of the middle meatus. Posterior cell development follows as evaginations in the superior meatal area. The ethmoid sinuses expand at their own expense and at the expense of the other sinuses until puberty or until the sinus walls reach a layer of compact bone. The lamellae prevent one group of cells from intermingling with another, but they do not prevent intramural expansion of one group into another. A concha bullosa results when posterior ethmoid cells extend intramurally to pneumatize the middle turbinate. This can result in a large obstructing turbinate or a focus of infection. There can also be extramural expansion of ethmoid cells outside the ethmoid to invade the frontal, maxillary, and sphenoid sinuses as well as the ascending process of the maxilla and lacrimal bone. Encroaching cells are the rule, and one can find any pattern of intramural and extramural expansion, which should be considered normal variations and not anomalies.[20]

There are some specific patterns of extramural spread that are of clinical significance (see also the discussion in Chapter 3). Anterior ethmoid cells can pneumatize the frontal process of the maxilla adjacent to the anterior attachment of the middle turbinate to the ethmoid crest of the ascending process of the maxilla. These are known as the aggar nasi cells, and they are located in relationship to the lacrimal bone. When present, they are the most accessible part of the ethmoid intranasally.[23] Anterior ethmoid cells can also pneumatize the roof of the orbit as supraorbital ethmoid cells. Failure to recognize disease in such cells may lead to failure of operations on the frontal sinus. On coronal images, if a bony septum is seen separating the ethmoid complex from the recess in the roof of the orbit, then the recess comes from the frontal sinus and not from the supraorbital ethmoid cells (see atlas axial and coronal Fig. 2-1B). A posterior ethmoid cell can invade the medial floor of the orbit, resulting in a Haller cell. These cells can be a source of persistent infection if overlooked.[22] A posterior ethmoid cell can also invade the sphenoid bone. Such an extension is usually superior and lateral and is known as an Onodi cell if it is related to the optic nerve.[20] A posterior ethmoid cell can invade the maxilla. When it does, the extension is posterior to the maxillary sinus, causing a double antrum.[24] This must be recognized so that the posterior wall of the maxillary sinus is opened to gain access to infection in that cell.

At birth the anterior ethmoid complex is about 5 mm high, 2 mm long, and 2 mm wide. The posterior cell group is 5 mm high, 4 mm long, and 2 mm wide. The sinuses have virtually reached their adult size by age 12 years. In the adult the ethmoid labyrinth is pyramidal in shape, with its base directed posteriorly. The average dimensions are 4 to 5 cm long, 2.5 to 3 cm high, 0.5 cm wide anteriorly, and 1.5 cm wide posteriorly.[23] Less commonly, the ethmoid can attain a flat, thin form in which the anterior and posterior dimensions are the same. This is important to recognize since the operating space will not increase as you go posteriorly.

The ethmoid bone resembles a cross in coronal section.[21] The horizontal part is represented by the cribriform plate. The vertical portion above the cribriform consists of the cristae galli. Below the cribriform plate the vertical portion consists of the perpendicular plate of the ethmoid, which contributes to the nasal septum. Attached to the lateral end of each cribriform plate is the actual ethmoid labyrinth.

From an anatomic standpoint, it is best to look at the ethmoid labyrinth as a box.[21] The superior surface, or roof, of the ethmoid is related to the anterior cranial fossa. Mosher calls this the tragedy surface because in inexperienced hands the ethmoid operation is one of the easiest operations with which to kill a patient.[23] The roof of the ethmoid is actually formed by the orbital process of the frontal bone. The underlying ethmoid cells bulge into this, producing a pitted surface called the fovea ethmoidalis. The fovea ethmoidalis descends 15° as it extends posteriorly. Thus, anteriorly the fovea ethmoidalis can be as much as 4 to 7 mm higher than the cribriform plate to which it is attached. This results in a thin ascending lamella of bone joining the lateral border of the olfactory fissure to the fovea ethmoidalis. This bone is extremely thin and is more commonly the site of surgical injury than is the cribrifrom plate.

The lateral wall of the ethmoid is related to the orbit. The posterior two thirds of this surface is formed by the lamina papyracea that covers the posterior ethmoid cells. These cells are related to the orbital contents, optic nerve, and medial rectus muscle. The lamina papyracea articulates with the frontal bone superiorly, the maxilla inferiorly, and the lesser wing of the sphenoid posteriorly. The anterior and posterior ethmoid foramina lie along the frontoethmoidal suture line that is just below the dural line. Thus, if during an external ethmoidectomy a surgeon remains below a line connecting these foramina, the anterior cranial fossa should not be entered. The ethmoidal vessels and nerves pass into the ethmoid complex via these foramina. Dehiscences can occur in the lamina papyracea, and mild degrees of hypoplasia can result in a lateral concavity to the lamina papyracea. This also occasionally results in a wide beveled opening in the lamina papyracea where the anterior and posterior ethmoidal canals are located. The anterior one third of the lateral wall of the ethmoid is formed by the lacrimal bone that covers the anterior ethmoid cells. These cells are thus related to the lacrimal apparatus and orbital contents. The lacrimal bone is thus the major landmark to the anterior ethmoid cells when approached externally.[23] The posterior surface of the ethmoid is formed by the lateral two thirds of the anterior face of the sphenoid sinus. This will be discussed further in the section on the sphenoid sinus. The medial wall of each ethmoid labyrinth is the turbinate surface from which project the middle, superior, and (when present) supreme turbinates. As discussed earlier, the support for the turbinates is the basal lamella. The attachment of the basal lamella of the middle and superior turbinates to the lamina papyracea and fovea ethmoidalis marks the entrance of the anterior and posterior ethmoid arteries into the ethmoid sinuses.[21] The middle turbinate is of paramount importance in intranasal surgery. It attaches anteriorly to the ethmoid crest of the ascending process of the maxilla and posteriorly to the ethmoid crest of the palatine bone (which is just anterior to the sphenopalatine foramen). The posterior half of the middle turbinate is loosely attached to the body of the ethmoid bone by the basal lamella, and only the posterior tip is firmly attached to the lateral nasal wall at the ethmoid crest of the palatine bone.[22]

The anterior half of the middle turbinate is more complex. Mosher divides it into an upper part called the superior overhang and a lower part called the inferior overhang.[23] The division point is a line drawn forward from the upper end of the superior meatus. The inferior overhang is also known as the tip of the middle turbinate and is at a lower level than the anterior insertion of the middle turbinate. The portion of the lateral wall of the nose between the anterior insertion and the tip of the middle turbinate is known as the atrium. The medial or nasal surface of the superior overhang consists of a medial lamella that inserts into the skull base at the lateral margin of the cribriform plate.[22] It conducts olfactory fibers and is thus part of the olfactory area. In addition, it serves as a major surgical landmark to the cribriform plate and should always be preserved as a landmark during operations on the ethmoid. The middle turbinate covers two elevations on the medial wall of the ethmoid. The more prominent elevation is the bulla ethmoidalis, which is more posterior and superior. It is an accessory turbinate pneumatized by anterior bulla air cells. The more anterior inferior elevation is the uncinate process. It is also an accessory turbinate and originates from the anterior point of attachment of the middle turbinate. It then runs parallel to the bulla ethmoidalis in an inferior posterior direction. The anterior insertion of the uncinate process overlaps the lacrimal bone and nasolacrimal duct and is a useful guide to the location of the nasolacrimal duct. This explains how the nasolacrimal duct can be injured by coming too far anteriorly when one is performing an infundibulotomy or middle meatal antrotomy.

The groove formed between the bulla ethmoidalis and the uncinate process is called the hiatus semilunaris. The hiatus semilunaris extends laterally to open into the infundibulum, which is lateral to the uncinate process. The depth of the infundibulum is thus dictated by the height of the uncinate process.[25] Anterior infundibular cells and occasionally the frontal sinus open into the anterior portion of the infundibulum, whereas the maxillary sinus opens into the posterior portion of the infundibulum. The lacrimal bone sits on the lacrimal process of the inferior turbinate and articulates superiorly with the frontal bone. Its anterior half covers the nasolacrimal duct, whereas its posterior half is related to the anterior ethmoid cells. It is frequently pneumatized in series with the aggar nasi cells and serves as a landmark to the nasofrontal duct.

The superior turbinate lies above and posterior to the middle turbinate. Since it lies behind the basal lamella of the middle turbinate, it marks the medial wall of the posterior ethmoid cells. Its posterior end abuts the face of the sphenoid. Occasionally there is a supreme turbinate that lies above the superior turbinate and, when present, marks the most posterior ethmoid cells.

The inferior surface of the ethmoid is related to the medial portion of the roof of the maxillary antrum below. The hiatus semilunaris marks the inferior extent of the ethmoid intranasally.[23] Thus the superior half of the lateral wall of the nose is formed by the ethmoid and the inferior half by the medial wall of the maxillary sinus.

The anterior end of the ethmoid is related to the posterior surface of the ascending process of the maxilla. It is the only solid boundary of the labyrinth.[23] This is an important landmark, as it defines the location of the nasofrontal duct and nasolacrimal duct. Intranasally it is defined by a line joining the insertion of the middle turbinate to the insertion of the inferior turbinate. The lacrimal bone lies between this ascending process of the maxilla and the anterior ethmoid cells.

The ethmoid sinuses receive their blood supply from nasal branches of the sphenopalatine artery and from the anterior and posterior ethmoidal arteries, which are branches of the ophthalmic artery. Thus the ethmoid sinuses receive blood from both the internal and external carotid arteries. The venous drainage is into the nose via the nasal veins or via the ethmoidal veins, which drain into the ophthalmic veins. This latter pathway is responsible for cavernous sinus thrombosis after ethmoid sinusitis. The sensory innervation of the ethmoid mucosa is via the ophthalmic and maxillary divisions of the trigeminal nerve. The nasociliary branch of the ophthalmic division supplies the anterior cells via the anterior ethmoidal nerve. The posterior ethmoid cells are supplied by the posterior ethmoidal nerve from the ophthalmic division and the posterolateral nasal branches of the sphenopalatine nerve from the maxillary division of the trigeminal nerve. The lymphatics drain into the submandibular lymph nodes (Level I nodes).[21, 26] The proximity of the posterior ethmoid cells to the orbital apex, optic canal, and optic nerve can lead to loss of vision as a complication of benign or malignant disease or surgery on these sinuses.

## Frontal Sinus

The frontal sinuses arise from one of several outgrowths originating in the region of the frontal recess of the nose. Their site of origin can be identified on the mucosa as early as 3 to 4 months in utero. Less commonly, the frontal sinus develops from anterior ethmoid cells of the infundibulum. The frontal sinuses are in effect displaced anterior ethmoid cells, and because they develop from a variable site, their drainage will be either via an ostium into the frontal recess or via a nasofrontal duct into the anterior infundibulum.[18, 20] In any instance, the opening or duct can be distorted by expansion of adjacent ethmoid cells. As noted earlier, the location of the nasofrontal duct is marked intranasally by the insertion of the middle turbinate or aggar nasi cells if present. Dissection in this area will lead to the ascending process of the maxilla, which will lead to the nasofrontal duct. From an external approach, the lacrimal bone is the preferred landmark to the nasofrontal duct.[23] Once the lacrimal bone is entered, the dissection proceeds anteriorly to the ascending process of the maxilla and hence to the nasofrontal duct.

Because on the average the frontal sinuses do not reach up into the frontal bone until about the age of 6 years, these sinuses are essentially the only paranasal sinuses that are absent at birth. Their development is quite variable but effectively appears to start only after the second year of life.[27] In otherwise normal individuals, both frontal sinuses fail to develop in 4% of the population. If there is persistence of a metopic suture, the frontal sinuses are small or absent. On the average, by the age of 4 years, the cranial extent of the frontal sinus reaches half the height of the orbit, extending just above the top of the most anterior ethmoid cells. By the age of 8 years the top of the frontal sinuses is at the level of the orbital roof, and by the age of 10 years the sinuses extend into the vertical portion of the frontal bone. The final adult proportions are reached only after puberty.[4, 27]

Based on a study of 100 normal frontal sinuses, the area of a patient's frontal sinuses correlates well with two lines that can be drawn on either a plain film or a coronal CT scan. One line extends vertically from the level of the highest point of the orbital roof to the most cranial margin of the sinus. The other line extends from the base of the crista galli obliquely to the most lateral margin of the sinus. On a Franklin-type head unit or on CT, the maximum length of each line is 63 and 74.5 mm, respectively. If either of these lengths is exceeded, the sinus is larger than the 99th percentile of the normal population and is considered abnormally enlarged.[28] The average frontal sinus has been described as being 28 mm high, 24 mm wide, and 20 mm deep. However, there is a wide range in frontal sinus size, and the frontal pneumatization may involve the vertical plate (squamosal portion) of the frontal bone, the horizontal plate (orbital roof) of the frontal bone, or both of these areas. Recognition of an orbital recess to the frontal sinus is particularly important if frontal sinus obliterative surgery is to be performed. If only the vertical portion of the sinus is obliterated because an orbital recess was not identified preoperatively, a mucocele eventually develops in the obstructed orbital recess.

Because the frontal sinus develops from a variable site, in approximately 40% of cases it drains into the ethmoidal infundibulum. In this case, the ethmoidal infundibulum can act as a channel for carrying the secretions (and infection) from the frontal sinus to anterior ethmoid cells and the maxillary sinus or vice versa. It is primarily in the patient whose nasofrontal duct opens directly in the frontal recess or above the infundibulum (85% of cases) that the frontal sinus is accessible to intranasal cannulation. The natural frontal sinus ostium is usually located in the posteromedial floor of the sinus.

As mentioned, the factors responsible for determining the extent of frontal sinus growth are poorly understood. One of the factors implicated in influencing frontal sinus size is a relationship between the cessation of frontal lobe growth and the development of the frontal sinus. Frontal lobe expansion normally ceases its anterior growth by 7 years of age, at which time the inner table of the frontal bone stops its forward migration. Any further development of the frontal bone occurs secondary to anterior growth of the outer frontal table and sinus pneumatization. The ipsilateral frontal sinus is abnormally enlarged in patients with the Dyke-Davidoff-Masson syndrome with an underdeveloped hemicerebrum and in cases of early childhood damage to the frontal lobe.[29, 30] In addition, a direct relationship between the mechanical stresses of mastication and frontal sinus enlargement has been demonstrated, as has a direct relationship with growth hormone, as seen in acromegaly.[5, 30]

In some patients a frontal bulla develops. This is an upward displacement of the frontal sinus floor caused either by encroachment from the opposite frontal sinus or, more frequently, by an underlying ethmoid cell. This bulla may influence frontal sinus drainage, and it has been implicated as a cause of chronic frontal sinusitis in some patients.[4]

Each frontal sinus is a single cavity, although rare duplication of a sinus has been reported.[4] Usually the frontal sinuses are asymmetric in size. Often the larger sinus extends across the midsagittal plane, so that a midline incision may inadvertently enter this sinus rather than the intended opposite smaller sinus. The normal sinus contour tends to be slightly scalloped, and intrasinus septa may extend into the sinus from one-half to one-third the height of the sinus cavity. Such septations can create recesses of the sinus that can be overlooked at surgery if preoperative imaging was not performed.

The larger the sinus cavity, the better the septations are developed. Conversely, in a hypoplastic frontal sinus, the sinus is usually a single, smoothly contoured cavity devoid of septations. As mentioned, the frontal sinus can pneumatize both the vertical and the horizontal (orbital) plates of the frontal bone. The deepest area of the vertical portion of the sinus is near the midline at the level of the supraorbital ridge, and the medial sinus floor and the caudal anterior sinus wall are thinnest in this area. As a result, the sinus is best approached for a trephination at this level. This thin anterior wall also permits the controlled fracture that is necessary in creating an osteoplastic flap of the frontal sinus.[21]

The intersinus septum is in reality the remaining frontal bone between the two frontal sinuses. It is usually in the midline at its base or lower portion; however, it may then deviate far to one side, depending on the differential growth rates of the frontal sinuses. Although the septum is almost always complete, focal areas of acquired or congenital dehiscence do occur, allowing intercommunication between the two frontal sinuses or herniation of the mucosa of one sinus into the contralateral sinus.[18] The normal well-developed frontal sinus abuts the superomedial orbital margin, but it does not encroach on the orbit and remodel it. Any flattening of this orbital margin should suggest the presence of an expanding frontal sinus process (mucocele, pneumocele, etc.).

Occasionally a central frontal sinus cavity is encountered, in the midline, just above the level of the nasion. This presumably is the result of a displaced ethmoid cell.

There is a rich sinus venous plexus (Breschet's canals) that communicates with both the diploic veins and the dural spaces. The main arterial supply to the frontal sinus is via the supraorbital and supratrochlear arteries derived from the ophthalmic artery. The venous drainage is primarily through the superior ophthalmic vein, and the sinus lymphatics drain across the face to the submandibular lymph nodes (level IB). The sensory innervation of the sinus mucosa is via the supraorbital and supratrochlear branches of the frontal nerve, which is a branch of the first division of the trigeminal nerve.

## Sphenoid Sinus

The sphenoid sinuses emerge in the fourth fetal month as evaginations from the posterior nasal capsule into the sphenoid bone. This occurs just above small crescent-shaped ridges of bone, the sphenoidal conchae, that projects from the undersurface of the body of the sphenoid bone. These conchae grow forward, fusing with the posterior ethmoid labyrinth. Complete absence of the sphenoid sinus is rare. The degree of pneumatization, however, varies considerably. The sinus starts its major growth in the third to fifth year of life, and by age 7 years the sinus usually has

extended posteriorly to the level of the anterior sella turcica wall. By the age of 10 to12 years the sinus usually has obtained its adult configuration.[20] The lack of any sinus pneumatization of the sphenoid bone by the age of 10 years should suggest the possibility of "occult" sphenoid bone pathology.[31] This is most commonly seen in diseases that require a large marrow demand to compensate for chronic anemia. Thus it is found in young patients with thalassemia and with chronic renal failure.

The average adult sphenoid sinus is 20 mm high, 23 mm long, and 17 mm wide. The posterior sinus development is variable. Depending on the degree of pneumatization, the sinus is classified as nonpneumatized, presellar, or sellar. In 60% of pneumatized sinuses, the sinus cavity extends posteriorly to the anterior sella turcica wall and lies under the sella floor (sellar). In 40% of sinuses, the sinus cavity extends only to the anterior wall of the sella turcica (presellar). In fewer than 1% of cases, the sphenoid sinuses do not develop posteriorly enough to reach the anterior sella wall (nonpneumatized). In this latter group of patients the thick, bony posterior sinus wall is a contraindication to transsphenoidal hypophysectomy.[32]

In 48% of people there are lateral recesses from the main sphenoid sinus cavity that extend into the greater sphenoid wing, where it forms the floor of the middle cranial fossa and the posterior orbital wall, the lesser sphenoid wing, or the pterygoid process. The pterygoid process is pneumatized in 25% of patients and is extensively pneumatized in 8% of patients.[33] It should be noted that there is considerable variation in the degree of pneumatization on the left and right sides of the sphenoid sinus. As a result of sphenoid pneumatization, the foramen rotundum may either be completely outside the sinus or bulge into the lower lateral sinus wall. Similarly, the vidian canal may either be within the sphenoid bone proper or elevated on a septum within the sinus cavity.

As mentioned earlier, the posterior ethmoid surface shares a common wall with the anterior face of the sphenoid sinus. The perpendicular attachment of the superior turbinate divides the face of the sphenoid into thirds.[23] The lateral two thirds form the common party wall with the posterior ethmoid cells. The medial one third of the sphenoid sinus's anterior wall is the free intranasal surface that is bounded by the superior turbinate laterally, the septum medially, the cribriform plate superiorly, and the upper surface of the posterior choanae inferiorly. The area bounded by the intranasal face of the sphenoid and the superior turbinate is called the sphenoethmoidal recess.[25] The ostia of the sinus is 2 to 3 mm in diameter and 2 to 5 mm from the midline and lies in the upper portion of the intranasal surface, 1.5 cm above the floor of the sinus. The normal drainage of each sphenoid sinus in the erect posture thus relies entirely on ciliary action. The ostium of the sphenoid can be located by passing a beaded probe 7 cm posterior to the anterior nasal spine upward at an angle of 30° to the floor of the nose.[34] The posterior wall of the sinus can lie up to 9 cm from the anterior nasal spine. If the probe goes beyond 9 cm, one must be concerned that the probe is intracranial. The sphenopalatine artery crosses the face of the sphenoid below the ostium. This must be cauterized or reflected inferiorly when approaching the sphenoid sinus.

The sphenoid sinus septum is usually in the midline anteriorly, aligned with the nasal septum. However, from this point it can deviate far to one side and even be twisted, creating two unequal sinus cavities. With the exception of the sinus roof, the other sinus walls are of variable thickness, depending on the degree of pneumatization. However, even in poorly developed sinuses the roof is thin, often measuring only 1 mm (planum sphenoidale). This wall is thus consistently vulnerable to perforation during surgery.

When the sphenoid sinuses are well developed, neighboring structures can be identified by their indentation into the sinus cavity. Thus, in addition to the already mentioned vidian or pterygoid canal and the foramen rotundum (maxillary nerve [$V_2$]), the optic nerve, the internal carotid artery, and the sphenopalatine ganglion all can be seen projecting toward the sinus cavity. Not only is knowledge of the anatomic relationships of the sphenoid sinus important because surgical complications may be avoided, but such knowledge can help explain unusual symptoms that arise from sphenoid sinus disease. Thus, from anteriorly to posteriorly, the sinus roof is related to the floor of the anterior cranial fossa, the optic chiasm, and the sella turcica. The lateral wall is related to the orbital apex, the optic canal, the optic nerve, the cavernous sinus, and the internal carotid artery. Situated posteriorly are the clivus, prepontine cistern, pons, and basilar artery. The sinus floor is the roof of the nasopharynx, and the anterior sinus wall is the back of the nasal fossa medially and the posterior ethmoid laterally. These anatomic relationships can present potential surgical hazards because fracture and removal of any sinus septations or indentations can lead to damage of the adjacent vessel or nerves. In addition, surgery in the sphenoid sinus can easily perforate the sinus walls and regions of the sphenoid sinus wall may be dehiscent.[35, 36] This is especially so with regard to the planum sphenoidale, the lateral sinus wall, and the medial roof of a lateral sinus recess into the greater sphenoid wing or pterygoid process. The latter area is frequently the site of spontaneous CSF leak into the sphenoid sinus, and in such cases this area should be carefully scrutinized.

There is a reciprocal relationship between the size of the sphenoid and the posterior ethmoid cells. When the posterior ethmoid invades the sphenoid it is usually in a posterior and superior direction, which will bring it into relationship with the optic nerve. It is thus important not to go further posteriorly than the face of the sphenoid when performing an ethmoidectomy. This can be accomplished by identifying the face of the sphenoid prior to performing the ethmoidectomy. The roof and lateral wall of the sphenoid sinus are continuous with the fovea ethmoidalis and laminae papyracea, respectively. Thus the sphenoid sinus is also an excellent surgical landmark from which to commence an intranasal ethmoidectomy.

The arterial supply of the sphenoid sinus is from branches of both the internal and external carotid arteries. The posterior ethmoidal branch of the ophthalmic artery may contribute vessels to the roof of the sphenoid sinus, and the floor of the sinus receives blood from the sphenopalatine branch of the maxillary artery. The venous drainage flows into the maxillary vein and the pterygoid venous plexus.

The sphenoid sinus is innervated from both the second and third divisions of the trigeminal nerve. The posterior ethmoid nerve from the nasociliary branch of the ophthalmic division supplies the roof of the sinus, and the sphenopala-

tine branches of the maxillary division supply the sinus floor.[36] The lymphatics drain into the retropharyngeal lymph nodes.[3]

## Maxillary Sinus

The maxillary sinus is the first of the paranasal sinuses to form. At approximately the seventieth day of gestation, after each nasal fossa and its turbinates are established, a small ridge develops just above the inferior turbinate, marking the future uncinate process. Shortly after this, an evagination just above this ridge, the uncibullous groove, is seen, which then proceeds to enlarge laterally from the nasal cavity. This is the site of the original maxillary sinus bud. By birth a rudimentary sinus, measuring up to $7 \times 4 \times 4$ mm or, on the average, about 6 to 8 cm$^3$ is present, with its longest dimension in the anteroposterior axis.[21] The developing maxillary sinus initially lies medial to the orbit. The annual growth rate of the maxillary sinus is estimated to be 2 mm vertically and 3 mm anteroposteriorly.[37] By the end of the first year, the lateral margin of the sinus extends under the medial portion of the orbit. The sinus reaches the infraorbital canal by the second year and passes inferolaterally to it during the third and fourth years. By the ninth year the lateral sinus margin extends to the malar bone. Lateral growth ceases by the fifteenth year.

In infancy the maxillary sinus floor lies at the level of the middle meatus. By the eighth to ninth year the sinus floor is near the level of the nasal fossa floor.[38] From this point there is considerable variation in the further growth of the lower recess of the sinus. If the sinus continues to grow downward, it reaches the actual plane of the hard palate by age 12 years. The final descent of the sinus, signaling the cessation of sinus growth, is not complete until the third molar has erupted. In 20% of adults the most dependent portion of the maxillary sinus is above the nasal cavity floor. It lies at the same level as the nasal floor in 15% of adults and below this level in 65% of adults.[38] The mean dimensions of the adult maxillary sinus are 34 mm deep, 33 mm high, and 25 mm wide. The average volume of the adult maxillary sinus is 14.75 ml.

For the most part the maxillary sinuses develop symmetrically, with only minor common variations. Unilateral hypoplasia and bilateral hypoplasia occur in 1.7% and 7.2% of people, respectively.[39, 40] Hypoplasia of the maxilla results from trauma, infection, surgical intervention, or irradiation to the maxillary that occurs during the development of this bone. These conditions can damage the maxillary growth center, producing a small maxilla and thus a "hypoplastic" sinus. Underdevelopment also occurs in first and second branchial arch anomalies such as Treacher Collins syndrome, mandibulofacial dysostosis, and thalassemia major when the demand for marrow prohibits sinus pneumatization.

The maxillary sinus lies within the body of the maxillary bone. Behind the inferior orbital rim, each sinus roof, or orbital floor, slants obliquely upward so that the highest point of the sinus is in the posteromedial portion, lying directly beneath the orbital apex. The groove and canal for the maxillary nerve lie in the middle third of the sinus roof. About 1 cm behind the inferior orbital rim, the canal dives downward to exit on the anterior face of the maxilla via the infraorbital foramen, which is about 1 cm below the inferior orbital rim. The medial antral wall is the inferolateral wall of the nasal cavity. The curved posterolateral wall separates the sinus from the infratemporal fossa. Each sinus has four recesses: the zygomatic recess, extending into the malar eminence or body of the zygoma; the palatine recess, which is usually small and variable, extending into the hard palate; the tuberosity recess, extending downward above and behind the third upper molar; and the alveolar recess, extending into the alveolar process of the maxilla. As discussed earlier, a posterior ethmoid cell can extend into the posterior maxilla and compartmentalize portions of the maxillary sinus. These uncommon septa usually divide the antrum into anterior and posterior sections, each of which may drain via accessory ostia into the nasal fossa. Rarely, a horizontal septum can divide the antrum into superior and inferior, or medial and lateral, portions.

The floor of the sinus is lowest near the second premolar and first molar teeth and usually lies 3 to 5 mm below the nasal floor. The roots of the three molar teeth often form conical elevations that project into the sinus floor. Less often the roots of the premolar and, even more rarely, the canine teeth project into the antrum. Occasionally there is dehiscent bone over the tooth roots, so that only sinus mucosa covers these roots and separates them from the main sinus cavity.[21] The lower expansion of the antrum is intimately related to dentition; when a tooth erupts, the vacated space becomes pneumatized, thus expanding the sinus lumen.

In the adult disarticulated skull the medial wall of the maxillary bone has a large hole, the maxillary hiatus, that exposes the interior of the maxillary sinus. However, in life, or in an articulated skull, this hole is partially covered by portions of four bones.[24] In addition to the portions of the ethmoid bone (to be discussed further), the perpendicular plate of the palatine bone covers part of the posterior maxillary hiatus, while the lacrimal bone covers the anterior and superior regions.

The inferior turbinate covers the inferior portion of the maxillary hiatus. It attaches anteriorly to the conchal crest of the ascending process of the maxilla and posteriorly to the conchal crest of the palatine bone. It has a thin maxillary process that articulates with the inferior rim of the maxillary hiatus. When performing an inferior meatal antrostomy, it is thus easier to enter the maxillary sinus through this thin bone in the upper part of the inferior meatus rather than through the thick bone of the maxilla in the lower part of the meatus. When performing an inferior meatal antrostomy, it is important to remember that the nasolacrimal duct terminates in the anterior superior portion of the inferior meatus.

The ethmoid bone is the last bone to help close the maxillary hiatus, as it rests above the line of attachment of the inferior turbinate as the uncinate process and ethmoid labyrinth. Below the uncinate process, the medial maxillary hiatus is covered by the opposing nasal and sinus mucosa. This membranous area is called the fontanelle. It is divided into a posterior and an anterior fontanelle by the ethmoidal process of the inferior turbinate, which extends superiorly to contact the uncinate process. This membranous area can break down secondary to infection, with the resultant formation of accessory ostia. In addition, this area of the middle meatus can be safely penetrated when the natural maxillary ostium cannot be clinically cannulated because of a large uncinate process or when it is believed that the orbit is at risk.[21] Above the uncinate process is the hiatus semilunaris and the remainder of the ethmoid labyrinth. The ostium of the maxillary sinus is on the highest part of the medial sinus wall and can be up to 4 mm in diameter. It does not open directly into the nasal fossa but rather into the posterior portion of the ethmoidal infundibulum, which, via the hiatus semilunaris, opens into the nasal cavity. The channel of the infundibulum is approximately 5 mm long and is directed upward and medially into the nasal fossa. The sinus ostial location dictates that sinus drainage in the erect position is accomplished by intact ciliary action. Thus a narrow infundibulum can interfere further with sinus drainage.

The location of the sinus ostium can be variable. When high, it lies just below the orbital floor. The ostium can also open further anteriorly in the infundibulum, bringing it even closer to the orbit. Thus, depending on the situation, the surgeon may elect to enter the maxillary sinus at a lower level such as the membranous fontanelle, as discussed earlier.

The maxillary sinus is vascularized via branches of the maxillary artery, and the supply is essentially topographic. Thus the infraorbital, greater palatine, posterosuperior alveolar, and anterosuperior alveolar arteries all contribute a blood supply. In addition, there are lateral nasal branches of the sphenopalatine artery and a small contribution from the facial artery. The venous drainage is anteriorly via the anterior facial vein and posteriorly via the maxillary vein. The maxillary vein joins the superficial temporal vein to form the retromandibular (posterior facial) vein, which drains into the jugular vein. However, the maxillary vein also communicates with the pterygoid venous plexus, which anastomoses with the dural sinuses through the skull base. It is through this latter pathway that maxillary sinusitis can lead to meningitis.[36]

The nerve supply to the antrum is via branches of the second division of the trigeminal nerve, namely, the branches of the superior alveolar nerves (posterior, middle, anterior), the anterior palatine nerve, and the infraorbital nerve. Of these, the posterior superior alveolar nerve pierces the posterior antral wall and runs forward and downward in a small canal to supply the molar teeth. The lymphatics of the main sinus drain into the lateral retropharyngeal and internal jugular nodes (levels II, III, and IV), and those of the lateral portion of the antrum drain into the submandibular nodes (level IB).

## PLAIN FILMS

In the present-day environment of emergency room medicine, there has been a resurgence of the use of plain film radiographs of the paranasal sinuses. In part this reflects their comparatively low cost, low radiation dose, and ready availability. These plain film studies are either the initial and only imaging study or, if clinically indicated, they may be followed by computed tomographic (CT) and/or magnetic resonance (MR) imaging studies. There are a number of plain film radiographic views available for evaluating the paranasal sinuses; however, only four of these projections are routinely employed. These consist of two frontal projections—the Caldwell and the Waters views—a base (submentovertex) view, and a lateral view. The most popular of the additional views include the oblique projection (Rhese view), other craniocaudal angulations of the frontal projection (transorbital, posteroanterior projections), the Towne view, the Granger view, and the modified Waters view.[27, 41]

If possible, the plain film examination should be performed with the patient sitting or standing erect so that any air-fluid levels can be clearly identified. If the patient cannot tolerate erect positioning, a cross-table lateral film with a horizontal beam should be obtained to visualize any potential air-fluid levels. If neither of these approaches can be used, on either supine or prone films any free sinus fluid will layer on the dependent sinus wall, and the sinus will appear as opacified rather than with an air-fluid level.

## PLAIN FILM VIEWS

### Horizontal Beam 5° Off-Lateral View

To achieve the horizontal beam 5° off-lateral view, the patient's head is positioned laterally relative to the cassette, and the nose is then rotated 5° toward the cassette from the true lateral position. If the patient is seated, the cassette is usually placed in the vertical position. If the patient is lying down in either the semiprone or the prone position, the cassette is positioned horizontally. The central ray enters perpendicular to the cassette and is centered at the outer

canthus of the eye in the middle of the film. The orbitomeatal line is parallel to the base of the film (Fig. 2-9). The purpose of using the 5° off-lateral view rather than the true lateral view is to rotate the posterior walls of the maxillary antra slightly so that they do not superimpose on one another. This permits individual evaluation of the integrity of the posterior antral bony margins.

### Modified Caldwell View

For the modified Caldwell view, the patient is positioned directly facing the cassette in either the sitting or the prone position. The midsagittal plane is perpendicular to the film. The orbitomeatal line is perpendicular to the cassette, and the central ray is angled 15° caudally as it enters the posterior skull. The central ray also serves as the centering point of the skull on the cassette. If the patient is properly positioned, this view projects the petrous pyramids in the lower third of the orbits (Fig. 2-10). The Caldwell view is the best projection for examining the frontal and ethmoid sinuses in the frontal projection.

### Modified Waters View

For the modified Waters view, the patient is positioned facing the cassette in either the erect or the prone position. The orbitomeatal line is angled 37° to the plane of the cassette. The central ray is centered on the film perpendicu-

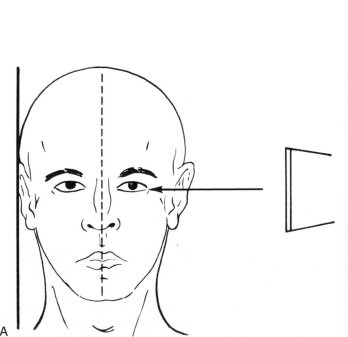

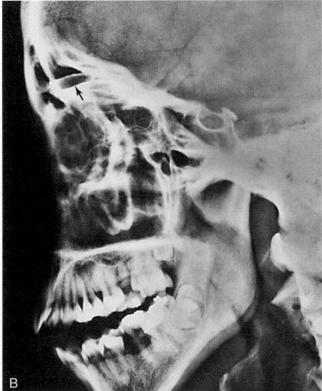

**FIGURE 2-9**   Lateral view. **A**, Positioning diagram. **B**, Sample radiograph. Note the extension of the frontal sinus into the orbital roof (*arrow*).

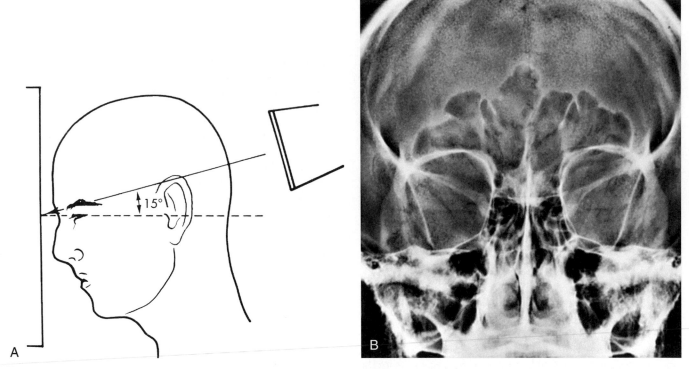

**FIGURE 2-10**    Modified Caldwell view. **A**, Positioning diagram. **B**, Sample radiograph.

lar to the cassette, emerging at the anterior nasal spine of the patient (Fig. 2-11A,B).

Variations in the positioning angle may be required to give the "perfect" Waters view. On the one hand, if the head is not sufficiently extended, the petrous pyramids are projected over the maxillary sinuses, thereby obscuring sinus detail. On the other hand, if the head is hyperextended, the maxillary sinuses become distorted and foreshortened, thus obscuring sinus disease. The "perfect" Waters view has the petrous pyramids projected just below the floor of the sinus cavities. This is the best single view for the evaluation of the maxillary antra in the frontal projection. Another variation is to use the Mahoney modification with the mouth open.[41] The open-mouth Waters view normally allows good visualization of the lower posterior sphenoid sinus margins (Fig. 2-11C).

## Modified Base (Submentovertical or Submentovertex) View

The modified base view was described by Schuller and Pfeiffer.[41] The reference line used is the infraorbital line, which runs from the infraorbital margin to the center of the external auditory meatus. The goal of the positioning is to have the infraorbitomeatal line parallel to the film plane. This projection is considerably easier to obtain with the patient in either the sitting (erect) or the prone position. Patients with cervical or thoracic degenerative disease, those with a short neck, or those who are obese have difficulty extending the head sufficiently if the examination is attempted with the patient supine. The central ray is directed

perpendicular to the infraorbitomeatal line and centered 1 inch anteriorly to the plane of the external auditory meatus (Fig. 2-12). A modification, with the centering 1½ inches in front of the external auditory meatus, has also been suggested.

A variation of the traditional submentovertex view is the Welin, or overangulated base, view. This view results in an average angle of 120° open posteriorly between the infraorbitomeatal line and the cassette. This overangulation is accomplished by tilting the top of the cassette toward the patient while the patient's head is fully extended, as in the modified base projection. The central ray is directed to the level of the frontal sinus. This position provides a useful adjunct view for evaluation of the anterior and posterior walls of the frontal sinuses (Fig. 2-13). It is also a good view for evaluating the lateral and, to a lesser extent, the medial walls of the maxillary antra. The sphenoid and ethmoid sinuses, with the nasal cavity superimposed, are thrown into relief with this projection.

## Rhese or Oblique View

The Rhese view is excellent for studying the posterior ethmoid air cells, which are otherwise obscured by superimposition of the anterior cells in the frontal views. Superimposition of the anterior right and left ethmoid cells in the Rhese view, however, tends to limit its usefulness in paranasal sinus examination. Correct positioning places the optic canal just off the midorbit in the lower outer quadrant. Each side is imaged separately, and then the images are compared. The patient is placed in either the seated erect position or the prone position. Then the median sagittal plane of the body is centered with the midline of the cassette. With the orbit centered in the portion of the cassette to be used, the flexion of the head is adjusted so that the canthomeatal line is perpendicular to the film. The patient's head is rotated so that the median sagittal plane forms an angle of 53° with the plane of the film. The central ray enters the skull posteriorly at an angle of 15° with the canthomeatal line and emerges at the midorbit (Fig. 2-14).[41] Short of sectional imaging, the oblique views coupled with a Caldwell view provide the least obscured images of the ethmoid cells.

## Nasal Bone Lateral View

To achieve the nasal bone lateral view, the patient is usually placed in a semiprone position, with the body rotated so that the median sagittal plane of the head is horizontal and parallel to the plane of the tabletop. The interpupillary line is also perpendicular to this plane. The flexion of the head ought to be such that the orbitomeatal line is parallel with the transverse axis at the tabletop. The jaw should be supported with a sandbag to prevent rotation. The film is placed under the frontonasal region and centered at the nasion. The focal-film distance should be 36 inches (Fig. 2-15).

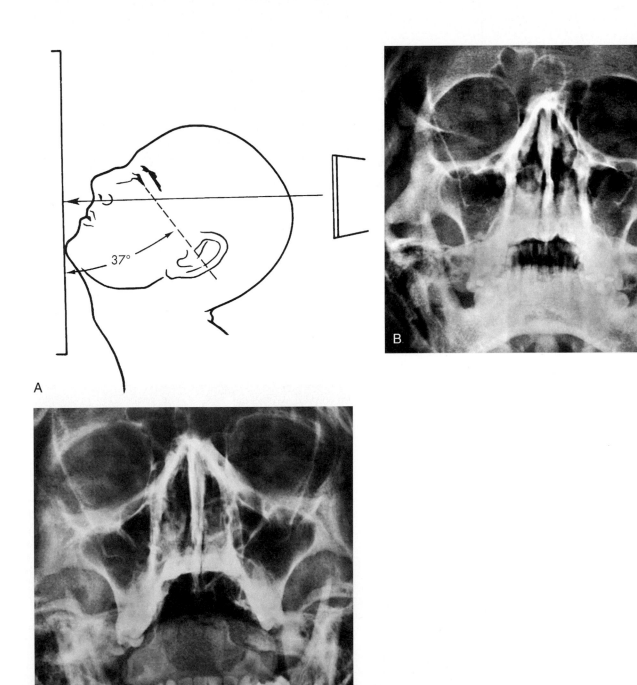

**FIGURE 2-11**   Modified Waters view. **A,** Positioning diagram. **B,** Sample closed-mouth radiograph. **C,** Sample open-mouth radiograph.

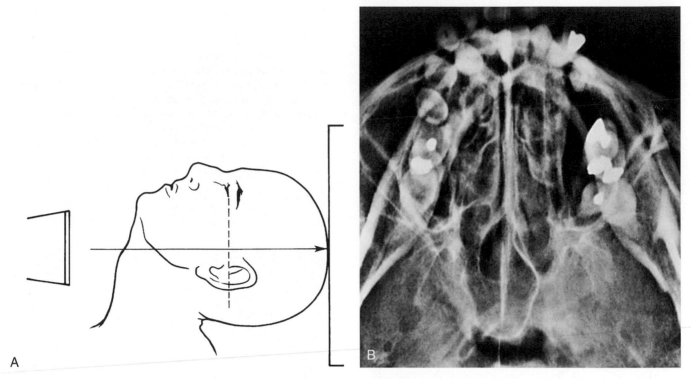

**FIGURE 2-12** Modified base view. **A**, Positioning diagram. **B**, Sample radiograph.

## Nasal Bone Axial View

The success of the nasal bone axial projection depends on either having the patient hold the occlusal film correctly between the front teeth or placing the larger film cassette under the patient's chin so that the plane of the film is at right angles to the glabelloalveolar line. The central ray should be directed along this line at right angles to the plane of the film (Fig. 2-16).

## IMAGING ANATOMY

Despite the most meticulous attention to technical detail, plain film examinations have substantial limitations. That is, even if interpreted by a knowledgeable radiologist, the full degree of both soft-tissue and bone disease may be consistently underestimated. In response to this limitation, in the recent decade and a half it has become popular to perform limited, low-cost, low-dose, coronal CT studies as

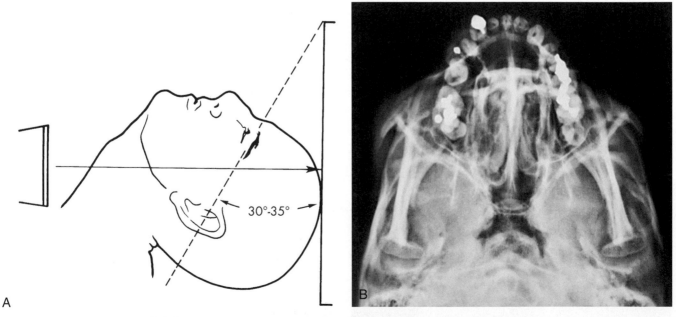

**FIGURE 2-13** Overangulated base view. **A**, Positioning diagram. **B**, Sample radiograph.

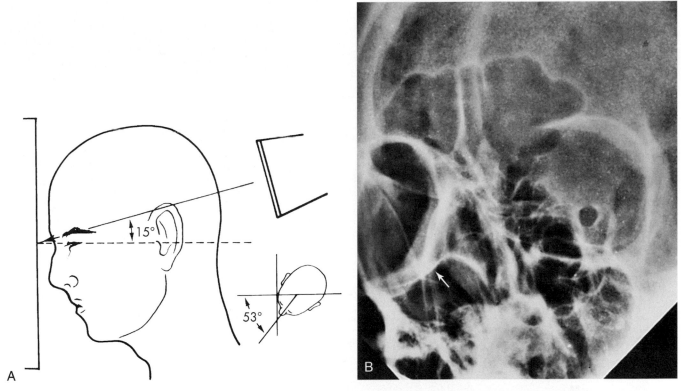

**FIGURE 2-14**    Rhese (oblique) view. **A**, Positioning diagram. **B**, Sample radiograph. Note the visualization of the right orbital floor (*arrow*).

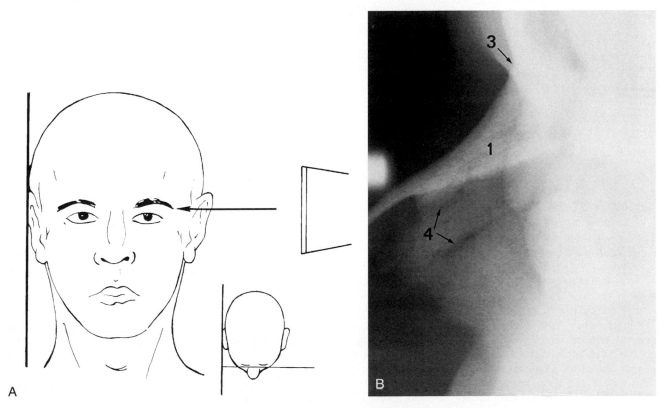

**FIGURE 2-15**    Lateral nasal bone view. **A**, Positioning diagram. **B**, Sample radiograph.

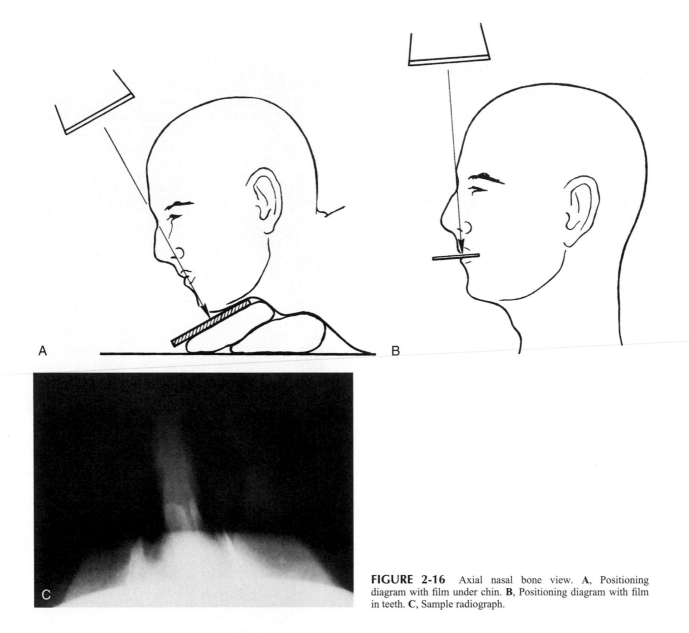

**FIGURE 2-16**    Axial nasal bone view. **A**, Positioning diagram with film under chin. **B**, Positioning diagram with film in teeth. **C**, Sample radiograph.

an alternative to the plain film examination. Although the radiation dose of these limited CT studies is lower than that of the routine CT examination, it usually is higher than that of a plain film series. This radiation dose and the frequency of these examinations represent a net radiation risk to the population. Thus the clinical setting for these studies should be carefully monitored so that patient dose and examination cost are balanced by the radiologist's choice of the best study to provide the information needed by the clinician determining the patient's management.

Patients who have signs and symptoms of acute sinonasal disease usually do not require any radiologic study, as most often they respond to conservative medical management. If the clinician is concerned that obstruction to sinus emptying has occurred, an erect plain film study will provide good visualization of any air-fluid level. The plain film examination also provides a gross assessment of sinus disease, usually all the information that is needed by the clinician at this initial stage of assessment. However, if the patient has associated signs or symptoms that suggest

extension of disease outside the boundaries of the sinonasal cavities, a more detailed examination such as either a contrast-enhanced CT scan or an MR imaging study should be performed to provide better disease mapping. Signs or symptoms that should signal CT or MR imaging include headache, retro-orbital pain, orbital pain, suboccipital pain, facial swelling, orbital inflammatory disease, and proptosis.

It is estimated that between one third and one half of patients with acute sinonasal inflammatory disease will progress to chronic disease. In these cases, it is probable that some type of surgical intervention will be a part of further treatment, and a preoperative CT scan should be obtained. Not only is disease mapping more complete on CT scans than on plain films, but normal anatomic variants can be identified that may influence surgery or aid the surgeon in avoiding an operative complication. That is, if sinus surgery is planned, a plain film examination can not only be avoided, but it should be considered inadequate as a preoperative study.

In the patient with signs and symptoms of sinonasal inflammatory disease, CT, not MR imaging, is the suggested initial examination because the details of the bone/soft tissue/air interface are better seen on CT and the CT examination costs less than an MR imaging study. In addition, on MR imaging, because air, desiccated secretions, calcifications, and ossifications all give signal voids, they may be indistinguishable from one another. However, with CT, such differentiation is routine. Lastly, if there are no symptoms to suggest the intracranial spread of inflammatory disease, contrast is not necessary for the CT study. Thus, for most patients with sinonasal inflammatory disease, a noncontrast CT study provides the most detailed information at the lowest cost.

However, if the clinician suspects that a sinonasal tumor is present, the examination of choice is MR imaging due to its better differentiation of soft tissues. Thus, compared to CT, MR imaging can distinguish better between tumor and adjacent obstructed secretions or inflammatory disease.

To identify the early manifestations of sinonasal disease, it behooves the radiologist to become fluent in sinonasal anatomy as it appears on plain films, CT, and MR imaging. That is, before mastery in the analysis of pathologic cases is possible, the radiologist must be able to move confidently through the visual thicket of normal radiographic anatomy and its variants. The important role of the radiologist in evaluating disease in the sinonasal cavities is better appreciated when it is considered that the clinician can directly observe only a small portion of the volume of interest. Clearly, imaging provides the most thorough noninvasive evaluation of the nasal cavities and paranasal sinuses.

The following section addresses the normal sinonasal anatomy as seen on plain films, CT scans, and MR images. The common denominator leading to the successful interpretation of these examinations is the anatomy itself, and once this is learned, its depiction as rendered by any specific modality will be clearly and easily approached. Thus, technology per se is irrelevant as long as it meets the final test of delineation of structure. There are 22 bones in the facial area and calvarium that are routinely seen on images or films through the facial region: 1 frontal, 2 parietal, 1 occipital, 2 temporal, 1 sphenoid, 2 zygoma, 2 maxilla, 2 palatine, 1 ethmoid, 2 lacrimal, 2 nasal, 2 inferior turbinates, 1 vomer, and 1 mandible.

The normal sinonasal anatomy is presented in two sections. The first section discusses the normal anatomy as seen on plain films and contains a presentation of anatomic variants and potential problems that are created by overlying soft-tissue structures and bones.[32, 42–46] The second section presents sectional anatomy and is illustrated with CT images in the axial, coronal, and sagittal projections.[47–51] Further discussion of the paranasal sinus anatomy is presented in Chapter 3.

## PLAIN FILM ANATOMY

### The Frontal Sinuses

The main or vertical portion of the frontal sinuses is best visualized in the Caldwell and Waters projections (Figs. 2-10B and 2-11B). On occasion the Rhese view can better

display some of the sinus contours, particularly in the smaller sinuses (Fig. 2-14B). The anterior and posterior sinus walls are best evaluated in the lateral and base (submentovertex) views (Figs. 2-9B and 2-17). However, in these projections, only those portions of the sinus walls that are parallel to the incident beam (perpendicular to the film plane) are visualized. The adjacent curvilinear surfaces are obliquely oriented to the incident x-ray beam and only contribute to the perceived density of the adjacent calvarium. Thus, on the lateral view, only the midsagittal anterior and posterior frontal sinus tables are visualized, and on the base view (depending on the angulation and the particular curvature of the skull), it is usually the caudal portions of the sinus walls that are identified. It is important to remember that only these limited areas of the frontal sinus anterior and posterior walls are seen routinely on these projections. One may not assume that the entire sinus table is normal simply because it appears intact on the lateral or base views. This is especially true in suspected fractures of the posterior table or if an erosion of this bone is in question. Sectional imaging clarifies this issue.

The horizontal portion of the frontal sinus is best seen in Caldwell (Fig. 2-18) and lateral (Fig. 2-9B) views. The depth of this recess can be best assessed by evaluating the posterior extent of pneumatization in the bony roof of the orbit, as shown on these projections.

Because the frontal sinuses develop independently from anterior ethmoid cells, asymmetry is the rule. Differential sinus growth is responsible for displacement of the intersinus septum to one side. However, this septum is usually near the midline at its caudal extreme, near the level of the glabella (Fig. 2-19). If the intersinus septum is displaced far to one side at this lower margin, an expansile process such as a mucocele within a frontal sinus should be suspected.

Unilateral or bilateral sinus aplasia or hypoplasia can occur. The smaller sinuses usually consist of a single, centrally concave recess (Fig. 2-20). Because of their small

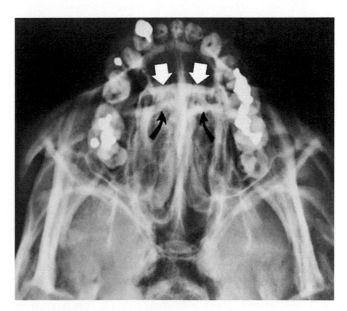

**FIGURE 2-17**   Overangulated base view with the anterior table of the frontal sinus (*large arrows*) and the posterior table (*curved arrows*) projected over the midpalate and nasal structures.

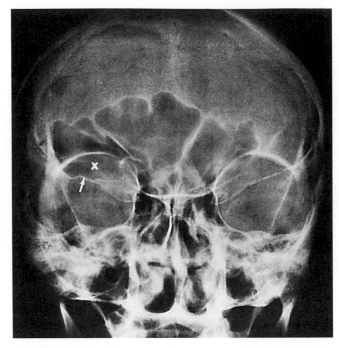

**FIGURE 2-18** Caldwell view shows well-developed frontal sinuses. On the right side, the sinus pneumatizes the roof of the orbit. This is seen as air (*x*) contained within a thin white sinus margin (*arrow*) that is projected through the orbit.

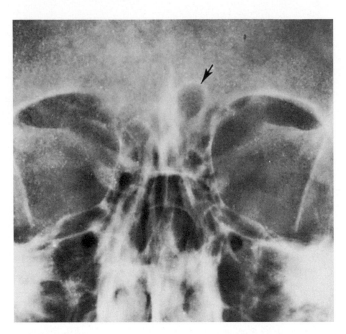

**FIGURE 2-20** Caldwell view shows an aplastic right frontal sinus and a hypoplastic left frontal sinus. Note the smooth contour of the hypoplastic sinus.

size, there is little sinus air compared with the amount of overlying bone, and these sinuses almost always appear somewhat ''clouded'' on plain films, even if they are disease free. As such, they are difficult to evaluate. Rhese and Waters views may help to evaluate these small sinuses (Fig. 2-21).

The normally developed frontal sinus is always less dense than the adjacent frontal bone. The frontal bone, as part of the calvarium, is composed of cortical bone (forming both its inner and outer tables) and medullary bone (middle table, or diploic space) interposed between the two cortices.

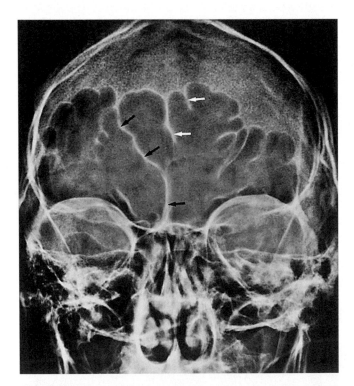

**FIGURE 2-19** Caldwell view shows a well-developed frontal sinus. Note the scalloped contour and the thin white mucoperiosteal line. Normal septations project into the sinus cavity (*white arrows*). The intersinus septum is to the right of the midline cranially but is near the midline caudally (*black arrows*). Despite the large size of the frontal sinuses, the orbital contours remain normal and are not encroached upon.

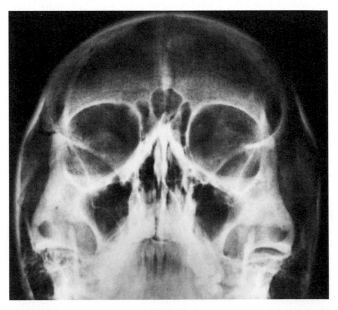

**FIGURE 2-21** Waters view shows hypoplastic frontal sinuses and a small central sinus cell, a not uncommon finding. This view complements the Caldwell projection for evaluating the frontal sinuses.

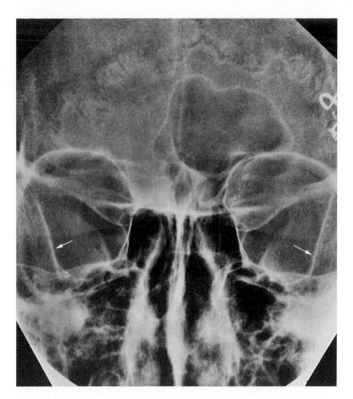

**FIGURE 2-22**   Caldwell view shows a moderately well-developed left frontal sinus. The right frontal sinus is aplastic. The perisutural sclerosis of the lambdoid suture is projected over the right frontal area and may mimic a clouded sinus contour. The "linea nominata" (*arrows*) is seen bilaterally. This line is formed by the greater wing of the sphenoid as it forms the calvarium in the anterior-most temporal fossa.

The margins of each frontal sinus are outlined by a thin (1 mm), dense rim, the mucoperiosteal (white) line, that separates the sinus from the adjacent frontal bone. If this line is not visualized, it could be the result of active infection, which is common, or bone destruction from tumor, which is rare. In the case of active inflammatory disease, there is increased mucosal vascularity that results in increased mobilization of the calcium in the surrounding bone, and this results in a loss of the mucoperiosteal white line. In chronic infection the thin, sharp white line is replaced by an unsharp, thick zone of sclerosis or reactive bone. This thickened white zone indicates only that the frontal sinus was exposed to previous chronic infection and does not necessarily imply that there is currently active sinus infection.

In the Caldwell view, the lambdoidal perisutural sclerosis of the occiput, a normal finding, can be projected over the region of the frontal sinus and can mimic a chronically thickened reactive margin of an opacified sinus (Fig. 2-22). Comparison of the Caldwell view to Waters or Rhese view permits correct interpretation.

On occasion, it is difficult to distinguish between a completely clouded (opacified) frontal sinus and an absent (aplastic) sinus. With good-quality films, some frontal sinus margin can almost always be identified, albeit poorly, on at least one of the plain films in the sinus series. If no such margin is seen, an aplastic sinus is the probable diagnosis. Sectional imaging will resolve any remaining issue.

On the lateral view a bone density area is usually seen at the base of the frontal sinuses anteriorly, near the nasion (Fig. 2-23). This represents the overlapping lower bony sinus walls and the superomedial orbital margins. The

The diploic space is made up of a bony latticework that is less dense than cortical bone but osseous nonetheless. Frontal sinus development proceeds by invagination of an air-containing mucosal sac into the diploic space, thus replacing the osseous latticework of the medullary bone. Because the air-containing sinus cavity is less dense than medullary bone, the sinuses invariably appear less dense than the adjacent frontal bone. In general, the density of the normal frontal sinus is comparable to that of the superior orbital fissure as seen on the Caldwell view.

The larger sinuses normally have scalloped margins with septations that can project well into the sinus cavity (Figs. 2-18 and 2-19). If these scallops and septations are not seen and instead a smooth sinus contour is present, the diagnosis of a mucocele should be considered. The mucocele creates the smooth contour by progressively eroding the septations and remodeling the sinus shape.

Normally the frontal sinuses never violate the orbital contour, no matter how large they become (Fig. 2-19). If there is a downward and lateral flattening of the superomedial orbital rim, a mucocele should be suspected.

The normal superomedial orbital margin often appears unsharp on Caldwell and Waters views. This is because this area curves not only from medially to laterally in the orbital rim, but also from vertically to horizontally as the bone of the forehead region merges into the bone of the orbital roof. Usually a repeat Caldwell view at a slightly different angulation or a Rhese view allows this orbital margin to be visualized intact so that erosion is not erroneously diagnosed.

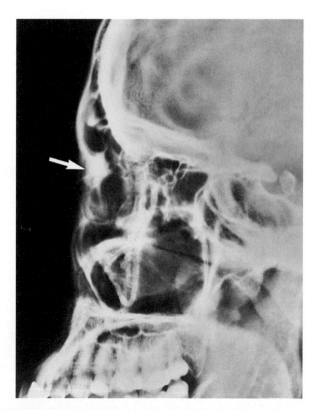

**FIGURE 2-23**   Lateral view shows normal bone density near the anterior base of the frontal sinuses (*arrow*). This "pseudo-osteoma" is not seen on either the Caldwell or Waters view.

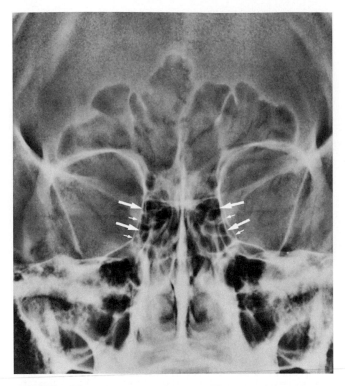

**FIGURE 2-24**    Caldwell view shows that the posterior ethmoid lamina papyracea (*small arrows*) is lateral to the more anterior lamina papyracea (*large arrows*). The medial orbital wall extends obliquely between them, reflecting the conical shape of the orbit. Also note the horizontally oriented normal ethmoid septa.

nasofrontal suture is usually situated just anteriorly. The dense bony area should not be confused with an osteoma. When seen from the front (Caldwell and Waters views), no osteoma is visualized and the bone in this region appears normal. Occasionally on the lateral view, small, bony ridges also are seen projecting from the anterior or posterior sinus walls. These are the sinus septa seen from the side.

## The Ethmoid Sinuses

The ethmoid sinuses are best evaluated on the Caldwell view. However, in every plain film projection, some ethmoid cells are superimposed on others. This reflects the fact that the ethmoid sinuses are not a single sinus cavity, as are the other paranasal sinuses, but rather are formed by 3 to 18 cells that are packed into the ethmoid bone. This superimposition can lead to confusion on the plain film examination when the patient has symptoms referable to these cells, and yet the ethmoid sinuses appear normal. This situation arises because an isolated group of cells can be totally opacified, while all of the adjacent cells remain normally aerated. The air in these normal cells nullifies the plain film "clouding" of the infected cells, and the net result is often a very unimpressive plain film appearance. In this clinical circumstance, sectional imaging identifies any localized ethmoid disease.

On the Caldwell view, the normal density of the ethmoid sinuses can be judged by comparing it with the air density around the inferior turbinate of the nasal fossae. This reflects

the fact that the ethmoid sinuses and the nasal fossae are of approximately the same anteroposterior depth, and thus the density of the air volume is about the same.

The thin lamina papyracea forms the lateral boundary of the ethmoid bone, separating it from the orbit. This medial orbital wall is oriented obliquely to an anteroposterior incident beam. Thus the majority of this oblique, thin, bony plate is not visualized on routine plain film studies. The straight or slightly concave lateral line that appears to form the medial orbital wall on a Caldwell view is in reality only the posterior ethmoid margin near the sphenoid bone. The anterior margin abutting the lacrimal bone is more medially placed and often is poorly seen (Fig. 2-24). It can be best localized by following the outline of the orbital rim from the superior aspect around to the superomedial margin and then caudally to the medial contour.

On the Waters view, only the most anterior ethmoid cells can be visualized, with the lacrimal bone separating them from the orbit (Fig. 2-25). The middle and posterior ethmoid cells are hidden from view by the nasal fossae structures. Similarly, the lateral and base views have so many overlapping structures that only gross localization of an ethmoid process can be achieved. On the base view the palate, nasal septum, turbinates, and anterior calvarium overlay the ethmoids, and on the lateral view the lateral orbital margins and even the frontal processes of the maxilla may project as vague dense zones overlying the ethmoid cells (Figs. 2-17 and 2-23). These should not be misinterpreted as sites of pathology. Although some isolation of the posterior ethmoid cells can be obtained on a Rhese view, some overlapping of ethmoid cells still occurs. Sectional imaging is indicated for proper mapping.

On the Caldwell view a small indentation, or groove, is often seen along the upper medial orbital wall. This is the anterior ethmoidal canal, and it transmits the vessels of the

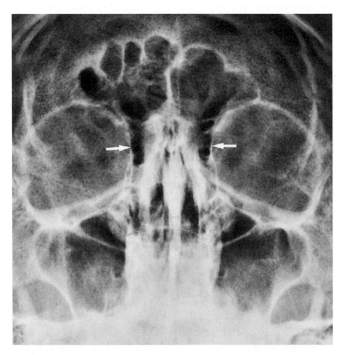

**FIGURE 2-25**    Waters view isolates the anterior ethmoid cells and the overlying lacrimal bones (*arrows*).

same name along with the nasociliary nerve (Fig. 2-26). Because the canal is formed from the ethmoid bone below and the frontal bone above, it represents the level of the floor of the anterior cranial fossa. Less often seen on plain films are the posterior ethmoidal canals, which transmit the posterior ethmoidal nerve and vessels.

The ethmoidomaxillary plate is the posteroinferior boundary between the ethmoid and maxillary bones. It is best seen in the Caldwell view and is a useful plain film landmark for localizing the spread of tumors (Fig. 2-27).

Supraorbital ethmoid cells are ethmoid sinus extensions into the orbital plate of the frontal bone. Unlike the frontal sinuses, the supraorbital ethmoid cells tend to be symmetric. If such a cell is present on one side, it should be present on the opposite side. If one of these supraorbital cells is not seen, opacification or destruction should be suspected. Sectional imaging performed in the coronal plane resolves any questionable case. On the Caldwell view the supraorbital ethmoid cells appear as slightly curvilinear lucent zones in the superomedial orbital roof (Fig. 2-28). Their posterior extent is best evaluated on either a Waters or a lateral view. It is clinically important to ascertain whether a pathologic process is in a supraorbital ethmoid sinus or in the frontal sinus because the surgical approaches to these sinuses differ.

## The Maxillary Sinuses

The maxillary sinuses are best evaluated by the Waters view. Unlike the frontal and sphenoid sinuses, the maxillary sinuses tend to be symmetric in size and configuration, with only minor variations being common. When some degree of hypoplasia is present, the roof of the smaller antrum has a greater downward slant on its lateral margin than does the larger sinus (Fig. 2-29). On plain films this may simulate a blowout-type orbital floor fracture. However, in the hypoplastic sinus, there usually is an identifiably thicker lateral bony sinus wall that results from the poorer than normal pneumatization of the maxilla. Although this may be misdiagnosed as thickened sinus mucosa, this confusion is

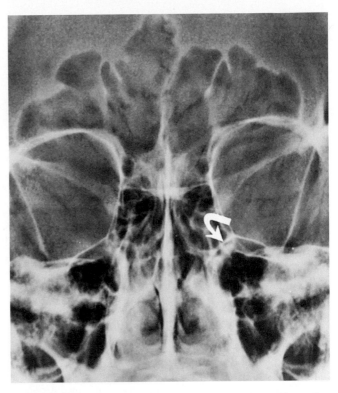

**FIGURE 2-27**   Caldwell view shows the ethmoidomaxillary plate (*curved arrow*). This is the boundary between the posteroinferior ethmoid bone and the maxillary bone.

not likely to be made by the radiologist who is aware of the appearance of a hypoplastic antrum.

A small sinus can also result from diseases of the sinus wall that cause bone expansion, with resultant encroachment into the antral cavity. Such diseases include fibrous dysplasia, "brown" tumors of hyperparathyroidism, Paget's disease, and rare giant cell tumors. In these cases, at least one dimension of the original sinus may be identified as being fully developed, and the "bony changes" can be

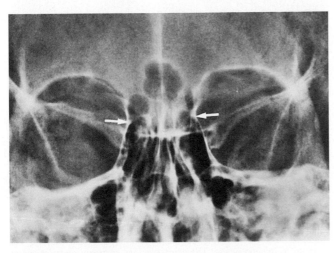

**FIGURE 2-26**   Caldwell view demonstrates medial indentations in the lamina papyracea (*arrows*) that represent the anterior ethmoidal canals. These canals mark the level of the floor of the anterior cranial fossa.

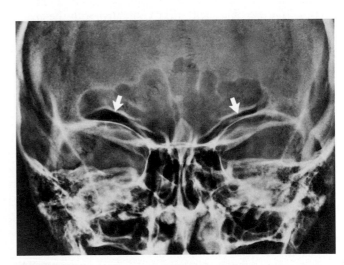

**FIGURE 2-28**   Caldwell view shows a curvilinear collection of air (*arrows*) just above each orbital margin. These areas appear darker than the frontal sinuses because the air in these supraorbital ethmoid cells is projected over the air in the frontal sinuses.

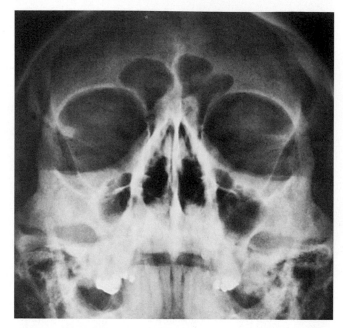

**FIGURE 2-29**   Waters view shows that the right maxillary sinus is smaller than the left. This hypoplasia is noted by the thicker lateral bony sinus wall and the more exaggerated downward slant of the sinus roof when compared with the left side. Also note that there is a suggestion of mucosal thickening in this normal hypoplastic right antrum due to its smaller sinus cavity and its thicker sinus walls when compared with the left side.

visualized bulging into the sinus, as well as being formed by abnormally textured bone. These changes differentiate these conditions from a simple hypoplastic antrum. Often sectional imaging may be necessary to resolve difficult cases.

Similarly, conditions that arrest the growth of the maxilla result in a small "hypoplastic" antrum. These childhood conditions include severe infection, trauma, tumor, irradiation, and congenital first arch syndromes.

The most lateral extension of the maxillary sinus is the zygomatic recess. This portion of the sinus hollows out the body of the zygoma, and when compared with the main antral cavity, it has less air and more surrounding bone. Because of this, the recess usually appears "clouded" on a Waters view and is often misinterpreted as representing mucosal thickening (Fig. 2-11B,C). True mucosal changes are best seen extending along the adjacent lower lateral antral wall.

On the lateral view, the anterior and posterior walls of the zygomatic recesses are seen as two overlapping V's projected over the main maxillary sinuses. These should be evaluated routinely to assess the possibility of early bone destruction in these recesses (Fig. 2-30). Also seen on the lateral view is the cranial continuation of the posterior wall of the zygomatic recess, the most anterior margin of the temporal fossa, which also represents the portion of the greater sphenoid wing that forms the oblique orbital line on the Waters and Caldwell views (Figs. 2-22 and 2-31).

The infratemporal maxillary sinus wall is a sigmoid-shaped, curved posterolateral surface. It is poorly seen on the Caldwell and Waters views. The most lateral extent (the back of the zygomatic recess) and the most medial margin (the anterior wall of the pterygopalatine fossa) can be

identified on the lateral view (Fig. 2-31). The base view provides the best visualization of the curved nature of this wall, as well as an en face projection of portions of the pterygopalatine fossa and pterygoid plates (Figs. 2-32 and 2-33).

The medial wall of the maxillary sinus is best seen on the Caldwell view. Unfortunately, the overlying nasal structures anteriorly and the sphenoid sinuses and skull base structures posteriorly obscure most detail. Only the inferior turbinates and the lower medial antral wall are identified consistently. The clinically important osteomeatal complex is well visualized only on coronal sectional imaging.

Slight asymmetry, minimal rotation, and the physiologic nasal cycle all contribute to making one nasal turbinate larger than the other. As long as some air can still be visualized around the contour of the turbinate, separating it from the lateral nasal fossa wall and the nasal septum, the turbinate is probably not pathologically enlarged. Asymmetry per se should not be overdiagnosed as pathology. On the lateral view, the posterior tips of the inferior conchae are often seen projecting over the posterior antra, and they should not be confused with a pathologic mass (Fig. 2-34). Also on the lateral view, air trapped under or above the inferior turbinate can produce a linear lucency that may mimic a fracture.

Little consistent detail about the middle turbinates is obtained from plain film studies, and sectional imaging is necessary to provide accurate information.

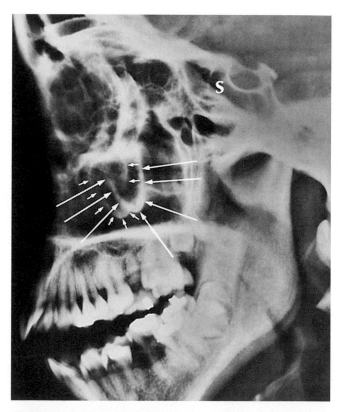

**FIGURE 2-30**   Lateral view with large arrows pointing to the zygomatic recess of one maxillary sinus and small arrows outlining the opposite zygomatic recess. These recesses are routinely seen on lateral views as overlapping Vs. The air around them is air in the main maxillary sinus cavities, which are located nearer the midline. The S is in the sphenoid sinus, with its posterior and superior limits clearly visible on this lateral film.

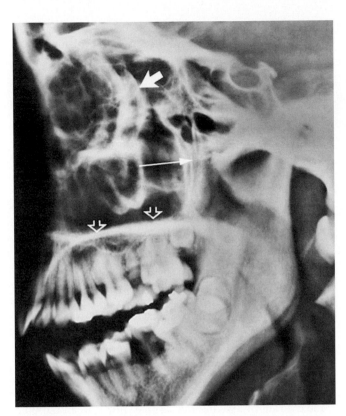

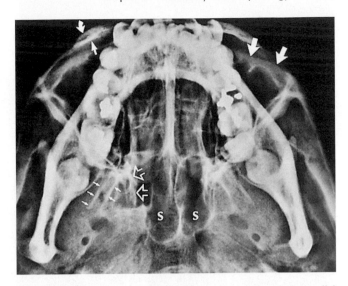

**FIGURE 2-33**  Base view with open arrows pointing to the medial pterygoid plate. Because the lateral pterygoid plate curves laterally as it descends from the skull base, the two small arrows point to the line of the lateral pterygoid plate near the skull base, and the three small arrows indicate the lateral pterygoid plate near the level of the hard palate. The large arrows point to the anterior wall of the left zygoma and maxilla. The frontal bone's anterior table (*curved arrow*) and posterior table (*small, straight arrow*) are also indicated on the right side. Each sphenoid sinus cavity (*S*) is seen well.

**FIGURE 2-31**  Lateral view with long arrows pointing to one posterior antral wall, which also forms the anterior margin of the pterygomaxillary fissure near the midline. The short arrow indicates the upward continuation of the posterior portion of one V that forms the zygomatic recess of one antrum (Fig. 2-30). The short arrow points to the bone just behind the orbit, which forms the anterior border of the temporal fossa. Open arrows indicate the upper, flat nasal fossa surface of the hard palate. The lower oral surface is slightly concave downward in configuration.

The anterior antral wall is not well seen on any view. Both the lateral and overangulated base views reveal only limited portions of this wall (Fig. 2-33).

The lateral view best delineates the inferior extension of the maxillary sinus and its relationship to the hard palate and teeth roots (Fig. 2-35). The sinus cortex of this alveolar recess can be elevated normally by unerupted molar teeth. Although this is well seen on the lateral view, its often broad upper surface can simulate an air-fluid level or a localized mass on a Waters view. This is especially notable in older children and teenagers.

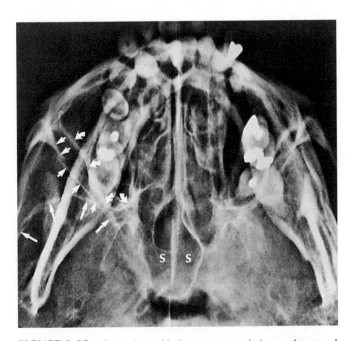

**FIGURE 2-32**  Base view with large arrows pointing to the curved anterior margin of the right middle cranial fossa (greater sphenoid wing). The small, straight arrows indicate the straighter posterior wall of the right orbit. The lateral margin is formed by the zygoma; the medial portion is formed by the greater sphenoid wing. The curved arrows outline the "sigmoid-shaped" posterior wall of the maxillary sinus. Each sphenoid sinus cavity (*S*) is seen well.

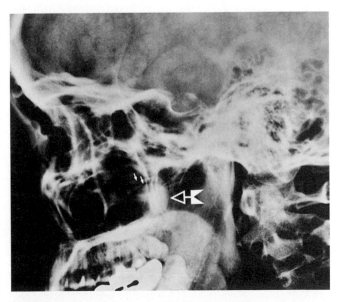

**FIGURE 2-34**  Lateral view with the large arrow pointing to the posterior tip of the normal inferior turbinate. Normal air just above the turbinates (*small arrows*) may mimic a fracture line.

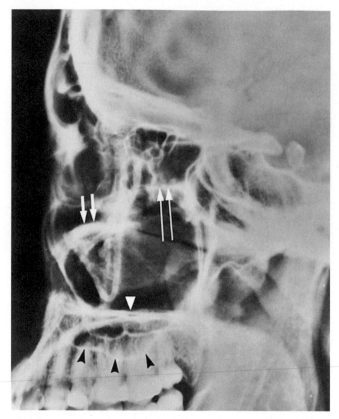

**FIGURE 2-35** Lateral view demonstrates maxillary sinus extension (*black arrowheads*) below the level of the hard palate (*white arrowhead*). The shorter arrows point to the anterolateral and most inferior orbital floor on one side, and the longer arrows point to the posteromedial and most superior orbital floor near the orbital apex.

The antral roof, or orbital floor, is flattest and lowest anterolaterally. It is also highest and most angulated posteromedially. The majority of the midportion of the antral roof is seen almost tangentially on a Caldwell view, and thus this large surface is usually seen as a single line in this projection. On the Caldwell view a second, smaller, more slanted line is seen superomedially in the orbital floor. This line represents the orbital apex floor; a notch at the lateral aspect of this line identifies the site of the infraorbital groove (Fig. 2-36).

On the lateral view the orbital floor is usually seen as two separate lines; one anteriorly, near the level of the inferior orbital rim, represents the lowest, most lateral, and flattest area of the floor; the second, located higher and more posteriorly, represents the medial orbital apex region. The slanting floor joining these two areas is not normally seen on the lateral view (Fig. 2-35). However, on a nonconed Rhese view (or optic canal view), the contralateral orbital floor is often seen extending from the anterior orbital rim almost to the orbital apex.

The Waters projection gives a better view of the inferior orbital rim. However, much of the orbital floor is seen obliquely en face, and small fractures, depressions, or erosions may not be detected. Three roughly parallel lines are seen near the inferior orbital margin in the Waters view. The most superior of these is the soft-tissue skin margin overlying the inferior orbital rim. The middle line is the actual bony inferior orbital rim, and the lowest line is the roof of the antrum located about 1 cm behind the rim, the lowest point of the orbital floor. About 1 cm below the middle third of the inferior orbital rim, the infraorbital foramen is seen. It transmits the second division of the trigeminal nerve to the cheek and nasal region (Fig. 2-37).

On the Waters view a small lucency is occasionally seen in the lateral antral wall. This is the canal for the posterior superior alveolar nerve and should not be confused with a fracture (Fig. 2-38).

On the Caldwell view the foramen rotundum is projected through the superomedial portion of the antrum (Fig. 2-36).

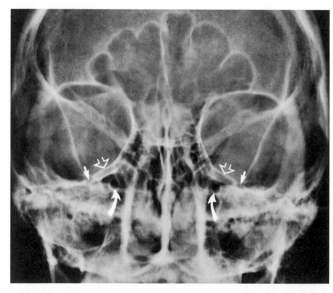

**FIGURE 2-36** Caldwell view with open arrowheads indicating posteromedial orbital floors. The straight arrows point to the posterior margin of infraorbital canals. The curved arrows point to each foramen rotundum.

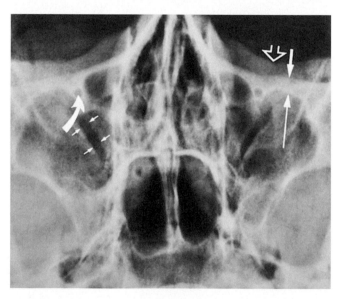

**FIGURE 2-37** Waters view with curved arrow pointing to the infraorbital foramen. The open arrow indicates a soft-tissue line over the inferior orbital rim. The short arrow points to the bony inferior orbital rim, while the long arrow indicates the lowest point of the orbital floor, which is about 1 cm posterior to the orbital rim. The small arrows outline the margins of the superior orbital fissure projected through the right antrum.

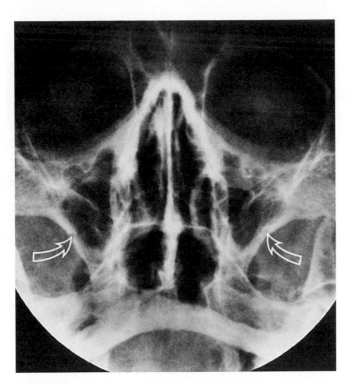

**FIGURE 2-38**   Waters view with arrows indicating the canals for the posterior and superior alveolar nerves.

The superior orbital fissure is easily identified and normally has a slightly concave lateral appearance ( Fig. 2-39). If the superior orbital fissure is followed inferiorly and slightly laterally, it points to the foramen rotundum. The maxillary

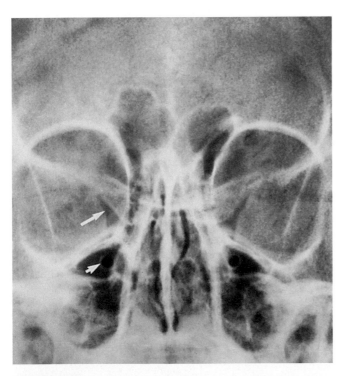

**FIGURE 2-39**   Caldwell view shows the superior orbital fissure (*large arrow*) and the foramen rotundum (*short arrow*), which is at the lower lateral margin of the superior orbital fissure.

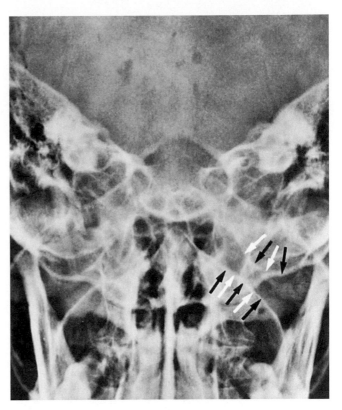

**FIGURE 2-40**   Towne view with arrows outlining the margins of the inferior orbital fissure. The superior line is formed by the sphenoid bone, and the inferior line is formed by the maxilla.

nerve ($V_2$) runs through this foramen, crosses the pterygopalatine fossa and retromaxillary fissure, enters the infraorbital fissure, exits via the infraorbital canal, and supplies the cheek and nasal regions.

The two foramina rotunda are usually symmetric in size and configuration. The superior orbital fissures, on the other hand, need not be as symmetric. The most important observation is that the bony cortical rims on either side of each fissure are thin and sharply defined. These fissures are narrower superolaterally and wider inferomedially. It is through this wider area that the veins and nerves traverse the fissure (Fig. 2-39). On the Waters view the lower portions of the superior orbital fissures are projected through the upper medial antra. These can simulate either a fracture of the inferior orbital rim or a septum of the antral roof (Fig. 2-37).

The infraorbital fissure can sometimes be seen on the Waters view as a pair of parallel thin cortical lines that are oriented anteroposteriorly. Their course is parallel, rather than divergent, and their configuration distinguishes them from the posteriorly located superior orbital fissure.

The inferior orbital fissure is poorly seen on the routine sinus views and can be best evaluated on the Towne view (Fig. 2-40).

The oblique orbital lines (linea innominata) are seen in both the Waters and Caldwell views. They represent the most anterior portions of the medial temporal fossa and usually are formed by the greater sphenoid wings. At the lower margin of each innominate line a sharp medial turn is seen, indicating the lower margin of the temporal fossa and the beginning of the infratemporal fossa. Occasionally

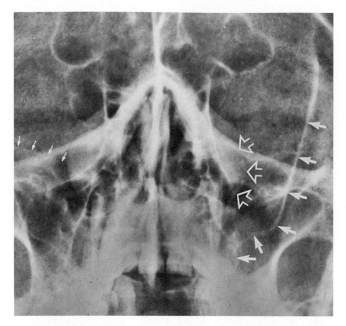

**FIGURE 2-41** Waters view with arrows pointing to the left oblique orbital line. At its lower margin the line bends medially at the level of the infratemporal fossa. The line then bends downward at the level of the lateral pterygoid plate. The small white arrows point to the upper rim of the right middle cranial fossa. The open arrows indicate the left nasal margin, which can mimic a cyst or polyp in the medial antrum.

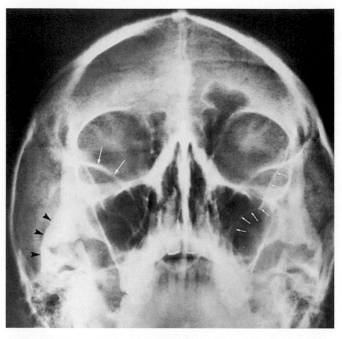

**FIGURE 2-42** Waters view with smaller arrows outlining the left oblique orbital line, its inferior extension to the infratemporal fossa, and finally the lateral pterygoid plate. The larger arrows point to the upper anterior margin of the right middle cranial fossa. The arrowheads outline the right zygomatic arch.

this line is seen to continue medially and then bend downward, outlining the lateral pterygoid plate (Figs. 2-41 and 2-42).

The superior bony margin of the middle cranial fossa is a concave posterior ridge that is formed medially by the lesser sphenoid wing and laterally by the posterior edge of the orbital plate of the frontal bone. The curved margin can be seen projected through the orbit and upper antrum on the Waters view (Figs. 2-41 and 2-42).

The body of the zygoma and the zygomatic arches are well seen in the Waters and base views (Figs. 2-17 and 2-42). Alternate views for this arch are the underpenetrated base view and the ''jug handle,'' or oblique zygomatic projection. The posterior portions of the arch are best seen on a Towne view. The zygomaticotemporal suture in the zygomatic arch is an obliquely oriented line that is seen routinely and should not be confused with a fracture. Occasionally the zygomaticofacial canal can be seen in the lateral body of the zygoma. It transmits the zygomaticofacial nerve.

On the Waters view the soft-tissue shadow of the upper lip is often seen traversing the lower antrum (Fig. 2-43). This shadow usually extends laterally to the lower maxillary sinus margin. Similarly, a mustache also can produce such a shadow. These soft-tissue densities should not be confused with true retention cysts of the lower antrum, which unlike the shadows just described can be identified as cysts on a lateral view. Similarly, the nasal alae can mimic cysts of the medial antral wall in the Waters view (Fig. 2-41).

Soft-tissue swelling of the cheek can mimic ''clouding'' of the antrum on a Waters view. This usually can be identified by elevation of the superior skin line over the inferior orbital rim. However, sectional imaging may be

necessary in some cases to isolate the maxillary sinus from the overlying swollen skin and subcutaneous tissues.

In the lateral view the coronoid processes of the mandible project over the inferoposterior maxillary sinuses. This is

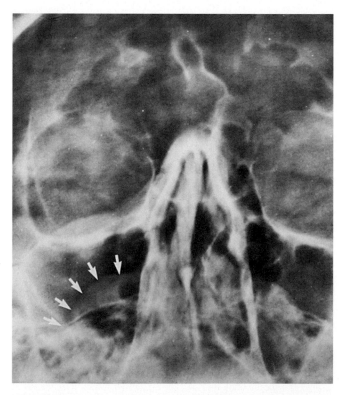

**FIGURE 2-43** Waters view with arrows outlining the shadow of the upper lip, which is projected over the lower maxillary sinus.

especially noted if the mouth is closed. If these coronoid processes are blunt or rounded, they may simulate retention cysts (Fig. 2-44). If the coronoid processes are sharply pointed, they may simulate a fractured bone segment or an unerupted tooth.

## The Sphenoid Sinuses

The sphenoid sinuses are probably the most difficult sinuses to evaluate by routine films because they are buried deep in the skull base and are surrounded by the facial bones, nasal cavity structures, and occiput on the frontal views; the mastoids and lateral skull base structures on the lateral view; and the calvarium and pharynx on the base views. The sphenoid sinuses are extremely variable in their configuration. About one half of the population has only a central sinus cavity, and the other half has, in addition, lateral recesses. These recesses can extend into the greater wings of the sphenoid, lesser wings, and pterygoid processes.

The central, or main, sphenoid sinus cavity is best evaluated on the lateral, base, and open-mouth Waters views (Figs. 2-30 and 2-33). The sinus roof (planum sphenoidale), the sella floor (lamina dura), and the posterior development of the sinus cavity are all well seen on the lateral view; the floor and anterior sinus walls, however, are partially obscured by the overlapping lateral skull base. The base view provides a means of evaluating the sinus depth and lateral extension. The open-mouth Waters view allows evaluation of the lower posterior sinus wall as it is projected through the mouth.

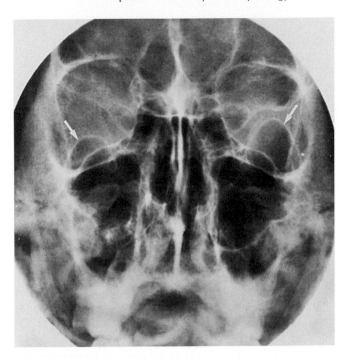

**FIGURE 2-45**    Caldwell view shows lateral sphenoid sinus pneumatization of the greater sphenoid wings as they form the posterior orbital walls (*arrows*). They are limited on all but their inferomedial margins (where they join the main sinus cavity) by the thin white mucoperiosteal line of the sinus margin.

The lateral sinus extensions into the greater wing of the sphenoid can go into the floor of the middle cranial fossa and up into the posterior orbital wall. These extensions are seen best on the Caldwell and Waters views. On the Caldwell view the "orbital recess" is seen as a "lytic" area in the lower lateral orbit. There is a thin cortical white line outlining its contour except in its lower, medial portion. It is at this margin that this sphenoid recess communicates with the main sinus cavity (Fig. 2-45). On the Waters view the lateral sphenoid sinus recesses in the floor of the middle cranial fossae are projected through the maxillary sinuses. They have a variable shape, depending on the configuration of the recess. They can appear as "dog ears" or can simulate compartments of the maxillary sinus (Fig. 2-46). Regardless of their shape, they always join the central sphenoid sinus medially and, when normal, are always rimmed by a thin white cortical line.

Pterygoid pneumatization results in a triangular lucency in the pterygoid plates in the lateral view and a round or oval lucency in the pterygoid process in the base view (Fig. 2-47). These recesses, when normal, are again outlined by a thin white cortical line.

The plain film appearances of all of these recesses are classic. Once they are mastered, the interpreter should not confuse them with pathologic processes.

In patients with a pituitary mass who may require a transsphenoidal surgical approach, special attention should be given to evaluating the posterior extent of the main sphenoid sinus cavity. If more than 1 or 2 mm of bone remains between the posterior margin of the pneumatized sinus and the anterior sella wall (less than 1% of the cases), most surgeons avoid a transsphenoidal hypophysectomy. This relationship is most easily seen in the lateral view.

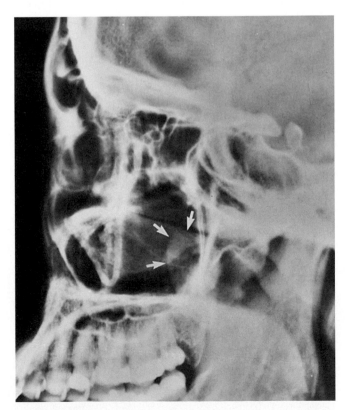

**FIGURE 2-44**    Lateral view with arrows pointing to the coronoid process of the mandible, which is projected over the lower posterior antrum in this closed-mouth view.

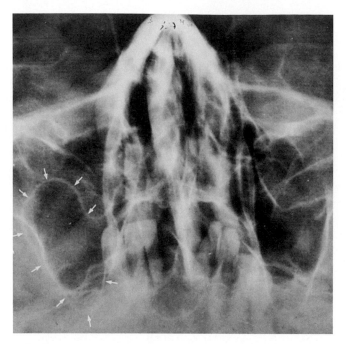

**FIGURE 2-46** Waters view shows lateral recesses of sphenoid sinuses extending into the greater sphenoid wings in the floor of the middle cranial fossa. The arrows outline the right "dog-ear-shaped" recess projected through the maxillary sinus. There is also a recess on the left side.

## Associated Structures Surrounding the Paranasal Sinuses

There are a number of important structures that surround the paranasal sinuses and project over them on the plain film examinations.

On the lateral view, the anterior walls of the middle cranial fossa are seen as paired curvilinear lines that project over the sphenoid sinus cavities and merge posteroinferiorly with the bone density of the skull base. The planum sphenoidale is clearly identified as a straight, bony line. The cribriform plate is not as well seen as it continues anteriorly from the planum sphenoidale. However, a line drawn connecting the nasion and the anterior planum very closely approximates the level of the cribriform plate. The fovea ethmoidalis (ethmoid sinus roofs) lie just lateral to and above the cribriform plates. They usually are identified as slightly concave, downward thin, bony lines positioned just above the plane of the cribriform plates. The orbital roofs are situated higher and more laterally than the fovea ethmoidalis. Thus one can roughly localize a lytic process on a lateral film by evaluating which of these lines is eroded. The more superior the line, the more lateral the process (Fig. 2-48). The midline crista galli is best seen on the Caldwell view. This intracranial structure rests on the midline upper surface of cribriform plates.

The bony nasal septum is not seen optimally on any plain film projection, but it is best evaluated on the Caldwell view. Only gross deviation of the bony septum can be appreciated. The cartilaginous septum is poorly seen on plain films and is well visualized only on sectional imaging.

In the lateral view the anterior nasal spine usually has a sharply triangular appearance. The film must often be "bright lighted" to properly evaluate the spine. Destruction of the anterior nasal spine should raise the question of prior surgery or trauma. Midfacial anomalies, Hansen's disease (leprosy), other infectious processes, and carcinomas can also result in nonvisualization of this spine.

The hard palate is best evaluated in the lateral view. Its upper nasal surface is flat and usually has a clear cortical margin. The lower oral surface is slightly concave downward, and it also has a good cortical margin (Fig. 2-31).

In the base view, three paired lines are consistently seen. The most posterior of these is concave posteriorly and represents the greater wings of the sphenoid bone as they form the anterior margin of the middle cranial fossae. The second and most often the anterior pair of lines are relatively straight, being obliquely oriented to the midsagittal plane and open-faced anteriorly. Each line is composed medially by the sphenoid bone as it forms the posterior orbital wall and laterally by the orbital surface of the zygoma. The suture between these bones often can be identified clearly. Medially these two sets of paired lines (each primarily formed by the sphenoid bone) join at the pterygoid processes. The third pair of lines are sigmoid (S-shaped) and represent the infratemporal or posterolateral antral walls. Depending on the angulation used to make the base view, the sigmoid line can be anterior to, overlapping and crossing, or posterior to the orbital lines (Figs. 2-32 and 2-33).

In the base view the pterygoid fossa is seen as a V-shaped space with its apex placed anteriorly. The pterygoid plates are usually seen as three thin, bony lines. The medial pterygoid plate is seen as a single line. However, the lateral pterygoid plate is seen as two separate lines, a lateral line that represents the most caudal end of the lateral pterygoid plate at the level of the hard palate and a central or medial

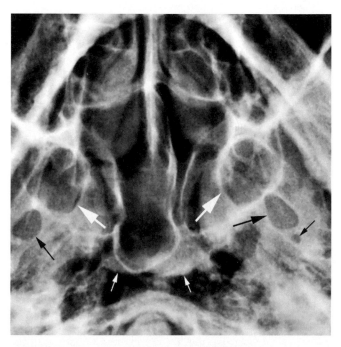

**FIGURE 2-47** Base view with large white arrows outlining the pneumatized pterygoid process. The small black arrows point to the foramen spinosum, and the large black arrow indicates the right foramen ovale. The small white arrows outline the posterior margin of the tongue.

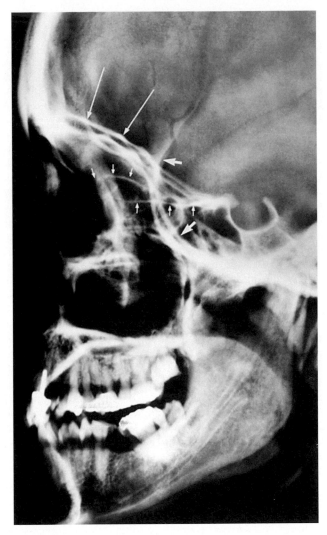

**FIGURE 2-48** Lateral view with small arrows pointing upward indicating the planum sphenoidale in the midline. The small arrows pointing downward outline the roof of the ethmoid sinuses (fovea ethmoidalis). The long arrows indicate the laterally positioned roofs of the orbit. The short arrows outline the curved anterior margins of the middle cranial fossa.

lines to the zygomaticomaxillary lines depends on the particular angulation used in the base view (Figs. 2-32, 2-33, and 2-49). In the more markedly angulated base view, the lacrimal canals can also be seen projected through the medial antral walls and hard palate.

The nasopharyngeal soft tissues should be carefully and routinely examined because disease can spread from this area into the sinonasal cavities and vice versa. This evaluation is best accomplished on the lateral view. The presence of a soft-tissue fullness in the roof and uppermost posterior wall of the nasopharynx may indicate adenoidal tissue, lymphoma, nasopharyngeal carcinoma, a Thornwalt cyst, or other lesions. If an ''adenoidal'' mass abuts on the upper surface of the soft palate, it may account for respiratory-related symptoms such as snoring or sleep apnea. Thus obliteration of the posterior nasal airway should always be noted in the radiologist's report.

On the base view the uvula, the posterior surface of the soft palate, and the back of the tongue all can cast transverse soft-tissue shadows across the skull base. In particular, the tongue base is often visualized extending transversely across the sphenoid sinuses. This should not be confused with sinus ''clouding'' and should be correlated with the lateral and open-mouth Waters views. The air in the nasopharynx and oropharynx is routinely seen as a low-density region projected over the central skull base. The degree of tube angulation and neck extension determines if this air shadow primarily represents the nasopharynx or the oropharynx. Thus a rectangular shadow with its greatest dimension extending from side to side suggests the nasopharynx, while a more square-shaped shadow suggests the oropharynx. On the routine base view, fullness in the region of the palatine tonsils can produce lateral soft-tissue

line that represents the lateral pterygoid plate near the skull base. The lateral pterygoid plate is seen as two lines because this plate has a curved, laterally tilted shape, which results in the main body of this plate being oblique to a craniocaudal incident beam. As a result, only the upper and lower bony margins are directly ''on end'' to the beam. Occasionally the hamulus of the medial pterygoid plate can be seen on the base view. The pterygoid fossa is thus the space, open posteriorly, between the medial and central pterygoid lines near the skull base and between the medial and lateral lines near the hard palate.

In the base view the frontal bone casts two transverse lines across the anterior portion of the ethmoid and maxillary sinuses. These lines correspond to the anterior and posterior cortices of the frontal bone. In addition, the anterior surface of the body of the zygoma and the anterior wall of the maxilla cast a transverse line across the anterolateral skull base. The relationship of the frontal table

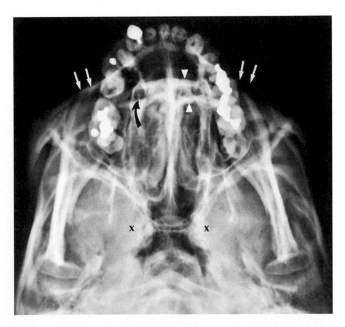

**FIGURE 2-49** Base view with arrows indicating the anterior wall margin of the maxilla and the zygoma. The curved arrow points to the nasolacrimal duct, which in this film is projected over the frontal bone's anterior and posterior margins (*arrowheads*). The soft-tissue shadows of the palatine tonsils (*X*s) can also be seen.

masses that overlie the posterior nasal fossae and pharyngeal airway (Fig. 2-49).

On the lateral view the pinna of the ear occasionally is projected over the sphenoid sinus and nasopharynx. This may simulate a mass and is usually seen on slightly underpenetrated films. It can be identified as an artifact by tracing out the entire ear lobe.

The nasal bones are best evaluated in the lateral view (Fig. 2-15B). The nasofrontal suture is identified easily at the level of the nasion. Also, the nasomaxillary sutures can often be seen. There are no normal sutures or bone segments that routinely traverse the midline nasal bones. However, several radiolucent lines are usually present in the lateral aspect of the nasal bones. These lines, which are the normal grooves for the nasociliary nerves and vessels, roughly parallel the plane of the midline nasal bones, and they should not be confused with fractures. As a general rule, there should be no lucent lines that extend across the midline nasal bones, and any such line or lines must suggest the diagnosis of a fracture. Medial depression of the nasal bones is best evaluated in the occlusal (axial) and Waters views. As mentioned, when evaluating the nasal bones, attention should also be paid to the anterior nasal spine.

In a patient with recent nasal trauma, clinical examination can usually determine whether a fracture is present. The examiner places the thumb and index finger on either side of the bridge of the nose and gently rocks the fingers from side to side. In cases of fracture the patient has exquisite local pain. By comparison, if there is only hemorrhage and edema (often markedly deforming the nasal contour) without fracture, the patient is only slightly tender. Thus, in such cases, strictly speaking the x-ray request for nasal films should read "Nasal fracture, please evaluate for the number of fractures and any displacement" rather than "Rule out a nasal fracture." The radiologist's report should include a comment on the number and location of the fractures and whether there is depression or elevation of the fracture segments. These nasal fractures are usually best seen on sectional imaging.

## SECTIONAL IMAGING TECHNIQUES

### Computed Tomography

The mucosal surfaces and the bony framework of the sinonasal cavities are well suited for investigation by CT. Because the radiologist and the clinician are as interested in soft-tissue disease as they are in bony changes, it would be convenient if each scan could be viewed at an appropriate window and center level that optimizes both subtle soft-tissue differences in attenuation as well as fine bony detail. Unfortunately, there is no one combination of window and center (level) settings that optimally accomplishes both of these aims. The soft tissues are best shown at narrow windows that allow easy discrimination between the attenuation values of muscle, fat, and tumor, as well as some distinction between entrapped secretions and cellular soft tissues. In addition, narrow windows allow prompt detection of any enhancement differences on contrast-enhanced CT scans. Such soft tissue settings have window values in the range of 150 to 400 HU.

Conversely, bone detail is best shown at wide window settings in the range of 3000 to 4000 HU. In addition, these wide window settings allow the most accurate evaluation of the air soft-tissue interfaces. This reflects the fact that almost all commercial vendor algorithms have difficulty handling abrupt transitions in attenuation values from very low (air) to very high (bone) attenuation regions. Thus, when the same images are viewed side by side at both narrow and wide window settings, the air spaces and the bones always appear larger at the narrower settings but are more accurately seen at the wider window settings (Fig. 2-50).

The appearance at wide window settings correlates accurately with the true measurements of the air spaces and the thickness of both soft-tissue disease and bone. In addition, at narrow window settings, volume-averaging errors allow a small soft-tissue mass to be obscured by surrounding sinus air and a focal area of abnormal bone to be obscured by adjacent normal bone.

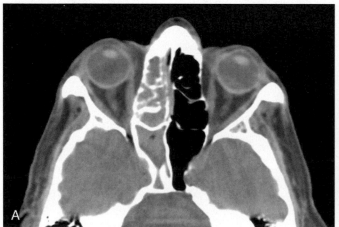
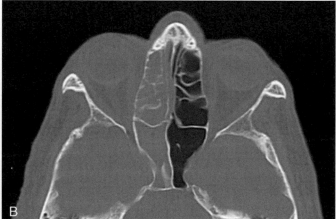

**FIGURE 2-50** **A,** Axial CT scan through the ethmoid and sphenoid sinuses viewed at narrow "soft-tissue" window settings shows opacification of these sinuses, with apparent sclerosis and thickening of the surrounding bone and ethmoid septae. **B,** Same image viewed at wide "bone" window settings shows that the bones are not sclerotic and thickened. The wide window views of the bone most closely reflect the actual bony changes.

In summary, the most accurate assessment of mucosal soft-tissue disease and bone is accomplished at wide window settings. However, the best distinction of watery sinonasal secretions from more viscous or desiccated secretions or a tumor requires narrow window settings.

Because of the popularity of endoscopic sinus surgery and its focus on the osteomeatal complex, the limited coronal CT study has become the most requested imaging examination of the sinonasal cavities. These studies best show the osteomeatal unit and are designed to limit the patient's radiation dose. Such limited CT examinations also are comparable in price to a plain film study. Although this approach is adequate for most patients, there are some pitfalls in interpreting such limited studies. Specifically, the anterior and posterior walls of the frontal, maxillary, and sphenoid sinuses are not well seen in the coronal view, and any abnormality or violation of these walls is most often overlooked or underestimated if only coronal views are available. In addition, because of varying patient compliance with the degree of neck extension, the coronal scan angle varies from patient to patient and often from examination to examination on the same patient. This alters the appearance of some anatomic landmarks and may make precise localization of ethmoid disease difficult. Such variation may soon be eliminated with the greater use of the multidetector CT scanners that allow precise coronal plane reconstructions from axial scans.

The axial studies provide the best CT evaluation of the anterior and posterior sinus walls. Thus, while a limited coronal CT study may be an adequate examination for most patients with suspected inflammatory sinonasal disease, the interpretation of such a study must be viewed with a caveat in mind. Namely, whenever there is total opacification of the frontal, maxillary, or sphenoid sinuses, a complete axial and coronal CT examination should be performed. In addition, if the patient has a suspected neoplasm, a complete axial and coronal examination ought to be performed to provide the most detailed analysis of the sinonasal cavities and the adjacent skull base.[52–54]

The axial examination is most often performed with the patient supine, the hard palate perpendicular to the table top, and the scanning plane parallel to the inferior orbitomeatal (IOM) line. The IOM line is readily identified on a lateral scout view. In addition, the cranial and caudal limits of the average scan (a level just above the top of the frontal sinuses and the bottom of the maxillary teeth, respectively) can be easily localized off the lateral scout view. The routine study should be obtained as 3 mm contiguous scans throughout the scan volume. Narrower slice thicknesses are usually unnecessary unless there is a specific region of interest. Spiral CT can also be performed at 3 mm intervals and reconstructed at 1 to 3 mm intervals.

Just as volume averaging may cause diagnostic difficulties in the coronal view, there are three levels in the axial view that may cause interpretive difficulties. These levels correspond to three bony planes, all of which are nearly parallel to the axial scan plane: the floor of the anterior cranial fossa, portions of the orbital floor, and the hard palate. Because knowledge of extension of disease across these bony planes is critical for the surgeon in determining some surgical procedures (for example, an antral tumor growing into the orbit, or a nasoethmoid or sphenoid tumor extending into the anterior cranial fossa), a coronal study must also be obtained whenever imaging of these bony planes is essential.

Because most adult patients have dental amalgams or metal bridges that cause considerable artifact, direct 90° coronal CT scans (to the IOM plane) are usually of limited diagnostic value because the involved teeth lie immediately below the sinonasal areas of interest. In addition, many patients cannot sufficiently extend their necks (because of pain, vertigo, arthritis, etc.) in either the supine or prone position to obtain such 90° coronal studies. In general, a scan plane is chosen that extends from a caudad margin just anterior to the dental fillings to a cranial point just posterior to the area of greatest interest (osteomeatal unit, orbit, sphenoid, etc.). These coronal studies are routinely obtained as 3-mm-thick contiguous slices.[55, 56] Spiral CT is now a viable alternative technique to the conventional multislice approach. This may be especially pertinent in the coronal view, where the faster spiral CT minimizes patient motion. In addition, the newer multidetector CT scanners allow excellent coronal images to be created at any desired scan angle from images made in the axial plane.

The routine CT study performed to evaluate sinonasal inflammatory disease does not require intravenous contrast administration. However, if one needs to determine if a nasal mass extends into an adjacent sinus or simply obstructs the sinus, or if there is suspected intracranial extension of disease, contrast should be given. In such instances, contrast CT is usually performed because the patient cannot have an MR study, as MR better visualizes mass/secretion interfaces and intracranial disease. There are a variety of methods for administering the CT contrast, and today a power injector is commonly used. If multiple serial CT slices are obtained, a small volume (10 to 20 ml) may be given as a bolus to "load" the patient and then the remaining contrast given at a slower rate throughout the examination. If spiral CT is used, the rapid scanning time allows the delivery of a larger effective bolus throughout the examination.

## Magnetic Resonance Imaging

As the era of MR imaging proceeds, new sequences and techniques are constantly being suggested. However, these approaches are primarily variations of facilitating the acquisition of basic T1-weighted and T2-weighted information. The advantage of imaging without ionizing radiation is occasionally outweighed by a claustrophobic patient's rejection of the procedure (about 10% of cases) or the presence of metal hardware, foreign bodies, or a pacemaker that abrogates the examination. Industry has responded to most of these problems by producing implantable nonmagnetic materials, nonparamagnetic support equipment for use with the more critically ill patient, and open MR units. Although bone is not directly imaged on MR, invasion of bone marrow and gross bone erosion can be easily identified.[57, 58] Fine bone alterations as well as focal calcifications are difficult, if not impossible, to see on MR imaging, and they are far better demonstrated on CT.

There stills remains some debate regarding the indications for the use of MR contrast material. Below the skull base, contrast enhancement occurs in most tumors and inflammatory tissue, as well as in some normal mucosa. As a result, the region of enhancement may contain a variety of normal as well as pathologic tissues, and the actual pathology may appear larger than it actually is. Despite this, some authors have recommended the use of double- and even triple-dose MR contrast agents to better assess the pathology visually. However, no new pathology was identified in such high-dose studies, and today single contrast dosing is the rule.[59] Actually, in day-to-day practice, pathology is often better mapped on noncontrast T1-weighted and T2-weighted images than on enhanced studies. However, if the pathology has spread intracranially, contrast-enhanced MR is superior to noncontrast studies in demonstrating an intracranial tumor margin and dural disease, as well as any intracranial complications of sinusitis such as meningitis, cerebritis, intracranial abscess, and orbital complications.[59, 60] Some radiologists firmly believe that fat suppression offers better visualization of contrast-enhanced areas. This is especially true when there is orbital involvement. However, other radiologists believe that the use of fat suppression techniques introduces unwanted artifacts that complicate image interpretation. Although most studies are done with fat suppression, the final decision is based on the preference of the radiologist.

MR contrast may also help in differentiating between entrapped secretions and a solid mass, as there is peripheral enhancement of uniformly thick, inflamed mucosa around secretions, while there usually is enhancement of a tumor nodule either centrally or along the margin of a neoplasm.[61, 62] Lastly, an MR contrast-focused study of the skull base and cavernous sinuses is the best way to identify perineural tumor spread. This topic is discussed in detail in Chapter 13.

The basic MR examination usually includes axial and coronal images. The scan thickness should be 3 to 5 mm, and a narrow interslice distance (1 mm) is suggested. Basic or equivalent T1-weighted and T2-weighted information should be obtained, whether by conventional spin echo or fast scan imaging. Fat suppression can be used in selected cases but is rarely necessary unless contrast-enhanced sequences are also obtained. The best study for an individual patient is often the one that is most confidently read by the radiologist. Thus sagittal images, though not necessary in the routine case, may help, especially in evaluating the cribriform plate region or the orbital floor. Gradient echo or FLAIR-type images can also be obtained to confirm the presence of hemorrhage.

Because there is no uniformity in the literature regarding the optimal TR and TE, these parameters can be varied to some degree to limit the total duration of the MR study, alter the resolution, or produce more scan slices in a single scan sequence. The greatest challenge for the imager is to tailor the examination to each patient so that all of the necessary information is gathered without unduly lengthening the examination. An additional benefit of this approach is that more patients can be examined in a given work day.

## SECTIONAL IMAGING ANATOMY

This section highlights the anatomy that can be seen on CT and MR imaging of the sinonasal cavities. The anatomy is divided into sections to help organize the anatomic detail. For specific anatomic descriptions of the sinuses, one should also review the previous sections dealing with plain film anatomy. Only the pertinent anatomic details are mentioned in the following sections. The reader is also referred to the images in the atlas section.

## The Nasal/Palatal Region

Far anteriorly on coronal images, the nasal bones and frontal processes of the maxilla form the upper outer nasal contour.[47] The upper nasal septum is formed by the perpendicular plate of the ethmoid bone above and the septal cartilage below. Inferiorly, the premaxilla is seen; anteriorly, at the level of the hard palate, is the anterior nasal spine. Within the hard palate and about 1 cm behind the anterior premaxilla is the incisive foramen. This foramen extends cranially as two separate incisive canals that open on either side of the base of the nasal septum. Together these canals and the foramen form a Y shape on coronal images. These canals transmit the terminal branches of the sphenopalatine arteries and their anastomoses with the terminal branches of the greater palatine arteries. The canals also transmit the nasopalatine nerves.

On coronal images, the palatine spines are seen on the oral surface of the hard palate. Lateral to the spines are the palatine grooves in which run the palatine vessels and nerves. The greater palatine foramen is seen posteriorly at the lateral junction of the lateral hard palate and the maxillary alveolus. The anterior surface of this canal is formed by the maxillary bone, the posterior surface by the palatine bone. Extending upward from the greater palatine foramen toward the pterygopalatine fossa is the pterygopalatine canal. The canal transmits the anterior palatine nerve and the descending palatine artery. Occasionally the lesser palatine foramen may be identified. It also extends to the pterygopalatine fossa and opens just posterior to the greater palatine foramen. The lesser palatine foramen transmits the posterior palatine nerve.

The anterior two thirds of the hard palate on each side is formed by the palatine process of the maxilla, the posterior one third by the horizontal process of the palatine bone. The most posterior medial wall of the antrum is formed by the vertical portion of the palatine bone.

## The Pterygopalatine Fossa

The pterygopalatine fossa is a small, thin rectangular space directly behind the perpendicular plate of the palatine bone and in front of the pterygoid process of the sphenoid bone. On axial images it appears that this space is directly posterior to the medial back wall of the maxillary sinus, this observation often leading to the false impression that the anterior wall of the pterygopalatine fossa is formed by the maxillary bone. In actuality, although the palatine bone cannot be separated on images from the maxillary bone, it is the ascending portion, or perpendicular plate of the palatine bone, that forms the anterior wall of the pterygopalatine fossa.

The pterygopalatine fossa communicates with five

anatomic areas: (1) the nasal fossa (via the sphenopalatine foramen), (2) the mouth (via the greater and lesser pterygopalatine canals, which open on the palate through the greater and lesser palatine foramina), (3) the infratemporal fossa (via the retromaxillary space or fissure), (4) the orbit (via the inferior orbital fissure), and (5) the intracranial compartment and skull base (via the pterygoid or Vidian canal and the foramen rotundum).

More specifically, the medial boundary of the fossa is formed by the sphenopalatine foramen, which is at the craniocaudal level of the posterior tip of the middle concha, about 1 cm dorsal to it. This foramen may be seen connecting the nasal fossa with the pterygopalatine fossa. Within the pterygopalatine fossa are the sphenopalatine ganglion, portions of the maxillary nerve, and the internal maxillary artery. It is actually the sphenopalatine artery (the terminal branch of the internal maxillary artery) that runs through this foramen. All of these structures are supported by fat, which fills the majority of the pterygopalatine fossa. The nasopalatine nerve (a branch of the sphenopalatine nerve, which is a branch of the maxillary nerve [$V_2$]), also passes through the sphenopalatine foramen.

Extending posteriorly into the middle cranial fossa via the skull base are two canals. The lower and more medial canal is the pterygoid or Vidian canal, while the upper and more lateral canal is the foramen rotundum/canal. The Vidian canal may be almost entirely within the sphenoid bone or sitting well within the sinus on a septum above the sinus floor. Similarly, the foramen rotundum may protrude into the lateral lower wall of the sphenoid sinus or may be completely lateral to the sinus. More posteriorly, the optic canal may protrude into the upper lateral sinus wall. These sphenoid sinus variations are discussed in detail in Chapter 3.[47]

## The Pterygoid Plates

The medial pterygoid plate is almost vertically oriented. The lateral plate is tilted so that its lower end, at the level of the hard palate, is more lateral than its cranial margin at the skull base. The pterygoid fossa lies between these plates. These relationships are often best appreciated on coronal images. The medial or internal pterygoid muscle arises from the medial side of the lateral pterygoid plate within the pterygoid fossa, and the lateral or external pterygoid muscle arises from the lateral side of the lateral plate. The tendon of the tensor veli palatini muscle passes around the laterally concave-shaped hamulus of the lower medial pterygoid plate to form part of the soft palate.

## The Nasal Septum

The nasal septum is formed anteriorly to posteriorly by the medial crura of the alar cartilages, the septal cartilage, the perpendicular plate of the ethmoid bone, and the vomer. Inferiorly, the nasal crests of the maxilla and palatine bones contribute to the base of the septum. The posterior edge of the vomer joins the undersurface of the sphenoid bone at the sphenoid rostrum, a prominent triangular ridge on the underbody of the sphenoid bone. In addition to deviations of the nasal septum, nasal spurs can occur on either side. These usually triangular bony excrescences occur at the level of the junction of the perpendicular plate of the ethmoid bone and the vomer.

## The Olfactory Recesses and Nasal Atrium

The olfactory recess is the narrow channel-like region of the nasal cavity on either side of the upper nasal septum. These spaces continue up to the cribriform plate. On either side, the olfactory recess widens posteriorly into the sphenoethmoidal recess. This marks the junction between the ethmoid and sphenoid bones.

In the anterior lateral nasal cavity, just below and medial to the agger nasi cells, is the region referred to as the nasal atrium. This atrium region is continuous with the more posterior nasal fossa (see Chapter 3).

## The Margins of the Orbit

On coronal images through the superior orbital rims, a localized notch, or foramen, can be seen along the medial orbital margin. This is the supraorbital notch (or foramen), and the supraorbital artery and nerve pass through it. Medial to the supraorbital notch is the frontal notch, which transmits the frontal artery and the frontal nerve. Although the orbital surface of the orbital roof is smooth, the intracranial margin of the orbital roof has bony ridges that, in a general way, reflect the impressions of the gyri of the base of the frontal lobes.

Along the medial orbital walls are the anterior ethmoidal canals, which are seen as medial indentations in the upper lamina papyracea. They transmit the anterior ethmoidal nerves and vessels. The lower margins of these canals are formed by the ethmoid bones, and the upper margins are formed by the frontal bones. More posteriorly are the similarly formed posterior ethmoidal canals, which transmit their respective vessels and nerves.

In the middle third of the orbital floor are the infraorbital foramen and canal. The canal extends from the inferior orbital fissure posteriorly to the anterior maxilla. This canal runs parallel to the orbital floor except in its most anterior portion, where, starting about 1 cm behind the inferior orbital rim, it turns downward to exit as the infraorbital foramen about 1 cm below the inferior orbital rim on the anterior face of the maxilla.

The inferior orbital fissure is about 2 cm long and is angled at about 45° (open anteriorly) with the midsagittal plane. This fissure is narrowest in its midportion and widens at both its medial and lateral margins. This fissure separates the lateral orbital wall from the orbital floor, and at the lateral posterior margin of the inferior orbital fissure the temporal fossa becomes the infratemporal fossa.

The circular configuration of the anterior orbit slowly changes to a more triangular shape in the posterior orbit. This change in shape occurs because the medial orbital floor elevates, and the lower lamina papyracea tilts laterally, as the larger posterior ethmoid cells are encountered.[47]

The thin lacrimal bone has a slightly concave lateral configuration, forms the anterior medial orbital wall, and overlies the anterior ethmoid cells. The ethmoid lamina papyracea, which lies just behind the lacrimal bone, tends to be even thinner and has a straighter configuration than the lacrimal bone.

## The Lacrimal Fossa and Nasolacrimal Duct

The fossa for the lacrimal gland is a shallow, smooth indentation in the frontal bone along the upper outer aspect of the orbital roof. The lacrimal groove is in the lower medial orbital wall and is related to the lacrimal sac of the nasolacrimal system. It is actually preseptal in location and not in the orbit, being anterior to the posterior lacrimal crest. The lacrimal groove is also anterior to the nasolacrimal canal, which lies in the medial antral wall. This reflects the anatomy of the nasolacrimal canal, which runs downward and posteriorly at about a $20°$ angle with the coronal plane. On imaging, the lacrimal groove creates a normal "dehiscence" in the medial orbital floor that should not be confused with a focal site of erosion. The caudal opening of the nasolacrimal canal is in the medial antral wall under the inferior turbinate (lateral wall of the inferior meatus). The medial wall of the nasolacrimal canal is formed superiorly by the lacrimal bone and inferiorly by the lacrimal process of the inferior turbinate. The lateral wall is formed entirely by the maxilla. See Chapter 10.

## The Sphenoid Sinus Septum

The sphenoid intersinus septum is usually in the midline anteriorly, but posteriorly it may be angulated sharply to one side. This creates two unequally sized sinuses, and once the scan plane moves posterior to such an angled septum, it will appear as if there is only one sphenoid sinus cavity. In the floor of the sinus runs the Vidian canal. This canal may lie entirely within the sphenoid bone or may be elevated by a septum and lie within the lower sinus cavity. The foramen rotundum anteriorly and the optic canal posteriorly can also be partially within the lateral sinus wall. If any of these canals do project into the sinus cavity, or if there is dehiscence of the bony wall separating the canal from the sinus, injury to the nerve can occur during sinus surgery. This topic is discussed further in Chapter 3.

## The Maxillary Sinus Walls

The medial wall of the maxillary sinus is partially bone and partially membrane. This membranous area forms a C shape, which is closed posteriorly and bridges the posterior attachment of the inferior turbinate. The anterior wall of the maxillary sinus has a slightly concave anterior configuration, with the concavity marking the site of the canine fossa. This fossa lies cranial to the lateral incisor and canine teeth and caudal to the infraorbital canal, and the caninus muscle arises in it. The posterior sinus wall is curved and sigmoid-shaped, and the infratemporal fossa fat abuts its posterior surface. Within the posterolateral antral wall there is a thin canal for the posterosuperior alveolar nerve. This canal should not be confused with a site of bone erosion or a fracture.

## THE INTEGUMENT OF THE FACE AND SCALP

The facial bones, calvarium, and contained spaces receive the primary attention of the imager. However, in a limited way, the overlying skin, muscles, nerves, and vessels that supply them are also seen on images of the sinonasal cavities and head. The following sections briefly review the muscles, nerves, arteries, and veins that involve the face and scalp.[6]

## The Facial Muscles

The facial muscles can be thought of as connecting bone and skin. These muscles are responsible for facial expression, and they create tension lines (Langer's cleavage lines) in the skin that are oriented at right angles to the plane of the muscle fibers. These tension lines, which deepen with age as the skin loses its elasticity, can be used to hide surgical incisions. These muscles are summarized in Table 2-1. The nasal muscles have already been discussed in the section on The Nose and Nasal Fossae[63, 64] under the heading of "Anatomy and Physiology."

An important concept to understand is that the mimetic muscles of the face, including the platysma, are interconnected by a fibrous aponeurosis called the superficial musculo-aponeurotic system (SMAS). This system divides the subcutaneous fat into two layers and acts as a tensor of the facial muscles (see also Chapter 34).

## Scalp and Forehead

On the scalp and forehead are the occipital and frontal bellies of the occipitofrontal (epicranius) muscle and the corrugator supercilii muscle. The occipital belly elevates the skin of the forehead, and the frontal belly pulls the skin toward the eyebrow. The corrugator supercilii draws the brow medially, creating frown lines near the glabella. There is the temporoparietalis muscle, which draws the skin back from the temple region and tightens the scalp. There are also small muscles (auriculares anterior, superior, and posterior) that are related to the ear and that retract and elevate the ear. The layers of the scalp include the skin, the superficial fascia or tela subcutanea (in which runs most of the blood vessels and cutaneous nerves), the epicranial aponeurosis or gala aponeurosis, loose connective tissue, and the cranial periosteum or pericranium.

## Orbit

About the eye is the orbicularis oculi, which is composed of a series of concentric muscular rings. Closure of the eye is the result of coordinated contraction of the entire muscle. Blinking involves only the palpebral region of the muscle. This palpebral portion of the muscle attaches posterior to the medial palpebral ligament and aids in pumping tears from the lacrimal sac.

## Cheek and Lips (Mouth)

In the region of the cheek and lips (mouth), the buccinator muscle serves to compress the cheeks, to help expel air, and to aid in mastication. As such, it is more a muscle of mastication than a muscle of facial expression. The orbicularis oris acts to compress, contract, and protrude the lips. Elevation of the upper lip is caused by the levator labii superioris and the levator labii superioris alaeque nasi muscles, while the levator anguli oris muscle elevates the angle of the lip. Similarly, the lower lip has the depressor labii inferioris (irony) muscle and the depressor anguli oris (grief) muscles. The lesser (minor) and greater (major) zygomaticus muscles elevate the angle of the mouth (laughing), and the lesser zygomaticus muscles help produce the nasolabial fold. The risorius muscle retracts the angle of the mouth (grinning). The mentalis muscle raises and protrudes the lower lip and wrinkles the skin (disdain). The transverse menti muscle is present in about 50% of people; it crosses the midline just under the chin. Lastly, the platsyma muscle assists in depressing the lower jaw and lip and tenses the skin of the neck. These facial muscles are summarized in Figure 2-51.

## Cutaneous Innervation of the Face

On a lateral projection of the head and face, a line drawn from the vertex of the head to the tip of the chin defines a plane. The cutaneous innervation of the skin and head by the trigeminal nerve is anterior and above this plane; the cutaneous distribution of the cervical nerves is posterior and below this line. The trigeminal distribution follows the major branches of this nerve. Thus, the first division supplies the upper nose to its tip, around the medial, upper, and lateral orbits, and the upper scalp. The second division of the trigeminal nerve supplies the lateral nose, upper lip, and skin between the nose and mouth. It also supplies the skin over the malar eminence of the zygoma and a tapering triangle of skin along the anterior side of the scalp. The third division supplies the lower lip, chin, lateral face to the level of the lower mandibular border, and lateral scalp up to the line drawn from the vertex to the chin tip. The superficial cervical plexus supplies the ear, periauricular region, and anterior neck. The posterior divisions of the cervical nerves supply the posterior scalp and neck. These cutaneous nerves derive from the second, third, and fourth cervical nerves as they form the cervical plexus. The superficial cutaneous branches include the smaller occipital nerve (C2), the greater auricular nerve (C2 and C3), the cervical cutaneous nerve (C2 and C3), and the supraclavicular nerve (C3 and C4). These areas are summarized in Figure 2-52.

## Arterial Supply of the Face and Scalp

The vascular supply of the face and head comes from branches of both the external and internal carotid arteries. The branches from the internal carotid artery are terminal branches of the ophthalmic artery, the supratrochlear and supraorbital arteries. They supply the upper periorbital region and immediate forehead. The major branches of the external carotid artery are the superficial temporal artery (supplies most of the forehead and scalp), the transverse facial artery (supplies the lateral face), the facial artery (supplies the central and lower portions of the face), the posterior auricular artery (supplies the back of the auricle or pinna and the periauricular region), and the occipital artery (supplies the posterior scalp, upper posterior neck, auricle, and a meningeal branch that enters the skull through the jugular foramen and supplies the dura of the posterior fossa).[63–65] These relationships are summarized in Figure 2-53.

## Venous Drainage of the Face and Scalp

The drainage of the face is primarily via the facial vein and the retromandibular vein. The frontal vein begins in a venous plexus in the forehead that anastomoses with the superficial temporal vein. The frontal vein then descends to the root of the nose, where the nasal arch vein joins the parallel frontal vein of the opposite side. The supraorbital vein runs down the forehead and anastomoses with the frontal vein near the medial canthus to form the angular vein. The angular vein runs down the side of the nose in the nasolabial fold to the level of the lower orbit or bottom of the nose, where it becomes the anterior facial vein, which drains the blood from the nose and lips. It then follows the course of the facial artery down across the face, over the mandible, to join the common facial vein that drains into the internal jugular vein near the level of the hyoid bone. The anterior facial vein is joined by the superior and inferior palpebral veins, the superior and inferior labial veins, the buccinator vein, and the masseteric vein.

The superficial temporal vein starts in the scalp in a venous plexus that communicates with the frontal and supraorbital veins, the opposite superficial temporal vein, and the posterior auricular and occipital veins. Frontal and parietal veins join and then are in turn joined above the zygomatic arch by the middle temporal vein, which receives tributaries from orbital veins. This vein is then joined by the maxillary vein draining the infratemporal fossa. The pterygoid plexus drains the sphenopalatine, middle meningeal, deep temporal, pterygoid, masseteric, buccinator, alveolar, and some palatine veins and communicates via the inferior orbital fissure with the ophthalmic vein. It also communicates with the facial vein and cavernous sinus. Together the superficial temporal vein and the internal maxillary vein form the retromandibular vein, which receives tributaries from the parotid and auricular veins and from the transverse facial vein. At the lower margin of the parotid gland, the retromandibular vein joins the common facial vein and also anastomoses with the external jugular vein. The posterior auricular vein communicates with the superficial temporal and occipital veins and descends behind the auricle to join the posterior facial vein and form the external jugular vein. The occipital vein begins as a plexus at the back of the vertex of the scalp and as a single vein descends into the suboccipital triangle, where it is joined by the deep cervical and vertebral veins. It can join the internal jugular vein directly or join the posterior auricular vein. The occipital vein receives the parietal emissary vein, which communicates with the superior sagittal sinus and the mastoid emissary vein, which communicates with the transverse sinus. The veins of the forehead and upper lids drain into the orbit and the inferior and superior branches of the ophthalmic vein.[63–65] The relationships are summarized in Figure 2-53.

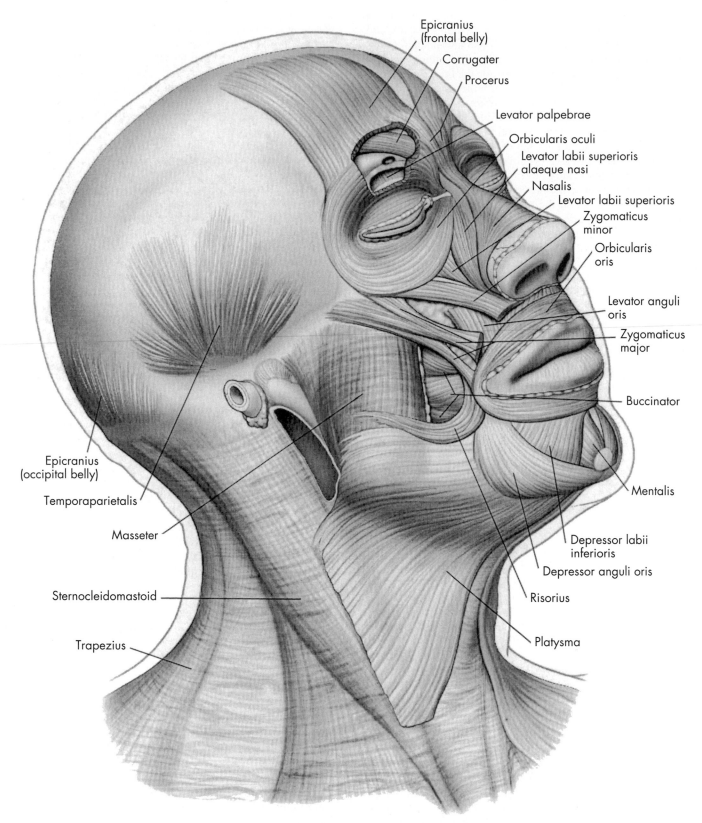

**FIGURE 2-51**   Drawing of the face and neck in the right lateral oblique view. The facial muscles and the superficial neck muscles are shown.

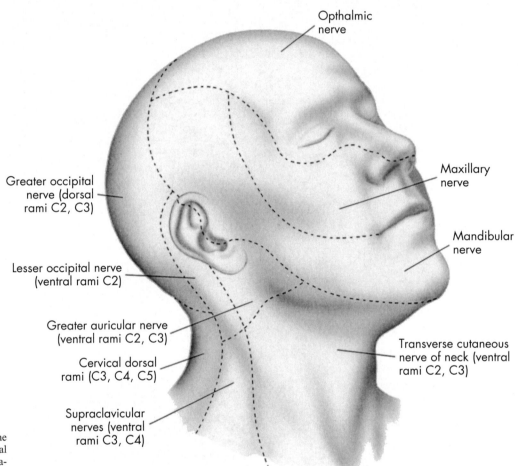

Opthalmic nerve

Maxillary nerve

Mandibular nerve

Transverse cutaneous nerve of neck (ventral rami C2, C3)

Greater occipital nerve (dorsal rami C2, C3)

Lesser occipital nerve (ventral rami C2)

Greater auricular nerve (ventral rami C2, C3)

Cervical dorsal rami (C3, C4, C5)

Supraclavicular nerves (ventral rami C3, C4)

**FIGURE 2-52** Drawing of the face and neck in the right lateral oblique view. The cutaneous innervation of the face and scalp is shown.

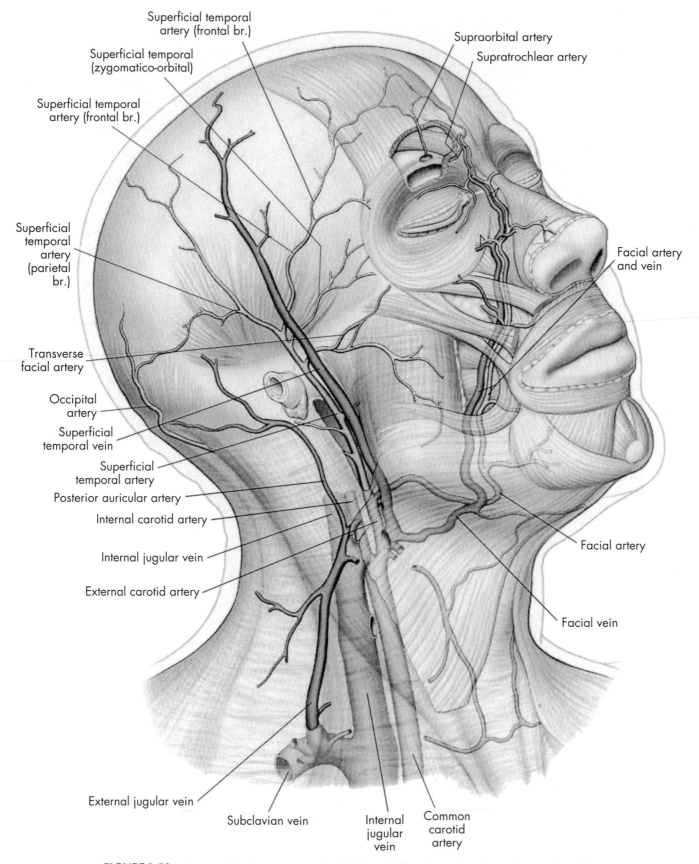

Superficial temporal artery (frontal br.)

Superficial temporal (zygomatico-orbital)

Superficial temporal artery (frontal br.)

Superficial temporal artery (parietal br.)

Transverse facial artery

Occipital artery

Superficial temporal vein

Superficial temporal artery

Posterior auricular artery

Internal carotid artery

Internal jugular vein

External carotid artery

Supraorbital artery

Supratrochlear artery

Facial artery and vein

Facial artery

Facial vein

External jugular vein

Subclavian vein

Internal jugular vein

Common carotid artery

**FIGURE 2-53** Drawing of the face and neck in the right lateral oblique view. The major arteries and veins of the face and upper neck are shown.

## ATLAS OF NORMAL ANATOMY
## OF THE PARANASAL SINUSES

| | |
|---|---|
| AEthCan | Anterior Ethmoidal Canal |
| Agger Nasi Cell | Agger Nasi Ethmoid Cell Deep to Lacrimal Bone |
| Alv Rec M | Alveolar Recess of Maxillary Sinus |
| Ant Clin Proc | Anterior Clinoid Process |
| AntCranFossa | Anterior Cranial Fossa |
| AntEth Can | Anterior Ethmoidal Canal |
| Ant Nas Spine | Anterior Nasal Spine |
| Att Inf Turb | Attachment of Inferior Turbinate |
| Basal Lam Mid Turb | Basal Lamella of the Middle Turbinate |
| Bas Nas Cav | Base of Nasal Cavity Above Hard Palate |
| Bas Nas Sep | Base of the Nasal Septum as it attaches to Hard Palate |
| Bulla | Bulla Ethmoidalis |
| Can | Canine Tooth |
| Car Can | Carotid Canal |
| Cen Inc | Central Incisor Tooth |
| CG | Crista Galli |
| Clivus | Clivus |
| Colum | Columella |
| Concha Bullos | Concha Bullosa Middle Turbinate |
| Cor Proc | Coronoid Process of Mandible |
| Cort Wt Line | Cortical Dense White Line Surrounding the Frontal Sinuses |
| Crib Plt | Cribriform Plate |
| Crista Galli | Crista Galli |
| DS | Dorsum Sellae |
| E | Ethmoid Sinus |
| F | Frontal Sinus |
| FB | Frontal Bone |
| Floor of Sella | Floor of Sella Turcica |
| For Lac | Foramen Lacerum |
| For Ovale | Foramen Ovale |
| For Rot | Foramen Rotundum |
| Fovea Eth | Fovea Ethmoidalis of Frontal Bone |
| F Proc Max | Frontal Process of Maxilla |
| FrontZyg Sut | Fronto-Zygomatic Suture |
| Fst Mol | First Molar Tooth |
| Fst Pre Mol | First Premolar Tooth |
| Gr Pal Can | Greater Palatine Canal |
| Great Wing Sph | Greater Wing of the Sphenoid Bone |
| Hamulus Med Pter Plt | Hamulus of the Medial Pterygoid Plate |
| Hard Pal | Hard Palate |
| Hor Plt Pal | Horizontal Plate of Palatine Bone |
| IC Lig | Interclinoid Ligament |
| Incis Can | Incisive Canal |
| Incis For | Incisive Foramen |
| Inf Meatus | Inferior Meatus |
| InfOrCan | Infraorbital Canal |
| InfOrFis | Inferior Orbital Fissure |
| InfOrFor | Infraorbital Foramen |
| InfTemFossa | Infratemporal Fossa |
| Inf Turb | Inferior Turbinate |
| Infra Or Canal | Infraorbital Canal |
| Infra Or For | Infraorbital Foramen |
| IOF | Inferior Orbital Fissure |
| Lac Bone | Lacrimal Bone |
| Lac Sac Fossa | Lacrimal Sac Fossa |
| Lam Dura Sella | Lamina Dura of Sella |
| LamPap | Lamina Papyracea of Ethmoid |
| Lat Inc | Lateral Incisor Tooth |
| Lat Pter Plt | Lateral Pterygoid Plate |
| Lat Rec S | Lateral Recess of Sphenoid Sinus |
| Lac Sac | Lacrimal Saccule |
| Les Pal Can | Lesser Palatine Canal |
| Less Wing Sph | Lesser Wing of the Sphenoid Bone |
| Limbus | Sphenoid Bone Limbus |
| LPap | Lamina Papyracea Ethmoid |
| M | Maxillary Sinus |
| Man Hd | Mandibular Head |
| Mand For and Can | Mandibular Foramen and Upper Canal |
| Mand Notch | Mandibular Notch |
| Max Alv | Maxillary Alveolus |
| Max Exost | Maxillary Exostosis |
| Max Pal Sut | Maxillary Palatine Suture |
| Max Teeth Rts | Maxillary Teeth Roots |
| MB | Maxillary Bone |
| Med Pter Plt | Medial Pterygoid Plate |
| Med Wall M | Medial Wall of Maxillary Sinus |
| MidCranFossa | Middle Cranial Fossa |
| Mid Meatus | Middle Meatus |
| Mid Sut Pal | Midline Suture Between Left and Right Halves of Hard Palate |
| Mid Turb | Middle Turbinate |
| MSept | Maxillary Sinus Septum |
| Nasal Cavity | Nasal Cavity Airway |
| Nasal Fossa | Nasal Fossa Air Space |
| Nasal Septum | Nasal Septum |
| NasoLac Duct | Nasolacrimal Duct |
| NasoFtl Sut | Nasofrontal Suture |
| NasoLac Can | Nasolacrimal Canal |
| NB | Nasal Bone |
| Nose | Nose Cartilages and Soft Tissues |
| Nostril | Nostril of Nose |
| NP | Nasopharynx |
| OC | Optic Canal |
| Olf Groove | Olfactory Groove |
| OlfRec | Olfactory Recess |
| Open Nasolac Duct | Opening of the Nasolacrimal Duct into the Middle Meatus |
| Opt Can | Optic Canal |
| Or | Orbit |
| Or Roof | Orbital Roof |
| Pal Proc Max | Palatine Process of Maxilla |
| Palatal Recesses Max | Palatal Recesses of the Maxillary Sinuses |
| PerpPlt Eth | Perpendicular Plate of the Ethmoid Bone |
| Pet Apex | Petrous Apex |
| PEthCan | Posterior Ethmoidal Canal |
| Plan Sphen | Planum Sphenoidale |
| Post Ant Cr Fossa | Posterior Edge of Anterior Cranial Fossa |

| | |
|---|---|
| PostEth Can | Posterior Ethmoidal Canal |
| PPF | Pterygopalatine Fossa |
| Pter Fossa | Pterygoid Fossa |
| Ptery Proc S | Pterygoid Process of Sphenoid |
| Pty Rec S | Pterygoid Recess of Sphenoid Sinus |
| Ramus Man | Ramus of Mandible |
| Rostrum Sphenoid | Rostrum of Sphenoid Bone |
| S | Sphenoid Sinus |
| SB | Sphenoid Bone |
| Sec Mol | Second Molar Tooth |
| Sec Pre Mol | Second Premolar Tooth |
| Sella | Sella Turcica |
| Septum | Septum Within a Sinus |
| SphenoEth Rec | Sphenoethmoidal Recess |
| Sph Sin Ostium | Sphenoid Sinus Ostium |
| SOF | Superior Orbital Fissure |
| S Sep | Sphenoid Sinus Septum |
| STSut | Sphenotemporal Suture |
| Styl Proc | Styloid Process |
| Supraor Can | Supraorbital Canal Tub |
| Supraor Grv | Supraorbital Groove |
| Sup Turb | Superior Turbinate |
| SZySut | Sphenozygomatic Suture |
| Thd Mol | Third Molar Tooth |
| Torus Pal | Torus Palatinus |
| Torus Tub | Torus Tubarius |
| Tub Sel | Tuberculum Sellae |
| Uncin Proc | Uncinate Process of Ethmoid |

| | |
|---|---|
| Vidian Can | Vidian Canal (Pterygoid Canal) |
| Vomer | Vomer |
| ZB | Zygomatic Bone |
| Zyg Arch | Zygomatic Arch |
| ZygoTemp Can | Zygomaticotemporal Canal |

Within the axial anatomic atlas, Figures 10A, B, and C show variations in the size of the sphenoid sinuses with lateral and pterygoid recesses. Figure 21A shows an alveolar recess of the maxillary sinus, with the sinus extending caudal to the hard palate. Figures 21B and C show the incisive canals and the incisor foramen.

Within the coronal anatomic atlas, Figure 10 shows variations in the pneumatization of the lower maxillary sinus. Figure 10A shows palatal recesses. Figure 10B shows lack of pneumatization of the maxillary alveolus. Figure 10C shows pneumatization of the inferior turbinate. Figure 11 shows a typical example of a torus palatinus and maxillary exostoses. Axial Figure 16A and coronal Figure 11B show pneumatization of the inferior turbinate by the maxillary sinus. Figures 14-17 show variations in sphenoid sinus configuration and the location of the foramen rotundum and Vidian canals near and within the sinus. Axial and coronal Figures 1B show frontal sinus pneumatization of the orbital roofs. The presence of bone between the ethmoid complex and the recess differentiates these from supraorbital ethmoid cells.

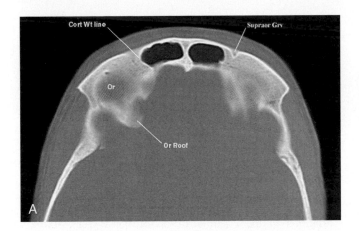

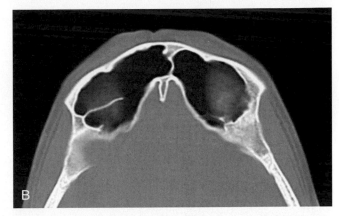

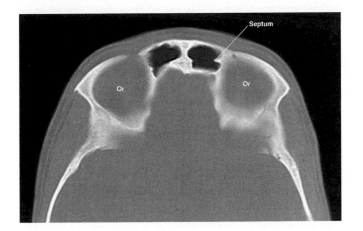

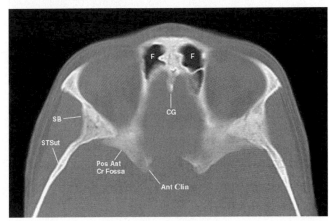

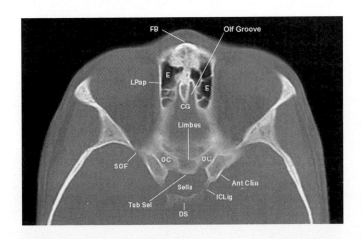

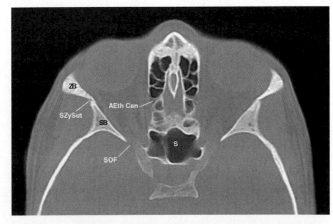

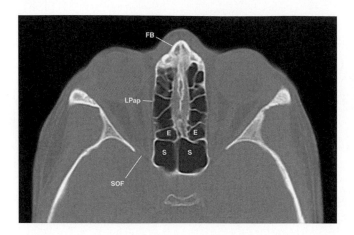

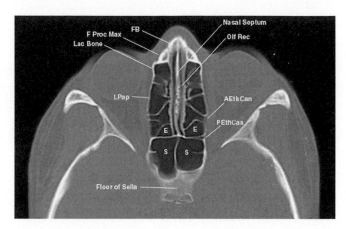

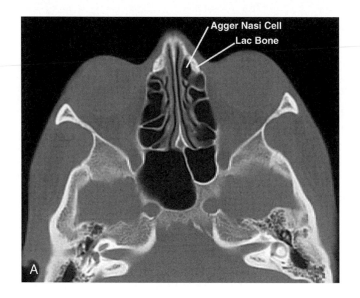

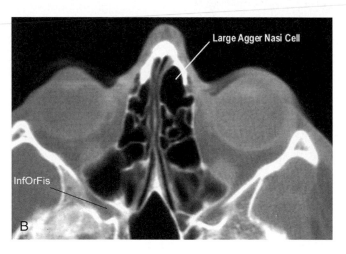

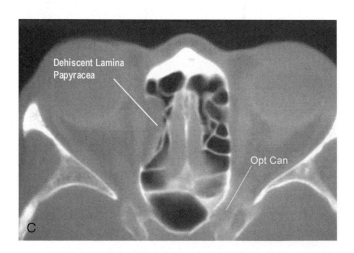

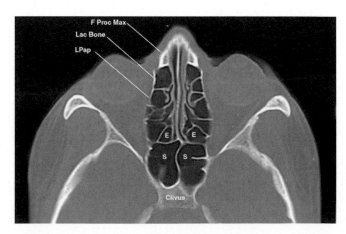

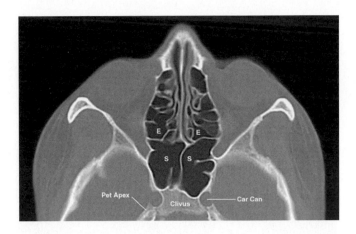

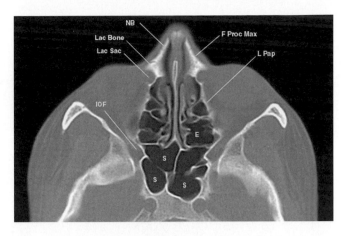

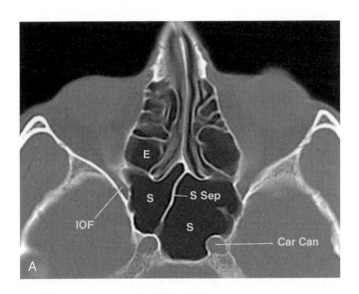

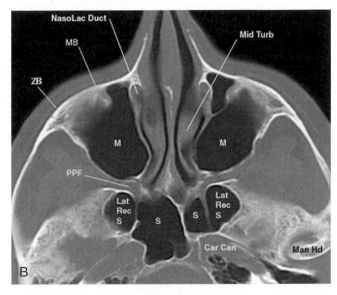

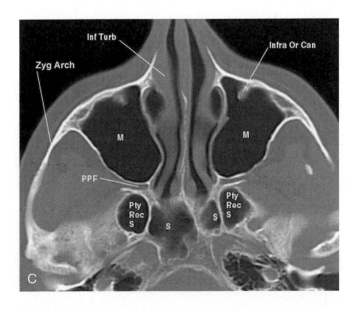

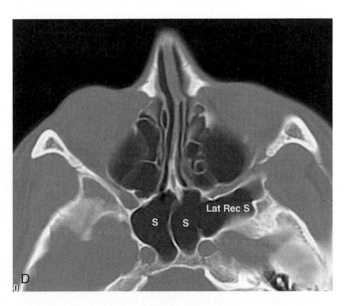

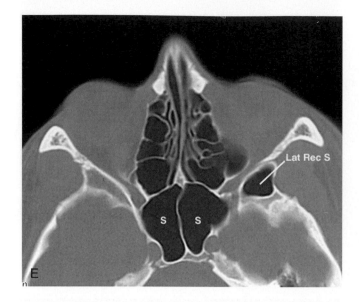

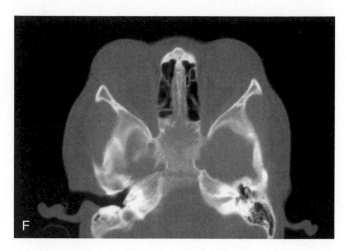

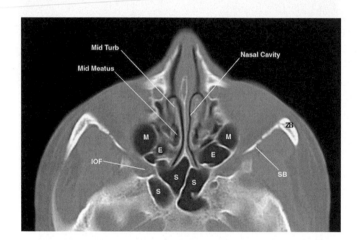

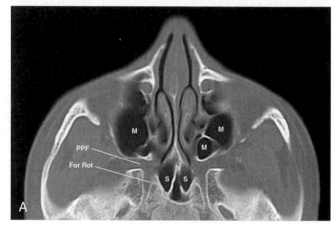

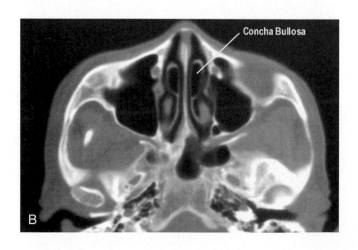

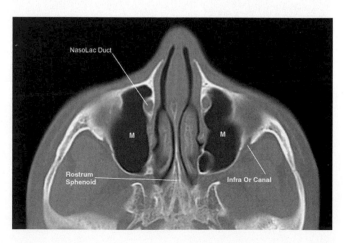

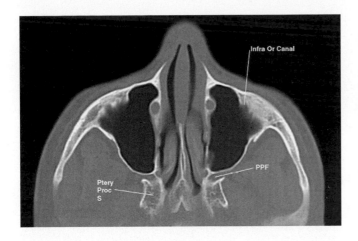

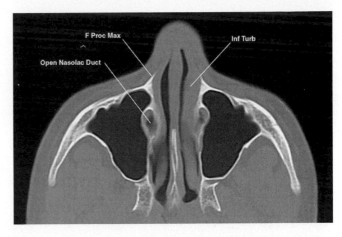

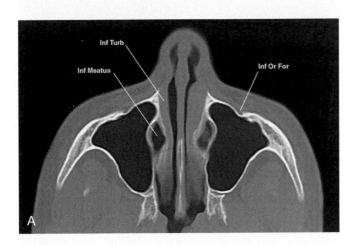

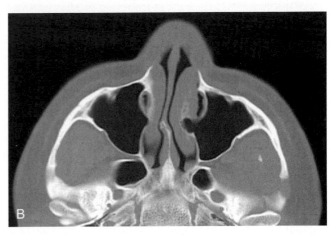

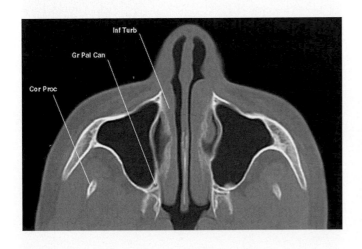

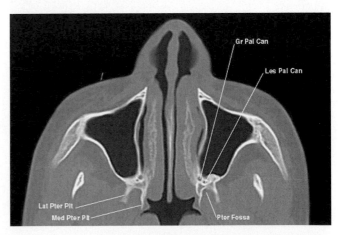

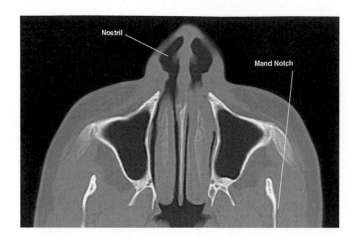

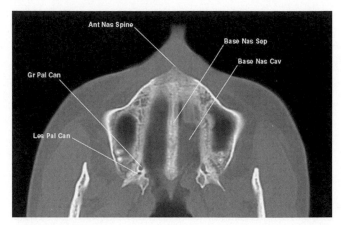

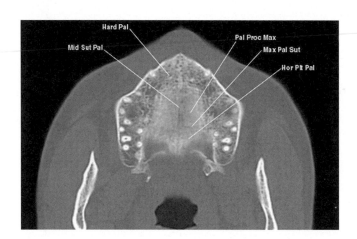

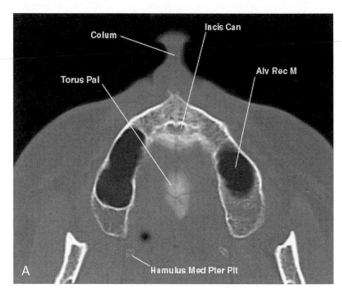

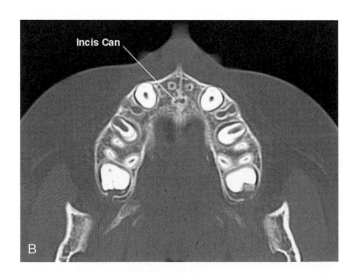

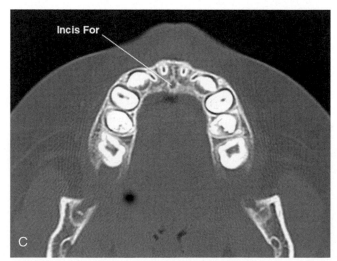

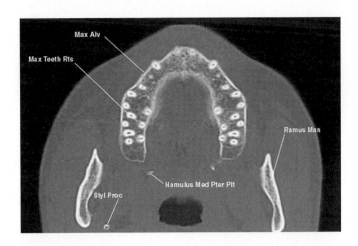

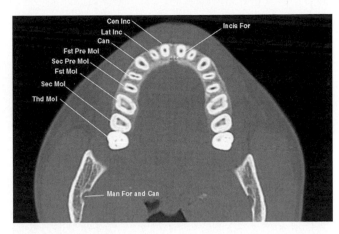

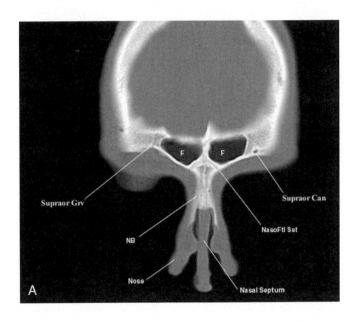

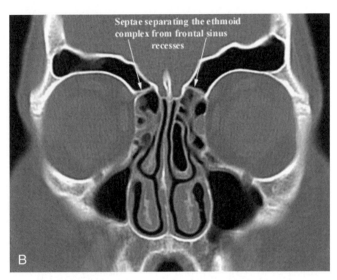

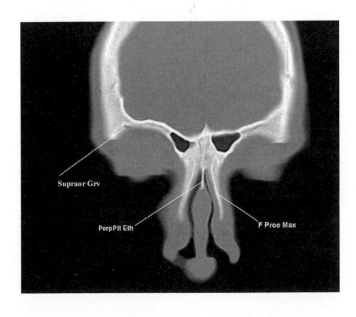

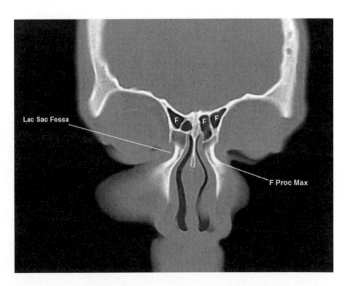

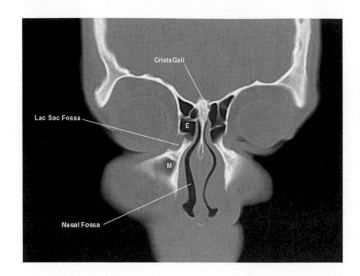

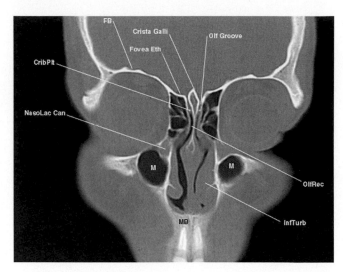

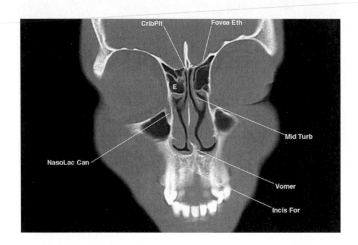

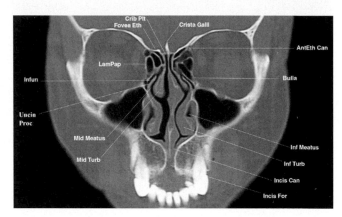

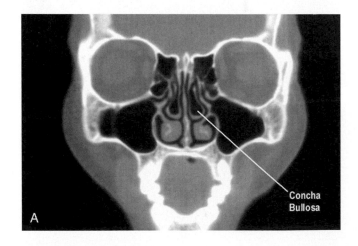

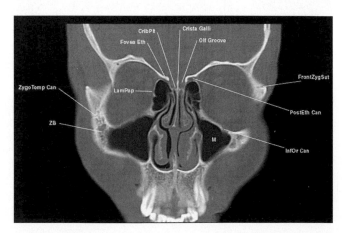

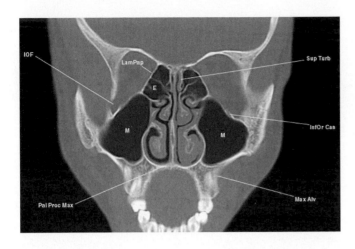

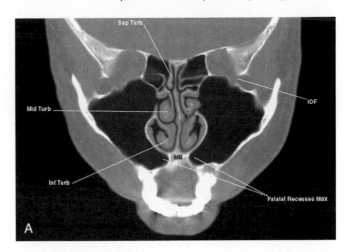

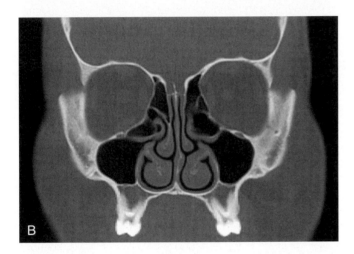

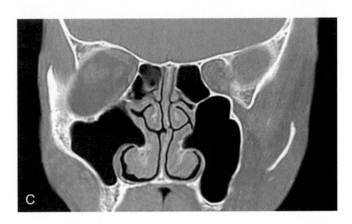

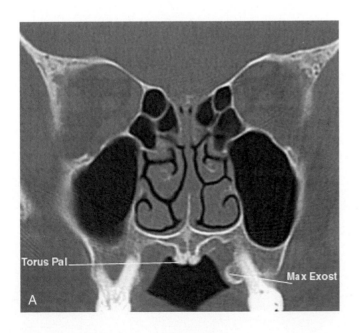

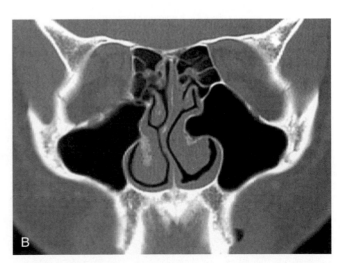

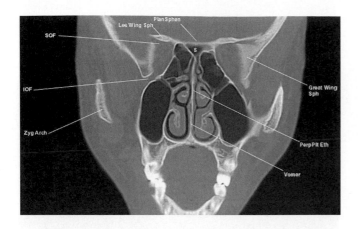

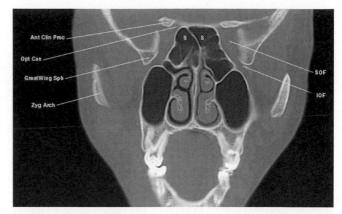

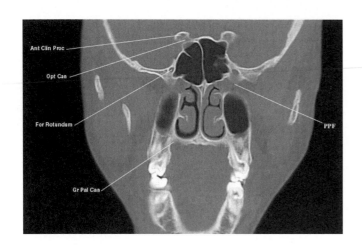

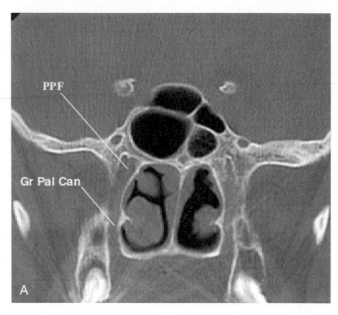

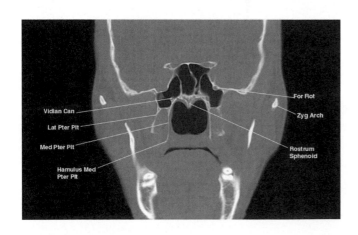

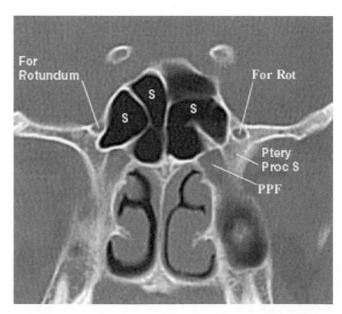

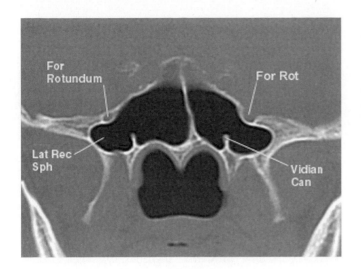

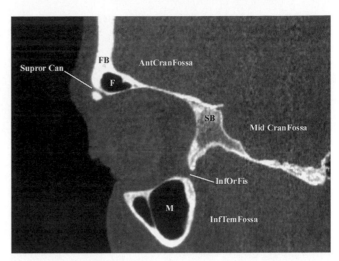

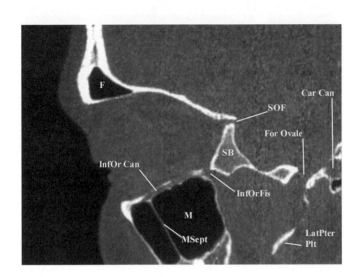

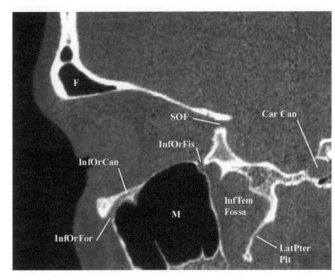

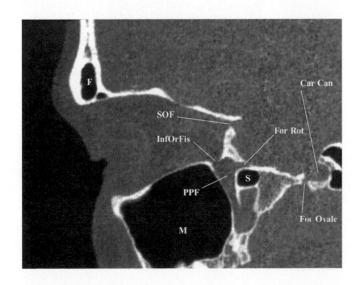

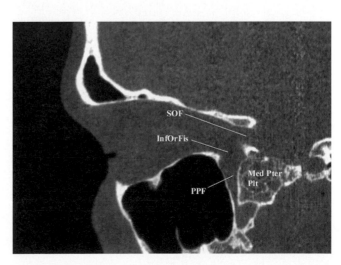

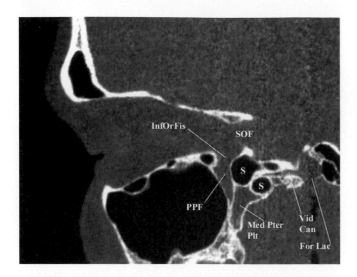

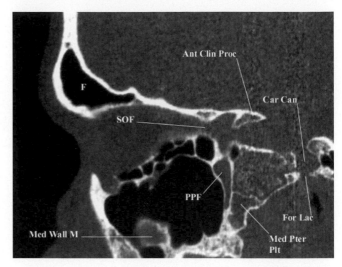

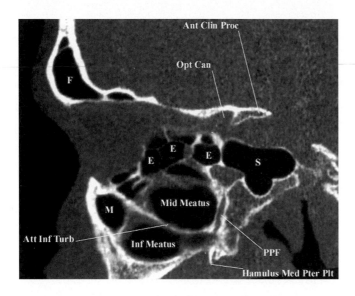

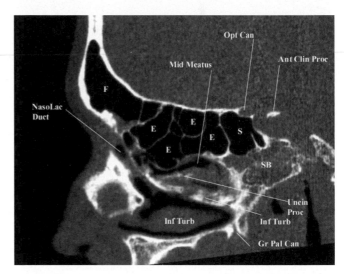

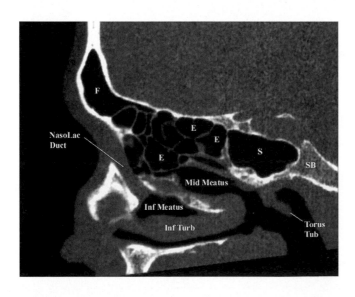

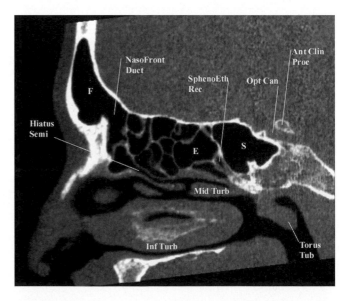

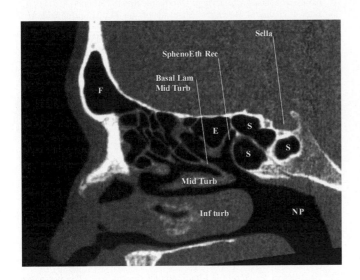

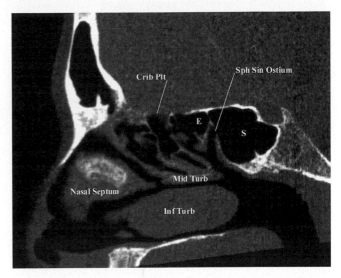

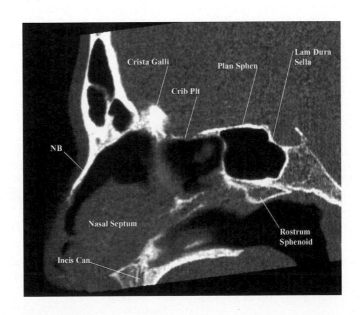

# REFERENCES

1. Tardy M, ed. Surgical Anatomy of the Nose. New York, NY: Raven Press, 1990;1, 47, 65.
2. Williams H. Basic science and related disciplines. In: Paparella M, Shumrick D, eds. Otolaryngology. Vol. 1. Philadelphia, WB Saunders, 1973;329–346.
3. Last R, ed. Anatomy Regional and Applied. 6th ed. Edinburgh and London: Churchill Livingstone, 1978;398–406.
4. Hollinshead W. The nose and paranasal sinuses. In: Hollinshead W, ed. Anatomy for Surgeons. Vol. 1. New York: Hoeber-Harper, 1954; 229–281.
5. Goss C, ed. Gray's Anatomy of the Human Body. 27th ed. Philadelphia: Lea & Febiger, 1963.
6. Graney D, Baker S. Anatomy. In: Cummings C, Fredrickson J, Harker L, Krause C, Schuller D, eds. Otolaryngology: Head and Neck Surgery, Vol 1. 2nd ed. St. Louis: CV Mosby, 1993;627–639.
7. Zinreich SJ, Kennedy DW, Kumar AJ, et al. MR imaging of normal nasal cycle: comparison with sinus pathology. J Comput Assist Tomogr 1988;12:1014–1019.
8. Phillips P, McCaffrey T, Kern E. Physiology of the human nose. In: Blitzer A, Lawson W, Friedman W, eds. Surgery of the Paranasal Sinuses. Philadelphia: WB Saunders, 1991;25–40.
9. Meyerhoff W. Physiology of the nose and paranasal sinuses. In: Paparella M, Shumrick D, eds. Otolaryngology. Vol 1. 2nd ed. Philadelphia: WB Saunders, 1980;297–318.
10. Kimmelman C. The problem of nasal obstruction. In: Kimmelman C, ed. The Otolaryngologic Clinics of North America. Vol 22. Philadelphia: WB Saunders, 1989;253–264.
11. Paff G, ed. Anatomy of the Head and Neck. Philadelphia: WB Saunders, 1973;183–203.
12. Leopold D. Physiology of olfaction. In: Cummings C, Fredrickson J, Harker L, Krause C, Schuller D, eds. Otolaryngology—Head and Neck Surgery. Vol 1. 2nd ed. St. Louis: CV Mosby, 1993; 640–664.
13. Abramson M, Harker L. Physiology of the nose. In: Bernstein L, ed. The Otolaryngologic Clinics of North America. Vol 6. Philadelphia: WB Saunders, 1973;623–635.
14. Hilger J, Hilger P. Physiology of the nose and paranasal sinuses. In: Goldman J, ed. Principles and Practice of Rhinology. New York: Wiley, 1987;15–25.
15. Yousem DM, Geckle RJ, Bilker WB et al. Posttraumatic olfactory dysfunction: MR and clinical evaluation. AJNR 1996;17:1171–1179.
16. Osborn A. The nasal arteries. Am J Roentgenol 1978;130:89–97.
17. Fried R. The Hyperventilation Syndrome: Research and Clinical Treatment. Baltimore: Johns Hopkins University Press, 1987.
18. Schaeffer J, eds. The Embryology, Development and Anatomy of the Nose, Paranasal Sinuses, Nasolacrimal Passageways and Olfactory Organs in Man. Philadelphia: P. Blakiston's Son, 1920.
19. Graney D. Anatomy. In: Cummings C, Fredrickson J, Harker L, et al, eds. Otolaryngology: Head and Neck Surgery. Vol 1. St. Louis: CV Mosby, 1993;845–850.
20. Van Alyea O. Nasal Sinuses: Anatomic and Clinical Considerations. 2nd ed. Baltimore: Williams & Wilkins, 1951.
21. Ritter R. The Paranasal Sinuses: Anatomy and Surgical Technique. 2nd ed. St. Louis: CV Mosby, 1978.
22. Wigand M. Endoscopic Surgery of the Paranasal Sinuses and Anterior Skull Base. New York: Thieme, 1990.
23. Mosher H. Symposium on the ethmoid. The surgical anatomy of the ethmoid labyrinth. Trans Am Acad Ophthalmol Otolaryngol 1929: 376–410.
24. Hajek N, ed. Pathology and Treatment of the Inflammatory Diseases of the Nasal Accessory Sinuses. 5th ed. Vols. 1, 2. St. Louis: CV Mosby, 1926.
25. Hollingshead W, ed. Anatomy for Surgeons. 3rd ed. Vol. 1. Philadelphia: Harper & Row, 1982.
26. Zinreich SJ, Mattox DE, Kennedy DW, et al. Concha bullosa: CT evaluation. J Comput Assist Tomogr 1988;12:778–784.
27. Dodd G, Jing B. Radiology of the Nose, Paranasal Sinuses and Nasopharynx. Baltimore: Williams & Wilkins, 1977;59–65.
28. Urken M, Som P, Lawson W, et al. The abnormally large frontal sinus. Part I: a practical method for its determination based upon an analysis of 100 normal patients. Laryngoscope 1987;97:602–605.
29. Enlow D. Handbook of Facial Growth. Philadelphia: WB Saunders, 1975;120–121.
30. Shapiro R, Schorr S. A consideration of the systemic factors that influence frontal sinus pneumatization. Invest Radiol 1980;15: 191–202.
31. Fujioka M, Young L. The sphenoidal sinuses: radiographic pattern of normal development and abnormal findings in infants and children. Radiology 1978;129:133–136.
32. Yanagisawa E, Smith H. Normal radiographic anatomy of the paranasal sinuses. Otolaryngol Clin North Am 1973;6:429–457.
33. Etter L. Atlas of Roentgen Anatomy of the Skull. Springfield, IL: Charles C. Thomas, 1955.
34. Goldman J. Intranasal sphenoethmoidectomy and antrostomy. In: Goldman J, ed. The Principles and Practice of Rhinology. New York: Wiley, 1987;403–411.
35. Graney D. Anatomy. In: Cummings C, Fredrickson J, Harker L, et al., eds. Otolaryngology: Head and Neck Surgery. 2nd ed. Vol 1. St. Louis: CV Mosby, 1993;901–906.
36. Pandolfo I, Gaeta M, Blandino A, Longo M. The radiology of the pterygoid canal: normal and pathologic findings. AJNR 1987;8: 479–483.
37. Proetz A. Essays on the Applied Physiology of the Nose. St. Louis: Annals Publishing, 1953.
38. Alberti P. Applied surgical anatomy of the maxillary sinus. Otolaryngol Clin North Am 1976;9:3–20.
39. Karmody C, Carter B, Vincent M. Developmental anomalies of the maxillary sinus. Trans Am Acad Ophthalmol Otolaryngol 1977;84: 723–728.
40. Sperber G. Craniofacial Embryology. 4th ed. London: Wright, 1989;144–146.
41. Merril V, ed. Atlas of Roentgenographic Positions. 3rd ed. St. Louis: CV Mosby, 1967.
42. Yanagisawa E, Smith H. Radiographic anatomy of the paranasal sinuses IV: Caldwell view. Arch Otolaryngol 1968;87:311–322.
43. Yanagisawa E, Smith H, Merrell R. Radiographic anatomy of the paranasal sinuses III: submentovertical view. Arch Otolaryngol 1968;87:299–310.
44. Yanagisawa E, Smith H, Thaler S. Radiographic anatomy of the paranasal sinuses II: lateral view. Arch Otolaryngol 1968;87:196–209.
45. Yanagisawa E, Smith H. Radiology of the normal maxillary sinus and related structures. Otolaryngol Clin North Am 1976;9:55–81.
46. Zizmor J, Noyek A. Radiology of the nose and paranasal sinuses. In: Paparella M, Shumrick D, eds. Otolaryngology. Vol. 1. Philadelphia: WB Saunders, 1973;1043–1095.
47. Potter G, ed. Sectional Anatomy and Tomography of the Head. New York: Grune & Stratton, 1971.
48. Gambarelli J, Greinel G, Chevrot L, et al. Computerized Axial Tomography: An Anatomic Atlas of Serial Sections of the Human Body, Anatomy-Radiology-Scanner. Berlin: Springer-Verlag, 1977.
49. Ferner H, ed. Pernkopf Atlas of Topographical and Applied Human Anatomy. Vol. 1. Baltimore: Urban and Schwarzenberg, 1980.
50. Schatz C, Becker T. Normal and CT anatomy of the paranasal sinuses. Radiol Clin North Am 1984;22:107–118.
51. Terrier F, Weber W, Ruenfenacht D, et al. Anatomy of the ethmoid: CT endoscopic and macroscopic. AJNR 1985;6:77–84.
52. Mafee M. Preoperative imaging anatomy of nasal-ethmoid complex for functional endoscopic sinus surgery. Radiol Clin North Am 1993;31:1–30.
53. Mafee M, Chow J, Meyers R. Functional endoscopic sinus surgery: anatomy, CT screening, indications, and complications. AJR 1993; 160:735–744.
54. Hudgins P. Complications of endoscopic sinus surgery: role of the radiologist in prevention. Radiol Clin North Am 1993;31:21–32.
55. Som P. Paranasal sinuses and pterygopalatine fossa. In: Carter B, ed. Computed Tomography. New York: Churchill Livingstone, 1985; 101–130.
56. Mancuso A, Hanafee W, ed. Computed Tomography and Magnetic Resonance Imaging of the Head and Neck. Baltimore: Williams & Wilkins, 1985;1–19.
57. Brant-Zawadzki M, Norman D. Magnetic Resonance Imaging of the Central Nervous System. New York: Raven Press, 1987.
58. Lloyd G, Lund V, PD P, et al. Magnetic resonance imaging in the evaluation of nose and paranasal sinus disease. Br. J Radiol 1987;60:957–968.

59. Vogl T, Mack M, Juergens M, et al. MR Diagnosis of head and neck tumors: comparison of contrast enhancement with triple-dose gadodiamide and standard-dose gadopentetate dimeglumine in the same patient. AJR 1994;163:425–432.

60. Yousem D, Kennedy D, Rosenberg S. Ostiomeatal complex risk factors for sinusitis: CT evaluation. J Otolaryngol 1991;20: 419–424.

61. Yousem D. Imaging of sinonasal inflammatory disease. Radiology 1993;188:303–314.

62. Lanzieri C, Shah M, Krauss D, et al. Use of gadolinium-enhanced MR imaging for differentiating mucocele from neoplasm in the paranasal sinuses. Radiology 1991;178:425–428.

63. Graney D, Baker S. Anatomy. In: Cummings C, Fredrickson J, Harker L, et al., eds. Otolaryngology: Head and Neck Surgery. 2nd ed. Vol. 1. St. Louis: CV Mosby, 1993;305–314.

64. Quiring D, Warfel J. The Head, Neck, and Trunk Muscles and Motor Points. 2nd ed. Philadelphia: Lea & Febiger, 1960.

65. Gray S, Skandalakis J. Embryology for Surgeons: The Embryological Basis for the Treatment of Congenital Defects. Philadelphia: WB Saunders, 1972.

# ATLAS OF NORMAL ANATOMY
# OF THE PARANASAL SINUSES

| | |
|---|---|
| AEthCan | Anterior Ethmoidal Canal |
| Agger Nasi Cell | Agger Nasi Ethmoid Cell Deep to Lacrimal Bone |
| Alv Rec M | Alveolar Recess of Maxillary Sinus |
| Ant Clin Proc | Anterior Clinoid Process |
| AntCranFossa | Anterior Cranial Fossa |
| AntEth Can | Anterior Ethmoidal Canal |
| Ant Nas Spine | Anterior Nasal Spine |
| Att Inf Turb | Attachment of Inferior Turbinate |
| Basal Lam Mid Turb | Basal Lamella of the Middle Turbinate |
| Bas Nas Cav | Base of Nasal Cavity Above Hard Palate |
| Bas Nas Sep | Base of the Nasal Septum as it attaches to Hard Palate |
| Bulla | Bulla Ethmoidalis |
| Can | Canine Tooth |
| Car Can | Carotid Canal |
| Cen Inc | Central Incisor Tooth |
| CG | Crista Galli |
| Clivus | Clivus |
| Colum | Columella |
| Concha Bullos | Concha Bullosa Middle Turbinate |
| Cor Proc | Coronoid Process of Mandible |
| Cort Wt Line | Cortical Dense White Line Surrounding the Frontal Sinuses |
| Crib Plt | Cribriform Plate |
| Crista Galli | Crista Galli |
| DS | Dorsum Sellae |
| E | Ethmoid Sinus |
| F | Frontal Sinus |
| FB | Frontal Bone |
| Floor of Sella | Floor of Sella Turcica |
| For Lac | Foramen Lacerum |
| For Ovale | Foramen Ovale |
| For Rot | Foramen Rotundum |
| Fovea Eth | Fovea Ethmoidalis of Frontal Bone |
| F Proc Max | Frontal Process of Maxilla |
| FrontZyg Sut | Fronto-Zygomatic Suture |
| Fst Mol | First Molar Tooth |
| Fst Pre Mol | First Premolar Tooth |
| Gr Pal Can | Greater Palatine Canal |
| Great Wing Sph | Greater Wing of the Sphenoid Bone |
| Hamulus Med Pter Plt | Hamulus of the Medial Pterygoid Plate |
| Hard Pal | Hard Palate |
| Hor Plt Pal | Horizontal Plate of Palatine Bone |
| IC Lig | Interclinoid Ligament |
| Incis Can | Incisive Canal |
| Incis For | Incisive Foramen |
| Inf Meatus | Inferior Meatus |
| InfOrCan | Infraorbital Canal |
| InfOrFis | Inferior Orbital Fissure |
| InfOrFor | Infraorbital Foramen |
| InfTemFossa | Infratemporal Fossa |
| Inf Turb | Inferior Turbinate |
| Infra Or Canal | Infraorbital Canal |
| Infra Or For | Infraorbital Foramen |
| IOF | Inferior Orbital Fissure |
| Lac Bone | Lacrimal Bone |
| Lac Sac Fossa | Lacrimal Sac Fossa |
| Lam Dura Sella | Lamina Dura of Sella |
| LamPap | Lamina Papyracea of Ethmoid |
| Lat Inc | Lateral Incisor Tooth |
| Lat Pter Plt | Lateral Pterygoid Plate |
| Lat Rec S | Lateral Recess of Sphenoid Sinus |
| Lac Sac | Lacrimal Saccule |
| Les Pal Can | Lesser Palatine Canal |
| Less Wing Sph | Lesser Wing of the Sphenoid Bone |
| Limbus | Sphenoid Bone Limbus |
| LPap | Lamina Papyracea Ethmoid |
| M | Maxillary Sinus |
| Man Hd | Mandibular Head |
| Mand For and Can | Mandibular Foramen and Upper Canal |
| Mand Notch | Mandibular Notch |
| Max Alv | Maxillary Alveolus |
| Max Exost | Maxillary Exostosis |
| Max Pal Sut | Maxillary Palatine Suture |
| Max Teeth Rts | Maxillary Teeth Roots |
| MB | Maxillary Bone |
| Med Pter Plt | Medial Pterygoid Plate |
| Med Wall M | Medial Wall of Maxillary Sinus |
| MidCranFossa | Middle Cranial Fossa |
| Mid Meatus | Middle Meatus |
| Mid Sut Pal | Midline Suture Between Left and Right Halves of Hard Palate |
| Mid Turb | Middle Turbinate |
| MSept | Maxillary Sinus Septum |
| Nasal Cavity | Nasal Cavity Airway |
| Nasal Fossa | Nasal Fossa Air Space |
| Nasal Septum | Nasal Septum |
| NasoLac Duct | Nasolacrimal Duct |
| NasoFtl Sut | Nasofrontal Suture |
| NasoLac Can | Nasolacrimal Canal |
| NB | Nasal Bone |
| Nose | Nose Cartilages and Soft Tissues |
| Nostril | Nostril of Nose |
| NP | Nasopharynx |
| OC | Optic Canal |
| Olf Groove | Olfactory Groove |
| OlfRec | Olfactory Recess |
| Open Nasolac Duct | Opening of the Nasolacrimal Duct into the Middle Meatus |
| Opt Can | Optic Canal |
| Or | Orbit |
| Or Roof | Orbital Roof |
| Pal Proc Max | Palatine Process of Maxilla |
| Palatal Recesses Max | Palatal Recesses of the Maxillary Sinuses |
| PerpPlt Eth | Perpendicular Plate of the Ethmoid Bone |
| Pet Apex | Petrous Apex |
| PEthCan | Posterior Ethmoidal Canal |
| Plan Sphen | Planum Sphenoidale |
| Post Ant Cr Fossa | Posterior Edge of Anterior Cranial Fossa |

| | |
|---|---|
| PostEth Can | Posterior Ethmoidal Canal |
| PPF | Pterygopalatine Fossa |
| Pter Fossa | Pterygoid Fossa |
| Ptery Proc S | Pterygoid Process of Sphenoid |
| Pty Rec S | Pterygoid Recess of Sphenoid Sinus |
| Ramus Man | Ramus of Mandible |
| Rostrum Sphenoid | Rostrum of Sphenoid Bone |
| S | Sphenoid Sinus |
| SB | Sphenoid Bone |
| Sec Mol | Second Molar Tooth |
| Sec Pre Mol | Second Premolar Tooth |
| Sella | Sella Turcica |
| Septum | Septum Within a Sinus |
| SphenoEth Rec | Sphenoethmoidal Recess |
| Sph Sin Ostium | Sphenoid Sinus Ostium |
| SOF | Superior Orbital Fissure |
| S Sep | Sphenoid Sinus Septum |
| STSut | Sphenotemporal Suture |
| Styl Proc | Styloid Process |
| Supraor Can | Supraorbital Canal Tub |
| Supraor Grv | Supraorbital Groove |
| Sup Turb | Superior Turbinate |
| SZySut | Sphenozygomatic Suture |
| Thd Mol | Third Molar Tooth |
| Torus Pal | Torus Palatinus |
| Torus Tub | Torus Tubarius |
| Tub Sel | Tuberculum Sellae |
| Uncin Proc | Uncinate Process of Ethmoid |

| | |
|---|---|
| Vidian Can | Vidian Canal (Pterygoid Canal) |
| Vomer | Vomer |
| ZB | Zygomatic Bone |
| Zyg Arch | Zygomatic Arch |
| ZygoTemp Can | Zygomaticotemporal Canal |

Within the axial anatomic atlas, Figures 10A, B, and C show variations in the size of the sphenoid sinuses with lateral and pterygoid recesses. Figure 21A shows an alveolar recess of the maxillary sinus, with the sinus extending caudal to the hard palate. Figures 21B and C show the incisive canals and the incisor foramen.

Within the coronal anatomic atlas, Figure 10 shows variations in the pneumatization of the lower maxillary sinus. Figure 10A shows palatal recesses. Figure 10B shows lack of pneumatization of the maxillary alveolus. Figure 10C shows pneumatization of the inferior turbinate. Figure 11 shows a typical example of a torus palatinus and maxillary exostoses. Axial Figure 16A and coronal Figure 11B show pneumatization of the inferior turbinate by the maxillary sinus. Figures 14-17 show variations in sphenoid sinus configuration and the location of the foramen rotundum and Vidian canals near and within the sinus. Axial and coronal Figures 1B show frontal sinus pneumatization of the orbital roofs. The presence of bone between the ethmoid complex and the recess differentiates these from supraorbital ethmoid cells.

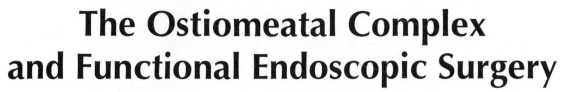

## 3

# The Ostiomeatal Complex and Functional Endoscopic Surgery

*S. James Zinreich, Sait Albayram,
Mark L. Benson, and Patrick J. Oliverio*

## HISTORIC PERSPECTIVE

Sinonasal inflammatory disease is a serious health problem that affects an estimated 30 to 50 million people in the United States.[1] Traditionally, plain films were the modality of choice in evaluation of sinus pathology. Clinical and radiographic emphasis was directed primarily to the maxillary and frontal sinuses. In recent years, it has become evident that sinusitis is primarily a clinical diagnosis. The role of imaging is to document the extent of disease, to answer questions regarding ambiguous cases, and to provide an accurate display of the anatomy of the sinonasal system.

Imaging now provides the surgeon with a detailed "road map" for guiding the functional endoscopic sinus surgery procedure. Today, computed tomography (CT) is the modality of choice for the imaging evaluation of the morphology in this area.

Although most patients with sinonasal inflammatory disease are initially treated medically, the disease often does not resolve. Patients with persistent disease usually require surgical intervention, and the surgical treatment of refractory inflammatory sinus disease has undergone revolutionary changes in the last 10 to 20 years. These advances are due to an improved understanding of the mucociliary clearance pathways in the nasal cavity and paranasal sinuses, improved endoscopes that afford direct access to nasal cavity and ethmoid sinus drainage portals, and the availability of high-resolution coronal CT images that provide an accurate display of the regional anatomy.

Functional endoscopic sinus surgery (FESS) was first described independently by both Messerklinger in the German literature and Wigand, Steiner, and Jaumann in the English literature in 1978.[2–4] FESS was introduced in the United States in 1984 by Kennedy et al., and subsequent evolution of the technique has occurred through innovations in both the surgical and radiologic fields.[5, 6]

This chapter will discuss the imaging modalities available for patients with surgically amenable inflammatory sinus disease and describe the pertinent imaging anatomy and anatomic variants of the paranasal sinuses and adjacent structures, review the radiographic appearance of inflammatory sinus disease and describe FESS procedures.

## TECHNIQUES OF EVALUATION

### Plain Films

The standard plain film sinus series usually consists of four views: lateral, Caldwell, Waters, and submentovertex. The anatomy displayed on each of these views is reviewed in Chapter 2.[7] Although the standard radiographs may be accurate in showing air-fluid levels, the degree of chronic inflammatory disease present is consistently and significantly underestimated. Furthermore, the superimposition of structures precludes the accurate evaluation of the anatomy of the ostiomeatal channels, with which the modern surgeon needs to be familiar.[6, 8–11]

### Computed Tomography

CT is currently the modality of choice in the evaluation of the paranasal sinuses and adjacent structures.[6, 8–11] Its ability to optimally display bone, soft tissue, and air provides an accurate depiction of both the anatomy and the extent of disease in and around the paranasal sinuses.[6, 8–11] In contrast to standard radiographs, CT clearly shows the fine bony anatomy of the ostiomeatal channels.

Many authors stress the importance of performing the initial CT scan after a course of adequate medical therapy to eliminate or diminish reversible mucosal inflammation. Several authors also suggest routine pretreatment with a sympathomimetic nasal spray 15 minutes prior to scanning in order to reduce nasal congestion (mucosal edema) and thus improve the display of the fine bony architecture and any irreversible mucosal disease.[12]

The coronal plane best shows the ostiomeatal unit (OMU), shows the relationship of the brain to the ethmoid roof, and correlates closely with the surgical orientation. Thus, the coronal plane should be the primary imaging orientation for evaluation of the sinonasal tract in all patients with inflammatory sinus disease who are endoscopic surgical candidates.[6–8, 11] This can be accomplished by direct coronal scanning or by reformatting data acquired in the axial plane into coronal plane images.

If direct scanning is done, the coronal study optimally should be performed in the prone position so that any remaining sinus secretions do not obscure the OMU. In patients who cannot tolerate prone positioning (children, patients of advanced age, etc.), the hanging head technique can sometimes be utilized. In this technique, the patient is placed in the supine position and the neck is maximally extended. A pillow placed under the patient's shoulders facilitates positioning. The CT gantry is then angled to be perpendicular to the hard palate. However, it is not always possible to obtain true direct coronal images with this technique.

Patients who are intubated or have tracheostomy tubes usually cannot tolerate positioning for coronal scans. Similarly, young children, patients with severe cervical arthropathy, and patients who are otherwise debilitated often cannot tolerate direct coronal positioning. In such patients, spiral scanning or thin section, contiguous axial CT images with coronal reconstructions are performed.

Axial images complement the coronal study, particularly when there is severe disease (opacification) of any of the paranasal sinuses and surgical treatment is contemplated. The axial studies are needed, as the posterior walls of various sinuses are not well seen, if at all, in the coronal plane. Axial images are particularly important in visualizing the frontoethmoid junction and the sphenoethmoid recess.

Today spiral CT offers the advantage of speed and the ability to generate very thin images. With the use of double spiral scanners or multidetector technology, the slice thickness can be reduced to 0.5 mm or less. For the pediatric, elderly, and debilitated patients who may not be able to remain still for prolonged periods of time, this technique offers the best opportunity to acquire a motion-free, high-quality study. The patient may be positioned prone with the head hyperextended or supine with the head in neutral position on the scanning table. Given the ability of spiral CT to generate very thin images, the quality of reconstructed coronal and/or sagittal images is virtually indistinguishable from that of images obtained in the primary scan plane. In phantom studies performed with the parameters outlined in Box 3-1, a lens dose of 14 mGy was measured for scanning the paranasal sinuses in either the axial or coronal position.[13]

The recent introduction of multidetector CT scanners has allowed even more refined reconstructions in planes other than the primary scan plane. Motion and reconstruction artifacts may still create very minor image degradation, but this is offset by the lack of obscuration of important anatomy by "spray" artifact from dental restorations. Since the original data set is acquired in the axial plane, the important

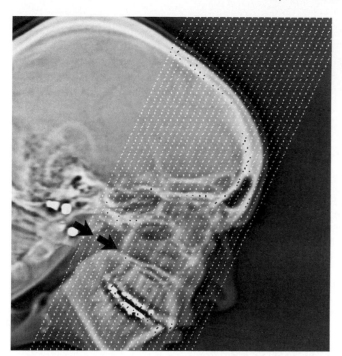

**FIGURE 3-1** CT lateral topogram shows the patient's position during the examination. Dotted lines represent the scanner gantry angulation, which should be as perpendicular as possible to the hard palate (*arrows*).

anatomy of the OMU is not imaged at the same time as the metallic restorations, so the artifact is projected well away from the crucial landmarks. This multidetector scanner most likely will become the scanner of choice for imaging the sinonasal cavities.

### Examination Protocol

For direct coronal scanning, the patient is placed prone on the scanner table, with the chin hyperextended. The scanner gantry is angled perpendicular to the hard palate (Fig. 3-1). The angulation of the scan plane is very important, as Melhem et al. noted that variations in scan angulation greater than 10° from the plane perpendicular to the hard palate result in significant loss of anatomic detail of the structures of the OMU.[14]

Scanning is performed as contiguous 3-mm-thick images from the anterior wall of the frontal sinus through the posterior wall of the sphenoid sinus. Contiguous scans are essential to avoid loss of information through "skipped" areas.[14] The field of view should be adjusted to include only the areas of interest. This not only helps reduce artifact from the teeth and associated metallic restorations, but magnifies the small anatomic structures of the nasal cavity and adjacent paranasal sinuses.[9]

The original exposure settings for sinus CT were 125 kVp, 450 mAs, and 5-second scan time. However, Babbel et al. showed that there was no compromise of image quality when the milliampere-second (mAs) setting was reduced to 200 mAs (2-second scan time), and recent work by Melhem et al. showed no significant loss of diagnostic quality with mAs settings of 160 or even 80 mAs (2-second scan time).[12, 14] It is therefore recommended that the exposure

---

**SUMMARY BOX 3-1**

**Parameters for Sinus CT**

| | |
|---|---|
| Patient position | Prone |
| Angulation | Perpendicular to hard palate |
| Field of view | 14 cm |
| Thickness | 3 mm, contiguous |
| Exposure | 125 kVp and 80–160 mAs |

---

settings be 125 kVp and 80 to 160 mAs. Box 3-1 summarizes the sinus CT examination protocol.[10]

### Radiation Exposure

To review briefly, the radiation exposure (dose) that a patient receives is known as the radiation-absorbed dose. This dose is a measure of the total radiation energy absorbed by the tissues, and it is expressed in an SI unit known as the *Gray* (Gy). One Gy is the amount of radiation needed to deposit the energy of 1 joule (J) in 1 kg of tissue (Gy = 1 J/kg). Formerly, the unit used to express the radiation-absorbed dose was the *rad* (1 rad = amount of radiation needed to deposit the energy of 100 ergs in 1 g tissue). The conversion of the rad to the Gy is: 1 Gy = 100 rad.[15, 16]

A more useful term is *radiation dose equivalent*, which takes into account the quality factor $Q$ of the radiation (radiation dose equivalent = radiation dose absorbed × $Q$). This quality factor accounts for the varying biologic effectiveness of different forms of ionizing radiation. For x-rays, $Q = 1$; thus, the radiation-absorbed dose is equivalent to the radiation dose equivalent. Currently the SI unit of radiation dose equivalent is the *Sievert* (Sv); the former unit was the *rem*. Therefore, for diagnostic x-rays, 1 Gy = 1 Sv and 1 Sv = 100 rem.[15, 16]

The radiation dose equivalent is dependant on the kilovolt peak (kVp) and mAs. For a given kVp, the radiation dose equivalent varies linearly with the mAs. At 125 kVp the radiation dose equivalent for a CT slice is approximately 1.1 to 1.2 cSv/100 mAs (1.1 to 1.2 rem/100 mAs). The actual dose varies slightly from machine to machine. Table 3-1 shows that the radiation dose equivalent for a CT slice can be considerably reduced using a low mAs technique.[10]

In contiguous CT imaging, the dose delivered to a particular region scanned (for example, the paranasal sinuses) is approximately equal to the per-slice dose. The dose delivered to a region is less than the per-slice dose if

**Table 3-1**
**RELATIVE RADIATION DOSE FOR SINUS CT**
**(UTILIZING 125 kVp)**

| mAs | Radiation Dose Equivalent |
|---|---|
| 450 | 4.95–5.40 cSv (4.95–5.40 rem) |
| 240 | 2.64–2.88 cSv (2.64–2.88 rem) |
| 160 | 1.76–1.92 cSv (1.76–1.92 rem) |
| 80 | 0.88–0.96 cSv (0.88–0.96 rem) |

Source: Zinreich S. Imaging of inflammatory sinus disease. Otolaryngol Clin North Am 1993;26(4):535–547.

**Table 3-2**
**ESTIMATED EFFECTIVE DOSE EQUIVALENT
OF COMMON EXAMINATIONS**

| Examination | Effective Dose Equivalent |
|---|---|
| Sinus series, four views | 7.0 mrem |
| Chest, PA and lateral | 7.2 mrem |
| Kidneys, ureters, bladder (KUB) | 8.7 mrem |
| Lumbar spine, five views | 125.1 mrem |
| CT, brain* | 112.0 mrem |
| CT, sinus (160 mAs)† | 51.2 mrem |
| CT, sinus (80 mAs)‡ | 25.6 mrem |

*120 kVp, 240 mAs, 10-mm slice thickness, contiguous.
†125 kVp, 160 mAs, 3-mm slice thickness, contiguous.
‡125 kVp, 80 mAs, 3-mm slice thickness, contiguous.
Source: Zinreich S. Imaging of inflammatory sinus disease. Otolaryngol Clin North Am 1993;26(4):535–547 and Zinreich S, Abidin M, Kennedy D. Cross-sectional imaging of the nasal cavity and paranasal sinuses. Operative Techniques Otolaryngol Head Neck Surg 1990;1(2):93–99.

there is a gap between slices, and the delivered dose is higher if there is overlap between slices.

### Image Display

The effective dose equivalent was developed as a way of representing the fraction of the total stochastic risk of fatal cancers and chromosomal abnormalities resulting from the irradiation of a particular organ or tissue when the body is uniformly irradiated.[15, 16] A system of weighting is used to take into account the individual sensitivity of the body's major tissues and organs.[15, 16] A full discussion of the effective dose is beyond the scope of this chapter. Suffice it to say that for a given examination, the effective dose to the patient is less than the dose (radiation dose equivalent) received by the area scanned. A list of effective dose equivalents for some common radiographic procedures is presented in Table 3-2.[15, 17]

Windows are chosen to highlight the air passages, the bony detail, and the soft tissues. Usually a window width of +2000 Houndsfield units (HU) and a level of −200 HU are good starting parameters. The window and level settings can then be manipulated manually to display optimally the anatomic detail of the uncinate process and ethmoid bulla.

Once this is accomplished, these settings can be used to film the entire study.[6, 8–11]

Sagittal reconstructions can be obtained for a morphologic orientation, and various distances and angles can be measured to aid in the passage of instruments during surgery. If only coronal scans are obtained, axial reconstructions can help display the position of the internal carotid arteries and optic nerves with respect to the bony margins of the posterior ethmoid and sphenoid sinuses.

## Magnetic Resonance Imaging

Although magnetic resonance (MR) imaging provides better visualization of soft tissue than CT, its disadvantage is its inability to display optimally the cortical bone–air interface.[9, 10] Because both cortical bone and air have signal voids, at times MR imaging is unable to discern the intricate anatomic relationships of the sinuses and their drainage portals. Thus, MR imaging cannot be reliably used as an operative road map to guide the surgeon during FESS.

## NASAL CYCLE

There is a side-to-side cyclic variation in the thickness of the nasal mucosa known as the nasal cycle (see Chapter 2), and the signal intensity of the mucosal lining of the nasal cavity and the ethmoid sinuses varies in concert with the nasal cycle.[18, 19] Thus, during the edematous phase of the nasal cycle, the mucosal signal intensity on T2-weighted images is similar to the appearance of mucosal inflammation, limiting the usefulness of MR imaging in these patients (Fig. 3-2).[11, 12] Interestingly, there is no cyclic variation of the mucosal signal in the frontal, maxillary, or sphenoid sinuses, and increased mucosal thickness and increased signal on T2-weighted images in these sinuses are always abnormal.[18, 19] To date, with respect to the paranasal sinuses, MR imaging has proven most helpful in the evaluation of the regional and intracranial complications of inflammatory sinus disease, in identifying complications of its surgical treatment, and in mapping neoplastic diseases (see Chapters 5 to 7).[20–24]

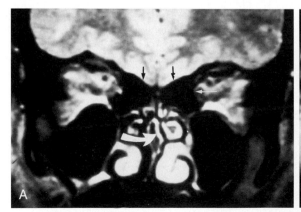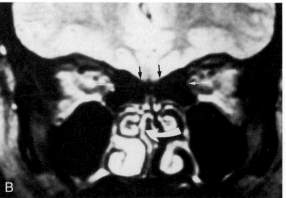

**FIGURE 3-2**    Nasal cycle on MR imaging. **A** and **B**, Coronal T2-weighted MR images of the anterior ethmoid sinuses show the changing edema of the nasal cavity (*curved arrow*), the ethmoid sinus mucosa, and the changing size of the turbinates. Note the lack of signal for definition of the ethmoid sinus roof and lamina papyracea (*arrows*).

# INTERPRETATION OF IMAGING STUDIES

In any imaging study, the radiologist must use a variety of skills to provide consistent, accurate interpretations. With regard to the paranasal sinuses, these skills include the following:

1. Detailed knowledge of the anatomy of the paranasal sinuses
2. Systematic reading pattern
3. Detailed knowledge of the common pathologies affecting the region
4. Working knowledge of the available surgical options and their radiographic appearance
5. Awareness of common operative complications and their radiographic appearance

# NORMAL ANATOMY

## Mucociliary Clearance

An understanding of the regional anatomy and the importance of the anterior ethmoid sinus structures is critical if one is to understand the flow pattern of the mucous blanket coating the paranasal sinuses. The movement of this mucous blanket is referred to as mucociliary clearance. Further, one must be acquainted with the concept that inflammatory sinus disease results primarily from interference of mucociliary clearance due to compromise of the drainage portals (ostiomeatal channels) of the individual sinus cavities.

The mucosa of the paranasal sinuses and nasal fossae is made up of a ciliated cuboidal epithelium that secretes mucus. This mucus covers the epithelium and, as such, is referred to as a mucous blanket. The cilia are in constant motion and act in concert to propel the mucus in each sinus toward the sinus ostium and then, once in the nasal fossae, back toward the pharynx (see also Chapter 2). The pattern of flow is specific for each sinus and persists even if alternative openings are surgically created in the sinus.[25–27] One of the reasons that FESS has gained such wide acceptance is that its goal is to restore sinus drainage via the normal anatomic drainage pathways, thus allowing normal mucociliary clearance.

In the maxillary sinus, mucous flow originates in the antral floor and is then directed centripetally toward the primary ostium. The mucus is then transported through the infundibulum to the hiatus semilunaris, whence it passes into the middle meatus and ultimately into the nasopharynx. This pattern of mucus movement persists even after a nasal antrostomy is created.[25–27]

In the frontal sinus, the mucus flows up along the medial wall, laterally across the roof, and medially along the floor. As the flow approaches the medial aspect of the floor, some is directed into the primary ostium and the remainder is recirculated. The cleared mucus travels down the frontal recess and then into the middle meatus, where it joins the flow from the ipsilateral maxillary sinus.[25–27]

The posterior ethmoid and sphenoid sinuses clear their mucus into the sphenoethmoidal recess. The flow then enters the superior meatus and subsequently the nasopharynx.

Thus, there are two main ostiomeatal channels. The anterior OMU includes the frontal sinus ostium, frontal recess, maxillary sinus ostium, infundibulum, and middle meatus. These channels provide communication between the ipsilateral frontal, anterior ethmoid, and maxillary sinuses. The posterior OMU consists of the sphenoid sinus ostium, the sphenoethmoidal recess, and the superior meatus. The imaging investigation of these regions should be directed to optimally display these ostiomeatal channels.

## Normal Anatomy (Ostiomeatal Unit)

Correct interpretation of sinonasal imaging studies requires an understanding of the anatomy of the lateral nasal wall and its relationship to adjacent structures (Fig. 3-3).[28, 29] The lateral nasal wall contains three bulbous projections: the superior, middle, and inferior turbinates (conchae). The turbinates divide the nasal cavity into three distinct air passages: the superior, middle, and inferior meati. Each respective meatus is lateral to its corresponding turbinate. The superior meatus drains the posterior ethmoid air cells and, more posteriorly, the sphenoid sinus (via the sphenoethmoidal recess). The middle meatus receives drainage from the frontal sinus (via the frontal recess), the maxillary sinus (via the maxillary ostium and subsequently the ethmoidal infundibulum), and the anterior ethmoid air cells (via the ethmoid cell ostia). The inferior meatus receives drainage from the nasolacrimal duct.

The imaging evaluation of the morphology of this area should focus on the anatomic structures surrounding three specific "tight spots." Anteriorly, the first area comprises the structures surrounding the frontal recess. The second area consists of the structures surrounding the infundibulum and middle meatus. The third and most posterior area includes the anatomic structures surrounding the sphenoethmoid recess. Summary Boxes 3-2, 3-3, and 3-4 outline the individual anatomic structures found in each of these tight spots.

On CT scanning, the first coronal images display the outline of the frontal sinuses (Fig. 3-4). The frontal sinuses have an overall funnel shape, and their aeration varies from patient to patient and from side to side in individual patients. Some sinuses are small and occupy only the diploic space of the medial frontal bone, while other sinuses can be large enough to extend through the floor of the entire anterior cranial fossa. In general, a central septation separates the left and right sides; however, often there may be several septations. The floor of the frontal sinus slopes inferiorly toward the midline.

Close to the midline, the primary ostium is located in a depression in the floor. The frontal recess is an hourglass-like narrowing between the frontal sinus and the anterior middle meatus through which the frontal sinus drains (Figs. 3-5 to 3-7).[8] It is not a tubular structure, as the term *nasofrontal duct* might imply, and therefore the term *recess* is preferred.

Anterior, lateral, and inferior to the frontal recess is the agger nasi cell. This cell is a remnant ethmoturbinal and is present in nearly all patients. It is aerated and represents the most anterior ethmoid air cell, usually lying deep to the lacrimal bone. It usually borders the primary ostium or floor of the frontal sinus, and thus its size may directly influence

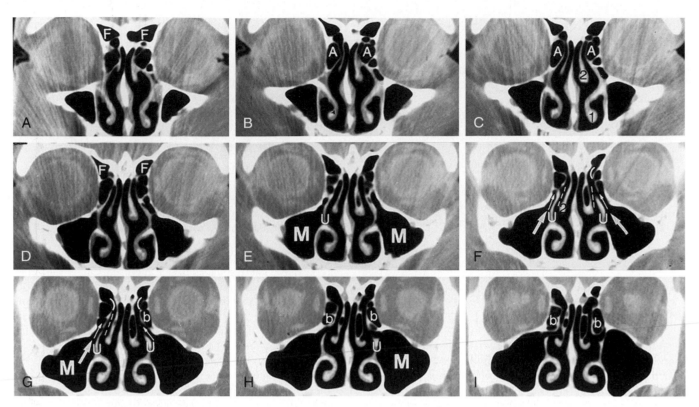

**FIGURE 3-3** Coronal CT display of paranasal sinus anatomy. **A** to **I**, Thin section coronal CT images of a cadaver specimen. Frontal sinus (*F*), agger nasi cell (*A*), ethmoid bulla (*b*), maxillary sinus (*M*), basal lamella (*black arrow*), sphenoid sinus (*S*), inferior turbinate (*1*), middle turbinate (*2*), superior turbinate (*3*). The anterior ostiomeatal unit is displayed in images **F** through **H**. Frontal recess (*small curved lines*), middle meatus (*dashed lines*), infundibulum (*small arrows*), and primary ostium of the maxillary sinus (*large white arrows*).

the patency of the frontal recess and the anterior middle meatus. The frontal recesses are the narrowest anterior air channels and are common sites of inflammation. Their obstruction subsequently results in loss of ventilation and mucociliary clearance of the frontal sinus.

## Frontal Cells

Frontal cells are invariably found in relation to the anterior ethmoid air cells and the agger nasi cell (Fig. 3-7). The recognition and subsequent definition of the appearance and etiology of frontal cells was initiated by J. Parson Schaeffer. During the course of his observations of the embryonic development of the sinuses, he discovered that it is possible, although infrequent, for one cell to aerate each half of the frontal bone, each with a separate communication to the frontal

recess. Schaeffer coined the term *frontal cell* to describe this phenomenon.[30, 31] Van Alyea subsequently defined the frontal cell as a cell encroaching on the frontal recess or frontal sinus.[32–34] He considered supraorbital ethmoid, agger nasi, and intersinus septal cells, as well as cells limited to the frontal recess, as frontal cells. Bent et al.[35] defined frontal cells more specifically as belonging to one of four categories, detailed in Table 3-3. They also stated that all frontal cells derive from the anterior ethmoid sinus behind the agger nasi cell and pneumatize the frontal recess above the agger nasi cell. Each type of frontal cell may obstruct the nasofrontal communication or the frontal sinus itself.

---

### SUMMARY BOX 3-2

**Frontal Recess "Tight Spot" Anatomy**

- Frontal sinus
- Frontal cell(s)
- Agger nasi
- Frontal recess
- Nasofrontal process
    *anterior bony beak
- Middle meatus

---

### SUMMARY BOX 3-3

**Infundibulum/Middle Meatus "Tight Spot" Anatomy**

- Ethmoid bulla
- Uncinate process
- Infundibulum
- Maxillary sinus
- Primary ostium of maxillary sinus
- Middle turbinate
- Middle meatus
- Hiatus semilunaris
- Retrobullar recess
- Basal lamella

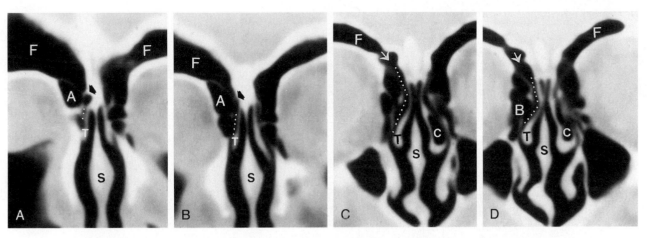

**FIGURE 3-4**   Anatomy of the frontal sinus. Coronal CT images of the frontal sinuses from anterior (**A**) to posterior (**D**) show the relationship between the frontal sinus (*F*) and the middle meatus (*dotted line*). Note that there is a bony strut (*heavy black arrow* in **A** and **B**) separating the frontal sinus and the anterior middle meatus. This separation is lost on the more posterior images (**C** and **D**) revealing the position of the frontal recess (*white arrow*). Note the position of the frontal cell (*A*) and its relationship to the frontal recess. Nasal septum (*S*), ethmoid bulla (*B*), middle turbinate (*T*), and concha bullosa (*C*).

The uncinate process is a superior extension of the lateral nasal wall (medial wall of the maxillary sinus).[8, 10] Anteriorly, the uncinate process fuses with the posteromedial wall of the agger nasi cell and the posteromedial wall of the nasolacrimal duct. The uncinate process has a "free" (unattached) superoposterior edge. Laterally this free edge delimits the infundibulum (Fig. 3-8). The infundibulum is the air passage that connects the maxillary sinus ostium to the middle meatus. Posterior to the uncinate process is the ethmoid bulla, usually the largest of the anterior ethmoid cells. The uncinate process usually courses medial and inferior to the ethmoid bulla. The ethmoid bulla is enclosed laterally by the lamina papyracea.

The gap between the ethmoid bulla and the free edge of the uncinate process defines the hiatus semilunaris. Medially, the hiatus semilunaris communicates with the middle meatus, the air space lateral to the middle turbinate.[8, 10] Laterally and inferiorly, the hiatus semilunaris communicates with the infundibulum, the air channel between the uncinate process (caudal border) and the inferomedial margin of the orbit (cranial border). The infundibulum serves as the primary drainage pathway from the maxillary sinus.[10, 11]

The structure medial to the ethmoid bulla and the uncinate process is the middle turbinate. Anteriorly it attaches to the medial wall of the agger nasi cell and the superior edge of the uncinate process. Superiorly it adheres to the lateral edge of the cribriform plate. As it extends posteriorly, the middle turbinate emits a number of posterolaterally coursing bony structures. The first such "laterally fanning" attachment to the lamina papyracea is the basal lamella, which is posterior to the ethmoid bulla (Figs. 3-9, 3-10). This bony structure serves to separate the anterior and posterior ethmoid cells.

In most patients, the posterior wall of the ethmoid bulla is intact, and an air space is usually found between the basal lamella and the posterior ethmoid bulla. This air space, the sinus lateralis, may extend superior to the ethmoid bulla and

---

### SUMMARY BOX 3-4

**Sphenoethmoid Recess "Tight Spot" Anatomy**
- Superior turbinate
- Posterior ethmoid sinus
- Primary ostium of sphenoid sinus
- Sphenoid sinus
- Optic nerve
- Carotid canal
- Foramen rotundum
- Vidian canal

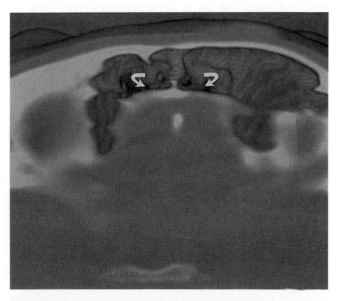

**FIGURE 3-5**   3D image of the floor of the frontal sinus. The roof of the frontal sinus is removed to demonstrate the floor of the frontal sinus, with emphasis on displaying the location of the frontal recess (*curved arrows*).

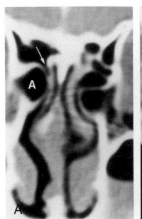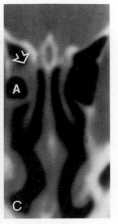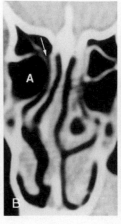

**FIGURE 3-6** Anatomy of the frontal recess. **A** and **B**, Coronal CT images reveal a patent frontal recess (*white arrow*) despite the presence of a large agger nasi cell (*A*). **C**, Coronal CT image in a different patient with an obstructed right frontal recess and mucoperiosteal thickening in the right frontal sinus (*open arrow*). Agger nasi (*A*).

communicate with the frontal recess (Fig. 3-11). Recently, the sinus lateralis has been renamed by an international surgeon's group and is now called the retrobullar recess cell.[36] If it extends above the ethmoid bulla, this extension would be called the suprabullar recess cell. A dehiscence or total absence of the posterior wall of the ethmoid bulla is common and may provide communication between these two usually separated air spaces.

The posterior ethmoid sinus consists of air cells between the basal lamella and the sphenoid sinus. The number, shape, and size of these air cells vary significantly from person to person.[8, 9, 11, 37]

The sphenoid sinus is the most posterior sinus. It is usually embedded in the clivus and is bordered superoposteriorly by the sella turcica. Its ostium is located medially in the anterosuperior portion of the anterior sinus wall and communicates with the sphenoethmoidal recess and the posterior aspect of the superior meatus. The sphenoethmoidal recess lies just lateral to the nasal septum and can sometimes be seen on coronal images, but it is best displayed in the sagittal and axial planes (Figs. 3-12, 3-13).[8, 10]

The relationship between the aerated portion of the sphenoid sinus and the posterior ethmoid sinus must be accurately demonstrated so that the surgeon can avoid operative complications (Fig. 3-14). Usually in the paramedian sagittal plane, the sphenoid sinus is the most superior and posterior air space. Horizontally oriented structures within the sphenoid sinus are actually separations between the posterior ethmoid sinus (Fig. 3-15). All sphenoid sinus septations are vertically oriented. This relationship is well demonstrated on axial and sagittal images. The number and position of the septations in the sphenoid sinus are quite variable, and of particular importance are septations that adhere to the bony canal wall covering the internal carotid artery, which often projects into the posterolateral sphenoid sinus. Less often, the canal of the vidian nerve (pterygoid canal) and the canal of the second division of the trigeminal nerve can project into the floor of the sphenoid sinus.

Anatomically, the paranasal sinuses are in close proximity to the anterior cranial fossa, the cribriform plate, the internal carotid arteries, the cavernous sinuses, the orbits and their contents, and the optic nerves as they exit the orbits.[38-42] The surgeon must be especially cautious when maneuvering instruments directed cranially and dorsally in order to avoid inadvertent penetration and damage to these structures.[6, 11, 40, 41]

## ANATOMIC VARIATIONS AND CONGENITAL ABNORMALITIES

Even though nasal anatomy varies significantly from patient to patient, there are some specific variations that occur repeatedly within the population. The prevalence of these variations, as reported by several groups of investigators, are outlined in Summary Box 3-5.[43-53] Certain anatomic variations are thought to be predisposing factors for the development of sinus disease or operative complications. Thus, it is necessary for the radiologist and surgeon to be cognizant of these variations, especially if the patient is a candidate for FESS.

### Variations of the Middle Turbinate

#### Paradoxic Curvature

Normally, the convexity of the middle turbinate bone is directed medially, toward the nasal septum. When paradoxically curved, the convexity of the bone is directed laterally toward the lateral sinus wall(Fig. 3-16). The inferior edge of the middle turbinate may assume various shapes with exces-

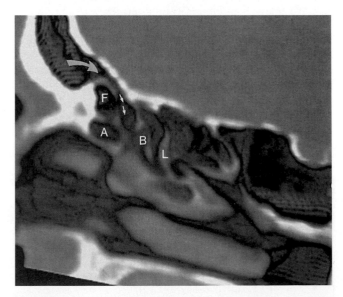

**FIGURE 3-7** Saggital 3D image of the frontal recess and adjacent anatomy. This three-dimensional image of the lateral nasal wall reveals the agger nasi cell (*A*) and the frontal cell (*F*). Note the frontal recess behind these structures (*large curved arrow, small arrows*). Ethmoid bulla (*B*), basal lamella (*L*).

**Table 3-3**
**FRONTAL CELL TYPES I–IV**

| | |
|---|---|
| **TYPE I** | Single frontal recess cell above agger nasi cell |
| **TYPE II** | Tier of cells in frontal recess above agger nasi cell |
| **TYPE III** | Single massive cell pneumatizing cephalad into frontal sinus |
| **TYPE IV** | Single isolated cell within the frontal sinus |

sive curvature, which in turn may narrow and/or obstruct the nasal cavity, infundibulum, and middle meatus. Because of this potential narrowing or obstruction, most authors agree that paradoxic middle turbinates can be a contributing factor to sinusitis. Certain authors have, however, found no significant relationship between paradoxically curved middle turbinates and recurrent sinusitis: Lloyd reported no correlation between the variant and increased incidences of asymptomatic sinusitis, and Calhoun et al. found no statistical correlation between paradoxical curvature of the middle turbinate and symptomatic sinusitis.[44, 54]

### Concha Bullosa

A concha bullosa is an aerated turbinate, most often the middle turbinate. Although it may be either unilateral or bilateral (Fig. 3-17), Lloyd et al. report it occurring bilaterally more frequently.[55] Less frequently, aeration of the superior turbinate may occur, and an aerated inferior turbinate is uncommon. Concha bullosae are classified according to the degree and portion of turbinate pneumatization. When the pneumatization involves the bulbous segment of the middle turbinate, the term *concha bullosa* applies. If only the attachment portion of the middle turbinate is pneumatized, and the pneumatization does not extend into the bulbous segment, it is known as a lamellar concha.

The reported prevalence of concha bullosa, or pneumatized middle turbinate, varies greatly. Two separate cadav-

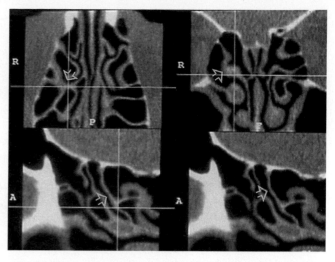

**FIGURE 3-9**   Triplanar display of the basal lamella (*open arrows*).

eric studies found concha bullosa in 8% and 20% of specimens, respectively.[51] The reported prevalence of the radiographic appearance of concha bullosa on coronal CT scans ranges from 14% to 53%.[44, 53] The significant discrepancy in the reported prevalence of concha bullosa is due to several possible factors. Attempts to determine the general prevalence of this variation have been characterized by the use of diverse study populations, different criteria for pneumatization, and analytic methods. These varying features have undoubtedly affected the results of the investigations.

Although middle turbinate pneumatization has been suspected as a potential cause of middle meatal obstruction and resultant sinusitis, the definitive relationship between concha bullosa and sinusitis continues to be debated. A concha bullosa involving the middle turbinate may enlarge

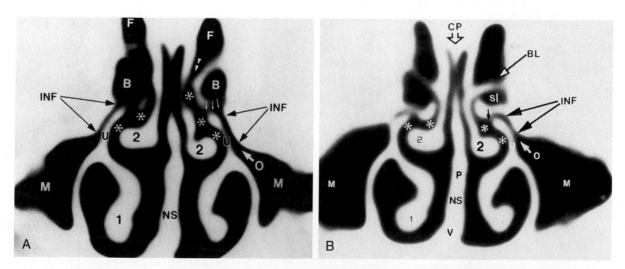

**FIGURE 3-8**   Anterior ostiomeatal channels. Coronal CT images through the anterior ethmoid sinuses show the air passages communicating with the frontal sinus (*F*), anterior ethmoid sinus, and maxillary sinus (*M*). The primary ostium (*O*) of the maxillary sinus communicates with the infundibulum (*INF*). The infundibulum is bordered medially by the uncinate process (*U*) and laterally by the orbit. In turn, the infundibulum communicates with the middle meatus (*asterisks*) through the hiatus semilunaris (*most medial white arrows in* **A**, *small black arrow in* **B**) The frontal recess (*white arrowheads*) is patent. The ethmoid bulla (*B*) is usually the largest air cell in the anterior ethmoid sinus. Note the vertical attachment of the middle turbinate (*2*) to the cribriform plate (*CP*) and its lateral attachment to the lamina papyracea, the basal lamella (*BL*). The air space between the basal lamella and the ethmoid bulla is the sinus lateralis (*sl*). Inferior turbinate (*1*), nasal septum (*NS*), vomer (*V*), and perpendicular plate of the ethmoid bone (*P*).

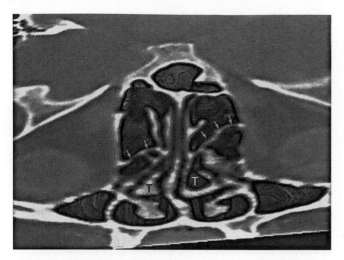

**FIGURE 3-10** 3D of the basal lamella. This three-dimensional image, viewed from superoanteriorly, reveals the anterior segment of the middle turbinates (*T*). Note the lateral attachment of the middle turbinate to the lamina papyracea—the basal lamella (*arrows*).

the turbinate, so that it obstructs the middle meatus or the infundibulum, and extensively pneumatized middle turbinates are associated with a higher prevalence of ipsilateral sinus disease.[43, 56] This is especially true when the concha bullosa exists in conjunction with another anatomic configu-

ration that may obstruct the ostiomeatal complex, such as an extensively pneumatized ethmoid bulla.[51]

The air cavity in a concha bullosa is lined with the same epithelium as the rest of the sinonasal cavities. Thus these concha bullosa cells can experience the same inflammatory disorders that affect the paranasal sinuses, and obstruction of the drainage of a concha may also lead to mucocele formation (Fig. 3-18). Isolated or smaller conchae bullosae, or those in which pneumatization is confined to the anterior or inferior aspect of the middle turbinate (farther from the ethmoid infundibulum), are less frequently associated with symptoms of sinusitis.[51]

### Other Variations

Additional variations of the middle turbinate can occur, including medial displacement, lateral displacement, lateral bending, L shape, and sagittal transverse clefts (Fig. 3-19). Medial displacement of the middle turbinate is the result of other middle meatal structures (i.e., polypoid disease, pneumatized uncinate process) encroaching upon the middle turbinate. Lateral displacement of the middle turbinate is usually due to the compression of the turbinate toward the lateral nasal wall by a septal spur or septal deviation. Either or these two variants may predispose to sinus disease.[51] L-shaped and lateral bending of the middle turbinate, as well as sagittal or transverse clefting, may also be observed; however, these variants are not associated with sinusitis.[51]

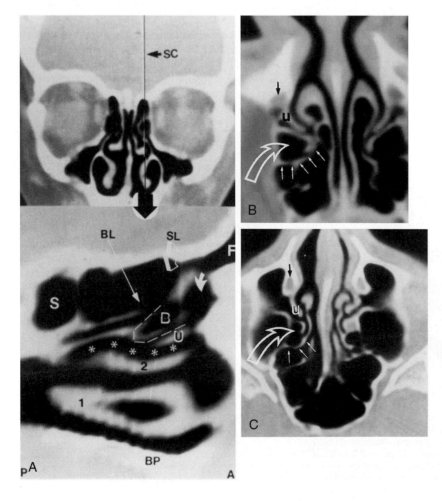

**FIGURE 3-11** Anatomy of the basal lamella and sinus lateralis. **A**, Sagittal reconstructed plane (*SC*) from direct coronal CT data shows the outline of the basal lamella (*BL*) and the position of the sinus lateralis (*SL*) between the basal lamella and the ethmoid bulla (*B*). The position of the hiatus semilunaris (*dashed U-shaped line*), the frontal recess, and the anterior middle meatus (*curved arrow*) are noted. Frontal sinus (*F*), sphenoid sinus (*S*), uncinate process (*U*), middle meatus (*asterisks*), inferior turbinate (*1*), middle turbinate (*2*), bony palate (*BP*), anterior (*A*), and posterior (*P*). **B** and **C**, Axial CT images show the orientation of the uncinate process (*u*) and its association with nasolacrimal duct (*small black arrow*). Note the attachment of the basal lamella (*small white arrows*) to the lamina papyracea. The ethmoid bulla (*curved arrow*) is the air cell anterior to the basal lamella, and in both of these patients the posterior wall of the air cell is incomplete, providing direct communication between the ethmoid bulla and the sinus lateralis.

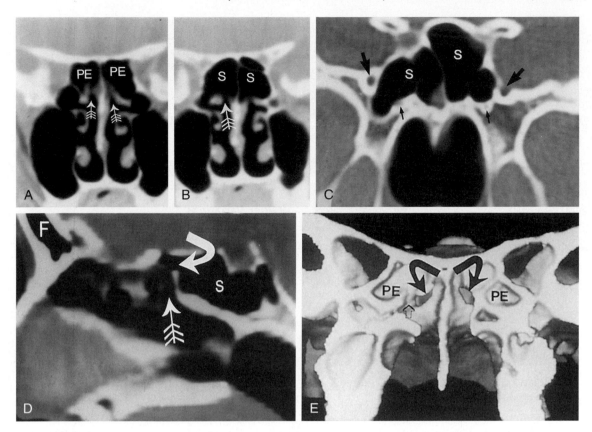

**FIGURE 3-12**   Sphenoid sinus anatomy. **A** and **B**, Coronal CT images show the boundary between the posterior ethmoid sinus (*PE*) and the sphenoid sinus (*S*). This boundary is best recognized by the position of the sphenoethmoidal recess (*feathered arrows*). It is relatively clear that the coronal image is through the anterior sphenoid sinus when only the inferior edge of the sphenoethmoidal recess is identified (**B**). **C**, Coronal CT image through the sphenoid sinus (*S*) shows the number and orientation of septations within the sinus, as well as the relationship to the foramen rotundum (*heavy black arrow*) and vidian canal (*fine black arrow*). **D**, Paramedial sagittal CT image shows the position of the sphenoid sinus ostium (*curved arrow*) and the sphenoethmoidal recess (*feathered arrows*). Frontal sinus (*F*), and sphenoid sinus (*S*). **E**, Three-dimensional CT image with a coronal cut–plane view through the posterior aspect of the posterior ethmoid sinus (*PE*) reveals the orientation of the sphenoethmoidal recess (*open arrow*) and position of the sphenoid sinus ostia (*curved arrows*).

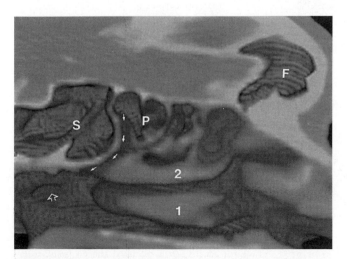

**FIGURE 3-13**   Saggital 3-D image of the sphenoethmoid recess. Three-dimensional image of the lateral nasal wall reveals the sphenoid sinus (*S*), the posterior ethmoid sinus (*P*), and the sphenoethmoid recess (*small arrows*). Inferior turbinate (*1*), middle turbinate (*2*), frontal sinus (*F*), fossa of Rosenmueller (*open arrow*).

## Nasal Septal Deviation

The nasal septum is fundamental to the development of the nose and paranasal sinuses. Nasal septal deviation is usually congenital but may be posttraumatic in some patients. Malalignment of the components of the adult nasal septum (septal cartilage, perpendicular ethmoidal plate, and vomer) may cause deviation of the nasal septum, deformity of the chondrovomerine articulation, or a septal spur. Asymptomatic septal deviation is observed in 20% to 31% of the population; however, more significant deviation, especially at the level of the chondrovomerine articulation, may contribute to sinusitis symptoms.[46, 48] Severe asymmetric bowing of the nasal septum may compress the middle turbinate laterally, narrowing the middle meatus (Fig. 3-20), and the presence of associated bony spurs may further compromise the OMU. Obstruction, secondary inflammation, swollen membranes, and infection of the middle meatus have all been observed as a result of severe nasal septal deviation.[57]

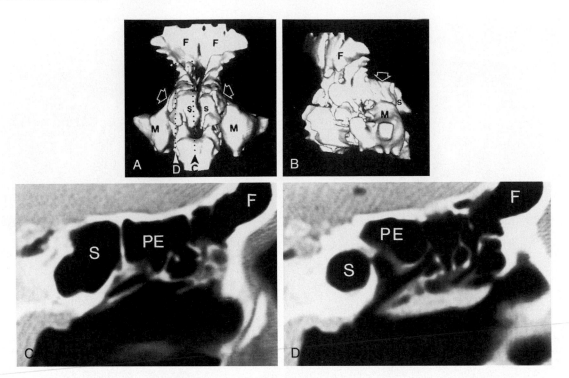

**FIGURE 3-14**   Anatomic relationship of the posterior ethmoid and sphenoid sinuses. **A** and **B**, Posterior (**A**) and anterolateral (**B**) views from three-dimensional CT images of a "cast" of the aerated nasal cavity, nasopharynx, and paranasal sinuses viewed from behind (**A**) and from the left side (**B**). Note that the posterior ethmoid sinus (*open arrows*) is wider and positioned more superiorly than the sphenoid sinus (*S*). The dotted lines denote the position of the sagittal planes displayed in **C** and **D**. Frontal sinus (*F*) and maxillary sinus (*M*). **C**, Paraseptal CT image of a cadaver head shows that the sphenoid sinus (*S*) is the most posterior and superior air space and that it is accessible from the posterior ethmoid sinus (*PE*). Frontal sinus (*F*). **D**, Sagittal CT image of a cadaver head performed approximately 1.5 cm lateral to the nasal septum shows that the sphenoid sinus (*S*) is inferior to the posterior ethmoid sinus (*PE*). Frontal sinus (*F*).

## Uncinate Process Variations

### Deviation

The uncinate process is one of the crucial bony structures of the wall of the lateral nasal cavity. Together with the ethmoid bulla, it forms the boundaries of the hiatus semilunaris and ethmoid infundibulum, the structures through which the frontal and maxillary sinuses drain. The course of the free edge of the uncinate process may be configured in a variety of ways. In most cases, it either extends slightly obliquely toward the nasal septum, with the free edge surrounding the inferoanterior surface of the ethmoid bulla, or it extends more medially to the medial surface of the ethmoid bulla. If the free edge of the uncinate is deviated in a more lateral direction, it may cause narrowing or obstruction of the hiatus semilunaris and infundibulum. Less frequently, a medial deviation or "curling" of the uncinate is encountered, which may result in the structure's contact and subsequent obstruction of the middle meatus (Fig. 3-21).

### Attachment

Normally, the upper tip of the uncinate process attaches to the lateral nasal wall in the location where agger nasi cells are commonly found. Anatomic variations of this attach-

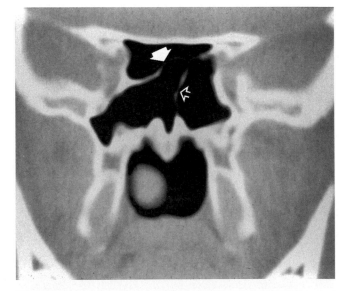

**FIGURE 3-15**   Relationship between the posterior ethmoid sinus and the sphenoid sinus. Coronal CT image through the middle sphenoid sinus reveals a horizontal bony membranous structure (*solid arrow*). This structure is not a septation; rather, it represents the separation from the sphenoid sinus inferiorly and the posterior ethmoid sinus superiorly. Septations (*open arrow*) are vertically oriented.

## SUMMARY BOX 3-5

### Reported Prevalences of Anatomic Variations

| | Agger Nasi Cell | Enlarged Ethmoid Bulla | Haller Cells | Pneumatized Uncinate Process | Deviated Uncinate Process | Paradoxical Middle Turbinate | Concha Bullosa | Nasal Septal Deviation | Onodi Cells |
|---|---|---|---|---|---|---|---|---|---|
| Zinreich et al. | Nearly all | 8% | 10% | 0.4% | 3% | 15% | 36% | 21% | |
| Bolger | 98.5% | | 45.1% | 2.5% | | 26.1% | 53% | 18.8% | |
| Lloyd | 3% | 17% | 2% | | 16% | 17% | 14% | | |
| Van Alyea | 89% | | | | | | | | 98% |
| Messerklinger | 10–15% | | | | | | | | |
| Lebowitz | 86% | | | | | | | 31% | |
| Scribano et al. | | 4% | 24% | 18%: combination of pneumatization and deviation | | | 67% | | |
| Wanamaker | | | 20% | | 45% | | 30% | 20% | |
| Driben et al. | | | | | | | | | 39% |
| Tonai & Baba | 86.7% | | 36% | | | 25.3% | 28% | | |
| Yousem | | | 10–45% | | | Less than 10% | 34–53% | | |
| Joe Weinberger et al. | | | | | 15% | 3% | 15% | | 14% |
| Perez-Pinas et al. | Nearly all | 0% | 3% | 0% | 4.5% | 10% | 73% | 80% | 11% |

ment include attachment to the lamina papyracea, the lateral surface of the middle turbinate, or the fovea ethmoidalis in the floor of the anterior cranial fossa (Fig. 3-22). It is necessary for the surgeon to be cognizant of any of these variations in the patient undergoing FESS, especially when an uncinatectomy is contemplated. In particular, if the uncinate process attaches to the ethmoidal roof or middle turbinate, the surgeon must take special care not to put aggressive traction or torque on the upper tip of the structure during uncinatectomy, as this could inadvertently damage the ethmoid roof and result in CSF rhinorrhea or other intracranial complications.

Sometimes the free edge of the uncinate process adheres to the orbital floor, or inferior aspect of the lamina papyracea. This is referred to as an atelectatic uncinate process (Fig. 3-23) and is associated with a hypoplastic, and often opacified, ipsilateral maxillary sinus due to closure of the infundibulum. For surgical planning, it is important to note this variant, as the ipsilateral orbital floor is low-lying as a result of the hypoplastic maxillary sinus, increasing the risk of inadvertent penetration of the orbit during surgery.

An additional variant of the uncinate process configuration is its extension superiorly to the roof of the anterior ethmoid sinus, causing the superior infundibulum to end as a "blind pouch." This continuation of the uncinate is referred to as the lamina terminalis. In these cases, the infundibulum drains via the posterior aspect of the middle meatus.

### Pneumatization

Pneumatization of the uncinate process, also referred to as an uncinate bulla, has been suggested as a predisposing factor for impaired sinus ventilation, especially in the anterior ethmoid, frontal recess, and infundibular regions (Fig. 3-24).[58] Functionally, the pneumatized uncinate process resembles a concha bullosa or an enlarged ethmoid bulla. The pneumatization of the uncinate process is believed to be due to extension of the agger nasi cell within the anterosuperior portion of the uncinate process.[21] The reported incidence of this variant is relatively low, ranging from 0.4% to 2.5% to 18%.[11, 43]

## Infraorbital Ethmoid Cells (Haller's Cells)

Infraorbital ethmoid cells are pneumatized ethmoid air cells that project along the medial roof of the maxillary sinus and the most inferior portion of the lamina papyracea, below the ethmoid bulla and lateral to the uncinate process (Fig. 3-25). These cells were first identified by Haller in 1765 and subsequently named after him; recently, however, the preferred term for these air cells has been changed to reflect both a growing trend that discourages the naming of structures after anatomists who first describe them, as well as the need for international standardization and descriptive nomenclature for anatomic terms.[36] Most often, infraorbital

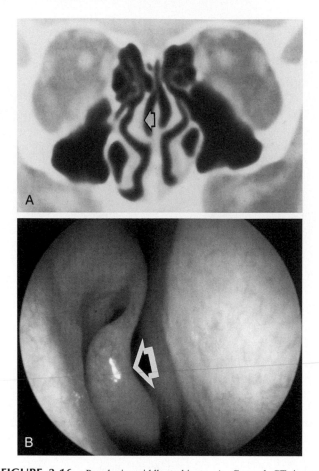

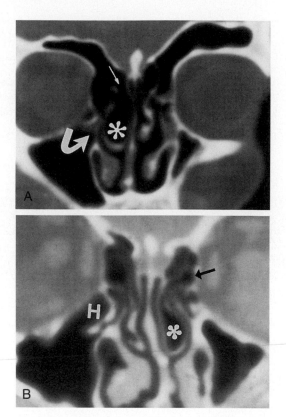

**FIGURE 3-16** Paradoxic middle turbinate. **A,** Coronal CT image demonstrates bilateral paradoxic middle turbinates. The right side is highlighted (*solid arrow*). **B,** Endoscopic view correlates with the CT findings (*arrow*).

**FIGURE 3-17** Concha bullosa in two different patients. **A,** Coronal CT image demonstrates a prominent right concha bullosa (*asterisk*) with communication to the frontal recess (*small arrow*). Note the obstruction of the right middle meatus (*curved arrow*). **B,** Coronal CT image demonstrates a left-sided concha bullosa (*asterisk*) with communication to the sinus lateralis (*small arrow*). Note the contralateral Haller (infraorbital ethmoid) cell (*H*).

ethmoid cells arise from the anterior ethmoid cells and are closely related to the infundibulum.[48] These cells contribute to the narrowing of the infundibulum and may also compromise the adjacent ostium of the maxillary sinuses. Consequently, many authors cite infraorbital ethmoid cells as a factor in recurrent maxillary sinusitis.[57, 58]

Some authors consider the existence of this variant a predisposing factor for recurrent maxillary sinusitis. How-ever, Bolger et al. reported an incidence of 45%, and their study found no statistical difference between the prevalence of infraorbital ethmoid cells in patients presenting with recurrent maxillary sinusitis and asymptomatic patients. This led these investigators to suggest that the role of infraorbital ethmoid cells in disease should be evaluated on an individual basis, depending on the size, placement, and evidence of inflammation in the cell.[43]

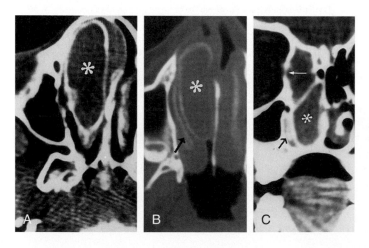

**FIGURE 3-18** Mucocele within a concha bullosa. Axial (**A** and **B**) and coronal (**C**) CT images show a prominent soft-tissue mass (*asterisk*) well circumscribed by a bony perimeter (the bony framework of the concha bullosa). The inferior turbinate is compressed against the medial wall of the maxillary sinus (*black arrow*). In the coronal image, the extent of the obstruction of the nasal cavity is apparent, as is the presence of a more superior mucocele, which erodes the lamina papyracea (*white arrow*).

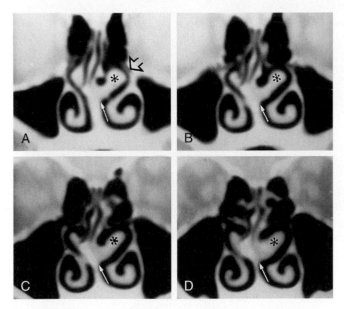

**FIGURE 3-19** Coronal CT scans. **A** to **D**, The free edge of the middle turbinate may also assume some other shapes. Note its prominent lateral curvature in this case (*asterisk*). It obstructs the nasal passage (*fine white arrows*) and contributes to the position of the uncinate process and, therefore, the prominent narrowing of the infundibulum (*open arrow*).

## Onodi Cells

Two primary definitions of Onodi cells have been presented in the literature. The first defines them as the most posterior ethmoid cells, being superolateral to the sphenoid sinus and closely associated with the optic nerve.[39, 59, 60] Another, more general description defines Onodi cells as posterior ethmoid cells extending into the sphenoid bone, situated either adjacent to or impinging upon the optic nerve.[36] The reported incidence of Onodi cells ranges from 3.4% to 51%.[52] This discrepancy is most likely due to the use of different criteria to define these cells. Onodi cells abut or may even surround the optic nerve, thereby placing this nerve at risk when surgical excision of these cells is performed.

Onodi cells are also a potential cause of incomplete sphenoidectomy. If a surgeon is operating in an Onodi cell, he or she may recognize landmarks traditionally associated with the sphenoid sinus (internal carotid artery, optic nerve) and thus mistakenly conclude that the sphenoid sinus has been entered.

## Ethmoid Bulla Variations

The ethmoid bulla is usually the largest and most constant anterior ethmoid air cell. Its appearance varies considerably, based on the extent of pneumatization; extensive pneumatization may obstruct the ostiomeatal complex. Elongated ethmoid bullae are usually the result of pneumatization that extends in a superior to inferior direction rather than in an anterior to posterior direction. Because such pneumatization does not extend in an anterior or posterior direction, elongated ethmoid bullae are relatively unlikely to obstruct the ostiomeatal complex.

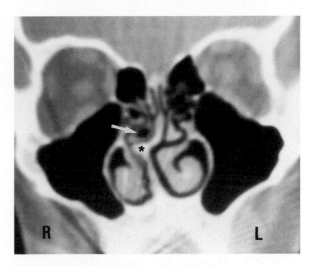

**FIGURE 3-20** Nasal septal deviation with spurring. Coronal CT image demonstrates that there is deviation of the nasal septum toward the right side, with a right-sided cartilaginous nasal "spur" (*asterisk*). Note the ipsilateral concha bullosa (*arrow*). Both of these anatomic variants contribute to marked narrowing of the right nasal cavity and ethmoid passages.

## Extensive Pneumatization of the Sphenoid Sinus

Although encountered infrequently, pneumatization of the sphenoid sinus that extends into the lesser wing and the anterior and posterior clinoid processes is important to note. A pneumatized anterior clinoid process is associated with Type 2 and Type 3 optic canal configurations (see below), making these nerves especially vulnerable to injury during FESS.[61] A more extensive description of the relationship between the posterior paranasal sinuses and the optic nerves, optic nerve configurations, and their reported incidence can be found in the sections discussing the systematic evaluation of paranasal sinus CT examinations (Fig. 3-26).

## Medial Deviation or Dehiscence of the Lamina Papyracea

Medial deviation or dehiscence of the lamina papyracea may be either congenital or the result of prior facial trauma. In either case, if the surgeon does not know about this

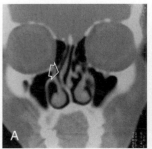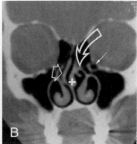

**FIGURE 3-21** Medially curved uncinate process. **A** and **B**, Coronal CT images through the ethmoid sinuses show a prominent right-sided deviation of the nasal septum (*straight open arrow*). Note the medially curved left uncinate process (*curved open arrow*), which is medially displacing the left middle turbinate (+) and obstructs the left middle meatus. A left-sided Haller (infraorbital ethmoid) cell is present (*small arrow*).

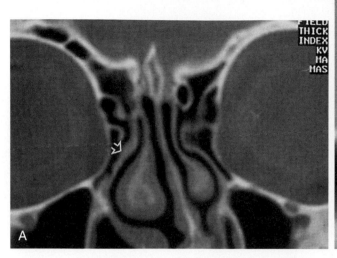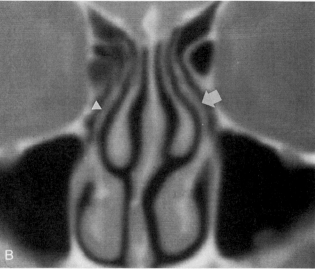

**FIGURE 3-22** Variations in the superior attachment of the uncinate process. **A**, Coronal CT image obtained at the level of the frontal recess reveals that the right uncinate process (*open arrow*) attaches to the superior right middle turbinate. **B**, Coronal CT image reveals that the left uncinate process (*solid arrow*) attaches to the roof of the ethmoid sinus. On the right side, the uncinate (*arrowhead*) adheres to the medial agger nasi cell and frontal cell.

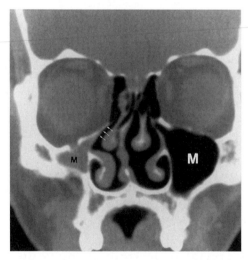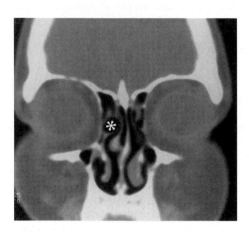

**FIGURE 3-23** Atelectatic uncinate process. Coronal CT scan shows that the right uncinate process is apposed to the inferomedial aspect of the orbit (*arrows*). The resultant obstruction of the infundibulum is usually the cause of the prominent inflammatory process in the ipsilateral maxillary sinus (*small black M*). Note that, in this case, as is often seen, this is associated with hypoplasia of the ipsilateral maxillary sinus compared with its counterpart (*large white M*).

**FIGURE 3-24** Uncinate bulla. Coronal CT image demonstrates an air cell within the right uncinate process (*asterisk*). The cell contributes to the narrowing of the right infundibulum and middle meatus.

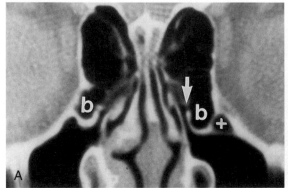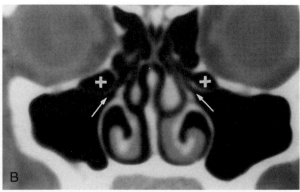

**FIGURE 3-25** Haller (infraorbital ethmoid) cell. **A**, Note the left Haller (infraorbital ethmoid) cell (+) with the ethmoid bulla ostia located medially (*b*), opening into the infundibula (*arrow*). **B**, Bilateral Haller (infraorbital ethmoid) cells (+). Note their close proximity to the uncinate process and their influence on the infundibula (*small arrows*).

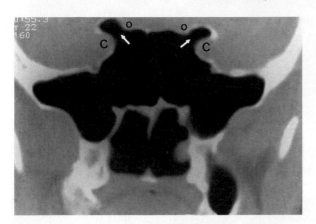

**FIGURE 3-26** Extensive pneumatization of the sphenoid sinus. Coronal CT image shows pneumatization of both anterior clinoid processes (*arrows*) and their relationship to the optic nerves (*o*) and internal carotid arteries (*C*). The presence of anterior clinoid pneumatization is an important indicator of optic nerve vulnerability during FESS.

situation preoperatively, the orbital contents are placed at risk during surgery, as the surgeon will not know that there is a restricted ethmoid complex in which to operate (Fig. 3-27). Both excessive medial deviation and bony dehiscence of the lamina papyracea occur most often at the site of the insertion of the basal lamella into the lamina papyracea, thus rendering this portion of the lamina papyracea most delicate.

## Aerated Crista Galli

When aeration of the normally bony crista galli occurs, the aerated cells may communicate with the frontal recess, and obstruction of this ostium can lead to chronic sinusitis and mucocele formation within the crista galli. To avoid unnecessary surgical extension into the anterior cranial vault, it is important to recognize an aerated crista galli and differentiate it from an ethmoid air cell prior to surgery.

## Cephalocele

Cephaloceles involving the anterior cranial fossa floor may be congenital, occur spontaneously, or be the result of previous ethmoid or sphenoid sinus surgery. Preoperative

coronal CT scanning is especially well suited to display the extent of any such areas of missing bone (Figs. 3-28, 3-29) (see also Chapters 1, 4, and 5).[62]

## Posterior Nasal Septal Air Cell

Air cells are commonly found within the posterosuperior portion of the nasal septum and, when present, communicate with the sphenoid sinus. As a result, any inflammatory disease that occurs within the paranasal sinuses may also affect these cells (Fig. 3-30). Such disease may opacify this cell, causing it to resemble a cephalocele. CT and MR imaging usually define the involved pathology and resolve any differential diagnostic problems.

## Asymmetry in Ethmoid Roof Height

It is important to note any asymmetry in the height of the ethmoid roof, as there is a higher incidence of intracranial penetration during FESS when this anatomic variation occurs. Intracranial penetration is more likely to occur on the side where the position of the roof is lower.[63]

## Systematic Radiographic Evaluation

### Routine Report

When interpreting sinus CT studies, it is helpful to use a systematic approach. In this regard, most radiologists progress from anterior to posterior when describing findings. As one reads the study, a mental checklist should be made of important structures for evaluation and comment. The reporting system normally includes three steps, which will now be described.

### Step One

Identify and describe the important structures of the paranasal sinuses (there are 14 such structures). The dictated report should mention the status of these structures on both the right and left sides. The structures to identify are as follows:

| | |
|---|---|
| Frontal sinus | Ethmoid bulla |
| Frontal recess | Basal lamella |
| Agger nasi cell and anterior ethmoid sinus | Sinus lateralis |
| Maxillary sinus | Posterior ethmoid sinus |
| Uncinate process | Sphenoid sinus |
| Infundibulum | Middle meatus |
| Ethmoid roof | Nasal septum and nasal turbinates |

**FIGURE 3-27** Medial deviation of the left lamina papyracea. Coronal CT images optimally demonstrate the outline of the lamina papyracea in relation to the anterior ostiomeatal channels. Medial deviation (*open arrow*), when present, should not be confused with an ethmoid bulla. Note that the medially deviated lamina papyracea lies in close proximity to the lateral attachment of the middle turbinate, the basal lamella (*white arrow*).

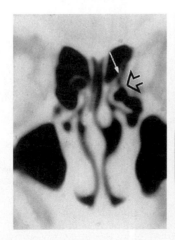
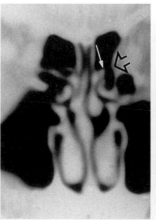
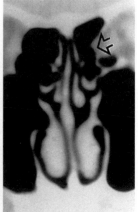

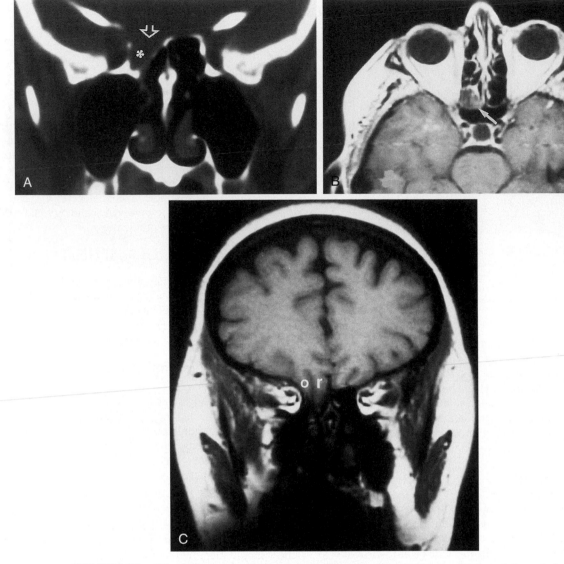

**FIGURE 3-28**    CT and MR imaging display of an encephalocele. Coronal CT image (**A**) through the posterior ethmoid sinus shows erosion of the roof of the posterior ethmoid sinus (*open arrow* and *asterisk*). Axial T1-weighted MR image (**B**) shows an isolated soft-tissue mass within the posterior ethmoid sinus (*arrow*), which on the coronal T1-weighted MR image (**C**) is confirmed to be an encephalocele. Gyrus rectus (*r*) and gyrus orbitales (*o*) are noted.

**FIGURE 3-29**    CT and MR imaging appearance of an encephalocele. **A**, Coronal CT image through the posterior ethmoid sinus shows a wide erosion of the ethmoid sinus roof (*open arrow*), with a soft-tissue mass penetrating into the ethmoid sinus (*asterisk*). Left (*L*), right (*R*). **B**, Sagittal T1-weighted sagittal MR image shows the outline of the brain tissue (*large arrows*), meninges, and cerebrospinal fluid (*small arrows*).

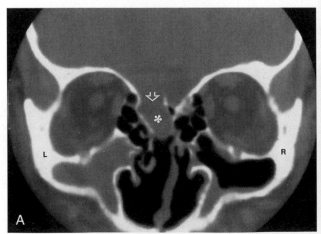

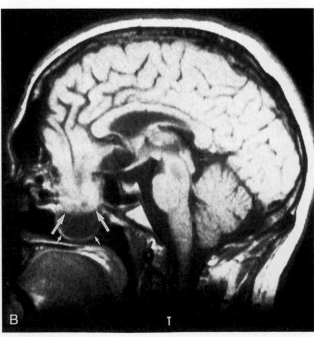

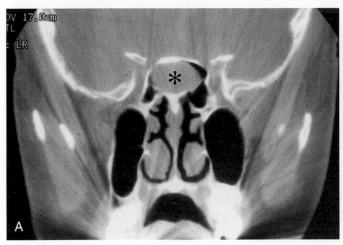
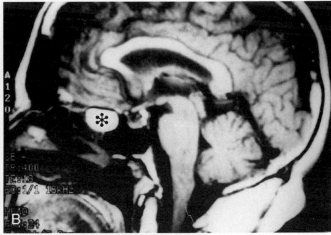

**FIGURE 3-30**   Nasal septal air cell. **A**, Coronal CT image demonstrates an expansile mass in the anterior sphenoid sinus (*asterisk*). **B**, Sagittal T1-weighted MR image displays the hyperintense inflammatory mass (*asterisk*), which is well separated from the intracranial compartment. This was proven to be a mucocele within a posterior nasal septal air cell.

*Step Two*

Evaluate the critical relationships. In addition to describing findings directly related to the diagnosis of inflammatory sinus disease, it is important for the radiologist to evaluate several critical areas that aid in surgical planning. The symmetry of the ethmoid roof should be noted. Careful attention should be paid to the status of the lamina papyracea, and any dehiscence or excessive medial deviation should be reported. The relationship of the sphenoid sinus and posterior ethmoid air cells with the internal carotid artery and optic nerves should be clearly mentioned. In particular, extensive expansion of the sinuses around the internal carotid artery or the optic nerve, as well as bony dehiscences adjacent to either structure, should be noted and reported to the referring surgeon (Fig. 3-31). The incidence of bony dehiscence around the presellar and juxtasellar portions of the internal carotid artery ranges from 12% to 22%.[61, 64, 65]

Frequently the carotid canal extends into the aerated portion of the sphenoid sinus, and in many such cases the sphenoid sinus septations adhere to the bony covering of the carotid canal. The surgeon must be made aware of this situation in order to prevent fracturing of the sphenoid sinus septum/carotid canal junction and puncturing of the carotid artery.

The relationship between the posterior paranasal sinuses and the optic nerves is crucial to note during the radiographic examination (Fig. 3-32). The optic nerves, carotid arteries, and vidian nerves develop prior to the paranasal sinuses, which accounts for their influence on congenital variations in the walls of the sphenoid sinus. Awareness of the intercommunication between the sphenoid sinus, posterior ethmoid cells, and optic nerves is paramount to avoid potentially devastating operative complications during FESS. Delano et al. described four discrete classifications of the various relationships that exist between the optic nerves and posterior paranasal sinuses.[61] Type 1 optic nerves include those that course immediately adjacent to the sphenoid sinus, without indentation of the wall or contact with the posterior ethmoid air cell. This is the most common type, occurring in 76% of patients. Type 2 nerves course adjacent to the sphenoid sinus, causing indentation of the sinus wall, without contact with the posterior ethmoid air cell. Type 3 nerves course through the sphenoid sinus, with at least 50% of the nerve surrounded by air. Type 4 nerves course immediately adjacent to the sphenoid sinus and posterior ethmoid sinus. The optic nerve is exposed without a complete bony margin in all cases where it travels through the sphenoid sinus (Type 3) and in 82% of cases where the nerve is impressed on the sphenoid sinus wall (Type 2).

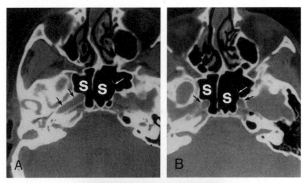
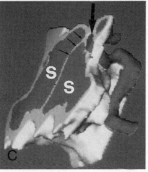

**FIGURE 3-31**   Relationship of the carotid canal to the sphenoid sinus. **A** and **B**, Axial CT images through the sphenoid and ethmoid sinuses show that the carotid canals (*small black arrows*) penetrate into the sphenoid sinus (*S*). An incomplete sphenoid sinus septum (*white arrow*) connects to the bony covering of the carotid canal. **C**, Three-dimensional images of the sphenoid sinus (*S*) and presellar and juxtasellar portions of the internal carotid artery (*black arrow*) graphically display the close relationship between the internal carotid artery and the sphenoid sinus septation (*small black arrows*).

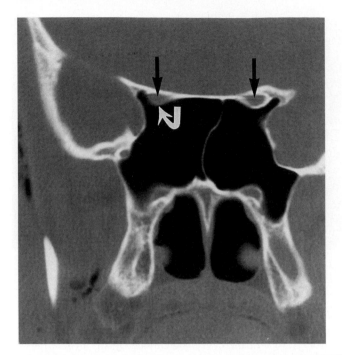

**FIGURE 3-32**   Relationship of the optic nerves to the sphenoid sinus. Type 3 optic nerves (*black arrows*) course through the sphenoid sinus, with more than 50% of the nerves surrounded by air. Note that there is dehiscence of the bone covering the right optic nerve (*curved white arrow*). This increases the risk of optic nerve damage during FESS.

Delano et al. also found that 85% of optic nerves associated with a pneumatized anterior clinoid process were of the Type 2 or Type 3 configuration, and 77% were dehiscent. Therefore the presence of anterior clinoid pneumatization is an important indicator of optic nerve vulnerability during FESS because of the frequent association of this pneumatization with both bony dehiscence and Type 2 and 3 optic nerve configurations.[61]

*Step Three*

Lastly, but just as important as steps one and two, is the evaluation of the ''character'' of the bony framework of the nasal vault and paranasal sinuses. It has been noted that a prominent thickening of the bone about a paranasal sinus may occur, especially in patients who have had several surgical procedures and in patients with repeated exacerbations of chronic inflammation (Fig. 3-33). Similar changes have been noted in patients with Wegener's granulomatosis and in patients who suffer from a prolonged chronic inflammation and have had no previous surgery. Unfortunately, to date there is no good pathophysiologic explanation of this finding. However, it is believed that this change is directly related to the underlying inflammatory process and periosteal stimulation.

Bone may not be visualized on CT for several reasons. Bone may have been removed during a prior surgical procedure and, therefore, a defect is noted. Evidence of prior surgery should be sought on the CT examination and established through a proper medical history. Bone may not be seen because it is deossified secondary to chronic pressure from a mucocele or because the bone is invaded and destroyed by tumor. The associated mass will suggest the etiology, and MR imaging may afford a distinction between these two processes (see Chapter 6). Lastly, bony dehiscences may be developmental, and in the absence of prior surgery or associated pathology, this diagnostic possibility should be considered.

## Radiographic Appearances of Inflammatory Sinus Disease

### *Acute Sinusitis*

Acute sinusitis usually is due to bacterial infection of an obstructed paranasal sinus. The obstruction is often the result of apposition of edematous mucosal surfaces from an antecedent viral upper respiratory tract infection. The edematous mucosa disrupts the normal mucociliary drainage pattern of the sinus, and obstruction of the sinus ostium results. This, in turn, alters the oxygen tension within the obstructed sinus and predisposes the sinus to a bacterial superinfection.[24, 43, 66] Acute sinusitis usually involves only a single sinus, with the ethmoid sinus being the most common location.[57, 66] There is an increased risk of regional

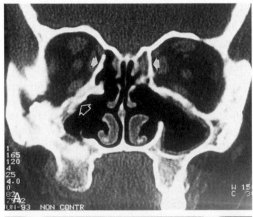

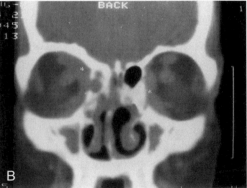

**FIGURE 3-33**   Osteitis of the paranasal sinus walls. **A**, Coronal CT image through the ethmoid sinus shows that the patient has had bilateral antrostomies, uncinectomies, and partial anterior ethmoidectomies. Note the pronounced thickening of the orbital floors bilaterally but more severely on the right side (*open arrow*). There is marked thickening of the lamina papyracea bilaterally (*solid arrows*). These changes are occasionally seen in patients who have undergone multiple surgical procedures in this area. **B**, Coronal CT image through the anterior ethmoid sinus in a patient with Wegener's granulomatosis. Note the diffuse, pronounced bony thickening of the perimeter of the maxillary sinuses and lamina papyracea, as well as the presence of soft-tissue masses (*asterisks*) within the orbits.

and intracranial complications, with involvement of the frontal, ethmoid, and sphenoid sinuses.[57] Acute sinusitis is rarely the result of a pure viral infection. A thorough discussion of sinusitis is presented in Chapter 5.

### Chronic Sinusitis

Chronic sinusitis is diagnosed when the patient has repeated bouts of acute infection or persistent inflammation.[57, 66] Staphylococcus, streptococcus, corynebacteria, bacteroides, fusobacteria, and other anaerobes and anerobes are more commonly involved in chronic sinusitis than in acute sinusitis.[43, 57, 66] The radiographic findings are quite variable and are discussed in Chapter 5.[67] The sinuses most commonly involved with chronic sinusitis are the anterior ethmoid air cells.

Opacification of the OMU has been found to predispose patients to the development of sinusitis. Zinreich et al. found middle meatus opacification in 72% of patients with chronic sinusitis. In this study, 65% of these patients had mucoperiosteal thickening within the maxillary sinus, and all of the patients with frontal sinusitis had opacification of the frontoethmoidal recess.[6, 8, 9] Opacification of the OMU without frontal, maxillary, or anterior ethmoid sinus inflammatory disease was rare.[6, 8, 9] Yousem et al. found that when the middle meatus was opacified, there were associated inflammatory changes in the ethmoid sinuses in 82% of patients and in the maxillary sinuses in 84% of patients.[68] Bolger et al. found that when the ethmoid infundibulum was free of disease, the maxillary and frontal sinuses were clear in 77% of patients.[43]

Babbel et al. reviewed 500 patients with screening sinus CT scans and defined five recurring patterns of inflammatory sinonasal disease.[69] The five anatomic patterns were infundibular, OMU, sphenoethmoidal recess, sinonasal polyposis, and sporadic or unclassifiable. The infundibular pattern (26% of patients) referred to focal obstruction within the maxillary sinus ostium and ethmoid infundibulum, which was associated with maxillary sinus disease. The OMU pattern (25% of patients) referred to ipsilateral maxillary, frontal, and anterior ethmoid sinus disease (Fig. 3-34). This pattern was due to obstruction of the middle meatus. Sparing of the frontal sinus was sometimes seen as a result of the variable location of the nasofrontal duct insertion in the middle meatus. The sphenoethmoidal recess pattern (6% of patients) resulted in sphenoid or posterior ethmoid sinus inflammation caused by sphenoethmoidal recess obstruction. The sinonasal polyposis pattern (10% of patients) was due to diffuse nasal and paranasal sinus polyps. Associated radiographic findings included infundibular enlargement, convexity (bulging) of the ethmoid sinus walls, and thinning of the bony nasal septum and ethmoid trabeculae.[28, 69, 70]

Certain anatomic variants, as described above, have been implicated as causative factors in the presence of chronic inflammatory disease. Stammberger and Wolf and Lidov and Som found that a large concha bullosa produced signs and symptoms of sinusitis.[58, 71] However, Yousem et al. found that the presence of a concha bullosa did not increase the risk of sinusitis.[68] This was corroborated by Bolger et al., who found that the presence of a concha bullosa, paradoxic turbinates, Haller cells, and uncinate process pneumatization were not significantly more common in patients with chronic

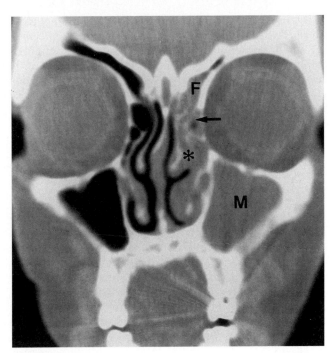

**FIGURE 3-34**   OMU pattern of sinusitis. Inflammatory changes obstruct the left middle meatus (*asterisk*), with resulting opacification of the left maxillary (*M*), frontal (*F*), and anterior ethmoid (*arrow*) sinuses.

sinusitis than in asymptomatic patients.[43] Yousem et al. found that the presence of nasal septal deviation and a horizontally oriented uncinate process was more common in patients with inflammatory sinusitis.[68] Although the presence of these variants may not necessarily predispose to sinusitis, it appears that the size of a given anatomic variant and its relationship to adjacent structures plays an important role in the development of sinusitis.[37]

### Fungal Sinusitis

Fungal sinusitis may be suspected clinically when the patient fails to respond to standard antibiotic therapy.[37, 57, 68, 72, 73] According to Som and Curtin, two circumstances can be seen that suggest the presence of fungal infections: soft tissue changes in the sinus associated with thickened, reactive bone with localized areas of osteomyelitis, and the association of inflammatory sinus disease with involvement of the adjacent nasal fossa and the soft tissues of the cheek.[21, 22] These signs of aggressive infection are atypical of bacterial pathogens. This topic is described in detail in Chapter 5.

### Allergic Sinusitis

Allergic sinusitis occurs in 10% of the population and typically produces a pansinusitis with symmetric involvement.[28, 69] CT often shows a nodular mucosal thickening with thickened turbinates; air-fluid levels are rare unless bacterial superinfection occurs.[28, 67] This topic is discussed in more detail in Chapter 5.

### Orbital Complications of Sinusitis

About 3% of patients with sinusitis have some form of orbital involvement. These complications are more common in children than in adults, and the orbital manifestations may be the initial clinical signs of sinus infection. Complicated sinusitis is the most common cause of orbital infection, accounting for 60% to 84% of cases.[38, 74–77] The origin of the infection most commonly is in the ethmoid sinuses. In decreasing order of frequency, the sources of the infection are the frontal, sphenoid, and maxillary sinuses. The ethmoid and maxillary sinuses are present at birth and therefore are the source in younger children. The topic of orbital infection is discussed in detail in Chapter 9.

## COMMON FESS TECHNIQUES

For the surgical treatment of inflammatory sinonasal disease, FESS has largely replaced more traditional sinus surgery techniques. It is now believed that obstruction of the drainage portals of the sinuses, particularly the anterior ethmoids, is the primary cause of recurrent sinusitis. The rationale for FESS is that these techniques allow restoration of the flow of sinus secretions through their native drainage portals, allowing the inflamed sinus to return to a normal state, thus hopefully alleviating the patient's symptoms.[26, 78, 79]

## Types of FESS

Panje and Anand have developed a classification system to standardize the type of FESS technique that is appropriate based on the preoperative extent of sinus disease as determined by CT imaging.[79] These authors outline the various types of FESS in the following manner:

### Type I
Uncinatectomy with or without agger nasi cell exenteration.
  **Indications**
  1. Isolated OMU thickening of mucous membrane
  2. Infundibular disease
  3. Patent maxillary sinus ostia without maxillary sinus membrane thickening or cysts
  4. Unsuccessful prior inferior maxillary sinus antrostomy or antrotomy with irrigation
  5. Prior septoplasty or adenoidectomy with continued paranasal sinus symptoms

### Type II
Uncinatectomy, bulla ethmoidectomy, removal of the sinus lateralis mucous membrane, and exposure of the frontal recess or frontal sinus.
  **Indications**
  1. OMU thickening of the mucous membrane
  2. Evidence of anterior ethmoid sinus opacification, including obstruction of the infundibulum
  3. Limited frontal recess disease
  4. Unsuccessful prior inferior maxillary sinus antrostomy or antrotomy with irrigation
  5. Prior septoplasty or adenoidectomy with continued paranasal sinus symptoms

### Type III
Type II plus maxillary sinus antrostomy through the natural sinus ostium.
  **Indications**
  Same as for Type II, with the following:
  1. Maxillary sinusitis, as evidenced by membrane thickening or sinus opacification
  2. Stenotic or edematous maxillary sinus ostium

### Type IV
Type III plus complete posterior ethmoidectomy.
  **Indications**
  Same as for Type III, with the following:
  1. Total ethmoid involvement
  2. Nasal polyposis with extensive ethmoidal and maxillary sinus disease
  3. Prior Type I or Type II FESS without a response or with progression of sinus disease

### Type V
Type IV plus sphenoidectomy and stripping of the mucous membrane.
  **Indications**
  Same as for Type IV, with the following:
  1. Evidence of sphenoid sinusitis
  2. Pansinusitis and rhinitis

In practice, Types II and III are the most commonly performed FESS techniques.

## RADIOGRAPHIC EVALUATION OF PATIENTS FOLLOWING FUNCTIONAL ENDOSCOPIC SINUS SURGERY

### Expected Findings

Evaluation of the postoperative patient is similar to that of the preoperative patient. Ideally, the CT scan should be performed in the coronal projection. Given the fact that a surgical procedure was performed, the type and extent of surgery must be established. Subsequently the emphasis is on the anatomy. The mental checklist should identify and mention the presence or absence of the 14 important structures discussed earlier in this chapter. A close look at the nasal cavity and paranasal sinus boundaries and the important relationships described previously should once again be observed and evaluated. Areas of bony thickening or dehiscence should be noted.

Areas that merit close scrutiny on follow-up (postoperative) CT scans are as follows:

  1. *Frontal recess.* The frontal recess should be identified to determine its patency. Postoperatively, one often finds that recurrence of disease is due to persistent obstruction in this area. It is the narrowest channel within the anterior ethmoid complex, and it is a structure that is very difficult to access surgically. Therefore, the frontal recess is the area most likely to be affected by inflammatory disease in a patient with a previous paranasal sinus surgical procedure. To this

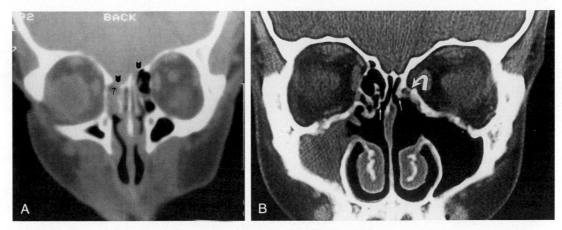

**FIGURE 3-35**   Anatomic landmarks to be evaluated in patients after FESS. **A,** Coronal CT image through the anterior ethmoid sinuses shows a prominent asymmetry in the position of the roof of the ethmoid sinuses (*solid arrowheads*). The intracranial penetrations (*fine black arrow*) are usually on the side where the roof is lower in position. **B,** Coronal CT image through the anterior ethmoid sinus in a patient after bilateral uncinatectomies and partial middle turbinectomies (*fine white arrows*). If there is an intraorbital complication during such a surgical procedure, it usually involves the lamina papyracea at the attachment of the basal lamella (*curved arrow*).

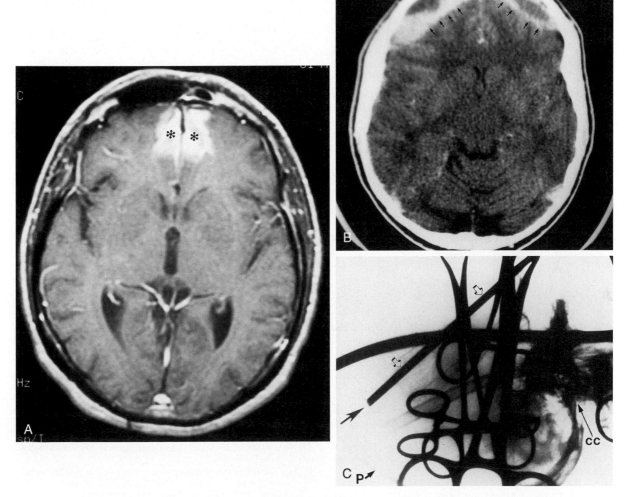

**FIGURE 3-36**   Intracranial complications from FESS. **A,** Axial T1-weighted MR image after gadolinium-DTPA administration shows abnormal bifrontal parenchymal enhancement (*asterisks*) caused by encephalitis from perforation through the cribriform plate. **B,** Axial CT image shows bilateral acute subdural hematomas (*arrows*) after FESS. **C,** Intraoperative cross-table lateral skull radiograph shows the intracranial extension of an endoscope (*open arrows*). Note the position of the endoscope in the deep portion of the posterior frontal lobe (*solid black arrow*). Overlying surgical instruments are noted. Craniocervical junction (*CC*) and parietal bone (*P*).

end, note should be made of the agger nasi cell (if it remains), because its persistence may continue to narrow the frontal recess.

2. *OMU*. Note should be made of the extent of the uncinatectomy and removal of the ethmoid bulla. The course of the infundibulum should be examined for persistent anatomic narrowing. The outline of the middle turbinate should be examined to determine whether a middle turbinectomy has been performed. If so, then careful attention should be paid to both the vertical attachment of the middle turbinate to the cribriform plate and the attachment of the basal lamella to the lamina papyracea. Traction applied on the vertical attachment and basal lamella of the middle turbinate during the course of a middle turbinectomy can cause a fracture of the lamina papyracea or the cribriform plate. These breaks in the continuity of the lamina papyracea and ethmoid roof are easily demonstrated on coronal images (Figs. 3-35, 3-36).

3. *Lamina papyracea*. Inspection of the entire course of the lamina papyracea should be carried out to evaluate the integrity of this structure. Postoperative dehiscences are commonly found just posterior to the nasolacrimal duct, and these may be caused by the uncinate resection (Figs. 3-13, 3-35).

4. *Ethmoid roof*. Asymmetry in the position of the roof (fovea ethmoidalis) of the ethmoid sinuses should be noted. Intracranial penetrations usually occur on the side where the position of the roof is lower. One should examine for a break in the continuity of this roof (Fig. 3-35).[63]

5. *Sphenoid sinus area*. The margins of the sphenoid sinus should be evaluated for bony dehiscence or cephalocele.

## Operative Complications

The topic of operative complications is discussed in Chapter 4.

## REFERENCES

1. Moss A, Parsons V. Current estimates from the National Health Interview Survey, United States, 1985. Hyattsville, Md: National Center for Health Statistics, 1986.
2. Messerklinger W. Endoscopy of the nose. Baltimore: Urban & Schwartzenberg, 1978.
3. Messerklinger W. Zur Endoskopietchnik des mittleren Nassenganges. Arch Otorhinolaryngol 1978;221:297–305.
4. Wigand ME, Steiner W, Jaumann MP. Endonasal sinus surgery with endoscopic control: from radical operation to rehabilitation of the mucosa. Endoscopy 1978;10:255–260.
5. Kennedy DW, Zinreich SJ, Rosenbaum AE, et al. Functional endoscopic surgery: theory and diagnostic evaluation. Arch Otolaryngol 1985;111:576–582.
6. Zinreich S, Kennedy D, Rosenbaum A, et al. Paranasal sinuses: CT imaging requirements for endoscopic surgery. Radiology 1987;163:769–775.
7. Som P. Sinonasal cavity. In: Som P, Bergeron T, eds. Head and Neck Imaging. St. Louis, Mosby-Year Book, 1991;51–168.
8. Zinreich S. Paranasal sinus imaging. Otolaryngol Head Neck Surg 1990;103:863–868.
9. Zinreich S. Imaging of chronic sinusitis in adults: x-ray, computed tomography, and magnetic resonance imaging. J Allergy Clin Immunol 1992;90:445–451.
10. Zinreich S. Imaging of inflammatory sinus disease. Otolaryngol Clin North Am 1993;26:535–547.
11. Zinreich S, Abidin M, Kennedy D. Cross-sectional imaging of the nasal cavity and paranasal sinuses. Operative Techniques Otolaryngol Head Neck Surg 1990;1:93–99.
12. Babbel R, Harnsberger HR, Nelson B, et al. Optimatization of techniques in screening CT of the sinuses. Am J Roentgenol 1991;157:1093–1098.
13. Bernhardt TM, Rapp-Bernhardt U, Fessel A, Ludwig K, et al. CT scanning of the paranasal sinuses: axial helical CT with reconstruction in the coronal direction versus coronal helical CT. Br J Radiol 1998;71:846–851.
14. Melhem ER, Oliverio PJ, Benson ML, et al. Optimal CT screening for functional endoscopic sinus surgery. Am J Neuroradiol 1996;17:181–188.
15. Beck, DSc T. Radiation Physicist, Dept. of Radiology, The Johns Hopkins Hospital, Baltimore. Personal communication.
16. Curry TS, Dowdey JE, Murry RC. Christensen's Physics of Diagnostic Radiology. 4th ed. Philadelphia: Lea & Febiger, 1990;372–391.
17. Jones DJ, Wall BF. Organ doses from medical x-ray examinations calculated using Monte Carlo techniques. NRPBR186. London: National Radiological Protection Board, 1985.
18. Zinreich SJ, Kennedy DW, Kumar A, et al. MR imaging of normal nasal cycle: comparison with sinus pathology. J Comput Assist Tomogr 1988;12:1014–1019.
19. Kennedy D, Zinreich S, Kumar A, et al. Physiologic mucosal changes within the nose and ethmoid sinus: imaging of the nasal cycle by MRI. Laryngoscope 1988;98:928–933.
20. Zinreich S, Kennedy D, Malat J, et al. Fungal sinusitis: diagnosis with CT and MR imaging. Radiology 1988;169:439–444.
21. Som P, Curtin H. Chronic inflammatory sinonasal diseases including fungal infections: the role of imaging. Radiol Clin North Am 1993;31:33–44.
22. Som P. Imaging of paranasal sinus fungal disease. Otolaryngol Clin North Am 1993;26:983–994.
23. Som P, Dillon W, Curtin H, et al. Hypointense paranasal sinus foci: differential diagnosis with MR imaging and relation to CT findings. Radiology 1990;176:777–781.
24. Weber A. Inflammatory diseases of the paranasal sinuses and mucoceles. Otolaryngol Clin North Am 1988;21:421–437.
25. Shankar L, Evans K, Hawke M, et al. An Atlas of Imaging of the Paranasal Sinuses. London: Martin Dunitz 1994;41–72.
26. Stammberger H. Functional Sinus Surgery. Philadelphia: B.C. Decker, 1991;273–282.
27. Kennedy DW, Zinreich SJ. The functional endoscopic approach to inflammatory sinus disease: current perspectives and technique modifications. Am J Rhinol 1988;2:89–93.
28. Harnsberger R. Imaging for the sinus and nose. In: Harnsberger R, ed. Head and Neck Imaging Handbook. St. Louis: Mosby-Year Book, 1990;387–419.
29. Hosemann W. Dissection of the lateral nasal wall in eight steps. In: Wigand ME, ed. Endoscopic Surgery of the Paranasal Sinuses and Anterior Skull Base. New York: Thieme Medical, 1990;36–41.
30. Schaeffer JP. The Nose, Paranasal Sinuses, Naso-lacrimal Passageways, and Olfactory Organs in Man. Philadelphia: P. Blakiston's Son & Co., 1920.
31. Schaeffer JP. The genesis, development, and adult anatomy of the nasofrontal region in man. Am J Anat 1916;20:125–146.
32. Van Alyea OE. Ethmoid labyrinth: anatomic study, with consideration of the clinical significance of its structural characteristics. Arch Otolaryngol 1939;29:881–902.
33. Van Alyea OE. Frontal cells: an anatomic study of their clinical significance. Arch Otolaryngol 1941;34:11–23.
34. Van Alyea OE. Sphenoid sinus: anatomic study, with consideration of the clinical significance of the structural characteristics of the sphenoid sinus. Arch Otolaryngol 1941;34:225–253.
35. Bent JP, Cuilty-Siller C, Kuhn FA. The frontal cell as a cause of frontal sinus obstruction. Am J Rhinol 1994;8:185–191.
36. Stammberger HR, Kennedy DW, Bolger WE, et al. Paranasal sinuses: anatomic terminology and nomenclature. The Anatomic Terminology Group. Ann Otol Rhinol Laryngol Suppl 1995;167:7–16.

37. Yousem D. Imaging of sinonasal inflammatory disease. Radiology 1993;188:303–314.
38. Buus D, Tse D, Farris B. Ophthalmic complications of sinus surgery. Ophthalmology 1990;97:612–619.
39. Hudgins P. Complications of endoscopic sinus surgery: the role of the radiologist in prevention. Radiol Clin North Am 1993;31:21–31.
40. Hudgins P, Browning D, Gallups J. Endoscopic paranasal sinus surgery: radiographic evaluation of severe complications. Am J Neuroradiol 1992;13:1161–1167.
41. Maniglia A. Fatal and major complications secondary to nasal and sinus surgery. Laryngoscope 1989;99:276–283.
42. Maniglia A. Fatal and other major complications of endoscopic sinus surgery. Laryngoscope 1991;101:349–354.
43. Bolger W, Butzin C, Parsons D. Paranasal sinus bony anatomic variations and mucosal abnormalities: CT analysis for endoscopic sinus surgery. Laryngoscope 1991;101:56–64.
44. Lloyd GAS. CT of the paranasal sinuses: study of a control series in relation to endoscopic sinus surgery. J Laryngol Otol 1990;104:477–481.
45. Messerklinger W. On the drainage of the normal frontal sinus of man. Acta Otolaryngol 1967;163:176–181.
46. Lebowitz RA, Brunner E, Jacobs JB. The agger nasi cell: radiological evaluation and endoscopic maagement in chronic frontal sinusitis. Operative Techniques Otolaryngol Head Neck Surg 1995;6:171–175.
47. Scribano E, Ascenti G, Loria G, et al. The role of the ostiomeatal unit anatomic variations in inflammatory disease of the maxillary sinuses. Eur J Radiol 1997;24:172–174.
48. Wanamaker HH. Role of Haller's cell in headache and sinus disease: a case report. Otolaryngol Head Neck Surg 1996;114:324–327.
49. Driben JS, Bolger WE, Robles HA, et al. The reliability of computerized tomographic detection of the Onodi (sphenoethmoid) cell. Am J Rhinol 1998;12:105–111.
50. Tonai A, Baba S. Anatomic variations of the bone in sinonasal CT. Acta Otolaryngol 1996;Suppl 525:9–13.
51. Joe JK, Ho SY, Yanagisawa E. Documentation of variations in sinonasal anatomy by intraoperative nasal endoscopy. Laryngoscope 2000;110:223–229.
52. Weinberger DG, Anand VK, Al-Rawi M, et al. Surgical anatomy and variations of the onodi cell. Am J Rhinol 1996;10:365–370.
53. Perez-Pinas I, Sabate J, Carmona A, et al. Anatomical variations in the human paranasal sinus regions studied by CT. J Anat 2000;197:221–227.
54. Calhoun KH, Waggenspack GA, Simpson CB, et al. CT evaluation of the paranasal sinuses in symptomatic and asymptomatic populations. Otolaryngol Head Neck Surg 1991;104:480–483.
55. Lloyd GA, Lund VJ, Scadding GK. CT of the paranasal sinuses and functional endoscopic surgery: a critical analysis of 100 symptomatic patients. Laryngol Otol 1991;105:181–185.
56. Zinreich SJ, Mattox DE, Kennedy DW, et al. Concha bullosa: a CT evaluation. J Comput Assist Tomogr 1988;12:778–784.
57. Laine F, Smoker W. The ostiomeatal unit and endoscopic surgery: anatomy, variations, and imaging findings in inflammatory diseases. Am J Roentgenol 1992;159:849–857.
58. Stammberger H, Wolf G. Headaches and sinus disease: the endoscopic approach. Ann Otol Rhinol Laryngol Suppl 1988;134:323.
59. Kainz J, Stammberger H. Danger areas of the posterior rhinobasis. An endoscopic and anatomical-surgical study. Acta Otolaryngol 1992;112:852–861.
60. Yeoh KH, Tan KK. The optic nerve in the posterior ethmoid in Asians. Acta Otolaryngol 1994;114:329–336.
61. Delano M, Fun FY, Zinreich SJ. Optic nerve relationship to the posterior paranasal sinuses: a CT anatomic study. Am J Neuroradiol 1996;17:669–675.
62. Laine FJ, Kuta AJ. Imaging the sphenoid bone and basiocciput: pathologic considerations. Semin Ultrasound CT MRI 1993;14:160–177.
63. Dessi P, Moulin G, Triglia JM, et al. Difference in height of the right and left ethmoidal roofs: a possible risk factor for ethmoidal surgery: prospective study of 150 CT scans. Laryngol Otol 1994;108:261–262.
64. Johnson DW, Hopkins RJ, Hanafee WN, et al. The unprotected parasphenoidal carotid artery studied by high-resolution computed tomography. Radiology 1985;155:137–141.
65. Kennedy DW, Zinreich SJ, Hassab MH. The internal carotid artery as it related to endonasal sphenoethmoidectomy. Am J Roentgenol 1990;4:7–12.
66. Evans F, Sydnor J, Moore W, et al. Sinusitis of the maxillary antrum. N Engl J Med 1975;293:735–739.
67. Gullane P, Conley J. Carcinoma of the maxillary sinus: a correlation of the clinical course with orbital involvement, pterygoid erosion or pterygopalatine invasion and cervical metastases. J Otolaryngol 1983;12:141–145.
68. Yousem D, Kennedy D, Rosenberg S. Ostiomeatal complex risk factors for sinusitis: CT evaluation. J Otolaryngol 1991;20:419–424.
69. Babbel R, Harnsberger H, Sonkens J, et al. Recurring patterns of inflammatory sinonasal disease demonstrated on screening sinus CT. Am J Neuroradiol 1992;13:903–912.
70. Scuderi A, Babbel R, Harnsberger H, et al. The sporadic pattern of inflammatory sinonasal disease including postsurgical changes. Semin Ultrasound CT MR 1991;12:575–591.
71. Lidov M, Som P. Inflammatory disease involving a concha bullosa (enlarged pneumatized middle nasal turbinate): MR and CT appearance. Am J Neuroradiol 1990;11:999–1001.
72. Moloney J, Badham N, McRae A. The acute orbit, preseptal, periorbital cellulitis, subperiosteal abscess, and orbital cellulitis due to sinusitis. J Laryngol Otol 1987;12:1–18.
73. Centeno R, Bentson J, Mancuso A. CT scanning in rhinocerebral mucormycosis and aspergillosis. Radiology 1981;140:383–389.
74. Osguthorpe J, Hochman M. Inflammatory sinus diseases affecting the orbit. Otolaryngol Clin North Am 1993;26:657–671.
75. Walters E, Waller P, Hiles D, et al. Acute orbital cellulitis. Arch Ophthalmol 1976;94:785–788.
76. Weber A, Mikulis D. Inflammatory disorders of the paraorbital sinuses and their complications. Radiol Clin North Am 1987;25:615–631.
77. Patt B, Manning S. Blindness resulting from orbital complications of sinusitis. Otolaryngol Head Neck Surg 1991;104:789–795.
78. Vinning EM, Kennedy DW. Surgical management in adults: chronic sinusitis. Immunol Allergy Clin North Am 1994;14:97–112.
79. Panje WR, Anand VK. Endoscopic sinus surgery indications, diagnosis, and technique. In: Anand VK, Panje WR, eds. Practical Endoscopic Sinus Surgery. New York: McGraw-Hill, 1993;68–86.

# 4

# Postoperative Complications of Functional Endoscopic Sinus Surgery

### Patricia A. Hudgins and Todd T. Kingdom

## SURGICAL COMPLICATIONS

### Major and Minor

The paranasal sinuses are flanked on all sides by important structures. Thus, only the delicate lamina papyracea separates the ethmoid complex from the orbit, the roof of the ethmoids (fovea ethmoidalis) separates these cells from the anterior cranial fossa, the fenestrated cribriform plate separates the roof of the nasal cavity from the anterior cranial fossa, a thin bony carotid canal may separate the cavernous internal carotid artery from the mucosa of the sphenoid sinus, and the optic canal may be surrounded by the sphenoid sinus when there is a pneumatized anterior clinoid process. In addition, glistening, moist, diseased mucosa may look identical to periorbita or even dehiscent, inflamed meninges. As a result of this compact anatomy, when performing functional endoscopic sinus surgery (FESS), it is the endoscopist's experience and anatomic knowledge of the many potential structural variations that may occur in this region that help avoid surgical catastrophes.[1–3]

Preoperative sinus computed tomography (CT) is essential to understand the individual's anatomy and thereby avoid intraoperative complications. However, ultimately, most surgical complications from the endoscopic approach are probably sporadic and are not specifically the result of variant anatomy. Nonetheless, the standard of care is that anatomic variants believed to predispose to surgical complications should be mentioned by the radiologist in the preoperative CT interpretation (see Chapter 3).[4]

Surgical complications can be divided into major and minor events. Complications that require further surgical intervention, or blood transfusion, or that result in a new patient deficit or death, are considered major and include cerebrospinal fluid (CSF) leak, optic nerve injury, ocular motility deficits, injury to the nasolacrimal duct, permanent anosmia, and major intraoperative or perioperative hemorrhage. The incidence of major complications ranges from 0.5% to 9% and the complication rate increases with an inexperienced surgeon, severity of disease (extensive polyposis can hinder the surgeon's visibility), the extensive nature of the surgery, prior FESS, and unusual anatomic variants.[5–9]

Minor complications include periorbital swelling or orbital emphysema, small orbital hematomas, temporary olfactory dysfunction, bleeding that does not require reoperation or blood transfusion (minor epistaxis), and tooth pain. Synechiae and scar formation associated with recurrent symptoms following surgery are reported to occur in 4% to 8% of cases. Usually, the synechiae develop between the lateral nasal wall and the lateral aspect of the middle turbinate, in which case there will be a lateral deviation of the nasal septum. Formation of synechiae in this area can cause middle meatal stenosis and inadequate sinus drainage. Synechiae may also occur between the inferior turbinate and the nasal septum or within the frontal recess.

Approximately 18% of patients reportedly develop recurrent inflammatory disease after a FESS procedure. Although this is not considered a true complication, such recurrent disease is usually mentioned along with the other complications of FESS. The recurrent inflammatory disease may be present because sinusitis is a complex disease that cannot be completely cured by surgery or because the recurrent disease reflects incomplete FESS that did not fully address the ostiomeatal obstruction. Failed FESS is probably underreported, and its exact incidence is not known.

### Hemorrhage and Vascular Injury

Hemorrhage requiring transfusion or postoperative packing is a major complication and fortunately is unusual. Extensive disease, especially polyposis, prior FESS, and chronic steroid or aspirin use are risk factors for significant hemorrhage. Bleeding from the internal maxillary artery branches is likely if the turbinates or nasal septum are involved, and injury to the sphenopalatine, anterior, and posterior ethmoidal arteries is the most common reason for hemorrhage.[1]

Posterior bleeding may result from injury to the sphenopalatine artery at the anterior wall of the sphenoid sinus.[10] Injury to the internal carotid artery (ICA) is the most devastating and, fortunately, the rarest complication.[7, 8, 11] (Fig. 4-1). The ICA is vulnerable when surgery is performed in or around the posterior ethmoid air cells and the sphenoid sinus, as absence of the bony carotid wall in the posterior ethmoid or sphenoid sinus is not uncommon. An autopsy series found 71% of ICAs bulging into the sphenoid sinus,

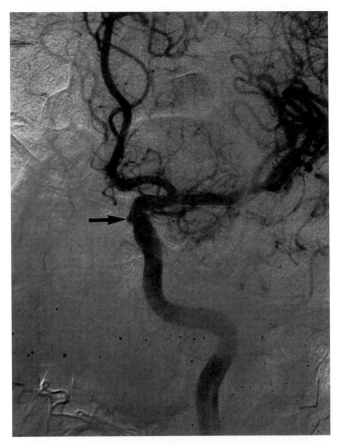

**FIGURE 4-1** Intraoperative hemorrhage during posterior ethmoidectomy. Conventional angiogram, lateral view of a left ICA injection, obtained several hours after massive intraoperative hemorrhage, shows a small pseudoaneurysm (*arrow*) of the left ICA. The patient underwent a test balloon occlusion, developed no neurologic deficits, and had permanent balloon occlusion.

with bone only microns in thickness protecting the carotid artery in many cases.[12] In a large CT series, 31.4% of patients had at least one ICA at risk, with extremely thin, bony wall seen on CT about the ICA in 17% of patients and no bony covering found in 14.4%.[13] On the traditional CT window settings used for preoperative sinus imaging, and without intravenous contrast, at times only an estimate of the ICA location can be made. When there is extensive superolateral pneumatization of the posterior ethmoid cell, termed the *Onodi cell*, the ICA and optic nerve may bulge into the pneumatized cell. Pneumatization of the anterior clinoids should be noted, as both the optic nerve and the ICA are theoretically placed at risk. Finally, intrasphenoidal bony sinus septums that insert on or near the carotid canal should be described in the radiology report. Although these septums are variable, they usually arise from the posterior or posterolateral sphenoid sinus wall and are attached at the level of the ICA. If there is a surgical attempt to resect such a septum, the twisting and applied torque may fracture the bone at the level of the ICA and inadvertently injure the vessel.[4] In summary, the ICA is vulnerable during FESS at the lateral wall of the sphenoid sinus if there is a bony septum abutting the lateral wall near the ICA canal, if Onodi cells are present, and if there is a pneumatized anterior clinoid process.

If intraoperative bleeding cannot be stopped with packing, immediate diagnostic conventional angiography is indicated. Perforation or pseudoaneurysm of the cavernous ICA can be assessed on diagnostic angiography, followed by transvascular treatment by the interventional neuroradiologist with endovascular balloon occlusion or coiling of the injured ICA. Temporary balloon occlusion is usually performed initially to determine whether there is an intact circle of Willis that will permit the patient to tolerate sacrifice of the ICA.

### Skull Base Injury, Including CSF Leak

Anterior skull base injury results in pneumocephalus, subdural hematoma, intracranial hemorrhage or contusion, cerebritis, or an abcess. There also may be focal encephalomalacia of the gyrus rectus when there has been perforation of the cribriform plate. Factors associated with such injury include dehiscence of the cribriform plate, ethmoid roof, or sphenoid roof (Fig. 4-2). CSF fistula occurs rarely in FESS, but FESS is one of the most common causes of CSF leak.[14] Subsequent development of meningitis or intracranial abscess is unusual, as the defect is generally detected intraoperatively by the surgeon and repaired immediately.[14, 15]

The roof of the ethmoid air cells may be unusually low on one side, potentially placing this ethmoid complex at risk for inadvertent surgical penetration of the anterior cranial fossa. Any asymmetry (especially if marked) in the height of the ethmoid roof on either side should also be noted in the radiology report. Any thinning or dehiscence of the ethmoid roof, cribriform plates, or roof of the sphenoid sinus (whether posttraumatic, congenital, or from prior surgery) is important preoperative information for the surgeon. Therefore, the position, symmetry, and integrity of the roof of the ethmoids, cribriform plate, and planum sphenoidale are always assessed by the radiologist prior to FESS to help avoid a surgical complication (also see Chapter 3). This is

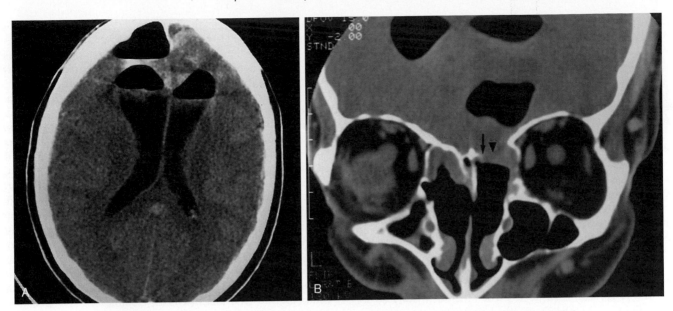

**FIGURE 4-2** Anterior skull base defect with pneumocephalus. The patient presented with headaches immediately following FESS. A CT scan was obtained several days after FESS, revealing pneumocephalus and an anterior skull base defect. **A,** Axial CT scan shows massive intracranial air, including intraventricular air. This implies that the surgical instruments went through the bony anterior skull base. **B,** Direct coronal CT scan shows resection of the entire left middle turbinate, cribriform plate (*arrow*), and roof of the ethmoids (*arrowhead*).

especially important for revision FESS, as previous FESS remains the single most important risk factor for iatrogenic CSF leak.[14]

The anterior vertical insertion of the middle turbinate lies along the lateral edge of the cribriform plate. It is an important surgical landmark, as medial to it is the cribriform plate and lateral lies the roof of the ethmoids. The anterior ethmoid artery (AEA) enters the olfactory fossa at this location, making the lateral cribriform plate, or lateral lamella of the olfactory groove, the thinnest portion and the area most "exposed" to perforation.[2] Thus, during FESS, the endoscope must remain lateral to the vertical insertion of the middle turbinate. The olfactory nerve fibers pass through the cribriform plate, and surgical injury to the olfactory mucosa or torque applied to the middle turbinate may injure these fibers as well as create a CSF leak.[3] If the entire vertical insertion of the middle turbinate has been partially or completely resected during prior surgery, it should be noted that an important surgical landmark is missing. Disturbance of olfactory function occurs in about 20% of the patients who have a CSF leak or an anterior skull base defect as a result of FESS.[16]

The posterior ethmoid roof at the border between the posterior ethmoids and sphenoid sinus is an underrecognized location of CSF leak.[1] This area should be scrutinized by the radiologist, especially prior to revision FESS. The posterior ethmoid roof is especially vulnerable to injury because it may be inadvertently misinterpreted during FESS as the anterior aspect of the sphenoid sinus.

When postoperative CSF rhinorrhea is suspected, the nasal secretions should be tested to confirm that CSF is present. Although the glucose-oxidase test was formerly used for this purpose, its high incidence of false-positive results led to the use of the β2-transferrin test. This test is highly sensitive and capable of detecting CSF in only a few millimeters of nasal secretions. If the β2-transferrin test is positive, imaging examinations are indicated.[15, 16]

For the diagnosis and localization of CSF leak following FESS, the literature does not express a definitive bias toward the use of either MR cisternography, high-resolution CT, or CT cisternography. Each has distinct advantages and disadvantages. MR and CT cisternography can identify the actual site of CSF leakage within the nasal cavity or paranasal sinuses, provided that there is an active CSF leak. The MR study, however, does not provide adequate bony detail. Plain high-resolution CT does provide a detailed display of the bone at the site of the leak; however, it does not show the flow of CSF into the sinus. In difficult cases, it is recommended that both techniques be utilized for accurate diagnosis or that a CT cisternogram study be performed. However, since the radiation dose that results from high-resolution CT is significant, MR cisternography is usually the first technique employed. The reported sensitivity of MR cisternography in the diagnosis of CSF fistulae ranges from 87% to 100%. If this examination does not provide adequate information, then high-resolution CT may be utilized. The sensitivity of high-resolution CT reportedly ranges from 71% to 92%. However, in some cases these results may be misleading, as congenital or other bony abnormalities seen may not be associated with the CSF leak.

In many institutions, a radionuclide CSF study is utilized as the initial radiologic screening examination for patients with suspected CSF leaks. Before beginning the study, the otolaryngologist places absorbent pledgets in the nasal cavity. Usually, three to four are placed on each side, and note is made of their location within the nasal cavity. Next, 400 to 500 Ci of [111]Indium-labeled ([111]In) DTPA is placed in the subarachnoid space by the radiologist via a cervical or lumbar puncture. The patient is imaged with a gamma camera at multiple intervals for up to 24 hours. Any position or activity known to provoke the leak is encouraged. Even if the images of the head and neck do not show evidence of a leak, indirect scanning evidence may confirm the presence of a leak by showing activity in the bowel. Such activity indicates that the patient is swallowing CSF as it leaks into the nasal cavity. At 24 hours, the nasal pledgets are removed and assayed. The results are compared with [111]In activity in a serum sample drawn at the same time. A ratio of pledget activity to serum activity is determined and expressed in terms of counts per gram. Pledgets showing activity 1.5 times greater than serum activity are considered positive. It is then possible to predict the general area of the leak based on which pledgets show increased activity. Even if none of the pledgets have increased activity, if there is increased activity over the abdomen the radionuclide test is considered positive.

The radiographic evaluation for CSF leak necessitates careful attention to technique and detail. On coronal CT imaging, CSF leak is suspected when there is a bony defect and a fluid level at the site of the defect. These two findings in the setting of a clinically suspected CSF leak strongly predict the presence of a leak. Because the defect may be only millimeters in size, thin-section CT in multiple planes is essential for small defects.

CT cisternography is useful to confirm the leak and can be performed on an outpatient basis. The study begins with a noncontrast thin-section 3-mm coronal CT scan of the sinuses and anterior skull base in the prone coronal position. In the axial plane, 5-mm-thick sections may be adequate. If there is a single bony defect, with or without sinus opacifica-

tion, in conjunction with a strong clinical history, no further imaging is needed to direct the surgical repair. If no bony defect is seen, the level of clinical suspicion determines whether further imaging is necessary. If the clinical suspicion of a leak is low, the study is deemed normal.

However, if the clinical suspicion of a leak is high, cisternography with intrathecal contrast can be performed. Usually, about 5 ml of nonionic contrast material is placed in the lumbar subarachnoid space, the fluoroscopy table is tilted head down for 1 to 2 minutes, and cranial flow of contrast is confirmed using fluoroscopy. Any maneuvers that provoke CSF rhinorrhea, such as a Valsalva maneuver, should be performed by the patient prior to rescanning. CT scans in the prone coronal and supine axial planes are then repeated. Visualization of contrast within a bony defect or contrast material within a sinus, air cell, or nasal cavity indicates a leak (Fig. 4-3). In subtle cases, there may be no visual suggestion of contrast accumulation, but region of interest (ROI) measurements in a sinus may be increased compared to ROI measurements obtained on the precisternogram CT. Sinus wall sclerosis or osteitis is seen commonly in patients with failed FESS, and the sclerosis might be misinterpreted as contrast extravasation if the precisternogram scan is not carefully compared to the postcontrast scan (Fig. 4-4). Images are best viewed magnified on a workstation, with varied window and level settings to improve detection of contrast accumulation.

Nuclear medicine cisternography can be performed at the same time as CT cisternography. It is especially helpful if the leak is questionable or subtle or if bilateral defects are seen and the site of the leak is not clear.

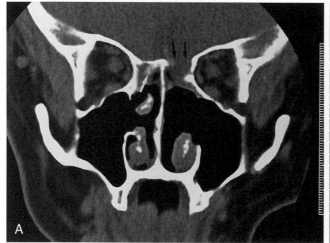 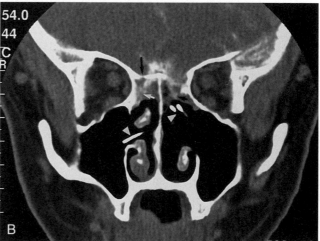

**FIGURE 4-3**   Persistent nasal discharge months after FESS. **A,** Precisternogram coronal CT scan, 3-mm slice thickness, intermediate window, shows obvious bony dehiscence at the posterior ethmoid roof on the left (*black arrows*). Postoperative findings include a thinned, straightened septum from prior septoplasty, widening of each maxillary sinus infundibulum including bilateral uncinectomies, complete resection of the left middle turbinate, and bilateral ethmoidectomies. There is high density within the right complex (*white arrow*), probably from osteitis. This bony sclerosis is often seen in chronic sinus inflammatory disease, especially following FESS. **B,** Postcisternogram coronal CT scan shows high-density nonionic contrast within the subarachnoid spaces. There is a collection of contrast within the soft tissue filling the left posterior ethmoid (*black arrow*) at the location of the bony dehiscence. Subtle contrast accumulation is also seen in the right ethmoid complex (*white arrow*) inferior to the osteitis. The smaller bony defect on the right (*long black arrow*) was not seen on the precisternogram portion of the study. Nasal pledgets, placed for the nuclear cisternogram, are seen bilaterally (*arrowheads*). These were removed at 24 hours to detect the presence of radiopharmaceutical. This additional portion of the study confirms the presence of a leak and is helpful in subtle cases. Also note that the window and level settings (window—500, level—40) are narrower than those used for screening sinus CT. The narrower settings improve visualization of contrast.

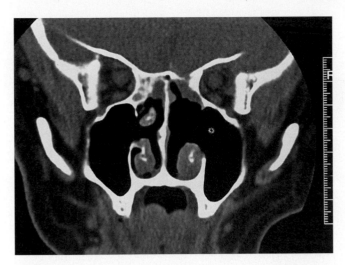

**FIGURE 4-4**  CSF rhinorrhea months following FESS. This precisternogram coronal CT scan shows the need for precontrast imaging. There is definite osteitis within the right posterior ethmoid complex, but the bony dehiscence is on the left. If only a postcisternogram CT scan had been obtained, the high density on the right might be misinterpreted as contrast accumulation, implying a right-sided leak.

Most iatrogenic skull base defects are detected intraoperatively at the time of injury, and 90% are successfully repaired during the FESS procedure at the first attempt.[14–16] A leak is suspected when there is pooling of clear fluid at the surgical site. A low dose of intrathecal fluorescein placed during or just prior to surgery, with subsequent visualization of the fluorescein at the suspected defect intraoperatively, confirms the leak.[17] A free patch repair involving fascia, mucoperiosteum from the turbinate or nasal septum, free fat, muscle, or fibrin glue may be used.[15] Endoscopic repair of CSF leak is the procedure of choice, with craniotomy reserved for the largest or most complicated defects.

CSF fluid leak, meningitis, or even meningoencephalocele, complications that are associated with FESS, present clinically days to years after surgery.[11, 18] Nonspecific symptoms of nasal obstruction, nasal discharge, or headaches may suggest recurrent sinus inflammatory disease; meningitis is rarely the presenting event. Because the symptoms of CSF leak and recurrent inflammatory disease are similar, careful radiographic assessment of the skull base is especially important in the patient with suspected FESS failure.

The rhinologist will suspect a skull base defect if there is pooling of clear fluid in the nasal cavity or if a frank intranasal mass is detected at nasal endoscopy. Cross-sectional imaging is essential to confirm the bony defect or leak (Fig. 4-2B), characterize the size and pinpoint the location of the bony defect, and determine if there is downward herniation of meninges or brain. The radiologic workup is complex, requiring more than one imaging procedure in subtle defects and MR imaging in large defects when pseudomeningocele (Fig. 4-5) or meningoencephalocele (Fig. 4-6) is suspected. A screening sinus CT scan alone is rarely enough to confirm and precisely characterize the defect.

Computer programs for intraoperative surgical guidance, now widely available, are useful in the workup of a CSF leak. These systems require preoperative CT imaging using a vendor-specific technique, which always includes extremely thin slice increments to allow high spatial resolution, multiplanar reformation capability. The CT data are loaded onto a computer system in the operating room, the data are registered to the patient using fixed fiducial markers, and the location of intranasal instruments is confirmed on the CT image by a system using either optical or electromagnetic detectors. When a CSF leak is strongly suspected, the surgeon may anticipate the need for CT surgical guidance, and the cisternogram can be performed using the required parameters. Thus, extremely thin axial CT sections, with multiplanar reformation capability, are used both for the diagnosis of a bony defect and for surgical guidance.[19] When a leak is detected, the multiplanar reformations allow precise defect localization and accurate measurement of both the depth and the width of the defect. In this regard, the thinner slices improve CSF leak detection.

When a soft-tissue mass is seen within the sinus, especially if it abuts the skull base, herniation of intracranial contents should be suspected. Meninges, CSF, or even the anteroinferior aspect of the frontal lobe can herniate downward through a skull base defect. MR imaging, including postgadolinium-enhanced images, is recommended to characterize the soft tissue within the sinus.[11]

### Orbital Complications

Orbital complications are also considered mild or severe and can be secondary to trauma to the nasolacrimal duct, inadvertent penetration of the lamina papyracea, or direct injury to the optic nerve.

Epiphora, or tearing due to interruption of the nasolacrimal duct, and dacryocystitis can result from injury to the duct. Fortunately, most ductal injuries heal spontaneously or remit by spontaneous fistularization into the middle meatus. However, stenosis or total occlusion of the nasolacrimal duct can result from more severe injury. The injury can occur during anterior enlargement of the infundibulum, usually when a backbiter is used to resect the uncinate process, enlarging the communication between the infundibulum and the middle meatus. Injury can also occur distally when an anterior maxillary antrostomy is performed near the inferior meatus.[20] In experienced surgical hands, the reported incidence of post–middle meatal antrostomy epiphora due to nasolacrimal duct injury is between 0.3% and 0.7%. Cross-sectional CT imaging can be used to assess the duct but is not commonly requested, as the duct can be directly explored by the surgeon.[21] Dacryocystography is another method used to assess the lumen of the nasolacrimal duct (see Chapter 10). Ductal dilatation with balloon dacryocystoplasty may be performed or a surgical dacryocystoplasty may be performed to restore the patency of the stenosed ductal segment.[21]

Predisposing anatomic features and variations in both major and minor orbital complications include unnoticed lamina papyracea dehiscences, medially deviated segments of the lamina papyracea (usually above or below the insertion of the basal lamella), prominent deviation of the nasal septum and large concha bullosa (which cause additional spatial limitations during the FESS ethmoidectomy procedure), and an uncinate process that adheres to the

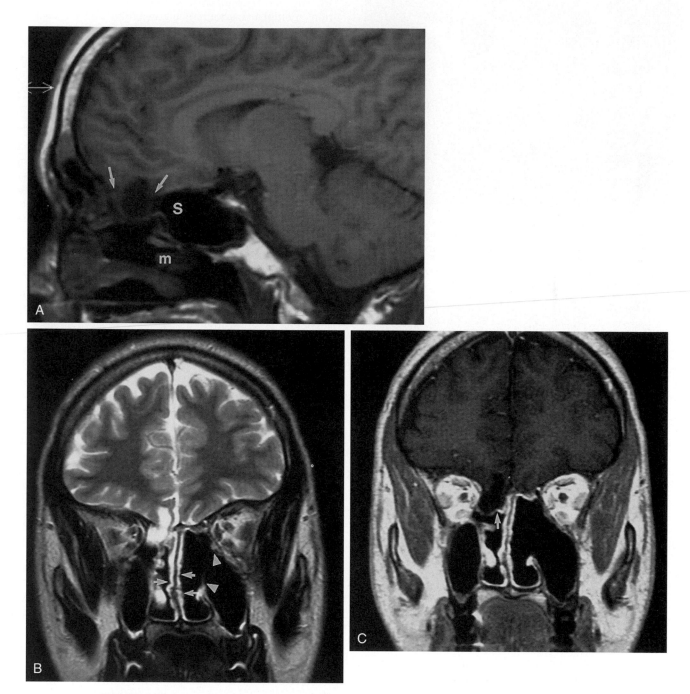

**FIGURE 4-5** Pseudomeningocele, right. Persistent "sinusitis" with nasal discharge was noted 1 year following FESS. **A,** T1-weighted sagittal MR image shows a large anterior skull base defect in the posterior ethmoid complex (*arrows*), immediately anterior to the sphenoid sinus (*S*), with intranasal herniation of meninges and CSF. Note that the midportion of the middle turbinate has been resected. The residual posterior middle turbinate is denoted by *m*. **B,** On the T2-weighted coronal MR image, the right intranasal pseudomeningocele is noted, and is clearly contiguous with a region of encephalomalacia in the anterior frontal lobe. Postoperative changes include an irregular septal contour following a septoplasty (*arrows*), total left ethmoidectomy, marked widening of the left maxillary ostium and infundibulum (*arrowheads*), and complete resection of the left middle turbinate, including the vertical insertion. **C,** T1-weighted coronal contrast-enhanced MR images show subtle enhancement of the inferior aspect of the pseudomeningocele (*arrow*) and normal mucosal enhancement of the nasal cavity.

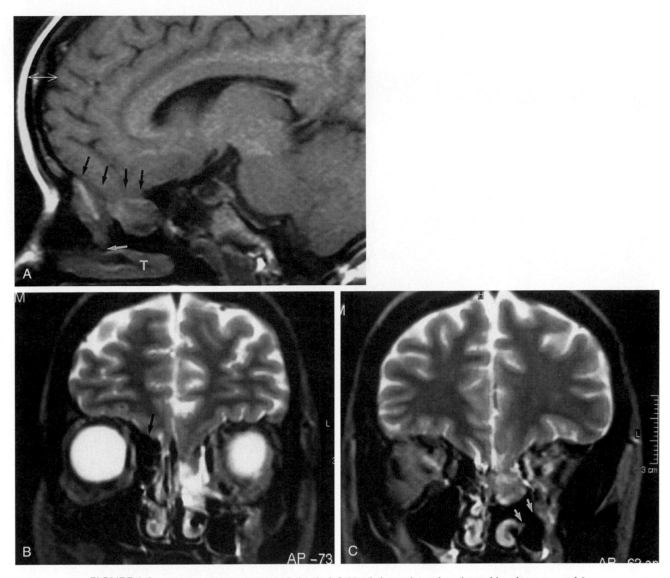

**FIGURE 4-6**   Postoperative meningoencephalocele, left. Nasal obstruction and persistent rhinorrhea was noted 6 months following FESS. **A,** On this T1-weighted sagittal MR image, note the defect in the anterior skull base (*black arrows*) and the complex large soft-tissue mass in the nasal cavity. The anterior portion of the mass abuts the inferior turbinate (*white arrow*). Inferior turbinate denoted by *T*. **B,** T2-weighted coronal MR image confirms that the mass is primarily fluid inferiorly, but there is intranasal herniation of the frontal lobe. The intact ethmoid roof on the right is denoted by the arrow. **C,** T2-weighted coronal MR image posterior to **B** shows that this portion of the meningoencephalocele is primarily brain tissue. Note the widened maxillary ostium and infundibulum on the left (*arrows*) following surgery and uncinectomy and resection of the left middle turbinate. No surgery had been performed on the right side.

inferior lateral orbit under the ethmoid bulla (atelectatic uncinate process).

When the lamina papyracea has been violated, mild complications may be periorbital ecchymosis, orbital emphysema, or a small orbital hematoma. For these minor injuries, treatment includes close observation for development of proptosis, orbital massage to decrease the intraocular pressure, and antibiotic treatment to prevent development of infection. Imaging is rarely required for these mild orbital FESS complications.

More severe orbital complications from medial orbital wall injury include a large orbital hematoma, edema and swelling of the orbital soft tissues, orbital abscess, injury to the superior or medial rectus muscle (Fig. 4-7), and injury to the optic nerve. The resulting symptoms include orbital pain, proptosis, diplopia, and vision loss.

Orbital hematoma occurs due to either rupture of the orbital ciliary veins or direct injury to the ethmoidal arteries.[21, 22] At the superior aspect of the lamina papyracea, near the level of the superior oblique and medial rectus muscles, the AEA runs within the anterior ethmoidal canal (AEC) and perforates the bony ethmoid wall (Fig. 4-8).[23] It is here that the vessel is most vulnerable. The AEC is often seen on screening sinus CT scans, especially if there is extensive pneumatization of supraorbital air cells. It may have a very thin or dehiscent bony canal, running exposed within the superior ethmoid complex (Fig. 4-9).[22] If the AEA is transected, it may retract into the orbit, the surgeon

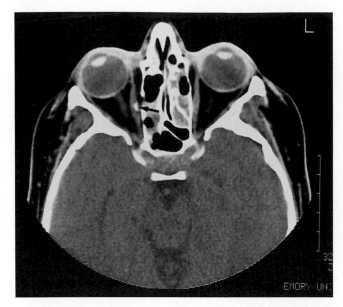

**FIGURE 4-7** Diplopia noted immediately after FESS. On this noncontrast axial CT scan, note the small bony fragment, from the lamina papyracea, within the medial rectus muscle on the right (*arrow*).

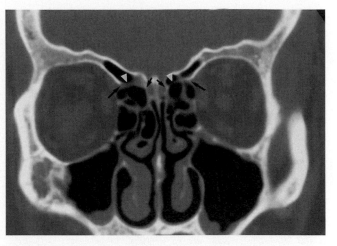

**FIGURE 4-9** Coronal CT scan. "Dehiscent" anterior ethmoidal arteries bilaterally. When the supraorbital ethmoid cells are well pneumatized, the AEA and AEC are well seen. Note the medial (*small arrows*) and lateral (*large arrows*) portions of the canals. No bone is seen around either the right or left AEA (*white arrowheads*).

will lose control of the artery, and an orbital hematoma will result.

Less often there can be injury to the posterior ethmoidal artery, which runs through the posterior ethmoidal foramen approximately 10 to 12 mm posterior to the anterior ethmoidal foramen. Injury to the posterior ethmoidal artery can also cause intraorbital hematoma. However, this artery is relatively close to the optic nerve, and due to this proximity, even small posterior ethmoidal hematomas can cause serious nerve damage, with resultant blindness.

The anterior lamina papyracea may be violated during uncinectomy or surgery of the agger nasi cell. Additionally, incidental lamina papyracea dehiscence, either from prior surgery (Fig. 4-10) or from a previous fracture, likely predisposes to orbital injury during FESS. Congenital

dehiscence of the lamina papyracea is rare but should be noted on a preoperative sinus CT report (Fig. 4-11).[24] Periorbital fat prolapsing through the defect into the ethmoid complex may be misinterpreted by the surgeon as hypertrophied or diseased mucosa or polypoid disease, and the forceps may tear the fat or injure the extraocular muscles.

Maxillary or ethmoid sinus hypoplasia and a laterally displaced uncinate process also predispose to orbital trauma during FESS. Normally, the medial wall of the orbit is in the same vertical plane as the maxillary ostium.[25] With ethmoid

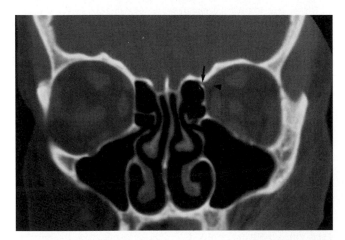

**FIGURE 4-8** Anterior ethmoidal artery canal. Coronal CT scan. Note the narrow bony canal (*arrow*) on the left at the superior aspect of the medial orbital wall, just medial to the superior oblique muscle (*arrowhead*). Visualization of the canal is variable and was not seen on the contralateral side in this patient.

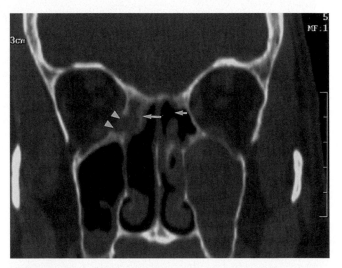

**FIGURE 4-10** Recurrent sinusitis and lamina papyracea dehiscence on the right. Axial CT scan data were acquired at 1-mm slice thickness, and this coronal reformatting was performed. There has been a prior septoplasty, ethmoidectomy bilaterally, resection of the inferior portion of the right middle turbinate with a residual superior portion (*long arrow*), and resection of the insertion of the left middle turbinate (*short arrow*), and there is recurrent mucosal thickening in the right maxillary antrum and opacification of the right ethmoid and left maxillary sinuses. Note the lamina papyracea dehiscence on the right (*arrowheads*), increasing the potential risk of orbital injury during revision FESS.

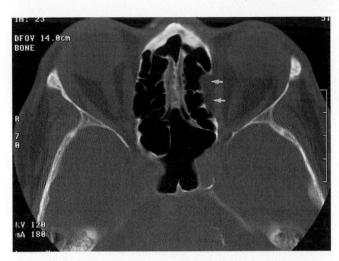

**FIGURE 4-11**   Lamina papyracea dehiscence, left. On this axial sinus CT scan, dehiscence of the left lamina papyracea with herniation of extraconal fat (*arrows*) into the ethmoid complex is seen. There was no history of prior trauma or surgery.

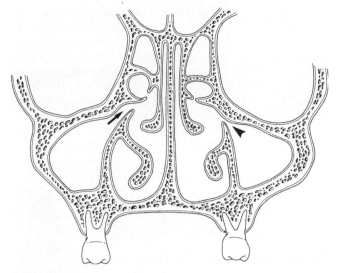

**FIGURE 4-12**   Maxillary sinus hypoplasia. Coronal diagram of the sinonasal cavity at the level of the osteomeatal unit. On the normal right side, the maxillary sinus opens into the infundibulum through the internal ostium (*arrow*). Note that the ostium is in the same vertical plane as the lamina papyracea. If the maxillary sinus is hypoplastic, as on the left, the medial antral wall is located laterally and the ostium (*arrowhead*) is lateral to the lamina papyracea. This variant predisposes to orbital penetration.

hypoplasia, the medial orbital wall is medial to the vertical plane of the maxillary ostium, presumably predisposing to orbital penetration during FESS.[4, 26] A similar anatomic relationship exists when there is a hypoplastic maxillary sinus; the medial orbital wall is located medially with respect to the maxillary ostium (Fig. 4-12). Uncinate process lateralization, hypoplasia, or even total absence is also associated with severe maxillary sinus hypoplasia.[27] Although most surgical injuries to the lamina papyracea are probably sporadic, the status of the bony orbital walls should be noted on the screening sinus CT report.

Postoperative orbital soft-tissue or osseous injury is best evaluated with direct coronal and axial CT imaging (or by using reformatted coronal images acquired from axial images using a multidetector scanner) with review of both soft-tissue and bone window settings. If orbital infection or abscess is suspected, the addition of intravenous contrast may facilitate the differentiation of phlegmon from frank abscess (Fig. 4-13). MR imaging is less sensitive in detecting small bony defects in the thin lamina papyracea, but it clearly delineates the orbital soft tissues, including the optic nerve.

Blindness from direct optic nerve injury is a rare but a devastating FESS complication. The optic nerve is vulnerable during dissection in the lateral recess of the sphenoid sinus and when there is a pneumatized superolateral recess of the sphenoid sinus. The sinus wall may be markedly thinned or even nonexistent, especially when the sphenoid sinus is excessively pneumatized.

As previously mentioned, pneumatization of the anterior clinoid process and resultant protrusion of the optic canal into the sphenoid sinus, which occurs in 8% of the population, is a potential risk factor and should be noted when seen on a preoperative sinus CT scan. The Onodi cell, a posterior ethmoid cell within the upper sphenoid sinus, occurs 3% to 15% of the time and may predispose to optic nerve injury when the FESS procedure involves the sphenoid sinus.[4] Surgical dissection in the sphenoid sinus is not commonly performed during most FESS procedures, but

occurs when there is extensive polyposis or isolated sphenoid sinus disease. Optic nerve injury, therefore, is rare, and if the intraorbital optic nerve is injured, the anatomic surgical landmarks were not appreciated by the surgeon. Sporadic reports of intraorbital optic nerve transection are rare.[28]

Radiographic evaluation of the patient presenting with post-FESS symptoms suggesting orbital complications should include a thin-section CT scan performed in the

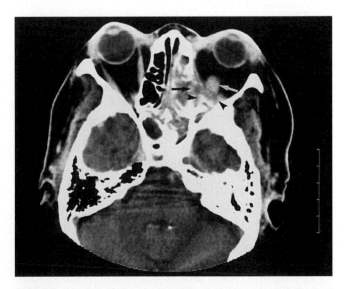

**FIGURE 4-13**   Orbital apex infection, left. Axial contrast-enhanced CT scan obtained 1 day following surgery. Proptosis, orbital pain, and decreased motility were noted. Note the bony defect in the lateral wall of the posterior ethmoid complex (*black arrow*), phlegmonous changes in the apex (*arrowheads*), and thickening of the inferior rectus muscle (*white arrow*). The diffuse sinus opacification may be seen immediately after surgery.

coronal and axial planes. On CT, penetration into the orbit through the lamina papyracea is indicated by proptosis, obliteration of orbital fat planes, orbital emphysema, retrobulbar hematoma, and distortion of the extraocular muscles or the optic nerve. Injury of the periorbital contents may be difficult to detect, but bony damage should be visible. The optic nerve should be traced in its entirety from the insertion at the posterior globe to the chiasm. The CT examination is usually diagnostic; however, if orbital and intracranial injury extent is unclear, MR imaging should also be performed.

## ENDOSCOPIC SINUS SURGERY

### Theory and Treatment Options

As discussed in Chapter 3, prior to the development of FESS, surgical sinus procedures were performed under the assumption that the sinus mucosa was the primary abnormality and that if the mucosa was stripped or resected, the chronic sinusitis would resolve. Poor outcomes necessitated reassessment of that theory. During the 1970s and 1980s, Messerklinger in Austria, Draf and Wigand in Germany, and Kennedy in the United States proposed that the mucosa was secondarily diseased and that a stenotic sinus ostium or a narrowed nasal cavity region obstructed the sinus, leading to hyperplastic, edematous mucosal changes.[29, 30] Stagnant sinus secretions then became infected, the mucosal changes became more severe, and the ostium was further obstructed. A cycle of mucosal swelling, sinus obstruction, infection, and worsening of mucosal swelling followed.[31] It has been shown that with improved sinus ventilation and drainage, the ciliated mucosal epithelium usually normalizes, with resolution of symptoms.[32]

Development of recurrent acute or chronic sinusitis is multifactorial, and ensuring ostial patency is only part of the treatment. Mucociliary function, transport, and clearance of secretions theoretically should normalize with the creation of a patent sinus ostium.[33] This concept likely oversimplifies treatment, as abnormal sinus ventilation, defective mucociliary function, and systemic conditions such as atopy, aspirin intolerance, and asthma also contribute to sinus inflammatory disease.

Disease or obstruction of the ethmoid sinuses is the primary event in chronic or recurrent acute sinusitis affecting the ethmoid complex, frontal sinuses, and maxillary sinuses.[34] Radiographic studies have shown that the ethmoids are the most common location for inflammatory disease. When the ethmoids are abnormal, the frontal and maxillary sinuses are more often abnormal; when the ethmoid complex is clear, the maxillary and frontal sinuses are generally normal.[31, 35-37]

Surgical procedures used in this region include widening of the ethmoid infundibulum and treating variants in the ostiomeatal complex. The most common procedure includes removal of the uncinate process and widening of the maxillary sinus ostium and infundibulum, resection of diseased mucosa in the frontal recess, unroofing the ethmoid bulla, and removing the bony septae in the anterior ethmoid complex. Total endoscopic sphenoethmoidectomy, a more extensive surgery often performed for sinonasal polyposis, involves exenteration of the ethmoid complex, opening the sphenoid sinus, and widening the ostiomeatal complex and the maxillary sinus infundibulum. Between these two procedures is a range of surgical treatments specific to each disease location (also see Chapter 3).

Endoscopic sinus surgery is individualized to each patient and to the specific sites of disease seen on nasal endoscopy and screening sinus CT. The procedure may be unilateral or bilateral and may be minimal, with only one or two sites treated (Fig. 4-14), or extensive, with multiple sites treated. In general, the trend with FESS is to operate conservatively and to do less surgery in order to preserve more mucosa.

### FESS Outcomes

The success of FESS, defined as significant clinical improvement of preoperative symptoms, normalization of the mucosa and sinus ostia seen during endonasal examination, or resolution of abnormal CT findings, ranges from 78% to 95%.[8, 38-41] From 10% to 20% of patients, therefore, may report no benefit or are worse after FESS.[40, 42] There may be discordance between subjective patient-reported symptoms and the objective endonasal and/or CT examination. Alternatively, resolution or significant improvement in symptoms may be reported by the patient, with only small changes in abnormalities found at physical examination or CT imaging. In turn, the physical and CT examinations may return to normal but the patient may report continued symptoms. Subjective symptomatic relief is the primary end result, regardless of the objective examinations. The post-FESS sinus CT results, therefore, supplement the

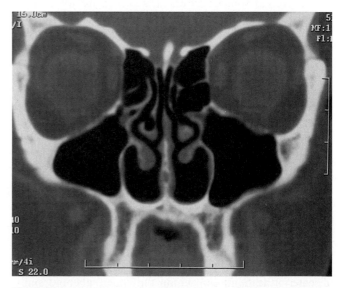

**FIGURE 4-14** Subtle post-FESS findings. On this coronal CT scan, note that the nasal septum is unusually straight, with loss of the normal mucosal contours. There has been minimal resection of the inferior turbinates. The surgery was performed to relieve symptoms of chronic nasal obstruction.

clinical data. Long-term outcome data on FESS have only recently become available. Most outcome data are short-term, with reexamination 3 months to 3–8 years after surgery. It is therefore difficult to report the efficacy of the procedure accurately, as it depends on which parameter is considered. Symptom reports are by definition subjective. The outcome depends on the degree of preoperative disease, the presence of polyposis, and which surgical procedure is performed. In summary, it is common for objective examinations to diverge from subjective patient reports, but FESS has been established as effective based on symptoms.

Recurrent acute sinusitis, chronic sinusitis, sinogenic headache, recurrent polyposis with infection or nasal obstruction, or nasal drainage are generally considered symptoms suggestive of surgical failure.[38] Sinogenic headache is defined as midface dull aching or pressure, often localized to the medial canthal region, which correlates with inflammatory disease in the ethmoid complex or ostiomeatal unit.[43] An abnormal nasal examination with mucopurulent rhinorrhea, erythema and edema of the mucosa, scarring at surgical sites, or recurrent or residual polyps, coupled with an abnormal sinus CT examination, are also considered surgical failures, especially when associated with patient symptoms.[39]

Indicators or predictors that suggest a higher likelihood of a poor outcome include smoking, allergy, asthma, aspirin intolerance, sinonasal polyps, cystic fibrosis and polyps, prior "classic" sinus surgery, and possibly gastroesophageal reflux disease.[40, 42, 44] Recurrent or residual sinonasal polyposis is common, occurring in about 30% to 40% of patients with polyps.[40, 42] In fact, recurrent or residual polyps are the most common endoscopic finding following FESS and one of the most common reasons patients return for revision surgery.[40, 45] As patients with polyposis, regardless of the etiology, represent a different population from patients without polyposis, outcome data for the two groups should be reported separately.

It is well established that the findings on preoperative CT images of the sinuses are not specific for sinonasal inflammatory disease, and there is no association between symptom severity and CT findings.[46, 47] The incidence of asymptomatic sinonasal mucosal thickening or opacification is high. The definition of sinusitis (adopted by the American Academy of Otolaryngology–Head and Neck Surgery, the American Academy of Otolaryngic Allergy, and the American Rhinologic Society) does not even include radiographic findings but relies solely on symptoms and physical examination findings.[48] Therefore, most surgeons would not operate on the basis of sinus CT abnormalities alone.

Sinus CT does appear to have prognostic significance for symptom resolution following FESS. The distribution and severity of disease on CT may predict the postoperative endoscopic appearance of the sinonasal region, the success of sinus surgery, and the likelihood of disease recurrence following FESS.[42, 49–51] Sinonasal polyposis with bilateral disease is the single best preoperative radiographic predictor of surgical failure.[51] Severe disease, as defined by bilateral ethmoid disease and involvement of one or two dependent sinus cavities, also is a strong predictor of FESS failure.[42]

Several objective staging systems for rhinosinusitis have been proposed and may be used to aid the patient and surgeon in making treatment decisions and predicting the surgical outcome.[42, 49, 50] The staging system at this time is an investigative tool used to quantify the degree of disease and to determine prospectively if the amount of disease correlates with surgical success. One system, termed the *Lund staging system for rhinosinusitis*, grades CT findings, anatomic variants, the surgical score, the symptom score, and the endoscopic appearance score.[52] With respect to the CT portion of the system, each sinus group is graded 0–2, with 0 indicating no abnormality, 1 partial opacification, and 2 total opacification. The ostiomeatal complex is graded 0 (not obstructed) or 2 (obstructed). Normal variants including absent frontal sinuses, concha bullosa, paradoxic middle turbinates, Haller cells, everted uncinate process or agger nasi cell pneumatization are graded 1 (present) or 0 (absent) (Table 4-1). Each side is considered separately. The CT outcome number is combined with the surgical and symptom scores for a total number to categorize the extent of rhinosinusitis and to aid the surgeon in objectively determining the need for surgery or revision FESS.

## Table 4-1
## LUND STAGING SYSTEM

Sinus
    0—normal
    1—partial opacification
    2—total opacification

Ostiomeatal complex
    0—no obstruction
    2—obstructed

Normal variants
    0—absent
    1—present
    Absent frontal sinuses
    Concha bullosa
    Paradoxical middle turbinates
    Haller cells
    Everted uncinate process
    Agger nasi cell pneumatization

## The FESS Procedure and Imaging Findings

### Overview of the FESS Procedure

When assessing a postoperative sinus CT study, it is helpful to begin the interpretation with a thorough discussion of the anatomic changes that resulted from the surgery, including which structures were resected and which structures remain intact. This is especially important for the FESS procedure, as there is no routine surgery, since each operation is carefully individualized for the specific patient. After that task, the scan is assessed for residual or recurrent sinus disease. Revision FESS carries the same potential complications as initial surgery, so review of the integrity of the lamina papyracea, cribriform plate, roof of the ethmoids, and sphenoid sinus pneumatization is as important as the first preoperative sinus CT interpretation. Injury to the nasolacrimal duct occurs at a slightly higher rate with revision surgery, especially when a radical ethmoidectomy is performed.[53]

Understanding the FESS procedure facilitates recognition of surgical changes on the CT study. Septoplasty is an adjunctive procedure often performed during FESS to gain surgical access or treat nasal obstruction. The deviated septum can obstruct the nasal cavity, restricting endoscopic access to the ethmoid complex and ostiomeatal unit. By resecting the deviated septum or a bony septal spur, the surgeon can more easily move the endoscope posteriorly through the nasal cavity. Also, a severe septal deviation or spur can result in nasal obstructive symptoms or chronic sinusitis due to mass effect in the middle meatus, stenosing the ethmoid recess or maxillary sinus infundibulum.[54, 55]

The next step is infundibulotomy by resecting the uncinate process. A large concha bullosa or polyp is resected if it blocks access to the uncinate. Once the uncinate has been removed, the surgeon has visual and surgical access to the maxillary ostium, frontal recess, and anterior ethmoid complex. The ostium of the maxillary sinus is inspected, and obstructing polyps or hyperplastic mucosa are resected to restore normal drainage. After uncinectomy, the maxillary sinus ostium may be extended posteriorly and inferiorly, but only the minimal amount of bony resection is performed. If indicated, an ethmoidectomy is performed from anterior to posterior. The extent of this procedure is determined by the CT scan and direct visualization of disease. The ethmoid bulla is taken down as the first step in any ethmoid procedure, especially if the bulla is diseased, deviates the middle turbinate, or is so large as to obstruct the hiatus semilunaris.

If there is disease in the frontal sinus or recess, the natural ostium is identified and obstructing polyps or mucosa are resected. This is one of the most difficult areas to access and treat surgically. A large agger nasi cell may obstruct identification of the frontal recess. Other important variants here include frontal cells or superior orbital cells. The AEA must be identified prior to further dissection. The recess may be extremely narrow and obliquely angled. Generally, once the ostium is isolated, polyps or cysts can be removed, but disease located laterally is not resected. Occasionally, the bony ostium may be widened.

The ground lamella, or the posterior horizontal insertion of the middle turbinate to the lamina papyracea, separates the anterior from the posterior ethmoid cells. When significant disease is seen in the posterior ethmoid complex, the surgical dissection will be extended to treat these locations. The posterior ground lamella is carefully perforated, and the posterior ethmoid cells are entered. The roof of the ethmoid complex is identified prior to any additional surgery to avoid injury to the skull base. Careful removal of polyps, diseased mucosa, or inflammatory debris is then performed.

The usual approach to the sphenoid sinus, if necessary, is through the nasal cavity to the natural ostium at the sphenoethmoidal recess, medial to the turbinates. To gain access, it may be necessary to resect the posterior aspect of the middle turbinate.[33] A second approach is transethmoidal. In these cases, the surgeon relies on the screening preoperative sinus CT scan to be familiar with the individual anatomy in this region. It is essential that the optic nerve and internal carotid artery, and their relationship to the posterior ethmoid and sphenoid sinuses, are well understood prior to the surgical procedure.

## Postoperative Findings: Expected and Complications

The postoperative CT scan reflects the surgical procedures that were performed. In the radiographic report, there should be a description of the surgical changes present and the presence of any recurrent soft tissue (likely related to scar and fibrosis), hyperplastic mucosal disease, or polyps. Radiographically, differentiation between scar, fibrosis, and diseased mucosa may not be possible.[56] One of the most common reasons for FESS failure is poor control of mucosal inflammation.[57] Recurrent symptoms following FESS are related to surgical undertreatment of a region, residual variants, restenosis from scar or adhesions, recurrent hyperplastic mucosa, or residual or recurrent polyposis. Two endoscopic findings that correlate best with a poor outcome are scarring of the ethmoids and scarring of the middle meatal antrostomy. The location of a scar or mucosal disease is particularly important to describe, especially if it occurs at a sinus ostium. Thus, significant mucosal thickening in a maxillary antrum may be secondary to recurrent stenosis at the maxillary sinus infundibulum due to a scar or a polyp. Given the theory of sinusitis, it is likely that mucosal thickening and outlet stenosis, although different in location, are causally related.

The most common CT finding in a patient with failed FESS is mucosal disease, with or without associated anatomic factors.[57] In descending order of frequency, recurrent mucosal disease is reported in the anterior ethmoid sinuses, the maxillary sinus, the posterior ethmoid sinuses, the frontal sinus, and the sphenoid sinus.[57, 58] Residual agger nasi cells, Haller cells, and ethmoid air cells are also seen in failed sinus surgery patients. Recurrent or residual polyps are commonly found, especially if polyposis was treated at the initial procedure.

The following is a location-specific description of the CT findings commonly seen when revision FESS for recurrent symptoms is being considered. These findings are summarized in Table 4-2. After septoplasty, the nasal septum on CT imaging appears straightened and the mucosa is thinned (Fig. 4-14). Bony spurs should no longer be seen. A complication of septoplasty is compromise of the septal arterial blood supply, which may lead to a septal perforation. Any bony septal interruption seen on CT should be reported by the radiologist.

The appearance of the middle turbinate is variable, depending on the extent of the surgical procedure. If a middle turbinate concha bullosa has been resected, this should be noted by the radiologist.

**Table 4-2**
**ANATOMIC VARIABLES THAT MAY PREDISPOSE TO RECURRENT DISEASE AFTER FESS**

Persistent septal deviation
Lateralized middle turbinate
Residual uncinate process
Residual ethmoid, frontal, or superior orbital cells
Scar at the maxillary infundibulum
Scar at the frontoethmoid infundibulum
Sinonasal polyposis
Residual variants—agger nasi cells, concha bullosa, Haller cells
Sinus wall osteitis

There is controversy in the surgical literature regarding whether middle turbinectomy is efficacious. Following partial middle turbinectomy, some authors report a lower incidence of recurrent frontal sinusitis, while others report a higher incidence.[59] Reasons not to resect the middle turbinate include its role in olfaction, the possible increased incidence of frontal sinusitis, and fear of mucociliary dysfunction. Most surgeons will not resect the entire middle turbinate, as the vertical insertion of the turbinate on the skull base is an important surgical landmark. As previously mentioned, a cardinal surgical rule is to stay lateral to the middle turbinate in order to avoid creating a CSF leak. If the entire turbinate is resected, this important surgical landmark is removed.

After partial turbinectomy, the middle turbinate may be intentionally opposed to the nasal septum (Fig. 4-15). Thus, the turbinate cannot narrow the middle meatus. This "medialized middle turbinate" contributes to maintaining a patent middle meatus and is a desired finding on postoperative CT or nasal examination. Lateralization of the middle turbinate, or scar formation between the turbinate and the lateral nasal wall, is associated with recurrent sinus inflammatory disease (Fig. 4-16).[57]

Widening of the maxillary sinus ostium and infundibulum is seen after uncinectomy, and different degrees of maxillary sinus opening are seen, depending on the extent of surgery. As described previously, only the uncinate process may be resected or there may have been a wider maxillary osteotomy. Subtotal resection of the uncinate process may be intentional, as total uncinectomy reportedly carries a risk of frontal recess scarring.[40] On the other hand, incomplete uncinectomy is a factor in recurrent sinus inflammatory disease. Any soft tissue at the maxillary ostium or infundibulum, or a residual total or partial uncinate process, should be noted by the radiologist. Synechiae or scar at the natural ostium are common postoperative findings (Figs. 4-15, 4-16).[40]

Middle meatal antrostomy is believed to contribute to the recirculation syndrome, which occurs when mucus that exits the natural maxillary sinus ostium enters the nasal cavity and reenters the maxillary sinus through a surgically created opening separate from the natural ostium (Fig. 4-17).[33, 40] The nasal antral window is an antrostomy surgically created immediately below the lateral insertion of the inferior turbinate and is not in continuity with the natural ostium. It was commonly performed in conjunction with the Caldwell-Luc procedure.[60] Widening or relieving obstruction of the natural ostium is currently preferred over the surgical creation of a new and separate opening in the medial wall of the maxillary sinus. Any medial maxillary sinus wall defect seen on the postoperative CT scan should be noted by the radiologist (Fig. 4-17B).

The most common CT appearance of the ethmoid complex after surgery is that of a common anterior ethmoid cavity with resection of multiple ethmoidal septations (Fig. 4-16). The ethmoidectomy may have been either partial or total, and the CT scan will reflect the procedure. Intact or residual ethmoid air cells, including the ethmoid bulla, should be reported by the radiologist, as residual cells are one of the major reasons for FESS failure (Fig. 4-18).[56] Scar formation at the ethmoid infundibulum, obstructing the sinus outflow, should be noted, as this finding is also

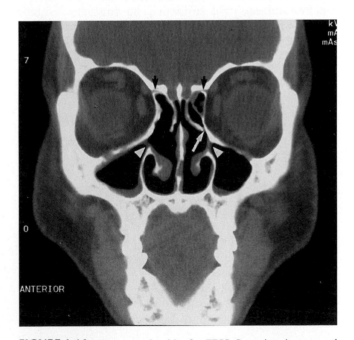

**FIGURE 4-16**    Recurrent sinusitis after FESS. Screening sinus coronal CT scan shows changes from septoplasty (straight septum with irregular mucosal contour), resection of the inferior aspect of both inferior and middle turbinates, total ethmoidectomy on the right, and partial ethmoidectomy on the left. There is soft-tissue scar or fibrosis at both maxillary sinus ostia (*arrowheads*), a lateralized left middle turbinate that is adherent to the lateral nasal wall (*white arrow*), and inflammatory changes in the left ethmoid complex. Minor mucosal thickening is seen in the alveolar recess of both maxillary sinuses, but the most important observation is soft tissue obliterating the anterior maxillary ostia (*arrowhead*) bilaterally. It is unclear whether this finding affects maxillary sinus clearance, but it should be mentioned by the radiologist. Incidental note is made of both anterior ethmoid arteries within anterior ethmoid canals (*black arrows*). Note the proximity of the lateral AECs near the superior oblique muscles.

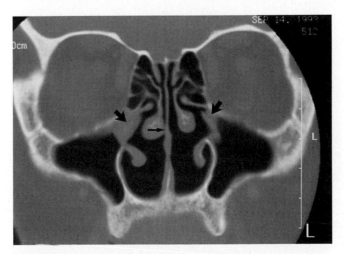

**FIGURE 4-15**    Recurrent symptoms, probably due to functional and flow changes after extensive FESS. Postoperative findings on this sinus coronal CT scan include a septoplasty, resection of most of the inferior turbinates, and a medialized right middle turbinate (*black arrows*). There is soft tissue in both maxillary sinus ostia (*thick arrows*). The soft tissue on the right is polypoid and probably represents recurrent polyps. On the left, it likely represents scar.

associated with failed FESS.[40] Most commonly, residual cells are located in the roof of the ethmoid complex and far posteriorly near the sphenoid sinus. Many surgeons leave these extreme cells intact in order to avoid perforation into the floor of the anterior cranial fossa or injury to the optic nerve.

Early frontal recess stenosis may be asymptomatic but should be noted, as it likely predisposes to future mucocele formation (Fig. 4-19).[42, 61] Causes of frontal sinus obstruction after FESS include residual agger nasi cells, residual frontal cells, and bony or soft-tissue obstruction of the infundibulum. Persistent ethmoid sinus disease is also a significant cause of recurrent frontal sinus disease, and prior ethmoidectomy is reported to be associated with frontal sinus disease.[42] Some of these outcomes appear discordant, and clearly long-term follow-up is necessary to understand and clarify what appear to be contradictory outcomes.

Recurrent frontal sinus disease following FESS is a difficult clinical problem. Resistant frontal sinusitis has been traditionally treated by an osteoplastic flap procedure, an external surgical approach that obliterates the sinus cavity (see Chapter 7).[62] Alternative transnasal endoscopic approaches to the frontal sinus have been proposed, and early results appear promising.[61, 63, 64] The most commonly performed procedure, termed a *Draf-type drill out* or *modified intranasal Lothrop procedure*, involves resecting all anterior ethmoid air cells and the uncinate process near the frontal recess and performing an endoscopic frontal sinusotomy. On CT, the frontal recess will appear widened and resection of the structures described will be seen. A more extensive Draf procedure will include resection of the inferior interfrontal sinus septum, the superior nasal septum, and the frontal sinus floor to the level of the orbit. This procedure, generally reserved for the most recalcitrant disease, creates a large anatomic opening with the goal of preventing recurrent stenosis.

The worst outcome based on symptoms, clinical examination, and the post-FESS CT scan, occurs in patients with extensive sinonasal polyposis. The failure rate in this group, reportedly as high as 75%, is so high that most series report diffuse polyposis outcomes separately from those in patients without polyps or with only a few polyps (Fig. 4-20).[42] Aspirin intolerance, asthma, and atopy are often seen with polyposis, suggesting a systemic but poorly understood association.[65] It has been proposed that polyposis is a systemic disease, thereby explaining the higher rate of recurrence.[38] The common CT findings seen in this group of patients are recurrent severe mucosal thickening and polyps in both operated and nonoperated sinuses and in the nasal cavity. These patients with sinonasal polyposis, with or without fungal involvement, often undergo multiple endoscopic procedures, and as the surgical risk rises with each operation, the radiologist should be particularly vigilant in assessing the lamina papyracea and anterior bony skull base.

Dense sclerotic new bone in a previously operated cavity is a common finding in patients who have failed FESS (Fig. 4-21). Similar changes may be seen in the bone of the middle

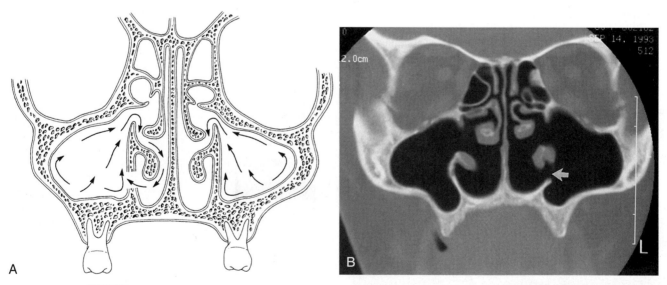

**FIGURE 4-17**  Recirculation syndrome. **A,** Coronal diagram of the sinonasal cavity at the level of the ostiomeatal unit. Middle meatal antrostomy is believed to contribute to the recirculation syndrome, which occurs when mucus that exits the natural maxillary sinus ostium enters the nasal cavity and reenters the maxillary sinus through a surgically created opening separate from the natural ostium (right side). The nasal antral window is an antrostomy surgically created immediately below the lateral insertion of the inferior turbinate and is not in continuity with the natural ostia. Any middle maxillary sinus wall defect seen on the postoperative CT scan should be noted. Note the normal mucociliary pattern on the left beating toward the natural ostium. **B,** Coronal CT scan. Note the patent middle meatal antrostomy on the left (*arrow*). There is also nearly complete resection of the inferior turbinates. No recurrent sinus inflammatory changes are noted. The meatal antrostomy, turbinate resection, and extensive loss of mucosa may contribute to abnormal sinus ventilation and function, resulting in nasal dryness and crusting simulating recurrent sinusitis.

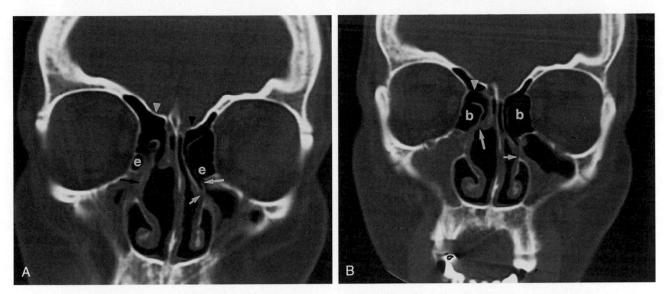

**FIGURE 4-18** Recurrent sinusitis, preoperative scan prior to revision surgery. **A,** Coronal CT scan. On the right side, note the residual uncinate process (*black arrow*) and inflammatory hyperplastic mucosa in the maxillary sinus. Hyperplastic mucosa is seen along the uncinate process and the residual anterior ethmoid air cell (*e*), contributing to infundibular stenosis. On the left side, the inferior aspect of the middle turbinate (*short white arrow*) is lateralized and adherent to the residual uncinate process (*long white arrow*). Note the residual ethmoid air cell (*e*). There is asymmetry of the ethmoid roofs, with the left roof (*black arrowhead*) 8 mm lower than the right (*white arrowhead*). **B,** Coronal CT scan posterior to **A.** There are residual ethmoid bullar cells (*b*) bilaterally, and infundibular stenosis with adhesions between the middle turbinate and the lateral nasal wall on the left (*short arrow*) and the bulla and lateral nasal wall on the right (*long arrow*). Incidental note is made of an unprotected anterior ethmoid artery (*arrowhead*), without a bony canal, in the right ethmoid roof.

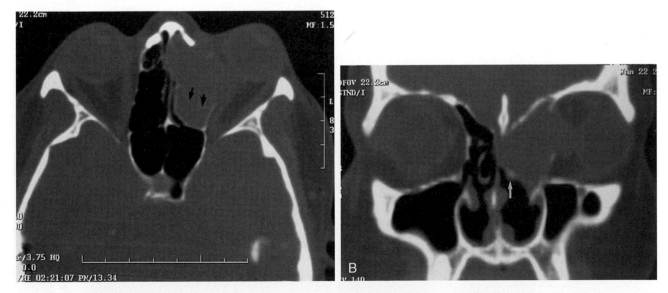

**FIGURE 4-19** Post-FESS frontoethmoidal mucocele, likely due to postoperative frontal recess stenosis. **A,** On the axial CT scan, 1-mm slice thickness, the left ethmoid sinus is airless and expanded. Deossification of the medial orbital wall results in poor visualization of the bony wall, and there is intraorbital, extraconal extension of the mucocele. Note the posterior displacement of the anterior wall of the posterior ethmoid sinus (*arrows*). **B,** The high-resolution coronal reformation shows a prior septoplasty, resection of both inferior turbinates, with only the inferior aspect of the left middle turbinate remaining (*arrow*), and the large mucocele. Recurrent frontoethmoidal recess stenosis from synechiae or mucosal disease likely led to the mucocele. The patient complained only of proptosis.

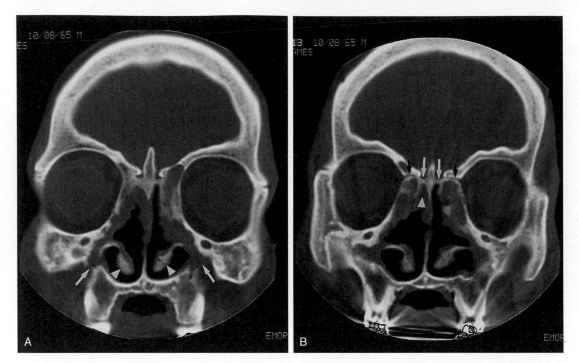

**FIGURE 4-20** Recurrent polyposis. **A,** On this coronal CT scan, note the maxillary sinus hypoplasia, prior Caldwell-Luc defects (*arrows*), and diffuse recurrent mucosal thickening. There is extensive osteitis involving all the sinus cavity walls and even the bone of the inferior turbinates (*arrowheads*). **B,** Coronal CT scan posterior to **A.** Inflammatory mucosal changes are seen medial to the right middle turbinate (*arrowhead*). This area is almost never approached surgically, as injury to the perforated cribriform plate (*white arrows*) can result in CSF leak. The sinus walls are so dense and sclerotic that the anterior ethmoid artery canals (*black arrows*) are well seen.

turbinate.[66] Histopathologic study reveals an increase in bone physiology with bone resorption, neogenesis, and fibrosis, similar to chronic osteomyelitis.[67] Chronic inflammatory changes are seen even when the overlying mucosa is normal. It is not clear whether this is a response to chronic infection or surgery or whether it is causal in the continuing cycle of sinusitis. These poorly understood osseous changes should be noted on screening sinus CT because of their frequent coexistence with chronic sinusitis. The bony changes may be isolated to a portion of a sinus, may be present throughout the sinus walls, or may be strategically located at the sinus ostium. This is an area of active basic research because of the potential implications for long-term antibiotic treatment.[67]

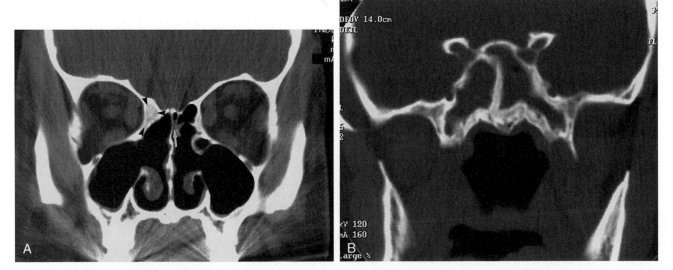

**FIGURE 4-21** Failed FESS, two separate patients with osteitis. **A,** Coronal CT scan. At this level the maxillary ostia and infundibulum are widely patent, and the residual left middle turbinate is adherent to the nasal septum (*arrow*), a desired postoperative result, as the ethmoid infundibulum is patent. Note that at this level the entire right middle turbinate, even the vertical portion, has been resected. This observation should be reported in the dictation, as an important surgical landmark is gone. The dense sclerosis within the right ethmoid complex (*arrowheads*) is seen and represents a new finding. The significance of this physiologic bony change is not well understood, but it likely relates to chronic osteitis and inflammatory changes and is a common finding in patients with recurrent symptoms after FESS. **B,** Coronal CT scan. In this patient with recurrent sphenoid sinusitis after FESS, note the sclerosis of the sinus walls and the intersphenoidal septum.

# REFERENCES

1. Stankiewicz JA. Complications of endoscopic intranasal ethmoidectomy. Laryngoscope 1987;97:1270–1273.
2. Stankiewicz JA. Complications in endoscopic intranasal ethmoidectomy: an update. Laryngoscope 1989;99:686–690.
3. Rontal M, Rontal E. Studying whole-mounted sections of the paranasal sinuses to understand the complications of endoscopic sinus surgery. Laryngoscope 1991;101:361–366.
4. Meyers RM, Valvassori G. Interpretation of anatomic variations of computed tomography scans of the sinuses: a surgeon's perspective. Laryngoscope 1998;108:422–425.
5. Maniglia AJ. Fatal and other major complications of endoscopic sinus surgery. Laryngoscope 1991;101:349–354.
6. Kinsella JB, Calhoun KH, Bradfield JJ, et al. Complications of endoscopic sinus surgery in a residency training program. Laryngoscope 1995;105:1029–1032.
7. Maniglia A. Fatal and major complications secondary to nasal and sinus surgery. Laryngoscope 1989;99:276–283.
8. Weber R, Draf W, Keerl R, et al. Endonasal microendoscopic pansinus operation in chronic sinusitis. II. Results and complications. Am J Otolaryngol 1997;18:247–253.
9. Keerl R, Stankiewicz J, Weber R, et al. Surgical experience and complications during endonasal sinus surgery. Laryngoscope 1999; 109:546–550.
10. May M, Levine HL, Mester SJ, Schaitkin B. Complications of endoscopic sinus surgery: analysis of 2108 patients—incidence and prevention. Laryngoscope 1994;104:1080–1083.
11. Hudgins PA, Browning DG, Gallups J, et al. Endoscopic paranasal sinus surgery: radiographic evaluation of severe complications. AJNR 1992;13:1161–1167.
12. Rhoton AL Jr, Renn WH, Harris FS. Microsurgical anatomy of the sellar region cavernous sinuses. In: Rand RW, ed. Microneurosurgery. 2nd ed. St. Louis: C.V. Mosby, 1978; •••.
13. Johnson DM, Hopkins, RJ, Hanafee WN, Fisk JD. The unprotected parasphenoidal carotid artery studied by high-resolution computed tomography. Radiology 1985;155:137–141.
14. Hegazy HM, Carrau RL, Snyderman CH, et al. Transnasal endoscopic repair of cerebrospinal fluid rhinorrhea: a meta-analysis. Laryngoscope 2000;110:1166–1172.
15. Senior BA, Jafri K, Benninger M. Safety and efficacy of endoscopic repair of CSF leaks and encephaloceles: a survey of the members of the American Rhinologic Society. Am J Rhinol 2001;15:21–25.
16. Weber R, Keerl R, Draf W, et al. Management of dural lesions occurring during endonasal sinus surgery. Arch Otolaryngol Head Neck Surg 1996;122:732–736.
17. Mattox DE, Kennedy DW. Endoscopic management of cerebrospinal fluid leaks and cephaloceles. Laryngoscope 1990;100:857–862.
18. Stankiewicz JA. Cerebrospinal fluid fistula and endoscopic sinus surgery. Laryngoscope 1991;101:250–256.
19. Caversaccio M, Bachler R, Ladrach K, et al. Frameless computer-aided surgery system for revision endoscopic sinus surgery. Otolaryngol Head Neck Surg 2000;122:808–813.
20. Lawson W. The intranasal ethmoidectomy: evolution and an assessment of the procedure. Laryngoscope 1994;104(Suppl 64):13–16.
21. Janssen AG, Mansour K, Bos JJ. Obstructed nasolacrimal duct system in epiphora: long-term results of dacryocystoplasty by means of balloon dilation. Radiology 1997;205:791–796.
22. Stankiewicz JA, Chow JM. Two faces of orbital hematoma in intranasal (endoscopic) sinus surgery. Otolaryngol Head Neck Surg 1999;120:841–847.
23. Chung S-K, Dhong HJ, Kim HY. Computed tomography anatomy of the anterior ethmoid canal. Am J Rhinol 2001;15:77–81.
24. Moulin G, Dessi P, Chagnaud C, et al. Dehiscence of the lamina papyracea of the ethmoid bone: CT findings. Am J Neuroradiol 1994;15:151–153.
25. May M, Sobol SM, Korzec K. The location of the maxillary os and its importance to the endoscopic sinus surgeon. Laryngoscope 1990;100: 1037–1042.
26. Driben JS, Bolger WE, Robles HA, et al. Maxillary sinus hypoplasia: classification and description of associated uncinate process hypoplasia. Otolaryngol Head Neck Surg 1990;103:759–765.
27. Bolger WE, Woodruff WW, Morehead J, Parsons DS. Maxillary

28. sinus hypoplasia: classification and description of associated uncinate process hypoplasia. Otolaryngol Head Neck Surg 1990;103: 759–765.
28. Stammberger H. Results, problems, and complications. In: Stammberger H, ed. Functional Endoscopic Sinus Surgery. Philadelphia: B.C. Decker, 1991;459–477.
29. Messerklinger W. On the drainage of the normal frontal sinus of man. Acta Otolaryngol 1967;63:176–181.
30. Kennedy DW, Zinreich SJ. Functional endoscopic approach to inflammatory sinus disease: current perspectives and technique modifications. Am J Rhinol 1988;2:89–96.
31. Stammberger H. Endoscopic surgery—concepts in treatment of recurring rhinosinusitis. Part I. Anatomic and pathophysiologic considerations. Otolaryngol Head Neck Surg 1986;115:143–146.
32. Guo Y, Majima Y, Hattori M, et al. Effects of functional endoscopic sinus surgery on maxillary sinus mucosa. Arch Otolaryngol Head Neck Surg 1997;123:1097–1100.
33. Waguespack R. Mucociliary clearance patterns following endoscopic sinus surgery. Laryngoscope 1995;105(Suppl 71):1–40.
34. Lawson W. The intranasal ethmoidectomy: evolution and an assessment of the procedure. Laryngoscope 1994;104(Suppl 64):13–16.
35. Havas TE, Motbey JA, Gullane PJ. Prevalence of incidental abnormalities on computed tomographic scans of the paranasal sinuses. Arch Otolaryngol Head Neck Surg 1988;114:856–859.
36. Zinreich SJ, Kennedy DW, Rosenbaum AE, et al. Paranasal sinuses: CT imaging requirements for endoscopic surgery. Radiology 1987; 163:769–775.
37. Bolger WE, Butzin CA, Parsons DS. Paranasal sinus bony anatomic variations and mucosal abnormalities: CT analysis for endoscopic sinus surgery. Laryngoscope 1991;101:56–64.
38. Levine HL. Functional endoscopic sinus surgery: evaluation, surgery, and follow-up of 250 patients. Laryngoscope 1990;100:79–84.
39. Rice DH. Endoscopic sinus surgery: Results at 2-year followup. Otolaryngol Head Neck Surg 1989;101:476–479.
40. Chambers DW, Davis WE, Cook PR, et al. Long-term outcome analysis of functional endoscopic sinus surgery: correlation of symptoms with endoscopic examination findings and potential prognostic variables. Laryngoscope 1997;107:504–510.
41. Lazar RH, Younis RT, Long TE, Gross CW. Revision functional endonasal sinus surgery. Ear Nose Throat J 1992;71(3):131–133.
42. Kennedy DW. Prognostic factors, outcomes, and staging in ethmoid sinus surgery. Laryngoscope 1992;102(Suppl 57):1–18.
43. Stammberger H, Wolf G. Headaches and sinus disease: the endoscopic approach. Ann Otol Rhinol Laryngol Suppl 1988;134:3–23.
44. King JM, Caldarelli DD, Pigato JB. A review of revision functional endoscopic sinus surgery. Laryngoscope 1994;104:404–408.
45. Hosemann W, Kuhnel T, Held P, et al. Endonasal frontal sinusotomy in surgical management of chronic sinusitis: a critical evaluation. Am J Rhinol 1997;11:1–9.
46. Bhattacharyya T, Piccirillo J, Wippold FJ II. Relationship between patient-based descriptions of sinusitis and paranasal sinus computed tomographic findings. Arch Otolaryngol Head Neck Surg 1997;123: 1189–1192.
47. Stewart MG, Sicard MW, Piccirillo JF, Diaz-Marchan PJ. Severity staging in chronic sinusitis: are CT scan findings related to patient symptoms? Am J Rhinol 1999;13:161–167.
48. Lanza DC, Kennedy DW. Adult rhinosinusitis defined. Otolaryngol Head Neck Surg 1997;117:51–57.
49. Gaskins RE. A surgical staging system for chronic sinusitis. Am J Rhinol 1992;6:5–12.
50. Friedman WH, Katsantonis GP, Bumpous JM. Staging of chronic hyperplastic rhinosinusitis: treatment strategies. Otolaryngol Head Neck Surg 1995;112:210–214.
51. Stewart MG, Donovan DT, Parke RB, Bautista MH. Does the severity of sinus computed tomography findings predict outcome in chronic sinusitis? Otolaryngol Head Neck Surg 2000;123:81–84.
52. Lund VJ, Holmstrom M, Scadding GK. Functional endoscopic sinus surgery in the management of chronic rhinosinusitis. An objective assessment. J Laryngol Otol 1991;105:832–835.
53. Kerrebijn JDF, Drost HE, Spoelstra HAA, Knegt PP. If functional sinus surgery fails: a radical approach to sinus surgery. Otolaryngol Head Neck Surg 1996;114:745–747.
54. Matthews BL, Smith LE, Jones R, et al. Endoscopic sinus surgery: outcome in 155 cases. Otolaryngol Head Neck Surg 1991;104: 244–246.

55. Elahi MM, Frenkiel S. Septal deviation and chronic sinus disease. Am J Rhinol 2000;14:175–179.

56. Katsantonis GP, Friedman WH, Sivore MC. The role of computed tomography in revision sinus surgery. Laryngoscope 1990;100: 811–816.

57. Chu TC, Lebowitz RA, Jacobs JB. An analysis of sites of disease in revision endoscopic sinus surgery. Am J Rhinol 1997;11:287–291.

58. Vleming M, de Vries N. Endoscopic paranasal sinus surgery: results. Am J Rhinol 1990;4:13–17.

59. Fortune DS, Duncavage JA. Incidence of frontal sinusitis following partial middle turbinectomy. Ann Otol Rhinol Laryngol 1998;107: 447–453.

60. Alusi HA. A new approach to the surgical treatment of chronic maxillary sinusitis. J Laryngol 1980;94:1145–1149.

61. Kuhn FA, Javer AR, Nagpal K, Citardi MJ. The frontal sinus rescue procedure: early experience and three-year follow-up. Am J Rhinol 2000;14:211–216.

62. Weber R, Draf W, Keerl R, et al. Osteoplastic frontal sinus surgery with fat obliteration: technique and long-term results using magnetic resonance imaging in 82 operations. Laryngoscope 2000;110:1037–1044.

63. Gross WE, Gross CW, Becker D, et al. Modified transnasal endoscopic Lothrop procedure as an alternative to frontal sinus obliteration. Otolaryngol Head Neck Surg 1995;113:427–434.

64. Weber R, Draf W, Kratzsch B, et al. Modern concepts of frontal sinus surgery. Laryngoscope 2001;111:137–146.

65. Jantti-Alanko S, Holopainen E, Malmberg H. Recurrence of nasal polyps after surgical treatment. Rhinology 1989;Suppl 8:59–64.

66. Biedlingmaier JF, Whelan P, Zoarski G, Rothman M. Histopathology and CT analysis of partially resected middle turbinates. Laryngoscope 1996;106:102–104.

67. Kennedy DW, Senior BA, Gannon FH, et al. Histology and histomorphometry of ethmoid bone in chronic rhinosinusitis. Laryngoscope 1998;108:502–507.

# 5

# Inflammatory Diseases

## Peter M. Som and Margaret S. Brandwein

## ACUTE RHINOSINUSITIS

Sinonasal inflammatory disease is a ubiquitous illness, and virtually everyone experiences multiple episodes of either a viral, bacterial, allergic, vasomotor-related, or reactive type of sinonasal inflammation. Of these, it is the common cold that is the most frequent infectious malady of the upper respiratory tract, and it is one of the major causes of absenteeism from work. The primary clinical

manifestations of this viral infection are clear, watery, profuse nasal discharge and nasal stuffiness that usually persist for less than a week. The evoked inflammatory changes are completely reversible. The most common causative agents are rhinoviruses, parainfluenza and influenza viruses, adenoviruses, and respiratory syncytial virus.[1]

The typical cold is rarely imaged and it remains primarily a viral rhinitis with little significant sinusitis. If imaging is obtained, it usually shows thickening of the nasal fossae mucosa, swelling of the turbinates, and little, if any, sinus mucosal disease.

If the clear nasal discharge becomes mucopurulent, a secondary bacterial infection has developed. This occurs when the swollen nasal or sinus mucosa causes obstruction of a sinus ostium. This causes the oxygen tension within the sinus to decrease and the normal bacterial flora becomes altered, resulting in a secondary-type acute bacterial sinusitis. Direct sinus puncture or open surgical biopsies yield the most accurate bacterial cultures for a sinusitis, as these procedures prevent contamination by the nasal flora.[2] The most commonly implicated pathogens from such studies are *Streptococcus pneumoniae* (pneumococcus), *Haemophilus influenzae*, and beta-hemolytic streptococcus. Rarely, *Staphylococcus aureus* and *Pseudomonas* infections occur.[3] Pathogenic anaerobes are rare in acute sinusitis. However, in cases of chronic sinusitis with persistently low intrasinus oxygen tensions, anaerobes predominate. These anaerobes include peptostreptococci, *Bacteroides sp. lanchnicus*, and fusobacteria.[4, 5] In the case of the maxillary sinus, it is estimated that 10% to 20% of the infections are secondary to dental infection or are the result of a complication of a tooth extraction.[6]

When imaging sinus mucosal inflammation from any cause, the inflamed mucosa enhances and there are variable amounts of submucosal edema and increased surface secretions (Fig. 5-1). There is no apparent prognostic relationship between the clinical response to the cause of the inflammation and the degree of submucosal edema or the amount of sinus secretions. An important point to note is that normal sinus secretions and submucosal fluid are each about 95% water. As these two fluids in varying amounts comprise the major response to sinonasal inflammation, inflammation is characterized by a water dominated response. This is important when MR imaging inflammation, where the signal intensities will be those of water.

If the sinus ostium is only transiently obstructed, with conservative treatment the bacterial sinusitis often resolves within 4 to 7 days. Sinusitis can cause pain over the affected sinus: cheek pain is associated with an antral infection, frontal pain may be caused by a frontal sinusitis, pain between the eyes may indicate an anterior ethmoid sinusitis, and suboccipital pain is often the result of a posterior ethmoid or sphenoid sinusitis. By comparison, a true headache is estimated to occur in only 3% of patients with sinusitis. Conversely, only 7% of headaches are the result of sinusitis.

Although a generalized headache can occur, it is unusual and may reflect intracranial spread of the sinonasal infection. Due to a rich venous emissary plexus between the posterior frontal sinus mucosa and the meninges, acute frontal sinusitis is most likely to spread intracranially, and clinical manifestations of this may be present in as few as 36 to 48 hours after initial presentation. Sphenoid and ethmoid sinusitis are the next most likely to progress to intracranial

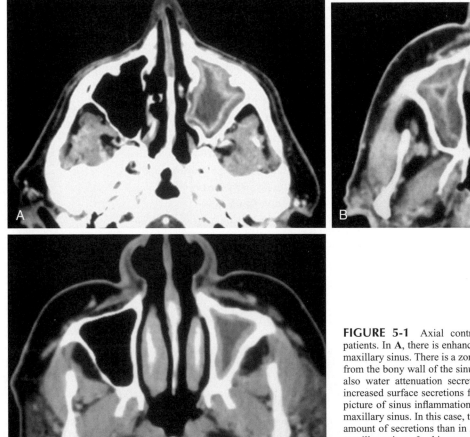

**FIGURE 5-1** Axial contrast-enhanced CT scans of three different patients. In **A**, there is enhancement of the inflamed mucosa within the left maxillary sinus. There is a zone of water attenuation separating this mucosa from the bony wall of the sinus. This zone is submucosal edema. There are also water attenuation secretions within the sinus cavity that represent increased surface secretions from the inflamed mucosa. This is the typical picture of sinus inflammation. In **B**, there is inflammation within the right maxillary sinus. In this case, there is more submucosal edema and a smaller amount of secretions than in **A**. In **C**, there is inflammation within the left maxillary sinus. In this case, there is little submucosal edema and a large amount of surface secretions. These three cases illustrate the variations in reactions to inflammation. They do not predict outcome.

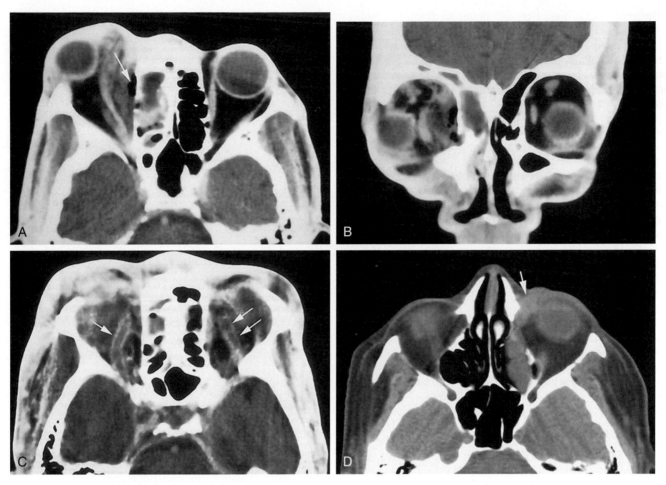

**FIGURE 5-2**   Axial (**A**) and coronal (**B**) contrast-enhanced CT scans on a patient with a right ethmoid sinusitis, a right orbital cellulitis, and air in an abscess (*arrow*). The globe is proptotic and laterally displaced. There is no gross defect in the right lamina papyracea. In **C**, a patient developed a right orbital cellulitis secondary to a right ethmoid sinusitis. The infection spread via the right superior ophthalmic vein (*arrow*) to the cavernous sinus, across the sella's vascular bed to the left cavernous sinus, and then retrograde into the left orbit via the left superior ophthalmic vein (*arrows*). In **D**, there is a left ethmoid sinusitis that spread through the lamina papyracea into the left lacrimal saccular area (*arrow*) and presented clinically as an acute dacryocystitis. This is a case of pseudodacryocystitis secondary to an ethmoid sinusitis.

infection. Intracranial extension from maxillary sinusitis rarely occurs.

Because headache may be the symptom most often suggesting intracranial extension of sinusitis, the causes of headache have been studied. In one study of 92 patients with headache, migraine was found to be the most frequent cause of headache. In decreasing order of occurrence, the other causes were tension-type headache, sinusitis, and epilepsy. The percentage of the findings relevant to headache on CT scans, MR studies, Waters' projections, and electroencephalograms were, respectively, 4.2%, 33.3%, 16%, and 25%. Observed imaging findings associated with headache included sinusitis, dilatation of the basal cistern, dilatation of the temporal horn of the lateral ventricle, pseudotumor cerebri, and mesiotemporal sclerosis. The conclusion of this study was that the most important points in evaluating these patients are taking a proper history of headache, obtaining a thorough physical and neurologic examination, and performing an MR imaging study.[7]

However, the cause of a headache may not be found on imaging studies. In another study on both HIV-seropositive and HIV-seronegative patients over a 2-year period, 50% of all subjects reported a headache. However, the frequency and characteristics of the headaches were not different between the two groups, and the headaches were neither more frequent nor different in HIV-seropositive individuals with advanced immunosuppression. There was no correlation between headache and abnormal CSF parameters, cranial MR imaging abnormalities, including the presence of sinusitis, or the use of zidovudine.[8]

Acute bacterial sinusitis is more likely to spread to the orbits than extend intracranially (Fig. 5-2A–C) (also see Chapter 9). The thin lamina papyracea and the absence of valves in the anterior and posterior ethmoidal veins allow unobstructed intraorbital spread of acute bacterial infection. Sphenoid and maxillary sinusitis are the next most likely to spread to the orbits, followed by frontal sinusitis. Older reports erroneously implicate frontal sinusitis as a major source of orbital infection. However, such cases are more likely the result of supraorbital ethmoid sinusitis. Of all orbital infections, nearly two-thirds arise secondary to sinusitis.

The contiguous spread of inflammation from infected ethmoid sinuses into the surrounding tissues of the lacrimal drainage system can produce symptoms easily confused with those of acute dacryocystitis (Fig. 5-2D) (also see Chapter 10). Cases of pseudodacryocystitis arising from anterior ethmoiditis have been reported, and the importance of differentiating these etiologies was noted, as the surgery of choice is an anterior ethmoidectomy rather than dacryocystorhinostomy when such pseudodacryocystitis proves unresponsive to antibiotic therapy.[9]

Acute bacterial sinusitis is the result of sinus ostial obstruction. Thus, bacterial sinusitis occurs as a sinus-by-sinus event rather than as a generalized systemic process. It is more common to find contiguous unilateral bacterial sinusitis than it is to encounter pansinusitis. Even with pansinusitis, one or more sinuses are usually more severely affected. Therefore, as a general rule, asymmetric sinusitis is a hallmark of bacterial disease. By comparison, diffuse, nonlocalized pansinusitis is more often found in allergic patients, presumably as a result of a systemic process rather than a localized obstruction.

With reference to acute maxillary sinus disease, periodontal disease is associated with a twofold increase in the risk of developing maxillary sinusitis. Recognition of this relationship is especially important in the clinical management of patients, particularly those planning to have implant surgery.[10]

Necrotizing fasciitis is a rare condition that usually affects the trunk, perineum, and limbs. Head and neck involvement is particularly rare, and in most cases it is secondary to orbital or dental infection. A case of craniofacial necrotizing fasciitis secondary to a maxillary sinusitis was reported. Although treated intensively and aggressively, the patient died 1 week after hospital admission. This report emphasizes the importance of early diagnosis and aggressive management in these cases.[11]

The relationship between acute sinusitis and ischemic stroke is also largely unexplored. However, the anatomic proximity of the paranasal sinuses and the internal carotid artery suggests that inflammation of the sinuses could easily extend to the intracranial vasculature. Four patients with acute ischemic stroke and extensive disease of the paranasal sinuses have been reported. All of these patients had strokes involving the cavernous internal carotid artery and all also had extensive sinus disease, especially involving the sphenoid sinus. This report suggests that, although rare, there may be a relationship between acute paranasal sinusitis, particularly sphenoid sinusitis, and ischemic stroke.[12]

Sphenoid sinusitis may also cause optic neuritis. Possible mechanisms of nerve damage include direct spread of infection, occlusive vasculitis, and bony deficiency in the wall of the sinus. Patients presenting with isolated optic neuritis and atypical headache should have a CT or MR study. An opaque sphenoid sinus in the context of decreased visual acuity should not be dismissed as coincidental, but considered as pathologic and the patient referred for drainage (Fig. 5-3).[13]

Evaluation of potential acute graft-versus-host disease (AGVHD) after bone marrow transplantation is becoming increasingly common. Imaging of the paranasal sinuses is part of the fever workup for these patients. In a retrospective case control study of 45 adults receiving allogeneic or

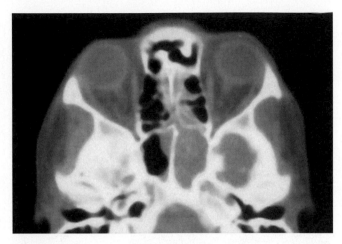

**FIGURE 5-3**    Axial CT scan of a patient with left optic neuritis and a chronic suboccipital headache. The brain was normal on CT and MR studies. There is opacification of the left sphenoid sinus, and minimal mucosal disease is present in the the right sphenoid sinus and in both ethmoid sinuses. The patient had no symptoms referable to the sinuses. Surgery revealed sinusitis, and in the immediately postoperative period the patient's headache and visual findings resolved. The walls of the sphenoid sinus were intact.

matched bone marrow transplantation, AGVHD developed in 28 (62%). All patients had paranasal sinus imaging with either CT or plain films for evaluation of possible sinusitis, and no direct correlation was found.[14] On the other hand, another study showed that CT of the paranasal sinuses is advised in patients suffering hemoblastoses, with an increased risk of infectious complications during the transplantation phase, because pathologic findings can be expected in 21% of these patients. The authors emphasized that the diagnosis of and therapy for an acute sinusitis are especially important prior to allogenous bone marrow transplantation.[15]

## AIR-FLUID LEVELS

Air-fluid levels are most common in the maxillary sinuses and are the result of acute bacterial sinusitis with obstruction of the sinus ostium. The obstruction does not allow normal sinus drainage to occur, and the sinus secretions accumulate within the sinus cavity. Although bacterial sinusitis is the most common cause of a paranasal sinus air-fluid level, it probably occurs in only 25% to 50% of patients with this disease (Figs. 5-4 to 5-6). In prior decades, when antral lavage was a common therapy for acute obstructive bacterial sinusitis, air-fluid levels could be seen within the sinus for 2 to 4 days after the lavage, reflecting the presence of residual saline that was used in the lavage. If lavage is performed, follow-up films should be obtained at least 7 days after the lavage. A persistent air-fluid level after 7 days indicates renewed sinus obstruction.

Nasogastric tube placement is common in patients with loss of consciousness, severe trauma, or who are post operative. Prolonged supine positioning, and irritation and edema caused by the tube, interferes with normal sinus drainage, and within 24 hours air-fluid levels can be seen in

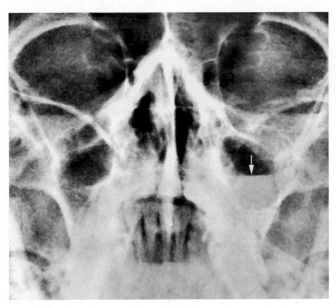

**FIGURE 5-4** Waters view shows a left maxillary sinus air-fluid level (*arrow*) with minimal mucosal thickening within the sinus. The remaining sinuses are normal. This patient had acute bacterial sinusitis.

any or all of the paranasal sinuses.[16] After several days the sinuses may become completely opacified with secretions, and imaging will reveal an apparent pansinusitis. These sinus opacifications usually clear within a few days after the nasal tube is removed and the patient has started to vary head position.

A mucosal tear or rent can occur with physical trauma, regardless of whether a sinus wall fracture occurred. Often, such a tear occurs after blunt trauma, and an air-fluid (air-blood) level usually indicates the presence of a mucosal tear. However, a coincidental acute sinusitis in the affected sinus may cause clinical confusion, which can be avoided by performing a CT or MR study. On CT, intrasinus blood is

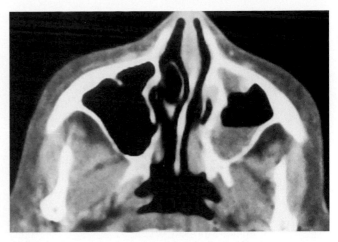

**FIGURE 5-6** Axial CT scan shows a left maxillary sinus mucoid attenuation air-fluid level with minimal mucosal thickening. The right maxillary sinus is normal. Clinically this patient had acute bacterial sinusitis.

denser than normal mucosal edema and inflammatory secretions, and since this is an acute process, desiccated secretions within the sinus are not a consideration (Fig. 5-7). On MR T1-weighted images, intrasinus blood (after 24 to 48 hours) has a high signal intensity (Fig. 5-8). By comparison, acute inflammatory related tissues have a low T1-weighted signal intensity. Thus sectional imaging can resolve questionable cases of sinus hemorrhage.[17, 18]

Barotrauma is a disorder that affects aviators, parachutists, divers, and caisson workers. It most often is associated with an upper respiratory tract infection (34%) accompanied by swelling of the mucosa around the sinus ostium. In these patients, this anatomic substrate prevents rapid pressure equilibration across this ostium, which creates a negative intrasinus pressure that causes rupture of submucosal vessels and sinus hemorrhage. Mucosal and submucosal hemorrhage occurs, usually associated with pain over the involved sinus. Epistaxis is the second most common symptom. The frontal sinus is involved in 68% of cases, the

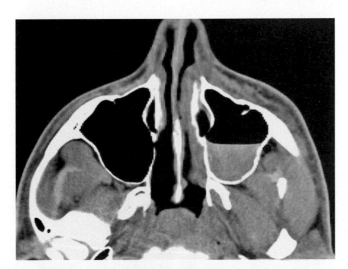

**FIGURE 5-5** Axial CT scan shows an air-fluid level in the left antrum in this patient with a clinically acute sinusitis. The attenuation of the fluid is that of watery "mucous secretions." Also note the slight cellulitis in the left facial soft tissues, as evidenced by thickening of the skin, subcutaneous fat, and facial musculature.

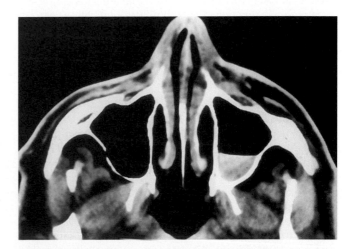

**FIGURE 5-7** Axial CT scan shows an air-fluid level in the left maxillary sinus. The fluid is dense compared to water attenuation (see Figs. 5-5 and 5-6) in this patient, who had received blunt facial trauma. This patient had sinus hemorrhage.

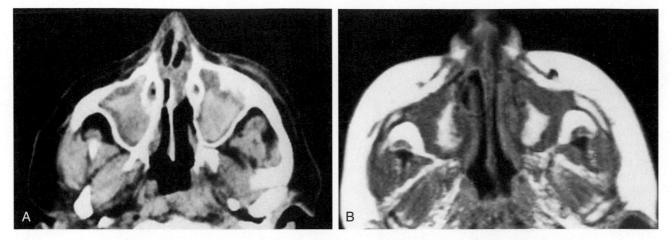

**FIGURE 5-8** In **A**, an axial CT scan shows central areas of increased attenuation in both maxillary sinuses, separated from the sinus walls by a thin zone of mucoid attenuation. This picture is consistent with either chronic sinusitis with desiccated sinus secretions, fungal sinusitis with a mycetoma, or sinus hemorrhage. In **B**, a T1-weighted MR image, the central area of each maxillary sinus has high signal intensity consistent with hemorrhage. The surrounding low signal intensity material is mucosa and fresh secretions.

ethmoid sinus in 16%, and the maxillary sinus in 8%. On plain film studies, mucosal thickening can be detected in the frontal sinuses (24%), the ethmoid sinuses (15% to 19%), and the antrum (74% to 80%); however, an air-fluid level (present in 12% of cases) appears to only be seen in the maxillary sinus.[19]

Hemorrhage can also result from bleeding disorders such as von Willebrand's disease, in which bleeding tends to occur at mucosal surfaces, and possibly Oler Weber Rendu syndrome. Hemophilia, on the other hand, tends to involve internal bleeding and is not associated with a sinus air-fluid level. Coagulation disorders and acute leukemia may also produce air-fluid levels. Rarely, chemically induced sinusitis can produce an air-fluid level. Chromates and other industrial pollutants have been implicated in such cases. Despite the rhinitis and rhinorrhea associated with allergy, few air-fluid levels are seen.

The significance of an air-fluid level varies, depending on the paranasal sinus involved. In the frontal sinuses an air-fluid level usually means acute bacterial sinusitis (Fig. 5-9). As previously mentioned, intracranial complications can occur readily, often within 48 hours (Fig. 5-10).[20] The clinician should be alerted immediately regarding a frontal sinus air-fluid level, as these patients require prompt, vigorous treatment, often including intravenous antibiotics. Failure of a clinical response and the beginning of resolution of the air-fluid level within another 48 to 72 hours after the onset of treatment usually mandates sinus trephination. Such aggressive therapy usually avoids any intracranial complications.

An ethmoid sinus air-fluid level is rare and usually is not associated with either trauma or acute infection. However, if an ethmoid mucocele ruptures and partially drains into the nasal fossa, an air-fluid level may result in what is invariably a mucopyocele. This unusual occurrence is the most common cause of an ethmoid air-fluid level (Fig. 5-11A).

In the sphenoid sinus an air-fluid level may indicate the presence of acute sinusitis or nasal cavity obstruction. An air-fluid level in a supine and/or unconscious patient may only indicate poor sinus drainage. In a trauma patient, a sphenoid sinus air-fluid level may also signify the presence of either hemorrhage or CSF from a skull base fracture.

Most often these fractures involve the floor of the anterior cranial fossa or the mastoid portion of the temporal bone, not the sphenoid sinus walls. In the case of anterior skull base fractures, because the dura is firmly attached to the bone, a fracture here is likely to cause a dural rent and resulting CSF rhinorrhea.[21] With the patient supine, the CSF drains back into the sphenoethmoidal recess and into the sphenoid sinus. In the case of a temporal bone fracture with an intact tympanic membrane, the CSF drains into the hypotympanum of the middle ear, escapes via the eustachian tube into the upper nasopharynx and nasal fossa, and then into the sphenoid sinus. Thus CSF rhinorrhea with or without a

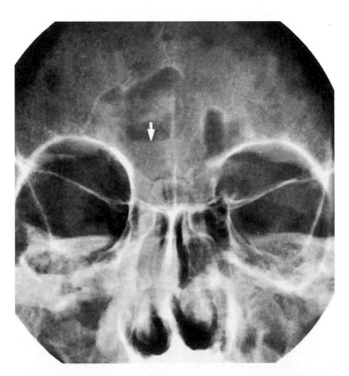

**FIGURE 5-9** Caldwell view shows soft-tissue clouding of both frontal sinuses and in the right ethmoid sinuses. There is also a right frontal sinus air-fluid level (*arrow*) in this patient with acute bacterial sinusitis.

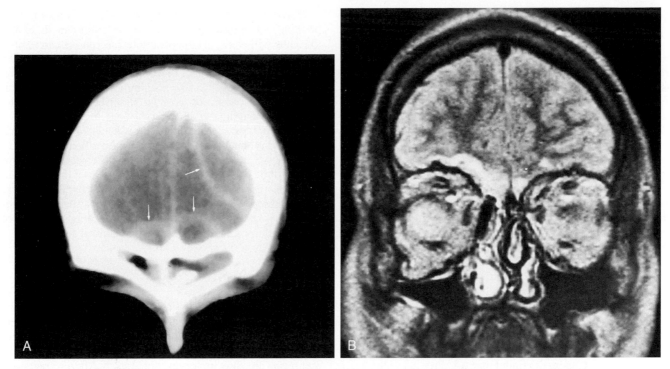

**FIGURE 5-10**   In **A**, a coronal CT scan, there is an osteoma obstructing the left frontal sinus and three epidural abscesses (*arrows*) that occurred within 48 hours of the initial frontal sinus symptoms. In **B**, a coronal T2-weighted MR image, there is an area of high signal intensity above the right orbit and in the base of the midline anterior cranial fossa. This patient had cerebritis secondary to frontal sinusitis.

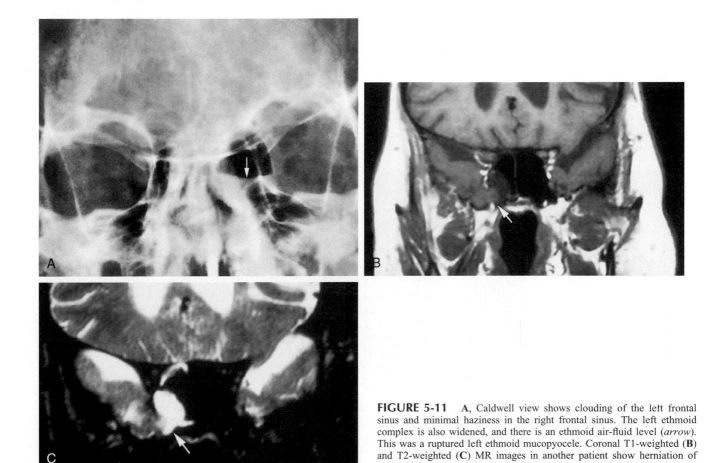

**FIGURE 5-11**   **A**, Caldwell view shows clouding of the left frontal sinus and minimal haziness in the right frontal sinus. The left ethmoid complex is also widened, and there is an ethmoid air-fluid level (*arrow*). This was a ruptured left ethmoid mucopyocele. Coronal T1-weighted (**B**) and T2-weighted (**C**) MR images in another patient show herniation of brain and CSF (*arrow*) into a lateral recess of the right sphenoid sinus.

sphenoid sinus air-fluid level may reflect a temporal bone fracture.

CSF fluid may also enter the sphenoid sinus spontaneously, usually through a dehiscence in the medial aspect of the roof of a lateral sinus recess (Fig. 5-11B,C). A CSF leak associated with a pituitary tumor or surgery is rare.

## CHRONIC SINUSITIS

Chronic sinusitis results from either persistent acute inflammation or repeated episodes of acute or subacute sinusitis. It is estimated that up to one third of patients with acute sinusitis develop some evidence of chronic sinusitis. The chronic disease can result in an atrophic, sclerosing, or hypertrophic polypoid mucosa. These varied mucosal changes most often coexist with one another and with areas of acute inflammation of either an infectious or allergic etiology. Because chronically inflamed and scarred mucosa loses some of its ciliary function, it becomes less resistant to future infection so that a vicious cycle of infection and reinfection may occur in patients with chronic sinusitis. The bony sinus walls surrounding a chronically infected sinus usually become thickened and sclerotic with reactive new bone formation. This bony response is found with all chronic inflammations regardless of etiology and presumably is a response to both the increased local blood flow associated with inflammation and periosteal involvement. However, on CT, care must be taken when viewing a sinus with mucosal disease at narrow "soft-tissue" windows, as bone appears denser and wider than it truly is. This is a problem of the algorithms of all CT manufacturers, and the actual bone density and size are best seen on wide window settings (Fig. 5-12).

Epithelial hyperplasia and mucosal infiltration of leukocytes are common features of chronic rhinosinusitis. It has been shown that the epithelium can produce chemoattractant cytokines that may contribute to leukocyte infiltration in rhinosinusitis. Mucosal IL-8 expression is increased in patients with chronic rhinosinusitis, and the level of expression directly correlates with disease severity.[22]

Chronically obstructed sinus secretions can result in four possible outcomes: (1) the sinus obstruction can abate and the sinus will clear, (2) the obstructed secretions can remain indefinitely within the sinus as watery secretions, (3) the entrapped secretions can become desiccated, or (4) the secretions can progressively accumulate and a mucocele can develop. These entities will be described further in the section on Imaging.

Nasal polyps are uncommonly associated with chronic inflammation and when present are most often solitary. By comparison, multiple nasal polyps are common with allergic-type rhinosinusitis. Although mucosal thickening in the nasal fossae, sphenoid, ethmoid, and frontal sinuses is more common in patients with acute asthma than in control subjects, maxillary sinus mucosal thickening is no more common in asthmatic patients than in control subjects.[23]

## Allergic Sinusitis

Nearly 10% of the population has allergic rhinosinusitis, which generally involves the sinuses symmetrically. The most common form is seasonal pollinosis, and the prevalent form in North America is ragweed allergy. Spores, molds, and mites are also important antigens.[24] Allergic reactions are manifestations of type I immunologic disorders, which reflect an IgE reagin-antibody reaction, with a resulting release of mediators that produce sneezing, nasal obstruction, and watery rhinorrhea. Profuse secretions associated with nasal obstruction can result in some retained secretions and eventual infection.[24] Thus the coexistence of bacterial and allergic sinusitis is not uncommon. The resulting hypertrophic, thickened, and redundant allergic sinus mucosa is often referred to as *hypertrophic polypoid mucosa*, which is less capable than normal mucosa of resisting subsequent infections. Rarely, in the maxillary sinus, hypertrophic mucosa can become so redundant that it prolapses into the nasal fossa, simulating an antrochoanal polyp.[25] The difference is that in these unusual cases the prolaped tissue is simply redundant mucosa rather than an actual polyp.

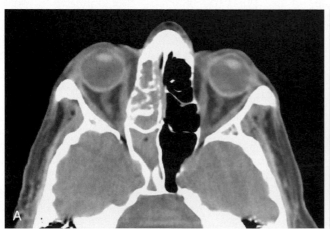
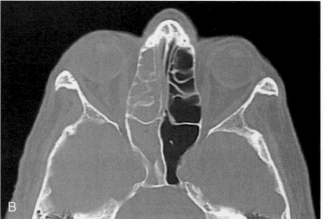

**FIGURE 5-12**    Axial CT scan (**A**) shows opacification of the right ethmoid and sphenoid sinuses. The ethmoid septae and the surrounding bone appear thickened and sclerotic on this narrow "soft-tissue" windowed image. This might imply a chronic process. However, in **B**, the same image viewed at wide "bone" window settings, the bone appears normal and similar to that on the left side. This is the more accurate assessment of the bone size and density in this patient with clinically acute sinusitis.

Tissue eosinophilia is a characteristic histologic feature of allergic sinusitis in children and adults, especially those with asthma. However, eosinophilia is not sensitive for allergic sinusitis and does not correlate with the severity of mucosal thickening, as seen on CT scans.[26]

As mentioned, infectious rhinosinusitis is caused by a variety of agents that produce both acute and chronic inflammation that may be associated with secondary polyp formation. These patients commonly have a secretory IgA deficiency.[27] There is evidence to suggest that fluctuating glucose levels occurring in concert with other factors (allergy, infection) may promote nasal polyps in patients with diabetes.[28] In general, nasal polyps in children are uncommon, and 29% of such cases are associated with cystic fibrosis. Between 10% and 20% of children with cystic fibrosis have nasal polyps. Thus, the presence of chronic sinusitis and nasal polyps in a child should prompt an investigation to rule out cystic fibrosis.[29, 30]

The triad (aspirin intolerance) of aspirin usage, nasal polyps (often highly destructive), and bronchial asthma is less commonly encountered, as the generalized use of acetaminophen products has replaced aspirin usage. This triad is associated with severe destructive-type nasal polyposis. In general, about 20% of patients with nasal polyps have asthma, and conversely, about 30% of asthmatic patients have polyps.[29–31] Nickel workers who have worked 10 years or more in nickel-refining facilities have a 4% incidence of inflammatory nasal polyps with squamous metaplasia and dysplasia. They are at increased risk of developing carcinomas in the lung, nasal fossa, and larynx.[32]

## Vasomotor Rhinitis

*Vasomotor rhinitis* refers to the symptoms of nasal congestion, watery discharge, and nasal polyps occurring in the absence of obstruction, ciliary dysfunction, or allergy. These patients do not have evidence of IgE-mediated disease and do not have positive skin tests. Instability of the autonomic nervous system has been implicated as the underlying problem. Vasomotor rhinitis can be stimulated by emotional stress, endocrine imbalance, atmospheric pressure changes, irritants, and as a reaction to medications. Among conditions associated with vasomotor rhinitis in some reports are antihypertensive medications, abuse of nasal sprays and drops, birth control pills, pregnancy and "premenstrual colds (estrogen related)," hypothyroidism (2% to 3% of patients), emotional stress, poor environmental temperature control, irritants (dust, gases, chemicals, aerosol cosmetics, and air pollutants such as sulfur dioxide and tobacco), recumbent position, nasal airway exclusion (postlaryngectomy, choanal atresia, marked adenoidal hypertrophy), Horner's syndrome, and systemic disorders such as superior vena cava syndrome, cirrhosis, and uremia.[33] When considering causes of nasal obstruction, vasomotor rhinitis is often a diagnosis of exclusion. Although no consistent imaging findings have been reported in patients with vasomotor rhinitis, one could expect at most to see mild swelling of the turbinates, some increased nasal secretions, and mild mucosal thickening within the sinuses.

## Fungal Sinusitis

A variety of fungal diseases involve the sinonasal cavities. These include aspergillosis, mucormycosis, candidiasis, histoplasmosis, cryptococcosis, coccidioidomycosis, North American blastomycosis, rhinosporidiosis, and myospherulosis.[34] There are four clinicopathologic classifications of mycotic sinonasal disease: (1) acute invasive fulminant disease, (2) chronic invasive infection, (3) noninvasive mycotic colonization ("fungus ball" or mycetoma), and (4) allergic mycotic sinusitis. These four types of infection can be seen with any fungus but are most commonly a result of *Aspergillus* infection. Not infrequently, the pathologic diagnosis of mycotic disease requires heightened clinicopathologic suspicion. From a pathologic viewpoint, hyphae may be sparse in allergic mycotic sinusitis, being found only beneath the mucosal surface or only within the mucin. In early invasive sinusitis, hyphae may be confined to the vessels. A thick sinonasal mucus of unusual color (green, brown, or black) should raise the clinical suspicion of a mycotic infection. Hyphal fragments may be impossible to classify without culture confirmation, and pathologic correlation is always necessary to distinguish clinical infection from laboratory contamination. The sinonasal fungal diseases can be classified as being either fungal hyphal diseases or fungal yeast forms (also see the section on imaging).

### Fungal Hyphal Diseases

Aspergillosis infection is caused by the fungus *Aspergillus*, a member of the Ascomycetes class. It is a ubiquitous organism frequently found in soil, decaying food, fruits, and plants. The spores are also common contaminants of the respiratory tract and the external auditory canal. *A. fumigatus* is the major human pathogen; however, *A. flavus* and *A. niger* can also cause human infections. Of the culture-confirmed cases of mycotic sinusitis, 87% contained some *Aspergillus* species as the sole pathogen or as a copathogen.[35]

Acute fulminant *Aspergillus* sinusitis occurs in the immunosuppressed, especially granulopenic patients with hematologic malignancies. Initial complaints are those of acute sinusitis such as nasal discharge, sinus pain, and/or periorbital swelling. Clinical examination of the nasal cavity and palate shows pale, ischemic tissue that may progress to gray and blackened, gangrenous tissue. The ability of *Aspergillus* to invade vessels is aided by its production of elastase and proteases. As the infection spreads through vascular and neuronal routes, orbital nerve invasion occurs, progressing to blindness. Treatment involves surgical debridement and antifungal agents. Treatment with antifungal medications usually includes itraconazole or one of the newer oral azoles (voriconazole).[36] The tissue at debridement is typically bloodless due to hyphal-related thrombosis. The prognosis for these patients is usually grave. *Aspergillus* sinusitis is not uncommon in immunocompromised patients and is unusual in immunocompetent patients.[37]

Chronic invasive *Aspergillus* sinusitis can be found in normal hosts living in highly endemic areas such as the Sudan or Saudia Arabia. Asymptomatic nasal colonization has also been demonstrated. The Middle Eastern cases are quite distinctive in that they occur in immunologically normal patients, probably because of prolonged exposure to large inocula of spores. In the United States, chronic invasive sinusitis is most commonly seen in mildly immunosuppressed patients such as diabetics. Most patients respond to surgical debridement and antifungal therapy.[38–40]

A mycetoma is the benign fungal hyphal colonization of a cavity or space. In the sinonasal tract, a mycetoma may develop in response to changes in the local microenvironment such as occur after surgery, radiotherapy, and anecdotally, in association with smoking marijuana. Patients with mycetomas may complain of chronic sinusitis, or they may be entirely asymptomatic. Therapy is conservative curettage, but benign recolonization may occur.

Patients with allergic mycotic sinusitis have a history of allergic sinusitis, polyposis, and possibly allergic asthma. Serum eosinophilia, elevated IgE, cutaneous sensitivity to fungal antigens, and the presence of fungus-specific serum precipitins support the diagnosis of allergic mycotic sinusitis. Conservative curettage and systemic steroid therapy are the recommended treatments.[41] Histopathologically, hyphae are sparse and noninvasive, and they may be seen only after special stains are examined. Culture confirmation is necessary because the hyphal fragments do not allow definitive identification. Because of the environmental prevalence of *Aspergillus*, it is the assumed cause of most allergic fungal sinusitis cases. However, the dematiaceous fungi may also cause allergic sinusitis.

Rhinocerebral mucormycosis (also phycomycosis or zygomycosis) is a disease caused by several genera of the fungi of the class Zygomycetes (formerly Phycomycetes) and the family Mucoraceae. The genera, in order of decreasing frequency, are *Rhizopus*, *Mucor*, and *Absidia*. The members of the class Zygomycetes can be found in decaying fruit (especially those with a high sugar content), vegetables, soil, old bread, and manure. The zygomycetes have been isolated sporadically in some studies of indoor environments. Various spices, herbal teas, and birdseed harbor *Rhizopus* and *Absidia*. Iatrogenic subcutaneous wound infections by *Rhizopus* can be caused by ElastoplastR brand bandages.

The Zygomycetes have a propensity for infecting uncontrolled diabetic patients as well as patients with hematologic malignancies (e.g., acute leukemia); chronic renal failure and acidosis; malnutrition; cancer; cirrhosis; and prolonged antibiotic, steroid, or cytotoxic drug therapy. *Rhizopus* grows favorably in an acidic, high-glucose environment, which relates to its elaboration of ketone reductase. The acidosis, in addition to providing a favorable growth environment, also further impairs polymorphonuclear leukocyte function.

Sinus mucormycosis occurs predominantly as an invasive rhinocerebral infection. The clinical course may be acute, invasive, and fulminant, just as in aspergillosis. The organism tends to spread rapidly from the nasal fossa to the paranasal sinuses and the fungus invades blood vessels, causing endothelial damage that initiates thrombosis, ischemic and hemorrhagic infarction, and purulent inflammation. Eventually the orbits and cavernous sinuses are invaded via the ophthalmic vessels. Invasion of the base of the brain is an end-stage event, and the entire progression of the disease can occur in only a few days. Perineural invasion can also occur, usually along the branches of the trigeminal nerve.[42]

Diabetic patients may develop a more chronic invasive sinusitis, which is amenable to debridement and antifungal therapy. In AIDS patients, whose neutrophil function is largely intact, mucormycosis is actually a rare infection.[43] Clinically, black, crusting, necrotic tissue is seen over the turbinates, septum, and palate. By comparison, in immunosuppressed patients, focal ischemic areas may be found instead of the more typical black crusts. In the cases occurring in nondiabetic patients, pulmonary and disseminated infections are more common. Among survivors there is a high incidence of blindness, cranial nerve palsies, and hemiparesis. The best therapy is adequate surgical debridement and systemic intravenous amphotericin B.[34]

Mucormycoses has been documented in nondiabetic, nonimmunosuppressed patients. A preexisting foreign body, marijuana use, or prior surgery or radiotherapy may be predisposing factors in these unusual cases.[44, 45]

Fungi from the order Entomophthorales, which are also Zygomycetes, may cause granulomatous rhinoentomophthoromycosis in normal hosts from tropical climates. Cases have been reported in U.S. inhabitants with no history of travel, and Entomorphthora species have been isolated from algae, ferns, insects, and reptiles (*Basidiobolus ranarum* and *B. haptosporus*). Entomophthorales infection begins as a submucosal nasal mass that slowly expands, causing enormous erosion, destruction, and deformity of the nasal and labial soft tissues. The rhinocerous-like midface expansion is similar to that seen in advanced cases of rhinoscleroma.

*Pseudallescheria boydii* (formerly called *Allescheria boydii*) is the current nomenclature for this fungus of the Ascomycetes family. It is a ubiquitous organism most commonly found in rural areas, and it is isolated from soil, poultry, cattle manure, and polluted waters. *P. boydii* sinusitis, which may be fulminant and lethal, has been reported in immunocompromised patients. It has also been described in normal patients and may resolve with adequate therapy. Like aspergillosis, this disease may be either saprophytic or invasive. *P. boydii* has been reported to involve the maxillary, ethmoid, and sphenoid sinuses. The present treatment of choice is miconazole, with surgical debridement if necessary.[46, 47]

### Fungal Yeast Forms

The yeasts of the genus *Candida* are part of the normal mucocutaneous flora. However, under certain circumstances, *Candida* may produce either a minor or a life-threatening disease. Minor infections may result as overgrowths in patients on antibiotic therapy. The more severe *Candida* infections occur almost exclusively in patients with compromised immune systems. Today, candidiasis represents the most common and most lethal of the opportunistic fungal infections among immunocompromised patients.[34] Most infections are caused by *Candida albicans*, but *C. tropicalis*, *C. stellatoidea*, and *C. krusei* may also cause disease. When the paranasal sinuses are affected, it is usually in otherwise healthy patients who have been on broad-spectrum antibiotics. The maxillary sinuses are almost exclusively involved, and orbital and intracranial complications are rare. Infections can also occur after maxillary trauma. The treatment of choice for the sinus disease is antral lavage with topical nystatin.[48]

*Histoplasma capsulatum* is present worldwide and is endemic in the midwestern, central, and southeastern regions of the United States. Exposure to *H. capsulatum* occurs through exposure to aerosolized bird or bat droppings and contaminated soil or fertilizers. As with most inhaled mycotic pathogens, the most common manifestation of histoplasmosis is a subclinical pulmonary infection, usually a function of a small exposure source and the state of patient immunity. Patients may develop acute pneumonia after massive inhalation. Chronic cavitating and fibrosing pulmonary infection, sclerosing mediastinitis, and disseminated infection with bone marrow and adrenal involvement (resulting in Addison's disease) are more serious sequelae of histoplasmosis.

Before the AIDS epidemic, disseminated histoplasmosis was rarely seen, and when it was encountered, it was usually in elderly patients or those immunosuppressed by chemotherapy or hematologic malignancy. Today, disseminated histoplasmosis and extrapulmonary histoplasmosis in the face of HIV seropositivity are included as one of the criteria for AIDS. Disseminated histoplasmosis presents with fever, septicemia, pneumonia, hepatic or renal failure, CNS infection, or skin lesions. It is thought to be due to reinfection from an endemic focus or, less frequently, reactivation of latent disease. Head and neck manifestations of disseminated disease in AIDS patients include cervical adenopathy, pharyngitis, tonsillitis, and ulcerating oral lesions. Non-AIDS patients may also develop histoplasmosis of the oral cavity and larynx. Rarely, there can be involvement of the nasal mucous membranes, resulting in edema and nasal obstruction. Even more rarely, pansinusitis can occur. The current treatment of choice is amphotericin B.[34, 49, 50]

*Cryptococcus neoformans* is a ubiquitous yeast of worldwide distribution. It is associated with pigeon excreta and pigeon nesting sites, and human infection results from inhalation of aerosolized droppings.[34] It may cause asymptomatic, localized pulmonary granulomata. Cryptococcal pneumonia or disseminated infection can develop in immunosuppressed patients. Cryptococcal meningitis occurring in the AIDS population is thought to follow respiratory infection, and the frontal and maxillary sinuses have been documented as primary sources of infection. Isolated sinonasal disease is uncommon but is identical to that of histoplasmosis, and the treatment is the same as for histoplasmosis.[51, 52]

Coccidioidomycosis is a disease caused by the dimorphic fungus *Coccidioides immitis*. The pathogenesis and clinical manifestations of the disease are almost identical to those of histoplasmosis. *C. immitis* is endemic in the southern United States and in northern Mexico, as well as a few sites in Central America and South America. It has been estimated that 20% of cases reported yearly are diagnosed outside the endemic areas, thus widening the relevance of this organism. *C. immitis* is extremely infectious. Illness ranges from subclinical infections to disseminated and often lethal infections, depending on the patient's immune status, infectious dose, nationality, and other factors such as pregnancy. Most of the head and neck disease affects the laryngotracheal axis, with or without concurrent pulmonary disease. Sinonasal involvement is rare.[53, 54]

Myospherulosis is not a fungal disease but rather an iatrogenic condition that is caused by the interaction of red blood cells with petrolatum, lanolin, or traumatized human adipose tissue.[34] Microscopically, large sporangium-like sacs filled with spherules are produced that can be mistaken for a fungus. The disease was first recognized as skin lesions in East Africans; however, in the United States the disease has involved the nose, paranasal sinuses, and middle ear. In these patients there was always prior surgery (i.e., the Caldwell-Luc procedure), and the surgical defect was packed with gauze impregnated with petrolatum. It is important to recognize this disease as an innocuous iatrogenic process so that it is not confused with a true fungal disease and given unwarranted therapy.

## CYSTS AND POLYPS

The most frequent complications of inflammatory rhinosinusitis are polyps and cysts. The retention cyst is the most common, being found incidentally on routine plain film examinations in about 10% to 35% of patients. A mucous retention cyst results from the obstruction of a submucosal mucinous gland, and the cyst wall is the duct epithelium and capsule of the gland itself.[55, 56] Although by strict pathologic criteria a retention cyst can be called a *mucocele*, the radiographic and clinical findings of these two entities are sufficiently different to merit distinction (see the section on mucoceles). Mucous retention cysts can occur in any paranasal sinus, along any wall, but are most commonly found in the maxillary sinus. As mentioned, they usually are an incidental imaging finding.

Serous retention cysts result from the accumulation of serous fluid in the submucosal layer of the sinus mucosal lining. These cysts tend to occur in the base of the maxillary sinuses, and the lining of a serous retention cyst is the elevated sinus mucosa. By contrast, as mentioned, the lining of a mucous retention cyst is the actual obstructed ductal epithelium.

By comparison to serous retention cysts, polyps result from an expansion of fluids in the deeper lamina propria of the Schneiderian mucosa in the nasal fossa and paranasal sinuses. These polyps may result from allergy, atopy, infection, or vasomotor impairment.[57] Paranasal sinus and nasal polyps have an identical histology. Allergic polyps tend to have a significant population of eosinophils, more than what is usually seen in inflammatory polyps, and such polyps may be associated with allergic mucin, comprised of a sea of eosinophils in mucin and Charcot-Leydin crystals, which are the result of eosinophil degranulation. As mentioned, the associated allergic sinusitis tends to cause diffuse symmetric disease rather than localized disease. It has been suggested that there is an interaction between eosinophils and fibronectin that may play a role in edema formation, which contributes to the growth of nasal polyps.[58]

Inflammatory and allergic polyps rarely bleed and are not damaged by manipulation or compression. However, fibrosis and neovascularization of polyps (especially nasal polyps) can result in a vascularized polyp that pathologically mimics an angiofibroma. Anatomic and imaging features that distinguish a vascularized polyp from an angiofibroma include the following: (1) the former is located in the nasal fossa rather than in the nasopharynx, (2) the polyp does not extend into the pterygopalatine fossa, and (3) the polyp is easily removed. These polyps are poorly vascularized, further distinguishing them from angiofibromas.[59]

As mentioned, nasal polyps are most often associated with allergy and, when found in this clinical setting, they are usually multiple. Histologically there are a number of secondary changes that can occur with these polyps: infarction, surface ulceration, mucoid liquefaction, stromal cell atypia, and metaplasia of the surface epithelium. Carcinoma arising from surface metaplasia is very rare and is almost always associated with an external carcinogenic promoter, either smoking or some occupationally related promoter. On the other hand, atypia of stromal cells may be misinterpreted as a malignancy because of its microscopic resemblance to rhabdomyosarcoma or myxoid sarcoma.[57, 60]

Polyps are the most common expansile lesions in the nasal cavity. Although they usually are small and cause little deformity, if left unattended in the presence of progression, they can become highly deforming. Eventually they may remodel, disrupt, and destroy the central facial region. They can destroy the medial antral walls, cause hypertelorism, and break through intracranially either via the roof of the nasal cavity and ethmoid complex or via the sphenoid sinus. This marked degree of destruction may be found among medically underserved patients with intractable allergic polyps (primarily aspirin intolerance) and patients with a high level of denial. Destruction secondary to polyposis is an indolent process, causing little if any pain. Although surgery is the treatment of choice for large polyps, in allergic patients desensitization has in some cases shown dramatic results in reducing the number and size of these polyps.[61] Etiologically, in addition to allergy, polyps have been associated with vasomotor rhinitis, infectious rhinosinusitis, diabetes mellitus, cystic fibrosis, aspirin intolerance, and nickel exposure.[61]

On occasion a maxillary sinus polyp may expand and prolapse through the sinus ostium, presenting as a nasal polyp. These are referred to as antrochoanal polyps, which represent 4% to 6% of all nasal polyps. Most are unilateral solitary lesions, but bilateral antral inflammatory disease is found in as many as 30% to 40% of cases. Almost 8% of these patients have additional nasal polyps, and 15% to 40% of patients have a history of allergy.[60–62] These latter statistics have prompted the suggestion that there is an etiologic relationship to allergy, but this theory has not been borne out. Most antrochoanal polyps occur in teenagers and young adults. If such polyps are surgically snared in the nasal fossa like routine nasal polyps, without regard to their antral stalk, 20% to 30% of them will recur, usually within 2 years.[61] The proper treatment is via a Caldwell-Luc or endoscopic intraantral approach.

Ethmoidochoanal and sphenochoanal polyps have also been described. The latter are rare. The etiology of these polyps appears to be similar to that of the antrochoanal polyp.[63]

## The Pediatric Patient

In the pediatric patient, there is little correlation between active infection and sinus opacification and mucosal thickening. This is particularly true in children less than 4 years of age and especially in children less than 2 years of age, in whom tears, retained secretions, and normal redundant mucosa may account for these findings.[16, 64–67] In all such pediatric patients, identification of thickened sinus mucosa should be carefully evaluated in the clinical setting prior to making a diagnosis of active infection. Tissue eosinophilia is characteristic of chronic pediatric sinusitis, especially in children with asthma. However, the presence of allergy does not predict tissue eosinophilia, and the degree of tissue eosinophilia does not correlate with the severity of mucosal thickening as seen on CT scans.[68]

Persistent sinusitis in a pediatric patient may indicate the presence of cystic fibrosis. In these patients, persistent nasal obstruction and sinusitis often lead to hypoplasia of the frontal sinuses, presumably secondary to insufficient aeration. Additional conditions to consider in children with repeated episodes of sinusitis include immune deficiency syndromes, HIV infection, allergic sinusitis, unusual allergies such as aspirin intolerance, and immobile cilia syndrome. In ruling out the latter syndrome, it may be useful to recommend that the clinician submit a brush biopsy specimen from the lateral nasal wall for electron microscopy. Brush biopsy specimens submitted in glutaraldehyde are superior to routine forceps specimens for visualizing the ultrastructure of ciliated cells. Lastly, children under the age of 10 years rarely develop allergic nasal polyps. Thus the presentation of a nasal polyp in the first few years of life should raise the suspicion of an encephalocele, while the appearance of nasal polyposis should suggest the diagnosis of cystic fibrosis.[69, 70]

## The HIV-Positive Patient

In recent decades, there has been considerable interest in the prevalence and type of paranasal sinus inflammatory disease in HIV-positive patients.[71] Minimal sinus inflammatory disease may be clinically significant for these patients, and early treatment should be initiated. HIV specifically affects T helper lymphocytes, as well as monocytes, macrophages, and other parenchymal cells. One of the many ripple effects of the loss of T helper cells is dysfunction of the B lymphocytes, which results in unusually severe bacterial infections. The B cells are unable to respond normally to antigenic stimulation due to the loss of lymphokine-induced stimulation. AIDS patients may develop sinusitis secondary to the usual bacterial agents (*H. influenzae*, *S. pneumoniae*, *S. viridans*, *Moraxella catarrhalis*, coagulase-negative staphylococci, *Staph. aureus*), plus other bacteria (*Pseudomonas aeruginosa* and *Legionella pneumophila*) that are considered opportunistic pathogens and rarely cause sinusitis in normal hosts.[72, 73]

## MUCOCELES

A mucocele is the most common expansile lesion to develop in a paranasal sinus. Pathologically, it is defined as a collection of mucoid secretions surrounded by mucus-secreting respiratory epithelium. Although histopathologically both lesions consisit of mucous secretions surrounded by an epithelial lining, mucoceles and retention cysts are distinguished by their clinical and imaging features.[74]

The retention cyst, as mentioned, is a spherical mucoid-filled cyst that develops when a mucous gland of the sinus mucosa becomes obstructed. The epithelium of the duct and gland capsule is the cyst wall. These cysts are common, usually incidental findings identified in at least 10% of people. They are within the sinus cavity, and almost always some surrounding sinus cavity air remains. Although these cysts can occur in any sinus, they are most common in the maxillary sinus and they rarely cause any remodeling of the sinus wall.

By comparison, a mucocele develops from the obstruction of a sinus ostium or a compartment of a septated sinus, and the wall of the mucocele is the sinus mucosa. The sinus is completely filled and airless, and the sinus cavity is expanded as the bony walls are remodeled outward. An expanded sinus cavity is critical to making the diagnosis of a mucocele, as without this finding, the sinus is properly referred to as an obstructed sinus. Mucoceles occur in all of the paranasal sinuses, with most developing in the frontal sinuses (60% to 65% of cases). Between 20% and 25% occur in the ethmoid sinuses, and 5% to 10% in each sinus occur in the maxillary and sphenoid sinuses.[75–77]

At first, the sinus cavity expansion results in remodeled, intact surrounding bone. However, at some point the sinus cavity may become so large that periosteal repair can no longer maintain sinus wall ossification and deossification occurs. On imaging these areas appear as absent bone, but they may be mistaken for areas of eroded bone.

Rarely, a retention cyst or polyp may become so large that it completely fills the antrum and widens the infundibular region, making distinction from an early mucocele impossible. However, this is of no clinical significance, as the surgical treatment of these lesions is the same.

The classic mucocele is a sterile lesion that presents with signs and symptoms resulting from the mass effect of the lesion. Thus, frontal sinus mucoceles are commonly associated with inferolateral proptosis, a superomedial orbit mass, frontal bossing, nasal obstruction (unilateral or bilateral), and nasal voice quality. Ethmoid mucoceles are associated with lateral proptosis, nasal stuffiness, and possibly a nasal quality to the voice. A supraorbital mucocele can cause downward proptosis, as these mucoceles arise in the mid-roof of the orbit. They also may cause a mass in the floor of the anterior cranial fossa. Maxillary mucoceles may present as a cheek mass, upward displacement of the eye, and nasal obstruction. Sphenoid mucoceles may present with decreased vision, suboccipital headache, and, rarely, fullness in the roof of the nasopharynx. Pain is uncommon and may indicate the presence of an infected mucocele or a pyocele (mucopyocele). Mucoceles have also been reported in an Onodi cell, a pneumatized anterior clinoid process, and a concha bullosa. The potential for vision loss in the two former cases must be noted.[78]

An atelectatic or silent sinus results in effects almost opposite to those of an antral mucocele. Clinically this entity is, as the name implies, asymptomatic, and is revealed only when the major ophthalmologic complication, enophthalmos, becomes evident. It is postulated that chronic sinusitis leads to ostial obstruction, which, in turn, leads to chronic negative pressure within the sinus. Eventually there is retraction of the maxillary sinus walls leading to collapse of the orbital floor and enophthalmia. The findings also include lateral bowing of the uncinate process and inward bowing of the posterior sinus wall. Awareness of this entity is important, as endoscopic osteal decompression of the sinus can avoid ophthalmologic complications.[79 80]

## CORRELATION OF IMAGING AND CLINICAL FINDINGS

Occasionally, some patients may have symptoms of sinonasal inflammatory disease and normal CT and MR imaging studies. Conversely, some patients may have identifiable mucosal thickening on imaging studies and be asymptomatic. In most adult patients, there is a fairly good correlation between significant mucosal disease as seen on imaging and clinical presentation. However, for patients with treated acute sinonasal inflammatory disease, clinical improvement may occur well ahead of resolution of mucosal disease as seen on CT and MR studies. Thus, it is always treacherous for a radiologist to definitively imply that the presence of sinonasal mucosal thickening accounts for the patient's symptoms. Conversely, the radiologist should not imply that a normal sinus imaging study means that the patient does not have symptoms or is a malingerer. The radiologist's report should identify the sinuses involved and assess the degree of mucosal disease in each sinus, and reference to specific clinical symptoms should not, in general, be given.

This reference to the clinical presentation also applies to the terms *acute disease* and *chronic disease*. The presence of an air-fluid level in a patient with acute symptoms of sinonasal infection correlates well. However, many patients with acute sinusitis will not have air-fluid levels, and their imaging appearance may be indistinguishable from that of someone with subacute or chronic disease. Similarly, thickening and sclerosis of a sinus wall implies chronic, recurrent disease. It does not indicate whether any mucosal thickening in that sinus is due to acute or chronic change. Thus, without good clinical correlation, the terms *acute mucosal disease* and *chronic mucosal disease* should not be used by the radiologist. If thickened, sclerotic bone is seen, it merely indicates that there has been a chronic process in that sinus at some time. A dictation might include a statement such as ''Thickening and sclerosis of the sinus wall suggests some chronicity to the disease affecting that sinus.'' It should not qualify the acute or chronic nature of the mucosal disease presently identified within that sinus. In fact, such a sinus may contain scarred, thickened mucosa without any inflammation.

With regard to the nasal cavity, as long as, on imaging, some airway can be identified around the turbinates and the nasal septum, patients rarely complain of nasal obstruction. This imaging rule applies even in the presence of slightly enlarged turbinates and varying degrees of nasal septal deviation.

## IMAGING "NORMAL" MUCOSA

The resolution of present-day CT and MR scanners is such that physiologic mucosal thickening from the nasal cycle can be routinely seen. Thus, unilateral swelling of the middle and inferior turbinates, with minimal ipsilateral ethmoid and maxillary mucosal thickening, usually reflects this physiologic event (see Chapter 3). This is true provided that the opposite middle and inferior turbinates appear small and almost crenated, and a thin airway around the swollen turbinates remains. Usually, normal sinus mucosa is so thin that it is not seen routinely on CT and MR imaging, probably because it is volume averaged out at the sinus air/bone interface. When mucosal thickening is seen incidentally on MR studies in an asymptomatic patient, the mucosa probably is minimally inflamed or scarred.

Brain MR imaging studies have confirmed the lack of imaging specificity for sinus mucosa, as mucosal thickening of up to 3 mm may be present in clinically normal patients. In addition, clinically silent focal areas of ethmoid mucosal thickening were found in 66% of patients.[81] In another series of 263 patients, clinically silent areas of mucosal thickening were found in nearly 25%.[82]

Generally, normal sinuses contain air that directly abuts the bony walls of the sinus. Thus, whenever sinus mucosa is seen at the interface between air and bone, that mucosa is thickened, and, as such, it should be mentioned by the radiologist. However, mucosal inflammation, fibrosis, or physiologic engorgement cannot be confidently distinguished. The overall evaluation of the sinus mucosa is more easily and thoroughly performed on CT and MR imaging than it is on plain films.

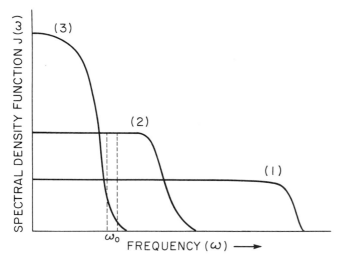

**FIGURE 5-13**  Diagram of a spectral distribution curve for physiologic solutions. The number of molecules at a specific frequency $J(\omega)$ is graphed against the range of frequencies ($\omega$). Curve (1) is for water and illustrates that a wide range of frequencies is present, but there is no preponderance of molecules at any one frequency. Curve (2) shows what happens as macromolecular proteins are added to the water system. A more limited number of frequencies is present due to the large number of more slowly tumbling macromolecular proteins and because the water molecules of higher frequencies drop out as they are magnetically bound to the large proteins. Curve (3) illustrates that when a large number of macromolecular proteins are added to the systems, most of the molecules have a very limited range of slower frequencies. $\omega 0$, Lamor frequency.

## MAGNETIC RESONANCE OF PROTEIN SOLUTIONS

For a specific solution, the concentration of macromolecular proteins affects the T1 and T2 relaxation times. The clinical relevance of this is that the T1-weighted and T2-weighted signal intensities of proteinaceous solutions may be quite varied for specific entities such as cysts, mucoceles, etc. Diagnostic problems in clinical interpretation can arise if this phenomenon is not understood and appreciated. Therefore, the following is a brief, simplified review of T1 and T2 relaxation times in macromolecular protein solutions.

The term *lattice* refers to the overall magnetic environment of the system being studied. A proton spin system can be excited by the addition of energy, and the most efficient way to transfer that energy to the protons is to choose an exciting pulse that is at the Larmor frequency. Once excited, the spin system tends to rid itself of the excess energy and return to an equilibrium state. The excess energy is absorbed by the lattice, and the time it takes for this process to occur is referred to as the spin-lattice or T1 relaxation time.

The most efficient transfer of this excess energy from the excited protons to the lattice occurs when the net molecular rotation of the lattice is at the Larmor frequency. Thus, if a system does not have many molecules rotating at the Larmor frequency, the energy absorption is inefficient and the T1 relaxation time is long. Conversely, if the system has most of its molecules rotating at or near the Larmor frequency, the T1 relaxation time is efficient and short. A study of the number of molecules in a system that are rotating at various frequencies yields a spectral distribution function that can be graphed as the number of molecules at a specific rotational frequency versus the range of frequencies (Fig. 5-13).

Analysis of pure water shows that these small molecules have a wide range of net rotational frequencies, but there is no preponderance of molecules at any one frequency, including the Larmor frequency. Thus pure water has a long T1 relaxation time. As large physiologic macromolecular proteins with relatively slow tumbling frequencies are added to pure water, for a variety of reasons the net rotational motion of the system slows. This effect continues as more macromolecular protein is added, until a protein concentration is reached at which there is a maximum number of molecules with a net rotation at the Larmor frequency. At this concentration the T1 relaxation time is the shortest for the system. As more macromolecular protein is added, the net rotational frequency of the system continues to slow and falls below the Larmor frequency. Consequently, for these more concentrated protein solutions, the T1 relaxation time is long. Thus, for such physiologic solutions, as one proceeds from low macromolecular protein concentrations to high concentrations, the T1 relaxation time goes from long to short to long (Fig. 5-14). This is reflected as the T1-weighted signal intensity goes from low to high to low.

With reference to the T2 relaxation time, initially, after the spin system has been excited, all of the protons can be considered as precessing at the same frequency. However, variations in the local magnetic environment of each proton cause the speed of precession to change by varying amounts, and the result of these magnetic inhomogeneities is that the

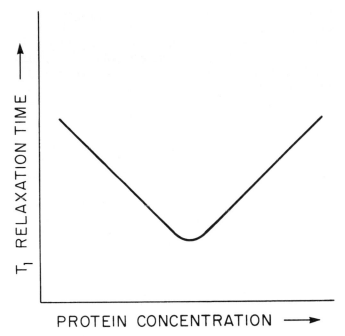

**FIGURE 5-14**   Graph of T1 relaxation time versus macromolecular protein concentration. As protein is added to a water system, the T1 relaxation slows until the net frequency of the lattice is that of the Lamor frequency. At that protein concentration the T1 relaxation time is the most efficient (shortest). As still more protein is added, the net frequency of the system slows below that of the Lamor frequency, and the T1 relaxation time again becomes less efficient.

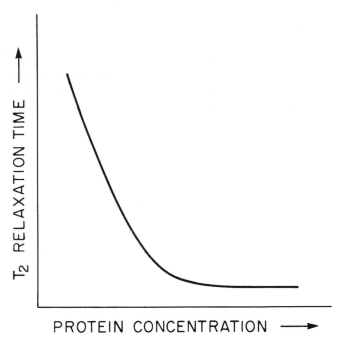

**FIGURE 5-15**   Graph of T2 relaxation time versus macromolecular protein concentration. The more protein added to the system, the lower (faster) the T2 relaxation time. This relationship holds until the system becomes a solid. In a solid, the T2 relaxation time is the fastest it can be, and it becomes a plateau.

protons start to precess at a wider and wider range of frequencies. This interaction is referred to as spin-spin relaxation or dipole-dipole dephasing, and the T2 relaxation time is a measure of this process. For pure water, all the molecules are the same, and they are moving so rapidly that they have little effect on the local magnetic fields of particular protons. Hence in pure water the excited protons precess in phase for a long time, and the T2 relaxation time is long. As macromolecular solute is added, the net frequencies slow so that there is more time for spin-spin interactions. In addition, more molecular inhomogeneity is introduced into the system. Thus, as the protein concentration increases, the T2 relaxation time decreases. However, in viscous solutions and solids, the T2 effects reach a maximum and the T2 relaxation time plateaus at its shortest time (Fig. 5-15). In fact, the T2 relaxation falls from the milliseconds range (thousandths of a second) for physiologic protein solutions to the microseconds range (millionths of a second) for solids. Such rapid dephasing does not allow any magnetic signal to be detected on MR imaging, and a signal void is observed. Lastly, when the T2 relaxation times are ultrashort in the microseconds range, this effect dominates any observed T1 relaxation, and signal voids are also observed on T1-weighted MR imaging. This phenomenon is often referred to as the *T2 effect on the T1 relaxation time*. With this simplified background, one can approach the MR signal intensities of sinonasal secretions (Fig. 5-16).

Normal sinonasal secretions form a complex solution that is in equilibrium with the interstitial fluids.[83] By weight, about 95% of these secretions is water and 5% is solids; virtually all of the solids are macromolecular proteins, predominantly (60%) mucous glycoproteins. Thus normal sinonasal secretions are predominantly water, and on MR

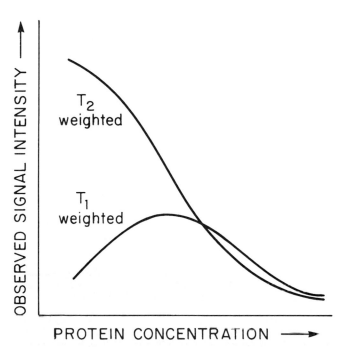

**FIGURE 5-16**   Graph of laboratory-observed T1-weighted and T2-weighted signal intensities versus macromolecular protein concentration. These curves reflect the relaxation times shown in Figures 5-14 and 5-15.

imaging they have long T1 and T2 relaxation times. These are observed as low T1-weighted and high T2-weighted signal intensities.

When normal sinonasal secretions become chronically obstructed, a number of predictable changes occur that alter the protein concentration, the amount of free water (that fraction of the water molecules that magnetically is independent of the effects of the macromolecular proteins), and the viscosity. These changes occur as a result of alterations in the composition and function of the obstructed sinus mucosa, which increases the number of goblet cells that are responsible for the production of the mucous glycoproteins. There is also decreased clearance of the mucous glycoproteins, and with time, the sinus mucosa also reabsorbs free water in the secretions. The result of these changes is an increase in the mucous protein concentration. The sinonasal secretions progressively change from primarily watery and serous to a thick mucus. Then they become a desiccated, stonelike mucous plug when the protein content is above about 35%.

These changes are predictable, but the rate of their evolution is highly variable, both between patients and within the various sinuses of a given patient. The protein concentration directly correlates with the T1-weighted and T2-weighted MR signal intensities of the secretions. This is shown by observing that the graphs of clinically observed T1-weighted and T2-weighted signal intensities reflect the laboratory signal intensities predicted in the prior discussion of the T1 and T2 relaxation times (Figs. 5-16 and 5-17).

As the protein content rises from 5% to about 25%, both the T1 and T2 relaxation times shorten as predicted. However, the T2 shortening is not seen on the MR images because the T2-weighted signal intensity remains high (white) throughout this range. The rise of the T1-weighted

signal intensity is more easily observed on the clinical scans.

Protein crosslinks occur at a protein concentration of about 25% to 30%. This correlates with the increased viscosity observed clinically. Crosslinking also slows the macromolecular motion, which in turn allows dipole-dipole dephasing to become a more significant factor. As a result, the T2 relaxation time and signal intensity plummet. The T1-weighted signal intensity falls back to a low value between the protein content range of 25% to 40%. Above a concentration of 35% to 40%, virtually all of the free water has been eliminated from the secretions and direct macromolecular protein-protein binding occurs. This results in a sudden increase in the viscosity of the secretions. These semisolid and solid protein mixtures have ultrashort T2 relaxation times. These are noted first as low T2-weighted signal intensities and then as signal voids on both T1-weighted and T2-weighted MR images.

Thus, the chronically entrapped secretions become progressively thickened and concentrated, and the MR signal intensities vary with the protein concentration. This may result in anatomically similar collections having variable signal intensities. A high protein concentration can produce signal voids on both T1-weighted and T2-weighted MR images, and thus appear indistinguishable from a normal aerated sinus on MR images (Figs. 5-18 and 5-19). Although the etiology of the signal voids is different (ultrashort relaxation times for the former versus paucity of protons for the latter), the observed imaging blackness is the same. Thus the radiologist can easily underestimate the presence of such chronic desiccated secretions, and therefore the severity of the sinus disease, if MR is the only imaging examination used. CT can distinguish an aerated sinus from a chronically obstructed sinus, as dried secretions are dense (high attenuation), reflecting their high protein concentration, while air is black. CT can also diagnose chronic bone changes and differentiate some radiodensities such as calcification, ossification, or a tooth. Therefore, CT, not MR, is recommended as the first modality for patients with suspected chronic inflammatory disease.[83–85]

## IMAGING

### Benign Sinonasal Mucosal Disease

On plain films the earliest sign of thickened mucosa is often a hazy or vaguely "clouded" appearance of the involved sinus. In such cases, a thickened mucosal margin per se may not yet be identified. If this appearance is not the result of technical or extrinsic factors (the entire film looks hazy, there is overlying swelling of the soft tissues of the cheek, etc.), then this sinus is abnormal. Most commonly this appearance is the result of a combination of retained secretions and minimal mucosal thickening (Fig. 5-20). Once the mucosa is thick enough to be distinctly identifiable on plain films, the mucosa usually appears as a uniformly thick soft-tissue density zone that separates the sinus air from the bone (Fig. 5-21).

There are several situations that may falsely cause a hazy sinus appearance. For instance, haziness is often seen on plain films in the maxillary zygomatic recesses. These areas

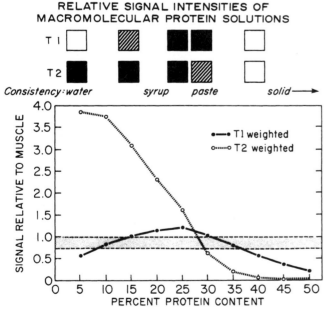

**FIGURE 5-17** Graph of clinically observed T1-weighted and T2-weighted signal intensities versus macromolecular protein concentration. The horizontal zone of gray represents the intermediate range of signal intensity compared with that of the brain. The relationship of the relative physical consistency of the solutions to the signal intensities is shown at the top of the graph. These curves parallel those in Figure 5-16.

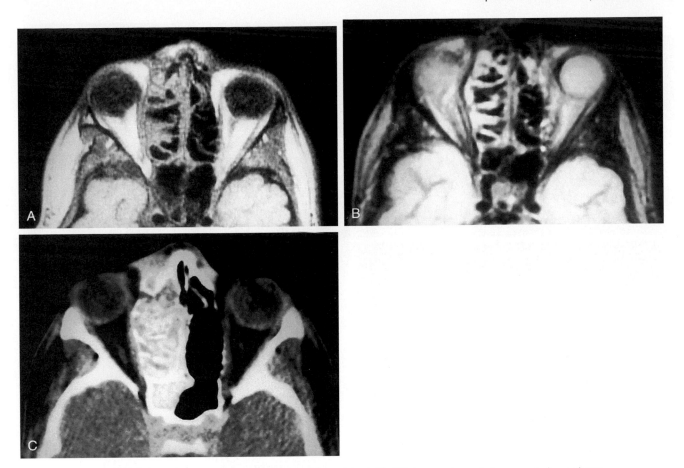

**FIGURE 5-18**   Axial T1-weighted (**A**) and T2-weighted (**B**) MR images show what appears to be moderate ethmoid sinusitis with residual aeration in scattered right ethmoid cells and in the right sphenoid sinus. In a CT scan (**C**) these sinuses are completely opacified, with desiccated secretions that are separated from the sinus walls by a thin zone of mucoid attenuation. This patient had chronic sinusitis.

of the antra have less air and thicker surrounding bone than the main sinus cavity and almost always appear slightly clouded when compared with the main body of the sinus.

Maxillary sinus hypoplasia is another cause of nonspecific sinus density on plain films. However, in most cases, the associated findings of a greater downward angulation of the lateral aspect of the orbital floor and a larger ipsilateral orbit (and often a larger superior orbital fissure) allow a diagnosis to be made. However, definitive evaluation of the mucosa within a hypoplastic sinus may be impossible without CT or MR imaging. In addition, axial sectional imaging clearly allows pathology in the soft tissues of the cheek to be separated from that in the maxillary bony wall or in the sinus mucosa.[86, 87]

The unique anatomy of the ethmoid complex can also lead to underdiagnosis of pathology, as resolution of the numerous closely packed ethmoid air cells is beyond the sensitivity of plain films. The increased density associated with mucosal thickening in an isolated group of ethmoidal cells may be almost completely nullified by air-containing surrounding cells and the adjacent sphenoid sinus.

The sensitivity of the plain film examination of the ethmoid sinuses may be increased by paying close attention to the appearance of the intrasinus septa. Poorly visualized septa may belie the presence of mucosal thickening or fluid

(Fig. 5-22). However, definitive diagnosis of minimal or focal ethmoid cell disease requires sectional imaging. The lack of visualization of these ethmoid septa with no obvious soft-tissue mass may also result from pneumosinus dilatans, mucocele, or previous ethmoidectomy.

In the sphenoid sinuses, minimal mucosal thickening is usually not identifiable on plain films because these sinuses are partially obscured by many overlapping bone and soft-tissue structures. Air-fluid levels can be identified on films taken in the erect position, but CT or MR is required in most cases to accurately identify mucosal disease.

Sinus opacification can be the result of a combination of mucosal thickening, increased sinus secretions, and submucosal edema. The mucosal thickening can vary from a few millimeters to a thick, hypertrophic, redundant mucosa. In some cases, increased mucosal secretions dominate, while in others, submucosal edema is dominant (Fig. 5-1). However, there seems to be no correlation between the dominant type of reaction and the clinical outcome. Rather, these various components seem simply to reflect differences in the individual response to an inflammatory insult, as previously mentioned. With reference to MR imaging, inflammation will have an impact on the MR signal intensities, as it is associated with increased sinus secretions and submucosal edema, both of which are about 95% water. Thus the presence of inflammation will be associated with the signal

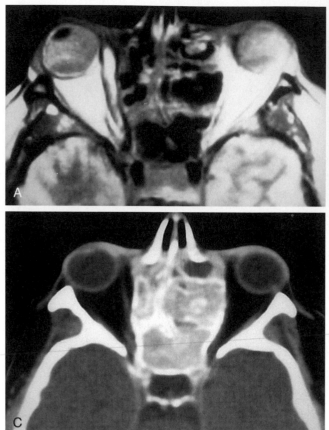

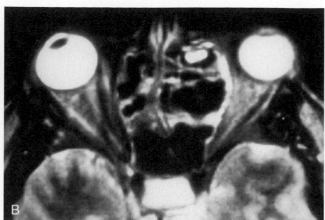

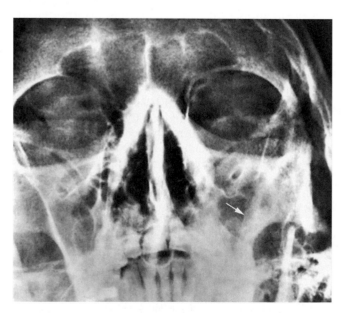

**FIGURE 5-19** Axial T1-weighted (**A**) and T2-weighted (**B**) MR images show expansion of the ethmoid complexes, with apparently moderate mucosal thickening in the ethmoid sinuses. The sphenoid sinuses appear aerated. However, a CT scan (**C**) shows that the expanded ethmoid and sphenoid sinuses are totally opacified, with desiccated secretions. This patient had chronic sinusitis.

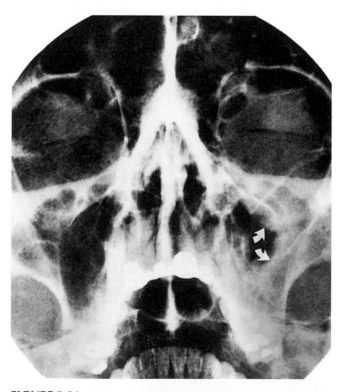

**FIGURE 5-20** Waters view shows a clouded or hazy right maxillary sinus without any identifiable mucosal thickening. The left antrum is also hazy, but there is a definite area of mucosal thickening along the lateral sinus wall (*arrow*). This patient had acute sinusitis.

**FIGURE 5-21** Waters view shows mucosal thickening (*arrows*) in the left antrum. As the mucosa becomes progressively thickened, it heaps up into polypoid masses. This patient had sinusitis.

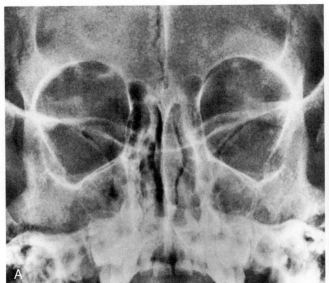
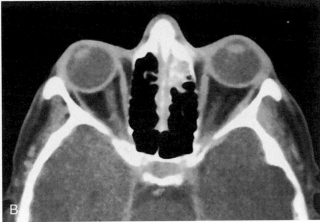

**FIGURE 5-22**   In a Waters view (**A**) there is opacification of a left hypoplastic frontal sinus, the left ethmoid sinuses, and both maxillary sinuses. An axial CT scan (**B**) on a different patient who had normal sinus plain films. There is localized inflammatory disease in the left anterior ethmoid cells. However, the left middle and posterior ethmoid cells and the left sphenoid sinus are well aerated. Because on a frontal film this air may negate the soft-tissue density of the anterior ethmoid disease, the frontal plain films may appear normal. Both of these patients had acute sinusitis.

intensities of water, namely, low T1-weighted and high T2-weighted signal intensities.

After several days of inflammation, increased calcium resorption from the sinus walls can be observed on plain films. The cause is unknown but may be the result of increased mucosal vascularity. Plain films show a "washing out" of the thin mucoperiosteal white line adjacent to each sinus cavity. This effect is most evident in the frontal and maxillary sinuses.

Conversely, when inflammation has been present for many months or years, the sinus walls become thickened by reactive bone (Fig. 5-23). In the maxillary sinus, this bone may become so thick as to decrease sinus cavity size, a finding confirmed on CT scans.

Chronic sphenoid sinusitis can also result in thickened, sclerotic surrounding bone. Often these patients complain of suboccipital pain or headaches (Fig. 5-24). Rarely, cavernous sinus thrombophlebitis and thrombosis can develop as a

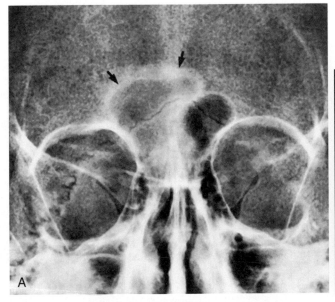
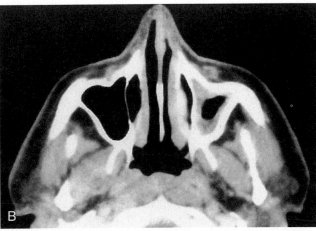

**FIGURE 5-23**   Caldwell view (**A**) shows a zone of reactive sclerosis around a clouded right frontal sinus (*arrows*). This suggests that there had been chronic disease in this sinus at one time. There also is minimal clouding of the right ethmoid sinuses. This patient had chronic sinusitis. In **B**, an axial CT scan shows thickening and sclerosis of the walls of the left maxillary sinus and mucosal thickening within this sinus. The mucosal disease may be acute sinusitis, noninfected edematous mucosa, or chronically scarred mucosa. The bone reaction indicates that there has been chronic inflammation in this sinus. This patient had chronic sinusitis.

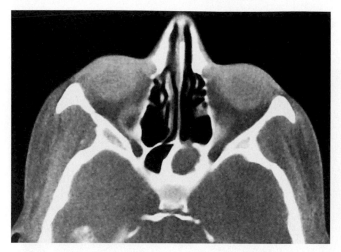

**FIGURE 5-24**  Axial CT scan shows an opacified left sphenoid sinus surrounded by thickened, sclerotic bone. This patient had chronic suboccipital headaches and chronic sinusitis.

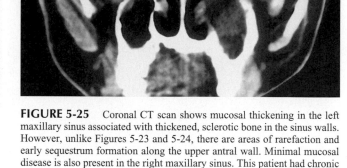

**FIGURE 5-25**  Coronal CT scan shows mucosal thickening in the left maxillary sinus associated with thickened, sclerotic bone in the sinus walls. However, unlike Figures 5-23 and 5-24, there are areas of rarefaction and early sequestrum formation along the upper antral wall. Minimal mucosal disease is also present in the right maxillary sinus. This patient had chronic sinusitis with osteomyelitis.

complication of sphenoid sinusitis that may lead to meningitis. Most patients with intracranial-type symptoms will initially have a CT or MR study. Such examinations should always include the skull base and paranasal sinuses to eliminate these as a source of the disease and symptoms.

Osteomyelitis of the bones of the face and paranasal sinuses is uncommon and is usually associated with localized pain. The involved bone has a mottled, irregular appearance on both plain films and CT. There may be sequestra, as well as areas of thickened and sclerotic bone (Fig. 5-25).

More commonly, osteomyelitis may be posttraumatic or iatrogenic. It is most often found following an osteoplastic flap procedure for frontal sinus inflammatory disease. A poorly vascularized and/or infected bone flap may result in osteomyelitis of the flap, a recognized complication of this procedure.

Postirradiation osteitis is rarely seen today in the facial bones because of megavoltage equipment and improved radiation treatment planning. Radiation osteitis is probably most commonly encountered in the mandible, usually in patients irradiated for carcinomas of the tongue and floor of the mouth. In patients irradiated for maxillary sinus carcinomas, the first manifestation of sinus osteomyelitis may be localized pain, swelling, and inflammation over the zygoma and maxilla, initially suggesting tumor recurrence. However, eventually a bone sequestrum is extruded, and symptoms temporarily improve. Multiple sequestra are usually extruded, and it is not uncommon for the osteitis to become clinically manifest up to 1 or 2 decades after irradiation. On CT the involved facial bones appear shattered, fragmented, and sclerotic (Fig. 5-26). Superficial sequestra should be specifically identified and localized to aid therapy.

When evaluating mucosal thickening on postcontrast CT scans, if the thickened mucosa does not enhance, it is probably not actively infected and usually is fibrotic and scarred. Active infection has a thin zone of mucosal enhancement with a variable zone of lower-attenuation submucosal edema (Fig. 5-1). If the sinus is opacified, the CT appearance shows roughly concentric rings or zones: an outer bony wall "ring," a water or mucoid attenuation (10 to 18 HU) submucosal ring, a thin infected mucosal enhancing ring, and a central zone of entrapped mucoid secretions (Fig. 5-1). Although most minimal to moderate mucosal thickening is seen as a fairly uniformly thick soft-tissue zone on sectional imaging, thicker, more redundant mucosa can appear almost nodular or "wavelike." In these instances, the disease tends to involve the sinus diffusely, unlike the focal nodularity often seen with tumors.

In all CT examinations, the sinuses should be viewed at wide window settings so that mucosal disease is not falsely interpreted as a hypoplastic or aplastic sinus (Fig. 5-27).

On MR imaging the thickened, inflamed mucosa typically has a low signal intensity on T1-weighted images, an intermediate intensity signal on proton density (PD) images, and a high signal intensity on the T2-weighted images (Figs. 5-18, 5-19, and 5-28). These changes reflect the high water content of the inflamed tissues. The high T2-weighted signal intensity is helpful in differentiating inflamed tissues from almost all sinonasal tumors. At most, such tumors tend to have an intermediate T2-weighted signal intensity. Dense scar or fibrosis has a low to intermediate signal intensity on all imaging sequences, a useful finding in differentiating it from inflammation and most tumors on the T2-weighted images. Unfortunately, both tumor and the vascularized scar tissue/granulation tissue that develops after surgery have similar signal intensities, and they cannot, at present, be confidently differentiated on MR imaging.

Unilateral swelling of the middle and inferior nasal turbinates, especially in the absence of concurrent paranasal sinus disease, probably reflects the normal nasal cycle. In these cases, a thin zone of air remains, separating the turbinates from the nasal septum and the lateral nasal wall. If this air space is not present, the turbinates probably are pathologically enlarged. Clinical correlation can help

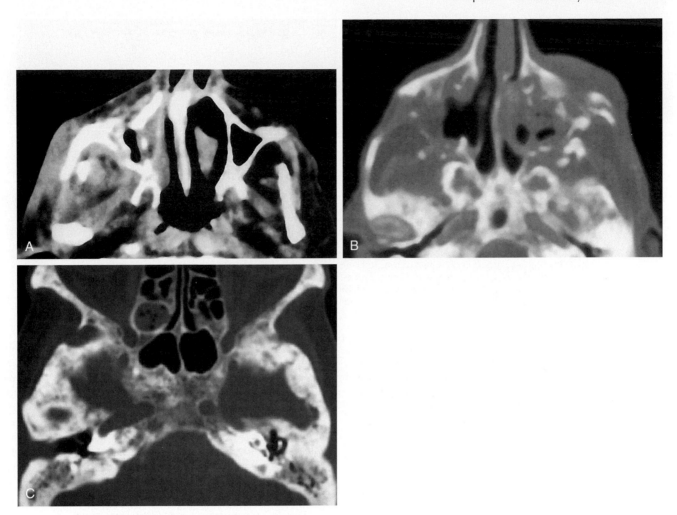

**FIGURE 5-26**   In **A**, an axial CT scan, there is fragmentation of the right maxillary sinus's bony walls, with sclerosis and thickening of the bone. Mucosal thickening is also present in the sinus. This patient had radiation osteitis and sinusitis. In **B**, an axial CT scan shows extensive sclerosis and fragmentation of the facial bones, with some of the osseous structures having been extruded as sequestra. This patient had radiation osteitis. In **C**, an axial CT scan shows areas of both dense bone and "washed-out," permeated-appearing bone in the skull base and posterior ethmoid and sphenoid sinus margins. Some secretions are also present in the most posterior right ethmoid cells. This patient had radiation osteitis after radiation therapy for a nasopharyngeal carcinoma.

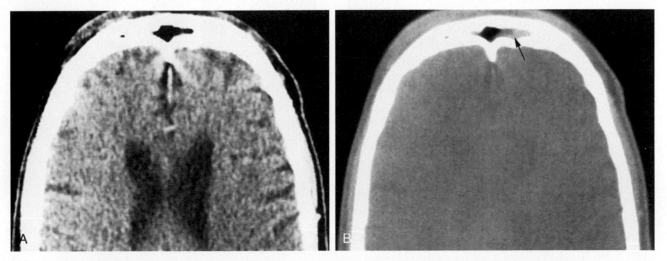

**FIGURE 5-27**   In **A**, an axial CT scan viewed at a "soft-tissue" window setting, the left frontal sinus appears well aerated. However, in **B**, inflammatory mucosal thickening in the left frontal sinus (*arrow*). This patient had a headache and acute sinusitis.

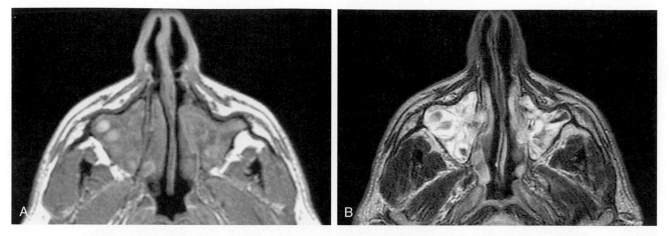

**FIGURE 5-28**    Axial T1-weighted (**A**) and T2-weighted (**B**) MR images show both maxillary sinuses filled with nonhomogeneous signal intensities. In **A**, the majority of the sinus content has a low to intermediate signal intensity, while in **B**, it has a high signal intensity. This represents heaped-up, inflamed mucosa and is the characteristic MR imaging appearance of inflammation. The areas of higher signal intensity in **A** and lower signal intensity in **B** are sites of desiccated secretions. This patient had chronic sinusitis.

resolve any issue.[88] On postcontrast CT and MR images, the turbinates will enhance whether enlarged physiologically or pathologically. On MR images they have low T1-weighted and high T2-weighted signal intensities (Fig. 5-29). Nasal turbinate swelling may also represent an allergy to contrast material on postcontrast CT scans. This is easily confirmed if the turbinates are normal on the initial noncontrast scan.[89]

## Polyps and Cysts

The intrasinus polyp and the retention cyst cannot be differentiated on either plain films or sectional imaging.

However, this is of little consequence, as both are common benign entities and any treatment is the same.

On all imaging, retention cysts and polyps are homogeneous soft-tissue masses with smooth, outwardly convex borders (Figs. 5-30 to 5-39). Multiple or single lesions may be present; most are small and clearly do not fill the entire sinus cavity. If a cyst or polyp occurs in the roof of the maxillary sinus in a patient with a history of recent trauma, the plain film examination may simulate a blowout fracture (Fig. 5-31). However, coronal CT or MR imaging will

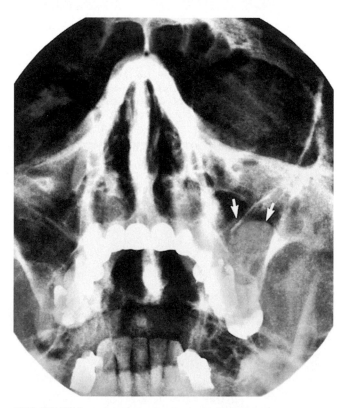

**FIGURE 5-29**    Coronal T2-weighted MR image shows swelling of the right inferior and middle turbinates, while the left turbinates have a shrunken appearance. In addition, there is some mucosal thickening in the right maxillary and ethmoid sinuses. This is an example of the normal nasal cycle in a symptomatic patient.

**FIGURE 5-30**    Waters view shows a solitary left antral retention cyst or polyp (*arrows*). This cyst typically has a smooth, outwardly convex contour. The remaining antrum and the other sinuses are normal.

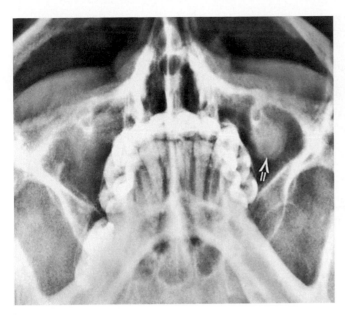

**FIGURE 5-31**   Waters view shows a retention cyst or polyp (*arrow*) in the roof of the left maxillary sinus. If there was a history of recent orbital trauma, this could be mistaken for part of a blow-out fracture. In this patient, coronal sectional images would have demonstrated an intact orbital floor.

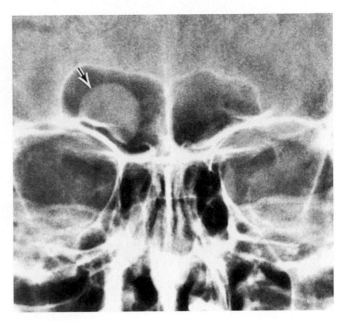

**FIGURE 5-32**   Caldwell view shows a retention cyst (*arrow*) in the right frontal sinus. Note that this sinus is otherwise normal.

demonstrate an intact orbital floor, with the cyst or polyp in the antral mucosa.

On the Waters view, a prominent infraorbital canal may mimic a cyst or polyp in the roof of the antrum. Similarly the nasal alae can simulate a medial wall antral cyst or polyp, and unerupted teeth, the lips, or a mustache can simulate a cyst or polyp on the floor of the maxillary sinus. The coronoid process of the mandible can simulate a cyst or polyp in the posterior floor of the antrum on a lateral plain film taken with the patient's mouth closed.

As a cyst or polyp enlarges to fill at least half of the antrum, it behaves like a water-filled thin balloon, the upper surface flattens out, and it resembles an air-fluid level (Fig. 5-40). A true air-fluid level is a fluid level throughout the entire involved sinus, with a concave upward meniscus at the margins of the fluid. Additionally the planar surface of the fluid will directly reflect gravity in every head position. On MR imaging these cysts or polyps usually have characteristics similar to those of mucosal inflammation, again reflecting the high water and low specific protein content. Thus, they tend to have low to intermediate T1-weighted and high T2-weighted signal intensities. If the protein content of the cyst or polyp fluid increases, either due to infection or the passage of time, the T1-weighted signal intensity may become high, reflecting the shortening of the T1 relaxation time.

Retention cysts and polyps are usually asymptomatic and are incidental radiographic findings. However, if they enlarge to fill the entire sinus, they may obstruct sinus drainage and become symptomatic. Rarely, these lesions can remodel the sinus walls and expand the sinus cavity. But in most cases on sectional imaging, small pockets of remaining sinus air can be identified overlying part of the convex margin of the lesion (Fig. 5-34). This distinguishes such a cyst or polyp from a mucocele, although when the lesion is large, the distinction is of more intellectual interest than clinical significance.

On sectional imaging, a typical antrochoanal polyp appears as a soft-tissue polyp that completely fills a maxillary sinus. Usually the infundibular region is widened, and there is a slight extrusion of the antral mass into the middle meatus. Alternatively, the polyp can extend through a secondary sinus ostium. At this stage, such an antrochoanal polyp can be confused with hypertrophic polypoid antral mucosa that has also extended through the sinus ostium. However, as the polyp grows, it fills the ipsilateral nasal fossa and extends back into the nasopharynx (Figs. 5-41 to 5-44). It may become sufficiently large to hang down into the oropharynx. Although the medial antral wall may eventually be deossified or destroyed, the remaining antral walls are rarely remodeled. This can be a difficult

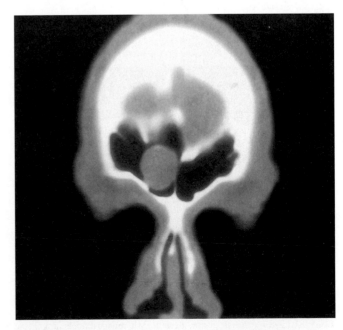

**FIGURE 5-33**   Coronal CT scan shows a solitary retention cyst or polyp in the right frontal sinus. The sinus is otherwise normal.

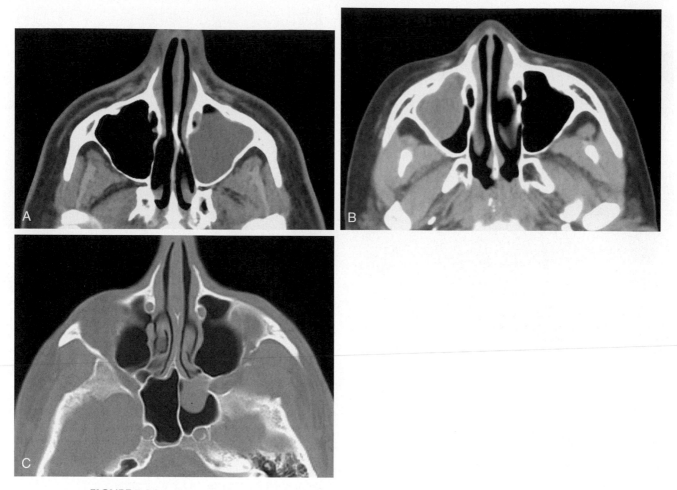

**FIGURE 5-34**    Axial CT scans. In **A**, there is a large retention cyst or polyp in the left maxillary sinus. A small amount of air is present over the upper surface of the lesion, and the sinus cavity is not enlarged. In **B**, there is a typical retention cyst or polyp in the right maxillary sinus. Note that the convex margin of the lesion is smooth and that the remaining sinus is normal. In **C**, there is a retention cyst or polyp in the left sphenoid sinus and minimal mucosal thickening in the right sphenoid sinus.

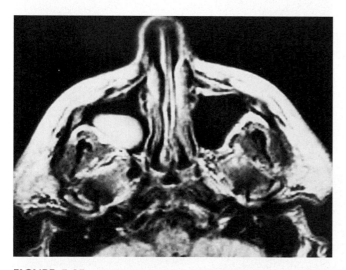

**FIGURE 5-35**    Axial proton density MR image shows a solitary retention cyst or polyp with a typically high signal intensity in the right antrum.

diagnosis on plain films, but it is rarely misdiagnosed on sectional imaging. Histologically, antrochoanal polyps differ from inflammatory polyps in that they are fibrotic, with minimal inflammation. The normal minor salivary tissue is obliterated. Of note, atypical fibroblasts may be seen within the lesion, mimicking a neoplastic process. Thus the radiologist may assist the pathologist in ruling out neoplasm by confirming a benign, slowly growing lesion.

On plain films, nasal polyps are often seen as a vague increased soft-tissue density within the nasal fossa. However, on sectional imaging they usually can be identified as discrete single or multiple broad-based soft-tissue masses (Figs. 5-45 to 5-59). On CT, more recent polyps tend to have a mucoid attenuation (10 to 18 HU), with mucosal enhancement occasionally seen at the polyp's surface. However, those polyps that have had sufficient time to develop stromal fibrosis plus desiccation of the secretions tend to have higher overall attenuation (20 to 35 HU). On MR imaging, typically the dominant feature is the high water and low protein content that gives the polyps low to intermediate T1-weighted and high T2-weighted signal intensities. When multiple polyps are present, often intermixed with mucoceles, the

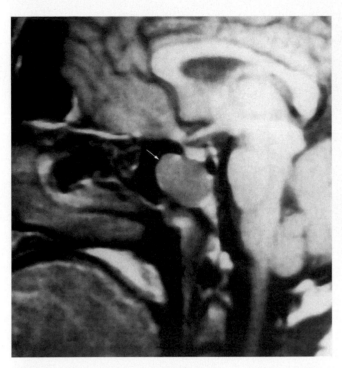

**FIGURE 5-36**  Sagittal T1-weighted MR image shows a solitary nonobstructing retention cyst or polyp (*arrow*) in the sphenoid sinus. This is the type of lesion that was formerly referred to as a *mucocele* in the older literature.

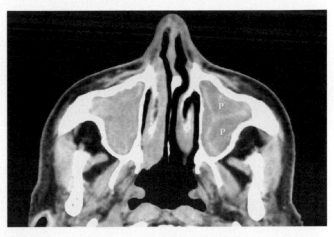

**FIGURE 5-37**  Axial CT scan shows both maxillary sinuses to be filled. On the right side, there is higher-attenuation material centrally within the sinus cavity representing desiccated secretions. However, on the left side, desiccated secretions form a thin curvilinear zone of higher attenuation, outlining the mucosal polyps (*P*) in this sinus.

entrapped secretions usually have variable T1-weighted and T2-weighted signal intensities (Figs. 5-56 and 5-57). It is this variable imaging appearance that distinguishes such polypoid masses from tumors, which tend to have more homogeneous signal intensities.[83, 90, 91]

On CT, when there are multiple polyps crowded within the nasal vault, they can form an overall conglomerate mass that may be difficult if not impossible to distinguish from a tumor. This is especially true of bulky lesions such as inverting papillomas and lymphomas that tend to remodel the surrounding bone. However, two findings typical of sinonasal polyps can reliably establish their diagnosis on CT studies. First, an ethmoid polypoid mucocele that involves

the ethmoid labyrinth unilaterally or bilaterally is characterized by widening of the ethmoid complex, with little if any destruction of the delicate ethmoid septa.[74, 92] The individual ethmoid cells are filled with polypoid mucosa and entrapped mucoid secretions. The CT appearance of each sinus cavity is that of a central high-attenuation region (desiccated secretions) separated from the bony sinus wall by a thin zone of lower mucoid attenuation. By comparison, a solid mass (either a single polyp, a mucocele, or a tumor) will destroy these septa, and in this latter circumstance it is impossible to distinguish a benign lesion from a low-grade malignant process. The preservation of ethmoidal septa, as seen in polypoid mucoceles, unequivocally signifies the presence of benign disease (Figs. 5-52 and 5-53).

Secondly, the finding of a unilateral or bilateral expansile sinonasal mass with cascading, looping, or curvilinear areas of fairly high attenuation (desiccated secretions) in a background matrix of mucoid attenuation (10 to 18 HU) is specific on CT for the presence of a benign process. Usually, these polypoid masses are separated from the adjacent bones by a thin zone of mucoid material (Figs. 5-50 to 5-53). This

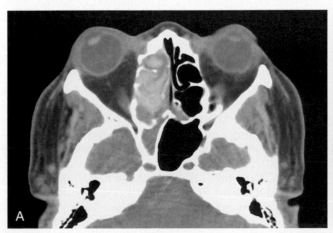

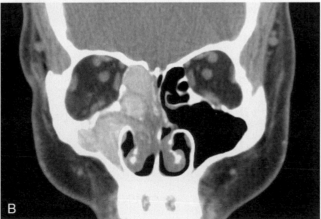

**FIGURE 5-38**  Axial (**A**) and coronal (**B**) CT scans show opacification of the right ethmoid, sphenoid, and maxillary sinuses. Within the ethmoid and maxillary sinuses are polypoid areas of higher attenuation representing desiccated secretions within chronic polyps. This patient had no history of allergies. Note that the left-sided sinuses are virtually normal.

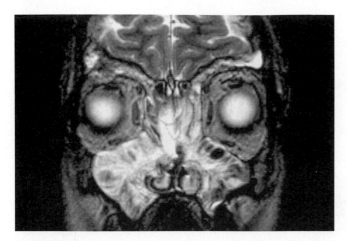

**FIGURE 5-39** Coronal T2-weighted MR image shows soft tissues opacifiying the ethmoid and maxillary sinuses. Overall, the signal intensity is high. However, there are multiple areas of lower signal intensity that represent partially desiccated secretions within polyps. This was an allergic patient with extensive polyposis.

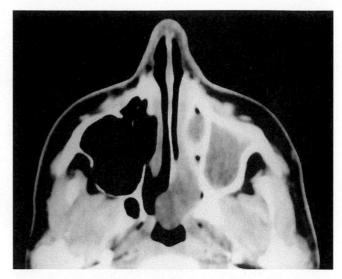

**FIGURE 5-41** Axial CT scan shows a mucoid density mass filling the left maxillary sinus. It extended through the infundibulum into the left nasal fossa and nasopharynx. This patient had an antrochoanal polyp.

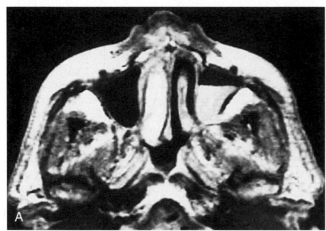

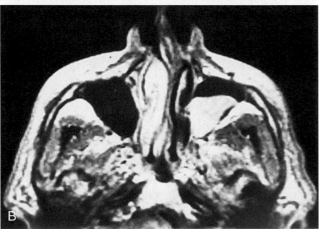

**FIGURE 5-40** Axial proton density MR images. In **A**, the image is through the lower sinus and there is an apparent air-fluid level. However, in **B**, the image is through the midsinus, and a convex margin is seen identifying this high signal intensity retention cyst or polyp. Because large cysts or polyps are essentially fluid-filled bags, gravity can flatten portions of large lesions to simulate an air-fluid level.

unique CT appearance is seen in about 20% of patients with nasal polypoid masses.

On MR, the signal intensity is determined by the degree of desiccation of the secretions entrapped within the sinuses and between and within the polyps. The resulting variable appearance of signal intensities is diagnostic of inflammatory disease. The primary diagnostic problem arises when semisolid or completely desiccated secretions are present. These dried secretions give signal voids on T2-weighted images and, depending on the degree of desiccation, either low signal intensity or signal voids on T1-weighted images. Possible confusion with an aerated sinus can occur unless a CT study is available for comparison (Figs. 5-18 and 5-19).

Sinonasal mucosa adjacent to polyps will enhance on MR imaging, while secretions and fluid within and around the polyps will not enhance. This appearance is distinctive from that of a neoplasm, which enhances more uniformly.

The CT finding of a high-attenuation central region separated from the sinus wall by a thin zone of mucoid attenuation material can be seen in three distinct cases in order of likelihood: chronic inspissated (desiccated) secretions, a mycetoma (usually from aspergillosis), and intrasinus hemorrhage (Figs. 5-8A and 5-60).[93] Although a specific diagnosis may not always be possible on CT, this appearance reliably indicates that the soft-tissue mass is not a tumor.[57] The MR imaging finding of a central intrasinus region of signal void or low T1-weighted and T2-weighted signal intensity can represent either desiccated secretions in chronic sinusitis, a mycetoma in a patient with sinus fungal disease, a sinolith, or an intrasinus tooth (antrum) (Figs. 5-18, 5-19, and 5-61 to 5-66).

The mycetomas are semisolid and have paramagnetic ions, both contributing to their low signal intensity or signal voids on all imaging sequences. Any inflammatory reaction around the mycetoma will have the typical MR imaging characteristics of infections or polyps.[94]

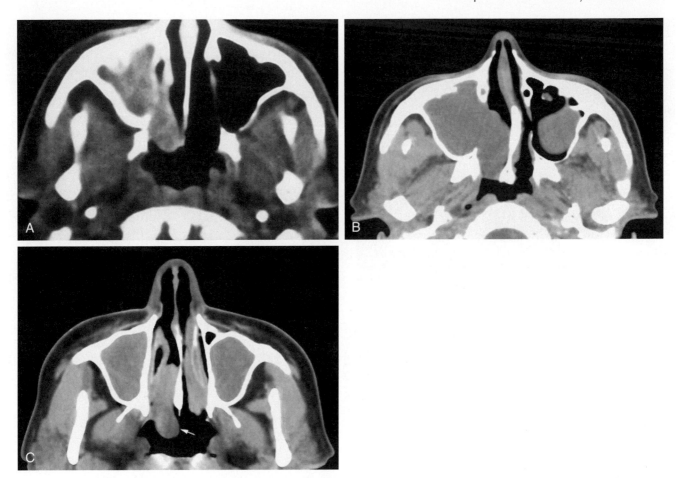

**FIGURE 5-42**   **A,** Axial CT scan shows a right maxillary sinus polypoid mass that has prolapsed into the posterior right nasal fossa. This patient had an antrochoanal polyp. Axial cranial (**B**) and caudal (**C**) CT scans on another patient show a polypoid mass in the right maxillary sinus that has extended into the right nasal fossa and prolapsed into the nasopharynx (*arrow*). This patient also had an antrochoanal polyp.

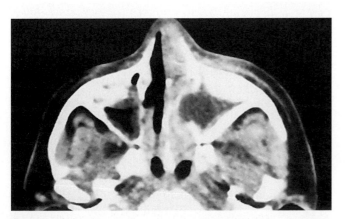

**FIGURE 5-43**   Axial contrast-enhanced CT scan shows a mucoid attenuation polypoid mass in the left maxillary sinus that bulges into the left nasal fossa. Inflammatory mucosal changes are seen in both nasal fossae, and there is enhancement of the mucosa around the polyp. This patient had an antrochoanal polyp.

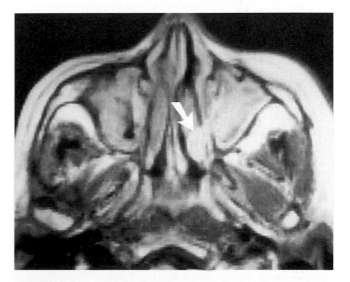

**FIGURE 5-44**   Axial proton density MR image shows inflammatory changes in both maxillary sinuses. On the left side, a polypoid mass fills the left maxillary sinus and extends into the nasal fossa (*arrow*). This patient had an antrochoanal polyp.

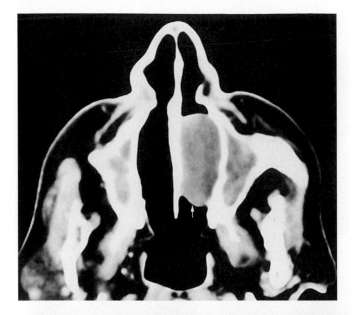

**FIGURE 5-45**   Axial CT scan shows a solitary mucoid attenuation left nasal mass (*arrow*). There are also secretions and inflammatory mucosal disease in both maxillary sinuses. This patient had a nasal polyp and sinusitis.

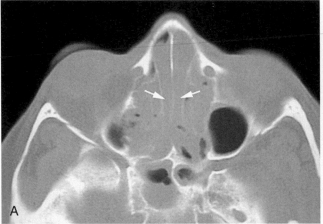
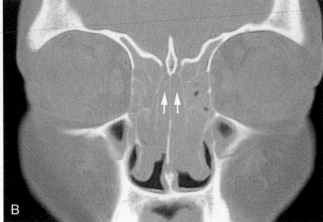

**FIGURE 5-46**   Axial (**A**) and coronal (**B**) CT scans show soft-tissue disease opacifying the ethmoid sinuses and inflammatory mucosal thickening in the sphenoid and maxillary sinuses. Polypoid soft tissues also fill both nasal fossae. Note that the normally thin olfactory recesses of the upper nasal fossae are widened (*arrows*). This suggests that the nasal masses are chronic nasal polyps.

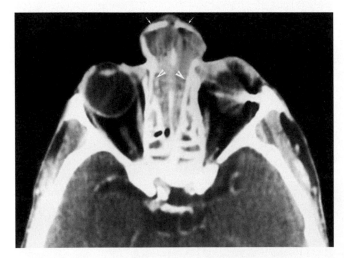

**FIGURE 5-47**   Axial contrast-enhanced CT scan shows bilateral nasal masses that have displaced the nasal bones anterolaterally (*small arrows*) and thinned part of the nasal septum. The upper nasal fossae are widened by the nasal masses, and the medial aspect of the each ethmoid complex has been displaced laterally (*arrowheads*). There are also secretions in both ethmoid sinuses. This patient had nasal polyposis and sinusitis.

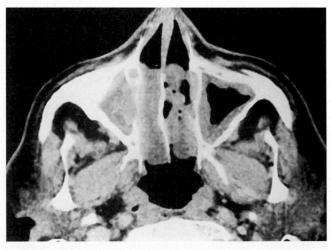

**FIGURE 5-48**   Axial CT scan shows multiple bilateral nasal polyps, inflammatory mucosal thickening in the left maxillary sinus, and opacification of the right maxillary sinus. This patient had nasal polyposis and sinusitis.

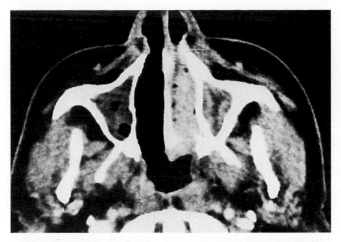

**FIGURE 5-49**  Axial contrast-enhanced CT scan shows an enhancing left nasal fossa polypoid mass. There are mucosal enhancement and secretions in the left maxillary sinus and mucoid secretions in the right maxillary sinus. This patient had nasal polyps and sinusitis.

An intrasinus hemorrhage initially has a low signal intensity on all imaging sequences. However, when the blood becomes oxidized to methemoglobin (by 24 to 48 hours after the trauma), it has a high T1-weighted and an intermediate T2-weighted signal intensity. Thus, with MR imaging, intrasinus hemorrhage can be distinguished in almost all cases from desiccated secretions and a mycetoma (Fig. 5-8).[17, 18] It should be noted that as long as some air remains in the sinus, it is rare to have any entrapped secretion desiccate enough to have high T1-weighted signal intensity.

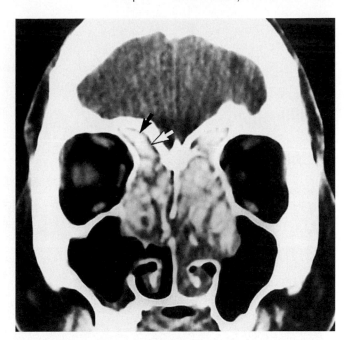

**FIGURE 5-50**  Coronal CT scan shows multiple high-attenuation soft-tissue masses extending from the ethmoid sinuses into the nasal fossae. Each polypoid mass is separated from the adjacent bone by a thin zone of mucoid attenuation material (*arrows*). The polyps are also embedded within a matrix of mucoid secretions. This patient had nasal and paranasal sinus polyposis.

## Mucoceles

On plain films a frontal sinus mucocele first appears as a slightly clouded sinus with a smooth, ovoid, or rounded contour, in contrast to the normal frontal sinus, which has a scalloped contour with septation extending into the sinus and a density similar to that seen in the superior orbital fissure. The normal thin mucoperiosteal white line becomes hazy. If chronic sinusitis predates mucocele development, a zone of dense reactive bone may surround the sinus. As the

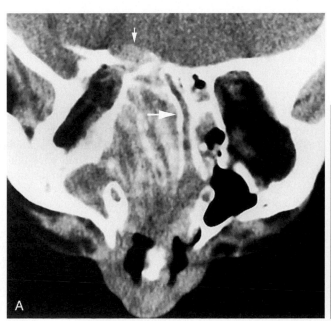

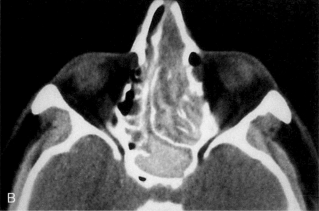

**FIGURE 5-51**  Coronal CT scan (**A**) shows an expansile right nasoethmoid mass that has displaced the nasal septum to the left (*large arrow*). The mass has also focally broken into the floor of the anterior cranial fossa (*small arrow*). Within the mass are discrete high-attenuation polypoid masses embedded within mucoid secretions. There are also inflammatory changes in the left ethmoid sinuses. This patient had polyposis. An axial CT scan (**B**) on another patient shows a high-attenuation soft-tissue mass in the sphenoid sinus that is separated from the sphenoid sinus's bony wall by a zone of mucoid attenuation. There also is an expansile left nasoethmoid mass that has discrete high-attenuation polypoid areas within mucoid secretions. This patient had polyposis and a sphenoid sinus polyp.

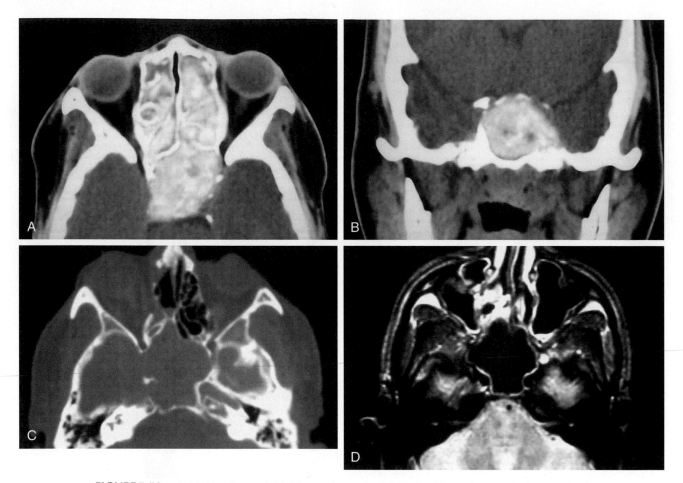

**FIGURE 5-52**    Axial (**A**) and coronal (**B**) CT scans show an expansile ethmoid complex mass that has remodeled the thin lamina papyracea laterally. The ethmoid sinuses are filled with high-attenuation material that is separated from the adjacent bone by a thin zone of mucoid attenuation. The sphenoid sinuses are also filled with dense material; however, the sphenoid sinus walls are deossified and appear destroyed. This patient had paranasal sinus polyposis. This case illustrates how the central facial bones can remodel in response to chronic pressure, while the central skull bones primarily deossify. **C,** Axial CT scan on another patient who had had a prior right external ethmoidectomy. Now the CT scan shows an opacified sphenoid sinus with apparent erosion of the skull base along the right side of the sinus. Axial T2-weighted MR image (**D**) shows high signal intensity in the inflammatory sphenoid sinus mucosa and no erosion of the adjacent skull base. This area of the skull base demonstrates pressure deossification from the mucocele. The dried sinus secretions seen in **C** have a signal void in **D** that could easily be overlooked if only MR was available.

mucocele erodes the sinus contour in the vertical plate of the frontal bone, it also slowly erodes the anterior and posterior frontal sinus tables. This results in a loss of bone density on frontal plain films that more than compensates for the soft-tissue density of the mucoid secretions. Thus a frontal sinus mucocele tends to maintain a radiodensity that is equal to or slightly less than that of the adjacent normal frontal bone. If one observes an expansile frontal sinus mass that is denser than the adjacent frontal bone, a fibroosseous lesion is a more likely diagnosis than a mucocele. As a frontal sinus mucocle enlarges, it tends to displace the superior-medial orbital margin downward and laterally, correspondingly displacing the eye (Figs. 5-67 to 5-70). A radiolucent frontal sinus mucocele is seen only when it becomes so large as to erode most of the sinus tables (Figs. 5-70 and 5-71).

A hypoplastic frontal sinus on plain films has a single, smooth, centrally concave border that may simulate a mucocele. The normally scalloped margins of larger sinuses are not present for assessment of possible erosion. However, regardless of the sinus capacity, the boundaries of a normal frontal sinus never violate the orbital contour. Any downward and outward displacement of the superomedial orbital rim (and a similar displacement of the eye) should be considered presumptive evidence of a frontal sinus mucocele until proved otherwise. Similarly the base of the frontal intersinus septum is normally in the midline, and any displacement of this portion of the septum to one side is also suggestive of a frontal sinus mucocele.

The midline segments of the anterior and posterior frontal sinus tables are seen on lateral plain films. Plain films are insensitive in detecting erosion of these tables off of the midline. It is important for the surgeon to know, prior to surgery, whether the posterior frontal sinus wall is intact. Sectional imaging of a suspected frontal sinus mucocele is then mandatory, and asymptomatic intracranial mucocele extention thus can be fortuitously discovered.

Mucoceles can extend posteriorly into the horizontal plate (orbital roof) of the frontal bone, as well as up into the vertical plate. Once in the orbital roof, a mucocele can extend both cranially into the floor of the anterior cranial

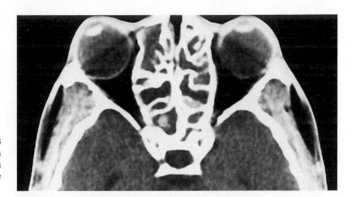

**FIGURE 5-53** Axial CT scan shows opacification of the ethmoid sinuses with widening of the anterior and middle ethmoid complexes. The lamina papyracea remains intact. Several discrete high-attenuation polyps are seen within the mucoid secretions filling the ethmoid cells. The delicate intercellular septa are intact. This patient had a polypoid mucocele.

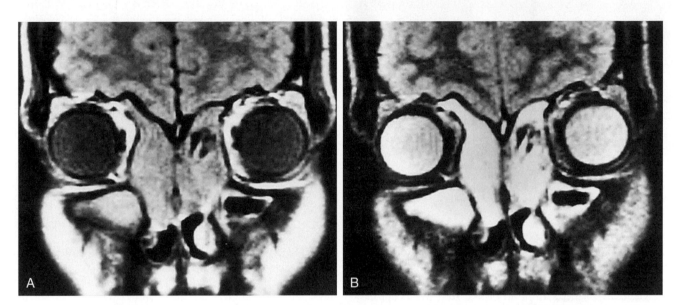

**FIGURE 5-54** Coronal proton density (**A**) and T2-weighted (**B**) MR images show bilateral nasoethmoidal expansile masses causing some hypertelorism. These masses have the signal intensities of inflammatory tissue. This patient had polyposis and sinusitis.

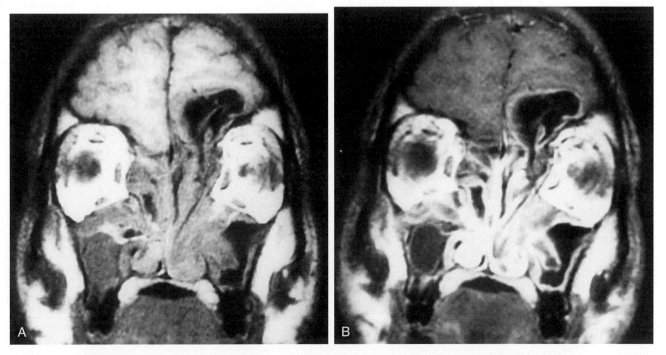

**FIGURE 5-55** Coronal T1-weighted MR images without contrast (**A**) and with contrast (**B**). There are polypoid masses in the nasal fossae, the maxillary sinuses, and the ethmoid complexes. The disease has broken intracranially on the left side. There are areas of high, intermediate, and low signal intensity. In **B**, the mucosal surfaces of the polyps enhance. This patient had polyposis.

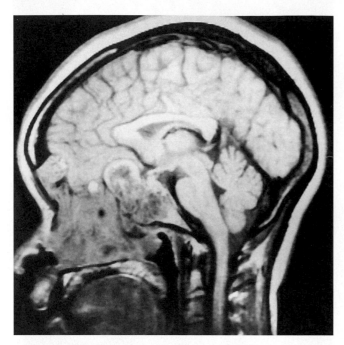

**FIGURE 5-56** Sagittal T1-weighted MR image shows a nonhomogeneous signal intensity polypoid mass in the sphenoid and ethmoid sinuses, breaking intracranially. Increased soft tissues are also present in the nasal fossae. This patient has polyposis.

fossa and caudally. If this orbital roof extension is not appreciated at the time of surgery, which is usually performed extracranially for the more obvious vertical plate disease, complications from an orbital roof mucocele may require a second operation and an intracranial approach. In the event that frontal sinus surgery was performed without preoperative sectional imaging, and retrospectively the plain films suggest the presence of horizontal recess disease, then postoperative CT or MR imaging is necessary to resolve this issue and provide an important prospective baseline study.

Ethmoid mucoceles usually arise from the anterior rather than the posterior ethmoid cells, presumably because the anterior ethmoid ostia are the smallest of any in the paranasal sinuses.[95, 96] Mucous viscosity also promotes mucoceles, as ethmoid mucoceles are common in patients with cystic fibrosis.[97] Ethmoid mucoceles are typically expansile, thinning and remodeling the lamina papyracea and bowing it laterally into the orbit, resulting in a laterally displaced globe. This may be very difficult to diagnose on plain films despite clinical evidence of a mass. The obliquely oriented lamina papyracea is not well seen on frontal films, and the air density of normal ethmoid cells surrounding the mucocele can partially nullify the soft-tissue density of the mucocele. An air-fluid level in the ethmoid complex can indicate an ethmoid mucocele rupture, with partial drainage into the nasal cavity and adjacent ethmoids. In these cases, a mucopyocele is usually present at the time of discovery (Fig. 5-11).[98]

Mucoceles also can arise in supraorbital ethmoid cells; these are best demonstrated on Caldwell films or coronal images. Infection or a polyp in the lower portion of the supraorbital cell can be the cause of obstruction that leads to these mucoceles, which typically erode through the middle third of the orbital roof and displace the globe inferiorly.

Polypoid mucoceles may involve the entire ethmoid complex, either unilaterally or bilaterally. Characteristically, sectional imaging confirms that ethmoid septa are preserved within the opacified, expanded ethmoid complex. The plain film findings may be only diffuse opacification of the ethmoid complex.

The typical antral mucocele totally opacifies the maxillary sinus and expands the sinus cavity (Fig. 5-72). Unchecked antral mucoceles may eventually overtake the osteoblastic ability of the outer maxillary periostium, resulting in frank bone destruction, thus making the distinction from neoplasia difficult on plain films (Fig. 5-73). If the orbital floor is elevated, the patient may experience diplopia. Rarely, if the mucocele spontaneously collapses after thinning the orbital floor, the globe may descend, causing enophthalmos and diplopia. If the antrum has been compartmentalized by a septum, a mucocele may be limited to only one of these sinus sections. Obviously,

*Text continued on page 228*

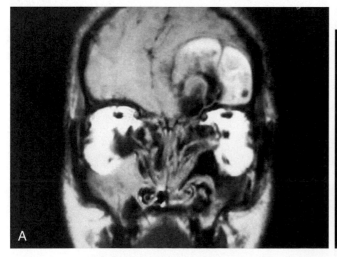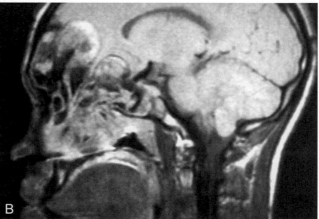

**FIGURE 5-57** Coronal (**A**) and sagittal (**B**) T1-weighted MR images show multiple sinonasal polypoid masses that have extended into the medial aspect of each orbit, broken through intracranially, and obstructed the maxillary sinuses. These are areas of high, intermediate, and low signal intensity throughout the lesion, as well as areas of signal void. This patient had polyposis from aspirin intolerance.

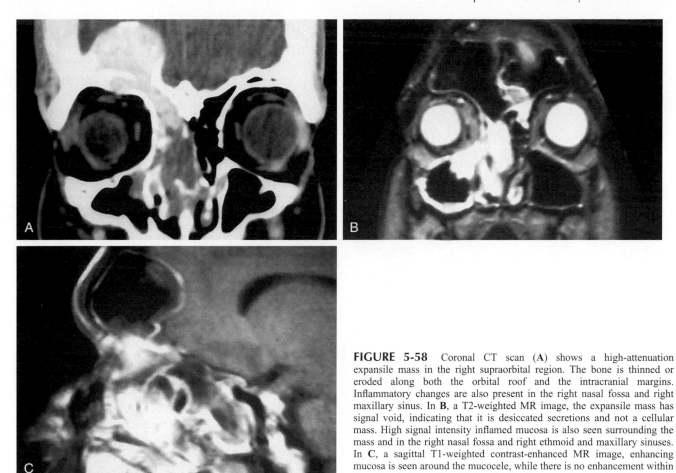

**FIGURE 5-58** Coronal CT scan (**A**) shows a high-attenuation expansile mass in the right supraorbital region. The bone is thinned or eroded along both the orbital roof and the intracranial margins. Inflammatory changes are also present in the right nasal fossa and right maxillary sinus. In **B**, a T2-weighted MR image, the expansile mass has signal void, indicating that it is desiccated secretions and not a cellular mass. High signal intensity inflamed mucosa is also seen surrounding the mass and in the right nasal fossa and right ethmoid and maxillary sinuses. In **C**, a sagittal T1-weighted contrast-enhanced MR image, enhancing mucosa is seen around the mucocele, while there is no enhancement within the entrapped secretions. This patient had a mucocele and sinusitis.

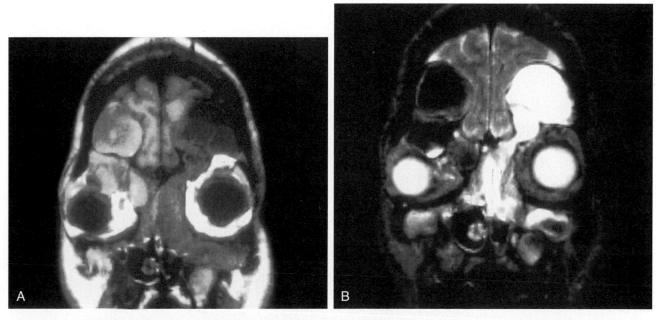

**FIGURE 5-59** Coronal T1-weighted (**A**) and T2-weighted (**B**) MR images show bilateral sinonasal polypoid masses that have broken intracranially, into the left superomedial orbit from the left frontal sinus, and down into the right superior orbit from a right supraorbital ethmoid cell. The signal intensities of the left-sided lesions are those of classical inflammation. The right-sided lesions contain thicker inspissated secretions and have intermediate T1-weighted and low T2-weighted signal intensities. This patient has polyposis.

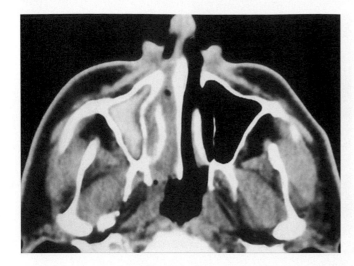

**FIGURE 5-60** Axial CT scan shows high-attenuation material within the right maxillary sinus, separated from the sinus bony wall by a thin zone of water attenuation. The most common cause of this CT appearance is desiccated secretions. A mycetoma in fungal sinusitis and intrasinus hemorrhage also can have this appearance. This patient had chronic sinusitis.

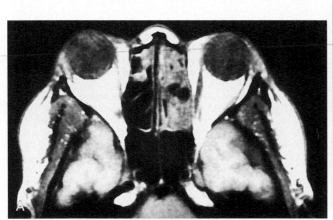
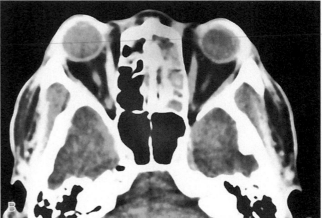

**FIGURE 5-61** Axial T1-weighted MR image (**A**) shows presumed inflammatory disease in the left ethmoid complex with apparent aeration of some middle ethmoid cells. However, the axial CT scan (**B**) shows total opacification of the left ethmoid sinuses. At surgery, the middle ethmoid cells were found to contain aspergilloma. This patient has aspergillosis.

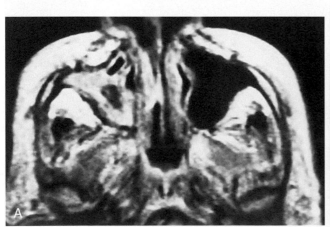
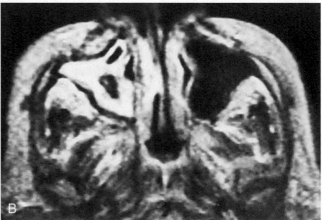

**FIGURE 5-62** Axial proton density (**A**) and T2-weighted (**B**) images show inflammatory-type mucosal thickening in the right maxillary sinus. In the center of the sinus is an ovoid mass with low signal intensity. This is an aspergilloma with surrounding inflammation. This patient had aspergillosis.

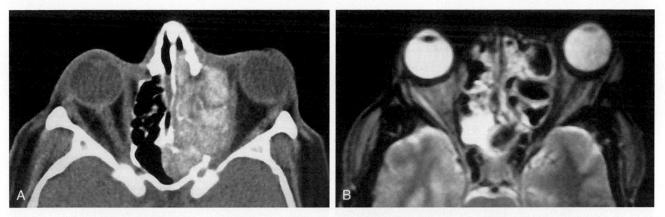

**FIGURE 5-63**   Axial CT scan (**A**) shows a mass in the left ethmoid and sphenoid sinuses that has broken out into the left orbit. There are discrete areas of high attenuation. The localized areas of high density on this non-contrast CT makes an inflammatory process likely, but not definite. However in **B**, a T2-weighted MR image, the areas of high attenuation in **A** have signal voids. This indicates that they are most likely either desiccated secretions or mycetomas. This patient had aspergillosis.

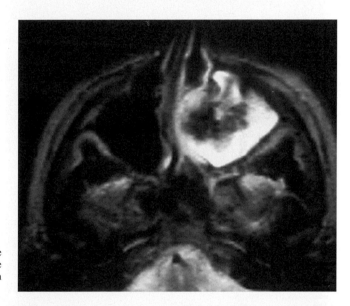

**FIGURE 5-64**   Axial T2-weighted MR image shows inflammatory disease with a high signal intensity in the left maxillary sinus. Centrally within the sinus is a region of both low signal intensity and signal void. This was an aspergilloma. This patient had aspergillosis.

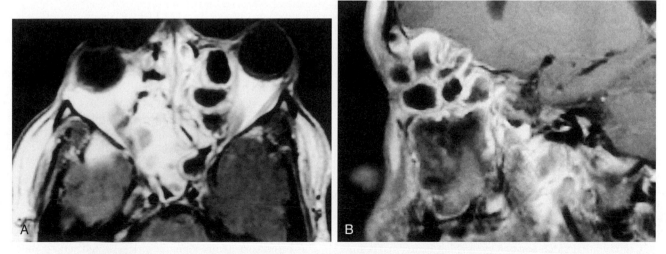

**FIGURE 5-65**   Axial (**A**) and sagittal (**B**) contrast-enhanced T1-weighted MR images show widening of the ethmoid complex by a mass that has also broken into the floor of the anterior cranial fossa and the left orbit. Enhancing mucosa is seen surrounding areas of signal void. The maxillary sinuses are also involved by the process. None of the sinuses were aerated on CT, and the areas of signal void were aspergillomas. This patient had aspergillosis.

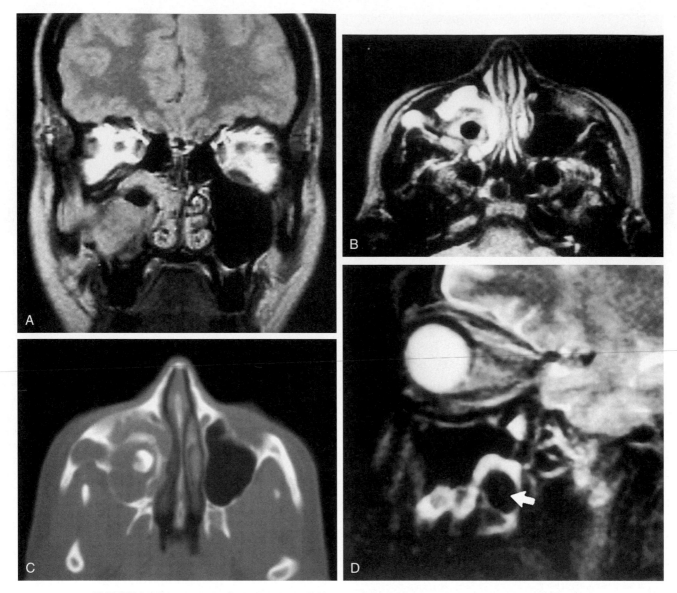

**FIGURE 5-66**    Coronal T1-weighted (**A**) and axial T2-weighted (**B**) MR images show a slightly expanded right maxillary sinus filled for the most part with inflammatory-type material. Within the sinus is an area of signal void. This could have been residual sinus air, desiccated secretions, a mycetoma, or a sinolith. An axial CT scan (**C**) shows that it was a tooth in a dentigerous cyst. A sagittal T2-weighted (**D**) image on another patient shows an area of signal void (*arrow*) just under the floor of the maxillary sinus. This patient had an undescended molar tooth.

there are significant clinical implications of an unexplored posterior compartmental mucocele. In such cases, the radiologist may be the only physician to detect this hidden mucocele and direct the surgeon to it (Fig. 5-74).[99]

Sphenoid sinus mucoceles have the highest incidence of surgical complication of all mucoceles. Due to their proximity to the optic nerve, blindness is the most serious major postoperative complication. Most sphenoid mucoceles expand anterolaterally into the posterior ethmoids and the orbital apex. Less commonly, expansion may occur upward into the sella turcica and cavernous sinuses or downward into the nasopharynx and posterior nares. In rare cases, intracranial extension can even result in areas of brain necrosis.[100, 101] Occasionally they may extend into the sphenoid sinus recesses in the greater wings and the pterygoid processes.[102] If sufficiently large, sphenoid sinus mucoceles may cause optic canal and orbital apex syndromes. The critical role of the radiologist is to accurately localize the relationship of the optic nerve to the mass, thereby guiding the surgeon during surgical decompression.

Multiple paranasal sinus mucoceles have been reported after facial fractures and in patients with severe allergies. Patients with aspirin intolerance seem to be particularly prone to develop multiple aggressive mucoceles that may extend intracranially.[103]

The finding on CT of an expanded, airless sinus cavity filled with fairly homogeneous mucoid attenuation (10 to 18 HU) secretions is diagnostic of a mucocele.[104] However, if the entrapped secretions are particularly viscid and proteinaceous, the attenuation can increase to 20 to 45 HU, similar to that of muscle. If the sinus is airless, filled with a mucoid density but not expanded, the diagnosis is that of an obstructed sinus, not a mucocele (Figs. 5-75 and 5-76). When a mucocele is present, the sinus walls are remodeled and may be of almost normal thickness, thinned, or partially eroded (Figs. 5-77 to 5-90). In the latter two cases, the sinus

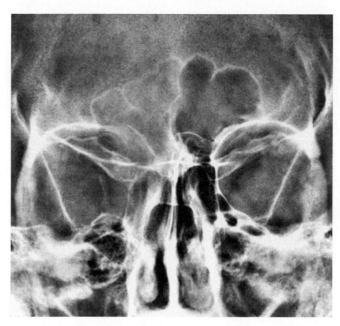

**FIGURE 5-67**   Caldwell view shows clouding of the right frontal and ethmoid sinuses. There is thinning and downward displacement of the right superomedial orbital rim. This patient has sinusitis and right frontal sinus mucocele.

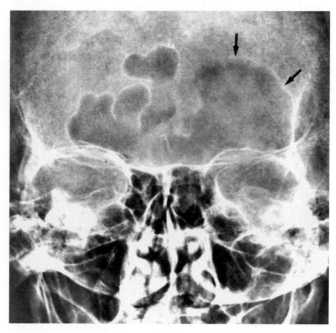

**FIGURE 5-69**   Caldwell view shows a loss of the normal left frontal sinus margin scalloping (*arrows*) and portions of the normal white mucoperiosteal line around the sinus and in the roof of the left orbit. This patient had a left frontal sinus mucocele.

mucosa and the sinus wall periostium are all that surround the mucous secretions. If a mucopyocele is present, the inflamed sinus mucosa is seen as a thin line of enhancement just inside the bony sinus walls, establishing the diagnosis of an infected mucocele (Fig. 5-91).[32]

Prior Caldwell-Luc procedures may result in a fibrous septum between the lateral margin of the anterior sinus wall surgical defect and the posterior sinus wall. Synechiae

can form and organize into a solid fibrous wall. The resulting septum can obstruct the drainage from the lateral portion of the sinus, while the sinus cavity medial to the septum drains normally. Thus an expansile mass in the lateral maxillary sinus is diagnostic of this condition. As it enlarges, a lateral antral mucocele may extend into the body of the zygoma and present in the cheek as a soft-tissue mass or it may extend into the lateral, inferior orbit (Figs. 5-92 and 5-93).

On MR imaging, the signal intensities of a mucocele are determined by the protein content of the entrapped secretions. As previously discussed, secretions become more con-

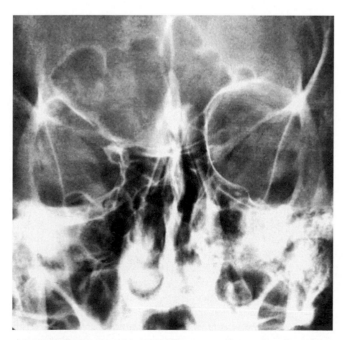

**FIGURE 5-68**   Caldwell view shows slight haziness in the right frontal sinus, as well as flattening and downward displacement of the right superomedial orbital rim. The frontal intersinus septum is also displaced to the left side. This patient had a right frontal sinus mucocele.

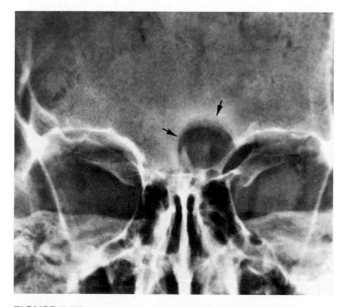

**FIGURE 5-70**   Caldwell view shows a left hypoplastic frontal sinus that has lost the normal thin mucoperiosteal white line. Instead, there is a thick zone of surrounding sclerosis (*arrows*). There is also erosion of the left superomedial orbital rim. This patient had a left frontal sinus mucocele.

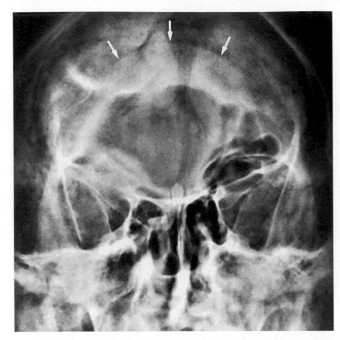

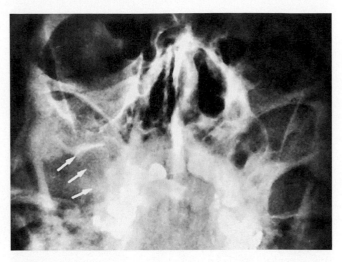

**FIGURE 5-73** Waters view shows an opacification of the right maxillary sinus, with apparent erosion of the lower lateral sinus wall (*arrows*). This looks like a carcinoma but is actually thinning of the bone secondary to a maxillary sinus mucocele.

**FIGURE 5-71** Caldwell view shows a smoothly contoured, enlarged frontal sinus. There is a surrounding zone of sclerosis, and only the most lateral portion of the left frontal sinus appears normal. There is erosion of the right superior and superomedial orbital rim, and a mound of soft tissue is seen above the mass (*arrows*). This patient had a frontal sinus mucocele that caused the forehead to bulge and resulted in right proptosis.

centrated and viscous over time and the T1-weighted and T2-weighted signal intensities vary. The relaxation-time shortening can be used to approximate the viscosity of the secretions, as shown in Figure 5-17 (Figs. 5-94 to 5-101).[83] On contrast-enhanced MR images, the sinus mucosa en-

hances and is seen as a uniformly thin zone surrounding the nonenhancing secretions. If a mucopyocele is present, the infection causes increased viscosity of the secretions, shorter relaxation times, and thickening of the mucosa.

If there is a mucoid collection in the antrum and a double bony wall is seen in the maxillary sinus, often at the most anterior or posterior margin of the sinus, it implies that the bony floor has been elevated by an odontogenic process (Fig. 5-102). This is important to recognize, as the surgical treatment of an odontogenic cyst differs from that of an antral mucocele.

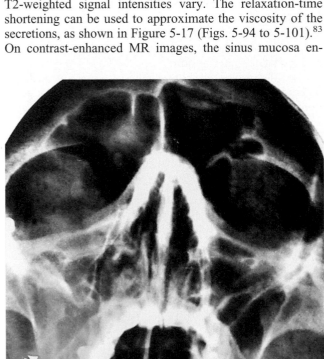

**FIGURE 5-72** Waters view shows opacification of the right maxillary sinus, with thinning of the lower lateral sinus wall (*arrow*) and some expansion of the sinus cavity. This patient had a right maxillary sinus mucocele.

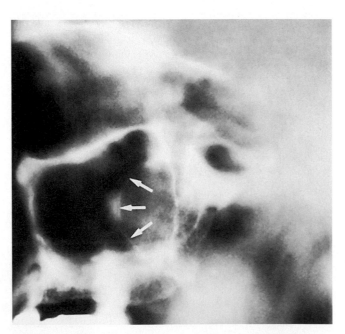

**FIGURE 5-74** Lateral view multidirectional tomogram shows an expanded compartment (*arrows*) in the posterior portion of the maxillary sinus. This patient had a mucocele in a posterior sinus compartment.

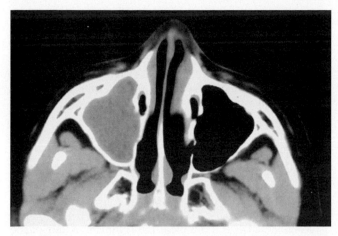

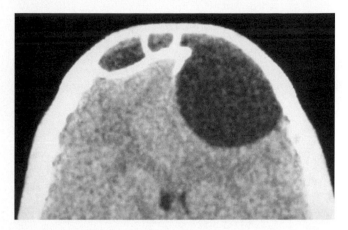

**FIGURE 5-75**   Axial CT scan shows an opacified right maxillary sinus. The attenuation of the material is approximately that of water. The sinus cavity is normal in size. This is an obstructed sinus, not a mucocele. In a mucocele, the sinus cavity must be enlarged.

**FIGURE 5-77**   Axial CT scan shows a large, expansile mucoid attenuation mass in the left frontal sinus that has thinned the posterior sinus table and bulged intracranially. A smaller mucocele that extended down into the orbit is also present on the right side. The left mucocele contents are separated from the brain by sinus mucosa, deossified bone, and the meninges. This patient had bilateral frontal sinus mucoceles.

## Fungal Diseases

Mycotic sinusitis has a highly variable appearance. During early infection, merely nonspecific mucosal inflammation in the nasal fossa or paranasal sinus(es) is seen.[105, 106] Most often either the maxillary sinus or ethmoid sinuses are involved. The sphenoid and frontal sinuses are only occasionally affected.[107] Air-fluid levels are uncommon and, when present, suggest a bacterial infection. The

surrounding bone in mycotic sinusitis may be thickened and sclerotic, eroded, or remodeled. Most often it is the combination of these bone changes that suggests either an unusual infection or fungal disease.[108]

Soft-tissue disease is often found both in the nasal fossa and the paranasal sinuses. In antral mycotic sinusitis, the nasal disease may act as a bridge for extension of infection into the cheek. This finding suggests an aggressive infection or fungal disease, as antral bacterial sinusitis rarely

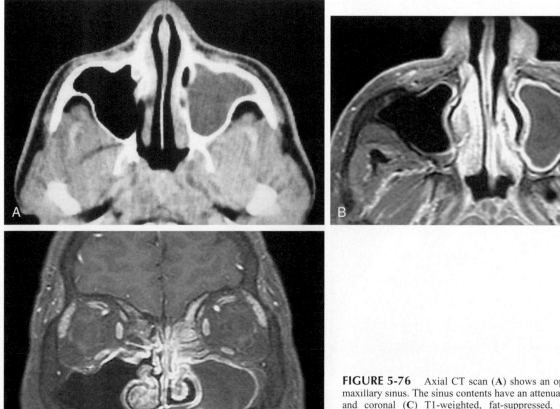

**FIGURE 5-76**   Axial CT scan (**A**) shows an opacified, obstructed left maxillary sinus. The sinus contents have an attenuation of water. Axial (**B**) and coronal (**C**) T1-weighted, fat-suppressed, contrast-enhanced MR images show an obstructed left maxillary sinus. The sinus mucosa enhanced about the secretions. There is also inflammatory disease in the left ethmoid sinuses.

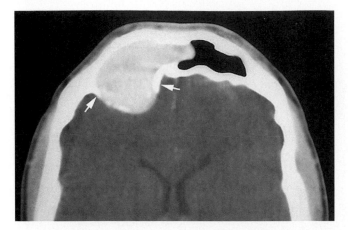

**FIGURE 5-78** Axial CT scan shows a high-attenuation, expansile right frontal sinus mass that has remodeled the margins of the posterior sinus table (*arrows*). However, most of the posterior sinus wall is deossified. This patient had a right frontal sinus mucocele.

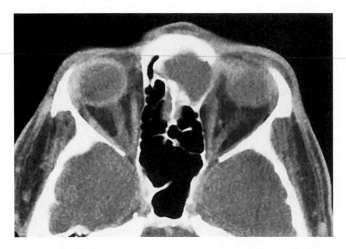

**FIGURE 5-79** Axial CT scan shows an expansile left frontal sinus mass that is bulging into the upper left medial orbit. There is primarily bone remodeling rather than bone destruction. This patient had a left frontal sinus mucocele.

extends into the facial soft tissues.[109] Intrasinus concretions within a mycetoma can be seen occasionally on plain films and CT (Figs. 5-103 to 5-105).[110, 111] As previously discussed, the signal void and adjacent sinus inflammation of a mycetoma mimic the MR imaging appearance of nonspecific chronic infection with desiccated secretions (Figs. 5-61 to 5-65).

# INFECTIOUS DESTRUCTIVE AND GRANULOMATOUS SINONASAL DISEASES

## *Actinomyces* and *Nocardia*

Actinomycosis is a commensural organism of human and bovine hosts; unlike most true fungi, they have not been identified as environmental saprophobes. The human pathogen, *Actinomyces israelii* (and, less often, *A. eriksonii*) is normally present around teeth, especially carious teeth, and in tonsillar crypts. It is classified as a filamentous bacterium rather than a fungus because (1) it reproduces by fission rather than by sporulation (as do perfect fungi) or filamentous budding (as do imperfect fungi), and (2) muramic acid is present in its cell walls and mitochondria are absent, both of which are features of bacteria.

*Actinomyces* has limited pathologic potential in the normal host. Antecedent trauma or other precursors are necessary predisposing factors for invasive infection. There are three forms: cervicofacial, thoracic, and abdominal; the cervicofacial is the most common form of infection. Soft-tissue abscesses and draining cervical fistulae develop as a result of secondary *Actinomyces* infection of periapical abscesses. Actinomycosis can also present in the neck without the characteristic sinus tracts. These sinuses can occasionally have long tracts, communicating with the soft tissues of the back and chest. Aspiration of oral *Actinomycetes* from carious teeth may lead to pulmonary abscess formation and pneumonia. Rarely, *Actinomyces* may be the cause of sinonasal, laryngeal, or pharyngeal disease.

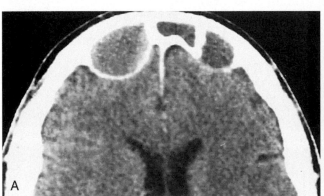
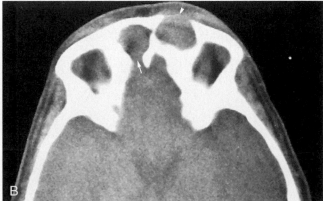

**FIGURE 5-80** Axial CT scan (**A**) shows bilateral frontal sinus expansile masses. Each mass has thinned and remodeled the posterior sinus wall, and each mucocele bulges intracranially. On the plain film, the posterior sinus wall appeared intact. This patient had bilateral frontal sinus mucoceles. Axial CT scan (**B**) on another patient shows an expansile mass in each of the left and right frontal sinuses. The left-sided mass has broken through the anterior sinus wall (*arrowhead*), and the right-sided mass has broken through the posterior sinus wall (*arrow*). This patient had bilateral frontal sinus mucoceles.

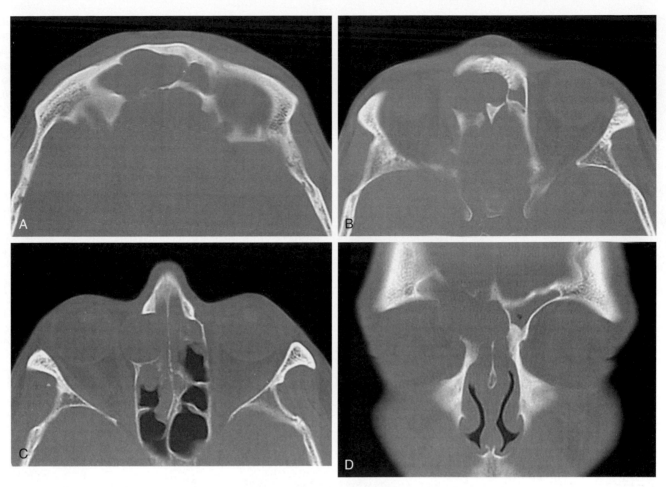

**FIGURE 5-81**    Serial axial CT scans from cranial (**A**) to caudal (**C**) and a coronal CT scan (**D**) show an expansile mass in the right frontal and ethmoid complex. There are areas of marked thinning of the surrounding bone. This patient had a right frontoethmoid mucocele.

The pale yellow ''sulfur granules'' or ''grains'' observed clinically are microcolonies of bacilli. On hematoxylin and eosin (H&E) stain, only blue amorphous masses are visible. The slender, filamentous nature of these bacilli is apparent on special stains. The filaments may mimic fungi in their tendency to branch. *Actinomycetes* are routinely not acid-fast, although occasionally they may be weakly acid-fast. This point can help distinguish *Actinomyces* on tissue sections from *Nocardia*. The latter filamentous

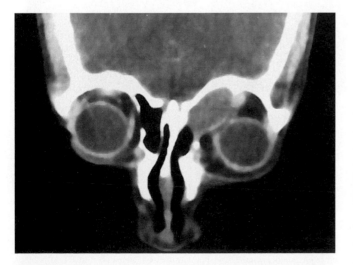

**FIGURE 5-82**    Coronal CT scan shows an expansile water attenuation mass in the superomedial left orbit. The globe is displaced downward and laterally. This is the typical direction of eye displacement from a frontal sinus mucocele.

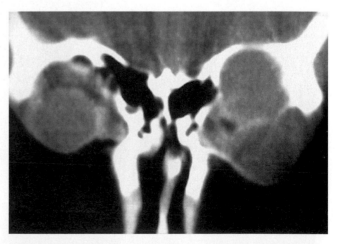

**FIGURE 5-83**    Coronal CT scan shows a water attenuation mass in the roof of the left orbit displacing the globe downward. This is the typical direction of eye displacement from a supraorbitial ethmoid mucocele.

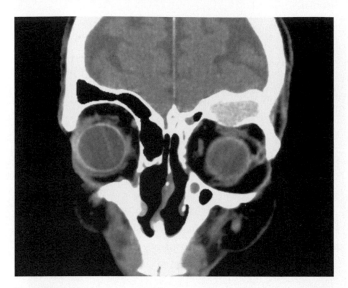

**FIGURE 5-84** Coronal CT scan shows a high-attenuation mass in the left orbital roof displacing the globe downward. There is thinning of the bone in the roof of the orbit, and some inflammatory disease is seen more proximally in the left ethmoid sinuses. This patient had a left supraorbital ethmoid mucocele.

bacterium does not stain well with H&E but does stain well with a modified Ziehl-Neelson stain. The distinction between these two filamentous bacteria is important because their sensitivity to antibiotics differs; penicillin is the drug of choice for *Actinomyces*, but *Nocardia* (most human infection is caused by *N. asteroides*) is unresponsive to penicillin and can be treated with sulfa drugs. The diagnosis of actinomycosis is confirmed by an aerobic culture.[34, 112–114]

Tuberculosis (TB) is caused by *Mycobacterium tuberculosis* and *M. bovis*, aerobic bacilli with a thick, multilayered capsule of complex lipids and waxes, which accounts for their staining and immunogenic properties. Once stained, they are resistant to decolorization by acid alcohol and hence are acid-fast. The disease has a worldwide distribution. *M. tuberculosis* is spread through aerosolized respiratory droplets from patients with cavitary TB. *M. bovis* and probably *M. tuberculosis* can cause infection via oral ingestion, although mucosal breaks are probably required. A definite resurgence has been reported in the United States as a result of (1) immigrant populations from endemic countries, (2) reactivation of disease in the elderly population, and (3) the AIDS pandemic. More than 25,000 cases were reported in the United States in 1993 (10 cases per

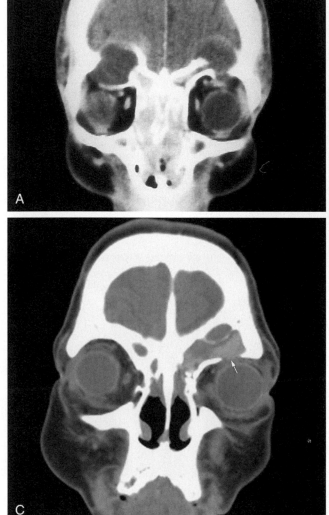

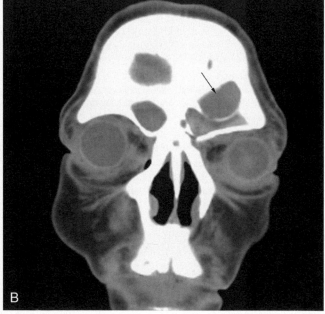

**FIGURE 5-85** Coronal CT scan (**A**) shows soft tissue attenuation material in both ethmoid sinuses and nasal fossae. In addition, there are "mucoid" density expanded areas in the roof of each orbit breaking both intracranially and intraorbitally. This patient had bilateral supraorbital ethmoid mucoceles and sinusitis. Coronal CT scans (**B** and **C**) on another patient show a water attenuation left frontal sinus mucocele (*black arrow*) and a higher-attenuation left supraorbital ethmoid mucocele (*white arrow*). It is important to identify both types of mucoceles, as the surgical approach for each is different.

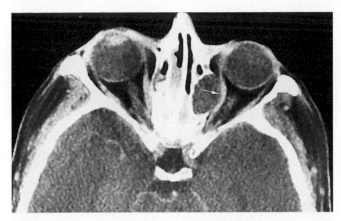

**FIGURE 5-86**   Axial CT scan shows an expansile water attenuation left ethmoid sinus mass that has extended into the orbit and displaced the medial rectus muscle laterally (*arrow*). This patient had a left ethmoid sinus mucocele.

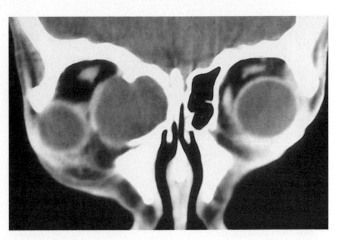

**FIGURE 5-88**   Coronal CT scan shows a water attenuation, expansile, right ethmoid sinus mass that bulges into the right orbit and displaces the eye laterally and slightly downward. This patient had a right ethmoid sinus mucocele.

100,000 people), a 14% increase over reported rates in 1985, which were at a nadir since national reporting began in 1953.[115] The common tuberculous pulmonary disease may be asymptomatic or cause fever, weight loss, and bloody sputum. Head and neck involvement in TB is rare and is thought to be the result of direct infection from expectorated sputum, as well as from hematogenous-lymphatic spread. The sinus disease may be nonspecific; however, when bone involvement occurs, the dominant symptom is pain. The treatment is prolonged antituberculous chemotherapy. Nasopharyngeal and sinonasal TB may clinically and histologically mimic Wegener's granulomatosis. This distinction has a grave consequence because administering the steroid and immunosuppressive agents indicated for active Wegener's granulomatosis may result in miliary progression of unrecognized TB. Also, nasopharyngeal TB can be accompanied by lymphadenopathy. This may clinically mimic nasopharyngeal carcinoma, especially in the Asian population at risk for this neoplasm.[116]

Syphilis is a worldwide disease that has been rising in incidence since the 1980s.[117] In 1977, the rate per 100,000 people in the United States was 10.4. The rate per 100,000 has been between 40 and 60 from 1988 to 1992, and more

than 110,000 cases were reported in the United States in 1992. Changing patterns of sexual promiscuity and prostitution have led to the disease resurgence. Syphilis is caused by *Treponema pallidum*, which is usually transmitted through sexual relations, although it can also be transmitted through blood transfusions. By contrast, *T. pertenue* is transmitted through nonvenereal, direct contact.

Syphilis may be divided clinically into three distinct phases: primary, secondary, and tertiary. The first two stages may escape clinical notice. Primary acquired syphilis develops within 1 week to 3 months following exposure. A characteristic chancre develops at the site of infection. Chancres can also develop after orogenital contact. Oral sites include the lips, palate, gingiva, tongue, and tonsil. Chancre has also been reported in the nose.[34, 118] Secondary syphilis occurs weeks to months after the primary chancre and is the result of systemic infection. There is a macular-papular rash that coalesces into warm, moist areas to form hyperplastic lesions: condyloma lata or flat condylomata. Head and neck manifestations of secondary syphilis include condyloma lata, which may occur in the larynx, ears, and nasolabial folds. Tertiary syphilis is a late manifestation seen years to decades after primary infection.

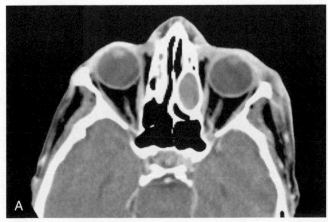

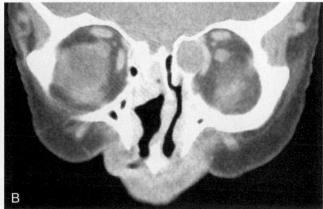

**FIGURE 5-87**   **A,** Axial CT scan shows an expansile, water attenuation, left ethmoid sinus mass that is minimally remodeling the lamina papyracea laterally. This patient had a left ethmoid mucocele. Coronal CT scan (**B**) on another patient shows an expansile right ethmoid sinus mucocele.

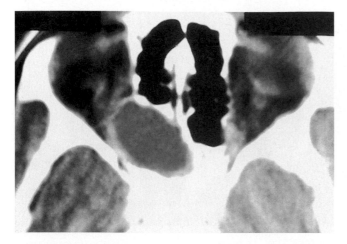

**FIGURE 5-89**   Axial CT scan shows a water attenuation, expansile mass in the right posterior ethmoid/sphenoid sinus area. The mass displaces the optic nerve and medial rectus muscle downward and laterally. This patient had a sphenoethmoidal mucocele. In these cases, the radiologist must carefully note the position of the optic nerve in relationship to the mass in order to help guide the surgeon away from intraoperative complications.

Ulcerated erosive gummas with indurated margins may develop. The gumma is a destructive, usually painless granulomatous process, which most likely represents a hypersensitivity reaction to *T. pallidum*, as well as progression of the disease to the tertiary phase. Gummas tend to develop in intramembranous bones such as those of the scalp, face, nose, nasal septum, and paranasal sinuses.[34, 118, 119] Without awareness of patient serology, the radiologist should be aware that syphilis can mimic Wegener's granulomatosis or sinonasal fungal disease. Mandibular resorption has been reported and may lead to spontaneous fracture. The treatment of choice remains penicillin.

Congenital syphilis may develop if transplacental infection occurs after the fourth fetal month (when immune competence develops) and within 2 years of the acquired maternal infection. The primary manifestations occur in the mucocutaneous tissues and bones; in the head and neck the

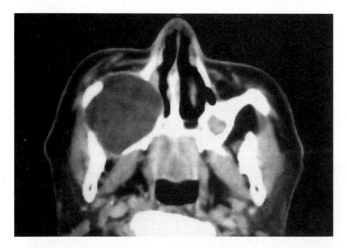

**FIGURE 5-90**   Axial CT scan shows a large, expansile mucoid attenuation right maxillary sinus mass. Portions of the bony wall are thinned. This patient had a right maxillary sinus mucocele.

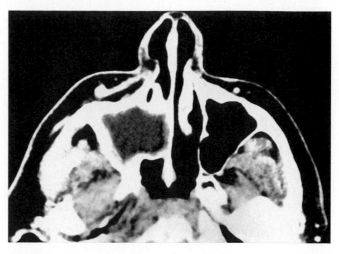

**FIGURE 5-91**   Axial contrast-enhanced CT scan shows an expansile right maxillary sinus mucoid attenuation mass that has a thin enhancing rim. This patient had a right maxillary sinus mucopyocele.

stigmata include frontal bossing (of Parrot), small maxilla, high palatal arch, Hutchinson's triad (Hutchinson incisors), interstitial keratitis, eighth nerve deafness, saddle nose, and mulberry molars.[34] The spirochete causes a periostitis that interferes with bone development.[120]

The differential diagnosis of syphilis includes yaws (*framboesia tropica*), a nonvenereally transmitted infection caused by *T. pertenue*, which occurs in children and young adults primarily in nongenital, unclothed areas. It is endemic in Central and West Africa and Southeast Asia. Uncommonly the late stages of the disease produce granulomas in the mucous membranes of the sinonasal cavities. These granulomas produce severe ulcerations of the nasal region (gangosa) and proliferative exostoses along the medial wall of the maxillary sinus (goundou). The treatment is penicillin. Histologically the spirochetes of *T. pertenue* tend to be more epidermotropic than those of *T. pallidum*, which can be present mainly at the dermal-epidermal junction and dermis. However, the clinical history is probably most helpful in distinguishing between syphilis and yaws.

Rhinoscleroma, which is caused by *Klebsiella rhinoscleromatis*, a gram-negative bacterium, is an infection that is endemic at tropical latitudes (Central America, Chile, and Central Africa), at subtropical latitudes (India, Indonesia, Egypt, Algeria, and Morroco), in temperate latitudes (Eastern and Central Europe), and in the Russian republics. *K. rhinoscleromatis* is an organism of low infectivity and is not a normal commensal organism. Human-to-human contact is assumed to be the only mode of transmission, and the infection results only after prolonged exposure.

Rhinoscleroma affects the nasal cavity and sinuses; however, it can involve the entire upper respiratory tract, so much so that the general name *scleroma* had been advocated. The natural course of this infection evolves through three stages. The early stage is the atrophic catarrhal stage; the involved mucosa is reddened and atrophic, with a foul purulent discharge and crusting. The clinical differential diagnosis in this early stage includes infection with *Klebsiella ozaenae*. The granulomatous stage may appear, months to years later, as waxy, ulcerating inflammatory masses that distend and deform the mucosal surfaces. The

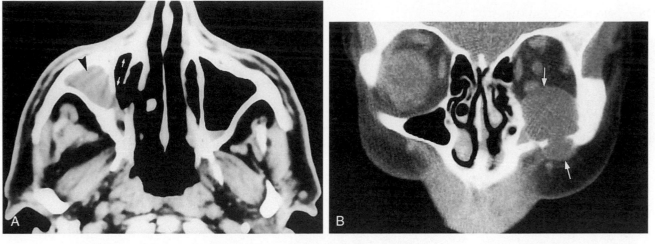

**FIGURE 5-92** Axial CT scan (**A**) on a patient who had had a right Caldwell-Luc procedure. There is an expansile mass (*arrowhead*) in the lateral portion of the sinus. The medial portion of the sinus (*small arrows*) is aerated. This patient had a right postoperative maxillary sinus mucocele. In **B**, a coronal CT scan on a different patient who had had a left Caldwell-Luc procedure, there is an expansile mass in the lateral portion of the left maxillary sinus that has broken into both the left orbit and the cheek (*arrows*). This patient had a left maxillary sinus postoperative mucocele.

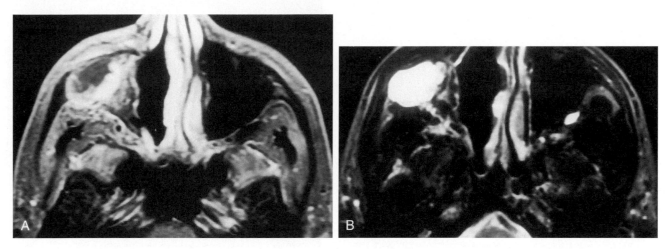

**FIGURE 5-93** Axial T1-weighted (**A**) and T2-weighted (**B**) MR images on a patient who had a right medial maxillectomy. There is a nonhomogeneous inflammatory-type collection in the zygomatic region of the remaining sinus cavity. The medial portion of this cavity remains well aerated. This patient had a postoperative right maxillary sinus mucocele.

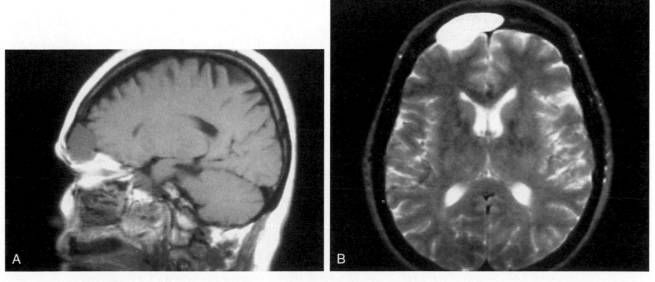

**FIGURE 5-94** Sagittal T1-weighted (**A**) and axial T2-weighted (**B**) MR images show an expanded, airless frontal sinus filled with material that has a low T1-weighted and a high T2-weighted signal intensity. The mass extends down into the upper medial orbit. The posterior sinus wall appears eroded but is only deossified by the chronic pressure of this right frontal sinus mucocele.

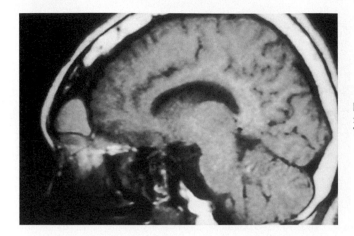

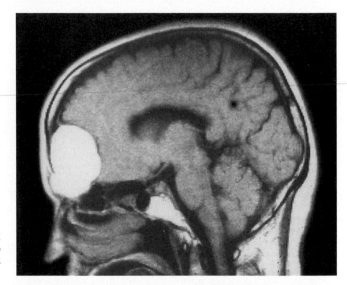

**FIGURE 5-95**  Sagittal T1-weighted MR image scan shows an expansile frontal sinus mass with an intermediate signal intensity. This mass had a high T2-weighted signal intensity. This patient had a frontal sinus mucocele.

**FIGURE 5-96**  Sagittal T1-weighted MR image shows an expansile frontal sinus mass with high signal intensity. The mass has extended both down into the medial orbit and back into the anterior cranial fossa. The mass also had a high T2-weighted signal intensity. This patient had a frontal mucocele.

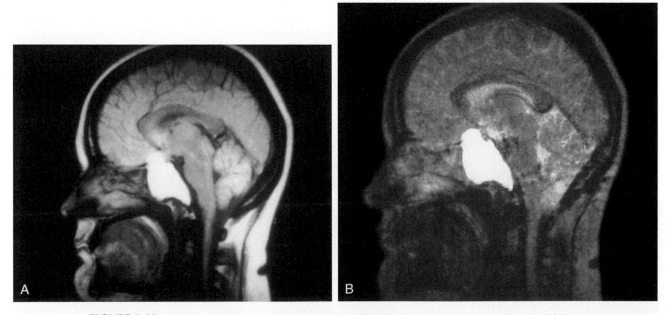

**FIGURE 5-97**  Sagittal T1-weighted (**A**) and T2-weighted (**B**) MR images show an expansile sphenoid sinus mass that has high signal intensity on both sequences. This patient had a sphenoid sinus mucocele.

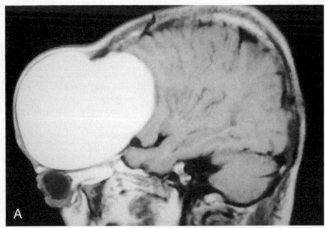

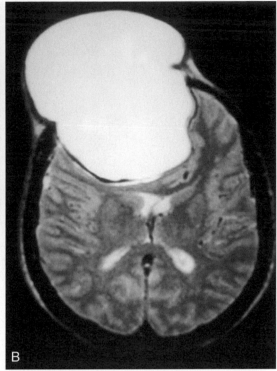

**FIGURE 5-98**   Sagittal T1-weighted (**A**) and axial T2-weighted (**B**) MR images show a huge expansile frontal sinus mass. There was no hemorrhage within this mucocele; the high signal intensity was due to the macromolecular protein concentration. (Case courtesy of Ilka Gerrero, M.D.)

inflammatory masses extend through the external nares in severe cases and may distort the soft tissues of the midface, resulting in a rhinoceros-like appearance. The clinical differential diagnosis includes leprosy and syphilis. The final sclerotic stage is characterized by fibrosis along with the inflammation, culminating in stenosis.[121]

Rhinosclerosis has been reported in AIDS patients, but the mucocutaneous infections do not appear to differ from those occurring in the usual hosts.[122] The treatment of choice is surgical excision to open the airway and long-term antibiotic therapy, usually with tetracycline.[34]

North American blastomycosis is caused by *Blastomyces dermatitidis*, and the disease is endemic in the Ohio and Mississippi River basins. The disease is not confined to North America and has been detected in South America and

Africa. A noted increase in blastomycosis has been seen among avid bird watchers. Based on point source case studies, it appears that closeness between the individual's face and soil (e.g., picking up objects from the ground to examine them) makes one more vulnerable to infection.

*Blastomyces* may cause disease either through inhalation or through traumatic inoculation into skin. Clinically, blastomycosis may present as the acute onset of pneumonia with fever, productive cough, and myalgias. Patients with insidious infection have symptoms such as weight loss, malaise, anorexia, and a chronic cough that may clinically mimic tuberculosis. Most of the head and neck lesions involve the skin, but involvement of the larynx and nasal

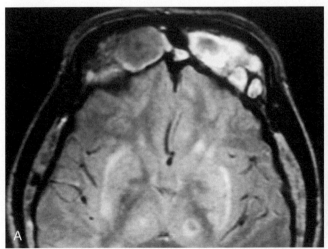

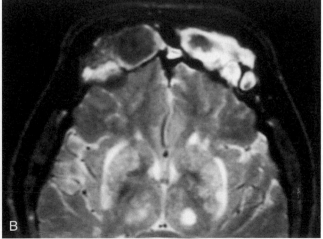

**FIGURE 5-99**   Axial T1-weighted (**A**) and T2-weighted (**B**) MR images show bilateral expansile, nonhomogeneous frontal sinus masses. On the right side, the mass has overall low to intermediate T1-weighted and low T2-weighted signal intensities. On the left side, the mass has an overall high signal intensity on both T1-weighted and T2-weighted images. This patient had bilateral frontal sinus mucoceles.

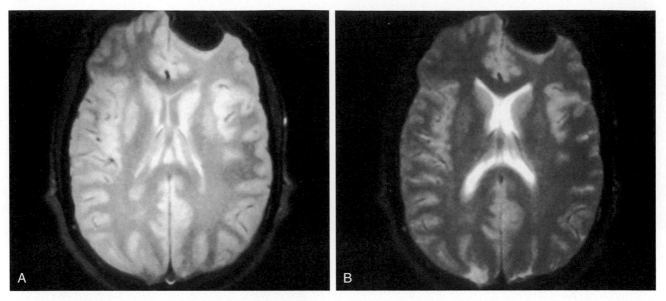

**FIGURE 5-100** Axial proton density (**A**) and T2-weighted (**B**) MR images show an expansile mass in the left frontal sinus that has signal voids on both sequences. This was a frontal sinus mucocele with dried, desiccated secretions.

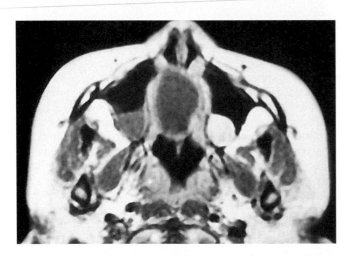

**FIGURE 5-101** Axial T1-weighted MR image shows an expansile process that arose in a pneumatized middle turbinate (concha bullosa). This mucocele has a low T1-weighted signal intensity and had a high T2-weighted signal intensity. Also present is a small retention cyst in the posterior recess of each antrum. On the right side the cyst has low T1-weighted signal intensity, while on the left side the cyst has intermediate signal intensity. This patient had a mucocele of a concha bullosa.

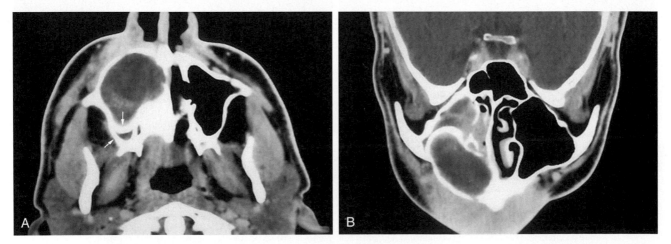

**FIGURE 5-102** Axial (**A**) and coronal (**B**) CT scans show a water attenuation expansile mass in the lower right maxillary sinus. In **A**, there are two bony walls seen posteriorly (*arrows*). In **B**, they can be seen to be due to elevation of the sinus floor by a cystic mass arising below the sinus. Obstructed secretions are also present within the right maxillary sinus. This patient had a right radicular cyst and maxillary sinusitis.

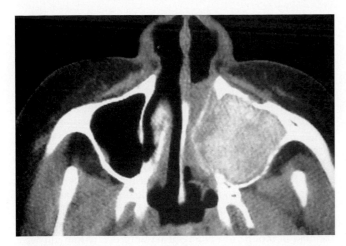

**FIGURE 5-103**   Axial CT scan shows a high-attenuation region in the left maxillary sinus separated from the bony walls of the sinus by a thin zone of mucoid attenuation material. There is also some remodeling of the medial maxillary sinus wall. This patient had aspergillosis with an aspergilloma.

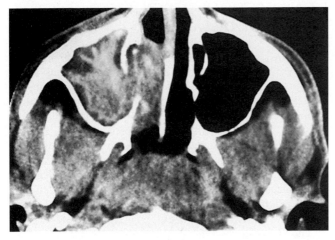

**FIGURE 5-104**   Axial CT scan shows a stellate high-attenuation soft-tissue mass in the right maxillary sinus and nasal fossa. The mass is separated from the bone by a thin zone of mucoid attenuation material. There is focal destruction of the medial antral wall. This patient had aspergillosis with an aspergilloma.

cavity has been reported. The laryngeal disease may appear clinically identical to carcinoma. Oral lesions may have associated draining sinuses, mimicking actinomycosis. The primary treatment of choice is amphotericin B.[34, 123]

South American blastomycosis (paracoccidioidomycosis) is caused by the dimorphic fungus *Blastomyces brasiliensis*. The disease is endemic to South America, especially Brazil, Colombia, Venezuela, Uruguay, and Argentina. As with coccidioidomycosis, a wide range of disease can be seen, from subclinical to clinical, in immunologically normal patients, patients who are immunosuppressed, and patients with AIDS. Aspiration with subsequent hematogenous dissemination is thought to be the mode of transmission because pulmonary involvement is common. It may produce painful, destructive granulomas of the alveolar process, gingiva, nasal cavity, and, rarely, the paranasal sinuses.[5, 123, 124] The primary treatment is amphotericin B, which cures more than 90% of the cases.[125]

Leprosy is caused by the pleomorphic acid-fast bacterium *Mycobacterium leprae*. The disease occurs in almost all tropical and warm temperate regions, including Latin America, South and Southeast Asia, Saharan Africa, the Mediterranean basin, and Northern Europe. In the United States, endemic states include Florida, Louisiana, Texas, California, and Hawaii. Leprosy affects more than 11 million people worldwide; the number of indigenous cases in the United States has remained stable (10 to 29 per year) over the last two decades. However, the number of imported cases reported in the United States has dramatically increased (up to 300 per year) since the late 1970s. This increase in imported cases did not lead to increased transmission among the U.S. population.

Leprosy is a disease of low infectivity transmitted through prolonged exposure either through nasal secretions or through injured skin. Immunologically, leprosy can be graded by the host response as tuberculoid leprosy (characterized by a robust immunologic response, with few bacilli and with the possibility of spontaneous cure), borderline leprosy, and lepromatous leprosy (characterized by anergy to the lepromin test and abundant bacilli). Clinically there is a widespread, symmetrical facial distribution of lesions lead-

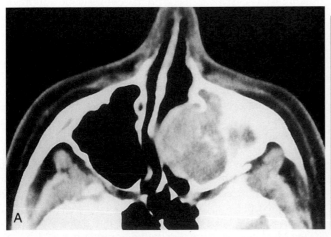

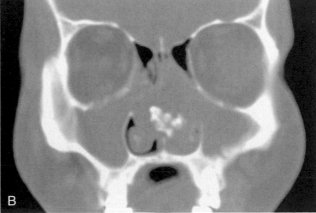

**FIGURE 5-105**   Axial CT scan (**A**) shows a soft-tissue mass in the left maxillary sinus that has thickened the posterior bony wall and thinned or destroyed the medial wall. Within the mass are several discrete calcifications. This patient had aspergillosis. Coronal CT scan (**B**) on a different patient shows soft-tissue disease in both ethmoid and maxillary sinuses and within both nasal fossae. In addition, there are calcifications in the nasal septum. This patient had aspergillosis.

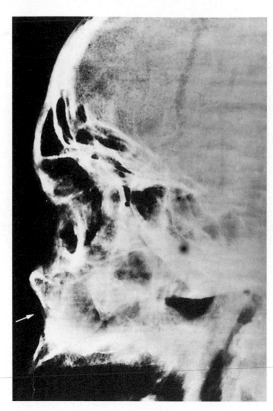

**FIGURE 5-106**  Lateral plane film shows erosion of the anterior nasal spine (*arrow*). There is also soft-tissue disease in the maxillary sinuses and nasal fossa. This patient had no prior surgery or trauma to this region. This patient had leprosy.

ing to a coarsening of features. The earlobes and nose are especially enlarged and infiltrated. Intranasal and paranasal sinus involvement is common and occurs after cutaneous nasal involvement. The changes in the sinonasal cavities are those of nonspecific chronic sinusitis and rhinitis. Later changes resemble those of a chronic granulomatous disease. A characteristic finding is progressive erosion of the anterior nasal spine. If previous surgery, trauma, and congenital maxillonasal dysplasia are not applicable to the patient, this finding is pathognomonic of leprosy (Fig. 5-106). Retrograde laryngeal involvement usually follows nasal disease. The treatment of choice remains the long-term administration of sulfone derivatives (dapsone).[125]

Rhinosporidiosis is caused by the fungus yeast *Rhinosporidium seeberi*.[126] The disease has a worldwide distribution but is endemic in places like India, Sri Lanka, Malaysia, Brazil, and Argentina. In the United States, cases have been reported in the rural South and West. Preceding mucosal trauma (e.g., by digital contamination or dust storms) is considered necessary in establishing the infection.[127] Patients with rhinosporidiosis generally are otherwise healthy. *Rhinosporidium* most commonly infects the conjunctiva and nasal cavity, with resultant friable, lobulated polyps that may cause obstruction of the nasal fossae and may be confused with neoplasms, especially cylindrical cell papilloma.[34] The nasal polyps are sessile, soft, pinkish, usually unilateral, and they may diminish aeration in the paranasal sinuses. The treatment of choice is surgical excision or electrocautery.

Glanders, or farcy, is caused by the bacterium *Pseudomonas mallei*. It is contracted by contact with horses, mules, or donkeys. In humans the disease is characterized either by an acute fulminant febrile illness that may lead to death or by a chronic indolent granulomatous disease. *Farcy* refers to the nodular abscesses found in the skin, lymphatics, and subcutaneous tissues.[125] The nasal manifestations of glanders are nasal cellulitis and necrosis that produce septal perforations. The treatment is with sulfonamides.

Leishmaniasis causes mucocutaneous infection (*Leishmania tropica*, known as Oriental sore or "Old World" sore; *L. mexicana* or *L. brasiliensis*, known as espundia or "New World" sore). The disease is endemic to Central and South America. After the initial primary cutaneous sores appear, satellite lesions develop in the nose and mouth; these sores are painful, mutilating erosions that can secondarily involve the sinuses.[125, 128] Scarring may eventually constrict the nose or mouth, producing gross deformities that interfere with swallowing. The majority of the oronasal diseases are caused by *L. brasiliensis*, and the treatment of this established oronasal disease is with amphotericin B.

## NONINFECTIOUS DESTRUCTIVE SINONASAL DISEASE

Wegener's granulomatosis is a necrotizing granulomatous vasculitis that usually affects the upper and lower respiratory tracts and causes a renal glomerulonephritis. A limited form of Wegener's granulomatosis may occur, with a more benign course in which only the sinonasal tract is affected. The initial disease may present as a chronic, nonspecific inflammatory process of the nose and sinuses and may remain as such for 1 to 2 years. Usually the nasal septum is first affected. The process becomes diffuse, and septal ulceration and perforations may result in a "saddle nose" deformity. Secondary bacterial infections complicate the clinical and imaging pictures.

The diagnosis of Wegener's granulomatosis may be difficult to establish early in the disease course or during periods of inactivity. The radiologist can suggest biopsy of the paranasal sinuses as opposed to the nasal cavity. Although this site is not as readily accessible as the nasal cavity, it has a greater yield of specific diagnostic features that aid the pathologist. Serum antineutrophil cytoplasmic antibodies (ANCA) are elevated during periods of active disease. In the absence of a specific diagnosis of Wegener's granulomatosis, it behooves the pathologist and the clinician to rule out other infectious and malignant causes of destructive sinonasal disease. Wegener's granulomatosis is probably autoimmune in origin, and the treatment of choice is cyclophosphamide, steroids, and possibly other cytotoxic drugs. Long-term remissions have been achieved; however, it is impossible to predict how long a remission will last.[125, 129]

Lethal midline granuloma, which was once classified as a granulomatous disease, was then reclassified as malignant midline reticulosis or polymorphic reticulosis.[129, 130] The disease is now classified as a lymphoma, and it is discussed in Chapter 6.

Sarcoidosis is a systemic, multisystem disease characterized by noncaseating epithelial granulomas.[131-133] An infectious etiology has been sought for these granulomas. Two decades ago, experimental data were presented suggesting the transmissibility of these granulomas, hence fulfilling one of Kock's postulates for an infectious etiology.

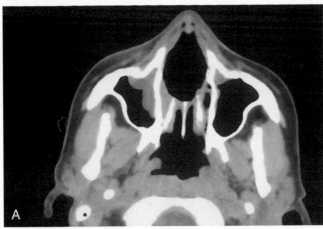
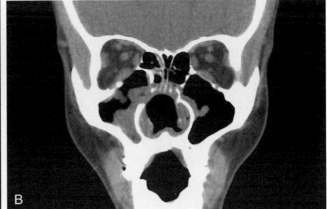

**FIGURE 5-107**   Axial (**A**) and coronal (**B**) CT scans show destruction of the nasal septum and portions of each medial maxillary sinus wall and the lower ethmoid complex. The distribution of disease suggests a granulomatous process. This patient was a chronic cocaine abuser.

Patients with sarcoidosis have elevated levels of antibodies to *Mycobacterium paratuberculosis*. However, direct inoculation of sarcoid tissue into a thymic mouse has failed to isolate an infectious agent, so at present no known agent has been directly implicated in the etiology of sarcoidosis.

Sarcoidosis has a predilection for the Scandinavian countries and for the rural southeastern United States. It is most common in African-American females with a median age of 25 years. Nasal sarcoidosis occurs in 3% to 20% of the patients with systemic sarcoidosis. When it occurs, there are multiple small granulomas of the nasal septum and turbinates. There may be nasal discharge, obstruction, and epistaxis. Polypoid degeneration of the nasal fossa mucosa may occur, but the paranasal sinuses are rarely affected. Sarcoidosis is not generally a destructive disease in the sinonasal tract; however, destruction of the nasal septum and turbinates can occur in unusual cases. Rarely, sharply defined lytic bone lesions may occur in the calvarium and facial skeleton. Steroid therapy may suppress the inflammatory reaction and provide symptomatic improvement, but fibrous organization of the granulomas may lead to organ dysfunction.[34, 134]

Exposure to beryllium may result in chronic granulomas of the nasal fossa. These granulomas may be indistinguishable from those of tuberculosis, leprosy, and sarcoidosis.[128] Chromate salts have been implicated as a cause of nonspecific granulomas of the nasal cavity; involvement of the paranasal sinuses is a late and unusual event. Cocaine abuse has become a major worldwide problem. Cocaine causes a necrotizing vasculitis and subsequent granuloma of the nasal septum, which with prolonged exposure usually results in septal erosion. Erosion of the nasal vault margins and the adjacent sinuses can occur in chronic abusers. A nonspecific mucosal inflammation may also occur in the nasal fossa. A mucosal reaction to the talc used to "cut" the cocaine can also occur.

## Imaging

In general, the destructive granulomatous diseases result in variable sinonasal mucosal changes, ranging from nonspecific inflammation with mucosal thickening and nasal secretions to a localized soft-tissue mass. Nasal cavity involvement usually precedes paranasal cavity disease. The nasal septum may be focally thickened by a bulky soft-tissue mass or septal erosion may be present. When the paranasal sinuses are involved, the maxillary and ethmoid sinuses are most often affected. The sphenoid sinuses are uncommonly involved, and the frontal sinuses are almost always spared. When the sinuses are affected, there is usually nonspecific inflammatory mucosal thickening. Air-fluid levels are rare. The bones of the nasal vault and affected paranasal sinuses may be thickened and sclerotic, reflecting the chronic nature of the inflammatory reaction. Sinus obliteration by reactive bone may also occur.[135] Similarly there may be areas of bony erosion, reflecting either osteomyelitis or necrosis. If the nasal disease becomes a bulky soft-tissue mass, there may, in addition, be remodeling of the adjacent bones (Figs. 5-106 to 5-111).[122]

On MR imaging, these diseases may have low T1-weighted and high T2-weighted signal intensities suggestive of an inflammatory disease. They also may have low to inter-

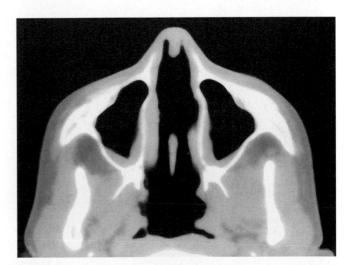

**FIGURE 5-108**   Axial CT scan shows a large erosion of the nasal septum and minimal mucosal thickening in the maxillary sinuses. This appearance suggests a granulomatous process. This patient was a chronic cocaine abuser.

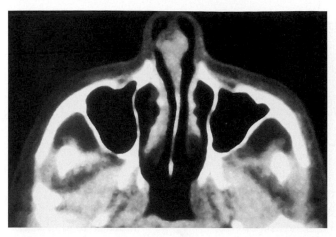

**FIGURE 5-109**   Axial CT scan shows localized soft-tissue thickening of the anterior nasal septum. This appearance suggests either granulomatous disease or a cartilaginous tumor. This patient had Wegener's granulomatosis.

## CHOLESTEATOMAS

Several entities in addition to mucoceles can cause sinus cavity enlargement. An epidermoid inclusion cyst (or cholesteatoma) is a cystic keratin-filled mass lined by stratified squamous epithelium. In the frontal bone, these cysts probably arise from a congenital inclusion rest or after traumatic implantation. They may develop either in the diplöe or, less frequently, in the outer table of the skull. On plain films they appear lucent when compared with the adjacent normal frontal bone. The margins may be slightly scalloped or smooth, and there is a thin, uniform white line that identifies the lesion's contour. These latter two findings help differentiate an epidermoid inclusion cyst from a mucocele (Fig. 5-112). Confusion with a mucocele may occur if an epidermoid inclusion cyst arises within or adjacent to the frontal sinus.[137, 138] These cysts may also rarely arise from other flat facial bones.[139]

In the antrum, invasion of buccal epithelium via an oroantral fistula has also been proposed as a possible etiology for an antral epidermoid inclusion cyst. A type of "cholesteatoma" or pseudocholesteatoma may develop within a chronically infected sinus after active infection has subsided. The breakdown products of the purulent exudate, as well as any blood, may contain cholesterol products that result in cholesteatomatous debris.[140–142]

An antral epidermoid inclusion cyst must also be differentiated from an odontogenic keratocyst. The latter is a benign cystic neoplasm arising from odontogenic rests that

mediate T1-weighted and T2-weighted signal intensities simulating malignancies. They all enhance with contrast.[136] However, not all septal masses represent granulomatous-type disease. In addition to chondroid tumors, a septal abscess can occur, usually following local trauma (Fig. 5-110B,C).

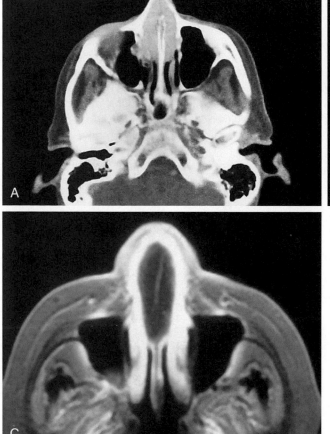

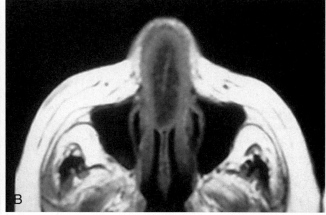

**FIGURE 5-110**   **A,** Axial CT scan shows a minimally enhancing bilateral nasal fossa mass that is centered on the nasal septum. There is some erosion of the anterior nasal septum. This patient had Wegener's granulomatosis. Axial T1-weighted (**B**) and T1-weighted, fat-suppressed, contrast-enhanced (**C**) MR images on another patient show an expansile nasal septal mass with enhancement of the surrounding mucosa. This patient had a septal abscess.

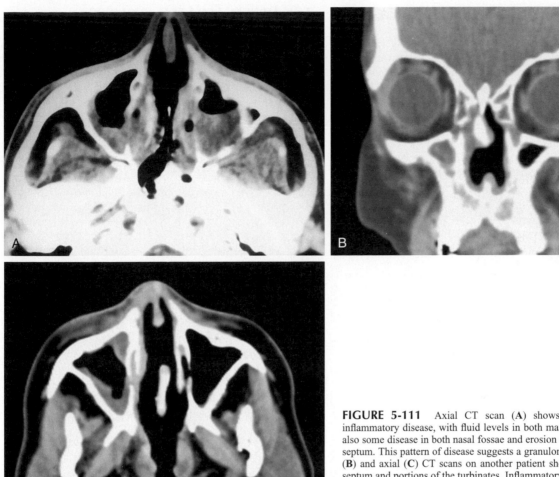

**FIGURE 5-111**   Axial CT scan (**A**) shows moderate degrees of inflammatory disease, with fluid levels in both maxillary sinuses. There is also some disease in both nasal fossae and erosion of a portion of the nasal septum. This pattern of disease suggests a granulomatous process. Coronal (**B**) and axial (**C**) CT scans on another patient show erosion of the nasal septum and portions of the turbinates. Inflammatory soft tissues are present in the ethmoid and maxillary sinuses. Both of these patients had sarcoidosis.

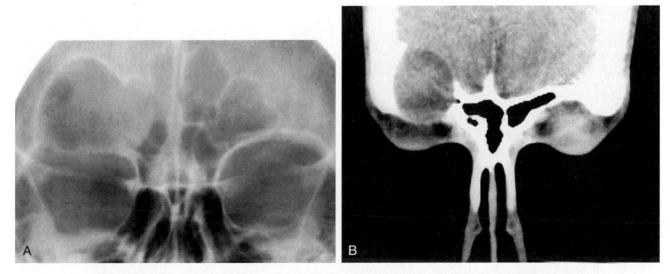

**FIGURE 5-112**   Caldwell view (**A**) shows a smoothly expansile lesion in the lateral right frontal bone, which is thinning and depressing the right orbital roof. A thin white mucoperiosteal line surrounds the mass. Coronal CT scan (**B**) shows the localized, expansile, homogeneously "mucoid" attenuation mass, which is depressing the right orbital roof. This patient has a cholesteatoma of the frontal bone.

may also remodel and expand the maxilla (see Chapters 6 and 17).

On CT, an epidermoid inclusion cyst or a cholesteatoma appears as an expansile lesion that has soft tissue, mucoid-like attenuation. If it occurs within a sinus cavity, it may be indistinguishable from a mucocele. On MR imaging, depending on the fatty components of the cholesterol, there can be an intermediate to high signal intensity on T1-weighted images and there usually is an intermediate to high signal intensity on T2-weighted images (Fig. 5-113).[143, 144]

## ENLARGED AERATED SINUSES

When evaluating a large sinus, there are no definitive measurements that define abnormal enlargement. Part of the problem is lack of pathologically confirmed etiologies for these processes. In one study, a sinus was judged to be abnormally large if its size exceeded that of 99% of the normal population.[145, 146] Using that criterion and taking into account magnification factors for films taken on a Franklin head unit (3.4%) or a standard 40-inch focal-

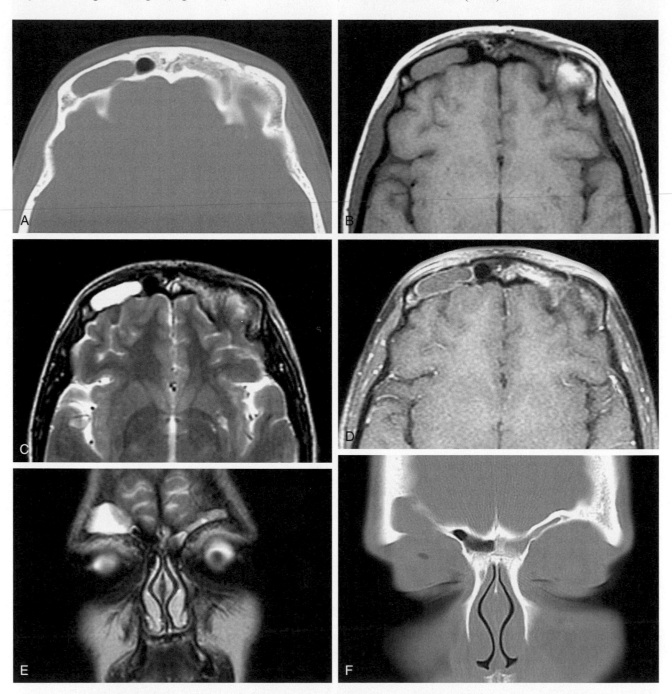

**FIGURE 5-113**    Axial CT scan (**A**) shows a smoothly marginated mass in the right frontal bone. The medial aspect of the mass abuts on the right side of the right frontal sinus. Axial T1-weighted (**B**) and T2-weighted (**C**) MR images show the mass to have an intermediate T1-weighted and high T2-weighted signal intensity. Axial T1-weighted, fat-suppressed, contrast-enhanced MR image (**D**) shows some enhancement around the margins of the mass. Coronal T2-weighted (**E**) MR image and coronal CT scan (**F**) show that the mass is adjacent to the right frontal sinus and has broken down into the roof of the right orbit. There is also some inflammatory disease in the left supraorbital sinus. This patient had a cholesteatoma of the right frontal bone.

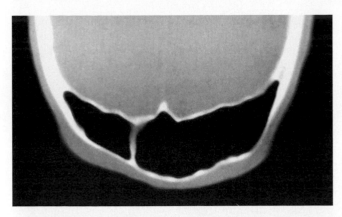

**FIGURE 5-114**   Coronal CT scan shows a very large, normally aerated frontal sinus. Despite its size, there was no bossing of the forehead or remodeling of the inner table. This patient had a hypersinus.

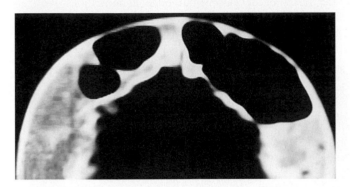

**FIGURE 5-115**   Axial CT scan shows large frontal sinuses in a patient with a dense cortical calvarium and hyperostosis interna. Despite the size of these sinuses, there was no deformity of the forehead or inner sinus table. This patient had hypersinuses.

distance Caldwell view (10.3%), if a line drawn from the base of the crista galli to a point of maximum distance along the perimeter of the sinus exceeds 74.4 mm (head unit) or 79.3 mm (posteroanterior skull film), the sinus is larger than 99% of normal frontal sinuses and may be referred to as a *hypersinus*. This term refers to an enlarged, aerated sinus that does not expand its normal bony contours (Figs. 5-114 and 5-115).

*Pneumosinus dilatans* refers to an aerated sinus that is abnormally expanded (either the entire sinus or a portion of the sinus). The sinus walls are intact and of normal thickness, but remodeled and outwardly displaced. Pneumosinus dilatans may result in frontal bossing, diplopia, or a nasal mass, depending on which portion of the sinus is expanded. Accordingly it is this extension of the sinus beyond the normal bony boundaries that differentiates pneumosinus dilatans from hypersinus. If the entire sinus is not involved, the remaining sinus dimensions are usually normal (Fig. 5-116).[147, 148]

*Pneumocele* refers to an aerated sinus with either focal or generalized sinus cavity enlargement and thinning of the bony sinus walls. It is the latter feature that differentiates pneumosinus dilatans from a pneumocele (Figs. 5-117 to 5-121). This distinction stems from the clinical literature, where the integrity, or lack of integrity, of the sinus wall was observed as a differentiating point. Although a "valve" theory has been suggested as an etiology for the delayed pressure equilibration that apparently occurs in pneumoceles, no such valve has been demonstrated physiologically.

At present there is no clear understanding of the factors that either influence the development of normal sinuses or signal the normal cessation of sinus growth. Consequently the etiology of excessive sinus aeration and growth that produces hypersinus, pneumosinus dilatans, and pneumocele is unclear.[146] The pneumocele's growth can be arrested by creating a surgical window (i.e., antrostomy, ethmoidectomy, sphenoid sinusotomy) to allow rapid pressure equilibration. The cosmetic deformity that may result from either a pneumosinus dilatans or a pneumocele can be dealt with surgically if necessary by collapsing the sinus.

In the sphenoid sinus, the planum sphenoidale may be bowed cranially by an overlying meningioma simulating pneumosinus dilatans on imaging.[149] However, a meningioma will bow primarily the sphenoid roof, sparing the other sinus walls. The intracranial component of the meningioma can then be confirmed on CT or MR imaging. The sphenoid bone is usually thickened and sclerotic adjacent to the neoplasm.

Enlarged, aerated frontal sinuses may also be seen in systemic conditions such as acromegaly, Dyke-Davidoff

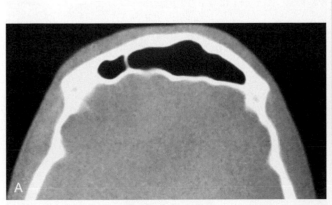 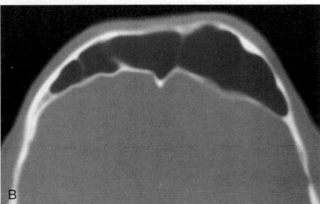

**FIGURE 5-116**   **A**, Axial CT scan shows an enlarged left frontal sinus that has not thinned the bone of either the anterior or posterior sinus walls. However, the anterior wall has been minimally bowed forward, causing a bulge in the forehead. This patient had a pneumosinus dilatans. **B**, Axial CT scan on another patient shows a very large frontal sinus with anterior bowing of the anterior sinus table. This patient also had pneumosinus dilatans.

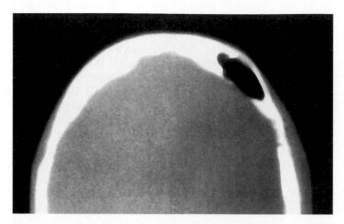

**FIGURE 5-117**   Axial CT scan shows the upper region of a large left frontal sinus with normal mucosa. A portion of the posterior sinus wall is thinned. This patient had a pneumocele.

Masson syndrome, Sturge-Weber syndrome, homocystinuria, lipodystrophy (lipoatrophic diabetes), Marfan's syndrome, myotonic dystrophy, and Turner's syndrome (Fig. 5-122).[150]

## SMALL OR ABSENT AERATED SINUSES

Small or absent but aerated sinuses are associated with a variety of abnormalities. A hypoplastic small sinus may be the result of developmental failure or encroachment from expanding sinus wall bone. Hypoplastic sinuses are associated with syndromes such as Binder's syndrome (maxillonasal dyplasia or maxillovertebral syndrome), Cockayne's syndrome, Down's syndrome, otopalatodigital syndrome (type 1), Prader-Willi syndrome, Schwarz Lélek syndrome, and Treacher Collins syndrome. Hypoplastic sinuses may also be the result of developmental bone abnormalities such as

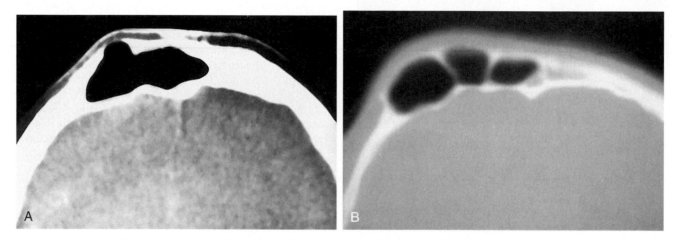

**FIGURE 5-118**   **A,** Axial CT scan shows a normal-sized right frontal sinus that has focally thinned the anterior sinus wall, causing a bulge in the forehead. This patient had a pneumocele. **B,** Axial CT scan on another patient shows a minimally expanded right frontal sinus with thinning of the anterior table. This patient also had a pneumocele.

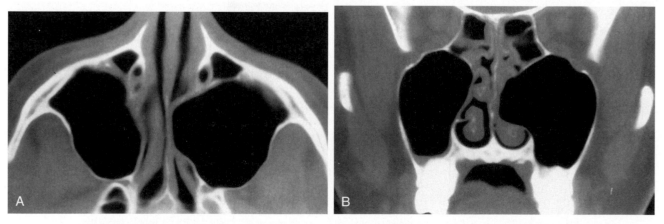

**FIGURE 5-119**   Axial (**A**) and coronal (**B**) CT scans show an aerated, expanded left maxillary sinus. The sinus walls are thinned. This patient had a pneumocele.

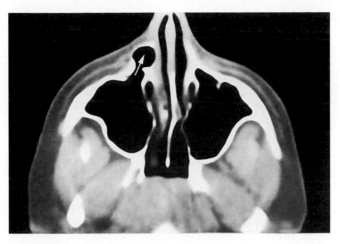

**FIGURE 5-120**   Axial CT scan shows a focal anterior enlargement of the right maxillary sinus (*arrow*) that has thinned the sinus wall and caused some cheek fullness. This patient had a pneumocele.

cleidocranial dysplasia, craniodiaphyseal dysplasia, craniometaphyseal dysplasia, fibrous dysplasia, frontometaphyseal dysplasia, frontonasal dysplasia, metaphyseal chondrodysplasia (Jansen type), osteodysplasty (Melnick needles), osteopathia striata with cranial sclerosis, osteopetrosis, pyknodysostosis, other conditions such as Paget's disease, and hematologic conditions that affect the marrow space such as sickle cell anemia and thalassemia. Hypoplastic sinuses may also be associated with endocrine diseases such as hypopituitarism and hypothyroidism.[150] Lastly, irradiation to a child's face can destroy the bony growth center and result in a hypoplastic bone. As a result of the small bone, the sinus cavity within the bone is small.

## COMPLICATIONS OF INFLAMMATORY PARANASAL SINUS DISEASE AFFECTING ADJACENT AREAS

In the present antibiotic era, most acute paranasal sinus infections are successfully treated. It is only in a few cases

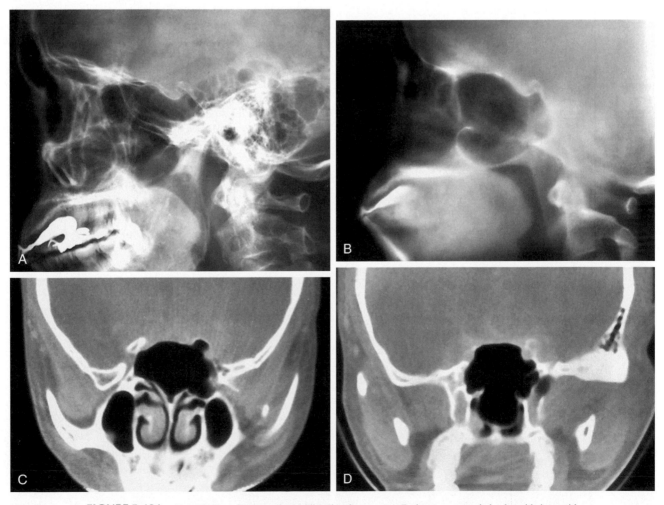

**FIGURE 5-121**   Lateral plane film **A** and multidirectional tomogram **B** show an expanded sphenoid sinus with thinned bony sinus walls. The sinus floor is displaced downward so that it rests atop the soft palate, the planum sphenoidale is elevated, and the posterior clivus is bowed backward. Coronal CT scans through the anterior **C** and the posterior **D** sphenoid sinus show the thinned bony walls and extension of the sinus into a pneumatized and expanded left anterior clinoid process. This patient had a pneumocele. When he traveled in an airplane, the sphenoid sinus expanded and compressed his left optic nerve, causing visual symptoms. He was cured by surgery.

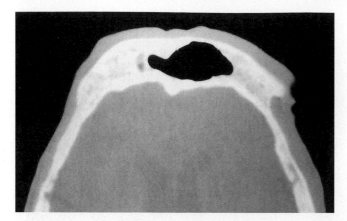

**FIGURE 5-122** Axial CT scan shows an expanded left frontal sinus in a patient with a thick, cortical-type calvarium. The sinus mucosa is normal. This patient had acromegaly.

that surgical intervention is required to help control an acute infection. However, a delay in initiating proper treatment, organisms resistant to the chosen antibiotics, or incomplete treatment regimens all can allow an initially localized infection to spread to adjacent regions.[151, 152]

About 3% of patients with paranasal sinusitis experience some related orbital or preseptal inflammatory disease. These various complications include retention edema of the eyelids, preseptal cellulitis, preseptal abscess, orbital cellulitis, subperiosteal orbital abscess, orbital abscess, and cavernous sinus thrombosis.[151, 153] Such orbital complications are discussed in Chapter 9. In addition, 15% to 20% of the cases of retrobulbar neuritis are secondary to posterior ethmoid and sphenoid sinusitis, and in some of these cases the neuritis can apparently occur without other manifestations of orbital inflammatory disease.[76, 154]

The ethmoid sinuses are clearly most often implicated as the source of infection for orbital complications. The thin lamina papyracea and the anterior and posterior valveless ethmoidal veins allow rapid access of infection into the orbit.[155] Sinusitis of the sphenoid, maxillary, and frontal sinuses are, in descending order, less likely to cause orbital infection.

Inflammatory pseudotumor (IMF), also referred to as *inflammatory myofibroblastic tumor*, is a fibro-inflammatory space-occupying lesion or, most likely, a number of entities with overlapping histologic features, the true nature of which is only beginning to be elucidated. The lung, liver, and gastrointestinal tract (omentum and mesentery) are the most common sites for IMF. Orbital inflammatory pseudotumors are a broad category of idiopathic, nonspecific, nonneoplastic, chronic inflammatory processes without identifiable local or systemic causes. On rare occasions, mucosal thickening in the nasal fossae and paranasal sinuses is seen in patients with concurrent orbital pseudotumor. These mucosal changes may be noninfectious and consistent with pseudotumor.[156] The association of the orbital and sinonasal diseases may suggest this diagnosis; however, more commonly, orbital pseudotumor is either an isolated finding or is associated with routine, unrelated sinonasal inflammatory disease.

Maxillary sinus pseudotumor can also occur without associated orbital complications. Unlike its orbital counterpart, which rarely involves the adjacent bone, antral pseudotumor usually presents with areas of bone erosion, sclerosis, and remodeling, often mimicking the imaging appearance of an aggressive fungal infection or an antral malignancy (Figs. 5-123 and 5-124).[157] The differential diagnosis of such orbital and sinonasal disease must also include Wegener's granulomatosis.

Occasionally sinusitis can lead to intracranial complications such as meningitis, epidural abscess, subdural abscess, cerebritis, and cerebral abscess (Fig. 5-10).[158] Only 3% of intracranial abscesses are the result of sinusitis, most commonly frontal sinusitis, followed in descending order by sinusitis in the sphenoid, ethmoid, and maxillary sinuses. The propensity for frontal sinusitis to spread intracranially is due to the rich emissary network (Beçhet's plexus) connecting the posterior sinus mucosa with the meninges.[151]

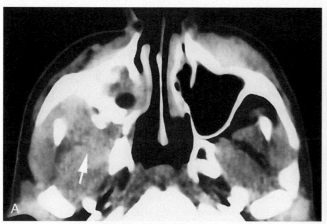
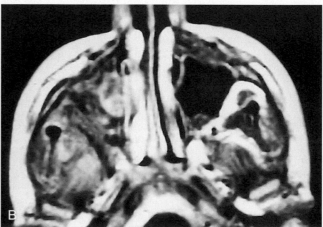

**FIGURE 5-123** Axial CT scan **A** shows an infiltrating lesion in the right infratemporal fossa (*arrow*), thickening of the right maxillary sinus bony walls, and soft-tissue disease in this sinus. An axial T1-weighted MR image **B** shows the soft-tissue disease; however, the thickened, sclerotic bone is almost undetected. This patient had an antral pseudotumor.

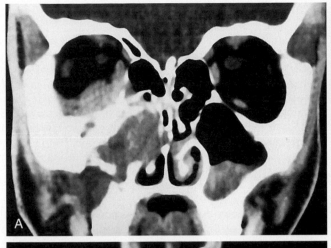

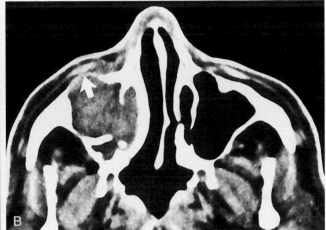

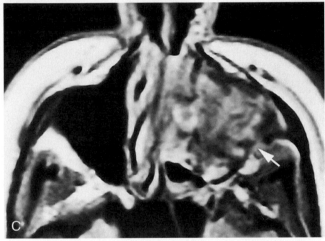

**FIGURE 5-124**   Coronal **A** and axial **B** CT scans show a soft-tissue mass in the right maxillary sinus. There are areas of bone thickening and sclerosis in the sinus roof, and there is a sequestration in the lateral sinus wall. Some bone remodeling is also present (*arrow* in **B**). Axial T1-weighted MR scan **C** on a different patient shows a nonhomogeneous soft-tissue mass in the left antrum, focally eroding the posterior wall (*arrow*) to extend into the infratemporal fossa. Both of these patients had antral pseudotumors.

Osteomyelitis can be a complication of chronic, smoldering bacterial or fungal sinusitis or sinusitis in patients with previous irradiation to the facial bones. The dominant clinical finding is persistent pain; the radiographic manifestations include focal rarefaction of bone, sequestrum formation, reactive thickening of the bone, bony sclerosis, and ultimately fragmentation of the bone.

Over the frontal sinus, a subgaleal abscess can form secondary to sinusitis. This occurs via osteothrombophlebitis and may or may not be associated with frank osteomyelitis. This subgaleal abscess is also called a Pott's puffy tumor.[159, 160]

Overall, intracranial and intraorbital complications are more likely seen with acute sinusitis, whereas osteomyelitis is more likely a complication of chronic sinusitis.

## THE NEED FOR PREOPERATIVE IMAGING

Chapters 2 and 3 discussed numerous anatomic variations between and within individuals. Some of these are incidental findings. However, if the surgeon is unaware of these variations prior to surgery, operative complications may occur. In addition, if preoperative imaging is not performed, unknown pathology that may influence treatment decisions can be overlooked (Fig. 5-125). Thus it is strongly recommended that prior to any sinus surgery, an imaging study should be performed.

## FOREIGN BODIES

A great variety of foreign bodies have been reported in the sinonasal cavities. Some are made of plastic materials (e.g., beads) or other nonradiopaque materials (e.g., gauze) that cannot be visualized on plain films, and others are radiodense (i.e., metallic) and can be localized easily on routine radiographic examinations (Fig. 5-126). If a foreign body is present for a sufficiently long time, it may act as a nidus and become encrusted with mineral salts. As such, these calcified masses are referred to as either rhinoliths or sinoliths, depending on whether they are located in the nasal fossa or a paranasal sinus, respectively (Figs. 5-127 to 5-129).[161, 162] If on CT a solitary calcification is seen within a sinus cavity, invariably it is the result of infection. Nearly 50% of the time that multiple discrete intrasinus calcifications are present, the cause is infection, often of a fungal etiology.[163] Tumors also account for about 50% of the cases of multiple sinonasal calcifications. The most likely lesions are olfactory neuroblastoms, inverted papilloma, or a chondroid tumor. Rarely, intrasinus ossification can occur, the implications being the same as those of calcifications.

## ANOSMIA

The two most common causes of anosmia are of an idiopathic origin and secondary to sinonasal inflammatory disease. Usually, imaging shows essentially normal sinuses or inflammatory mucosal thickening obliterating the nasal olfactory recess(es). Intracranial disease may also result in anosmia, for instance Kallman's syndrome, which consists of a primary eunuchoidism, secondary to hypogonatropic hypogonadism, and associated congenital anosmia, usually with absence of the olfactory bulbs and tracts. Coronal MR images best show the absence of these olfactory structures and allow differentiation of this syndrome from the other more common causes of anosmia (Fig. 5-130).[164–167]

## SYNDROMES AND SINUSITIS

Sinusitis may be associated with numerous clinical syndromes, which are briefly reviewed in this section.

## Kartagener's Syndrome

Kartagener's syndrome is an autosomal recessive inherited disease characterized by the clinical triad of bronchiectasis, sinusitis, and situs inversus. It is caused by an ultrastructural defect in the cilia that results in impaired mucociliary clearance. It is usually diagnosed during childhood, with only a small number of cases discovered in adults. Prompt, appropriate treatment of respiratory infections can minimize irreversible lung damage.[168]

## Primary Ciliary Dyskinesia Syndrome

Primary ciliary dyskinesia, also known as immotile cilia syndrome and dyskinetic cilia syndrome, is the generic term for a heterogeneous group of inherited diseases with motility

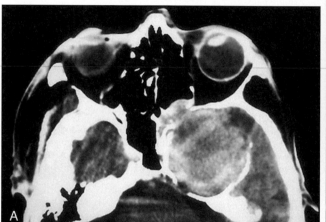

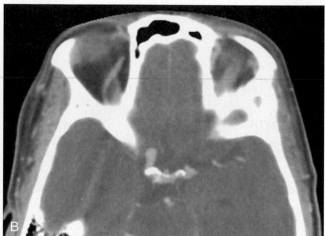

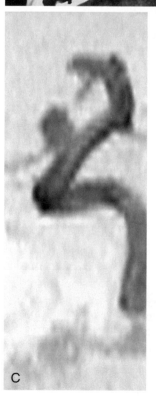

**FIGURE 5-125**    **A,** Axial contrast-enhanced CT scan shows a large mass with a partially calcified rim in the left middle cranial fossa. The mass has eroded through into the left sphenoid and posterior ethmoid sinuses. These sinuses simply looked "clouded" on plane films, suggesting inflammatory disease. This patient had a giant intracranial aneurysm that had eroded into the paranasal sinuses. Axial contrast-enhanced CT scan (**B**) performed to evaluate sinusitis on another patient shows an unsuspected aneurysm in the right supraclinoid region. **C,** MR angiogram image confirms the presence of the aneurysm.

disturbance resulting from defective ciliary ultrastructure. It is an autosomal recessive disorder with no sex predilection. Diagnostic criteria include chronic bronchitis, otitis, and childhood-onset sinusitis. Additionally, one or more of the following criteria must be present: Kartagener's syndrome, a dextrocardia situation, markedly reduced frequency in ciliary motility, or an essential ultrastructural deviation in more than 20% of the square cuts (e.g., reduced number of dynein arms). Vital microscopy and electron microscopy of the ciliated mucosa can distinguish primary and secondary ciliary dyskinesia and the rare case of primary ciliary dyskinesia without ultrastructural abnormalities. In special cases, establishing the cell tissue culture may allow for better ciliary evaluation and may be necessary for diagnosis.[169] Certain specific defects in the ciliary axoneme can be found, which are pathognomonic of the syndrome. The defects include missing dynein arms, abnormally short dynein arms, spokes with no central sheath, missing central microtubules, and displacement of one of the nine peripheral doublets. The most pronounced clinical manifestations are chronic paranasal sinusitis (52%) and chronic bronchiectasis (52%), followed by bronchopneumonia (26%), chronic bronchitis (21%), and nasal polyps (15%).[170, 171] Treatment with clarithromycin can be clinically useful in these patients.[172]

## Young's Syndrome

Young's syndrome, also known as sinusitis infertility syndrome and Barry Perkins Young syndrome, is mani-

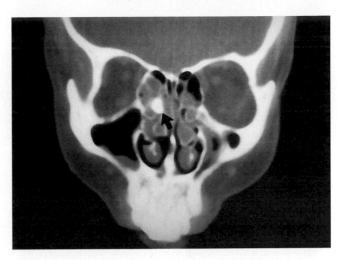

**FIGURE 5-127**   Coronal CT scan shows mucosal thickening in both ethmoid and maxillary sinuses, in the upper nasal fossae, and in both concha bullosa. In addition, there is a calcified rhinolith (*arrow*) in the right nasal fossa. This patient had sinusitis and a rhinolith.

fested by obstructive azoospermia and chronic sinopulmonary infection. Evaluation of nasal mucociliary transport reveals mucociliary stasis or decreased clearance. Ciliary ultrastructure is normal, but with decreased ciliary density, goblet cell hyperplasia, and low ciliary density. This is a chronic syndrome, which is less severe than syndromes with primary failure of mucociliary transport such as cystic fibrosis and primary ciliary dyskinesia. Young's syndrome should be considered in the differential diagnosis of patients suffering from chronic rhinosinusitis, particularly with cystic fibrosis and primary ciliary dyskinesia syndrome.[150, 173]

## Sertoli-Cell-Only Syndrome

The association of repeated sinus-bronchial-pulmonary infection and male infertility is well known in the literature in association with conditions such as cystic fibrosis, immotile cilia syndrome, and Young's syndrome. It is rarely seen otherwise. However, a patient with sinusitis, bronchiectasis, and sterility due to Sertoli-cell-only syndrome has been reported. Testicular biopsy showed absence of spermatogones and other germ cells, and nonspecific alterations were found in nasal cilia axonemes in the presence of DNA branches. A sweat test was negative. Recent studies have shown an increase in the prevalence of Sertoli-cell-only syndrome.[174]

## Hyperimmunoglobulinemia E Syndrome

Hyperimmunoglobulinemia E syndrome, also known as hyper IgE syndrome, Job's syndrome, Buckley's syndrome, and HIE syndrome, is an autosomal recessive disease characterized by eczematoid dermatitis, recurrent suppurative skin infections, chronic purulent sinusitis, otitis media, pneumonia, impaired neutrophil chemotaxis, and high levels of serum IgE. There are also depressed specific cell-

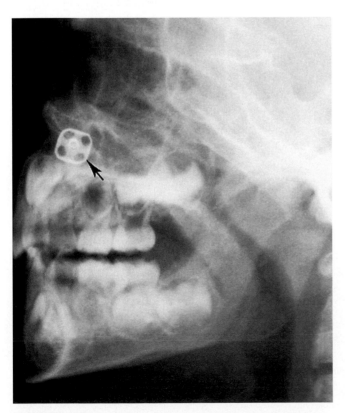

**FIGURE 5-126**   Lateral plane film shows a metallic snap foreign body in the nasal fossa (*arrow*).

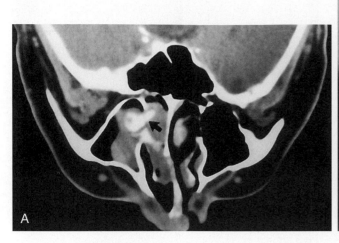
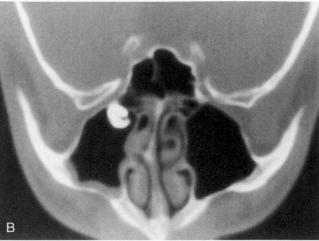

**FIGURE 5-128** **A,** Coronal CT scan shows inflammatory mucosal thickening in the right maxillary sinus and nasal fossa. A calcified rhinolith or sinolith is also present in the infundibulum (*arrow*). This patient had sinusitis and a sinolith/rhinolith. **B,** Coronal CT scan on another patient shows an intrasinus maxillary sinus tooth. This situation can occur when there is a highly situated, unerupted maxillary molar tooth.

mediated immune responses and a deficient antibody response.[150]

## Churg-Strauss Syndrome

The Churg-Strauss syndrome is a rare multisystem disease classified among the various vasculitides. It occurs primarily in adults and is rare in children. The initial symptoms are usually bronchial asthma and allergic rhinitis and sinusitis, which may progress to pulmonary, cardiac, and renal manifestations. Typical symptoms include fever, weight loss, sinusitis, myalgia and arthralgia, testicular pain, pulmonary infiltrations, asthma, pericardial effusion, peripheral neuropathy, seizure, and eosinophilia. Biopsies reveal necrotizing arteritis with eosinophilia.[175] The Churg-Strauss syndrome should be considered in the differential diagnosis if bronchial asthma and resistant sinusitis occur coincidentally. It is often difficult to establish the diagnosis, and frequently the syndrome is diagnosed only after several

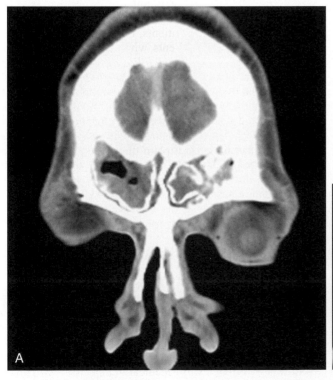
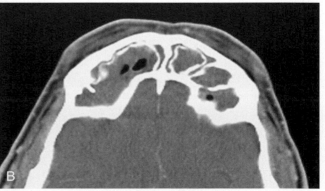

**FIGURE 5-129** Coronal (**A**) and axial (**B**) CT scans show extensive calcifications within the frontal sinuses. These were dystrophic calcifications in chronically obstructed sinuses, and they could be called sinoliths.

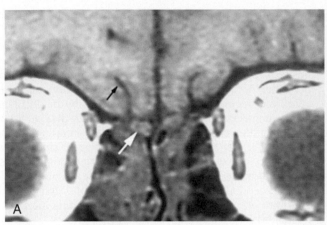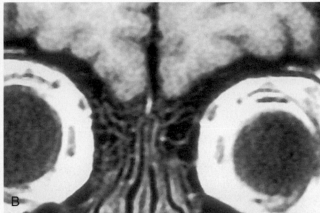

**FIGURE 5-130**   Coronal T1-weighted MR images. In **A**, a normal patient, the olfactory bulb (*white arrow*) and olfactory sulcus (*black arrow*) are well seen bilaterally. In **B**, a patient with anosmia, olfactory bulbs and sulci are absent in this patient with Kallman's syndrome. (Case courtesy of David Yousem, M.D.)

years. The therapy of choice is treatment with steroids, sometimes supplemented by cytotoxic drugs.[176] The long-term prognosis is good and does not differ from that of polyarteritis nodosa, although most patients need low doses of oral corticosteroids for persistent asthma even many years after clinical recovery from vasculitis.[177] However, the presence of severe gastrointestinal tract or myocardial involvement is significantly associated with a poor clinical outcome.

## Nijmegen Paragraph Signbreakage Syndrome

Patients with nijmegen paragraph signbreakage syndrome (NBS) have microcephaly with decreased size of the frontal lobes and narrow frontal horns, agenesis of the posterior part of the corpus callosum with colpocephaly and temporal horn dilatation, callosal hypoplasia with abnormal CSF spaces and wide cerebral cortex, and pachygyria. The invariable sinusitis associated with NBS is a result of primary immunodeficiency. Like patients with ataxia telangiectasia and other breakage syndromes, those with NBS show an inherited susceptibility to malignancy and hypersensitivity to X and gamma radiation. CT is therefore contraindicated in these patients, and MR imaging should be the method of choice for diagnostic imaging.[178]

## Croup

The etiology and clinical features of croup were studied in 132 children aged 3 months to 7 years. A diagnosis of laryngotracheobronchitis was made in 93.2%, and the pathogens identified included parainfluenza viruses, respiratory syncytial viruses, influenza A viruses, *Mycoplasma pneumoniae*, and adenoviruses. Bacterial tracheitis was present in 5.3% of cases, due to *S. viridans* and *Staph. aureus*. Fever of more than 3 days' duration was noted in 71% of children with bacterial tracheitis and in 28% of children with laryngotracheobronchitis. Among children with laryngotracheobronchitis, complications of pneumonia,

acute otitis media, or sinusitis were more frequently observed when there was a fever for more than 3 days (40% versus 17% for those with fever of shorter duration). Thus children with fever of long duration and more severe manifestations of airway obstruction probably have bacterial croup syndrome or a complication thereof.[179]

## Acquired Immune Deficiency Syndrome

Sinusitis is relatively rare among HIV-seropositive patients (3.3%) and may be clinically masked by other infections such as meningitis. Cure is difficult, relapses are frequent in spite of suitable treatment, and these are associated with a decline in immunocompetence.[180]

There is an amazing gamut of exotic agents that can cause sinusitis in seropositive patients, from algae to mushrooms. Bacterial sinusitis in patients with AIDS is caused by *P. aeruginosa* and *L. pneumophilia*, which are considered opportunistic bacterial pathogens that rarely cause sinusitis in normal hosts. Rare cases of *Microsporidium*-associated chronic sinusitis in HIV-seropositive patients have been reported, as have cases of *Septata intestinalis*–associated sinusitis. It appears that functional defects in local mucosal immunity may partially explain the acquisition of opportunistic mucosal infections in many HIV-seropositive patients.[181]

## Aspirin Triad Syndrome

The aspirin triad syndrome is defined as aspirin sensitivity, asthma, and chronic sinusitis with polyposis. The sinusitis associated with this disease is often fulminant and difficult to treat. Surgical treatment may be necessary to control the sinusitis in the majority of these patients, and multiple procedures may be necessary for some patients. Controlling the sinusitis may alleviate the asthmatic symptoms and reduce the need for steroids. Long-term follow-up and aggressive medical management of chronic sinusitis will decrease the risk of orbital and other complications.[182, 183]

## Silent Sinus Syndrome

Silent sinus syndrome was discussed earlier in this chapter. In response to chronic maxillary sinusitis, it is believed that a negative pressure develops within the obstructed sinus and, with time, the sinus walls collapse, allowing enophthalmus to occur.

## Toxic Shock Syndrome

Toxic shock syndrome may occasionally be associated with sinusitis. A patient was described who presented with *S. pneumoniae* sinusitis, severe sepsis syndrome, and a desquamative rash.[184]

## Cyclic Vomiting Syndrome

Although it remains a mysterious disorder since its description over a century ago, cyclic vomiting syndrome appears to be more prevalent than has been appreciated. Children are primarily affected, with vomiting that can range from an explosive, intermittent cyclic pattern to a low-grade, daily, chronic pattern. The etiologies causing a cyclic vomiting pattern include abdominal migraine, chronic sinusitis, intracranial neoplasm, anomalies of and mucosal injury to the gastrointestinal tract, urologic abnormalities, and metabolic and endocrine disorders. The cyclic pattern of vomiting is a symptom complex that can be induced by heterogeneous disorders that either cause or contribute to the vomiting. Once the cyclic vomiting pattern is identified, systematic diagnostic testing is warranted to look for these underlying disorders.[185, 186]

## Yellow Nail Syndrome

Onset of the symptoms of yellow nail syndrome, also known as *yellow nails-bronchiectasis-lymphedema syndrome*, occurs in adults. It is characterized by thickened, smooth yellow- or green-colored nails with transverse ridging and excessive curvature, onycholysis, primary lymphedema due to lymphatic hypoplasia, chronic cough, pleural effusions, bronchiectasis, sinusitis, and a propensity to develop malignancies.[150, 187]

## (P)FAPA Syndrome

The (P)FAPA syndrome (periodic fever, adenitis, pharyngitis, and aphthous stomatitis) was described in 1987. The etiology of this periodic syndrome remains unknown. In these children, this is an exclusionary diagnosis for a condition in which various treatments (antibiotics, antipyretics, nonsteroidal anti-inflammatory agents) have proved ineffective. The repetition of the periodic bouts of fever results in depressive disorders, absenteeism from school, and a drop in weight. In two of three patients there was chronic sinusitis, polyposis, and increased levels of immunoglobulin A. In all three patients, cimetidine was well tolerated and resulted in a disappearance of the periodic fever.[188]

## Ataxia Telangiectasia Syndrome

Ataxia telangiectasia syndrome (Louis-Bar syndrome, Boder-Sedgwick syndrome, cephalo-oculocutaneous telangiectasis syndrome, sinopulmonary infectious syndrome) is either a familial (50%) or sporadically occurring autosomal recessive disease characterized by oculocutaneous telangiectasias, progressive cerebellar ataxia, and a defect in the cellular immunity of the immunoglobulin system. The last condition results in recurrent sinusitis and pulmonary infections. These patients have a predisposition to develop malignancies, endocrine disturbances, a high susceptibility to irradiation, and mental deficiency in one-third of cases. The onset of symptoms occurs in childhood.[150]

## Wiskott-Aldrich Syndrome

Wiskott-Aldrich syndrome, also known as Wiskott-Aldrich-Huntley syndrome and eczema-thrombocytopenia syndrome, is as an X-linked recessive disorder that occurs in males. The onset of symptoms is in infancy or early childhood, and characteristically there is eczema, bloody diarrhea, recurrent infections (otitis, sinusitis, pneumonia), purpura, congenital thrombocytopenia, cellular and humoral immune deficiencies (without adenoidal development), anemia, and a predisposition to develop malignancies.[150]

## REFERENCES

1. Potsic W, Wetmore R. Pediatric rhinology. In: Goldman J, ed. The Principles and Practice of Rhinology. New York: Wiley, 1987;801–845.
2. Carpenter J, Artenstein M. Use of diagnostic microbiologic facilities in the diagnosis of head and neck infections. Otolaryngol Clin North Am 1976;9:611–629.
3. Fried M, Relly J, Strome M. Pseudomonas rhinosinusitis. Laryngoscope 1984;94:192–196.
4. Evans F, Sydnor J, Moore W, et al. Sinusitis of the maxillary antrum. N Engl J Med 1976;293:735–739.
5. Frederick J, Braude A. Anaerobic infection of the paranasal sinuses. N Engl J Med 1974;290:135–137.
6. Van Alyea O. Nasal Sinuses: Anatomic and Clinical Considerations. 2nd ed. Baltimore: Williams & Wilkins, 1951.
7. Aysun S, Yetuk M. Clinical experience on headache in children: analysis of 92 cases. J Child Neurol 1998;13:202–210.
8. Berger JR, Stein N, Pall L. Headache and human immunodeficiency virus infection: a case control study, Eur Neurol 1996;36:229–233.
9. Remulla HD, Rubin PA, Shore JW, Cunningham MJ. Pseudodacryocystitis arising from anterior ethmoiditis. Ophthalmol Plast Reconstr Surg 1995;11:165–168.
10. Abrahams JJ, Glassberg RM. Dental disease: a frequently unrecognized cause of maxillary sinus abnormalities? AJR 1996;166:1219–1223.
11. Raboso E, Llavero MT, Rosell A, Martinez-Vidal A. Craniofacial necrotizing fasciitis secondary to sinusitis. J Laryngol Otol 1998;112:371–372.
12. Perez Barreto M, Sahai S, Ameriso S, Ahmadi J, Rice D, Fisher M. Sinusitis and carotid artery stroke. Ann Otol Rhinol Laryngol 2000;109:227–230.
13. Moorman CM, Anslow P, Elston JS. Is sphenoid sinus opacity significant in patients with optic neuritis? Eye 1999;13:76–82.
14. Deutsch JH, Hudgins PA, Siegel JL, et al. The paranasal sinuses of patients with acute graft-versus-host disease. AJNR 1995;16:1287–1291.

15. Oberholzer K, Kauczor HU, Heussel CP, Derigs G, Thelen M. [Clinical relevance of CT of paranasal sinuses prior to bone marrow transplantation]. Rofo Fortschr Geb Rontgenstr Neuen Bildgeb Verfahr 1997;166:493–497.
16. Odita J, Akamaguna A, Ogisi F, et al. Pneumatization of the maxillary sinus in normal and asymptomatic children. Pediatr Radiol 1986;16:365–367.
17. Zimmerman R, Bilaniuk L, Hackney D, Goldberg H, Grossman R. Paranasal sinus hemorrhage: evaluation with MR imaging. Radiology 1987;162:499–503.
18. Som P, Shugar J, Troy K, et al. The use of MR and CT in the management of a patient with intrasinus hemorrhage. Arch Otolaryngol 1988;114:200–202.
19. Fagan P, McKenzie B, Edmonds C. Sinus barotrauma in divers. Ann Otol Rhinol Laryngol 1976;85:61–64.
20. Remmier D, Boles R. Intracranial complications of frontal sinusitis. Laryngoscope 1980;90:1814–1824.
21. Tamakawa Y, Hanafee W. Cerebrospinal fluid rhinorrhea: significance of an air-fluid level in the sphenoid sinus. Radiology 1980;135:101–103.
22. Rhyoo C, Sanders SP, Leopold DA, Proud D. Sinus mucosal IL-8 gene expression in chronic rhinosinusitis. J Allergy Clin Immunol 1999;103:395–400.
23. Crater SE, Peters EJ, Phillips CD, Platts-Mills TA. Prospective analysis of CT of the sinuses in acute asthma. AJR 1999;173:127–131.
24. Stahl R. Allergic disorders of the nose and paranasal sinuses. Otolaryngol Clin North Am 1974;7:703–718.
25. Nino-Murcia M, Rao V, Mikaelian D, et al. Acute sinusitis mimicking antrochoanal polyp. AJNR 1986;7:513–516.
26. Baroody FM, Suh SH, Naclerio RM. Total IgE serum levels correlate with sinus mucosal thickness on computerized tomography scans. J Allergy Clin Immunol 1997;100:563–568.
27. Ballenger J, ed. Diseases of the Nose and Throat. Philadelphia: Lea & Febiger, 1977;105–114, 155–167.
28. Smith M. Dysfunction of carbohydrate metabolism as an element in the set of factors resulting in the polysaccharide nose and nasal polyps (the polysaccharide nose). Laryngoscope 1971;81:636–644.
29. Schramm VJ, Effron M. Nasal polyps in children. Laryngoscope 1980;90:1488–1495.
30. Jaffe B, Strome M, Khaw K, et al. Nasal polypectomy and sinus surgery for cystic fibrosis: a 10 year review. Otolaryngol Clin North Am 1977;10:81–90.
31. Moloney J. Nasal polyps, nasal polypectomy, asthma and aspirin sensitivity: their association in 445 cases of nasal polyps. J Laryngol Otol 1977;91:837–846.
32. Torjussen W. Rhinoscopical findings in nickel workers, with special emphasis on the influence of nickel exposure and smoking habits. Acta Otolaryngol (Stockh) 1979;88:279–288.
33. Fairbanks D, Raphael G. Nonallergic rhinitis and infection. In: Cummings C, Fredrickson J, Harker L, Krause C, Schuller D, eds. Otolaryngology Head and Neck Surgery. 2nd ed. Vol. 1. St. Louis: Mosby Year Book, 1993;775–785.
34. Myerowitz R, Guggenheimer J, Barnes L. Infectious diseases of the head and neck. In: Barnes L, ed. Surgical Pathology of the Head and Neck. Vol 2. New York: Marcel Dekker, 1987;1771–1822.
35. Waxman J, Spector J, Sale S, et al. Allergic aspergillus sinusitis: concepts in diagnosis and treatment of a new clinical entity. Laryngoscope 1987;97:261–266.
36. Swift AC, Denning DW. Skull base osteitis following fungal sinusitis. J Laryngol Otol 1998;112:92–97.
37. Moss RB, Beaudet LM, Wenig BM, et al. *Microsporidium*-associated sinusitis. Ear Nose Throat J 1997;76:95–101.
38. Daghistani K, Jamal T, Zaher S, et al. Allergic aspergillus sinusitis with proptosis. J Laryngol Otol 1992;106:799–803.
39. Milroy C, Blanshard J, Lucas S, et al. Aspergillosis of the nose and paranasal sinuses. J Clin Pathol 1989;42:123–127.
40. Kameswaran M, Al-Waddei A, Khurana P, et al. Rhinocerebral aspergillosis. J Laryngol Otol 1992;106:981–985.
41. Blitzer A, Lawson W. Fungal infection of the nose and paranasal sinuses. Part I. Otolaryngol Clin North Am 1993;26:1007–1035.
42. McLean FM, Ginsberg LE, Stanton CA. Perineural spread of rhinocerebral mucormycosis. AJNR 1996;17:114–116.
43. Blatt S, Lucey D, DeHoff D, et al. Rhinocerebral zygomycosis in a patient with AIDS. J Infect Dis 1991;164:215–216.
44. Tyson J, Gittelman P, Jacobs J, et al. Recurrent mucormycosis of the paranasal sinuses in an immunologically competant host. Otolaryngol Head Neck Surg 1992;107:115–119.
45. Pafrey N. Improved diagnosis and prognosis of mucormycosis: a clinicopathologic study of 33 cases. Medicine 1986;65:113–123.
46. Mader J, Ream R, Heath P. *Petriellidium boydii (Allescheria boydii)* sphenoidal sinusitis. JAMA 1978;239:2368–2369.
47. Travis L, Roberts G, Wilson W. Clinical significance of *Pseudallescheria boydii*: a review of 10 years experience. Mayo Clin Proc 1985;60:531–537.
48. Chapnick J, Bach M. Bacterial and fungal infections of the maxillary sinus. Otolaryngol Clin North Am 1976;9:43–54.
49. Wheat L, Conolly-Stringfield P, Baker R, et al. Disseminated histoplasmosis in AIDS: clinical findings, diagnosis and treatment, and review of the literature. Med 1990;69:361–374.
50. Oda D, McDougal L, Fitsche T, et al. Oral histoplasmosis as a presenting disease in AIDS. Oral Surg Oral Med Oral Pathol 1990;70:631–636.
51. Browning D, Schwartz D, Jurado R. Cryptococcosis of the larynx in a patient with AIDS: an unusual cause of fungal laryngitis. South Med J 1992;85:762–764.
52. Lynch D, Naftolin L. Oral *Cryptococcus neoformans* infection in AIDS. Oral Surg Oral Med Oral Pathol 1987;64:449–453.
53. Boyle J, Coulthard S, Mandel R. Laryngeal involvement in disseminated coccidioidomycosis. Arch Otolaryngol Head Neck Surg 1991;117:433–438.
54. Fish D, Ampel N, Galgiani J, et al. Coccidioidomycosis during HIV infection. A review of 77 patients. Medicine 1990;69:384–390.
55. Fascenelli F. Maxillary sinus abnormalities: radiographic evidence in an asymptomatic population. Arch Otol Laryngol 1969; 90:190–193.
56. Zizmor J, Noyek A. Inflammatory diseases of the paranasal sinuses. Otolaryngol Clin North Am 1973;6:459–485.
57. Som P, Sacher M, Lawson W, et al. CT appearance distinguishing benign nasal polyps from malignancies. J Comput Assist Tomogr 1987;11:129–133.
58. Nakagawa T, Yamane H, Shigeta T, Takashima T, Nakai Y. Interaction between fibronectin and eosinophils in the growth of nasal polyps. Laryngoscope 1999;109:557–561.
59. Som P, Cohen B, Sacher M. The angiomatous polyp and the angiofibroma: two different lesions. Radiology 1982;144:329–334.
60. Batsakis J. The pathology of head and neck tumors: nasal cavity and paranasal sinuses. Part 5. Head Neck Surg 1980;2:410–419.
61. Barnes L, Verbin R, Gnepp D. Diseases of the nose, paranasal sinuses and nasopharynx. In: Barnes L, ed. Surgical Pathology of the Head and Neck. Vol 1. New York: Marcel Dekker, 1985: 403–451.
62. Smith C, Echevarria R, McLelland C. Pseudosarcomatous changes in antrochoanal polyps. Arch Otolaryngol 1974;99:228–230.
63. Weissman J, Tabor E, Curtin H. Sphenochoanal polyps: evaluation with CT and MR imaging. Radiology 1991;178:145–148.
64. Towbin R, Bundar J. The paranasal sinuses in childhood. Radiographics 1982;2:253–279.
65. Glasier C, Ascher D, Williams K. Incidental paranasal sinus abnormalities on CT of children: clinical correlation. AJNR 1986;7: 861–864.
66. Glasier C, Mallory GJ, Steele R. Significance of opacification of maxillary and ethmoid sinuses in infants. J Pediatr 1989;114:45–50.
67. Kronemer KA, McAlister WH. Sinusitis and its imaging in the pediatric population. Pediatr Radiol 1997;27:837–846.
68. Baroody FM, Hughes CA, McDowell P, Hruban R, Zinreich SJ, Naclerio RM. Eosinophilia in chronic childhood sinusitis. Arch Otolaryngol Head Neck Surg 1995;121:1396–1402.
69. Shugar J. Embryology of the nose and paranasal sinuses and resultant deformities. In: Goldman J, ed. The Principles and Practice of Rhinology. New York: Wiley, 1987;113–131.
70. Johnson J. Infections. In: Cummings C, Fredrickson J, Harker L, Krause C, Schuller D, eds. Otolaryngology Head and Neck Surgery. Vol 1. St Louis: CV Mosby, 1986;887–900.
71. Chong W, Hall-Craggs M. Prevalence of paranasal sinus disease in HIV infection and AIDS on cranial MR imaging. Clin Radiol 1993;47:166–169.
72. O'Donnell J, Sorbello A, Condoluci I, et al. Sinusitis due to *Pseudomonas aeruginosa* in patients with HIV infection. Clin Infect Dis 1993;16:404–406.

73. Schlanger G, Lutwick LI, Kurzman M, Hoch B, Chandler FW. Sinusitis caused by *Legionella pneumophila* in a patient with the acquired immune deficiency syndrome. Am J Med 1984;77: 957–960.

74. Som P, Shugar J. The CT classification of ethmoid mucoceles. J. Comput Assist Tomogr 1980;4:199–203.

75. De Juan E, Green W, Iliff N. Allergic periorbital mycopyocele in children. Am J Ophthalmol 1983;96:299–303.

76. Finn D, Hudson N, Baylin G. Unilateral polyposis and mucoceles in children. Laryngoscope 1981;91:1444–1449.

77. Zizmor J, Noyck A. Cysts, benign tumors and malignant tumors of the paranasal sinuses. Otolaryngol Clin North Am 1973;6:487–508.

78. Lim CC, Dillon WP, McDermott MW. Mucocele involving the anterior clinoid process: MR and CT findings. AJNR 1999;20:287–290.

79. Hazan A, Le Roy A, Chevalier E, et al. [Atelectasis of the maxillary sinus. Analysis of progression stages. Apropos of 4 cases]. Ann Otolaryngol Chir Cervicofac 1998;115:367–372.

80. Gillman GS, Schaitkin BM, May M. Asymptomatic enophthalmos: the silent sinus syndrome. Am J Rhinol 1999;13:459–462.

81. Rak K, Newell JI, Yakes W, et al. Paranasal sinus on MR images of the brain: significance of mucosal thickening. AJR 1991;156:381–384.

82. Moser F, Panush D, Rubin J, et al. Incidental paranasal sinus abnormalities on MRI of the brain. Clin Radiol 1991;43:252–254.

83. Som P, Dillon W, Fullerton G, Zimmerman R, Rajagopalan B, Marom Z. Chronically obstructed sinonasal secretions: observations on T1 and T2 shortening. Radiology 1989;172:515–520.

84. Dillon W, Som P, Fullerton G. Hypointense MR signal in chronically inspissated sinonasal secretions. Radiology 1990;174:73–78.

85. Som P, Dillon W, Curtin H, et al. Hypointense paranasal sinus foci: differential diagnosis with MR imaging and relation to CT findings. Radiology 1990;176:777–781.

86. Bassoiouny A, Newlands W, Ali H, et al. Maxillary sinus hypoplasia and superior orbital fissure asymmetry. Laryngoscope 1982;92:441–448.

87. Modic M, Weinstein M, Berlin A, et al. Maxillary sinus hypoplasia visualized with computed tomography. Radiology 1980;135:383–385.

88. Kennedy D, Zinreich S, Kumar A, et al. Physiologic mucosal changes within the nose and ethmoid sinus: imaging of the nasal cycle by MRI. Laryngoscope 1988;98:928–933.

89. Brock J, Schabel S, Curry N. CT diagnosis of contrast reaction. J Comput Tomogr 1981;5:63–64.

90. Som P, Dillon W, Sze G, MW L, Biller H, Lawson W. Benign and malignant sinonasal lesions with intracranial extension: differentiation with MR imaging. Radiology 1989;172:763–766.

91. Som P, Curtin H. Chronic inflammatory sinonasal diseases including fungal infections: the role of imaging. Radiol Clin North Am 1993;31:33–44.

92. Jacobs M, Som P. The ethmoidal "polypoid mucocele." J Comput Assist Tomogr 1982;6:721–724.

93. Naul L, Hise J, Ruff T. CT of inspissated mucus in chronic sinusitis. AJNR 1987;8:574–575.

94. Zinreich S, Kennedy D, Malat J, et al. Fungal sinusitis: diagnosis with CT and MR imaging. Radiology 1988;169:439–444.

95. Lloyd D, Bartram C, Stanley P. Ethmoid mucoceles. Br J Radiol 1974;47:646–651.

96. Ritter R. The Paranasal Sinuses: Anatomy and Surgical Technique. 2nd ed. St. Louis: CV Mosby, 1978.

97. Canalis R, Zajtchuck J, Jenkins H. Ethmoid mucoceles. Arch Otolaryngol 1978;104:286–291.

98. Zizmor J, Ganz AR. Mucoceles of paranasal sinuses. NY State J Med 1972 Jul 1; 72(13):1710–1715.

99. Som P, Sacher M, Lanzieri C, et al. The hidden antral compartment. Radiology 1984;152:463–464.

100. Close L, O'Connor W. Sphenoethmoidal mucoceles with intracranial extension. Otolaryngol Head Neck Surg 1983;91:350–357.

101. Osborn A, Johnson L, Roberts T. Sphenoidal mucoceles with intracranial extension. J Comput Assist Tomogr 1979;3:335–338.

102. Chui M, Briant T, Gray T, et al. Computed tomography of sphenoid sinus mucocele. J Otolaryngol 1983;12:263–269.

103. Price H, Batnitzky S, Karlin C, et al. Multiple paranasal sinus mucoceles. J Comput Assist Tomogr 1981;5:122–125.

104. Perugini S, Pasquini U, Menichelli F, et al. Mucoceles in the paranasal sinus involving the orbit: CT signs in 43 cases. Neuroradiology 1982;23:133–139.

105. Demaerel P, Brown P, Kendall B, et al. Case report: allergic aspergillosis of the sphenoid sinus: pitfall on MRI. Br J Radiol 1993;66:260–263.

106. Chang T, Teng M, Wang S, et al. Aspergillosis of the paranasal sinuses. Neuroradiology 1992;34:520–523.

107. Romett J, Newman R. Aspergillosis of the nose and paranasal sinuses. Laryngoscope 1982;92:764–766.

108. Centeno R, Bentson J, Mancuso A. CT scanning in rhinocerebral mucormycosis and aspergillosis. Radiology 1981;140:383–389.

109. Shugar J, Som P, Robbins A, et al. Maxillary sinusitis as a cause of cheek swelling. Arch Otolaryngol 1982;108:507–508.

110. Kopp W, Fotter R, Steiner H, et al. Aspergillosis of the Paranasal Sinuses. Radiology 1985;156:715–716.

111. Stammberger J, Jakse A, Beaufort F. Aspergillosis of the paranasal sinuses: x-ray diagnosis, histopathology and clinical aspects. Ann Otol Rhinol Laryngol 1984;93:251–256.

112. Richtsmeier WJ, Johns ME. Actinomycosis of the Head and Neck. CRC Crit Rev Clin Lab Sci 1979 Nov;11(2):175–202.

113. Bhatia P, Obafunwa J. Rare infections of the nose and paranasal sinuses. Trop Geograph Med 1990;42:289–293.

114. Kingdom T, Tami T. Actinomycosis of the nasal septum in a patient infected with HIV. Otolaryngol Head Neck Surg 1994;71:675–677.

115. MacGregor R. A year's experience with tuberculosis in a private urban teaching hospital in the post-sanatorium era. Am J Med 1975;58:221–228.

116. Bath A, O'Flynn P, Gibbin K. Nasopharyngeal tuberculosis. J Laryngol Otol 1992;106:1079–1080.

117. Control CFD. Annual summary. Morbid-Mort Weekly Rep 1981;19:3.

118. McNulty J, Fassett R. Syphilis: an otolaryngologic perspective. Laryngoscope 1981;91:889–905.

119. Olansky S. Syphilis Rediscovered. Chicago: Year Book Medical Publishers, 1967. Disease-a-month; 1–30.

120. Larsen S. Syphilis. Clin Lab Med 1989;9:545–557.

121. Andraca R, Edson R, Kern E. Rhinoscleroma: a growing concern in the US? Mayo Clin Proc 1993;68:1151–1157.

122. Becker T, Shum T, Waller T, et al. Radiological aspects of rhinoscleroma. Radiology 1981;141:433–438.

123. Lazow S, Seldin R, Soloman M. South American blastomycosis of the maxilla: report of a case. J Oral Maxillofac Surg 1990;48:68–71.

124. Sposto M, Scully C, Almeida O, et al. Paracoccidioidomycosis. A study of 36 South American patients. Oral Surg Oral Med Oral Pathol 1993;75:461–465.

125. Beeson P, McDermott W. Textbook of Medicine. 14th ed. Philadelphia: WB Saunders, 1975:164–539.

126. Lasser A, Smith H. Rhinosporidiosis. Arch Otolaryngol 1974; 102:308.

127. Thianprait M, Thagerngpol K. Rhinosporidiosis. Curr Top Med Mycol 1989;3:64–85.

128. Harrison T. Harrison's Principles of Internal Medicine. 9th ed. New York: McGraw-Hill, 1987.

129. Fauci A, Wolff S. Wegener's granulomatosis and related diseases. Dis Month 1977;23:1.

130. Harrison D. Midline destructive granuloma: fact or fiction? Laryngoscope 1987;97:1049–1053.

131. Gordon W, Cohn A, Greenberg S, et al. Nasal sarcoidosis. Arch Otolaryngol 1976;102:11–14.

132. Fredricks DN, Relman DA. Infectious agents and the etiology of chronic idiopathic diseases. Curr Clin Top Infect Dis 1998;18: 180–200.

133. Johns CJ, Michele TM. The clinical management of sarcoidosis. A 50-year experience at the Johns Hopkins Hospital. Medicine (Balt) 1999;78:65–111.

134. Mailland A, Geopfert H. Nasal and paranasal sarcoidosis. Arch Otolaryngol 1978;104:197–201.

135. Paling M, Roberts R, Fauci A. Paranasal sinus obliteration in Wegener's granulomatosis. Radiology 1982;144:539–543.

136. Le Hir P, Marsot-Dupuch K, Bigel P, et al. Rhinoscleroma with orbital extension: CT and MRI. Neuroradiology 1996;38:175–178.

137. Zizmor J, Noyek A. Radiology of the nose and paranasal sinuses. In: Paparella M, Shumrick D, eds. Otolaryngology. Vol 1. Philadelphia: WB Saunders, 1973;1043–1095.

138. Taveras J, Wood E. Diagnostic Neuroradiology. Baltimore: Williams & Wilkins, 1964;141–142.

139. Wax M, Briant T. Epidermoid cysts of the cranial bones. Head Neck 1992;14:293–296.

140. Dodd G, Jing B. Radiology of the nose, paranasal sinuses and nasopharynx. Baltimore: Williams & Wilkins, 1977;59–65.

141. Verbin R, Barnes L. Cysts and cyst-like lesions of the oral cavity, jaws and neck. In: Barnes L, ed. Surgical Pathology of the Head and Neck. Vol 2. New York: Marcel Dekker, 1985;1278–1281.

142. Kunt T, Ozturkcan S, Egilmez R. Cholesterol granuloma of the maxillary sinus: six cases from the same region. J Laryngol Otol 1998;112:65–68.

143. Koenig H, Lenz M, Sauter R. Temporal bone region: high resolution MR imaging using surface coils. Radiology 1986;159:191–194.

144. Latack J, Kartush J, Kemink J, et al. Epidermoidomas of the cerebellopontine angle and temporal bone: CT and MR aspects. Radiology 1985;157:361–366.

145. Urken M, Som P, Lawson W, Edelstein D, McAvay G, Biller H. The abnormally large frontal sinus. Part I: a practical method for its determination based upon an analysis of 100 normal patients. Laryngoscope 1987;97:602–605.

146. Urken M, Som P, Lawson W, et al. The abnormally large frontal sinuses II: nomenclature, pathology and symptoms. Laryngoscope 1987;97:606–611.

147. Dross P, Lally J, Bonier B. *Pneumosinus dilatans* and arachnoid cyst: a unique association. AJNR 1992;13:209–211.

148. Benedikt R, Brown D, Roth M, et al. Spontaneous drainage of an ethmoid mucocele: a possible cause of pneumosinus dilatans. AJNR 1991;12:729–731.

149. Lombardi G. Radiology in Neuro-Ophthalmology. Baltimore: Williams & Wilkins, 1967.

150. Taybi H. Metabolic disorders. In: Taybi H, Lachman R, eds. Radiology of Syndromes, Metabolic Disorders, and Skeletal Dysplasias. 4th ed. St. Louis: CV Mosby, 1996;635–637.

151. Kutnick S, Kerth J. Acute sinusitis and otitis: their complications and surgical treatment. Otolaryngol Clin North Am 1976;9:689–701.

152. Carter B, Bankoff M, Fisk J. Computed tomographic detection of sinusitis responsible for intracranial and extracranial infections. Radiology 1983;147:739–742.

153. Zimmerman R, Bilaniuk L. CT of orbital infection and its cerebral complications. Am J Roentgenol 1980;134:45–50.

154. Rothstein J, Maisel R, Berlinger N, et al. Relationship of optic neuritis to disease of the paranasal sinus. Laryngoscope 1984;94:1501–1508.

155. Bilaniuk L, Zimmerman R. Computer assisted tomography: sinus lesions with orbital involvement. Head Neck Surg 1980;2:293–301.

156. Eshaghian J, Anderson R. Sinus involvement in inflammatory orbital pseudotumor. Arch Ophthalmol 1981;99:627–630.

157. Som P, Brandwein M, Maldjiian C. Inflammatory pseudotumor of the maxillary sinus: CT and MR ftndings in six cases. Am J Roentgenol 1994;163:689–692.

158. Kaufman D, Litman N, Miller M. Sinusitis: induced subdural empyema. Neurology 1983;33:123–132.

159. Williams H. Infections and granulomas of the nasal airways and paranasal sinuses. In: Shumrick D, ed. Otolaryngology. Vol 3. Head and Neck. Philadelphia: WB Saunders, 1973;27–32.

160. Babu RP, Todor R, Kasoff SS. Pott's puffy tumor: the forgotten entity. Case report. J Neurosurg 1996;84:110–112.

161. Price H, Batnitzky S, Karlin L, et al. Giant nasal rhinolith. AJNR 1981;2:271–273.

162. RSNA. Case of the day: case IV, rhinolith. Radiology 1983;146:251–252.

163. Som P, Lidov M. The significance of sinonasal radiodensities: ossification, calcification, or residual bone? AJNR 1994;15:917–922.

164. Yousem D, Turner W, Snyder P, et al. Kallmann's syndrome: MR evaluation of olfactory system. AJNR 1993;14:839–843.

165. Knon J, Ragland R, Brown R, et al. Kallmann syndrome: MR findings. AJNR 1993;14:845–851.

166. Li C, Yousem D, Doty R, et al. Neuroimaging in patients with olfactory dysfunction. AJR 1994;162:411–418.

167. Yousem D, Geckle R, Bilker W, McKeown D, Doty R. MR evaluation of patients with congenital hyposmia or anosmia. AJR 1996;166:439–443.

168. Gomez de Terreros Caro FJ, Gomez-Stern Aguilar C, Alvarez-Sala Walther R, Prados Sanchez C, Garcia Rio F, Villamor Leon J. [Kartagener's syndrome. Diagnosis in a 75 year-old woman]. Arch Bronconeumol 1999;35:242–244.

169. Dombi VH, Walt H. [Primary ciliary dyskinesia, immotile cilia syndrome, and Kartagener syndrome: diagnostic criteria]. Schweiz Med Wochenschr 1996;126:421–433.

170. Min YG, Shin JS, Choi SH, Chi JG, Yoon CJ. Primary ciliary dyskinesia: ultrastructural defects and clinical features. Rhinology 1995;33:189–193.

171. Armengot M, Carda C, Basterra J. [Incomplete ciliary axonema: another cause of ciliary dysmotility syndrome?]. Acta Otorrinolaringol Esp 1998;49:57–59.

172. Nishi K, Mizuguchi M, Tachibana H, et al. [Effect of clarithromycin on symptoms and mucociliary transport in patients with sino-bronchial syndrome]. Nihon Kyobu Shikkan Gakkai Zasshi 1995;33:1392–1400.

173. Armengot M, Juan G, Carda C, Montalt J, Basterra J. Young's syndrome: a further cause of chronic rhinosinusitis. Rhinology 1996;34:35–37.

174. Carrion Valero F, Ferrer Gomez C, Pascual Izuel JM. [Sino-bronchial infections and male sterility. Presentation of a new variant]. Arch Bronconeumol 1998;34:405–408.

175. Louthrenoo W, Norasetthada A, Khunamornpong S, Sreshthaputra A, Sukitawut W. Childhood Churg-Strauss syndrome. J Rheumatol 1999;26:1387–1393.

176. Trittel C, Moller J, Euler HH, Werner JA. [Churg-Strauss syndrome. A differential diagnosis in chronic polypoid sinusitis]. Laryngorhinootologie 1995;74:577–580.

177. Guillevin L, Cohen P, Gayraud M, Lhote F, Jarrousse B, Casassus P. Churg-Strauss syndrome. Clinical study and long-term follow-up of 96 patients. Medicine (Balt) 1999;78:26–37.

178. Bekiesinska-Figatowska M, Chrzanowska KH, Sikorska J, et al. Cranial MRI in the Nijmegen breakage syndrome. Neuroradiology 2000;42:43–47.

179. Chiu TF, Huang LM, Chen JG, Lee CY, Lee PI. Group syndrome in children: five-year experience. Chung Hua Min Kuo Hsiao Erh Ko I Hsueh Hui Tsa Chih 1999;40:258–261.

180. Martinez-Subias J, Dominguez LJ. Urpegui A, Sancho E, Royo J, Valles H. [Sinus manifestations of the acquired immunodeficiency syndrome]. Rev Neurol 1997;25:1620–1623.

181. Moss RB, Scott TA, Goldrich M, et al. Nasal mucosal cells in human immunodeficiency virus type 1-seropositive patients with sinusitis. J Clin Lab Anal 1996;10:418–422.

182. McFadden EA, Woodson BT, Massaro BM, Toohill RJ. Orbital complications of sinusitis in the aspirin triad syndrome. Laryngoscope 1996;106:1103–1107.

183. McFadden EA, Woodson BT, Fink JN, Toohill RJ. Surgical treatment of aspirin triad sinusitis. Am J Rhinol 1997;11:263–270.

184. Friedstrom SR, Awad J. Toxic-shock-like-syndrome due to *Streptococcus pneumoniae* sinusitis. Scand J Infect Dis 1999;31:509–510.

185. Li BU. Cyclic vomiting: the pattern and syndrome paradigm. J Pediatr Gastroenterol Nutr 1995;21:S6–S10.

186. Li BUK, Murray RD, Heitlinger LA, Robbins JL, Hayes JR. Heterogeneity of diagnoses presenting as cyclic vomiting. Pediatrics 1998;102:583–587.

187. Luyten C, Andre J, Walraevens C, De Doncker P. Yellow nail syndrome and onychomycosis. Experience with itraconazole pulse therapy combined with vitamin E. Dermatology 1996;192:406–408.

188. Pillet P, Ansoborlo S, Carrere A, Perel Y, Guillard JM. [(P)FAPA syndrome: value of cimetidine]. Arch Pediatr 2000;7:54–57.

# 6

# Tumors and Tumor-like Conditions

*Peter M. Som and Margaret S. Brandwein*

## GENERAL CONSIDERATIONS

The sinonasal tract plays host to an enormous variety of neoplasms derived from a multitude of tissue types. Sinonasal neoplasias can be broadly classified as either epithelial or mesenchymal. Epithelial neoplasia may arise from the Schneiderian lining mucosa (e.g., papillomas, squamous carcinomas, intestinal-type adenocarcinoma), minor salivary tissue (which includes the whole array of benign and malignant minor salivary tumors), neuroendocrine tissue (e.g., sinonasal neuroendocrine carcinoma), or olfactory mucosa (olfactory neuroblastoma). Each of the mesenchymal tissues of the sinonasal tract can give rise to benign and malignant neoplastic counterparts. Thus one can expect an array of tumors with benign, malignant, or unknown biologic potential, recapitulating their tissue of derivation (bone, cartilage, fibroblasts, smooth and skeletal muscle, vessels, etc.).

By comparison to the ubiquitous nature of sinonasal inflammatory disease, neoplasms affecting the paranasal sinuses and nasal cavities are rare. Carcinomas are by far the most common neoplasm, yet they comprise only 0.2% to 0.8% of all malignancies and about 3% of all malignant tumors that arise in the head and neck.[1] In the SEER (surveillance, epidemiology, and end results) data of the National Institutes of Health, which followed more than 50,000 upper aerodigestive tract malignancies from 1973 to 1987, only 3.6% of these tumors occurred in the sinonasal tract.[2]

Despite their statistically low incidence, sinonasal malignancies are a clinically significant group of neoplasms with an overall grave outlook. They usually present at an advanced tumor stage, and often surgeons are reluctant to be appropriately aggressive for fear of creating either an undesirable cosmetic deformity, prolonged morbidity, or gross dysfunction. Furthermore the complex, compact anatomy of the region often limits the extent of surgical resection and contributes to serious radiotherapeutic complications.[3, 4] Although surgery remains the primary treatment modality, combined chemotherapy and radiation therapy now play a significant role for these patients, especially for those who present with advanced disease.

Sinonasal tumors can remain clinically silent until they reach an advanced stage. In addition, coexisting infection can overshadow the clinical presentation, further delaying diagnosis. Patients with antral and ethmoidal cancers have an average delay of 6 months between the onset of symptoms and the establishment of a final diagnosis.[3] Pain secondary to malignancy usually signifies an advanced tumor stage and possible perineural tumor invasion, especially with adenoid cystic carcinoma. Tooth or gum pain may indicate an antral tumor, whereas a headache may signify skull base invasion and intracranial extension. Inexplicably, pain is not often associated with the bone destruction that accompanies these tumors. Common complaints of patients with sinonasal tumors include diplopia, decreasing vision, proptosis, nasal stuffiness, anosmia, nasal-quality voice, epistaxis, and a facial mass. Maxillary sinus tumors cause trismus, epiphora, orbital pain, proptosis, or trigeminal or sphenopalatine ganglion–related deficits secondary to dorsal tumor spread. Ethmoid tumors usually cause nasal stuffiness, orbital complaints, and headache from intracranial tumor spread. Frontal sinus tumors may deform the face, spread intracranially, or extend into the orbits, while sphenoid sinus tumors can extend into the nasopharynx, intracranially (especially to the cavernous sinuses), and into the orbit.

With improved imaging technology, superior tumor mapping and staging are now available, and this accurate information permits more realistic treatment planning with regard to cure versus palliation.[5] Surgical techniques have also improved, and better tumor extirpation can be achieved with less morbidity and facial deformity. In addition, enhanced tumor mapping equates with more accurate

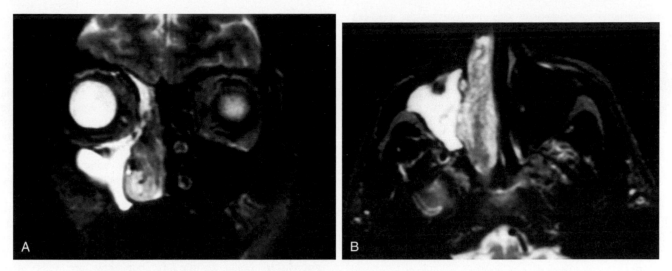

**FIGURE 6-1**   Coronal (**A**) and axial (**B**) T2-weighted MR images show a polypoid, nonhomogeneous right nasal fossa mass that has intermediate signal intensity. The right maxillary sinus, the right lateral ethmoid sinuses, and the lower nasal fossa have high signal intensity material that represents obstructed secretions. The tumor does not extend directly to the orbital margin. Such a high degree of tumor mapping was not possible on CT, where the secretions and tumor had similar attenuations. This patient had an inverted papilloma and obstructed secretions.

placement of radiation fields. To provide the tumor mapping necessary for decisions regarding resectability and curability, the radiologist must be aware of the critical areas of tumor extension that will alter a surgical or irradiation treatment plan. These areas include tumor extension into the floor of the anterior and middle cranial fossae, the pterygopalatine fossae, the orbits, and the palate.[6] The proximity of the paranasal sinuses and their structural communication via the nasal fossae allow tumor spread between sinuses. Thus the radiologist must describe in detail the sinus and the precise areas within each sinus that are apparently affected by neoplasm. Although primarily a communication tool with clinicians, gray scale and color 3D reconstructions allow the tumor to be visualized within the framework of the facial bones and skull base. Newer treatment-planning computers are now able to utilize the raw data of these images to help prepare treatment plans.[7]

Nodal metastasis from sinonasal carcinomas is one of the gravest prognostic signs. The retropharyngeal nodes are the primary lymph nodes draining the paranasal sinuses and nasal vault. However, these nodes or their lymphatic channels are frequently obliterated by repeated childhood infections. Accordingly, for adults, sinonasal malignancies often metastasize to the secondary nodes in levels I and II (see Chapter 36). Such nodal metastases occur in approximately 15% of patients and are associated with tumor extension to the skin, alveolar buccal sulcus, or pterygoid musculature, often as demonstrated on CT and MR studies.[4] Thus the radiologist should be thorough and precise in reporting tumor extension in these sites. The presence of cervical nodal disease is predictive of distant metastases, which have been found in 34% of autopsied patients.[6]

One of the major imaging problems of precise tumor mapping is distinguishing tumor from adjacent inflammatory disease. Basing this distinction on routine CT attenuation values is fraught with inaccuracies. Contrast-enhanced CT can improve the results; however, MR imaging is superior in making this distinction. Inflammatory secretions

and tissues have high water content and thus have high T2-weighted signal intensities (see Chapter 5). By comparison, virtually all sinonasal tumors are highly cellular, with relatively little intracellular and intercellular water, and the majority of these tumors have an intermediate signal intensity on T2-weighted images (Figs. 6-1 and 6-2).[8, 9] Thus, the mainstay of the MR imaging distinction between tumor and adjacent inflammatory tissues is the T2-weighted MR sequence. It is rare for sinonasal tumors to have inherently high T2-weighted signal intensities, which may be seen with benign or low-grade minor salivary gland tumors, schwannomas, rare hemangiomatous lesions, and polypoid tumors such as inverted papillomas. Therefore these tumors may not be as amenable to accurate T2-weighted tumor mapping.

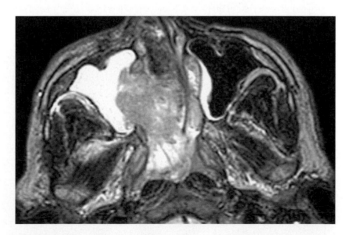

**FIGURE 6-2**   Axial T2-weighted MR image shows a large right-sided nasal fossa mass that has destroyed most of the medial wall of the right maxillary sinus and extends back into the nasopharynx. The mass has areas of high signal intensity that represent sites of necrosis. The right maxillary sinus is obstructed, and inflammatory mucosal thickening is seen in the left antrum. This patient had a squamous cell carcinoma and obstructed secretions.

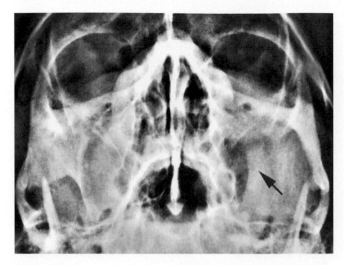

**FIGURE 6-3** Waters view shows that the lateral wall of the left maxillary sinus is totally destroyed (*arrow*). The right lateral antral wall is intact. This is an example of aggressive bone destruction. This patient had a squamous cell carcinoma of the left antrum.

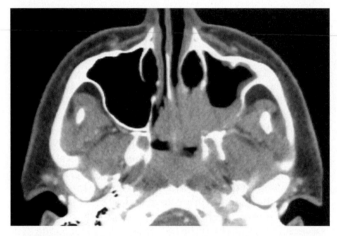

**FIGURE 6-4** Axial CT scan shows a destructive mass in the left posterior nasal fossa that has destroyed portions of the medial and posterior left maxillary sinus walls. There is also some destruction of the left pterygoid process, and tumor extends into the left retromaxillary fat. This patient had a squamous cell carcinoma.

Small tumors may often elude clinical and radiologic detection. Unfortunately, it is at this early stage that tumors may be most curable.[4] Small sinonasal tumors often have MR characteristics indistinguishable from those of adjacent inflammation. In addition, radiologists are reluctant to diagnose a tumor in the absence of adjacent bone involvement. Thus, on imaging, many small tumors are often misdiagnosed as inflammatory polypoid disease. Bony changes are seen in larger tumors and allow for a more definitive imaging diagnosis of neoplasm. The pattern of bone involvement (either aggressive bone destruction or bone remodeling) can aid in generating a radiographic differential diagnosis.[10–12]

Squamous cell carcinoma is associated with aggressive bone erosion, usually with only small bony fragments remaining (Figs. 6-3 to 6-6). Metastatic carcinomas, as well as some sarcomas and lymphomas, can also cause aggressive bone destruction, but they are less often encountered. By comparison, most sinonasal mucoceles, polyps, inverted papillomas, and rarer lesions such as minor salivary gland tumors, schwannomas, extramedullary plasmacytomas, most lymphomas, olfactory neuroblastomas, most sarcomas, and hemangiopericytomas tend to primarily remodel rather than aggressively destroy bone (Fig. 6-7).

For most tumors, one of these patterns of bone involvement appears to be dominant. Although the bony pattern is not sufficiently specific to predict histology, the radiologist can still use the type of bone involvement to occasionally question some histologic diagnoses. Thus, if a patient has a unilateral polypoid nasal mass and a microscopic diagnosis of a "large cell lymphoma," but the radiographic pattern of bone destruction is predominantly aggressive, the radiologist might question this diagnosis and recommend ancillary diagnostic tests such as immunohistochemistry. This might lead to a diagnosis such as "sinonasal undifferentiated carcinoma" (SNUC), which is in the pathologic differential diagnosis of large cell lymphoma. In fact, immunohistochemistry is routinely performed for all sinonasal "round cell" tumors to distinguish between SNUC, sinonasal neuroendocrine tumor (SNEC), olfactory neuroblastoma, malignant lymphoma, embryonal rhabdo-

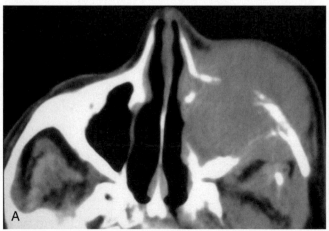
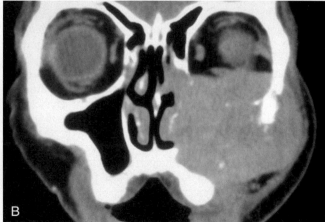

**FIGURE 6-5** Axial (**A**) and coronal (**B**) CT scans show a large left maxillary sinus mass that has destroyed most of the sinus walls and the body of the zygoma. The tumor extends into the left lower ethmoid complex, the left orbit, and the left retromaxillary fat in the infratemporal fossa. This patient had a squamous cell carcinoma.

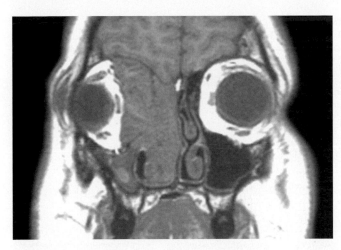

**FIGURE 6-6** Coronal T1-weighted MR image shows a large intermediate signal intensity mass that fills the right ethmoid complex and nasal fossa. The tumor extends into the right orbit, and there is erosion of part of the roof and medial floor of the right orbit, the fovea ethmoidalis, and the right cribriform plate, as evidenced by the loss of the bone signal void in these areas. The right maxillary sinus is obstructed by the tumor. This patient had a squamous cell carcinoma.

myosarcoma, extramedullary plasmacytoma, olfactory neuroblastoma, and amelanotic melanoma. Immunohistochemistry may be performed on unstained slides from the original biopsy (Table 6-1).

Tumor biology and prognosis are multifaceted issues. Host immune surveillance may limit tumor growth for a variable period of time, sometimes for many years. Successive activation of tumoral oncogenes or additional loss of tumor suppressor genes correlates with tumor progression or the acquisition of aggressive features (see Chapter 44), but the lethal propensity of certain tumors is, unfortunately, poorly understood. In addition to tumor biology, the critical anatomic location of the neoplasm has prognostic significance. Thus a lesion confined to the antrum generally has a better prognosis than one located in the pterygopalatine fossa or central skull base. However, certain tumors are highly aggressive regardless of location and despite a noninfiltrating imaging appearance. For example, a nasal fossa melanoma usually has a benign polypoid imaging appearance, yet the 5-year survival prognosis is abysmal (Fig. 6-8). Thus, the invasive, or lack of invasive, margins of a tumor cannot always be used to predict biologic aggressiveness. Clearly, the pathologic diagnosis is more important in predicting prognosis than the imaging appearance of a tumor. Yet, the radiographic tumor mapping may also predict survival if critical anatomic areas are involved that are not readily amenable to treatment.

Sclerotic bone is usually not seen with neoplastic processes and is more commonly seen with bacterial inflammatory disease or more aggressive infection (e.g., fungal disease) or granulomatous disease. Frank sinonasal osteomyelitis usually appears as foci of bone rarefaction and sclerosis, often with sequestra. Radiation osteitis also can produce a similar bone reaction. Tumor invasion rarely causes osteoblastic bony sclerosis, but it can occur with

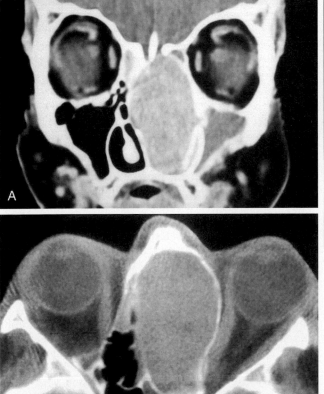

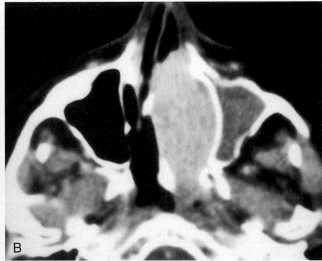

**FIGURE 6-7** Coronal (**A**) and axial (**B**) contrast-enhanced CT scans show a primarily expansile left nasal fossa mass that has obstructed the left antrum and some of the remaining upper left ethmoid cells, which are filled with lower-attenuation secretions. There is focal bone erosion of the left cribriform plate. This patient had an olfactory neuroblastoma. (**C**) Axial CT scan on another patient who has an expansile nasal fossa and left ethmoid sinus mass around which the facial bones are remodeled. This is not the appearance expected of a typical squamous cell carcinoma. This patient had a schwannoma.

## Table 6–1
## IMMUNOHISTOCHEMICAL ANALYSIS OF ENT MALIGNANCIES

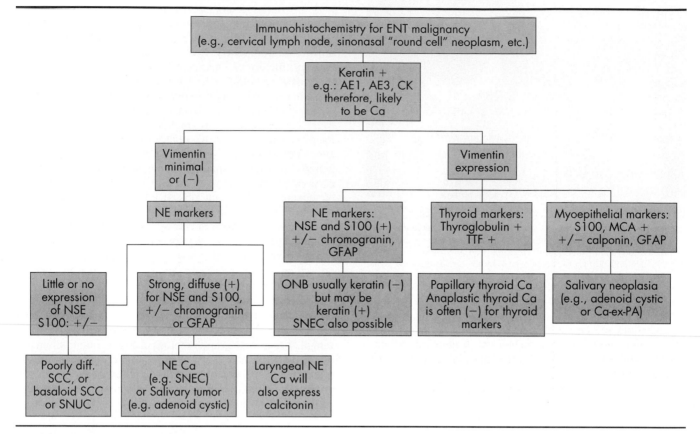

AE1, AE3, CK = low- and high-molecular weight keratins
Ca = carcinoma
Calponin = a marker of late smooth muscle differentiation
GFAP = glial fibrillary acidic protein
Keratin = a structural protein of epithelial differentiation
MCA = muscle cell actin
NE = neuroendocrine
NSE = neuron specific enolase

ONB = olfactory neuroendocrine carcinoma
S100 = a protein expressed in myriad neuronal and mesenchymal tissues
SCC = squamous cell carcinoma
SNUC = sinonasal undifferentiated carcinoma
SNEC = sinonasal neuroendocrine carcinoma
TTF = thyroglobulin transcription factor
Vimentin = an intermediate filament

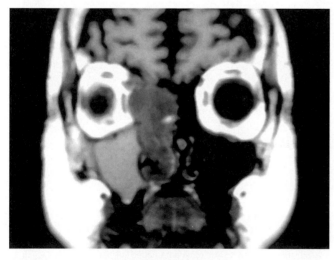

**FIGURE 6-8** Coronal T1-weighted MR image shows a low signal intensity mass in the right ethmoid complex and nasal fossa. The tumor has broken into the right orbit, but the tumor interface with the orbital fat is smooth and not infiltrative. The right maxillary sinus is chronically obstructed with intermediate signal intensity secretions. This patient had a melanoma.

anaplastic carcinoma, nasopharyngeal carcinoma, and osteosarcoma. Fibrous dysplasia and ossifying fibroma both result in characteristic dense, expanded bone. The sclerotic facial bone changes of Paget's disease may be indistinguishable from those of osteoblastic metastatic prostate cancer, but the presence of associated pagetoid calvarial disease allows differentiation. Osteoblastic metastases from breast carcinoma can occur; however, such lesions are usually a mixed blastic and lytic process. Dense osteoblastic bone may also be found as a reaction to meningiomas.

Tumoral calcifications in the sinonasal cavities are uncommon. Discrete solitary or multiple calcifications within a mass usually signify a chronic inflammatory process, either bacterial or fungal. Such calcifications have also been reported with osteoblastomas, osteochondromas, chondromas, chondrosarcomas, and olfactory neuroblastomas. "Calcifications" can be seen in inverted papillomas; however, these radiodensities are actually foci of residual bone. Diffuse calcifications within a lesion with invasive margins auger a sarcoma rather than a carcinoma, usually either a chondrosarcoma, an osteosarcoma, or an undifferentiated sarcoma.

Despite the long list of diagnostic possibilities, a unilateral polypoid nasal mass with "calcifications" is most likely to be either an olfactory neuroblastoma or an inverted papilloma. A nasal septal mass with calcifications is most likely to be either a chondroid tumor or the result of fungal disease.

As mentioned, although the radiologist is constantly tempted to offer pathologic diagnoses, there are only rare instances in which the CT and MR imaging is specifically pathognomonic. Therefore, the primary radiographic contribution is accurate tumor mapping, with awareness of the critical anatomic sites that will influence treatment planning. Final treatment planning must await pathologic diagnosis.

## BENIGN AND MALIGNANT EPITHELIAL TUMORS

### Papilloma

The term *Schneiderian mucosa* refers to the ectodermally derived lining of the nasal cavity and paranasal sinuses, composed generally of stratified ciliated columnar cells, loose abundant lamina propria, and minor salivary glands and on their ducts. This unique mucosa may give rise to three distinct histomorphologic papillomas: fungiform, inverted, and oncocytic, collectively called Schneiderian papillomas.[1, 13] Schneiderian papillomas are uncommon, representing only 0.4% to 4.7% of all sinonasal tumors, which are 25 to 50 times less common than the pedestrian polyp.[13] These papillomas are not the result of allergy, chronic infection, smoking, or other noxious environmental agents, as they are almost invariably unilateral. It has been suggested that their rarity in children mitigates against a viral etiology.[14-16] However, many sensitive and specific viral studies confirm the association of fungiform and inverted papillomas with human papilloma virus.[17, 18]

Fungiform papillomas (septal, squamous, or exophytic) comprise 50% of Schneiderian papillomas. They usually occur in males between the ages of 20 to 50 years, and 95% arise on the nasal septum. They are solitary (75%) and unilateral (96%), have a warty or verrucous appearance, and are quite unlikely to undergo malignant transformation.[13, 14, 19] Histologically, fungiform papillomas have stratified keratinized squamous mucosa on fibrovascular stalks.

Inverted papillomas (endophytic papillomas) comprise 47% of Schneiderian papillomas and most commonly occur in males between the ages of 40 to 70 years. Characteristically, they arise from the lateral nasal wall near the middle turbinate and extend into the sinuses. This secondary extension involves the maxillary and ethmoidal sinuses, but extension into the sphenoid and frontal sinuses has been documented.[13, 14, 20] Rarely, an isolated inverted papilloma may arise within a sinus without any nasal involvement. Inverted papillomas rarely arise from the nasal septal wall, and fewer than 4% occur bilaterally.[13, 14] The most common presenting symptoms are nasal obstruction, epistaxis, and anosmia. Secondary sinusitis and tumor extension into the sinuses and orbits can cause pain, purulent nasal discharge, proptosis, diplopia, and a nasal vocal quality.

Macroscopically, inverted papillomas appear as hard white polyps with a wrinkled, prune-like surface. Microscopically, hyperplastic squamous epithelium can be seen replacing seromucinous ducts and glands, resulting in an endophytic growth pattern (Fig. 6-9). The surrounding mucosa usually reveals squamous metaplasia and hyperplasia, considered incipient changes. For this reason, mere polypectomy results in high recurrence rates that vary from 27% to 73%.[13] Lateral rhinotomy with en bloc resection of the lateral nasal wall and mucosa is the preferred procedure for all but the smallest localized lesions. This more extensive surgical approach has decreased recurrence rates to 0% to 14%, with most relapses occurring within 2 years.[13, 14] However, there has been a controversial trend over the last decade of more conservative endoscopic management, which is indicated only for the treatment of more limited lesions with planned surveillance. Thus, the radiologist may assist the surgeon in choosing the optimal surgical approach by not only mapping the lesion but noting its size.[21, 22]

Carcinoma-ex-inverted papilloma has been reported in 3% to 24% (average, 13%) of cases. Carcinoma may be concurrent with, or develop subsequent to, inverted papilloma. Most reported malignancies are squamous cell carcinomas, but verrucous carcinoma, mucoepidermoid carcinoma, spindle cell carcinoma, clear cell carcinoma, and adenocarcinomas may also occur.[13]

Oncocytic Schneiderian papillomas (cylindric cell papillomas) represent only 3% of the Schneiderian papillomas. They are similar to inverted papillomas in their affinity for the lateral nasal wall, age of onset, and predominance in males. On gross examination, they are beefy red and soft, mimicking malignancy. Microscopically, there are stratified, tall (cylindrical) oncocytic cells with numerous small intraepithelial cysts filled with mucin and neutrophils (Fig. 6-10). The cysts occasionally cause confusion with rhinosporidiosis, but slightly more than superficial perusal at high power can end this confusion.[13]

The imaging findings for all of these papillomas can vary from a small nasal polypoid mass to an expansile nasal mass that has remodeled the nasal vault and extended into the sinuses, causing secondary obstructive sinusitis[23] (Figs. 6-11 to 6-13). The MR and CT findings are nonspecific.[24, 25]

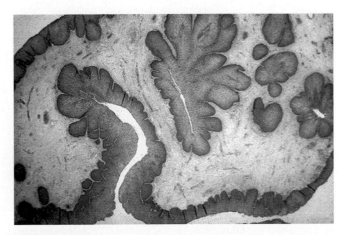

**FIGURE 6-9**   Inverted papilloma. Nonkeratinizing squamous epithelium proliferates within this loose stroma, forming ribbons and invaginating islands.

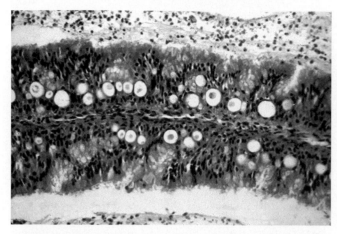

**FIGURE 6-10**    Oncocytic Schneiderian papilloma (cylindrical papilloma). This unusual form of Schneiderian papilloma is composed of tall oncocytes with a microglandular pattern. It can resemble, and may contain areas of, inverted papilloma.

Although apparent calcifications have been reported within the inverted papillomas, these radiodensities are in reality residual bone fragments.[21, 26] Nonetheless, the imaging differential diagnosis of a unilateral polypoid mass with apparent calcifications must include inverted papilloma (Fig. 6-14). The nasal septum usually remains intact, but it may be bowed to the opposite side by the mass. In patients with prior surgery including a medial antrectomy for an inverted papilloma, any polypoid mass that bridges the antral-nasal border on imaging must be considered a recurrence. A unilateral mass localized to the lateral nasal wall and the middle meatus region is predictive of inverted papilloma. A lobulated surface pattern, also typical, was noted in 19 of the 29 CT scans of cases.[27] Although a septal-based solitary polypoid mass could be any of these papillomas, the location most strongly suggests a fungiform papilloma. When an area of aggressive bone destruction is seen along the margin of an inverted papilloma, the radiologist must raise the possibility of an associated carcinoma.

## Squamous Cell Carcinoma

Overall, cancer of the nasal cavity and paranasal sinuses is uncommon. In the United States, the incidence is reported to be 0.75 per 100,000 people.[28] From 25% to 58% of the sinonasal carcinomas arise in the antrum, 25% to 35% arise in the nasal cavity, 10% arise in the ethmoid complex, and only 1% arise in the sphenoid and frontal sinuses.[1, 13] Secondary extension to the maxillary sinus is common, occurring in 80% of patients with sinonasal carcinoma. A number of occupations have been epidemiologically linked to sinonasal malignancies. Workers exposed to nickel have a 40–250 times greater chance of developing squamous cell cancer.[29] Workers involved in the production of wood furniture, chromium, mustard gas, isopropyl alcohol, and radium are also at risk for developing carcinomas of the nasal cavity and paranasal sinuses. The latency period from onset of occupational exposure to tumor discovery may be up to three decades. Some 15% to 20% of the patients have a history of chronic sinusitis and polyposis; however, a causal relationship is doubtful.[13] Coexistent inverted and cylindric cell papillomas, previous irradiation, and immunosuppression (i.e., lack of immune surveillance) may increase the risk of developing sinonasal carcinoma.[13, 30] Metachronous or synchronous tumors are seen in 15% of patients with sinonasal carcinomas; 40% of the secondary tumors occur in the head and neck, and 60% occur below the clavicles in the lungs, gastrointestinal tract, and breasts.[13]

Histologically, squamous cell carcinoma (SCC) can be recognized as infiltrating broad bands, nested islands, or small clusters of malignant cells, which have a variable amount of eosinophilic cytoplasm. Keratin formation within cells, and between groups of cells (keratin pearls) belies the tumor's mucosal origins. Intercellular bridges may also be seen, appearing as fine hair-like connections between malignant cells (Fig. 6-15). Poorly differentiated or undifferentiated SCC produce little or no keratin by light microscopy. These cells can appear as oval malignant cells with little cytoplasm and large nucleoli, mimicking large cell lymphoma. They may be confirmed as

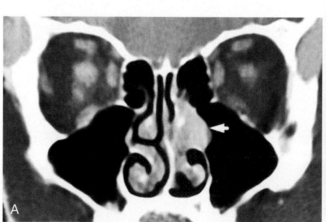
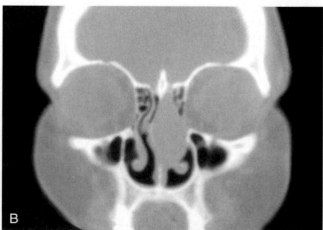

**FIGURE 6-11**    **A,** Coronal CT scan shows a small polypoid mass in the left nasal fossa (*arrow*) obliterating the middle meatus. There is no associated bone destruction. This patient had an inverted papilloma. **B,** Coronal CT scan on another patient shows an expansile left nasal fossa polypoid mass that bows the nasal septum to the right. There is no gross bone erosion. This patient had an inverted papilloma.

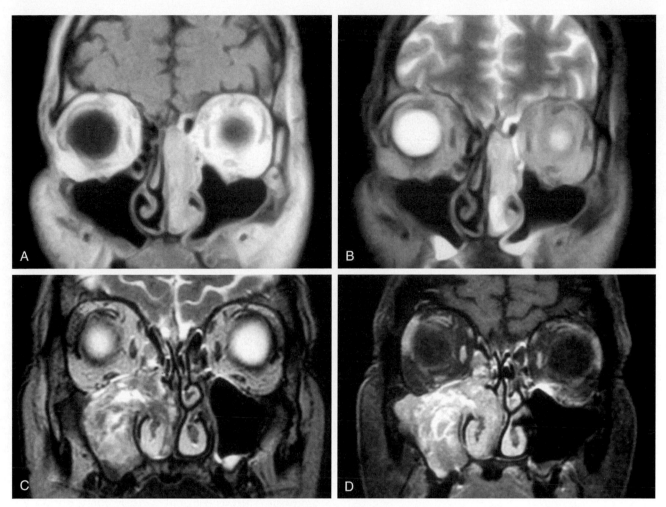

**FIGURE 6-12**   Coronal T1-weighted (**A**) and T2-weighted (**B**) MR images show a left nasal fossa and an ethmoid sinus mass. There is no gross infiltrative bone destruction, and there are obstructed secretions in the upper and most lateral left ethmoid cells. This patient had an inverted papilloma. Coronal T2-weighted (**C**) and T1-weighted (**D**), fat-suppressed, contrast-enhanced MR images show an expansile right maxillary sinus mass that extends into the right nasal fossa and ethmoid complex. The mass has highly irregular mixed signal intensity, possibly suggesting a disorganized-type tumor. This patient had an inverted papilloma and illustrates the poor correlation that often exists between the MR appearance of tumor organization and the actual pathology of the lesion.

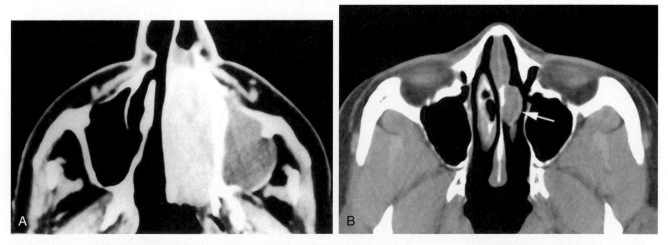

**FIGURE 6-13**   Axial CT scan (**A**) shows a large, expansile, enhancing mass in the left nasal fossa that has obstructed the left maxillary sinus, causing a mucocele to form, as noted by the modeled left antral wall. The nasal vault bones are intact. This patient had an inverted papilloma. Axial CT scan (**B**) on another patient shows a polypoid mass arising from the left side of the nasal septum (*arrow*). No erosion of the septum is seen. This patient had a fungiform papilloma.

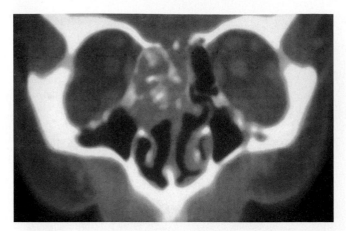

**FIGURE 6-14** Coronal CT scan shows a right ethmoid sinus and an upper nasal fossa mass. The right lamina papyracea is intact, and there is thinning or erosion of the cribriform plate. There are also apparent calcifications within the tumor. This patient had an inverted papilloma. The radiodensities were pieces of residual bone and not tumoral calcifications.

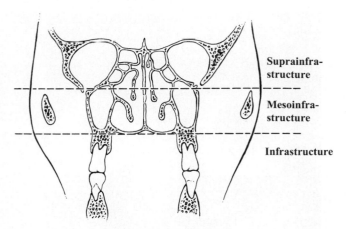

**FIGURE 6-16** Diagram of a coronal view of the sinonasal cavities. The lines divide the maxillary sinuses into three zones: suprastructure, mesostructure, and infrastructure. Tumors limited to and below the mesostructure usually can be resected by a partial or total maxillectomy without an orbital exenteration. Tumors involving the suprastructure usually need an orbital exenteration to reduce the chance of tumor recurrence.

SCC by immunohistochemistry, which reveals keratin expression.

Carcinomas of the nasal cavity tend to occur in males between 55 and 65 years of age. Most are low-grade tumors arising on the nasal septum near the mucocutaneous junction. The middle turbinate is also a common site. Patient prognosis relates to tumor stage rather than exact site within the nasal cavity.[30, 31] The treatment may be surgery, irradiation, or both. Local recurrences are found in 20% to 50% of the cases, and about 80% of these develop within the first year. Only 15% develop nodal metastases and only 10% have distant metastases. The overall 5-year survival rate is 62%.

Carcinoma of the maxillary sinus has been the most extensively studied of the sinonasal malignancies. The specific site of origin of antral carcinomas is thought to have prognostic significance and is important in planning therapy and in comparing the treatment results of various medical centers. Historically, the antrum was divided into an infrastructure and a suprastructure; however, this classification was soon modified into an infrastructure, a mesostructure, and a suprastructure, with the lines of division being

drawn on a coronal view of the sinuses through the antral floor and the antral roof (Fig. 6-16).[32] Using this system, tumors limited to the mesostructure and infrastructure require a partial or total maxillectomy, whereas tumors that involve the suprastructure require a total maxillectomy and possible orbital exenteration. Ohngren divided the antrum into posterosuperior and anteroinferior segments by drawing a line on a lateral view of the face from the medial canthus to the angle of the mandible (Fig. 6-17). He suggested that tumors limited to the anteroinferior segment had a better prognosis.[32] It was not until the early 1960s that the TNM

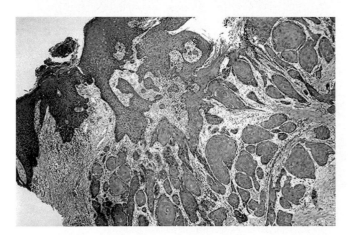

**FIGURE 6-15** Squamous cell carcinoma: Irregularly shaped infiltrating islands of carcinoma are present below the surface mucosa. The eosinophilia of these islands indicates keratinization.

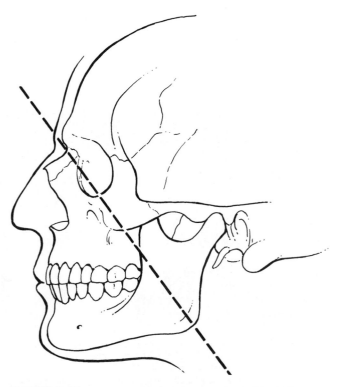

**FIGURE 6-17** Diagram of the lateral view of a skull with Ohngren's line drawn. Tumors anterior to this line tend to have a better prognosis.

system was first applied to antral cancers, and in 1976 the American Joint Committee on Cancer (AJCC) developed a TNM system based on Ohngren's line.[32] Harrison has criticized this TNM classification because it does not correspond to the clinical experience with these tumors.[33] He suggested that T-1 tumors should be defined as those neoplasms that are limited to the antral mucosa, without bone erosion and without regard to Ohngren's line, because clinically it is often impossible to determine where this line occurs. A T-2 tumor has bone erosion but no extension beyond the bone, and a T-3 tumor has extension to the orbit, ethmoid complex, or facial skin. Finally, a T-4 tumor extends to the nasopharynx, sphenoidal sinus, cribriform plate, or pterygopalatine fossa. In 1997, the AJCC modified its staging definitions as follows: TX = the primary tumor cannot be assessed; T0 − no evidence of disease; Tis = carcinoma in situ; T1 = tumor limited to the antral mucosa, with no erosion or destruction of bone; T2 = tumor causing bone erosion or destruction, except for the posterior antral wall, including extension into the hard palate and/or the middle nasal meatus; T3 = tumor invasion of any of the following: bone of the posterior wall of the maxillary sinus, subcutaneous tissues, skin of the cheek, floor or medial wall of the orbit, infratemporal fossa, pterygoid plates, or ethmoid sinuses; T4 = tumor invasion of orbital contents beyond the floor or medial wall including any of the following: the orbital apex, cribriform plate, base of the skull, nasopharynx, sphenoid, or frontal sinuses.[34]

Antral carcinomas are almost twice as common in men as in women, and nearly 95% occur in patients over age 40 years.[13, 35] The radioactive contrast medium Thorotrast is clearly established as an etiologic factor in antral carcinoma.

When the tumors are small, they often are misdiagnosed as chronic sinusitis, nasal polyposis, lacrimal duct obstruction, tic douloureux, or cranial arteritis. At diagnosis, 40% and 60% of patients have facial asymmetry, a tumor bulge in the oral cavity, and tumor extension in the nasal cavity. At least one of these findings is present in almost 90% of

cases.[36] Surgery plus adjuvant radiotherapy is the treatment of choice. Despite controversy in the literature, neoadjuvant radiation therapy provides no survival advantage compared to postoperative radiation therapy; the latter is associated with fewer complications.[13] Orbital exenteration is performed only if orbital periosteum is involved with tumor, as documented during surgery, either by gross examination or frozen section evaluation. Curative surgery generally is not attempted if there is central skull base destruction, tumor in the pterygopalatine fossa, tumor extension into the nasopharynx, regional or generalized metastases, advanced patient age, poor general patient health, or patient refusal to accept treatment.[13, 37] The 5-year survival rate varies from 20% to almost 40%, with mean figures ranging from 25% to 30%.[38] The main cause of failure is local recurrence, and 75% of these occur within 5 months of initial treatment.

Although more than 100 cases of primary frontal sinus carcinoma have been reported, it is still a rare entity. The presenting symptoms are similar to those of acute frontal sinusitis; patients have pain and swelling over the frontal sinus. However, in patients with frontal sinus carcinoma the frontal bone erodes rapidly, and few patients survive for more than 2 years.[4, 39]

Primary sphenoid sinus carcinoma is also rare. It is often difficult to distinguish primary sphenoid carcinoma from secondary extension from a posterior ethmoid or nasal fossa carcinoma. As with frontal sinus carcinomas, few of these patients survive longer than 1 or 2 years. Intracranial extension of squamous carcinoma is relatively common; however, an associated subarachnoid hemorrhage is rare.[40]

Poorly differentiated squamous cell carcinoma can be confused histologically with rhabdomyosarcoma, melanoma, large cell lymphoma, SNEC, and anaplastic plasmacytoma.[41] As mentioned, immunohistochemistry can confirm the diagnosis (Table 6-1).

On plain films, all patients with paranasal sinus carcinoma have a soft-tissue sinus mass, and 70% to 90% have evidence of bone destruction (Fig. 6-18).[35, 42] The primary reason to perform sectional imaging on these patients is to

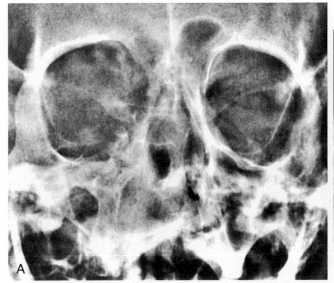
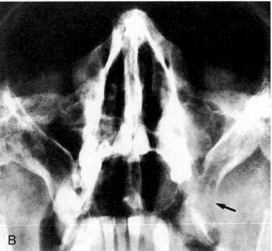

**FIGURE 6-18**   **A,** Caldwell view shows clouding of the right ethmoid and maxillary sinuses, with destruction of the right lamina papyracea and a portion of the floor of the right orbit. Squamous cell carcinoma. **B,** Waters view shows destruction of the lower lateral wall of the left maxillary sinus (*arrow*).

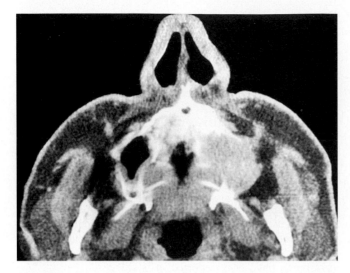

**FIGURE 6-19**   Axial CT scan shows an aggressively destructive lesion of the lower left antrum and palate. This patient had a squamous cell carcinoma.

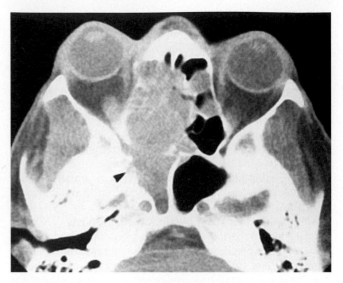

**FIGURE 6-21**   Axial CT scan shows a destructive lesion of the right ethmoid sinus that has extended into the nasal fossa and the sphenoid sinus. There is focal erosion of the skull base (*arrowhead*). This patient had a squamous cell carcinoma.

better visualize the extent of spread beyond the sinus cavity. On contrast-enhanced CT, carcinomas have a variable but slight enhancement. On MR imaging, these tumors have an intermediate T1-weighted and a slightly higher T2-weighted signal intensity. Carcinomas also enhance with contrast. Sinus carcinomas are fairly homogeneous; however, larger tumors may have areas of necrosis and hemorrhage (Figs. 6-5 and 6-19 to 6-37). The characteristic imaging feature of these carcinomas is their strong tendency to destroy bone aggressively, regardless of tumor differentiation. Bone remodeling is uncommon. Usually the area of bone destruction is substantial compared with the size of the soft-tissue tumor mass. However, the imaging findings are not specific.[43]

*Basaloid squamous carcinoma* refers to an aggressive, poorly differentiated variant of squamous carcinoma that may be confused with adenoid cystic carcinoma. We have seen a case in which there was CT and MR evidence of extensive bone destruction of the margins of the orbit, the floor of the middle cranial fossa, the right cavernous sinus,

and much of the calvaria. There was considerable dural disease and tumor in the right orbit, paranasal sinuses, and scalp, as well as mucoceles of the left ethmoidal sinus with desiccated secretions (Fig. 6-36).[44]

## Adenocarcinoma (Intestinal-Type Adenocarcinoma)

Approximately 10% of all sinonasal tumors are of glandular origin.[13] Sinonasal adenocarcinomas can be classified as either minor salivary gland tumors (e.g., adenoid cystic carcinomas, mucoepidermoid carcinomas, acinic cell carcinomas, and benign and malignant pleomor-

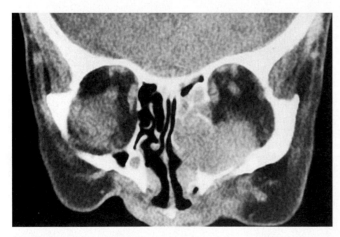

**FIGURE 6-20**   Coronal CT scan shows a destructive lesion of the left ethmoid sinus that has extended into the orbit. This patient had a squamous cell carcinoma.

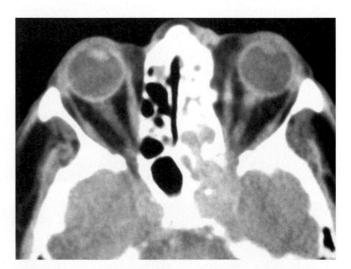

**FIGURE 6-22**   Axial contrast-enhanced CT scan shows a destructive mass in the sphenoid sinus and posterior ethmoid complex. The tumor erodes into the medial orbital apex and extends into the left cavernous sinus. This patient had a squamous cell carcinoma.

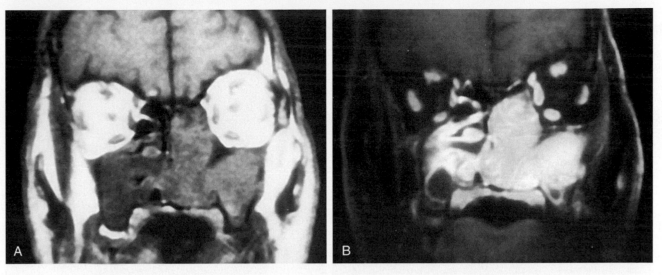

**FIGURE 6-23**    Coronal T1-weighted MR scans without contrast (**A**) and with contrast (**B**) show a mass in **A** of intermediate signal intensity that has destroyed some of the left antral walls and fills the left nasal fossa. Lower signal intensity material (secretions) fills the right antrum and nasal fossa. This appearance accurately reflected the findings at surgery. In **B**, the tumor enhances, the inflamed mucosa enhances, and some normal right ethmoid mucosa enhances. This presents a falsely large impression of the tumor size. This patient had a squamous cell carcinoma.

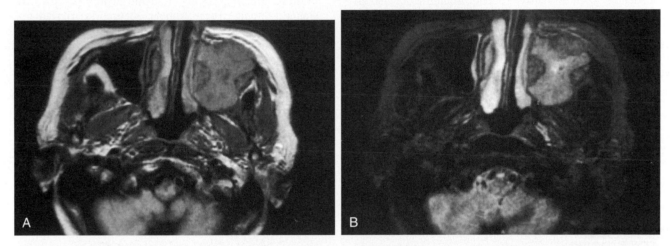

**FIGURE 6-24**    Axial T1-weighted (**A**) and T2-weighted (**B**) MR images show a destructive lesion in the left maxillary sinus that extends into the left infratemporal fossa and left cheek. The tumor has an intermediate signal intensity on both images but appears to brighten on the T2-weighted image. This is typical of most cellular tumors. Note that the tumor does not have as high a T2-weighted signal intensity as the turbinates or the inflamed mucosa along the medial wall of the right antrum. Such tumors almost never have a signal intensity that is lower on T2-weighted images than on T1-weighted images. This patient had a squamous cell carcinoma.

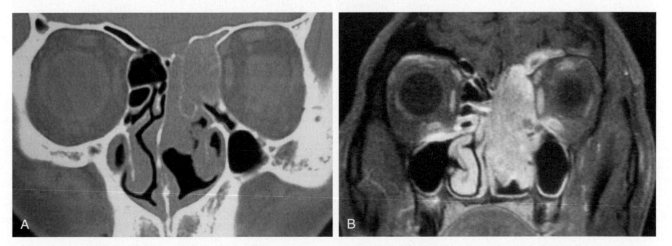

**FIGURE 6-25**    Coronal CT scan (**A**) shows a mass in the left ethmoid complex and upper nasal fossa. The bone in the region of the left cribriform plate and medial fovea ethmoidalis appears permeated but not completely destroyed. From this image, one might conclude that there is no intracranial disease. However, in **B**, a coronal T1-weighted, fat-suppressed, contrast-enhanced image, the enhancing tumor is seen to extend along the left floor of the anterior cranial fossa. This patient had a squamous cell carcinoma.

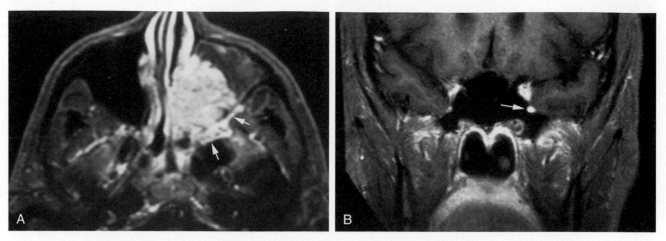

**FIGURE 6-26** Axial (**A**) and coronal (**B**) T1-weighted, fat-suppressed, contrast-enhanced images. (**A**) A destructive mass in the left nasal fossa and maxillary sinus with tumor in the left pterygopalatine and infratemporal fossae (*arrows*). In **B** the left second division of the trigeminal nerve (*arrow*) is enlarged and enhanced, signifying perineural tumor extension. This patient had a squamous cell carcinoma.

phic adenomas), intestinal-type adenocarcinomas, or sinonasal neuroendrocrine carcinomas.

Sinonasal *intestinal-type adenocarcinoma* (ITAC) was so named because of its histologic resemblance to various intestinal tumors, ranging from the benign polyp to frank adenocarcinoma. These tumors occur primarily in males (75% to 90% of cases) between 55 and 60 years of age. These tumors were first recognized among workers in the

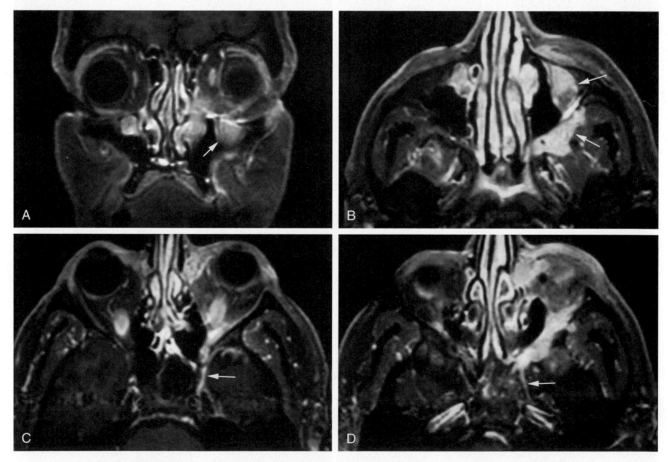

**FIGURE 6-27** A series of T1-weighted, fat-suppressed, contrast-enhanced MR images. In a coronal view (**A**), a tumor mass is seen in the upper medial lower left maxillary sinus, the left ethmoid complex, and the orbit. Tumor also is seen in the infraorbital nerve (*arrow*). An unrelated inverted papilloma is also present in the upper medial right antrum. In an axial view (**B**) the tumor is seen extending along the course of $V_2$ (*arrows*). In an axial view (**C**) the tumor extends along $V_2$ in the left cavernous sinus (*arrow*). In an axial view (**D**) the tumor extends along the vidian nerve (*arrow*). This patient had a squamous cell carcinoma.

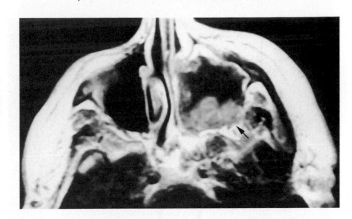

**FIGURE 6-28**   Axial T1-weighted, contrast-enhanced MR image shows a destructive lesion in the posterior left antrum. The tumor has extended into the infratemporal fossa (*arrow*). This patient had a squamous cell carcinoma.

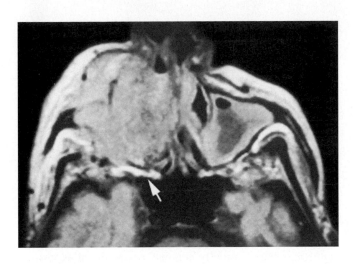

**FIGURE 6-29**   Axial proton density MR scan shows a large, destructive tumor in the right antrum. The zygoma and the soft tissues of the cheek have been invaded. However, the fat (*arrow*) in the pterygopalatine fossa remains intact. The lack of invasion of the central skull base greatly improves this patient's chance of cure. Incidentally noted are obstructed secretions in the left antrum. This patient had a squamous cell carcinoma.

**FIGURE 6-30**   Coronal T1-weighted (**A**) and sagittal (**B**) MR images show an intermediate signal intensity mass destroying the walls of the left maxillary sinus. There is minimal invasion of the orbital floor that was clinically silent. Incidental inflammatory mucosal thickening is present in the right antrum. This patient had a squamous cell carcinoma.

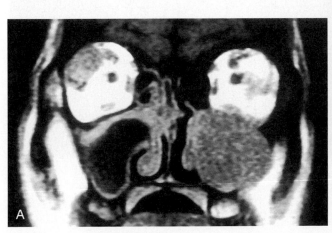

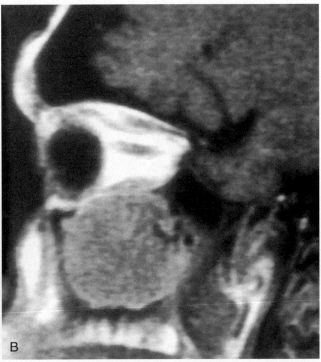

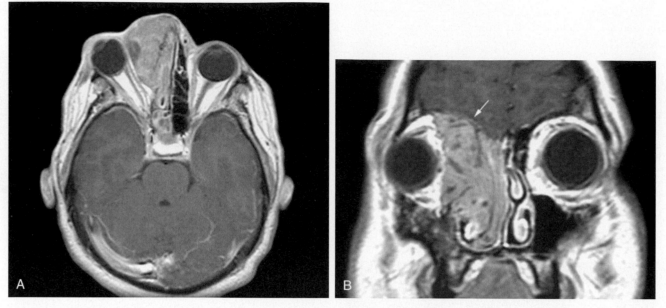

**FIGURE 6-31** Axial (**A**) and coronal (**B**) T1-weighted, fat-suppressed, contrast-enhanced MR images show a large tumor in the right ethmoid complex with extension into the orbit. The medial rectus muscle has been invaded, and the globe is laterally displaced and flattened by the tumor. In addition, in **B**, dural enhancement is seen (*arrow*), indicating tumor invasion. This patient had a squamous cell carcinoma.

hardwood and shoe industries and in people who use certain carcinogenic snuffs, particularly Bantus.[45, 46] Workers exposed to wood dust have an almost 900 times greater relative risk of developing adenocarcinoma and a 20 times greater relative risk of developing squamous carcinoma.[47, 48] ITAC can be classified as either low-grade or high-grade tumors. The papillary variant is invariably associated with low-grade cytology (grade I) and has a distinctly favorable prognosis (Fig. 6-37). The high-grade colonic or signet cell types especially resemble colonic and gastric carcinomas. In these cases, it is wise to rule out metastases from these gastrointestinal sites. Such an event is rare; only 6% of all metastases to the sinonasal cavities are from primary gastrointestinal tract tumors (the most common tumors that metastasize to the head and neck are tumors of the kidney, lung, breast, testis, and gastrointestinal tract).[13, 49] Patients with sporadic ITAC tend to have shorter survival times than those with occupational exposure–related tumors. The reason for this is related to the initial tumor stage at the time of discovery. Sporadic tumors, not associated with inhaled promoters, are more likely to occur in the maxillary sinus. By contrast, occupational exposure–associated ITAC are more likely to occur in the nasal cavity and ethmoids. The maxillary sinus tumors are more likely to become symptomatic and to be diagnosed at an advanced stage, unlike the nasal cavity and ethmoid tumors, which may become symptomatic before they invade local structures.[47, 48]

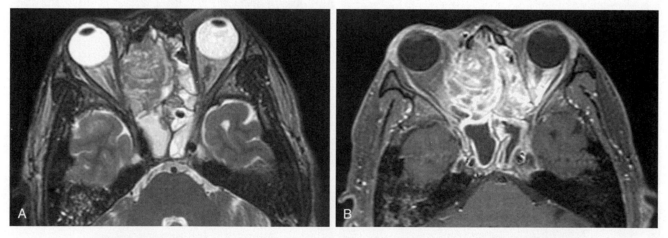

**FIGURE 6-32** Axial T2-weighted (**A**) and T1-weighted, fat-suppressed, contrast-enhanced MR images show a destructive mass in the right ethmoid complex and right orbit. Tumor extends into the left ethmoid complex. In **B**, there is poor separation of the tumor and any obstructed secretions in the left ethmoid cells. However, in **A**, this distinction is clear. There was no invasion of the left orbit. The sphenoid sinuses were obstructed. This patient had a squamous cell carcinoma.

The imaging characteristics of these tumors are nonspecific and are indistinguishable from those of squamous cell carcinoma.

## Salivary Tumors

### *Adenoid Cystic Carcinoma*

Salivary gland tumors can arise anywhere within the sinonasal cavities, but most commonly arise in the palate and then extend into the nasal fossae and paranasal sinuses. The most common diagnoses, in order of decreasing frequency, include adenoid cystic carcinoma, pleomorphic adenoma, mucoepidermoid carcinoma, adenocarcinoma not otherwise specified (NOS), acinic cell carcinoma, carcinoma ex-pleomorphic adenoma, and oncocytoma.[50]

Adenoid cystic carcinomas (ACC) account for about 35% of minor salivary gland tumors.[51] Of the primary sinonasal lesions, 47% arise in the maxillary sinuses, 32% involve the nasal fossae, 7% reside in the ethmoidal sinuses, 3% occur in the sphenoidal sinuses, and 2% are found in the frontal sinuses.[13] ACC usually arise in Caucasians between 30 and 60 years of age, although these neoplasms have been reported in an age range of 4 days to 86 years. Symptoms last an average of 5 years and relate to the mass effect and neural involvement of the tumor. A dull pain signals

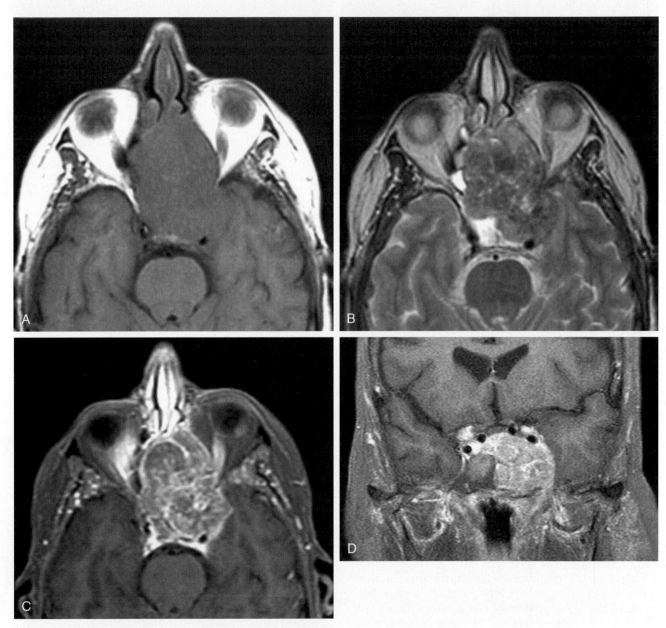

**FIGURE 6-33**   Axial T1-weighted (**A**), T2-weighted (**B**), and T1-weighted, fat-suppressed, contrast-enhanced (**C**) MR images show a destructive mass in the ethmoid sinuses, nasal fossae, and left cavernous sinus. The tumor has also broken into the left orbit. Note that in **B** there are obstructed secretions (high signal intensity) in the few remaining left ethmoid and sphenoid sinuses. In **C**, the tumor extension into the cavernous sinus and left temporal lobe is better seen. This is confirmed in **D**, a coronal T1-weighted, fat-suppressed, contrast-enhanced MR image. This patient had a squamous cell carcinoma.

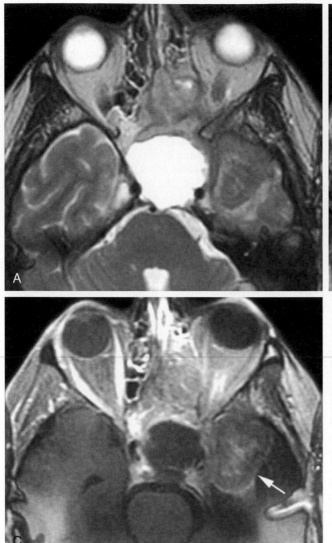

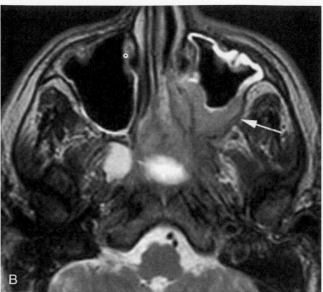

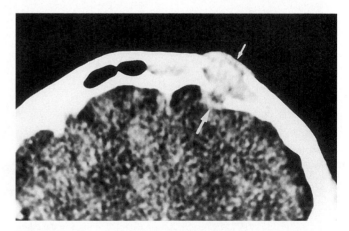

**FIGURE 6-34** Axial T2-weighted (**A** and **B**) and T1-weighted, fat-suppressed, contrast-enhanced (**C**) MR images show a mass involving the left ethmoid complex, the left orbit, the anterior wall of the sphenoid sinuses, and the posterior nasal fossa. The tumor has obstructed the sphenoid sinuses, and a mucocele has developed. In **B**, the tumor extends through the skull base, the pterygopalatine fossa, and the infratemporal fossa (*arrow*). Although the tumor extension into the medial left temporal lobe is seen in **A**, it is better seen in **C** (*arrow*).

perineural tumor invasion, which is characteristic of this tumor (see Chapter 13).

Histologically, ACC is composed of basaloid epithelial cells and myoepithelial cells. ACC forms three different architectural patterns: tubular, cribriform, and solid, with elaboration of a basement membrane and a collagenous matrix (Fig. 6-38). ACC that is predominantly tubular is considered well differentiated. If 30% or more is composed of cribriform patterns, it is classified as moderately differentiated. A poorly differentiated ACC is composed of 30% or more of the solid pattern. A temporal progression of patterns (grades) may be observed.[52]

"Skip lesions" within nerves are known to occur; thus, negative surgical margins have little prognostic significance. The local postsurgical recurrence rate is 62% within 1 year and 67% to 93% within 5 years.[13] The local recurrence rate for ACC is highest in the sinonasal tract (63%). While the rate of local recurrence is highest within the first 5 years, a significant number of patients develop locoregional recurrence after 10, 15, and 20 years. The 5-, 10-, and 15-year survival rates for 36 patients with sinonasal ACC (treated

**FIGURE 6-35** Axial CT scan shows an enhancing mass in the left frontal sinus that has eroded both the anterior (*small arrow*) and posterior (*large arrow*) sinus walls. This patient had a rare frontal sinus squamous cell carcinoma.

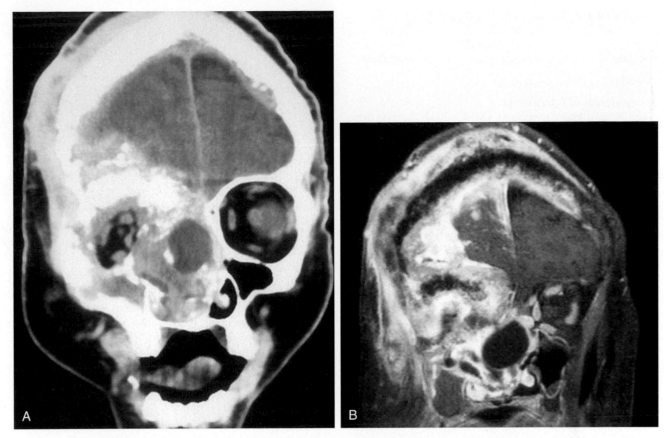

**FIGURE 6-36**   Coronal contrast-enhanced CT scan (**A**) and coronal T1-weighted, fat-suppressed, contrast-enhanced MR image (**B**) show a highly destructive tumor involving the nasal cavity, the right ethmoid and maxillary sinuses, the orbit, the right calvaria, dura, brain, and scalp. This highly aggressive tumor growth would be unusual for a typical squamous cell carcinoma. This patient had an adenosquamous carcinoma.

between 1962 and 1985) were 70%, 55%, and 55%.[53] Another report of 24 patients with sinonasal ACC (treated between 1962 and 1985) had similar survival rates at 5, 10, and 15 years (82%, 55%, and 43%).[54] As a result, 5-year survival data may give an erroneous indication of the absolute survival rate.[55] Some authorities have stated that no matter how long these patients have a disease-free interval,

they will eventually die of ACC. A solid or basaloid pattern is associated with a poorer outcome. Antral tumors have the worst prognosis; 46% of patients are alive at 5 years, but only 15% are disease free.[13] About half of the sinonasal tumors have distant metastases, primarily to the lungs, brain, cervical lymph nodes, and bone.

Wide surgical excision is the treatment of choice. ACC

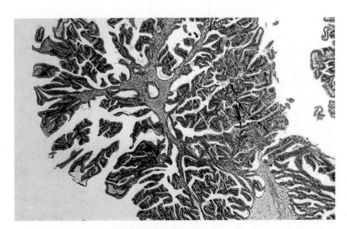

**FIGURE 6-37**   Intestinal-type adenocarcinoma (ITAC): This papillary tumor is composed of thin fronds lined by bland columnar epithelium. Although histologically bland, this low-grade ITAC is capable of local invasion.

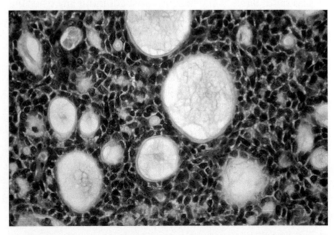

**FIGURE 6-38**   Adenoid cystic carcinoma (ACC): This high-power view shows a carcinoma composed of basaloid cells, here producing a cribriform (Swiss cheese) pattern.

are radiosensitive, but they are not curable with radiation therapy alone. Despite the fact that overall patient survival may not be affected by radiation treatment, better local tumor control may be achieved if postoperative irradiation is given.

### Mucoepidermoid Carcinoma

Mucoepidermoid carcinomas (MEC) rank third in frequency among sinonasal malignancies of the minor salivary glands after ACC and adenocarcinomas NOS. Most of these tumors involve the antrum and nasal cavity. Almost all minor salivary gland MEC are of the high-grade or intermediate-grade variety.[50]

Histologically, MEC is composed of epidermoid cells (squamous, keratin-producing cells), intermediate cells (large, clear, non-mucin-producing cells), and goblet or mucinous cells. Grading of MEC is more predictive when histologic features of aggression are taken into account, rather than basing grading on the relative proportion of solid, epidermoid areas to cystic, mucinous components.

The biologic activity of these high-grade and intermediate-grade lesions resembles that of the adenocarcinomas. Surgical resection with negative margins is the treatment of choice for sinonasal MEC. Adjuvant radiotherapy should be considered for inadequately resected cases. Tumor grade is a very important prognosticator for MEC, and preoperative knowledge of the tumor grade can be helpful in planning for a lymphatic dissection. While inadequately resected tumors will recur, a fully low-grade tumor acts no differently than a benign tumor; its ability to metastasize appears almost nil. There is not much data available concerning survival of patients with sinonasal MEC.

### Pleomorphic Adenoma

Benign mixed tumors of the sinonasal cavities are rare; most lesions occur within the nasal fossa. Usually they arise from the nasal septum, although one-fifth of the cases originate from the lateral nasal wall. The nasal septal location is curious because the septal submucosa is sparsely populated with minor salivary glands compared with the remainder of the sinonasal tract. A series of 41 cases of nasal cavity pleomorphic adenomas revealed that 90% of the cases originated from the septum and 10% (4 cases) arose in the lateral nasal wall.[56] The second most common site of origin is the maxillary sinus. Overall, pleomorphic adenoma is statistically the third most common minor salivary gland neoplasm.

Histologically, pleomorphic adenomas consist of epithelial and myoepithelial cells. The epithelial component produces ductal and glandular patterns, solid areas, and commonly undergoes squamous metaplasia. The myoepithelial component produces the abundant chondroid and myoid matrix so typical of these tumors (Fig. 6-39).

Intranasal and paranasal pleomorphic tumors are more cellular than their major salivary gland counterparts, and often the minor salivary gland lesions consist almost entirely of epithelial cells with little or no mesenchymal stroma.[55] Wide surgical excision usually prevents recurrences; however, recurrence of the tumor may be delayed well beyond the traditional 5-year period. Malignant change in a sinonasal pleomorphic adenoma is rare.[57] Benign metastasizing pleomorphic adenoma, or metastasizing pleomorphic

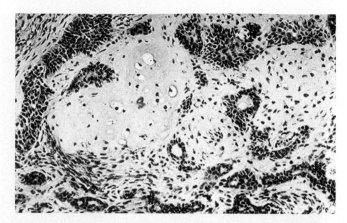

**FIGURE 6-39**   Pleomorphic adenoma: Glandular ductal elements are interspersed with a mesenchyme-like matrix produced by myoepithelial cells. In the center, a chondroid matrix is seen.

adenoma, is an infrequent tumor that metastasizes, despite benign histology, usually to the lungs and soft tissues. A benign metastasizing nasal septal pleomorphic adenoma reportedly spread to an ipsilateral submandibular node.[56, 58]

On imaging of salivary tumors, typically, pleomorphic adenomas remodel bone. Often, the nasal tumors develop as a spherical mass rather than the more typical polypoid lesion associated with most other tumors. When such a spherical configuration is seen, either a salivary gland tumor or a rare schwannoma should be considered in the imaging differential diagnosis. On CT, the less cellular salivary tumors may appear nonhomogeneous because of mesenchymal stroma, cystic degeneration, necrosis, or serous and mucous collections.[50] The highly cellular tumor tends to have a homogeneous appearance and may cause some bone erosion. On MR imaging, these tumors tend to have an intermediate signal intensity on T1-weighted images. The T2-weighted signal intensity depends on the cellularity of the neoplasm; highly cellular types usually have an intermediate signal intensity, while the stromal or less cellular variety have a high T2-weighted signal intensity (Figs. 6-40 to 6-53).[59]

The imaging characteristics of malignant pleomorphic tumors are nonspecific and are similar to those of SCC. Occasionally, they may have grossly less invasive margins on imaging than an SCC. Although this may allow an imaging diagnosis to be suggested, it is not a sufficiently reliable finding to truly differentiate these lesions.

### Epithelial-Myoepithelial Carcinoma

Epithelial-myoepithelial carcinoma is an uncommon, low-grade epithelial neoplasm composed of variable proportions of ductal cells and large, clear-staining myoepithelial cells arranged around the periphery of the ducts. About 120 cases have been reported in the world literature, most of which were located in salivary glands, especially the parotid gland. A few cases have occurred in unusual locations such as the breast, lacrimal gland, nose, paranasal sinus, trachea, bronchus, and lung. A case was reported in the nasal cavity with extension to the nasopharynx. The recurrence and metastatic rates of epithelial-myoepithelial carcinoma varied from 35% to 50% and from 8.1% to 25%, respectively, for all sites.[60]

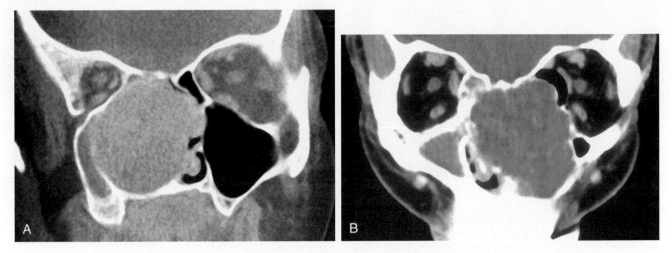

**FIGURE 6-40** **A,** Coronal CT shows an expansile right nasal fossa mass that has remodeled most of the surrounding bone. It also has obstructed what remains of the right maxillary sinus. This patient had a low-grade mucoepidermoid carcinoma. **B,** Coronal CT scan on another patient shows a primarily expansile mass filling the nasal fossae and the left ethmoid and maxillary sinuses. The right antrum is obstructed by the mass. This patient had a low-grade mucoepidermoid carcinoma.

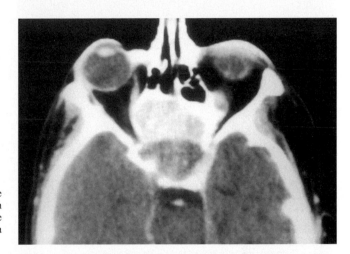

**FIGURE 6-41** Axial CT scan shows an enhancing expansile mass in the posterior ethmoid sinuses. The sphenoid sinuses are obstructed with lower-attenuation secretions. Some bone remodeling is also present in the lamina papyracea. This patient had a mucoepidermoid carcinoma and a sphenoid mucocele.

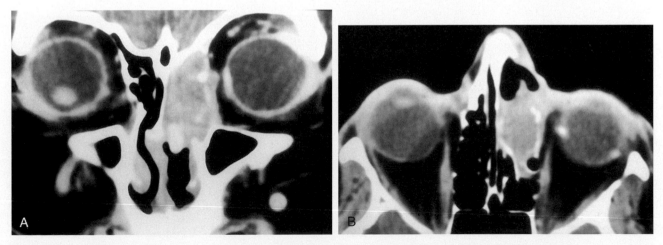

**FIGURE 6-42** Coronal (**A**) and axial (**B**) CT scans show a slightly expansile mass in the left ethmoid sinuses. Although there is some destruction of the lamina papyracea with minimal invasion of the orbit, there is also an element of widening or remodeling of the ethmoid complex. This patient had a mucoepidermoid carcinoma.

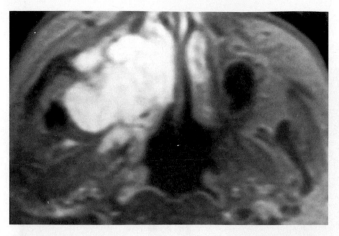

**FIGURE 6-43** Axial T2-weighted MR image shows an expansile right maxillary sinus mass that extends into the infratemporal fossa. The tumor has high signal intensity, suggesting that it contains water-like products such as mucoid secretions. This patient had a mucoepidermoid carcinoma.

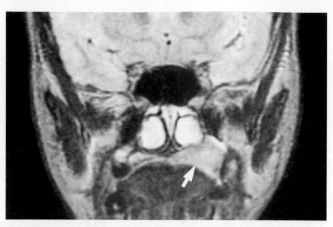

**FIGURE 6-44** Coronal proton density MR image shows a mass (*arrow*) in the left palate with extension to the lower left antrum. This patient had a high-grade mucoepidermoid carcinoma.

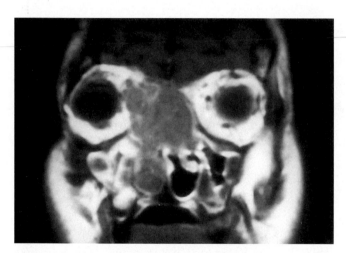

**FIGURE 6-45** Coronal T1-weighted, contrast-enhanced MR image shows a nodular, destructive lesion in the nasal fossae and both ethmoid sinuses. The tumor has invaded the right orbit and skull base. Inflammatory disease is present in both antra. This patient had an adenocarcinoma.

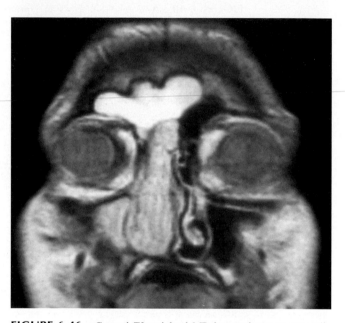

**FIGURE 6-46** Coronal T2-weighted MR image shows an expansile right nasoethmoid mass that extends into the base of the right frontal sinus. The lesion obstructs the right frontal and right maxillary sinuses. This patient had an adenocarcinoma.

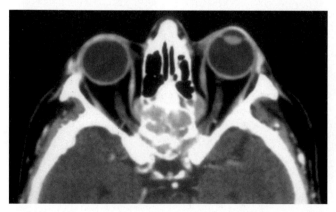

**FIGURE 6-47** Axial contrast-enhanced CT scan shows a partially expansile and destructive mass in the posterior ethmoid complexes, nasal fossae, and anterior sphenoid sinuses. The tumor has broken into both orbits; however, the margins of the tumor with the orbital fat are not grossly invasive. This patient had an adenocarcinoma.

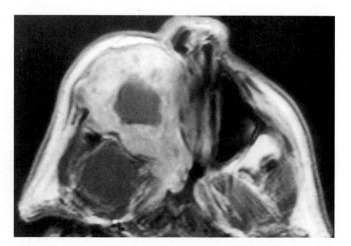

**FIGURE 6-48** Axial T1-weighted, contrast-enhanced MR image shows a large, destructive tumor in the right maxillary sinus that has invaded the overlying skin, the nasal fossa, the infratemporal fossa, and the central skull base. This appearance is similar to that of a squamous cell carcinoma; however, this patient had an adenoidcystic carcinoma.

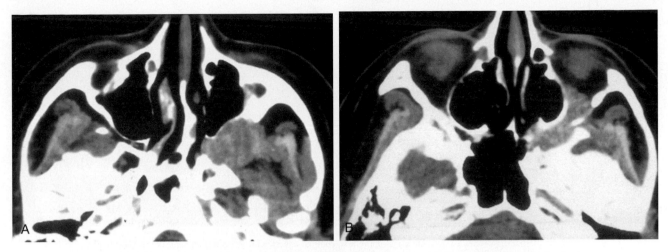

**FIGURE 6-49**   Axial CT scans show a mass in the left pterygopalatine and infratemporal fossae that has both thinned and remodeled the posterior antral wall (**A**). The tumor has extended up into the left orbital apex and the skull base (**B**). This patient had an adenoidcystic carcinoma.

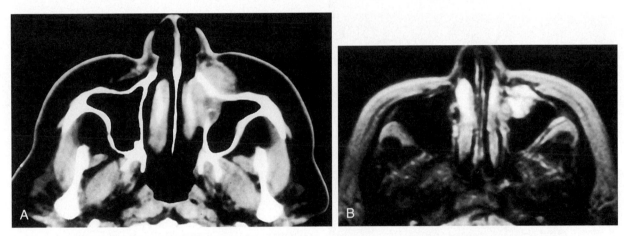

**FIGURE 6-50**   Axial CT scan (**A**) shows a mass in the anteromedial left maxillary sinus and the adjacent left cheek. There is some destruction of the medial antral wall. In **B**, a T2-weighted MR image, the mass has high signal intensity. This patient had an adenoidcystic carcinoma.

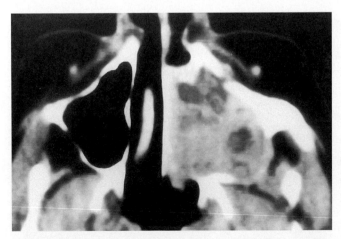

**FIGURE 6-51**   Axial CT scan shows a partially expansile, partially destructive, nonhomogeneous tumor in the left maxillary sinus. The lesion has extended into the nasal fossa and the infratemporal fossa. This patient had an adenoidcystic carcinoma.

# BENIGN AND MALIGNANT NEUROECTODERMAL, NEURONAL, NERVE SHEATH, AND CENTRAL NERVOUS SYSTEM TUMORS

## Paraganglioma

Primary paragangliomas in the sinonasal tract are extraordinarily rare. The diagnosis of a paraganglioma in this region almost always represents a large glomus jugulare tumor that has usually extended into the sphenoid and ethmoid sinuses (Fig. 6-54).[61, 62] However, at least two cases of sinonasal paraganglioma have been reported.[63, 64] Histologically, paragangliomas are composed of nests of epithelioid, neuroendrocrine cells ensheathed by Schwannian sustentacular cells.

Treatment may include surgery and radiotherapy. In one case, 22 years later the tumor recurred and showed rapid

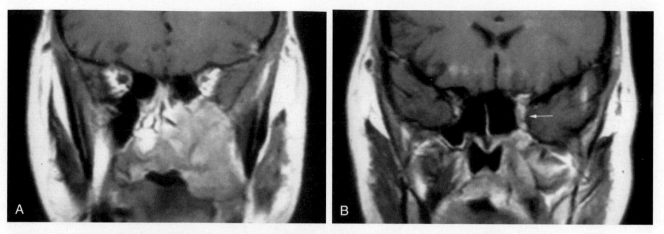

**FIGURE 6-52** Coronal T1-weighted, fat-suppressed, contrast-enhanced MR ventral (**A**) and dorsal (**B**) images show a large mass in the left antrum, lower nasal fossa, and hard palate. The tumor has extended back through the pterygopalatine fossa and invades the left cavernous sinus (*arrow*). This patient had an adenoidcystic carcinoma.

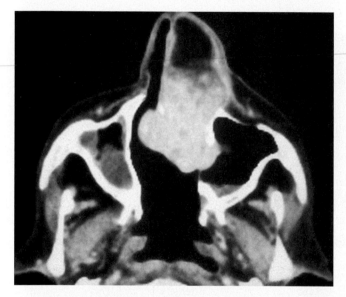

**FIGURE 6-53** Axial CT scan shows a bulky nodular mass arising in the nasal septum and laterally displacing the left nose and medial antral wall. This patient had a pleomorphic adenoma.

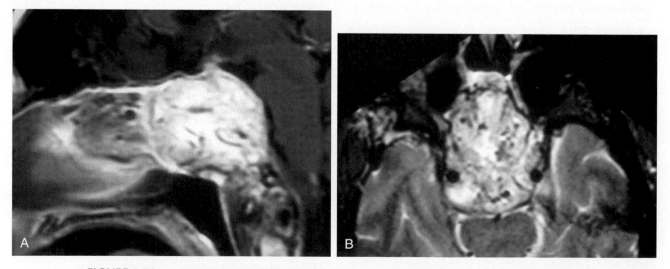

**FIGURE 6-54** Sagittal (**A**) and axial (**B**) T1-weighted, fat-suppressed, contrast-enhanced MR images show an enhancing mass in the sphenoid sinus. There is invasion of the clivus, and there are flow voids within the tumor. This patient had a paraganglioma of the sphenoid sinus.

growth due to malignant transformation that may have been related to the radiotherapy.[63]

On imaging, these tumors are usually expansile, enhanced, and may have vascular signal voids on MR imaging. These lesions are discussed in more detail in Chapter 39. When a primary paraganglioma is encountered, it is more likely that the true diagnosis is a well-differentiated sinonasal neuroendocrine carcinoma.

## Olfactory Neuroblastoma

Olfactory neuroblastoma (ONB) (historically referred to as esthesioneuroblastoma) is a neural crest–derived neoplasm arising from the olfactory mucosa in the superior nasal fossa. It occurs with a bimodal age distribution, peaking in the second and sixth decades, and representing 16.8% and 22.8% of all sinonasal tumors for these age groups, respectively. However, the age of these patients ranges from 3 to 88 years.[65, 66] ONB usually presents as a solitary soft-tissue nasal polyp that may bleed profusely on biopsy. It may also occur as a bilateral nasal mass; this usually happens in medically neglected patients.

Histologically, ONB is composed of small, relatively bland round malignant cells with scanty cytoplasm. A fibrillary background is characteristic of ONB, and ultrastructurally corresponds to neuronal processes formed by the most differentiated tumor cells. Groups of tumor cells that are centripetally aligned around tangles of neurofibrillary processes appear by light microscopy as Homer-Wright rosettes. An abundance of these rosettes indicates a well-differentiated tumor. Flexner-Wintersteiner rosettes represent evidence of true olfactory differentiation and are seen as gland-like structures formed by columnar or cuboidal tumor cells.

The term *ganglioneuroblastoma* refers to ganglionic maturation within a neuroblastoma. This may be seen at initial tumor presentation (referred to as differentiating neuroblastoma) and is associated with an improved prognosis. Ganglionic maturation may also be seen after a chemotherapeutic response of neuroblastoma. This type of de novo or secondary ganglionic differentiation is not seen in ONB. This may reflect inherent distinctions between olfactory neuroepithelium (a direct extension from CNS neurons) and the postsynaptic sympathetic neuroblasts that give rise to neuroblastomas.

Hyams introduced a four-tier grading system of ONB: grade I ONB represents the most differentiated tumor, with rosette formation and no pleomorphism, mitotic figures, or necrosis, while grade IV ONB reveals no histologic evidence of neuronal/neuroendocrine differentiation, and the findings of pleomorphism, mitotic activity, and necrosis are present. Hyams was able to correlate tumor grade with prognosis. More recently, the question has been raised if grade IV ONB tumors are actually not ONB, but better classified as sinonasal neuroendocrine carcinomas (see below). Additionally, the less differentiated an ONB appears to be, the greater the need to rule out other diagnoses such as undifferentiated carcinoma (sinonasal undifferentiated carcinoma), large cell lymphoma, melanoma, extramedullary plasmacytoma, and embryonal rhabdomyosarcoma. Immu-

nohistochemistry has become the standard adjunctive test to resolve these issues.

The Kadish staging system is a clinically based staging system for sinonasal tumors. Those lesions confined to the nasal cavity are stage A, those with disease in the nasal cavity and one or more paranasal sinuses are stage B, and those with disease extending beyond the nasal cavity and paranasal sinuses are stage C.[67] Both the Hyams grading system and the Kadish staging system can be used as independent predictors of outcome.[68] In the Kadish staging system, the 5-year survival rates for patients with stage A, B, and C tumors are 75%, 68%, and 41.2% respectively.[66, 67] Craniofacial resection can be curative for up to 90% of patients, as this approach addresses microscopic disease at the cribriform plate and in the olfactory bulbs, which are below the detection threshold of current radiographic imaging.[69] By contrast, a recurrence rate of nearly 50% can be seen after an extended lateral rhinotomy for stage A and stage B patients. The 5-year survival rate for all patients is 69%.[70] A more recent report indicates 80.4% disease-free survival at 8 years.[71] When survival is stratified for tumor grade, the 5-year disease-free survival for patients with low-grade and high-grade tumors is 80% and 40%, respectively.[72] Locoregional and distant metastasis occurs in up to 38% of patients.[73] Late recurrences or metastatic disease can occur up to two decades after initial presentation. Negative prognostic factors include female sex, age over 50 years at presentation, tumor recurrence, metastasis, high tumor grade, and Kadish stage C at presentation.[72]

Preoperative imaging is crucial to tumor mapping and planning the extent of surgery. On CT, ONBs usually are homogeneous, enhancing masses that primarily remodel bone. They commonly extend into the ipsilateral ethmoid and maxillary sinuses and rarely involve the sphenoid sinuses. When large, they can extend to involve both sides of the nasal cavity and the paranasal sinuses. Gross calcifications can occur within the tumor mass, and they can also be seen histologically.[74] On MR imaging these tumors have an intermediate signal intensity on all imaging sequences, with the T2-weighted signal intensity being higher.[75] They also enhance with contrast (Figs. 6-55 to 6-61). When imaging these tumors, the radiologist must carefully evaluate the floor of the anterior cranial fossa for tumor extension into this region. If intracranial tumor extension is seen, the imager should attempt to distinguish between tumor that remains extraaxial (with only dural disease) and tumor that has invaded brain, as such a differentiation alters surgery. In some of the larger tumors that have intracranial extension, peripheral tumor cysts can occur at the margins of the intracranial mass. These cysts have their broadest base on the tumor, and when seen, they strongly suggest the imaging diagnosis of this tumor.[76]

## Sinonasal Neuroendocrine Carcinoma and Sinonasal Undifferentiated Carcinoma

Sinonasal neuroendocrine carcinoma (SNEC) and sinonasal undifferentiated carcinoma (SNUC) were first described in the 1980s, but remarkably few series of either have been reported. SNEC and SNUC can be conceptualized

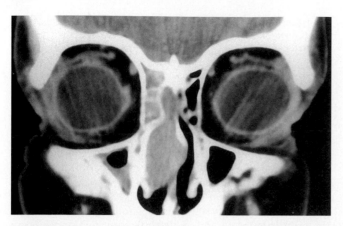

**FIGURE 6-55**   Coronal CT scan shows an expansile right nasal fossa mass obstructing the right ethmoid and maxillary sinuses. The lesion is limited to the sinonasal cavities. This patient had an olfactory neuroblastoma.

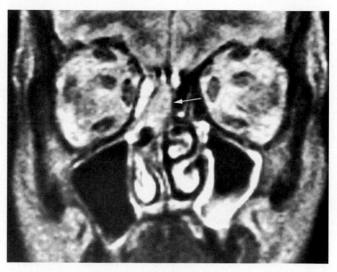

**FIGURE 6-56**   Coronal T2-weighted MR image shows a small right nasoethmoid mass (*arrow*) of intermediate signal intensity with inflammatory changes in the lateral right ethmoid complex and both maxillary sinuses (high signal intensity). The tumor extends through the cribriform plate. This patient had an olfactory neuroblastoma.

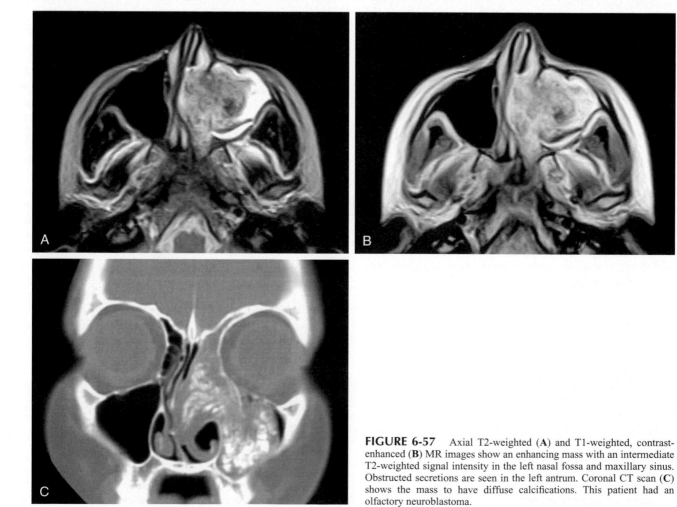

**FIGURE 6-57**   Axial T2-weighted (**A**) and T1-weighted, contrast-enhanced (**B**) MR images show an enhancing mass with an intermediate T2-weighted signal intensity in the left nasal fossa and maxillary sinus. Obstructed secretions are seen in the left antrum. Coronal CT scan (**C**) shows the mass to have diffuse calcifications. This patient had an olfactory neuroblastoma.

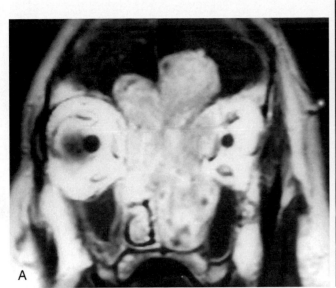

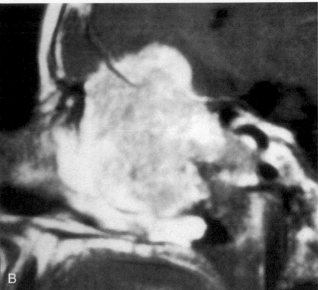

**FIGURE 6-58**    Coronal (**A**) and sagittal (**B**) T1-weighted, contrast-enhanced MR images show a large, enhancing nasal fossa mass that has broken through the floor of the anterior cranial fossa and displaced the frontal lobes upward. The tumor has also extended into each orbit and into the left maxillary sinus. This patient had an olfactory neuroblastoma.

as being part of a spectrum of neuroendocrine-type tumors, with ONB representing the most specialized and differentiated neuroendocrine tumors and SNUC having dubious or weak neuroendocrine qualities.

SNEC was first proposed in 1982, when it became clear that some tumors were less differentiated than ONB but still retained neuroendocrine features.[77] Many had been buried in the literature as oat cell carcinoma, atypical carcinoid,

malignant paraganglioma, or anaplastic or undifferentiated carcinoma. SNEC is defined as a malignant neoplasm with evidence of neurosecretory granules. Lacking evidence of a neurofibrillary background by light microscopy, as is seen in ONB, it is less differentiated and more ''carcinomatous'' than ONB. The term *sinonasal undifferentiated carcinoma* was first coined by Frierson and colleagues to define a group of sinonasal tumors with no obvious differentiation that

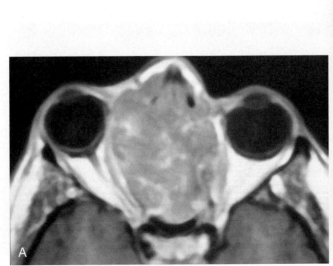

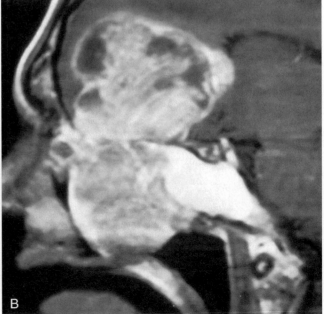

**FIGURE 6-59**    Axial (**A**) and sagittal (**B**) T1-weighted, contrast-enhanced MR images show an enhancing mass in the ethmoids and nasal fossa. The mass has extended into the anterior cranial fossa, and several small cystic areas are seen within the intracranial portion of the tumor. The mass has also extended into both orbits, and the sphenoid sinus is obstructed. This patient had an olfactory neuroblastoma.

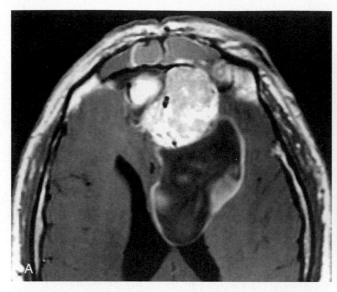

**FIGURE 6-60**    Axial (**A**) and sagittal (**B**) T1-weighted, fat-suppressed, contrast-enhanced MR images show a large, enhancing sinonasal mass that obstructs the frontal and sphenoid sinuses and extends intracranially. There is a large cyst at the intracranial margin of the tumor. This patient had an olfactory neuroblastoma.

were united by their obviously aggressive clinical course.[78] These tumors were previously diagnosed as "anaplastic" or "undifferentiated." A possible etiologic relationship to heavy metal exposure, coal mining, the chemical industry, and shoemaking has been reported.[78, 79]

Few demographic or prognostic comparisons can be made between SNUC, SNEC, and ONB due to their rarity. In the group reported by Silva et al., 20 patients diagnosed with SNEC were compared with 9 patients with ONB.[77] The mean age of the patients with SNEC was 50, while that of the patients with ONB was 20. However, other studies of larger groups of ONB patients reflect the true bimodal age peak of ONB, with a median age of 49.[78] Gallo et al. found that the mean age of patients with SNUC was 56.7 for men

and 68 for women.[79] Most cases of SNEC/SNUC occur in the same sites as ONB (superior nasal cavity, superior turbinates, ethmoids). Presenting symptoms relate to a sinonasal tumor: nasal obstruction, epistaxis, decreased visual acuity, diplopia, and pain.

The radiographic findings of SNEC and SNUC are usually indistinguishable from those of SCC: an aggressive soft-tissue mass that erodes and invades adjacent bone rather than remodeling it (Fig. 6-62). In contrast, the CT and MR imaging findings of ONB are usually those of an expansive mass. In smaller SNEC lesions, the mass is usually polypoid and confined to one nasal fossa, often with involvement of a surrounding ethmoid or medial maxillary sinus margin. Larger lesions may extend into adjacent structures such as the orbit and the cranium.

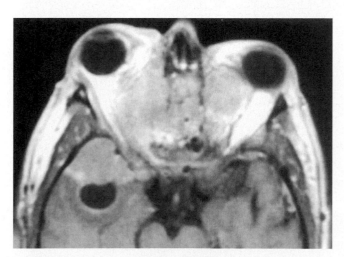

**FIGURE 6-61**    Axial T1-weighted, contrast-enhanced MR image on a patient who previously had a craniofacial resection for an olfactory neuroblastoma. There is a large enhancing recurrence extending into the orbits and the anterior cranial fossa. Note the small, broad-based cyst at the intracranial margin of the tumor. Such a cyst is highly suggestive of the diagnosis. This patient had an olfactory neuroblastoma.

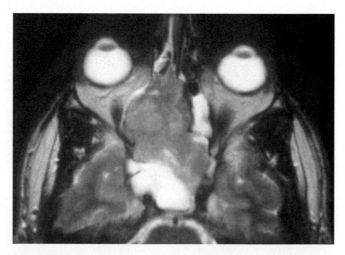

**FIGURE 6-62**    Axial T2-weighted MR image shows a destructive mass in the nasal fossae and both ethmoid complexes. The tumor has extended into the right orbit and the sphenoid sinus, which contains obstructed secretions. Both cavernous sinuses are also invaded. This patient had an olfactory carcinoma.

Histologically, SNEC is composed of cells with fine "salt and pepper" chromatin, with a variable amount of cytoplasm. Architecturally, classic neuroendocrine patterns can be seen: nesting, organoid, trabecular, and/or a ribboning pattern. Glandular-type differentiation may be seen. SNUC is composed of cells with little cytoplasm and large nuclei. No histologic tendency toward neuroendocrine architecture is seen. However, SNEC/SNUC and ONB may also appear quite similar histologically; immunohistochemistry is crucial for sorting out these entities.

In terms of clinical course, the prognosis of SNEC and SNUC seems to be related to the stage at the time of diagnosis. Silva et al. reported 5- and 7-year survival rates of 100% and 88%, respectively, for his cohort of 20 patients with SNEC but noted a propensity for early metastases and local recurrence. They reported evidence of metastases to lymph nodes, brain, and spine in all cases of theirs in which metastatic disease was present, except for one where the lungs and femur were involved.[77] Similarly, in our study, 7 of the 10 patients developed metastatic disease, either to cervical lymph nodes (2 cases), pelvis (2 cases), thoracic spine (1 case), brain (1 case), or skeletal bones (1 case). In our study, two patients with SNEC died of disease at 14 and 41 months. The other two patients in our series with SNEC were alive, with no evidence of disease, at 31 and 108 months. Outcomes for SNUC have been reported to be generally poor.

## Malignant Melanoma

Melanocytes in the sinonasal tract migrate from the neural crest during embryonic development.[13] The etiology of sinonasal melanomas is unknown, but they represent less than 3.6% of sinonasal neoplasms. Less than 2.5% of all malignant melanomas occur in the sinonasal cavities. These melanomas are two or three times more common in the nose than in the sinuses and most frequently arise from the nasal septum.[80, 81] Occasionally, they develop around the inferior and middle turbinates. The antrum is involved in 80% of paranasal sinus cases, usually in conjunction with the nasal cavity. Rare cases develop in the ethmoid sinuses. The frontal and sphenoid sinuses are virtually never involved as primary sites.[13, 80–82] Sinonasal melanomas generally develop in patients 50 to 70 years of age. The most common complaints are nasal obstruction and epistaxis, with pain occurring as an initial complaint in only 7% to 16% of patients.[13, 80, 81] Satellite tumor nodules are common.

Wide local surgical excision with or without postoperative radiation therapy is the treatment of choice. Up to 40% of patients with sinonasal melanomas present with positive neck nodes.[83, 84] Up to 65% of patients with melanoma have a local recurrence or metastases within the first year after surgery. Metastatic disease usually follows local recurrence.

Metastases tend to affect the lungs, lymph nodes, brain, adrenal glands, liver, and skin. Treatment of recurrences yields surprisingly good results.[13] The median survival time is 18 to 34 months.[83, 84] Occasional cases may be mysteriously dormant for up to a decade before there is an explosive recurrence. Nasal cavity melanomas have a better prognosis than tumors originating in the paranasal sinuses; the average survival time of all of these patients is 2 to 3

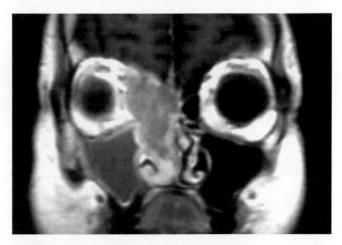

**FIGURE 6-63**   Coronal T1-weighted, contrast-enhanced MR image (on the same patient as in Fig. 6-8) shows an enhancing mass in the right ethmoid complex and nasal fossa. The tumor has broken into the right orbit but has a smooth interface with the orbital fat. The right antrum is obstructed by the mass. This patient had a melanoma.

years, and the 10-year survival rate is 0.5%. The differential diagnosis of melanoma includes undifferentiated carcinoma, lymphoma, embryonal rhabdomyosarcoma, ONB, and extramedullary plasmacytoma.[41]

Melanomas tend to remodel bone, although elements of frank bone erosion also may be present. Because of their rich vascular network, melanomas enhance well on contrast-enhanced CT and MR scans, and their MR imaging appearance is usually that of a homogeneous mass of intermediate signal intensity on all imaging sequences. However, some melanomas have high T1-weighted signal intensity primarily because of the presence of hemorrhage and, to a lesser degree, paramagnetic melanin (Figs. 6-8 and 6-63 to 6-67). These melanomas may have a deceptively noninvasive border on imaging, suggesting that they are low-grade lesions. Such lesions emphasize the lack of correlation between the imaging evidence of a noninvasive

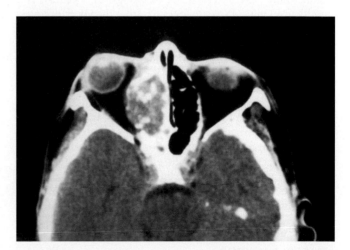

**FIGURE 6-64**   Axial CT scan shows an expansile mass in the right ethmoid complex that is bulging into the right orbit. Most of the lamina papyracea and ethmoid septations are destroyed or thinned. Radiodensities within the mass were residual pieces of bone. This patient had a melanoma.

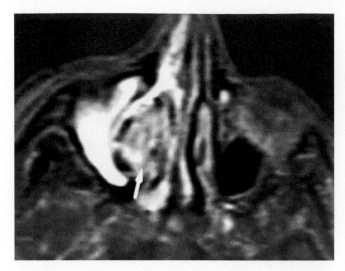

**FIGURE 6-65**    Axial T2-weighted MR image shows an expansile right nasal fossa mass (*arrow*) that obstructs the right antrum. The tumor has a low to intermediate signal intensity, and the obstructed secretions have a high signal intensity. This patient had a melanoma.

tumor margin and the biologic aggressiveness of the tumor. Most of these tumors occur in the nasal fossa. However, a rare case was reported to arise in the frontal sinus in a patient who presented with forehead swelling and progressive confusion.[85]

Pathologically, melanomas are known as the "great mimickers," as they produce myriad patterns composed of varying cell types. Melanomas may be epithelioid, sarcomatoid, plasmacytoid, or clear cell. Pink nucleoli, intranuclear holes, and cytoplasmic melanin can be seen (Fig. 6-68). The diagnosis can be confirmed immunohistochemically by the expression of S100 and HMB-45.

## Melanotic Neuroectodermal Tumor of Infancy

This is an extremely rare neuroectodermal tumor that occurs almost exclusively prior to the age of 1 year. It is a rapidly growing soft-tissue mass of either the upper or lower jaws, the CNS, or the orbit. The anterior maxilla is the most common site, accounting for 71% of all cases. Bone invasion may occur. Histologically, these tumors are distinctive, with tubular or alveolar formations of large melanin-containing cells around nests of smaller neuroblastic cells. A series of 20 cases has been reported by Kapadia and colleagues, 5 of 12 (45%) patients with follow-up developed recurrence within 4 months of diagnosis, but none metastasized.[87] Treatment is usually local excision. Only two or three malignant cases have been reported, with metastases to lymph nodes, liver, bones, adrenal glands, and soft tissues.[65, 86, 87]

## Primitive Neuroectodermal Tumor and Ewing's Sarcoma

Ewing's sarcoma (ES) is a highly malignant small, round cell tumor that accounts for 5% to 10% of all primary bone

malignancies. About 60% of cases occur in the lower extremities and pelvis.[88] Almost 90% of patients are between 5 and 30 years of age at diagnosis. Only 1% to 4% of all ES occur in the bone and soft tissue of the head and neck, most commonly the mandible, followed by the maxilla, calvaria, and cervical vertebrae.[89] ES rarely arises from the nasal cavity/paranasal sinuses and has been seen as a complication of radiation therapy for retinoblastoma.[90–92]

Primitive neuroectodermal tumor (PNET) is a malignancy of childhood and early adulthood that is closely related to ES. PNET occurs most commonly as a soft tumor of the lower truck or lower extremities. Association with a major nerve trunk has been seen in one third of the cases. PNET does occur in the head and neck, usually in the sinonasal cavities (Fig. 6-69) and has also been reported in patients who have survived retinoblastoma.[93–96] Patients with ES/PNET typically present with pain and localized swelling.

Radiographically with ES, a destructive soft-tissue lesion is seen with a typical "onion skin" type of periosteal reaction. Less often with both ES and PNET, a "sunburst" type of periosteal reaction can be seen.

Pathologically, ES and PNET appear as malignant "small blue round cell tumors" that are relatively bland in appearance. The distinction between these two neoplasms is based on immunophenotypic and ultrastructural findings. PNET shows some evidence of neuroendocrine differentiation, such as neurosecretory granules and cellular processes by electron microscopy (EM) and evidence of expression of two or more neuroendocrine markers (this neuroendocrine differentiation is quantitatively much less than that seen in ONB). ES, on the other hand, reveals no evidence of any kind of differentiation. Both tumors are associated with chromosomal translocation (11;22) (q24;q12) that forms the fusion protein EWS/FLI-1; EWS/ERG.

The treatment of choice for ES and PNET is local excision, with radiation therapy for the incompletely excised

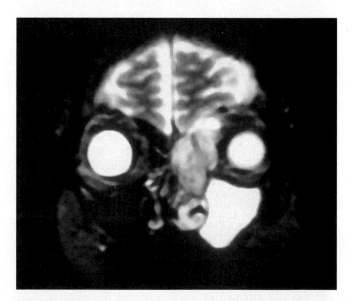

**FIGURE 6-66**    Coronal T2-weighted MR image shows a mass in the left ethmoid complex and nasal fossa. The tumor has extended into the left orbit and has a smooth interface with the orbital fat. The adjacent sinuses are obstructed. This patient had a melanoma.

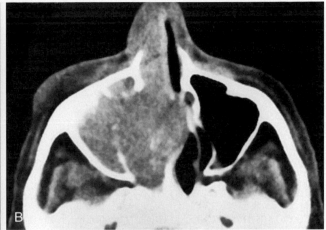

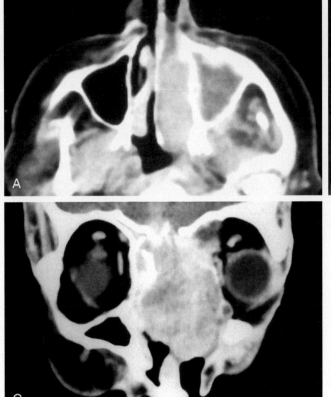

**FIGURE 6-67**   Axial CT scan (**A**) shows an enhancing, expansile polypoid mass in the left nasal fossa. The left antrum is obstructed. There is virtually no bone destruction associated with this benign-appearing lesion. Axial CT scan (**B**) on another patient shows a primarily expansile right nasal fossa mass that obstructs the right antrum. There is a greater element of bone destruction than in **A**. Coronal CT scan (**C**) on a third patient shows a primarily destructive mass in the nasal fossae, ethmoid sinuses, and left maxillary sinus. The tumor has invaded the left orbit and the floor of the anterior cranial fossa. All of these patients had melanomas. These three cases illustrate the variation of the imaging appearance of this tumor.

**FIGURE 6-68**   Melanoma: Gross specimen (**A**) shows a polypoid pigmented tumor of the superior nasal cavity. In **B**, brown melanin pigment is seen within these highly malignant cells.

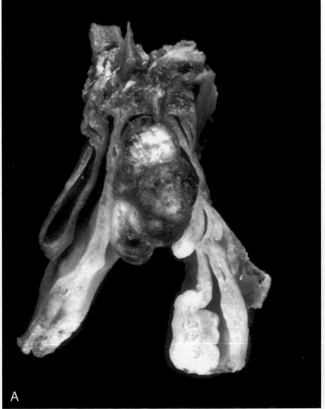

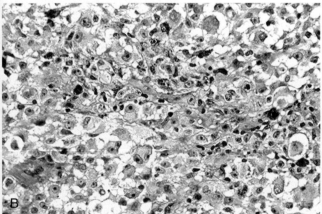

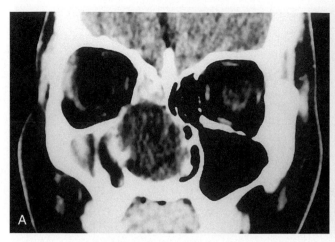
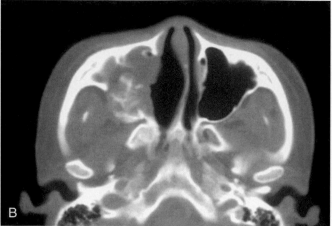

**FIGURE 6-69** Coronal CT scan (**A**) shows a mucoid attenuation mass expanding the right nasal fossa. Bony thickening is present along the adjacent right nasal vault wall. Axial CT scan (**B**) taken after biopsy of the mass shows irregular tumoral bone within the right antrum bulging into the infratemporal fossa. This patient had a primitive neuroectodermal tumor.

lesions. Micrometastases, which are present in 15% to 30% of patients, are treated with chemotherapy. The 5-year survival rates have risen from less than 10% in the prechemotherapy era to the current 60% to 79%. ES recurs locally in 13% to 20% of patients (65% at postmortem), usually coinciding with the completion of chemotherapy. The tumors metastasize to the lungs (86%), skeleton (69%), pleural cavity (46%), lymph nodes (46%), dura and meninges (27%), and CNS (12%). Because of its rarity in the facial area, ES of the sinonasal cavities probably should be considered a metastasis from an infraclavicular primary tumor until proven otherwise. The significance of the distinction between ES and PNET is that PNET is somewhat more chemosensitive than ES and is associated with a longer mean survival after multimodality therapy.

## Peripheral Nerve Sheath Tumors

### Schwannoma

*Peripheral nerve sheath tumors* is the currently preferred term for benign and malignant neoplasms that arise from neuronal axons and/or their supporting cells (Schwann cells and fibroblasts). Confusing terminology has arisen in the literature, with many names representing the same lesion. One of the difficulties in discussing neurogenic neoplasms is that there is also controversy regarding whether nerve sheath tumors arise from Schwann cells or neuroectodermal perineural cells.[65] Today most investigators use the term *Schwann cell* to describe both of these cells. The terms *schwannoma, neurinoma, neurilemoma,* and *perineural fibroblastoma* all refer to the same tumor.[1] Peripheral nerve sheath tumors are common in the head and neck. Up to 40% of these tumors occur in head and neck sites. Only 4% of these tumors occur in the sinonasal cavities.[97–99]

A schwannoma is defined as a tumor composed entirely of nerve-supporting cells, without neuronal elements. It is a benign, encapsulated, slowly growing tumor that occurs in patients 30 to 60 years of age. It is two to four times more common in females than in males. The most common sites are the vagus nerve in the neck and the eighth cranial nerve. Only about 65 cases have been reported in the sinonasal cavities, and most of these occurred in the nasal fossa, maxillary sinuses, and ethmoidal sinuses.[1, 65, 100] In rare cases, a schwannoma can occur in the olfactory bulbs (Fig. 6-70). This is a distinctly different entity than ONB. The most common complaint is a painless mass.

Schwannomas rarely undergo malignant change. At surgery, the nerve of origin may occasionally be found to be stretched over the tumor. In these cases, the surgeon may be able to extirpate the lesion while preserving the nerve. By contrast, neurofibromas are defined as having neuronal elements as an integral part of the tumor. They appear as swellings arising directly from the nerve, and the nerve must be sacrificed to excise the lesion.[65]

Histologically, schwannomas have two major components: the Antoni A areas, characterized by a compact arrangement of elongated spindled cells, and the Antoni B areas, characterized by a loose myxoid stroma with few spindled cells. This variation is reflected in their CT appearance, which ranges from a variably enhancing homogeneous ovoid mass to a primarily cystic lesion.[101] On contrast-enhanced CT, about one third of the cases enhance more than muscle, one third have attenuation values similar to that of muscle, and one third are primarily cystic.[99] The enhancement on CT and MR images occurs presumably because of extravascular extravasation of the contrast into a poorly vascularized tumor matrix. The MR imaging characteristics of schwannomas are those of an intermediate T1-weighted and a variable T2-weighted signal intensity that reflect whether the lesion is highly cellular (intermediate signal intensity) or cystic and stromal (nonhomogeneously high signal intensity). All schwannomas are roughly ovoid shaped, noninfiltrating, bone-remodeling lesions, and any site of aggressive bone destruction should raise the possibility of a malignancy rather than a schwannoma (Figs. 6-71 to 6-74).

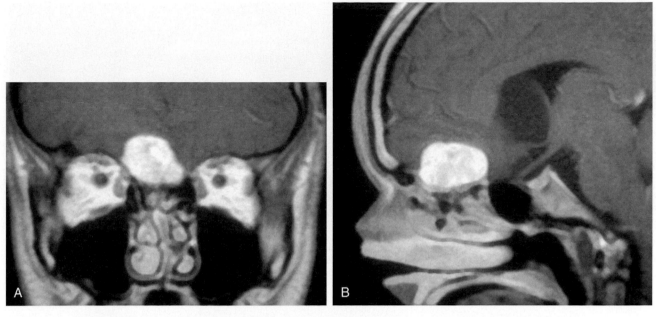

**FIGURE 6-70**   Coronal (**A**) and sagittal (**B**) T1-weighted, contrast-enhanced MR images show an ovoid mass sitting on the cribriform plate region and minimally displacing both the fovea ethmoidalis and the cribriform plate caudally. This was a rare schwannoma of the olfactory bulbs of the first cranial nerve. (Case courtesy of Dr. Geoffrey Parker.)

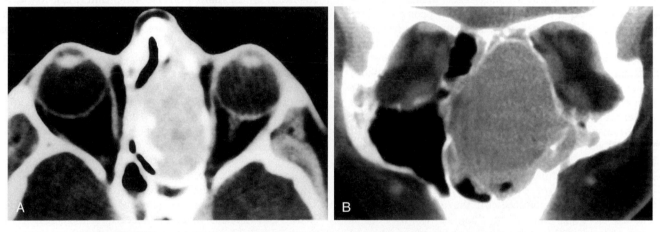

**FIGURE 6-71**   Axial CT scan (**A**) shows an expansile, homogeneous mass in the left ethmoid sinuses that has remodeled the surrounding bone. Coronal CT scan (**B**) on another patient shows a large, expansile mass in the left nasal fossa and ethmoid sinuses. The left antrum and right ethmoid sinuses are obstructed by the mass. The surrounding bone is remodeled rather than destroyed. Both of these patients had a schwannoma. Also see Fig. 6-7C.

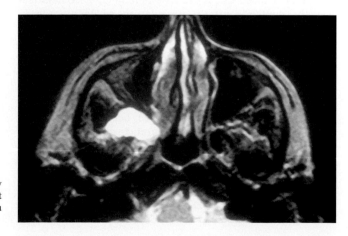

**FIGURE 6-72**   Axial T2-weighted MR image shows a high signal intensity mass in the right pterygopalatine and infratemporal fossae. The adjacent posterior antral wall has been remodeled anteriorly. This patient had a schwannoma.

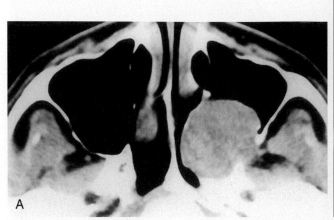
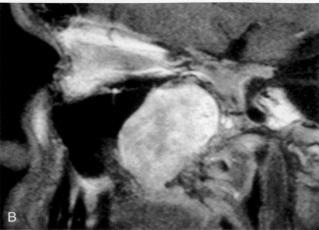

**FIGURE 6-73** Axial CT scan (**A**) and sagittal T1-weighted, fat-suppressed, contrast-enhanced MR image (**B**) show an expansile mass in the pterygopalatine fossa that has remodeled the posterior maxillary sinus wall anteriorly. This patient had a schwannoma.

### Neurofibroma

Neurofibroma is a benign, fairly well-circumscribed, but nonencapsulated nerve sheath tumor. Histologically, it is relatively uniform, composed of fibroblastic cells and neuronal elements within a collagenized matrix. Neurofibromas may occur as a solitary tumor or as multiple tumors. Neurofibromas, especially in a young patient, may herald the onset of other tumors with neurofibromatosis (von Recklinghausen's disease). This disease is transmitted as an autosomal dominant trait with variable penetrance. It is characterized by café au lait spots, multiple neurofibromas, and characteristic bone lesions.[102] Multiple neurofibromas are more likely to be associated with neurofibromatosis (Fig. 6-75).[99] Approximately 8% (5% to 15%) of these tumors may have malignant degeneration.[103, 104] The clinical appearance of a plexiform neurofibroma is considered pathognomonic of neurofibromatosis even in the absence of other signs. This tumor usually remains within the confines of the perineurium and resembles a "giant nerve," a "bag of worms," or a "string of beads."[65]

Neurofibromas can have a variable CT appearance, depending in part on the degree of cystic degeneration and fatty replacement present within the lesion. On contrast-enhanced CT, these tumors may enhance homogeneously, contain multiple cystic areas, or have predominantly fatty attenuation. The degree of fatty replacement within some neurofibromas is far more extensive than that ever seen in schwannomas and may at times cause the radiologist to suggest the diagnosis of lipoma. Neurofibromas remodel bone and do not cause aggressive bone destruction. They are roughly ovoid in shape and have noninvasive margins. If bone has been destroyed, the possibility of a malignant degeneration should be considered. On MR imaging they usually are nonhomogeneous tumors with overall intermediate T1-weighted and high T2-weighted signal intensities. The plexiform lesions in particular often have a fairly high T2-weighted signal intensity and have a "bag of worms" configuration rather than a solitary ovoid shape.

### Traumatic Neuroma

Traumatic neuroma is not a true neoplasm but a reparative lesion that occurs after disruption of a peripheral nerve. If the proximal portion of the nerve cannot reestablish contact with the distal portion, the proliferating Schwann cells and axons grow haphazardly and form a traumatic neuroma. Excision with approximation of the nerve endings is the treatment of choice.[65]

### Malignant Peripheral Nerve Sheath Tumor

*Malignant peripheral nerve sheath tumor* (MPNST), a term that has replaced *malignant schwannoma,* refers to a neuroectodermal sarcoma that is the malignant counterpart of a neurofibroma.[105] Up to half of MPNSTs occur in patients with neurofibromatosis (von Recklinghausen disease). The typical solitary MPNST occurs in adults, usually between the third and sixth decades of life. Only 9% to 14% of MPNSTs are found in the head and neck. The cranial nerves, large cervical nerves, sympathetic chain, and inferior alveolar nerve are the most commonly involved nerves. Symptoms include an enlarging mass, occasional pain, paresthesia, muscle weakness, and atrophy.[65]

Schwann cells are modified fibroblasts that produce collagen and have a spindled morphology. Some MPNSTs can then be confused histologically with fibrosarcomas.[65] Association with a nerve trunk, immunohistochemical expression of S-100, and ultrastructural evidence of redundant basement membrane and cellular processes aid in establishing the correct diagnosis. MPNSTs associated with neurofibromatosis behave more aggressively than isolated lesions. The 5-year survival rates are 15% to 30% with neurofibromatosis and 27% to 75% without it. Tumors that exceed 7 cm in size, have more than 6 mitoses per 10 high-power fields, and are located near the central body axis have a poorer prognosis. Local recurrences and hematogenous pulmonary metastases are common, whereas lymph node metastases are rare.[106] Their imaging characteristics may be similar to those of SCC (Fig. 6-63).

### Granular Cell Tumor

Granular cell tumors (histologically referred to as myoblastomas) are uncommon benign tumors that are most commonly seen in the dermis and subcutis as single or multinodular lesions. In the head and neck, they occur as subcutaneous tumors of the skin of the nose, eyelids, forehead, scalp, and neck. They also may develop in the lips, floor of the mouth, lateral tongue, palate, pharynx, larynx, and trachea. Granular cell tumors rarely occur in the paranasal sinuses. Most occur in patients 35 to 40 years old. There is a general female predominance, and a disproportionate number of cases occur in African-American patients.

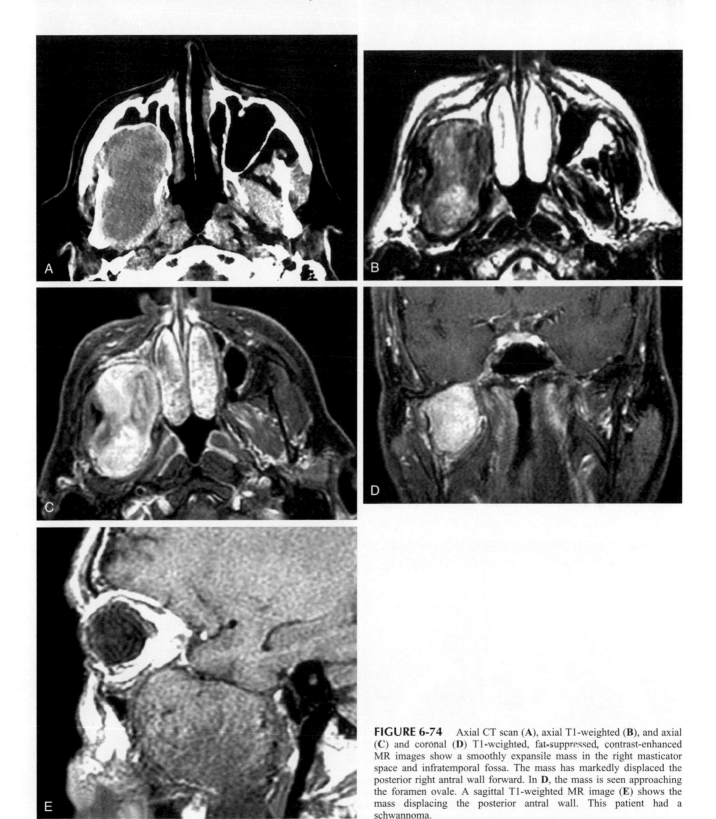

**FIGURE 6-74**   Axial CT scan (**A**), axial T1-weighted (**B**), and axial (**C**) and coronal (**D**) T1-weighted, fat-suppressed, contrast-enhanced MR images show a smoothly expansile mass in the right masticator space and infratemporal fossa. The mass has markedly displaced the posterior right antral wall forward. In **D**, the mass is seen approaching the foramen ovale. A sagittal T1-weighted MR image (**E**) shows the mass displacing the posterior antral wall. This patient had a schwannoma.

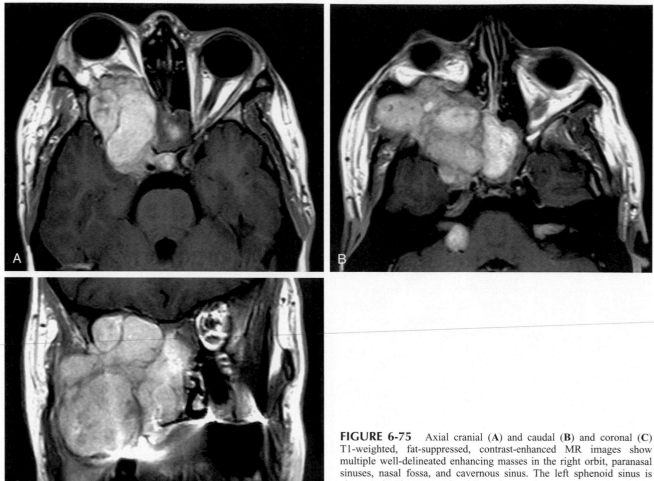

**FIGURE 6-75**    Axial cranial (**A**) and caudal (**B**) and coronal (**C**) T1-weighted, fat-suppressed, contrast-enhanced MR images show multiple well-delineated enhancing masses in the right orbit, paranasal sinuses, nasal fossa, and cavernous sinus. The left sphenoid sinus is obstructed. There are also bilateral acoustic neuromas. These were neurofibromas in a patient with neurofibromatosis.

However, in this latter group, laryngeal granular cell tumors do not occur.

Most granular cell tumors reach a size of 1 to 5 cm and are composed of polyhedral cells with eosinophilic granular cytoplasm and round to oval nuclei. Histologically, there are "packettes" of histiocyte-like cells with abundant eosinophilic granular cytoplasm and small round to oval nuclei (Fig. 6-77). If an association with a nerve can be seen, it indicates tumor origin rather than potential aggressiveness. Cellular pleomorphism, necrosis, or mitotic figures should

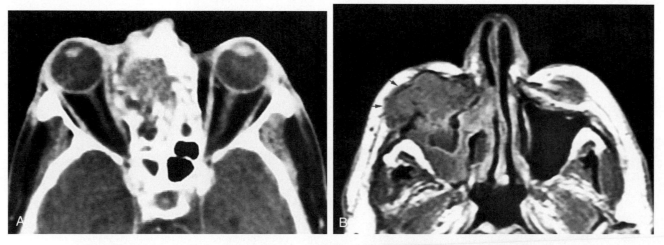

**FIGURE 6-76**    Axial CT scan (**A**) shows an expansile right anterior ethmoid mass that erodes the lamina papyracea and bulges into the right orbit. This patient had a malignant schwannoma. Axial T1-weighted MR image (**B**) on another patient shows a destructive lesion originating in the roof of the right maxillary sinus (*arrows*). The mass has a low T1-weighted signal intensity and an intermediate T2-weighted signal intensity. This patient had a malignant schwannoma of $V_2$.

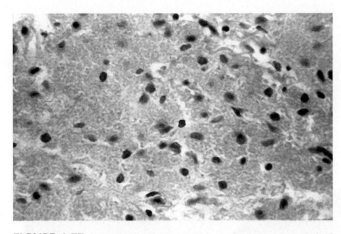

**FIGURE 6-77**   Granular cell tumor: This neoplasm is composed of bland cells with abundant granular cytoplasm and small nuclei. The granules correspond to lysosomes containing myelin.

not be present.[65] Ultrastructurally, cytoplasmic granules can be seen as autophagolysosomes containing myelin-like structures. This confirms the Schwannian lineage. Excision is curative, even for those tumors that may be incompletely excised. Rarely, malignant granular cell tumors may be encountered. Malignant granular cell tumors are either large yet histologically benign and metastatic, or they are histologically malignant and metastatic.[107] On imaging, they usually have slightly irregular margins and are located in the subcutaneous fat, deep to the skin line (Fig. 6-78).

## Meningioma and Craniopharyngioma

Meningiomas are benign, slowly growing tumors arising from rests within the arachnoid villi, usually in relation to the major dural sinuses. They comprise 13% to 18% of all primary intracranial tumors and are two to four times more common in females than in males; their incidence peaks near 45 years of age.[65] These tumors can extend from or arise outside of the neuroaxis; however, this is uncommon. When meningiomas are encountered outside of the neuroaxis, about two thirds are actually direct extensions from an intracranial or intraspinous lesion.[108, 109] Primary extracranial meningiomas are quite rare, comprising less than 1% of cases.[110] Most of these extraneuroaxis meningiomas occur in the head and neck, and also have been reported in the calvarium, orbit, nose, paranasal sinuses, oral cavity, middle ear, skin of the scalp, and cervical soft tissues.[65, 111, 112] Very rarely, an extracranial meningioma might represent a metastasis from an intracranial meningioma.[113]

The imaging characteristics of these sinonasal meningiomas are those of an enhancing, expansile mass with bone remodeling. Most lesions lie in the nasal vault, and adjacent sclerotic, reactive bone may be a dominant feature. This reactive bone radiographically mimics fibrous dysplasia. If the tumor has spread extracranially, the skull base remodeling and the sinonasal tumor extension are best seen on coronal images. On MR imaging, these tumors have signal intensities similar to those of the brain on all imaging sequences. They enhance, and vascular flow voids are rarely observed (Figs. 6-79 to 6-81).

Craniopharyngioma is a rare, histologically benign, expansile intracranial neoplasm derived from retained embryonic odontogenic rests within Rathke's pouch. It occurs in children and adults as solid and cystic calcifying tumors. Histologically, these epithelial tumors resemble ameloblastomas. A case of craniopharyngioma invading the nasal cavities and paranasal sinuses was reported in a patient who presented with nasal obstruction. Imaging showed a destructive mass of the skull base with involvement of the sinonasal cavities.[114] In another report, a 7-year-old boy complained of intermittent epistaxis for several months. CT scans showed a mass in the left ethmoid sinus and

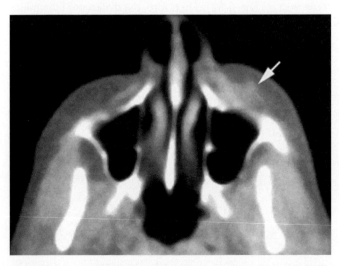

**FIGURE 6-78**   Axial CT scan shows a small soft tissue mass in the left cheek (*arrow*). The mass is within the subcutaneous tissues, adjacent to the anterior maxillary sinus wall. There was no bone erosion. This patient had a malignant granular cell tumor.

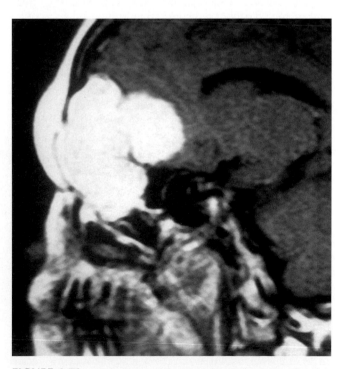

**FIGURE 6-79**   Sagittal T1-weighted MR image shows an enhancing anterior cranial fossa mass that extends caudally into the sinonasal cavities. The epicenter of this tumor is above the level of the cribriform plate, suggesting the intracranial origin of the lesion. This patient had a meningioma.

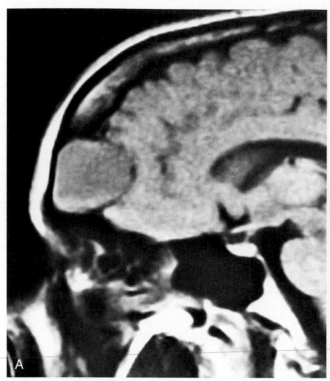

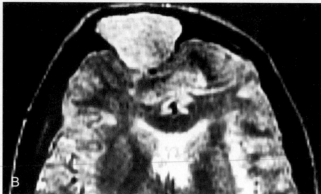

**FIGURE 6-80** Saggital T1-weighted (**A**) and axial T2-weighted (**B**) images show an expansile mass in the right frontal sinus that extends intracranially. The mass has low to intermediate, slightly nonhomogeneous signal intensity in **A** and high signal intensity in **B**. This patient had a frontal sinus meningioma.

endoscopic sinus surgery removed the mass completely, which was a craniopharyngioma[115] (see also Chapter 12).

## Chordoma

Chordomas are indolent, invasive tumors arising from embryonic notochord remnants representing about 1% of all primary malignant bone tumors.[116] The majority of tumors present either in the spheno-occipital (primarily clivus) area (30%) or in the sacrococcygeal area (51%). A smaller percentage may occur in other sites along the cervical or thoracic spine (19%). Rare chordomas have been reported in the ethmoid, maxilla, and mandible.[117, 118] In these cases, the tumor presumably arises in notochordal remnants that

separated from the main notochord during the extreme mesodermal movements of the face that take place in early embryogenesis. These ectopic rests can be located in the paranasal sinuses.[117, 119]

There is a broad age range for chordomas of the head and neck, from the first through the eighth decades of life, with a broad peak incidence in the third to fifth decades. Presenting symptoms include visual changes, cranial nerve deficits, and headache, symptoms for the most part referable to a skull base mass.

Histologically, chordomas are composed of strands and islands of cleared epithelial cells, some of which have a characteristic "soap bubble" (physilliferous cells) appearance. These cells produce an abundant myxoid/chondroid-type matrix (Fig. 6-82). Therefore, the differential diagnosis

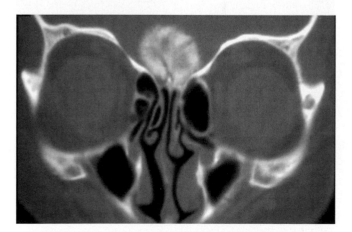

**FIGURE 6-81** Coronal CT scan shows a heavily calcified ovoid mass in the anterior cranial fossa resting on the cribriform plate. This patient had an old "burnt-out" meningioma.

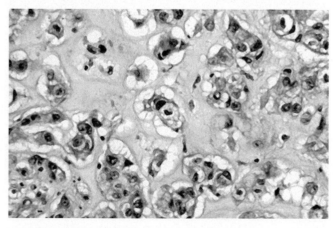

**FIGURE 6-82** Chordoma: The "physilliferous" cells of chordoma contain bubble-like cytoplasmic vacuoles. Nests of tumor cells are present in lacunar spaces within a myxoid stroma.

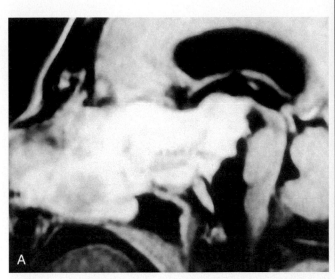
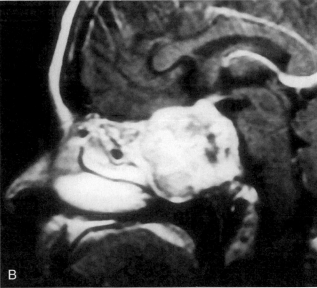

**FIGURE 6-83**   Sagittal T1-weighted, contrast-enhanced MR image (**A**) shows a large, enhancing mass that replaces almost the entire clivus and extends forward to fill the sinonasal cavities. There is also a large dorsal extension of this tumor. This is an unusually large chordoma with uncharacteristic exuberant ventral and dorsal growth. Sagittal T1-weighted, contrast-enhanced MR image (**B**) shows a bulky, nonhomogeneously enhancing mass in the clivus and sphenoid sinus. This is a more characteristic MR appearance of a chordoma than that shown in **A**.

of chordomas in the sinonasal tract includes chondroma, chondroblastic osteosarcoma, chondrosarcoma, and pleomorphic adenoma, all of which are fairly uncommon at this site.[120–122] Immunohistochemically, chordoma cells express cytokeratin, thus excluding tumors such as chondroma, chondroblastic osteosarcoma, and chondrosarcoma. As chordomas routinely express S-100, the differential diagnosis of a salivary tumor (namely, pleomorphic adenoma) is best excluded on light microscopy.

Chordomas have traditionally been treated by surgery plus adjuvant radiotherapy; however, recent data indicate an improved local control rate with higher-energy proton beam therapy.[123] Generally, patients with cranial chordomas have a lower metastatic rate (6.6%) than those with sacral tumors, but the former are obviously more likely to suffer morbidity/mortality due to the lack of tumor control.

On contrast-enhanced CT, the classic chordoma is a minimally enhancing, destructive lesion that has areas of dystrophic calcification and residual bone fragments. On MR imaging, chordomas are extremely variable in appearance, and they can have anywhere from low to high signal intensity on any sequence (Figs. 6-83 and 6-84).[124] Only rarely does a classic chordoma arising within the clivus grow sufficiently large to involve the posterior nasal vault and the paranasal sinuses. The only reported case in the maxillary sinus mimicked a mucocele (Fig. 6-85).[117] Recurrences of clival chordomas along the margins of the surgery have been reported to occur in the nasal soft tissues, the nasal septum, and the maxilla (Fig. 6-86)[125] (see also Chapter 12).

## Choristoma

The term *choristoma* refers to histologically normal mature tissue present in an ectopic site, such as salivary

tissue within the external auditory canal or thyroid tissue within the tongue base. Choristomas usually produce small incidental masses. Sinonasal or nasopharyngeal choristomas have been reported, albeit rarely.[126–128]

### Nasal Glioma

A nasal glioma is also, by definition, a choristoma and not a true neoplasia, as the term *glioma* might imply. It presents

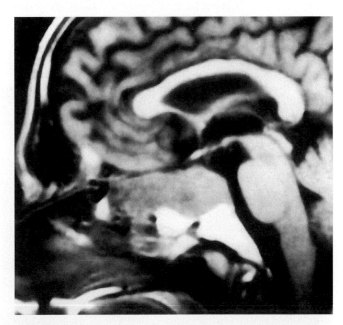

**FIGURE 6-84**   Sagittal T1-weighted MR image shows an intermediate signal intensity mass in the upper clivus, the sphenoid sinuses, and the ethmoid sinuses. There is little intracranial extension. This patient had a chordoma.

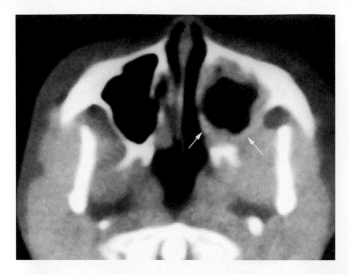

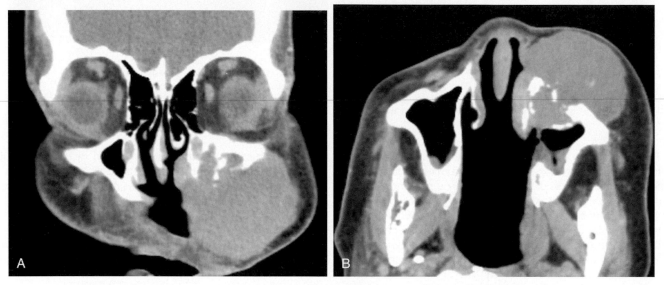

**FIGURE 6-85** Axial CT scan performed after surgical drainage of a presumed mucocele shows thinning or destruction of the medial and posterior antral walls (*arrows*), with fairly uniform soft tissues lining the antrum. This patient had a rare chordoma of the maxillary sinus.

**FIGURE 6-86** Coronal (**A**) and axial (**B**) CT scans through the paranasal sinuses show a destructive soft tissue mass in the left maxillary sinus. Part of the nasal septum had been removed at the time of prior surgery. This patient developed a recurrent chordoma along the course of the original operative procedure for a skull base chordoma.

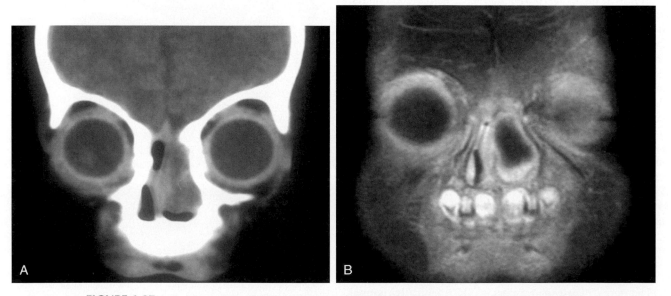

**FIGURE 6-87** Coronal CT scan (**A**) and T1-weighted, fat-suppressed, contrast-enhanced MR image (**B**) on a newborn show a cystic, expansile mass in the left nasal cavity. No intracranial communication was demonstrated. The central floor of the anterior cranial fossa was intact. This region is not yet ossified in the newborn. This patient has a nasal glioma.

as a subcutaneous mass of the nasal bridge with intranasal extension (60%) or as a polyp confined to the nasal vault. Radiographically, an intracerebral extension or a cribriform plate defect needs to be ruled out. If an intracerebral communication, in particular a CSF communication, is found, this lesion is better classified as a cephalocele (Fig. 6-87) (see also Chapter 1). Histologically, a glioma is composed of disorganized glial and fibrous tissue.

### Ectopic Pituitary

Nelson's syndrome is defined as the presence of an enlarging pituitary tumor, elevated fasting plasma ACTH, and hyperpigmentation after bilateral adrenalectomy in patients with Cushing's disease. Ectopic functioning pituitary tissue within the sphenoid sinus is a rare occurrence. The development of Nelson's syndrome presenting as a sphenoid mass was described in a young woman whose only functioning hypophyseal tissue was within the sphenoid sinus.[129]

# LYMPHOPROLIFERATIVE AND HEMATOPOIETIC DISORDERS

## Lymphoma

About half of all patients with malignant lymphoma clinically present with disease in the head and neck, most often as cervical lymphadenopathy. Only 10% of head and neck lymphomas are extranodal, usually involving the tonsils, sinonasal tract, and thyroid. The last usually develops in association with Hashimoto's thyroiditis.[130, 131]

Sinonasal lymphoma (SNL) is more common in Asian than in Western populations, where it represents the second most frequent group of extranodal lymphomas after gastrointestinal lymphomas. It has previously been referred to in the literature as lethal midline granuloma, malignant midline reticulosis, or polymorphic reticulosis. These are clinically inexact terms that imply a lack of definitive pathologic diagnosis. These terms have been replaced by microscopic and phenotypic classifications.[132] SNL can be classified as either B-cell, T-cell natural killer cell (T/NK-cell), or T-cell natural killer precursor cell (T/null-cell) phenotypes. The Revised European and American Lymphoma classification (REAL) is presented in Table 6-2, which includes SNL within the classification of extranodal lymphomas.

Some pertinent clinicopathologic distinctions can be made between B-cell and T-cell SNL.[133-137] B-cell phenotype SNL typically involves the paranasal sinuses, with a slight predominance in Western countries. Presenting symptoms relate to paranasal sinus involvement; patients may present late with pain, a facial or palatal mass, or ocular symptoms. These lymphomas are more likely to be associated with ocular symptoms and are more likely to have orbital extension than T/NK-cell phenotype SNL. T-cell SNL is most common in Asian and South American countries. The majority of T-cell SNLs have the natural killer T-cell phenotype T/NK-cell, however, a small

percentage lack this phenotype and are classified as T/null-cell SNL. These tumors are typically located in the nasal cavity and have an aggressive, angioinvasive growth pattern that often results in necrosis and bony erosion. The term *angiocentric T-cell lymphoma* refers to those T-cell lymphomas that grow around and into vessels and are associated with necrosis. Patients with T-cell SNL are younger, with a lower male-to-female ratio than those with B-cell SNL. T-cell SNL is more commonly associated with the Epstein-Barr virus (EBV) than is B-cell SNL.[138-141] Typically, T-cell SNL, especially angiocentric

**Table 6-2**
**REVISED EUROPEAN AND AMERICAN LYMPHOMA (REAL) CLASSIFICATION**

**B-Cell Neoplasms**
I. Precursor B-cell neoplasm
　1. B-lymphoblastic leukemia/lymphoma
II. Peripheral B-cell neoplasms
　1. B-cell chronic lymphocytic leukemia/small lymphocytic lymphoma
　2. Lymphoplasmacytoid lymphoma/immunocytoma
　3. Mantle cell lymphoma
　4. Follicle center lymphoma, follicular
　　• Provisional cytologic grades: small cell, mixed small and large cell, large cell
　　• Provisional subtype: diffuse, predominantly small cell type
　5. Marginal zone B-cell lymphoma
　　• Extranodal (MALT type +/− monocytoid B cells)
　　• Nodal (+/− monocytoid B cells)
　　• Splenic (+/− villous lymphocytes)
　6. Hairy cell leukemia
　7. Plasmacytoma/myeloma
　8. Diffuse large cell B-cell lymphoma
　　• Subtype: primary mediastinal (thymic) B-cell lymphoma
　9. Burkitt's lymphoma
　10. Provisional category high-grade B-cell lymphoma, Burkitt's-like

**T-Cell and Putative Natural Killer (NK) Cell Neoplasms**
I. Precursor T-cell neoplasm
　1. T precursor lymphoblastic lymphoma/leukemia
II. Peripheral T-cell and NK-cell neoplasms
　1. T-cell chronic lymphocytic leukemia/prolymphocytic leukemia
　2. Large granular lymphoproliferative (LGL) disorder
　　• T-cell type
　　• NK-cell type
　3. Mycosis fungoides/Sézary's syndrome
　4. Peripheral T-cell lymphoma (small cell, mixed small and large cell, large cell)
　　• Provisional subtype: lymphoepithelioid cell lymphoma
　5. Angioimmunoblastic T-cell lymphoma (AILD)
　6. Angiocentric lymphoma
　7. Intestinal T-cell lymphoma (+/− enteropathy associated)
　8. Adult T-cell lymphoma/leukemia (ATL/L)
　9. Anaplastic large cell lymphoma (ALCL), CD30+, T- and null-cell types

**Hodgkin's Disease**
1. Lymphocyte predominance
2. Nodular sclerosis
3. Mixed cellularity
4. Lymphocyte depletion
5. Provisional category: lymphocyte-rich classic Hodgkin's disease
6. Provisional category: anaplastic large cell lymphoma, Hodgkin's disease–like

**Unclassifiable**
1. B-cell lymphoma, unclassifiable (low grade/high grade)
2. T-cell lymphoma, unclassifiable (low grade/high grade)
3. Malignant lymphoma, unclassifiable

## Table 6-3
## COMPARISON OF THE DEMOGRAPHICS AND SURVIVAL OF SEVERAL RECENT SERIES OF B-CELL AND T-CELL SNL PATIENTS

| Author | Year | Country | Total Cases | Med Age | B-Cell Cases |
|---|---|---|---|---|---|
| Ko | 2000 | Korea | 48 | | |
| Quraishi | 2000 | UK | 24 | 72 | 21/24 (87%) |
| Rodriguez | 2000 | USA | 26 | 44 | 13 |
| Aviles | 2000 | Mexico | 108 | | |
| Lei | 1999 | Hong Kong | 25 SNL 19 NPL | | NSL: 4/16 (25%) NPL: 11/16 (69%) |
| Yang | 1997 | Taiwan | 34 | 60 | 2/20 (10%) |
| Nakamura | 1997 | Japan | 32 | | |
| Harabuchi | 1996 | Japan | 18 | 18 | |
| Davison | 1996 | USA | 30 | 44.5 | |
| Liang | 1995 | Hong Kong | 100 | 50 | 8/45 (33%) |
| Abbondanzo | 1995 | USA | 120 | 59 | 101/120 (84%) |
| Arber | 1993 | Peru | 14 | | 2 (14%) |
| Kojima | 1992 | Japan | 20 | | 9 (45%) |

Abbreviations: AWD = alive with disease, DID = died of intercurrent disease, DOD = died of disease, EBV = Epstein-Barr virus, NED = no evidence of disease, NPL = nasopharyngeal lymphoma, SNL = sinonasal lymphoma, YR = years, YS = year survival.

References: Abbondanzo, SL, Wenig BM. Non-Hodgkin's lymphoma of the sinonasal tract. A clinicopathologic and immunophenotypic study of 120 cases. Cancer 1995;75:1281–1291.

Arber DA, Weiss LM, Albujar PF, Chen YY, et al. Nasal lymphomas in Peru. High incidence of T-cell immunophenotype and Epstein-Barr virus infections. AMJ Surg Pathol 1993;17:392–399.

Aviles A, Diaz NR, Neri N, et al. Angiocentric nasal T/natural killer cell lymphoma: a single centre study of prognostic factors in 108 patients Clin Lab Haematol 2000;22(4):215–220.

Davison SP, Habermann TM, Strickler JG, et al. Nasal and nasopharyngeal angiocentric T-cell lymphomas. Laryngoscope 1996; 106(2 Pt 1):139–143.

Harabuchi Y, Imai S, Wakashima J, et al. Nasal T-cell lymphoma causally associated with Epstein-Barr virus: clinicopathologic, phenotypic, and genotypic studies. Cancer 1996;77(10):2137–2149.

Ko YH, Ree HJ, Kim WS, et al. Clinicopathologic and genotypic study of extranodal nasal-type natural killer/T-cell lymphoma and natural killer precursor lymphoma among Koreans. Cancer 2000;89(10):2106–2116.

lymphomas, may present with, or progress to involve, numerous extranodal sites such as skin, liver, larynx, kidney, breast, testis, and prostate. In addition to the development of extranodal disease, T/NK-cell SNL may be associated with hemophagocytic syndrome, a fatal complication that may be associated etiologically with EBV reactivation.[142]

SNL is treated with a combination of local irradiation and chemotherapy with an anthracycline-based regimen. B-cell SNL is usually responsive, whereas in Asian studies, T/NK-cell SNL is less responsive and has a worse prognosis. Table 6-3 compares some recent series of B-cell and T-cell SNL patients regarding demographics and survival. Generally, survival is dependant upon tumor stage and grade rather than phenotype.

On CT and MR imaging, lymphomas in the sinonasal cavities tend to be bulky soft tissue masses that enhance to a moderate degree.[143, 144] These tumors also tend to remodel bone, although occasionally aggressive bone invasion is seen.[145–148] Most often the disease is located in the nasal fossae and maxillary sinuses.[149] Less often, lymphoma is found in the ethmoid sinuses, and only rarely is it found in the sphenoid and frontal sinuses. On MR imaging, it tends to have an intermediate intensity signal on all imaging sequences and it enhances after contrast administration (Figs. 6-88 to 6-93).

## Granulocytic Sarcoma

Granulocytic sarcoma, or chloroma, is a rare complication of acute and chronic myeloid leukemia. It represents a soft-tissue infiltrate of immature myeloid elements that develops in 3% of patients with acute and chronic myeloid leukemia. The term chloroma describes the green hue seen when these tumors are sectioned. The color, caused by the cytoplasmic enzyme myeloperoxidase, fades after exposure to air. The mean patient age is 48 years, and most patients (85%) present with a solitary lesion. In the head and neck, osseous lesions have been reported in the skull, face, orbit,

**Table 6-3** (*Continued*)

| T-Cell Cases | Overall Survival | Notes |
|---|---|---|
| 45, plus 3 NK precursor neoplasms | 1 YS 41% | Strong association with EBV<br>Progression to extranodal disease |
| 3/24 (13%) | 5 YS 40%, 10 YS 33% | |
| 13 | 4 NED 1, 2, 3, 9 YR | Progression to extranodal disease |
| 108 (100%) | 8-year overall and disease-free survival ranged from 79% to 90% | |
| NSL: 12/16 (75%)<br>NPL: 5/16 (31%) | Overall 5 YS (33% versus 82%) and disease-free 5 YS (36% versus 76%) and worse in NSL than NPL patients, correlating with age and bulky disease | |
| 18/20 (90%) | Mean survival 84.2 months<br>Overall 5 YS 63% | |
| 32 (100%) | Overall 5 YS 49% | Strong association with EBV |
| 18 (100%) | Median survival 6 months | Strong association with EBV<br>Extranodal involvement |
| 30 (100%) | 10/30 (33%) NED<br>12/30 (40%) DOD<br>6/30 (20%) DID | Strong association with EBV |
| 35/45 (77%) | Improved survival correlated with age (<60), stage I disease, and absence of clinical (B) symptoms | |
| 19/120 (16%) | 24/66 patients (36.4%) DOD<br>17/66 (25.7%) NED<br>13/66 (19.7%) AWD<br>12/66 (18.2%) DID or unknown | Extranodal involvement |
| 11 (78%) | | Strong association with EBV |
| 9 (45%) | 2 YS was poorer for T-cell than B-cell lymphomas<br>Survival correlated with stage | |

Kojima M, Hosomura Y, Kurabayashi Y, et al. Malignant lymphomas of the nasal cavity and paranasal sinuses. A clinicopathologic and immunohistochemical study. Acta Pathol Jpn 1992;42(5):333–338.

Lei KI, Suen JJ, Hui P, et al. Primary nasal and nasopharyngeal lymphomas: a comparative study of clinical presentation and treatment outcome. Clin Oncol (R Coll Radiol) 1999;11(6):379–387.

Liang R, Todd D, Chan TK, et al. Treatment outcome and prognostic factors for primary nasal lymphoma. J Clin Oncol 1995;13(3):666–670.

Nakamura S, Katoh E, Koshikawa T, et al. Clinicopathologic study of nasal T/NK-cell lymphoma among the Japanese. Pathol Int 1997;47(1):38–53.

Quraishi MS, Bessell EM, Clark D, et al. Non-Hodgkin's lymphoma of the sinonasal tract. Laryngoscope 2000;110(9):1489–1492.

Rodriguez J, Romaguera JE, Manning J, Ordonez N, et al. Nasal-type T/NK Lymphomas: a clinicopathologic study of 13 cases. Leuk Lymphoma 2000;39:139–144.

Yang Y, Gau JP, Chang SM, et al. Malignant lymphomas of sinonasal region, including cases of polymorphic reticulosis: a retrospective clinicopathologic analysis of 34 cases. Chung Hua I Hsueh Tsa Chih (Taipei) 1997;60(5):236–244.

and paranasal sinuses, whereas extramedullary tumors have been reported in the nasal cavity, paranasal sinuses, nasopharynx, tonsil, mouth, lacrimal gland, salivary glands, and thyroid gland.[150] An associated myeloproliferative disease is found in 48% of patients, and acute myeloid leukemia occurs in 22% of the cases. However, 30% of patients with granulocytic sarcoma have no hematologic disease at the time of initial diagnosis. The onset of granulocytic sarcoma may be a harbinger of the development of acute blast crisis within a few months of the diagnosis. The prognosis of patients with acute myeloid leukemia is not altered by the development of a chloroma; however, in patients with chronic myeloid leukemia and other myeloproliferative disorders, the granulocytic sarcoma is an ominous sign because it is associated with the acute or blastic phase of the disease.[150–152] On CT, chloromas are enhancing, homogeneous masses, usually with slightly infiltrative margins.[153] On MR imaging, they have intermediate to high signal intensities on all imaging sequences, and they enhance with contrast administration.

## Multiple Myeloma

Multiple myeloma (MM) is the most common member of a group of diseases known collectively as plasma cell dyscrasias. These diseases, including Waldenstrom's macroglobulinemia, heavy chain disease, and primary amyloidosis, all have a malignant proliferation of plasma cells or lymphocytoid plasma cells with monoclonal immunoglobulin or immunoglobulin fragments in the patient's urine. The proliferation of neoplastic cells is associated with bone destruction and involves the bone marrow of the axial skeleton. However, the soft tissues can also be involved. MM usually affects patients over the age of 40 (mean age is 63) and has a roughly equal sex distribution. The most frequent complaints are bone pain (63%), weakness (23%), and weight loss (15%). Extraosseous plasmacytoma is the initial manifestation of MM in only 5% of patients.[150] In the head and neck, soft-tissue masses occur primarily in the nose, paranasal sinuses, nasopharynx, and tonsils. Patients may have oronasal

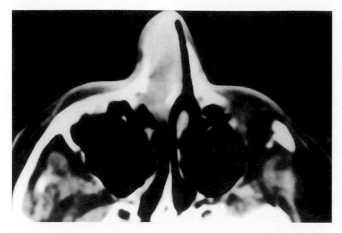

**FIGURE 6-88**   Axial CT scan shows a soft-tissue mass in the right nose and anterior nasal fossa. There is widening of the involved right side, and there is no bone erosion. This patient had a large cell lymphoma.

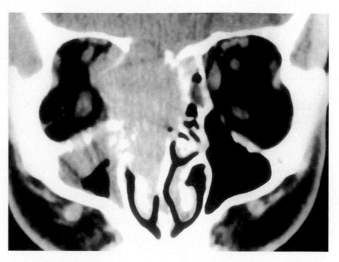

**FIGURE 6-90**   Coronal CT scan shows a bulky soft-tissue mass in the right ethmoid and nasal cavity. The tumor has invaded the right orbit and the floor of the anterior cranial fossa. There is also obstruction of the right antrum. This is a more aggressive appearance of a large cell lymphoma and, based on the imaging appearance, could be a carcinoma.

bleeding as a primary manifestation of hyperviscosity. Skeletal lytic lesions are found in 85% of patients, and a combination of lytic bone lesions, osteoporosis, and pathologic fractures is found in 63% of patients at disease onset.[148] Paraosseous tumor extension through destroyed cortical bone is found in 50% of patients at autopsy. In 10% to 12% of patients with MM, amyloidosis is present. Infection and renal failure are the primary causes of death. With the use of alkylating agents, steroids, and local irradiation, the median survival time is 20 months; 66% of patients are alive after 1 year, 32% after 3 years, and 18% after 5 years.[153] The imaging characteristics appear to be similar to those of lymphomas.

## Extramedullary Plasmacytoma

Extramedullary plasmacytoma (EMP) is a rare soft-tissue malignancy composed of plasma cells. Eighty percent of these tumors occur in the head and neck, 28% occur in the nasal cavity, and 22% occur in the paranasal sinuses.[150]

They represent 3% to 4% of all sinonasal cavity tumors.[154, 155] About 20% of head and neck EMPs are initially associated with MM. The tumors are four times more likely to occur in males than in females, and 90% of the patients are white; 95% of the tumors occur over the age of 40 years (mean is 59 years).[150] The most common presenting symptoms are a soft-tissue mass (80%), airway obstruction (35%), epistaxis (35%), local pain (20%), proptosis (15%), and nasal discharge (10%). The mean duration of symptoms is 4½ months.

Histologically, plasmacytomas range from well-differentiated cells indistinguishable from mature, benign

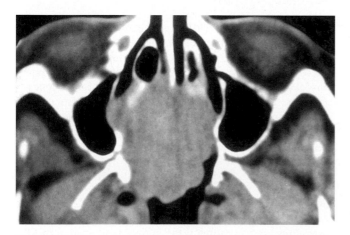

**FIGURE 6-89**   Axial CT scan shows a bulky, lobulated posterior nasal fossa mass centered on the nasal septum. There is minimal thinning of the medial right antral wall. The dominant finding is expansion of the nasal vault. This patient had a large cell lymphoma.

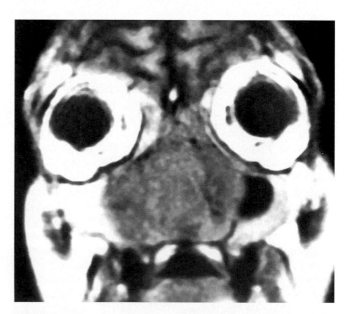

**FIGURE 6-91**   Coronal T1-weighted MR image shows an expansile bilateral nasal cavity mass that extends into the ethmoid and maxillary sinuses. The mass has a low to intermediate signal intensity and had a slightly higher T2-weighted signal intensity. This patient had a large cell lymphoma.

plasma cells to poorly differentiated tumor cells. The former can be distinguished from a benign plasma cell infiltrate by the demonstration of immunoglobulin clonality via immunohistochemistry. Poorly differentiated anaplastic plasmacytoma can also be distinguished from anaplastic carcinoma, ONB, melanoma, and large cell lymphoma by immunohistochemistry.[150, 156] Radiation therapy and surgery are the treatments of choice; alkylating agents and steroids help patients with painful bone lesions and patients with systemic disease. Eventually, 35% to 50% of patients with primary EMP develop MM. Local bone destruction and persistent primary tumors after radiation therapy are not necessarily poor prognostic indicators. Between 31% and 75% of patients are alive after 5 years; however, the median length of survival after the onset of MM is less than 2 years.[150]

On CT, EMPs of the sinonasal cavities are homogeneous, enhancing polypoid masses that remodel surrounding bone.[157, 158] On MR imaging they have an intermediate signal intensity on all imaging sequences, they enhance, and because they are highly vascular, they may have vascular flow voids (Figs. 6-94 to 6-97).

## Langerhans' Cell Granulomatosis

Langerhans' cell granulomatosis (LCG or histiocytosis X) is the current term for a group of childhood diseases including eosinophilic granuloma (EG), Hand-Schuller-Christian (HSC) disease, and Letterer-Siwe (L-S) disease. EG is a more localized form of LCG, often manifesting as a solitary bone lesion, whereas HSC disease and L-S disease are multifocal or disseminated diseases that involve the lymph nodes, skin, liver, spleen, lung, head and neck, or gastrointestinal tract. The etiology is unknown; however, some researchers suggest that all forms of LCG are clonal.[159, 160] Others, however, believe LCG to be a benign, possibly reactive process.[161]

The head and neck are frequently involved in LCG, usually the flat bones of the skull or the jaws. Patients often present with otitis media and/or destructive temporal bone lesions. Sinonasal involvement is virtually unreported, but sphenoid involvement has been seen.[150, 163, 164]

The histology of LCG is distinctive, but immunohistochemical confirmation is important.[161, 165] LCG is characterized by a polymorphous cellular infiltrate of mononuclear

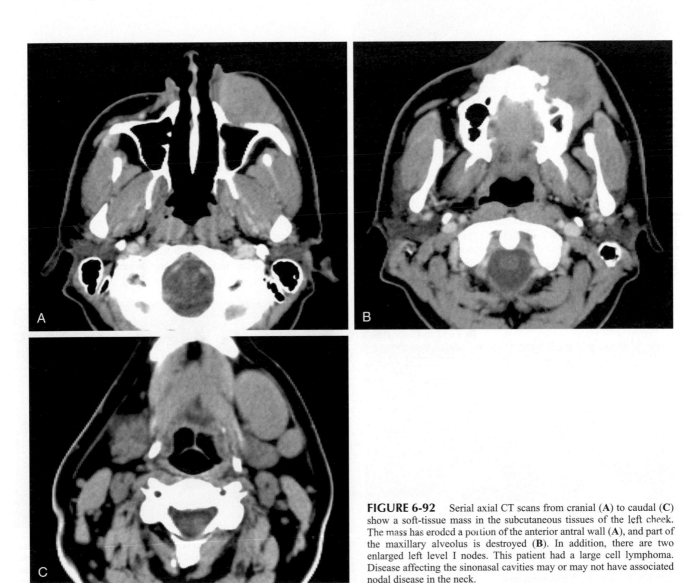

**FIGURE 6-92** Serial axial CT scans from cranial (**A**) to caudal (**C**) show a soft-tissue mass in the subcutaneous tissues of the left cheek. The mass has eroded a portion of the anterior antral wall (**A**), and part of the maxillary alveolus is destroyed (**B**). In addition, there are two enlarged left level I nodes. This patient had a large cell lymphoma. Disease affecting the sinonasal cavities may or may not have associated nodal disease in the neck.

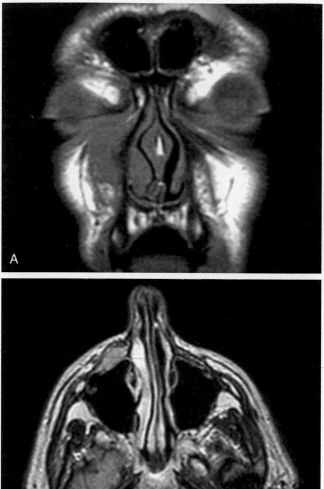

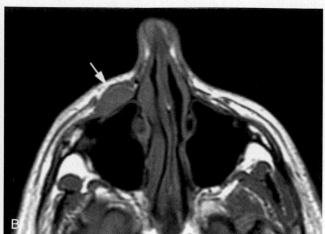

**FIGURE 6-93** Coronal (**A**) and axial (**B**) T1-weighted and axial T2-weighted (**C**) MR images show a soft-tissue mass in the medial right cheek lying against the anterior antral wall (*arrow*). There may be thinning of the wall immediately adjacent to the mass. The mass has a low to intermediate T1-weighted signal intensity and a higher intermediate T2-weighted signal intensity. This patient had a large cell lymphoma.

or multinucleated histiocytes (Langerhans' cells), with lobated or grooved (clefted) nuclei, mixed with varying numbers of eosinophils, granulocytes, and lymphocytes.[161, 165] Immunohistochemically, Langerhans' cells are typically positive for S-100 protein and, more specifically, CD1a. Intracytoplasmic Birbeck granules are diagnostic of LCG cells on ultrastructural analysis.[166]

The mixed infiltrate of histiocytes and eosinophils, and the presence of phagocytosis in LCG, may be mistaken for reactive histiocytosis, Hodgkin's disease, and sinus histiocytosis with massive lymphadenopathy (SHML or

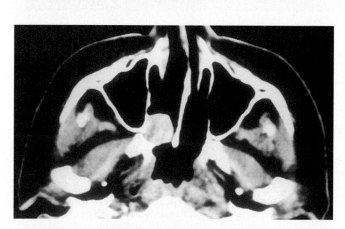

**FIGURE 6-94** Axial CT scan shows a small polypoid mass along the right posterior lateral nasal wall. There is no associated bone erosion. This patient had an extraosseous plasmacytoma.

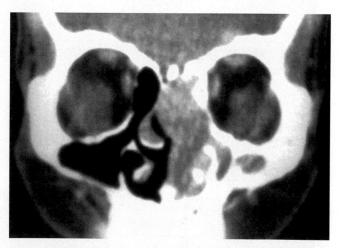

**FIGURE 6-95** Coronal CT scan shows a soft-tissue mass filling the left nasal cavity and left ethmoid sinuses and obstructing the left antrum. There is focal erosion of the cribriform plate region; otherwise, the marginal bone about the mass is intact. This patient had an extramedullary plasmacytoma.

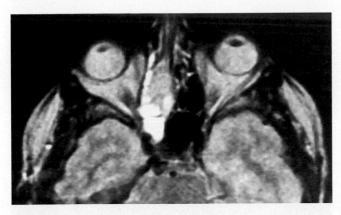

**FIGURE 6-96**   Axial proton density MR image shows a right ethmoid and nasal mass that has a low to intermediate signal intensity. Surrounding the mass are chronically obstructed secretions with high signal intensity. This is a nonspecific imaging appearance. This patient had an extramedullary plasmacytoma.

Rosai Dorfman disease). The characteristic feature of SHML is prominent lymphophagocytosis (emperipolesis). SHML cells lack the typical nuclear features of LCG cells and, furthermore, lack the characteristic intra-

cytoplasmic Birbeck granules seen on ultrastructural analysis.[166]

Treatment of LCH is based on the degree of disease involvement.[161] Biopsy or curettage of osseous lesions and, at times, low-dose radiation therapy are the treatments of choice for localized LCG. Aggressive or refractory disease may require chemotherapy. Generally, the greater the degree of organ involvement, the worse the prognosis. Alessi and colleagues subclassified 28 children with LCG as having either type I (monostotic disease—7 children), type II (multiple sites without visceral involvement—15 children), or type III (presentation with disseminated disease including visceral involvement—6 children).[162] Patients with type I disease had an excellent prognosis after local curettage, whereas patients with type III disease all died despite chemotherapy. A poor prognosis was associated with polyostotic bone disease, additional soft-tissue lesions of the skin, lymph node involvement, hepatosplenomegaly, diabetes insipidus and hypothalamic dysfunction, and disseminated bone marrow involvement.

On CT, bone involvement can vary from a well-localized destructive process to an infiltrative mass. Enhancement after contrast administration is seen on CT and MR imaging. Soft-tissue involvement is nonspecific, and again can vary

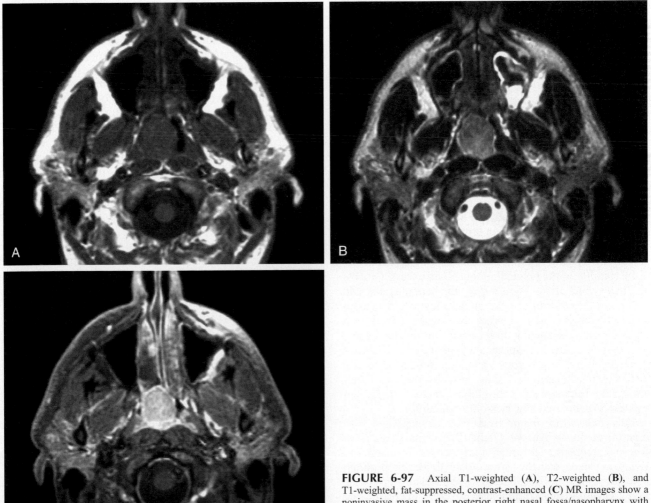

**FIGURE 6-97**   Axial T1-weighted (**A**), T2-weighted (**B**), and T1-weighted, fat-suppressed, contrast-enhanced (**C**) MR images show a noninvasive mass in the posterior right nasal fossa/nasopharynx with fairly low T1- and T2-weighted signal intensity. The mass enhances. This patient had an extramedullary plasmacytoma.

from a fairly well defined mass to one that has infiltrative margins. On MR imaging, there usually is an intermediate T1-weighted signal intensity and an intermediate to high T2-weighted signal intensity.[167] As mentioned, there is marked enhancement after contrast administration. Overall, MR imaging is usually better in assessing bone marrow invasion and any soft-tissue disease, while the actual bone disease is often better seen on CT.

## Rosai-Dorfman Disease

Rosai-Dorfman disease (massive lymphadenopathy with sinus histiocytosis) is a rare idiopathic benign histiocytic proliferation usually seen in young patients. The massive lymphadenopathy most commonly involves the cervical lymph nodes, with a predominant infiltration of sinusoidal histiocytes. Nearly half of the patients have extranodal involvement, the majority of which (75%) occur in sites in the head and neck. Paranasal sinus involvement has been reported, usually in conjunction with cervical adenopathy and multifocal extranodal lesions.[168–171] On CT, the paranasal sinus disease was a bulky, homogeneous mass similiar in appearance to lymphoma.

The clinical presentation depends upon the involved site. Patients may present with nasal obstruction, stridor, proptosis, decreased visual acuity, facial pain or tenderness, cranial nerve deficits, mandibular tenderness, dermal infiltrates, and mass lesions.

Rosai-Dorfman disease can be self-limiting. In other cases, surgery for locoregional lesions can result in long-term disease control. Sinonasal disease can be managed by endoscopic resection, although refractory cases may require chemotherapy, radiotherapy, steroids, or more extensive surgery. The imaging findings are nonspecific.

## Thalassemia

Thalassemia is a hereditary anemia characterized by defective hemoglobin synthesis and ineffective erythropoiesis caused by reduction and abnormalities in globin chain synthesis. Disease severity correlates with homozygosity and with the ensuing relative decrease in globin production and the stability of the residual globin chain excess. Patients with thalassemia minor syndromes are heterozygous and develop mild anemia and persistent microcytosis. Thalassemia intermedia is a homozygous state characterized by a moderate hemolytic anemia that presents during physiologic stressors such as infection, pregnancy, or surgery. Thalassemia major is a homozygous state that produces severe, life-threatening anemia; it can be classified as beta-thalassemia (diminished beta-globin chains) or alpha-thalassemia (decreased alpha-chain production).

Alpha-thalassemia major usually is incompatible with life and presents as hydrops fetalis. Beta-thalassemia is an autosomal recessive disorder that occurs primarily in patients of Mediterranean origin. The defect in β-globin synthesis results in imbalanced globin chain synthesis, delayed erythroid maturation, and severely decreased red cell survival.

Patients become symptomatic early in life, requiring

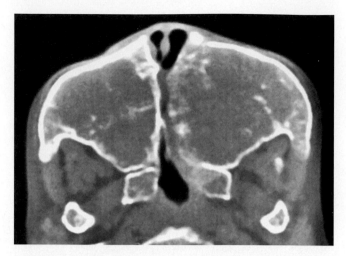

**FIGURE 6-98** Axial CT scan at a wide window setting shows a markedly expanded maxilla with no development of the maxillary sinuses. The surrounding cortical bone is intact. The central portions of each maxilla are filled with expanded marrow. This patient had thalassemia.

chronic transfusion therapy. Iron overload, due to increased gastrointestinal absorption and blood transfusion, is the major cause of tissue damage, morbidity, and death.

The radiographic features of beta-thalassemia are due in large part to compensatory bone marrow expansion. A markedly expanded marrow space leads to various skeletal manifestations in the spine, skull, facial bones, ribs, etc. The classic radiographic changes of thalassemia in the skull include a thickened calvarium and a "hair-on-end" appearance. In the facial area, sinus pneumatization is delayed and the maxilla is expanded secondary to marrow expansion, which can result in both malocclusion and a cosmetic deformity. On CT, soft-tissue density material (marrow) is seen filling and expanding the maxillae, and this process may extend into the central skull base and mandible (Figs. 6-98 and 6-99).[172] Because sinus pneumatization only occurs in a bone once red marrow has converted to yellow marrow, often the frontal, sphenoid, and maxillary sinuses are poorly developed, and the only sinuses seen are the ethmoids.

Advances in the management of thalassemia major (bone marrow transplantation, iron-chelating therapy) have greatly improved the prognosis.[173, 174]

## BENIGN AND MALIGNANT PRIMARY SOFT-TISSUE TUMORS

### Vascular

#### Angiofibroma

The nasopharyngeal angiofibroma (juvenile angiofibroma) is an uncommon, highly vascular, nonencapsulated polypoid mass that is histologically benign but locally aggressive. It represents 0.05% of all head and neck neoplasms and occurs almost exclusively in males.[13] However, a few cases have been documented in females, and it has been suggested that when such a diagnosis is made, sex chromosome studies should be performed to investigate the possibility of genetic mosaicism.[175] The typical patient is a male between 10 and 18 years of age, although the lesion may occasionally present in older patients.[13] The presenting symptoms include nasal obstruction, epistaxis, facial deformity, proptosis, nasal voice, sinusitis, nasal discharge, serous otitis media, headache, and anosmia. Almost all angiofibromas originate from the posterior choanal tissue near the pterygopalatine fossa and sphenopalatine foramen and fill the nasopharynx. Tumor growth is asymmetric, and one side is always the primary site of involvement. Extension into the pterygopalatine fossa occurs in 89% of the cases and results in widening

of this fossa, with resultant anterior bowing of the posterior ipsilateral antral wall.[176] Although there are other slowly growing lesions that may also similarly widen the pterygopalatine fossa (e.g., lymphomas, lymphoepitheliomas, schwannomas, and fibrous histiocytomas), the vast majority of antral bowing is caused by nasopharyngeal angiofibromas.[177] The sphenoid sinus is involved by extension through the roof of the nasopharynx in 61% of cases. Angiofibromas also spread into the maxillary and ethmoid sinuses in 43% and 35% of cases, respectively.[175] Intracranial extension occurs in 5% to 20% of cases and

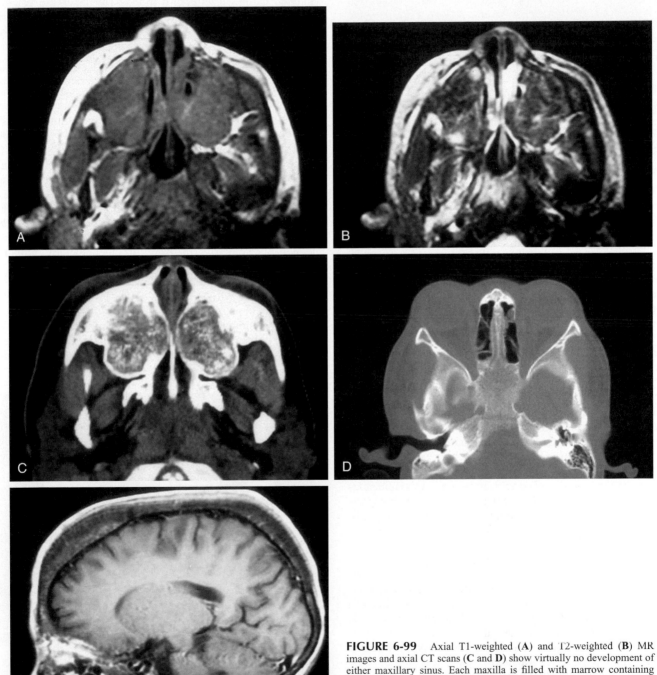

**FIGURE 6-99**   Axial T1-weighted (**A**) and T2-weighted (**B**) MR images and axial CT scans (**C** and **D**) show virtually no development of either maxillary sinus. Each maxilla is filled with marrow containing bone. Only the ethmoid sinuses are developed. No sphenoid sinus development is present. Sagittal T1-weighted MR image (**E**) shows a thickened calvaria. This patient had thalassemia.

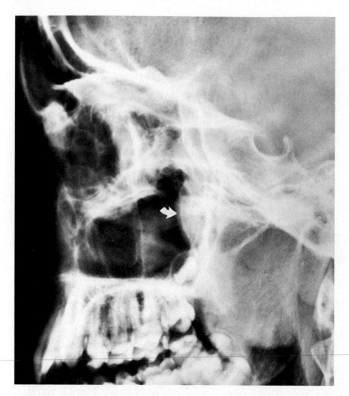

**FIGURE 6-100** Lateral view shows a large nasopharyngeal mass that has displaced the posterior antral wall anteriorly (*arrow*). The mass also extends into the sphenoid sinuses. This patient had an angiofibroma.

primarily involves the middle cranial fossa.[13] Most often this extension progresses from the pterygopalatine fossa into the orbit (through the inferior orbital fissure) and then intracranially through the superior orbital fissure. Direct intracranial extension from the sphenoid or ethmoid sinuses is uncommon. Biopsy should not be attempted in an outpatient or office facility because of tumor vascularity. Sectional imaging and angiography are sufficient to establish the diagnosis.[178] Histologically, thick-walled vessels are embedded in densely collagenized fibrous stroma. The differential diagnosis includes a fibrosed antrochoanal or nasal polyp and an angiomatous polyp.

Plain film findings of an angiofibroma include a soft-tissue nasopharyngeal mass, widening of the pterygo-palatine fossa with anterior bowing of the ipsilateral posterior antral wall, and opacification of the sphenoid sinus (Fig. 6-100). A polypoid nasal mass may cloud the ipsilateral ethmoid and maxillary sinuses. If the superior orbital fissure is widened, intracranial extension will be present.

Contrast-enhanced CT shows an enhancing mass with the anatomic distribution described above (Figs. 6-101 and 6-102). Intraorbital or intracranial extension is much better visualized on CT than on plain films. On contrast-enhanced CT, the imaging must be done while contrast material is flowing freely. If scanning is delayed, the rich vascular tumor network will wash out the contrast medium. Dynamic scanning also identifies the highly vascular nature of these tumors.[179] MR imaging reveals a mass of intermediate signal intensity on T1-weighted and T2-weighted sequences, with multiple-flow voids that represent the major tumor

vessels (Figs. 6-102 and 6-103). The primary imaging tasks are mapping the lesion for the surgeon and documenting any intracranial spread.[180–182] These tumors tend to deossify the adjacent skull base; however, the imaging may suggest aggressive erosion. Most often, the cavernous sinus is displaced rather than invaded, and current skull base surgical techniques usually allow such tumor extension to be resected.

Angiography demonstrates that the major feeding vessels are the internal maxillary artery and the ascending pharyngeal artery on the dominant side (Fig. 6-104). Cross-circulation from contralateral branches of the external carotid artery and occasional feeding branches from the internal carotid arteries are found. The latter are usually associated with intracranial tumor extension. Subselective angiography is usually necessary to identify all of the feeding vessels. Preoperative embolization of the external carotid artery's nutrient branches greatly reduces the blood loss at surgery.[13]

The treatment of choice is surgery. Unresectable intracranial disease, if present, can be irradiated. Control rates of 78% using a dose of 30 to 35 Gy have been reported, and an additional 15% of the cases can be controlled by a second course of radiotherapy.[183] Although the radiation affects tumor vascularity, the fibrous tumor component remains unchanged and a residual mass will be seen on imaging indefinitely. Experts disagree about the effect of estrogen therapy on angiofibromas. Although some cases of decreased tumor size and vascularity have been reported after estrogen therapy, this response is not achieved in most patients.[13] Similarly, the role of chemotherapy remains unclear.

### Angiomatous Polyp

The angiomatous polyp is a fibrosed, vascularized nasal polyp, presumably the response to minor trauma.[184] A choanal polyp may become quite vascularized and is termed an *angiomatous polyp*. The significance of this lesion is that

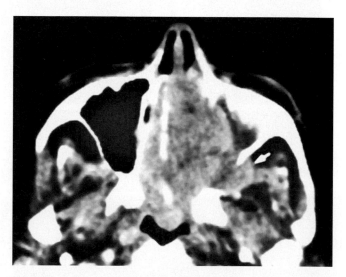

**FIGURE 6-101** Axial contrast-enhanced CT scan shows a left nasopharyngeal and nasal fossa enhancing mass that has extended into the left antrum, widened the left pterygopalatine fossa, and extended into the left infratemporal fossa (*arrow*). There were only obstructed secretions in the right nasal fossa. This patient had an angiofibroma.

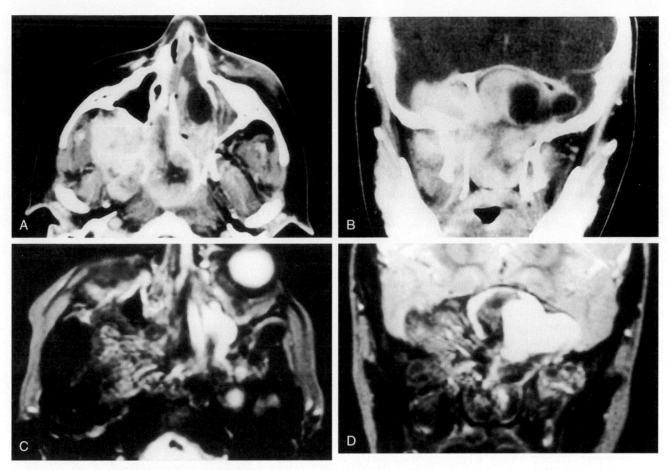

**FIGURE 6-102**   Axial **(A)** and coronal **(B)** CT scans show a large enhancing mass that fills the nasopharynx and nasal fossae, bows the posterior wall of the right maxillary sinus forward, and extends into the right infratemporal fossa. The tumor has also destroyed the floor of the sphenoid sinus and the right middle cranial fossa. There is a nonenhancing region in the vicinity of the left sphenoid sinus. Axial T2-weighted **(C)** and coronal **(D)** proton density MR images show that the mass is filled with serpiginous signal voids, reflecting its highly vascular nature. The left sphenoid sinus is filled with high T2-weighted fluid. This patient had a large angiofibroma with a left sphenoid sinus mucocele. The skull base was not destroyed, but only deossified from the chronic pressure of the tumor. Both cavernous sinuses were intact but were elevated by the mass.

histologically it can be confused with a nasopharyngeal angiofibroma.[176] Several points differentiate these two lesions: (1) the angiomatous polyp is located primarily in the nasal fossa and not in the nasopharynx; (2) the polyp does not extend into the pterygopalatine fossa and only rarely protrudes into the sphenoid sinuses. In these cases, the tumor enters the sinus through the anterior wall and not the sinus floor, as with angiofibromas; (3) these polyps do not extend intracranially; (4) on angiography the polyps have only a few demonstrable feeding vessels compared with the rich vascular supply of the angiofibroma; (5) on CT the angiomatous polyp does not enhance as well as the angiofibroma; (6) vascular flow voids are usually not seen on MR imaging, as they are in angiofibroma; (7) these polyps are easily "shelled out" surgically, as are routine nasal polyps, whereas the nasopharyngeal angiofibroma is difficult to remove from its primary attachment site; and (8) angiography and embolization are not necessary in patients with angiomatous polyps (Fig. 6-105).

The pathologic distinction between an angiomatous polyp and an angiofibroma may be difficult, and hence the

pathologist may need to rely on the radiologist's impression in arriving at a correct diagnosis.

### Hemangioma

Hemangiomas of the nasal cavity occur most commonly on the septum (65%), lateral wall (18%), and vestibule (16%). Most arise in the anterior septum near Kisselbach's plexus, and most are of the capillary type. Lesions arising on the lateral wall usually are of the cavernous type. Epistaxis and nasal obstruction are the most common patient complaints. Simple excision is generally curative for these lesions, which rarely exceed 2 cm in their greatest dimension. In the nasal cavity, hemangiomas also tend to develop in the inferior and middle turbinates. These lesions are diagnosed when small because they cause dramatically severe epistaxis. Rarely, intranasal hemangiomas may develop in the second trimester of pregnancy. Most of these lesions spontaneously regress within 4 to 8 weeks after delivery.[185] Hemangiomas of the paranasal sinuses are very rare; two have been described in the maxillary sinuses and two in the sphenoid sinuses. The sphenoid sinus cases showed destruction of the skull base.[185]

On CT, these hemangiomas enhance, and in the nasal cavity they are usually inseparable from the middle or inferior turbinates. Hemangiomas have an intermediate signal intensity on all MR imaging sequences they enhance, and vascular flow voids occasionally may be present (Figs. 6-106 to 6-108).

Hemangiomas can also occur as solitary lesions in bone. These tumors account for only 0.7% of all primary bone tumors. In the head and neck, the most common sites are the skull (53%), mandible (10.7%), nasal bones (9%), and cervical vertebrae (6%). Although many patients have a history of local trauma, a causal relationship remains doubtful. The lesions occur twice as often in females as in males; the average age of onset is 31 years. Most commonly, patients experience a firm, nonpainful swelling that is associated with a pulsating sensation. Actual bruits are rarely heard. When hemangiomas involve the facial bones and mandible, angiograms have revealed that the blood supply is from the facial artery or the internal maxillary artery. The inadvertent surgical violation of an intraosseous hemangioma can be associated with exceptionally rapid blood loss, often as much as 3500 ml. Even so, surgery is the primary treatment of choice. Embolization may greatly reduce operative blood loss, provided that the operation is performed shortly after embolization, before a collateral circulation can develop.[116]

Radiographically these lesions have a "sun ray," "soap bubble," or "honeycomb" appearance and enhance on contrast-enhanced CT scans. On MR imaging, they have low to intermediate T1-weighted and high T2-weighted signal intensity. They also enhance (Fig. 6-109).

### Angiosarcoma

*Angiosarcoma* refers to malignant neoplasia derived from vascular tissue. The term includes other vascular

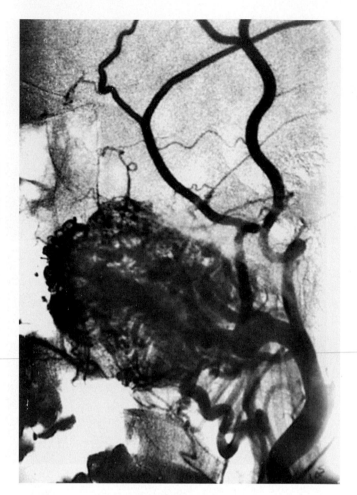

**FIGURE 6-104** Lateral subtraction angiogram shows the typical highly vascular tumor appearance of an angiofibroma.

tumors, such as hemangioendothelioma, in which endothelial differentiation is more prominent, or lymphangiosarcoma, derived from lymphatic tissue. Angiosarcomas account for only 2% to 3% of all soft-tissue sarcomas. Approximately half of all angiosarcomas occur in the skin and subcutaneous tissues of the head and neck, particularly the scalp, legs, and trunk. A smaller percentage of angiosarcomas occur in the breast (particularly after radiotherapy for breast carcinoma), liver (particularly after Thorotrast exposure), bone, and spleen.[186, 187]

Cutaneous angiosarcomas occur over a wide age range but are most common in the seventh decade of life. There is a male predominance. Cutaneous and osseous angiosarcomas may present as raised or flat, spreading blue or red masses that can have a bruise-like appearance, causing dull local pain and swelling of the affected region.

Sinonasal and nasopharyngeal angiosarcomas are extremely uncommon, comprising 11% of head and neck angiosarcomas.[187–189] They present with epistaxis, nasal obstruction, headaches, and proptosis.[190] Angiosarcomas can also occur as primary intraosseous tumors and represent less than 1% of all primary bone malignancies. Head and neck angiosarcomas comprise 15% of solitary osseous angiosarcomas, arising most frequently in the mandible and skull.

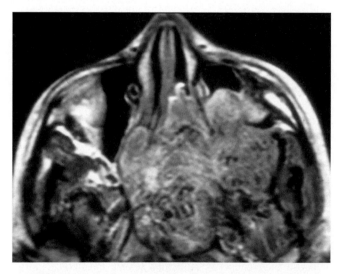

**FIGURE 6-103** Axial T1-weighted MR image shows a large left nasopharyngeal and nasal fossa mass that extends into the left antrum. The mass also extends into the infratemporal fossa via the pterygopalatine fossa, which is widened and destroyed. The tumor further extends laterally to involve the left pterygoid muscles. There are multiple vascular-type flow voids within the mass. This patient had a large angiofibroma.

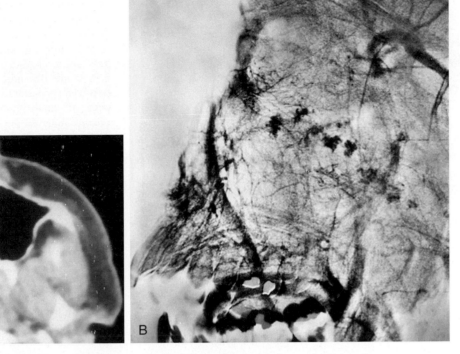

**FIGURE 6-105** Axial CT scan (**A**) shows a right nasal fossa polypoid mass that extends back into the nasopharynx but does not arise there. The mass does not extend into the pterygopalatine fossa or the sphenoid sinus. A biopsy specimen was interpreted as an angiofibroma. **B,** A lateral subtraction angiogram shows only focal areas of increased vascularity, without the typical vascular appearance of an angiofibroma. This patient had an angiomatous polyp.

The histologic appearance of angiosarcoma varies dramatically with the tumor grade. Well-differentiated angiosarcoma (malignant hemangioendothelioma, hemangiosarcoma) produces obvious blood-filled vascular spaces. There is a combination of "closed" lumina, which are finite and delineated, as well as serpiginous "open" lumina, which are insidiously infiltrating interanastomosing spaces. Low-grade angiosarcomas produce abundant open vascular lumina, and have a minimal solid component and a low-grade cytology. High-grade angiosarcomas are densely cellular, infiltrative sarcomas. The amount of malignant vascular lumen formation varies and may be focal. Cytologically, these tumors are frankly malignant, with nuclear pleomorphism and atypical mitotic figures. Immunohistochemistry may be necessary to distinguish high-grade tumors from other sarcomas, namely the demonstration of Ulex, CD31 and CD34 expression.

Surgical resection is indicated as the primary treatment for angiosarcomas. However, the insidious infiltrating pattern of angiosarcoma may render complete resection impossible; therefore, adjuvant radiotherapy may be necessary. Local recurrences are common. The rate of cervical lymph node metastasis reported for cutaneous angiosarcomas varies from 10% to 41%, and the reported

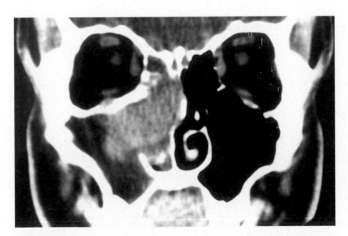

**FIGURE 6-106** Coronal CT scan shows a mass in the right nasal cavity, maxillary sinus, and ethmoid complex. Obstructed secretions are present in both the right antrum and ethmoid sinuses. Most of the bone around the margin of the tumor is intact. This patient had a hemangioma.

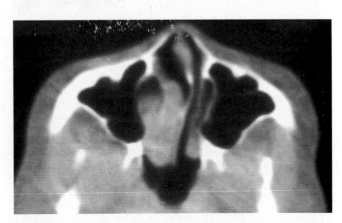

**FIGURE 6-107** Axial CT scan shows a mass in the right inferior turbinate, with incidental bowing of the nasal septum convexity to the left. This patient had a hemangioma.

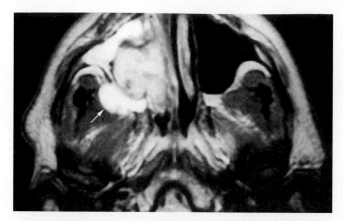

**FIGURE 6-108**   Axial T2-weighted MR image shows the tumor to have a high signal intensity, but not as high as the signal intensity of the obstructed secretions in the right antrum. The chronic antral obstruction has led to the development of a mucocele (*arrow*), which bulges into the right infratemporal fossa. This patient had a hemangioma.

rate of distant metastasis ranges from 33% to 63%.[191] The 5-year survival rate is poor, ranging from 41% to 18%.

The prognosis for intraosseous angiosarcomas varies with the tumor grade. Grade I lesions recur locally but do not metastasize, as do grade II and III lesions. For patients with solitary tumors, there is a 20% 5-year survival rate. The 5-year survival rate for patients with multifocal osseous tumors is 36%, reflecting the predominance of grade I tumors in this group. Inexplicably, sinonasal tumors appear to have a better prognosis than skin, soft-tissue, and osseous tumors, with a lower recurrence rate, a higher salvage rate, and a lower metastatic rate. Barnes reported that 6 of 10 patients with sinonasal angiosarcomas were recurrence free after 0.5 to 5 years (median, 29 months), and an additional patient was disease free at 12 years after one recurrence at 8 years.[188–191] On CT and MR imaging these tumors are aggressive, bone-destroying lesions with considerable enhancement.

## Hemangiopericytoma

Hemangiopericytomas (HPCs) are uncommon vascular lesions that arise primarily in the lower extremities, retroperitoneum, and pelvis. However, 15% occur in the head and neck, and of these, 55% arise in the nasal cavity.[193] HPCs are thought to be derived from Zimmerman's pericytes, contractive cells that surround the outer aspect of small vessels. The lower extremities and the retroperitoneum-pelvis are the most common sites for HPCs. The head and neck is the third most common site; tumors occur in the neck, the perioral soft tissues, and, lastly, the sinonasal tract. Sinonasal hemangiopericytomas (SNHPCs) present as gray to tan, spongy, vascular, polypoid masses. Nasal obstruction and epistaxis are common presenting symptoms.[194, 195] Other presenting complaints include watery rhinorrhea, serous otitis media, proptosis, infraorbital anesthesia, and facial pain. SNHPCs generally involve the nasal cavity along with one or more sinuses. A review of the literature revealed an overall recurrence rate of 19% (22 of 115 cases). The majority of recurrences (19 of 22) were single (16%), and most (14 of 19) occurred within the first 5 years after resection. However, first recurrences after the first 10 years have occurred. Multiple recurrences were a rarer finding, seen in only 4 of 115 cases. Overall, three patients (2.6%) developed metastases (usually locoregional sites and local lymph nodes). Four patients (3.5%) ultimately died of disease (usually from a lack of local control). This confirms the general low-grade malignant potential of this neoplasm. It appears that no single feature of SNHPC can predict the course of this basically low-grade neoplasm. The prognosis of SNHPC most likely strongly depends on the tumor stage at initial presentation and on the completeness of primary resection. Features such as mitotic rate, necrosis, and nuclear pleomorphism are probably significant for high-stage or incompletely resected tumors.[196] The diagnosis of SNHPC remains one of histologic pattern recognition, and traditionally, immunohistochemistry has aided in excluding other diagnoses. Vimentin has been consistently expressed by the tumor spindle cells of HPC. However, recent studies have shown that factor XIIIa is also expressed by HPC (as well as by tumors of fibrohistiocytic

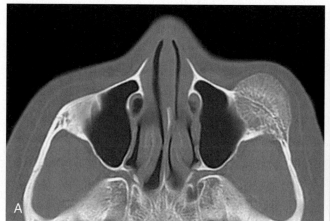
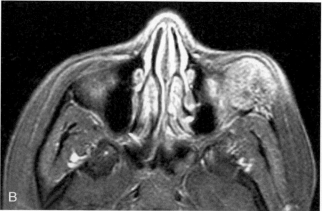

**FIGURE 6-109**   Axial CT scan (**A**) viewed at a wide window setting shows a 2.5 cm round lesion in from the left zygoma. The inner and outer cortices, although thinned, are preserved. The trabeculae radiate in a spoke wheel pattern. Axial T1-weighted, contrast-enhanced, fat-suppressed MR image (**B**) shows the enhancing, without evidence of large regional vessels. This patient had an intraosseous hemangioma.

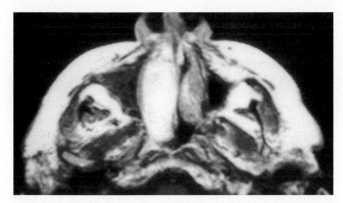

**FIGURE 6-110**   Axial T1-weighted MR image shows a high signal intensity expansile mass in the right nasal cavity. Obstructed inflammatory disease is present in the right antrum. This patient had a hemangiopericytoma.

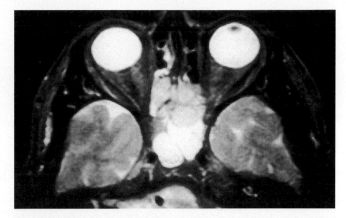

**FIGURE 6-112**   Axial T2-weighted MR image shows an intermediate signal intensity mass in the posterior ethmoid sinuses and anterior sphenoid sinuses. The remaining obstructed sphenoid sinuses are filled with high signal intensity secretions. This patient had a hemangiopericytoma.

differentiation) and hence may be yet another helpful positive marker in establishing an immunohistochemical profile. The role of chemotherapy is still evolving, but initial reports show promise.[185, 194, 197]

Microscopically, fusiform or spindle cells can be seen, forming short fascicles and bundles that become more dense around vessels. The abundant vessels have typical cuffs of perivascular hyalinization. Staghorn vessels may be rare. Nuclear pleomorphism is not normally present in SNHPCs.

On CT, HPCs are expansile, bone-remodeling lesions with a variably enhancing, fairly homogeneous appearance (Figs. 6-110 to 6-112). On MR imaging, they enhance and have low to intermediate T1-weighted and higher T2-weighted signal intensity. They tend to occur in the nasal fossa and in the maxillary sinus.[198]

### Kaposi's Sarcoma

The classic form of Kaposi's sarcoma (KS) is an indolent tumor that occurs most commonly as soft red nodules on the lower limbs and, less commonly, on the upper limbs. Lesions may be multicentric and coalescent, but they rarely

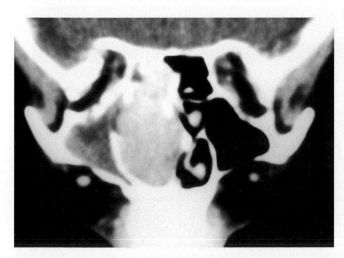

**FIGURE 6-111**   Coronal CT scan shows an enhancing right nasal fossa mass that extends into the right ethmoid sinuses. The right antrum is obstructed. There is primarily bone remodeling about the mass. This patient had a hemangiopericytoma.

exceed 2 cm. Patients with classic KS are usually over the age of 50 at the time of tumor diagnosis, although 3% to 4% of the cases of the classic form are diagnosed in patients less than 15 years old. Patients with classic KS usually have long survival periods and die of something other than KS.

From the literature and the files of the Armed Forces Institute of Pathology (AFIP), Gnepp, Chandler, and Hyams compiled a total of 83 cases of classic KS, which affected the head and neck.[199] Of all the classic KS cases, 8% affected cutaneous sites on the head and neck, and only 2% affected the mucosal surfaces. Mucosal sites included the conjunctiva, palate, tongue, gingiva, and tonsil. Dermal sites included the eyelids, nose, ears, and face. By comparison, HIV-associated KS very commonly affects the skin of the head and neck (32%) and upper airway mucosal surfaces (19%). Common sites include the palate, gingiva, buccal mucosa, tongue, larynx, trachea, nasal cavity, and paranasal sinuses. These patients tend to be decades younger than patients with the classic cases (mean age, 38 years), though there is overlap among the two age groups.[199–204] The imaging findings are not diagnostic and usually show a noninfiltrating soft-tissue mass.

## Muscle

Malignant soft-tissue sarcomas (STSs) represent approximately 1% of all newly diagnosed malignancies in the United States.[205] The 1991 NCI (National Cancer Institute) SEER (Surveillance, Epidemiology, and End Results) data report that the U.S. incidence of reported new sarcomas for that year represented 5700 cases.[206] The majority of primary STSs originate within the extremities (59%), followed by the trunk (19%), retroperitoneum (13%), and head and neck (9%).[207] Sarcomas occur over a wide age range, starting in the first decade of life; however, the peak incidence occurs after the sixth decade of life.[208]

### Leiomyoma and Leiomyosarcoma

Sinonasal smooth-muscle neoplasia are derived from the perivascular smooth-muscle tissue that is abundant in the sinonasal tract. Both leiomyomas and leiomyosarcomas are rare occurrences. Fu and Perzin identified only two leiomyomas and six leiomyosarcomas from 256 nonepithelial sinonasal tumors.[209]

Leiomyomas have been reported to arise from the nasal septum, turbinates, vestibule, and choanae.[210–213] As the vascular component may be prominent, leiomyomas may present with epistaxis. Sinonasal leiomyosarcomas are rare, with fewer than 50 reports in the literature.[214, 215] On occasion, leiomyomas may present as more extensive lesions involving multiple sinuses.[216] The AFIP reported on nine cases of sinonasal tract leiomyosarcoma, which constitute the largest such series.[217] Either the nasal cavity alone or contiguous paranasal sinuses were involved. There is an equal sex distribution and an average age incidence of 50 years.[218] The sinonasal symptoms are nonspecific; patients complain of unilateral nasal obstruction, bleeding, and pain.

Leiomyomas are benign smooth-muscle tumors, the vast majority of which affect the female genital tract. In a compiled series of 257 head and neck leiomyomas, the most common sites of occurrence were the cervical esophagus (36%), subcutis (23%), and oral cavity (20%). The nasal cavity and sinuses were affected in only eight (3%) cases;

the turbinate was a site of preference.[219] Five of these eight cases could be subclassified as angioleiomyomas; in all likelihood they were derived from the nasal erectile vasculature, which has thick vascular walls. Angioleiomyomas have been associated clinically with sharp knife-like pain, which probably relates to vascular constriction.

Histologically, leiomyomas are composed of bland whorls of spindled cells with blunt cigar-shaped nuclei. Immunohistochemistry confirms the expression of smooth muscle markers (actin, desmin). Angioleiomyomas have a prominent vascular component that may be compressed or thick-walled. The absence of nuclear pleomorphism, necrosis, and a prominent mitotic rate separates leiomyomas from leiomyosarcomas. Leiomyosarcomas are distinguished from leiomyomas by the presence of more than 10 mitoses per high-power field, atypia, and necrosis. The malignant cells of the epithelioid variant appear less spindled and more cuboidal. This variant is more likely to arise in the stomach or the mesentery but has been found in head and neck sites.[217]

On imaging, these tumors, like most sarcomas, tend to be homogeneous masses, often primarily expansile rather than invasively destructive (Fig. 6-113). They tend to have high

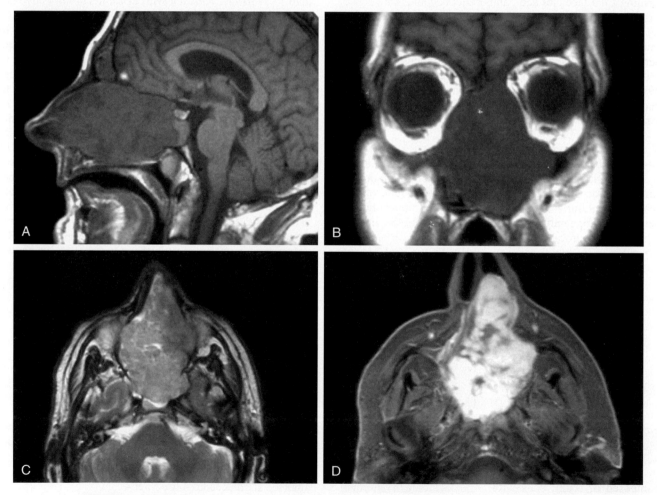

**FIGURE 6-113** Sagittal (**A**) and coronal (**B**) T1-weighted MR images and axial T2-weighted (**C**) and T1-weighted, fat-suppressed, contrast-enhanced (**D**) MR images. In **A** and **B**, there is a fairly homogeneous, expansile nasal fossa mass that has elevated the floor of the anterior cranial fossa and bowed the lamina papyracea laterally. The medial floor of the left orbit is also elevated. There was no gross intracranial invasion or invasion of either orbit. The mass is nonhomogeneous on the T2-weighted and contrast-enhanced images. This patient had a leiomyosarcoma.

T2-weighted signal intensity, and they enhance after contrast administration.

Both leiomyomas and leiomyosarcomas are treated primarily by surgery. Resection can be conservative for leiomyomas, as these are curable. Sinonasal leiomyosarcomas require a wider surgical approach, as they are locally aggressive tumors. About 75% of patients have a local recurrence and 35% develop metastases. At least 50% of patients die of the disease, usually within 2 years of diagnosis.[218] Adjuvant radiotherapy or chemotherapy has no proven efficacy.[217] Tumor stage and distribution have been found to affect disease-free survival. Kuruvilla and colleagues found that of 30 patients with sinonasal leiomyosarcomata, 10 had tumors confined to the nasal cavity, none of which recurred.

### Rhabdomyoma

Rhabdomyomas are rare benign tumors with skeletal muscle differentiation. They represent about 2% of all skeletal muscle tumors.[219] Clinically, rhabdomyomas can be classified as either cardiac or extracardiac.

Cardiac rhabdomyomas are most commonly associated with tuberosclerosis. Extracardiac rhabdomyomas are rare but have a tendency to affect head and neck sites such as soft tissues of the face and neck, the oral cavity, and the larynx. Histologically, rhabdomyomas can be classified as either fetal type (myxoid versus cellular types), adult type, or juvenile-intermediate type; histologically, the last type lies between the fetal and adult types. In a compiled series of 46 head and neck fetal rhabdomyomas, about half of the patients were in their second decade of life or older at diagnosis, and there was a male predisposition.[219] Five of these cases (11%) originated in the nasopharynx.[220, 221]

### Rhabdomyosarcoma

Rhabdomyosarcoma (RMS) is a soft-tissue sarcoma of skeletal muscle derivation. It comprises 20% of all soft-tissue sarcomas, and it is the most common soft-tissue sarcoma in children (75%). It is the seventh most common pediatric malignancy following leukemia, CNS tumors, lymphoma, neuroblastoma, Wilms' tumor, and osteogenic sarcoma.[221] The majority of patients with RMS (78%) are under 12 years of age, and 43% of patients are under 5 years of age. Only 7% of cases occur in the second decade of life, and 2% to 4% of cases occur in each subsequent decade. In the head and neck, the most common sites for all RMSs are the orbit (36%), nasopharynx (15.4%), middle ear and mastoid (13.8%), sinonasal cavities (8.1%), face (4.5%), neck (4.1%), larynx (4.1%), and oral cavity. Sinonasal RMS may occur over a wide age range and commonly presents with nasal obstruction.[223–226]

Histologically, RMS can be classified as embryonal, botryoid (a variant of embryonal RMS), alveolar, and pleomorphic types based on the growth pattern, differentiation, and shape of tumor cells. The majority of head and neck RMSs can be classified as either the embryonal type or its botryoid variant, or alveolar. Embryonal RMS (ERMS) is composed of round cells with darkly staining hyperchromatic nuclei, scant cytoplasm, short, spindled cells with central elongated nuclei, tapered ends, and eosinophilic or amphophilic cytoplasm. Botryoid ERMS (5% of cases) is a noteworthy subtype that has a characteristic polypoid ''bunch of grapes'' clinical appearance. It is associated with

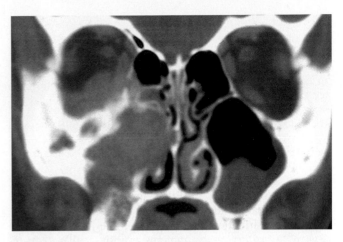

**FIGURE 6-114**   Coronal CT scan shows a soft-tissue mass in the right maxillary sinus. The medial sinus wall and portions of the antral roof are destroyed, and the tumor extends into the right orbit, ethmoid sinuses, and right nasal cavity. Despite these local areas of destruction, there are large areas where there is intact bone adjacent to the tumor. This patient had a rhabdomyosarcoma.

the most favorable prognosis of all RMSs. Histologically, it grows as a polypoid tumor with a prominent myxoid stroma in which hypocellular and more cellular areas are seen with a subepithelial condensation of tumor cells, the *cambium layer*. Most RMSs arise from skeletal or cardiac muscle cells.

The general approach to RMS is resection plus adjuvant therapy. Regional lymph node sampling is appropriate; however, prophylactic lymph node dissection is not necessary. Resection followed by chemotherapy is the mainstay of therapy. Radiation therapy is not necessary after complete surgical resection with adequate margins.[227] Survival depends on the site (orbit better than parameningeal), histologic type (botryoid and embryonal better than alveolar), and stage. Tumors at nonorbital and nonparameningeal sites also have a favorable prognosis.

On imaging, RMSs usually have elements of both bone remodeling and bone destruction. On contrast-enhanced CT, these tumors enhance moderately and generally homogeneously. On MR imaging, they also tend to be remarkably homogeneous, they have intermediate signal intensities on all imaging sequences, and they enhance with contrast (Figs. 6-114 to 6-116). They can also appear on imaging as indistinguishable from SCC.

## Lipoblastic

### Lipoma and Lipoma-Like Lesions

These lesions, which include the ordinary lipoma, myxoid lipoma, angiolipoma, pleomorphic lipoma, spindle-cell lipoma, myelolipoma, hibernoma, and lipoblastoma, have various reported frequencies; however, they have not been reported to arise within the sinonasal cavities. The lipomas are discussed in Chapter 41.

### Liposarcoma

Liposarcoma is one of the most common soft-tissue sarcomas of adulthood, usually occurring in the lower extremities and retroperitoneum. The head and neck region

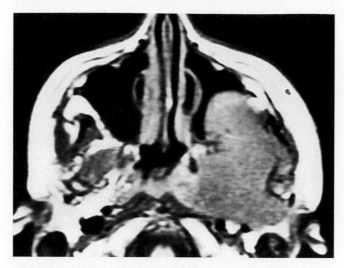

**FIGURE 6-115**   Axial T1-weighted MR image shows a homogeneous mass in the left infratemporal fossa extending into the left antrum and the skull base. The mass has an intermediate signal intensity. This patient had a rhabdomyosarcoma.

is involved in (5.6%) of liposarcomas.[186] The soft tissues of the neck, scalp, and face are the most common sites for liposarcomas above the clavicles, comprising 54% of head and neck cases.[228] Hypopharyngeal and laryngeal sites were affected in 38% of 76 cases of head and neck liposarcoma reviewed from the Royal Marsden Hospital over a 50-year period.[228] The sinonasal tract is an extremely rare site for either liposarcoma or lipoma.[185]

Liposarcomas can be polypoid pedunculated tumors that are soft and yellow/tan/gray upon sectioning. A spectrum of histology is seen, ranging from low-grade (lipoblastic liposarcoma, lipoma-like, sclerosing liposarcoma, or atypical lipoma) or intermediate to high-grade (myxoid liposarcoma, pleomorphic liposarcoma, round cell liposarcoma, dedifferentiated liposarcoma). Low-grade tumors are characterized by an abundance of mature, histologically benign adipose tissue coursed by collagenous fibrous tissue. Lipoblasts may be focal. They have characteristic ''chicken claw''–shaped nuclei that are indented by cytoplasmic fat globules. Their chromatin is usually dense and pyknotic, but enlarged nucleoli may be found. Myxoid liposarcoma is a common histologic pattern generally seen in soft-tissue liposarcoma. The stromal background is loose and myxoid, perforated by a fine ''chicken-wire'' meshwork of arborizing vessels. The lipoblasts appear as univacuolated signet ring cells and multivacuolated cells.

Generally, liposarcomas are properly treated by resection with adequate margins. Radical neck dissection is not usually warranted for low-grade tumors, but high-grade liposarcomas may develop locoregional metastases. The rarity of this tumor in the sinonasal tract precludes discussion of specific disease-free survival.

Based on the general experience with liposarcomas elsewhere in the body, on CT these lesions have an overall low (fatty) attenuation value (-65 to -110 HU), and irregular areas of soft-tissue density are seen within the lesion. The tumor margins may infiltrate adjacent soft tissues. MR imaging shows a nonhomogeneously high T1-weighted and an intermediate T2-weighted signal intensity.[229]

## Fibroblastic

### Fibrosarcoma (Including Desmoid Tumor)

Fibrosarcomas (desmoid tumors, aggressive fibromatoses) are infiltrative, nonmetastasizing, unencapsulated fibroblastic tumors that account for 12% to 19% of all soft-tissue sarcomas (STSs). They occur most often in the lower extremities and trunk; only 15% occur in the head and neck. Most head and neck tumors involve the sinonasal cavities (18.3%), larynx (14.8%), and neck (sternocleidomastoid) (6.1%). Fibromatoses (desmoid tumors, grade I fibrosarcomas) are more likely to occur in the pediatric population. Higher-grade fibrosarcomas (grades II/III) usually arise in patients between 20 and 60 years of age,[185] but may also occasionally occur in the pediatric population.[209, 230]

Grade II or III head and neck fibrosarcomas are more likely to present as bony jaw tumors than as STSs. Those occurring in the older population (30%) are usually the secondary jaw sarcomas, arising in previously irradiated or diseased bone such as bone with fibrous dysplasia, Paget's disease, giant cell tumors, bone infarcts, and osteomyelitis.

Fibromatoses (desmoid tumors) are histologically very bland and well differentiated, and appear as densely cellular spindle cell malignancies producing a collagenous matrix. The fascicles or bundles of tapered spindle cells grow in a variable intersecting pattern, seen on cross-section as ''herringbone'' areas. The diagnosis is firmly established on biopsy when the pathologist can identify the bland fibroblasts insidiously infiltrating host tissue. Examination during surgery shows that this white-tan scar-like tumor sends out innumerable tentacles, making complete extirpation virtually impossible. Positive resection margins are the rule. Nuclear pleomorphism, a significant mitotic rate, and necrosis are generally not seen, and, when present, indicate transformation to a higher grade (grade II or III fibrosarcoma).

Complete surgical excision with ample margins is the treatment of choice. Recurrences after resection are common, and in some series recurrence rates are as high as 90%.[208, 231] Progression to higher-grade fibrosarcoma may occur in occasional cases, usually after radiotherapy. Grade II and grade III fibrosarcomas develop local recurrences within 18 months of treatment and metastases within 2 years of recurrences.[185] The overall prognosis depends on the adequacy of the surgical resection, sarcoma grade, size, and location, male sex, and the presence of pain or cranial nerve symptoms. Of these parameters, sarcoma grade and resection margin status are probably the most important. Only 1% to 11% of patients develop positive regional lymph nodes; however, the 5-year survival rates are only 33% to 69%.[185]

Bony fibrosarcomas tend to spread more aggressively than their soft-tissue counterparts. Most grade II or grade III jaw fibrosarcomas have 5-year survival rates ranging from 27% to 40%. Metastases occur to the lungs and to other bones; only 3% spread to regional lymph nodes.[232] In addition, the younger the patient is when the tumor appears, the better is the prognosis. Although the local recurrence rate of pediatric fibrosarcoma is similar to that for adults (17% to

47%), younger patients have metastases in only up to 14% of cases, and they have a higher 5-year survival rate of 85%.[185] In a series of sinonasal fibromatoses, five patients (21%) (four adults and one child) developed single or multiple recurrences within 6 to 34 months.[155, 233]

The imaging findings are nonspecific. On CT, fibrosarcomas have a generally homogeneous, minimally enhancing appearance. They also tend to remodel bone (Fig. 6-117). On MR imaging, they have low to intermediate signal intensities on all imaging sequences and enhance minimally.

### Malignant Fibrous Histiocytoma

Malignant fibrous histiocytoma (MFH) is one of the most common soft-tissue sarcomas below the clavicles. While it has been recognized that MFH has become a "waste-

basket" category for some sarcomas, there is a group of sarcomas that truly reveal both fibroblastic and histiocytic phenotypes. Only about 3% occur in the head and neck, and most of these occur in the skin, orbit, or sinonasal cavities.[185, 234, 235]

A number of histologies, either uniform or a mixture of patterns, may be seen in MFH, which can be histologically classified as myxoid, angiomatoid, inflammatory, and giant cell type. Most MFHs have a storiform/pleomorphic pattern. Whorls and fascicles of malignant fibroblastic spindle cells forming a "rush-mat" or radiating "star-like" (storiform) pattern characterize MFH. The putative "histiocytic" component is composed of plump epithelioid cells and larger multinucleated giant cells that have bizarre nuclei. If a prominent myxoid background is present, these sarcomas

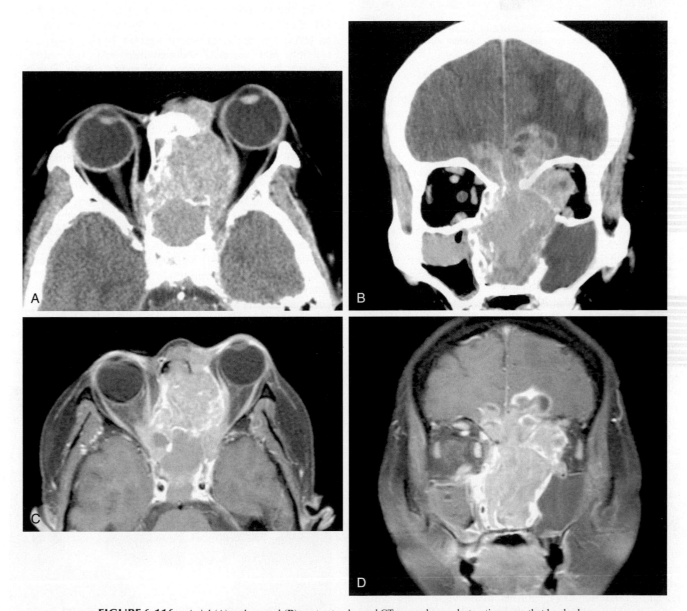

**FIGURE 6-116**   Axial (**A**) and coronal (**B**) contrast-enhanced CT scans show a destructive mass that has broken into the anterior cranial fossa and invaded the brain. The tumor also has extended into both orbits and obstructed the left antrum. Incidental inflammatory disease is present in the right maxillary sinus. Axial (**C**) and coronal (**D**) T1-weighted, contrast-enhanced MR images confirm the disease mapping and the presence of a sphenoid sinus mucocele. Statistically, in a 45-year-old male, this imaging appearance should suggest the diagnosis of squamous cell carcinoma. This patient had a rhabdomyosarcoma.

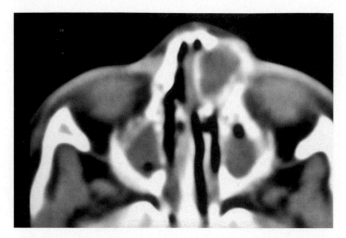

**FIGURE 6-117**   Axial CT scan shows a soft-tissue mass in the left lacrimal duct region bulging into the left nasal fossa. The bone has been remodeled around the lesion. Incidentally noted are inflammatory secretions in both maxillary sinuses. This patient had a low-grade fibrosarcoma.

can be classified as myxoid MFH. As with other sarcomas, focal metaplastic mesenchymal elements such as cartilaginous or osseous differentiation may be seen in MFH. A marked inflammatory infiltrate may be present, thus warranting the designation of *inflammatory MFH.*

MFHs express vimentin diffusely; other markers, such as desmin, may be seen focally. The immunohistochemical pattern of MFH also has many nonspecific markers: antibodies to lyzozyme, alpha-1 antitrypsin, and acid phosphatase mark some MFHs. Nemes and colleagues have shown that FXIIIa, a marker of histiocytes and pericytes, can be expressed in MFH and in HPC.[236] Therefore, strong, diffuse expression of FXIIIa in the right circumstances may support the diagnosis of MFH.[237]

The 2-year survival rate for all MFHs is 60%. Local recurrences develop in 27% of cases, 75% within 2 years of diagnosis. Cervical nodal metastases occur in 12% and distant metastases in 42% of cases. Of the eight nasopharyngeal carcinoma survivors with secondary sinonasal MFH, none were disease free at follow-up and six died of disease without distant metastasis within 30 months.[185]

On contrast CT, these tumors usually enhance moderately and either aggressive bone destruction or bone remodeling can occur, making the CT characteristics nonspecific (Fig. 6-118).[238, 239] On MR imaging, fibrous histiocytomas usually have intermediate signal intensities on all imaging sequences, and contrast enhancement may be nonhomogeneous.

### Benign Fibrous Histiocytoma

Benign fibrous histiocytoma (dermatofibroma) is a histologically benign lesion with fibroblastic and histiocytic components that most commonly occurs in the dermis and subcutis. It has been reported anecdotally as a sinonasal lesion.[240] Histologically, fibrous histiocytomas are composed of whorls of benign fibroblastic cells with a radiating, storiform pattern admixed with multinucleated giant cells. They can be distinguished from MFH, as they are less cellular and lack nuclear pleomorphism, abnormal mitotic figures, and necrosis.

### Inflammatory Myofibroblastic Tumor

Inflammatory myofibroblastic tumor (IMFT) (also referred to as inflammatory pseudotumor and plasma cell granuloma) is a poorly understood "emerging" entity that manifests as a space-occupying lesion composed of a benign lymphoplasmacytic and myofibroblastic infiltrate. In the head and neck, IMFT most often affects the periorbital and orbital soft tissue. It has also been described in the supraglottic larynx and the salivary glands. At least 17 cases have been reported involving the sinonasal tract, nasopharynx, pterygomaxillary space, and parapharyngeal space. These have occurred over a wide age range from childhood (3 years) to old age (the ninth decade). In the sinonasal tract, they present as polypoid masses causing nasal obstruction. Maxillary sinus involvement may result in a soft tissue mass with bony erosion and remodeling.

In the parapharyngeal and pterygomaxillary spaces, IMFT can cause trismus and pain. Systemic symptoms such as fever, weight loss, malaise, anemia, hypergammaglobulinemia, and elevated sedimentation rate may also be present. It is quite common for patients with IMFT to undergo multiple biopsy procedures in order to establish a diagnosis.[241–248]

On biopsy evaluation, IMFT appears to be a diagnosis of exclusion. Excised tumors have been described as fleshy, whorled, and firm or myxoid. The polymorphous appearance of IMFT may reflect its variable etiology or its shifting histology during disease course. Lymphocytes, plasma cells, histiocytes, fibroblasts, and myofibroblasts are the basic components of IMFT, with mutable proportions. Four basic histologic patterns have emerged: (1) a dominant lymphoplasmacytic infiltrate, (2) a dominant lymphohistiocytic infiltrate, (3) a predominantly "young and active" myofibroblastic process, and (4) and a predominantly collagenized process with a lymphoplasmacytic infiltrate. Lymphoplasmacytic IMFT consists of a mature lymphoid infiltrate with germinal centers and a rich plasma cell infiltrate—hence the name plasma cell granuloma. Lymphohistiocytic IMFT most closely resembles an infectious process, as foamy histiocytes are prominent. The "young and active" IMFT has a

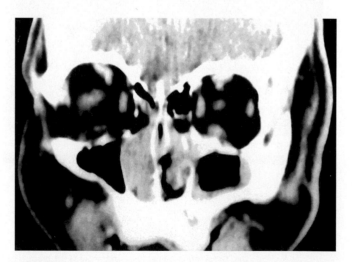

**FIGURE 6-118**   Coronal CT scan shows an expansile polypoid mass in the right nasal fossa (*arrowhead*). There is no bone erosion, and the nasal septum is intact. Inflammatory disease is present in the left antrum and nasal cavity. This patient had a fibrous histiocytoma.

densely cellular fascicular and storiform pattern resembling that of fibrous histiocytoma, except for the inflammatory infiltrate or nodular fasciitis (see Chapter 41 for a discussion of nodular fasciitis, which characteristically arises from superficial fascia and presents as a freely movable subcutaneous nodule). Overlapping histologic features between IMFT, nodular fasciitis, and fibrous histiocytoma corroborate the place of these entities in the pathologic spectrum between reactive and neoplastic processes. Collagenized IMFT is paucicellular and resembles a desmoid tumor, but with a prominent inflammatory infiltrate, and a zonation/maturation effect may be observed. Progression of patterns may also be seen in some long-standing cases necessitating multiple procedures.[241–248]

IMFTs of solid organs (e.g., lung, liver) are resected for diagnostic purposes and so effectively treated. Coffin et al. reported single or multiple recurrences in 25% of patients after initial excision; two cases progressed to sarcomatous transformation. However, the recurrent or transformed cases still showed a tendency to remain localized.[244] Recurrence was more often seen in patients with mesenteric or retroperitoneal tumors. In head and neck sites, including the sinonasal tract, most IMFTs do resolve/regress with excisional biopsy and steroid therapy; however, some IMFTs may persist and worsen, requiring more aggressive therapy such as radiotherapy.[241–248]

### Solitary Fibrous Tumor

Solitary fibrous tumor (SFT) is an uncommon spindle-cell neoplasm derived from primitive mesenchymal or fibroblast-like cells. First recognized as a pleural neoplasm (fibrous mesothelioma), SFT has gained greater recognition and has been described in other soft tissues, including the head and neck.[249–251]

In the sinonasal tract, SFT presents as a firm, polypoid, well-circumscribed or encapsulated soft-tissue neoplasm. Histologically, SFT is composed of bland spindle cells arranged in a "pattern-less pattern"; focally storiform or fascicular growth patterns or hemangiopericytoma-like vascular patterns are seen. Collagen deposition to the point of keloid-like hyalinization can be seen. Myxoid areas and rich vascularity are present, with hyalinized vessels. The tumor boundary may be circumscribed or infiltrative. Immunohistochemically, SFT expresses vimentin, CD34, and CD99. SFT is usually cured by resection; recurrences or progression to higher-grade tumors (mitotic figures, necrosis, pleomorphism, increased cellularity) are rare.

### Fibromyxoma and Myxoma

A number of other benign or low-grade neoplasms can develop from pleuripotential mesenchymal cells, producing fibromyxoid and myxoid tumors. These tumors are related to fibroosseous lesions; however, they contain no osseous or odontogenic matrix. Fibromyxomas and myxomas tend to occur during the second and third decades of life.

Radiographically, fibromyxomas are soft-tissue, primarily expansile masses when they involve the sinuses, although focal areas of aggressive bone destruction may be present. These lesions usually have flecks or thin strands of calcification dispersed within the tumor substance (Figs. 6-119 and 6-120).

Histologically, one sees bland stellate fibroblastic cells

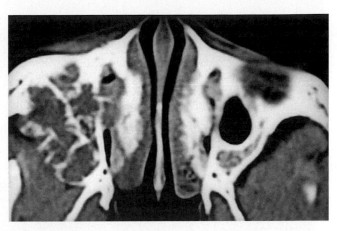

**FIGURE 6-119** Axial CT scan shows a partially destructive and partially expansile mass in the right maxillary sinus. The lesion contains lacelike areas of calcification. This patient had a fibromyxoma.

producing myxoid stroma. A variable collagenizing component may be present. Sinonasal fibromyxomas can be locally aggressive, with a significant recurrence rate, especially if treated by curettage.[219] Therefore, complete surgical excision is the treatment of choice.

A myxoma is a benign mesenchymal tumor composed of undifferentiated stellate cells producing a myxoid stroma. These tumors are generally uncommon and have been reported in the heart (atrial myxoma), subcutaneous tissues, bone, genitourinary tract, and skin. Head and neck myxomas are usually intraosseous; those of the jaws represent 40% to 50% of all head and neck myxomas. Mandibular myxomas have been presumed to arise from odontogenic tissue and hence are also called odontogenic myxomas. Those that arise from the maxillary bone may extend to the maxillary sinus and nasal cavity.[252] On CT they are cystic-appearing lesions that do not enhance (Fig. 6-121).[253]

## BENIGN AND MALIGNANT OSSEOUS LESIONS AND TUMORS (INCLUDING FIBROOSSEOUS LESIONS)

Of the nonepithelial tumors that involve the sinonasal cavities, nearly 25% are osseous or fibroosseous lesions. These lesions and tumors can be categorized as lesions of abnormal bone development causing tumoral masses (Paget's disease, fibrous dysplasia, cemento-ossifying dysplasia, cherubism, giant cell reparative granuloma), benign osseous tumors (osteoma, osteochondroma, exostosis, osteoid osteoma, osteoblastoma, ossifying fibroma, chondroma, giant cell tumor), and malignant tumors (chondrosarcoma, osteogenic sarcoma).

## Benign Tumors

### Osteoma and Exostosis

Osteoma is a benign expansile proliferation of mature bone that occurs within bone. Exostosis is a benign, expansile proliferation of mature bone that occurs on the surface of bone. When an exostosis projects intracranially from the calvarium, it is also referred to as an enostosis. Osteomas are found almost exclusively within the membranous bones of the skull and face, most commonly within the frontal sinuses, followed by the ethmoid sinuses. Maxillary and sphenoid sinus osteomas are rare. The high prevalence of frontal and ethmoid sinus osteomas may be related to the fact that these sites represent the junction of membranous and enchondral development of the frontal and ethmoid bones.[254]

Osteomas of the sinuses are not uncommon and may be seen in up to 1% of radiographs obtained for sinus symptoms. Sinus osteomas may be asymptomatic, or patients may complain of headache, sinus symptoms, or a frontal mass. They obstruct the frontal sinus in 17% of cases, resulting in the need for immediate surgery (Fig. 6-122).[209] They can also obstruct the lacrimal apparatus.[255] Almost all osteomas remain confined to the sinuses, often conforming to the contour of the sinus. However, osteomas are also the

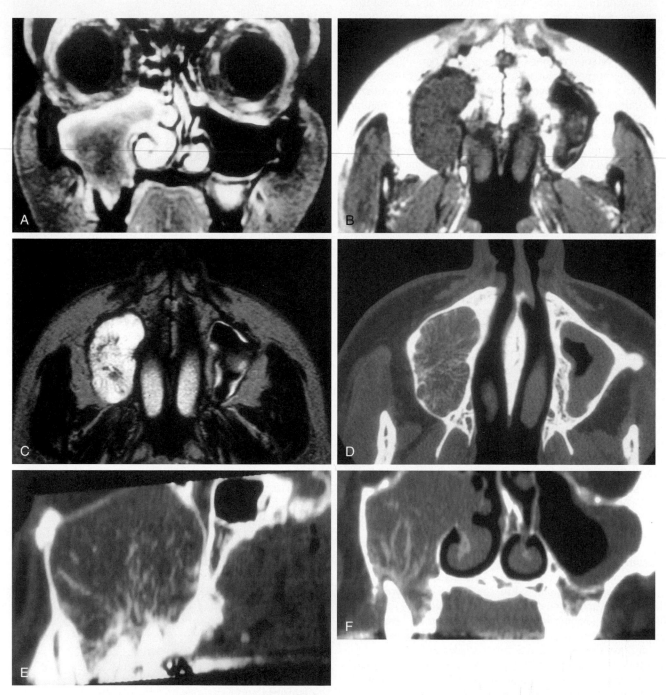

**FIGURE 6-120**   Coronal T1-weighted (**A**), axial T1-weighted (**B**), and T2-weighted (**C**) MR images, axial CT scan (**D**), and reformatted sagittal (**E**) and coronal (**F**) CT scans show an expansile low signal intensity mass filling the right maxillary sinus. Minimal nonhomogeneity is seen in **B**. Very fine lacelike signal voids are seen in **C**. Entrapped high signal intensity secretions are present around the lesion. The CT scans show that within the lower portion of the mass there are thin, lacelike calcifications. This patient had a fibromyxoma.

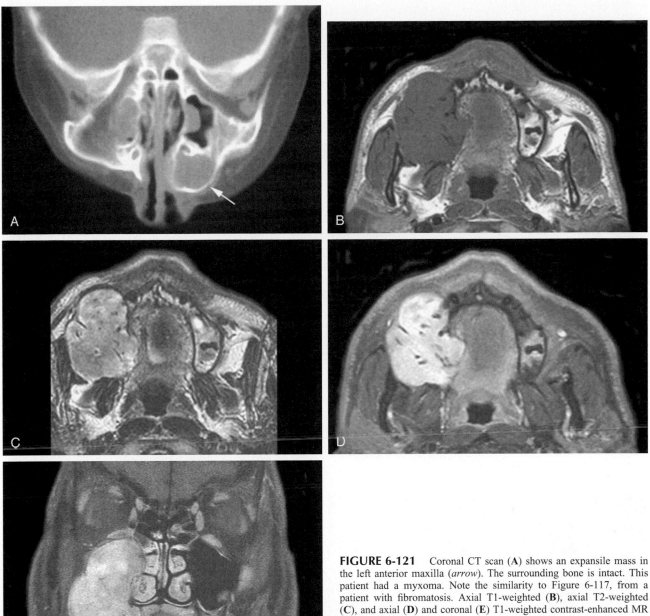

**FIGURE 6-121**   Coronal CT scan (**A**) shows an expansile mass in the left anterior maxilla (*arrow*). The surrounding bone is intact. This patient had a myxoma. Note the similarity to Figure 6-117, from a patient with fibromatosis. Axial T1-weighted (**B**), axial T2-weighted (**C**), and axial (**D**) and coronal (**E**) T1-weighted contrast-enhanced MR scans on a different patient show a large mass destroying part of the right maxillary alveolus and expanding and filling the left maxillary sinus, elevating and thinning the orbital floor. There is no infiltration of the orbit. The teeth roots are exposed by the tumor, and the tumor is fairly homogeneous in signal intensity. This patient had a myxoma.

most common benign paranasal sinus tumors associated with spontaneous CSF rhinorrhea, pneumocephalus, and tension pneumocephalus (Figs. 6-123 and 6-124).[256–258] Osteomas tend to grow slowly; the mean growth rate has been estimated at 1.61 mm/yr (range, 0.44 to 6.0 mm/yr) in a series of 13 patients with successive sinus radiographs.[259]

Multiple osteomas can be a manifestation of Gardner's syndrome, a very rare autosomal dominant transmitted disorder consisting of (1) intestinal polyposis with progression to intestinal adenocarcinoma, (2) benign skin and subcutaneous neoplasia, such as epidermoid inclusion cysts and desmoid tumors, and (3) multiple osteomas, with a proclivity for the mandible. These osteomas can arise within the second decade of life and precede intestinal polyps,

which are usually diagnosed after the third decade of life (Figs. 6-125 and 6-126).

Exostoses occur in the external auditory canal ("swimmer's ear") or on the palate or mandible (torus palatini or torus mandibularis). The latter usually presents as a painless bulging of the alveolus, possibly causing dentures to fit poorly (Fig. 6-127). Torus palatinus (Fig. 6-128) is seen in the hard palate, at the junction of the left and right horizontal plates of the palatine bones and the palatine processes of the maxilla.

Osteomas usually are small, incidental findings on plain films, where they have a variable bone density, ranging from very dense and sclerotic, for the ivory-type osteoma, to a progressively less dense and less ossified lesion for the

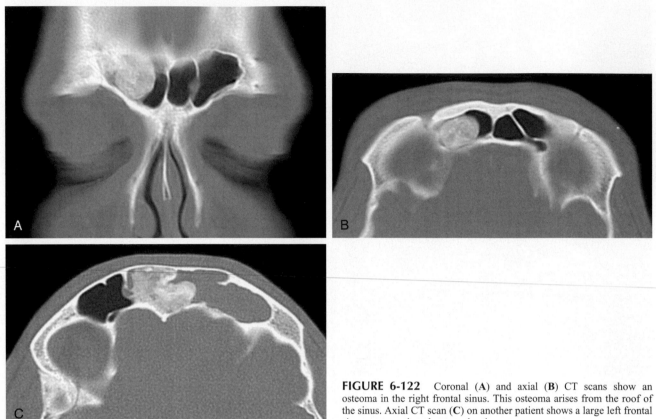

**FIGURE 6-122** Coronal (**A**) and axial (**B**) CT scans show an osteoma in the right frontal sinus. This osteoma arises from the roof of the sinus. Axial CT scan (**C**) on another patient shows a large left frontal sinus osteoma that obstructs the sinus.

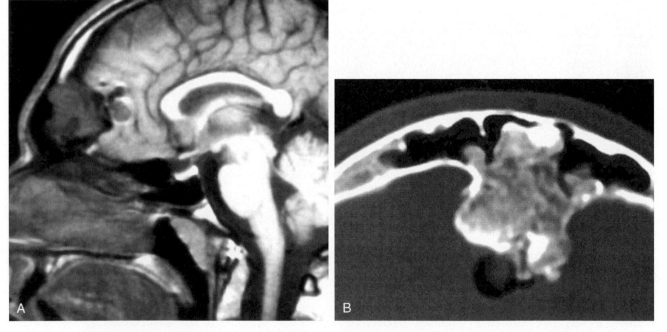

**FIGURE 6-123** Sagittal T1-weighted MR image (**A**) and axial CT scan (**B**) show an osteoma arising from the posterior frontal sinus wall and extending intracranially. A small amount of air is seen in the adjacent frontal lobe region. Notice how much more clearly this diagnosis can be established on CT. In **A**, this could just as easily be a nonossified cellular tumor.

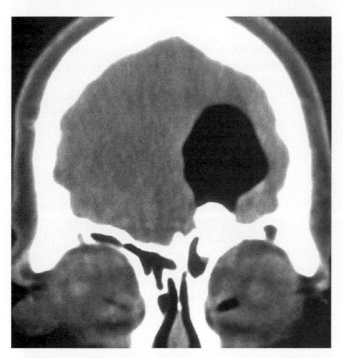

**FIGURE 6-124**   Coronal CT scan shows an osteoma in the roof of the left frontal sinus with a large collection of intracranial air.

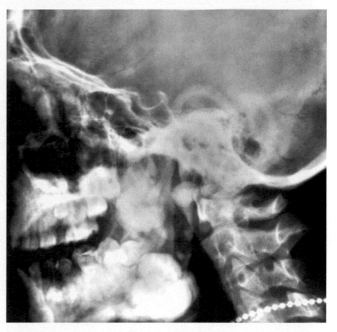

**FIGURE 6-125**   Lateral view shows multiple osteomas of the facial bones, mandible, and calvaria. Gardner's syndrome.

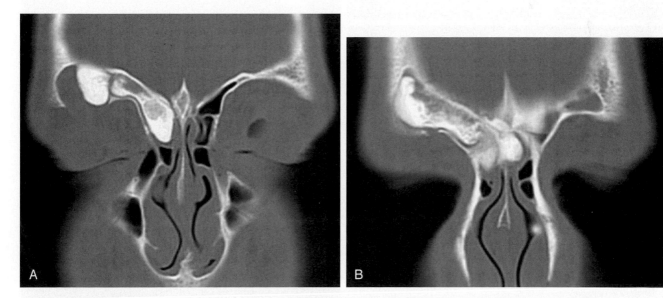

**FIGURE 6-126**   Coronal CT scans (**A** and **B**) through the frontal sinuses show multiple osteomas in the right frontal sinus and supraorbital ethmoid sinuses. A supraorbital mucocele has developed in the most lateral aspect of this sinus. This patient had Gardner's syndrome.

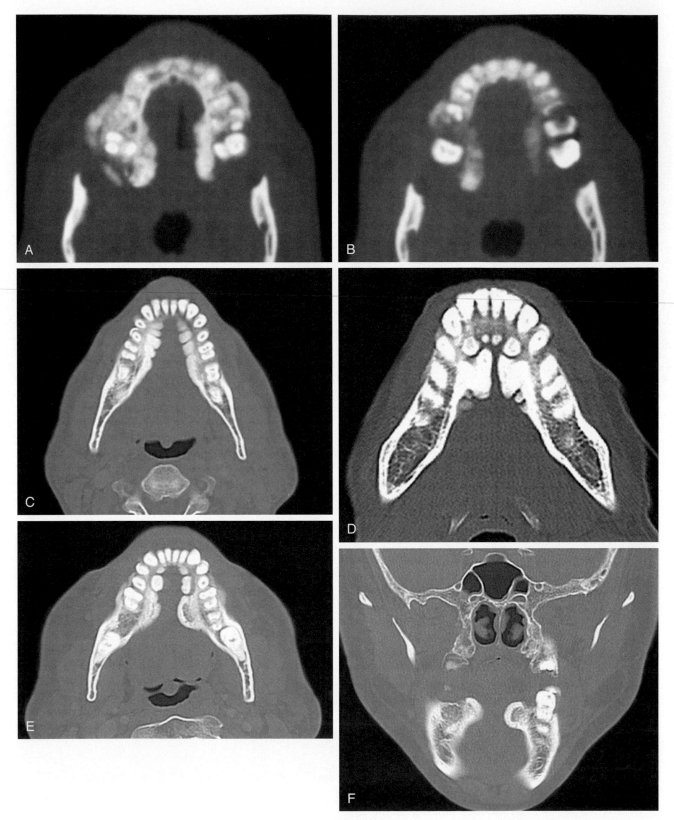

**FIGURE 6-127**    Axial CT scans (**A** and **B**) show multiple exostoses along both the buccal and lingual cortices of the maxillary alveolus. This patient has maxillary exostoses. In **C**, an axial CT scan shows multiple mandibular exostoses along the lingual cortices. In **D**, an axial CT scan shows exuberant exostosis in this patient with mandibular exostoses. Axial (**E**) and coronal (**F**) CT scans show extensive mandibular exostoses. Notice how these exostoses narrow the volume of the floor of the mouth.

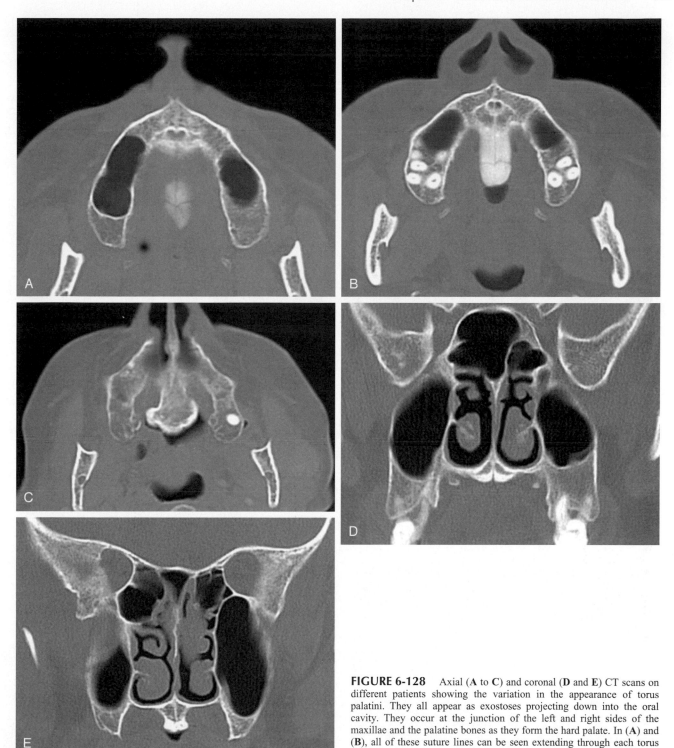

**FIGURE 6-128**   Axial (**A** to **C**) and coronal (**D** and **E**) CT scans on different patients showing the variation in the appearance of torus palatini. They all appear as exostoses projecting down into the oral cavity. They occur at the junction of the left and right sides of the maxillae and the palatine bones as they form the hard palate. In (**A**) and (**B**), all of these suture lines can be seen extending through each torus palatinus.

fibrous osteoma (Figs. 6-129 to 6-133). In fact, some fibrous osteomas may be confused on plain films with a retention cyst or polyp. On CT, osteomas arise from one of the sinus walls or the intersinus septum. The differences between the compact, cancellous, and fibrous types of osteoma correlate with the degree of bone matrix density seen within the lesion. On MR imaging these lesions give a nonhomogeneous, low to intermediate signal intensity on all imaging sequences. Based purely on MR imaging findings, their osseous nature may go undetected (Fig. 6-123).

Pathologically, osteomas are composed of dense, hard, mature bone, with only small amounts of fibrous tissue. The cancellous, or mature, osteoma has sparse intertrabecular spaces that may be empty or filled with fat, fibrous tissue or hematopoietic elements. Fibrous osteomas contain abundant mature lamellar bone, with greater amounts of intertrabecu-

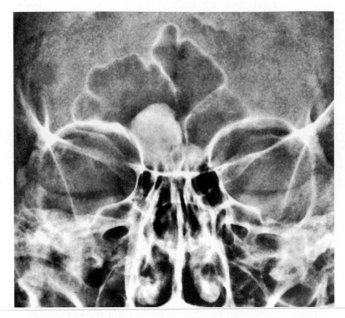

**FIGURE 6-129** Caldwell view shows an ivory-type osteoma in the base of the right frontal sinus. The sinus is not obstructed.

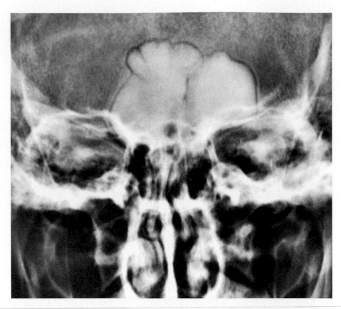

**FIGURE 6-131** Caldwell view shows bilateral frontal sinus osteomas. Note that in this patient the osteomas have remained within the contour of the frontal sinuses, and a thin rim of air is seen outlining each osteoma.

lar fibrous tissue. Exostoses are seen as compact layers of dense cortical bone without a medullary component.

### Osteochondroma

An osteochondroma is a benign cartilage-capped osseous growth arising from the surface of bone. They represent 35% to 50% of benign osseous lesions and 8% to 15% of all osseous tumors.[254] They are believed to represent a developmental abnormality rather than a neoplastic process. Osteochondromas arise from any bone developing via enchondral ossification. Because the craniofacial bones are membranous, sinonasal osteochondromas are rare. The mandible (coronoid process and condyle) was the most common site (52%) of 63 head and neck "osseous" osteochondromas reported in the literature.[254] They have also been reported rarely in the sphenoid bone, maxillary tuberosity, zygomatic arch, and nasal septum. Most osteochondromas have a limited growth potential; expansion ceases with axial skeletal maturation. However, some osteochondromas may continue to grow after skeletal maturation.

Radiographically, these tumors tend to have a pedunculated mushroom shape. The cartilaginous cap is often not visible and, when seen, may be focally calcified. On MR imaging, the tumors have a nonhomogeneous low to intermediate signal intensity on all imaging sequences (Figs. 6-134 and 6-135).

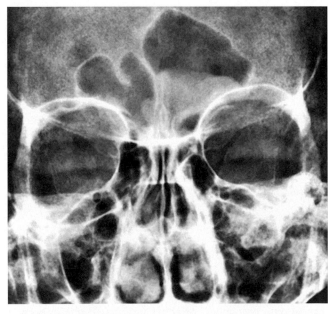

**FIGURE 6-130** Caldwell view shows a left polypoid mass that is slightly denser than the adjacent frontal bone. This patient had a fibrous-type "soft" osteoma. PA view shows bilateral frontal osteomas. Note how the osteomas have conformed to the sinus contour.

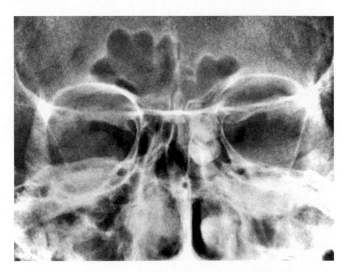

**FIGURE 6-132** Caldwell view shows an osteoma in the left ethmoid complex.

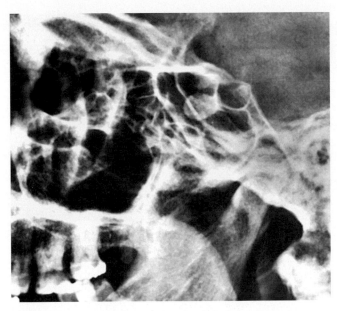

**FIGURE 6-133** Lateral view shows an osteoma in the sphenoid sinuses.

Pathologically, cortical and cancellous bone, with a cartilaginous "cap," are seen. This "cap" may become atrophic with time. Simple resection is the treatment of choice, and only 1% to 2% of lesions recur. Similarly, only 1% to 2% of solitary osteochondromas undergo malignant change, usually to chondrosarcomas.

### Chondroma

Chondromas are completely benign cartilaginous tumors. The definition of chondromas may vary with the tumor site, and there may be no absolute criteria distinguishing chondromas from grade I chondrosarcomas in some confined areas, such as the larynx. However, no diagnosis of "chondroma" should be accompanied by radiologic evi-

dence of destruction or histologic evidence of pleomorphism. It is well appreciated that lack of pleomorphism on a limited biopsy does not rule out the possibility of a grade I or higher chondrosarcoma. The majority of head and neck chondromas (70%) have been reported in the nasal cavity and ethmoids. Others may occur in the maxilla, sphenoid sinuses, palate, and nasopharynx. There is no sex predilection, and about 60% occur in patients less than 50 years of age.[254] Wide surgical excision with negative margins is the treatment of choice.[260, 261]

On CT, calcifications within the tumor matrix are not always seen. These lesions tend to be expansile, remodel bone, and have an attenuation less than that of muscle but greater than that of fat.[262, 263] They do not provoke sclerotic bone at their margins. On MR imaging, they usually have low T1-weighted and high T2-weighted signal intensities, and they enhance. The imaging findings are not specific.

### Osteoid Osteoma and Osteoblastoma

Osteoid osteoma is a benign expansile neoplasm characteristically associated with nocturnal pain. It represents 11% of benign bone neoplasms, with a male-to-female ratio of 2:1. The majority of patients are diagnosed between 5 and 25 years of age, and the femur and tibia are the most commonly affected bones. In 26 culled literature cases of the head and neck, the mandible and cervical vertebrae were the most common sites.[254] Osteoid osteomas have been rarely reported in the frontal, ethmoid, and maxillary bones. Patients describe a dull pain that usually worsens at night, intensifies with activity, and is relieved by rest and aspirin.

On plain films and CT, the classic lesion is a dense cortical ovoid mass with a 1 to 2 mm low-density nidus. However, the nidus also may be dense and difficult to identify radiographically.[254] Histologically, the nidus is recognized as a tangled array of new osteoid bony trabecula surrounded by reactive bone. The intertrabecular tissue is vascular and fibrotic. Simple excision or curettage is curative.

Osteoblastoma (giant osteoid osteoma) is a benign expansile lesion representing only 3% of all benign bone tumors. There is a peak incidence in the second decade of life, with a male-to-female ratio of 2:1. The most common

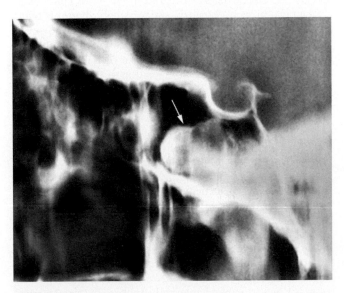

**FIGURE 6-134** Lateral multidirectional tomogram shows a partially ossified, pedunculated mass in the sphenoid sinus (*arrow*). This patient had an osteochondroma.

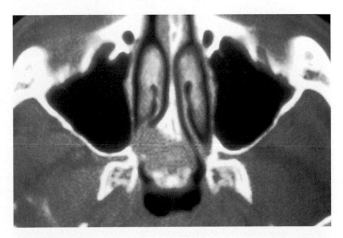

**FIGURE 6-135** Axial CT scan shows an expansile, partially calcified mass in the posterior nasal septum. This patient had an osteochondroma.

sites of occurrence are the vertebral column (34%) and the long bones of the appendicular skeleton (30%). However, osteoblastomas are more likely to involve the head and neck (15% of 364 cases) than are osteoid osteomas.[264] The mandible is the most common site (usually the mandibular body), followed by the cranium and maxilla. Ethmoid and sphenoethmoid osteoblastomas have also been reported.[254] Patients present with a painful mass; however, the pain does not have the consistent pattern encountered with osteoid osteoma (nocturnal and relieved with aspirin).

Radiographically, osteoblastomas tend to be expansile and remodel adjacent bone. They range from 2 to 10 cm in diameter; in contrast, the nidus of osteoid osteomas is invariably less than 1 cm. Osteoblastomas have a variable radiographic appearance; some lesions have large, discrete areas of organized bone density, and others have a mixed osseous and fibrous appearance. The latter tends to be more nodular and more coarsely organized than most ossifying fibromas and some fibrous dysplasias (Figs. 6-136 and 6-137).[256, 265, 266]

Pathologically, osteoblastomas are virtually identical to osteoid osteoma. Histologically, one sees interconnecting trabeculae of osteoid or woven immature bone. The term *aggressive osteoblastoma* (juvenile aggressive osteoblastoma) is reserved for recurrent tumors or those with histologic atypia. Histologically, these lesions have a denser population of epithelioid osteoblasts, with prominent mitotic activity and multifocality.[267] At times, the distinction between aggressive osteoblastoma and a well-differentiated osteogenic sarcoma may be difficult. Conservative surgery, consisting of local excision or curettage, cures 80% to 90% of the cases of benign osteoblastoma. Aggressive osteoblastomas recur locally but do not metastasize.[254]

### Ossifying Fibroma (Cemento-Ossifying Fibroma)

Ossifying fibroma (OF) is a benign expansile tumor occurring most commonly in tooth-bearing regions in the

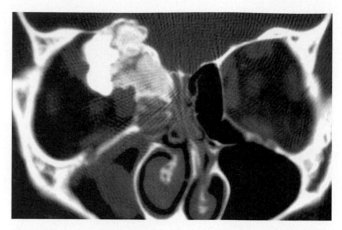

**FIGURE 6-137**  Coronal CT scan shows a bone-density lesion in the right frontal and ethmoid bones. The bone is expanded, and the cortices are intact. Part of the lesion has a "ground glass" appearance; however, the lateral portion of the mass has very dense bone production. This patient had a benign osteoblastoma.

second or third decade of life, with a female predominance. OF arises from the periodontic ligament, most commonly in the molar or premolar regions of the mandible, followed by the maxilla.[254] Many synonyms exist for this tumor (cemento-ossifying fibroma, fibroosseous lesion, psammomatoid ossifying fibroma, etc.), reflecting its ability to produce a variable matrix. Patients present with a painless, solitary expansile mass.

OF can also arise in the nasal cavity, usually from the lateral nasal wall or ethmoid complex. If it is sufficiently large, OF can affect the frontal, sphenoid, and maxillary sinuses.

Radiographically, OF appears as an expansile, circumscribed tumor with well-defined borders. The surrounding bone appears normal. The internal organization of OF reveals discrete zones of either variable osseous or fibrous tissue. CT usually reveals large, nonossified areas of fibrous tissue density, in contrast to fibrous dysplasia (FD).[255] Ideally, FD can be distinguished from OF by its noncircumscribed nature, as it "blends" into relatively abnormal bone, and its propensity for multiostotic involvement. However, some cases of OF may be indistinguishable from FD on CT imaging. The MR imaging appearance of OF can be quite variable, depending on the composition of this lesion.[268]

Pathologically, OF is composed of densely cellular, well-circumscribed fibrous tumor. Ossification, or cemento-ossification, commences at the periphery. The ossification is composed of immature woven bone that matures into lamellar bone. This is unlike FD, in which bony trabeculae are produced throughout the lesion but are highly atypical, without maturation or normalization. Cementum formation is seen as acellular coalescing spherical calcifications that have distinctive basophilic perimeters.

OF is optimally treated by conservative surgical excision, although larger tumors may require more aggressive resection. Compared with the clinical behavior of FD, which can remain stable, OF has a greater tendency to behave aggressively (grows faster and recurs more quickly after surgery) and to expand internally toward the orbits, nasal fossae, and sinus cavities rather than to deform the outer surface bones (Figs. 6-138 to 6-141).[269] Tension pneu-

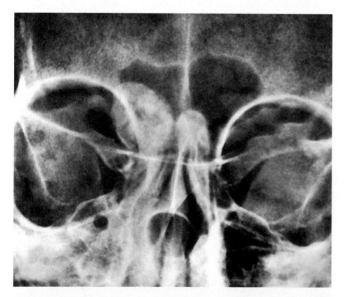

**FIGURE 6-136**  Caldwell view shows bone density masses in the ethmoid sinuses that project into the anterior cranial fossa. There is also disease-increased density in both ethmoid sinuses. This patient had a benign osteoblastoma.

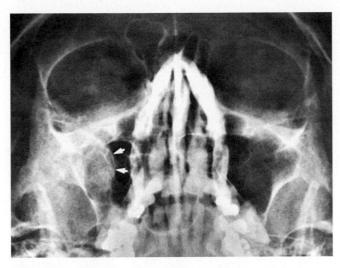

**FIGURE 6-138** Waters view shows an expansile bony mass in the lateral wall of the right maxillary sinus. The mass has displaced the lateral sinus wall toward the midline (*arrows*). This patient had an ossifying fibroma.

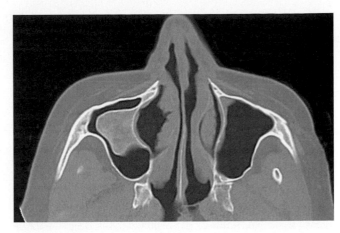

**FIGURE 6-139** Axial CT scan shows a "ground glass" bony mass projecting into the right maxillary sinus cavity. There is a surrounding cortex. This patient had an ossifying fibroma.

mocephalus has been reported as an uncommon complication of an OF.[270]

## Tumor-Like Conditions and Giant Cell–Rich Lesions

### Fibrous Dysplasia

Fibrous dysplasia (FD) is an idiopathic skeletal disorder in which medullary bone is replaced by poorly organized, structurally unsound fibroosseous tissue. Most patients are under 30 years of age at diagnosis.[271] The majority of cases (75% to 80%) are limited to the monostotic form (MFD), which most often involves the ribs or femur. The craniofacial bones may be involved in monostotic FD in up to 25% of cases; most commonly affected are the maxilla and mandible.[272] Polyostotic FD (PFD) comprises 20% to 25% of all cases. Usually there is unilateral bone involvement, but in severe cases bilateral disease can occur. The craniofacial bones are more often (40% to 50%) involved in PFD.[271, 272]

Albright's syndrome consists of PFD plus pigmented skin macules and sexual precocity. This syndrome is relatively rare. It is 40 times less common than MFD, and it occurs almost exclusively in females. The skin pigmentations have irregular margins ("coast of Maine"), as opposed to the smoother-bordered pigmentations ("coast of California") of neurofibromatosis.

Patients with craniofacial FD involvement usually present with asymmetric cheek swelling.

Encroachment into the paranasal sinuses, nasal fossae, orbit, or neurovascular canals can lead to nasal obstruction, headaches, and visual disturbances. Recently, it has been appreciated that involvement of the frontal and sphenoid sinuses by FD can result in mucoceles. Extensive maxillary involvement results in facial distortion, referred to as leontiasis ossea ("lion face").

New FD lesions usually do not develop after the growth plates have fused. Some lesions, however, continue to grow after skeletal maturation.

Histologically, FD appears as irregular, disformed bony trabeculae of immature woven bone, which are thinned, C-

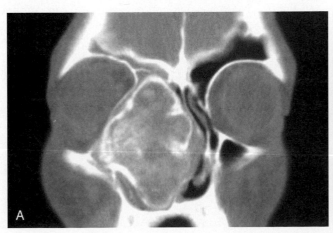
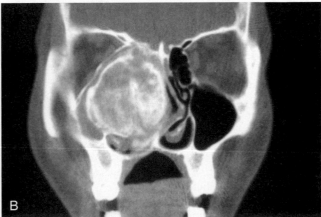

**FIGURE 6-140** Coronal CT scans (**A** and **B**) show an ovoid expansile mass projecting into the right nasal fossa and the right ethmoid and maxillary sinuses. Obstructed secretions are present in the remaining right antrum. Surrounding the partially ossified mass is a cortex. This patient had an ossifying fibroma.

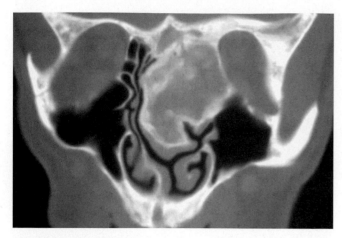

**FIGURE 6-141** Coronal CT scan shows a mass in the left ethmoid complex and nasal fossa. There is a cortex surrounding a primarily nonossified mass. This patient had an ossifying fibroma.

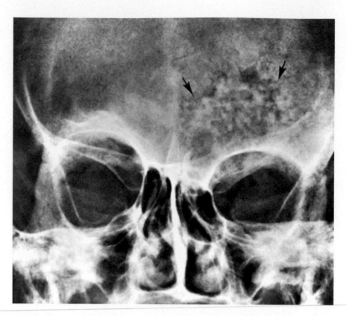

**FIGURE 6-142** Caldwell view shows a mixed "lytic" and "blastic" expansile lesion in the left frontal bone (*arrows*) that has depressed the superior orbital margin. This patient had fibrous dysplasia.

or S-shaped, and referred to as *Chinese characters*. The trabeculae are embedded in, and blend into, vascularized fibrous tissue lacking the osteoblastic rimming of normal bone. Serial biopsies over time do not reveal maturation of this woven bone into lamellar bone.[271] Surgery is used only to correct deformities, relieve pain, correct functional problems, decompress a mucocele, or resect sarcomas. FD recurs in 20% to 30% of cases, usually within 2 to 3 years of initial therapy.[271]

Malignant transformation of bone with FD is very rare (less than 1% of cases). In a review of 83 sarcomas complicating FD, 57% of the patients had MFD and 43% had PFD. The craniofacial bones are most commonly involved, and irradiation may promote malignant transformation. The average latency period from diagnosis of FD to development of malignancy is 13½ years. The majority of these tumors are osteogenic sarcomas, followed by fibrosarcomas and chondrosarcomas.[271]

The radiologic appearance varies according to the degree of fibrous tissue present. Thus, the bone texture can range from a nonhomogeneous mixture of bone and fibrous tissues to a predominantly fine, bony "ground glass" appearance. The disease expands the diploic or medullary space and widens the bone. A thin, intact rim of cortical bone is often seen over the margins of the involved bone. MR imaging usually shows a low to intermediate signal intensity on all imaging sequences, and often the cortical bone overlying the medullary disease can be identified as a zone of low signal intensity. There usually is intense enhancement with contrast. If areas of high T2-weighted signal intensity are present within an obstructed or involved sinus, the presence of a mucocele should be considered (Figs. 6-142 to 6-153).[273, 274] Because there is often an overlap in the imaging appearance of FD and ossifying fibroma, the term *benign fibroosseous lesion* has been suggested to describe the imaging findings of both lesions.[275]

### Cemento-Ossifying Dysplasia

There are a number of cementum-containing lesions that may affect the jaws. Periapical fibrous dysplasia (periapical cemental dysplasia) produces lytic and then blastic expan-

sile periapical lesions, usually affecting the lower anterior jaw. The etiology is unknown. It is usually seen in patients more than 20 years of age and is more prevalent in African Americans.[271] The lesions are usually smaller than 1 cm. Radiographically, early lesions appear as periapical radiolucencies. As cementum or osteoid is produced, central calcification is seen radiographically, which becomes more

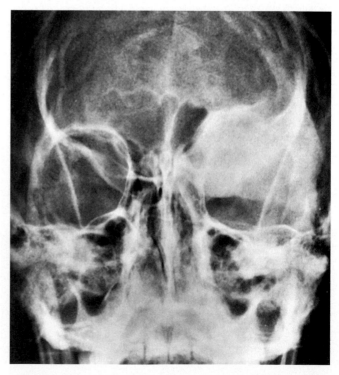

**FIGURE 6-143** Caldwell view shows a dense expansile lesion of the left frontal and zygomatic bones that has encroached on the left orbit. This patient had fibrous dysplasia.

dense and uniform as the lesion matures. Focal cemento-osseous dysplasia is characterized by the formation of an expansile cystic lesion, which usually occurs in the posterior mandible. It may occur in dentulous or edentulous bone.

There is a pronounced female predominance, with a peak incidence in the fourth and fifth decades. Radiographically, one sees an expansile cystic lesion that may or may not be associated with a tooth and can be either lucent, opaque, or mixed density, possibly with a sclerotic rim.

Florid cemento-osseous dysplasia appears to be a diffuse form of periapical cemental dysplasia. It is characterized by the development of multiple expansile jaw tumors containing cementum or osteoid. These lesions affect the lower jaw more commonly than the upper jaw and may be symmetric. Black middle-aged women are most commonly affected. Radiographically, the lesions are cystic, mixed lytic/blastic.

### Cherubism

Cherubism (familial multilocular cystic disease of the jaw, hereditary fibrous dysplasia) is a nonneoplastic disease limited to the jaws and characterized by bilateral, painless jaw enlargements that are said to give the patient a cherubic appearance. Cherubism may appear sporadically or be familially transmitted. It is inherited in an autosomal dominant fashion, with high (nearly 100%) penetrance in males and variable (50% to 75%) penetrance in females. The disease appears between the ages of 6 months and 7 years and is characterized by bilateral fullness of the jaws. The eyes appear to look up as the lower sclera are exposed. The disease often develops rapidly until age 7 years and then gradually regresses. The mandible is involved first, followed by the maxilla in about two thirds of the cases. Most of the radiographic changes occur in the mandible, where expansile cystic masses are seen in the angles and ramus. As the disease progresses to the maxilla, the sinus opacifies and the orbital floor may be bulged upward. The latter finding is one

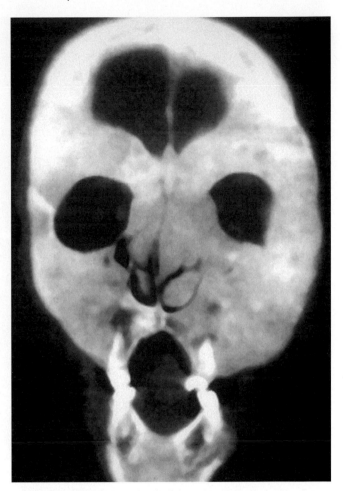

**FIGURE 6-145**  Coronal CT scan show a "ground glass" density expansile bony process that has encroached on the orbits and obliterated the frontal, ethmoid, and maxillary sinuses and portions of the nasal fossae. This patient had fibrous dysplasia.

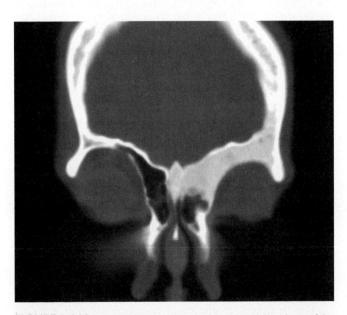

**FIGURE 6-144**  Coronal CT scan shows that the medullary bone of the left frontal and ethmoid bones is expanded; however, the cortices are intact. The medulary space has a "ground glass" appearance. This patient had fibrous dysplasia.

of the causes of the upward-looking eye of cherubism.[276] Pathologically, one sees proliferating fibrous connective tissue with numerous multinucleated giant cells indistinguishable from those of giant cell reparative granuloma. The disease is self-limited and is usually diagnosed after the age of 2 years. Treatment is usually not necessary, but if embarked on for cosmetic or other reasons, it will not provoke regrowth of lesional tissue.[277-279]

### True Giant Cell Tumor

Giant cell tumor (GCT) of bone (previously referred to as osteoclastoma) is an uncommon, benign, yet potentially locally aggressive tumor that comprises up to 5% of all primary bone neoplasia. More than 75% of these tumors are located in the epiphyseal region of long bones, half of them occurring about the knee. There is a female predisposition, and the majority of affected patients are beyond the second decade of life. GCT of the head and neck is extraordinarily rare.[271, 280] Huvos identified 3 GCTs of the cranium and maxilla out of 265 GCTs treated at the Memorial Sloan-Kettering Cancer Center.[280] Kujas and colleagues identified only seven cases of true GCT of the skull and cervical vertebrae after reviewing neuropathology specimens collected over 50 years.[281] An association

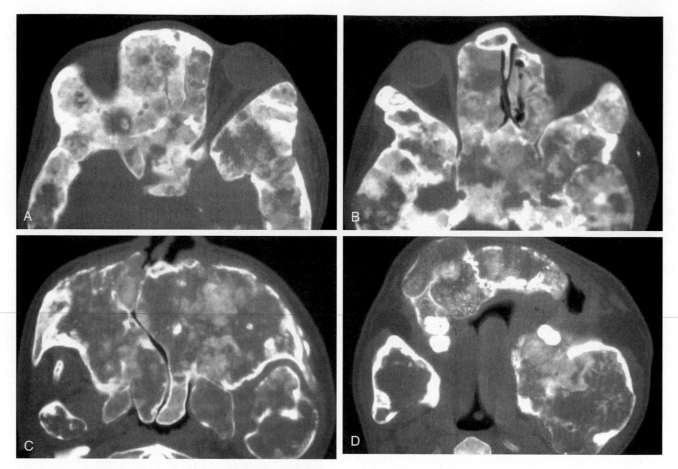

**FIGURE 6-146** Axial serial CT scans (**A** through **D**) through the facial region show that all of the facial and skull base bones are greatly expanded, with intact cortices. Their medullary spaces are filled with ossified and nonossified regions. The skull base foramina, orbital apices, and paranasal sinuses are all obliterated. The mandible is also affected. This patient had fibrous dysplasia.

between GCT of the jaws and Paget's disease has also been noted.[280]

Histologically, GCTs are characterized by a diffuse population of osteoclastic giant cells spread across a

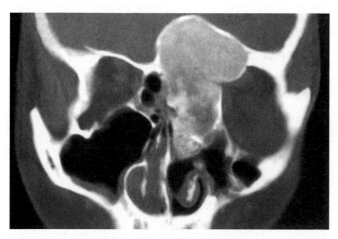

**FIGURE 6-147** Coronal CT scan shows a localized region of expanded bone in the left frontal and ethmoid bone. The medullary space has a "ground glass" appearance, and the cortices are intact. This patient had fibrous dysplasia.

background of short spindled cells with nuclei identical to those within the giant cells. This latter point allows for distinction between GCT and the myriad other osteoclastic giant cell–rich lesions that may affect bone. There may be dozens to hundreds of nuclei within the osteoclastic giant cells. Identification of these gargantuan benign giant cells also aids in establishing the diagnosis. Hemorrhage and hemosiderin deposition are not prominent features of GCTs. Reactive bone may be seen in the periphery of the tumor, as the ossified cartilage may undergo some remodeling. The differential diagnosis of GCT of the head and neck includes central giant cell reparative granuloma (CGCRG), "brown tumor" of hyperparathyroidism, or, more rarely, giant cell–rich osteogenic sarcoma. The distinctions between these entities may be impossible to make on a biopsy without radiographic and clinical correlation (Fig. 6-154).

There is considerable demographic (age of diagnosis) and histologic overlap between GCT and CGCRG, so that these two entities may represent a spectrum of a single disease process that is modified by patient age and site of occurrence.[282, 283]

The treatment of choice is complete surgical excision or curettage. The recurrence rate for GCT at all sites is 30% to 50% after curettage. Most local failures occur within 2 years of initial therapy.[284] Approximately 10% to

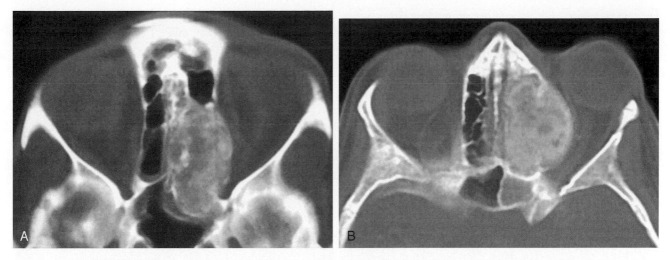

**FIGURE 6-148**   Axial CT scan (**A**) shows a "ground glass"-appearing bony process in the left ethmoid and sphenoid bones. There is encroachment into the left orbit. This patient had fibrous dysplasia. Axial CT scan (**B**) shows an expansile "ground glass"-appearing bony process in the left ethmoid complex. The left sphenoid sinus is obstructed by the process. Notice the similarity to **A**. This patient had an intraosseous meningioma.

15% of GCTs show clinical or histologic evidence of malignancy. Malignancy can occur de novo or as secondary transformation. Almost all secondary malignant transformations have been previously irradiated. Radiation therapy should be reserved for surgically inaccessible tumors, as GCTs are generally not radiosensitive and as radiation therapy is accompanied by the threat of malignant transformation.

On CT the tumors enhance moderately, and they tend to destroy and remodel bone.[285, 286] On MR they usually have fairly low signal intensity on all sequences, and they enhance.

### Giant Cell (Reparative) Granuloma

Giant cell (reparative) granuloma (GCG) is an entity of uncertain etiology that may affect either the jaw bones

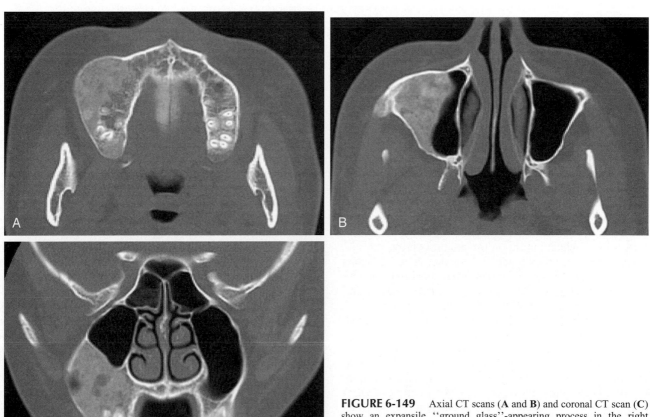

**FIGURE 6-149**   Axial CT scans (**A** and **B**) and coronal CT scan (**C**) show an expansile "ground glass"-appearing process in the right maxilla. The lesion affects the maxillary alveolus as well as the sinus walls. The sinus cavity is reduced by the encroachment of the bony process. This patient had fibrous dysplasia.

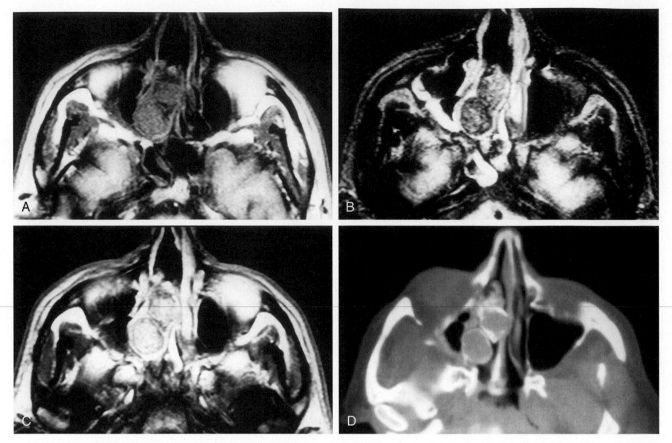

**FIGURE 6-150**   Axial T1-weighted (**A**), T2-weighted (**B**), and T1-weighted, contrast-enhanced MR images (**C**) and an axial CT scan (**D**) show a polypoid right posterior nasal cavity mass that has low T1-weighted and intermediate T2-weighted signal intensity and diffusely enhances. The CT scan shows the lesion to have an intact bony cortex and nonossified central regions. This patient had fibrous dysplasia.

(central giant cell granuloma [CGCG]) or the intraoral soft tissues (peripheral giant cell granuloma [PGCG]). The term *reparative* was originally introduced by Jaffe, but recently this modifier has been dropped from the name, as there is no evidence to support this function. PGCG is four times more common than CGCG. PGCG presents as an expansile mass of the gingiva or alveolar mucosa that rarely extends to the underlying bone. It occurs over a broad age range, with a peak incidence in the fourth decade of life. PGCG may occur after tooth extraction or with ill-fitting dentures and therefore may be related to trauma. There is a female predisposition, which implies hormonal sensitivity.

CGCG presents as an expansile, destructive intraosseous jaw mass. There is also a female predisposition, but the majority of patients present prior to the fourth decade of life. There is no association with prior trauma.

Radiographically, PGCG rarely is clearly visualized. However, CGCG typically appears as a multiloculated, expansile lytic lesion on plain film (Fig. 6-155).[185, 285–288] On CT, CGCG is bulky and enhancing and can be seen to aggressively erode the maxillary sinus walls or to have an expansile, remodeling apearance. On MR imaging, CGCG has an intermediate signal intensity on both T1-weighted and T2-weighted images. As such, the MR appearance may mimic that of SCC.[241]

Pathologically, GCG characteristically has a hemor-

rhagic, fibroblastic background with innumerable osteoclastic giant cells. This background is helpful in distinguishing GCRG from GCT. The latter lacks the diffuse hemorrhage, hemosiderin, and fibroblasts, and the background cells are identical to the nuclei of the osteoclastic giant cells. The giant cells of GCT are diffusely and evenly dispersed throughout the tumor. In contrast, the brown tumor of hyperparathyroidism has uneven clumps of osteoclasts, perivascular hemorrhage, and hemosiderin deposition.

It is useful to know the serum calcium and parathyroid hormone levels when dealing with any giant cell lesion. In hyperparathyroidism the calcium level is elevated unless the patient is already severely calcium depleted. Serum parathyroid homone (PTH) is elevated with a brown tumor of hyperparathyroidism and is normal with other GCTs. PTH is also normal in tumor-induced osteomalacia, which radiologically can mimic severe hyperparathyroidism.[289] Giant cell granuloma arising in the skull base is discussed in Chapter 12.

### Aneurysmal Bone Cyst

An aneurysmal bone cyst (ABC) is neither an aneurysm nor a true cyst, but it does occur in bone. Rather, it is a benign, nonneoplastic, expansile osseous lesion. ABC occurs mainly in females over the age of 20 years and represents only 1% to 2% of all primary bone tumors. It can present as a slowly or rapidly enlarging mass with nonthrobbing pain. ABCs may occur de novo; however, they may be "engrafted upon" (occur in conjunction with) another primary osseous tumor. This process may be pathologically identified in as many as one third of ABCs; the most common findings are GCT, unicameral bone cyst, or nonossifying fibroma.[284] Between 3% and 12% of ABCs occur in the head and neck, and they have also been reported in the maxilla, orbit, ethmoid, and frontal bones.[290] In a review of 64 reported cases of jaw ABC, the ratio of mandibular to maxillary cases was 2.4:1, with a predisposition for the posterior mandible. There was a wide age range, with a median age of 17 years.[291] Primary paranasal sinus/nasal cavity ABC has rarely been described and has been seen in conjunction with preexisting primary bone pathology.[292, 293]

Histologically, ABCs are composed of large, variably sized, blood-filled cystic and sinusoidal nonendothelium-lined spaces traversed by fibroblastic cells. New bone formation is evident; osteoid formation, osteoclast giant cells, and plump background spindle cells are seen. Hemorrhage and hemosiderin deposits are present. Surgical resection or curettage is the treatment of choice; in the jaws,

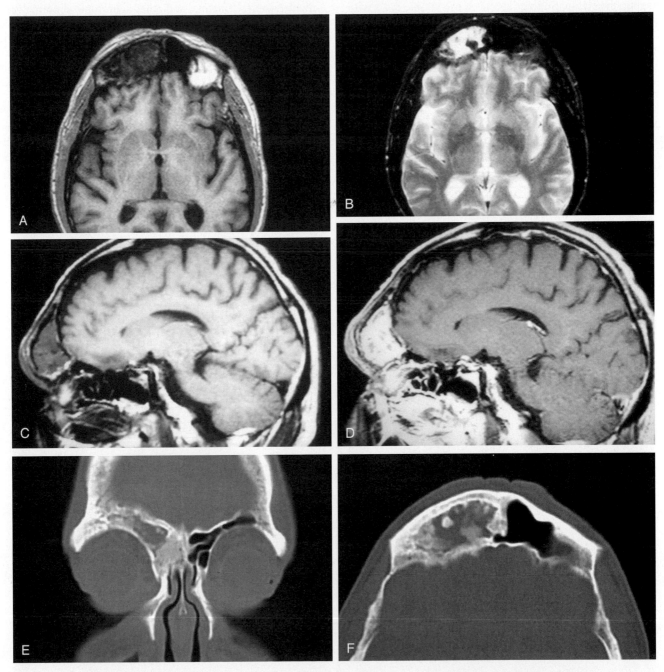

**FIGURE 6-151** Axial T1-weighted (**A**), T2-weighted (**B**), sagittal T1-weighted (**C**), and T1-weighted, contrast-enhanced (**D**) MR images and coronal (**E**) and axial (**F**) CT scans show a nonhomogeneous right frontal sinus mass that has low signal intensity in **A**, high signal intensity in **B**, and diffusely enhances in **D**. The CT scans show the bone to be expanded, with intact cortices and a medullary space filled with ossified and nonossified regions. This patient had fibrous dysplasia.

currettage has a somewhat higher recurrence rate (20% to 38%) than resection (11% to 25%).[284]

Radiographically, this lesion may be unilocular or may demonstrate a multilocular "soap bubble" or "honeycomb" radiolucency (Fig. 6-156). Kaffe and colleagues found that the majority of cases were radiolucent (87%), mixed (11%), or radiopaque (2%); the radiographic appearance was less common.[291] Fifty-three percent were multilocular, 43% were unilocular, and 3% were not loculated. The peripheral bone margins were defined but not corticated in 39%, well defined in 33%, and diffuse in 28%. Bony remodeling and destruction can be seen (Fig. 6-157). On MR imaging, the classic findings are those of multiple cysts with fluid-fluid levels (Figs. 6-158 and 6-159).

### Paget's Disease

Paget's disease (osteitis deformans) is a bone disorder of unknown etiology. Increased osteoclastic and osteoblastic activity results in the disorderly production of abnormally dense yet mechanically fragile bone. The disease usually occurs in patients over 50 years old, and its incidence increases with age, ranging from 3% to 5% of people older than 40 years to 11% of those older than 80 years.[294] There is a male predominance and some familial predisposition.

The disease is usually (90%) polyostotic and involves the vertebrae (76%), calvaria (65%), pelvis (43%), femur (35%), and tibia (3%). In the head and neck, the clavaria, maxilla, and mandible are most commonly affected.[295] In 80% of patients, the degree of skeletal involvement is limited and found fortuitously on radiographic studies or at autopsy. The facial bones are rarely involved; however, whenever the maxilla and mandible are affected, the calvarium is invariably also involved.[295] Advanced calvarial involvement may lead to a characteristically enlarged head, and the reduced size of the cranial cavity secondary to calvarial and skull base bony ingrowth can lead to altered mental status, dementia, and other neurologic abnormalities. Platybasia is associated with cranial nerve deficits. Encroachment into the orbits, neurovascular canals, and sinonasal cavities has led to proptosis, visual loss, neurologic deficits, facial deformity, and nasal congestion. Despite the thickness of the bone, it is extremely vascular and fragile and may be prone to fracture.

The initial radiographic and CT appearance of Paget's disease of the calvarium often reveals a lytic phase that produces osteoporosis circumscripta, usually involving the frontal region to the greatest degree. A "mixed" phase may follow. This phase shows foci of sclerotic, woven bone

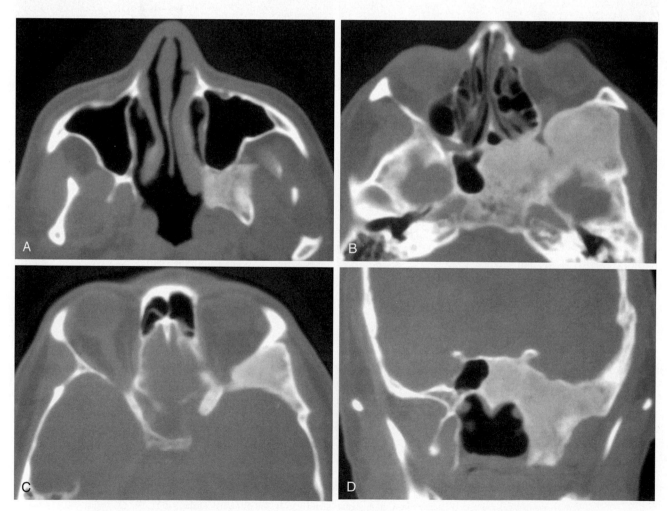

**FIGURE 6-152** Serial axial CT scans (**A** through **C**) and coronal CT scans (**D**) show a "ground glass" expanded left sphenoid bone. The left sphenoid sinus is obliterated, and all portions of the bone are affected.

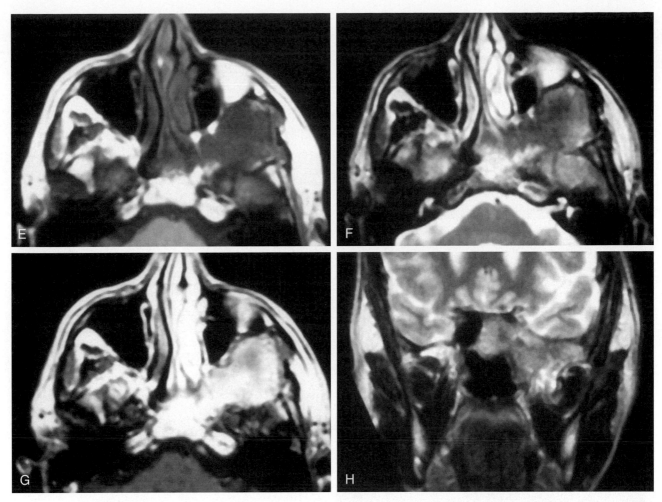

**FIGURE 6-152**  *Continued.* Axial T1-weighted (**E**), T2-weighted (**F**), and T1-weighted, contrast-enhanced (**G**) MR images and a coronal T2-weighted (**H**) MR image show the low to intermediate T1-weighted and T2-weighted signal intensity and the marked enhancement of the process. This patient had fibrous dysplasia.

within areas of lower density, which represent sites of fibrous myeloid production. The remaining bone often gives a moderately diffuse radiopacity producing a ''cotton wool'' appearance. Eventually, there can be a sclerotic phase, with poor corticomedullary differentiation. The calvarium itself is thickened; usually the greatest degree of thickening is anterior, and one side of the skull tends to be more affected than the other. Inner table irregularity is usually greater than that of the outer surface. It is the sclerotic form of Paget's disease that usually affects the facial bones. This results in a thickened, dense bone with slightly irregular cortical surfaces and poor corticomedullary differentiation (Figs. 6-160 to 6-163).[295]

On MR imaging, the dense foci of bone give rounded foci of signal void on all imaging sequences. The marrow tissues give high T1-weighted and fairly high T2-weighted signal intensities, reflecting the fat and blood protein in these regions. The background matrix gives an intermediate signal intensity on all imaging sequences. The facial area demonstrates a mixed, low to intermediate signal intensity on all imaging sequences. The lesion usually enhances nonhomogeneously.[295]

Histologically, pagetoid bone reflects an erratic resorption pattern and new production of bone that fails to mature

normally. This is seen as predominantly woven mosaic bone, with increased osteoclastic and osteoblastic activity.

Sarcomas may develop in 5% to 10% of patients with multifocal Paget's disease and in less than 2% of patients with limited bone involvement. The prognosis of Paget's sarcoma is grave; most patients die within 2 years. The development of multiple tumors is frequent; autopsy studies suggest a multicentric rather than a metastatic origin for these tumors. Most Paget's sarcomas are osteogenic sarcomas (50% to 60%) or fibrosarcomas (20% to 25%).[296] In the facial area, benign GCTs can also occur. On plain films and CT, GCTs usually appear as sharply localized, nonosseous masses. Because the bone seen in Paget's disease, as well as in the sarcomas, tends to give an intermediate signal intensity on all MR imaging sequences, it is often more difficult to diagnose and map these malignancies or tumors on MR imaging than on CT (Fig. 6-163).[295]

## Sarcomas

### Osteogenic Sarcoma and Chondrosarcoma

Primary bone sarcomas occur over a wide age range; osteogenic sarcoma (OS) occurs most commonly after the

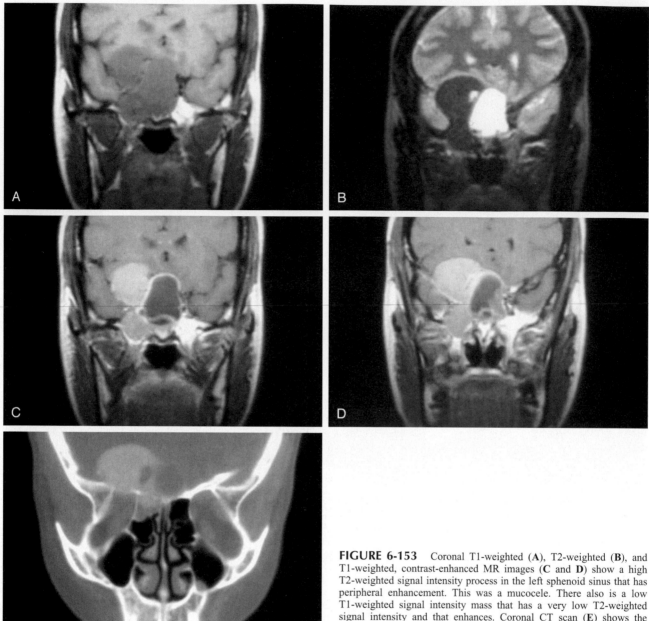

**FIGURE 6-153**   Coronal T1-weighted (**A**), T2-weighted (**B**), and T1-weighted, contrast-enhanced MR images (**C** and **D**) show a high T2-weighted signal intensity process in the left sphenoid sinus that has peripheral enhancement. This was a mucocele. There also is a low T1-weighted signal intensity mass that has a very low T2-weighted signal intensity and that enhances. Coronal CT scan (**E**) shows the mucocele and the ''ground glass'' expanded bone of fibrous dysplasia. This patient has fibrous dysplasia causing a left sphenoid sinus mucocele.

first decade of life, whereas chondrosarcoma (CS) occurs most commonly after the fourth decade. Primary OS, that is, OS in the absence of previous irradiation or Paget's disease, most commonly occurs prior to closure of the growth plates within the distal femur. Huvos reported on over 1000 cases of OS from Memorial Sloan-Kettering Cancer Center and found that half of them occurred around the knee, and that the femur was the most common bone affected.[297] Only 7% of these OSs occurred in the head and neck, usually in the jaws (55 of 77 cases in the head and neck, followed by craniofacial bones and calvaria).

Primary CSs occur most commonly in the pelvic region and femur.[298]

In a series of almost 500 CSs from Memorial Sloan-Kettering Cancer Center, only 5% (25 cases) occurred in the head and neck. Secondary CS of the head and neck can be seen after radiation therapy or in the setting of Maffucci syndrome or Ollier disease.[299] In a review of 56 craniofacial CSs, 25 (44.6%) involved the alveolar maxilla and maxillary sinus; 23 (41.1%) involved the nasal septum, ethmoid, and sphenoid; 6 (10.7%) involved the mandible; and 2 (3.6%) involved the nasal tip.[300–302]

Histologic diversity characterizes OS. OS, by definition, is a tumor in which the malignant cells produce an osteoid matrix. Histologic subtypes of OS include (1) osteoblastic OS, which produces abundant osteoid matrix; (2) chondroblastic OS, which produces abundant chondroid matrix, yet the osteoid present merits the classification of OS rather than CS; (3) telangiectatic OS, a highly vascular sarcoma with a lytic radiographic appearance; (4) fibroblastic (fibrosarco-

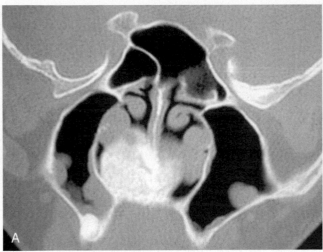

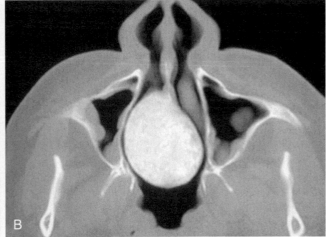

**FIGURE 6-154**   Coronal (**A**) and axial (**B**) CT scans show a densely ossified mass in the nasal septum. Two months earlier, this was a nonossified mass. This patient had a healed brown tumor from hyperparathyroidism.

matous) OS, composed predominantly of malignant fibroblast-like cells with some osteoid production; (5) fibrohistiocytic (malignant fibrous histiocytoma [MFH]) OS, which contains malignant multinuclear tumor giant cells in addition to the fibrosarcomatous component; and (6) round cell OS, composed predominantly of small round malignant cells with occasional osteoid production (Fig. 6-164). Many OSs display multiple histologic patterns,

thereby precluding neat categorization. Despite the wealth of clinicopathologic data, there is little to indicate that histologic subclassification for OS has prognostic significance over classic tumor staging and grading (Broder's grading) schemata.

CS is generally more histologically uniform than OS. Abundant chondroid matrix is the rule. CS is graded (I, II, III) according to tumor cellularity and cytologic atypia.

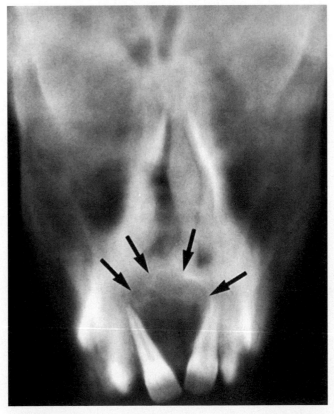

**FIGURE 6-155**   Coronal multidirectional tomogram shows an expansile lesion in the maxillary alveolus and hard palate (*arrows*). This patient had a central-type giant cell granuloma.

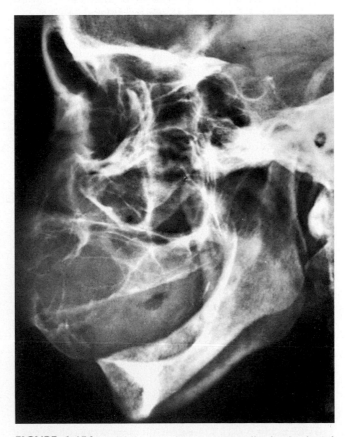

**FIGURE 6-156**   Lateral view shows an expansile, loculated, and destructive lesion of the maxilla. This patient had an aneurysmal bone cyst.

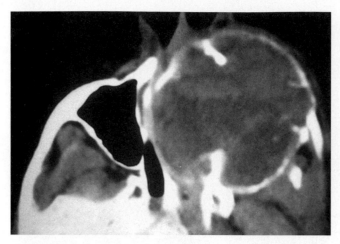

**FIGURE 6-157** Axial CT scan shows an expansile mass in the left maxillary sinus. The surrounding bone is remodeled and not eroded. This patient had an aneurysmal bone cyst. (Courtesy of Dr. Revel and Dr. Vanel.)

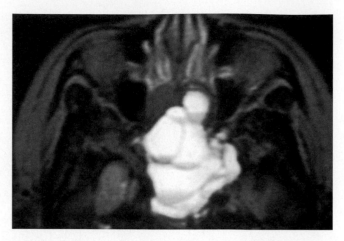

**FIGURE 6-159** Axial T2-weighted MR image shows a mass in the sphenoid bone and sphenoid sinus. This lesion is composed of multiple cystic areas, each with a fluid-fluid level. This patient had an aneurysmal bone cyst.

Grade I CS is composed of invasive lobulated tumor producing abundant matrix, with binucleate chondrocytes (Fig. 6-165). Distinguishing it from a benign chondroma may not be possible with limited material and requires radiographic correlation to establish an aggressive, invasive growth pattern. Grade II CS has greater cellularity and pleomorphism than a grade I tumor and is easily identified as both malignant and chondroid in nature. A grade III neoplasm is very cellular and pleomorphic. The chondroid matrix may be limited. Spindle cell CS (so-called dedifferentiated CS) is an unusual variant in which a high-grade undifferentiated sarcoma "springs forth" from a lower-grade CS.

Surgery and adjuvant chemotherapy is indicated for OS. Establishing a preoperative diagnosis of OS allows for neoadjuvant chemotherapy. The chemotherapeutic effect can then be histologically assessed based on postoperative (postchemotherapy) tumor viability, and thus the postoperative completion of chemotherapy can be tailored based on the observed response. Complete surgical resection is

indicated for CS; adjuvant chemotherapy and radiotherapy have not been shown to improve survival. Proton beam therapy may be considered as primary therapy for unresectable cases. Survival of patients with head and neck OS and CS is dependent upon tumor stage, grade, and site. Jaw OS has a 5-year disease-free survival rate of between 30% and 50%. The prognosis for OS in Paget's disease, as mentioned, is known to be particularly poor. The 5-year disease-free survival rate for craniofacial CS is around 40%.[303] Fu and Perzin emphasize that sinonasal CS is less amenable to resection than CS at other sites.[209] For both OS and CS, the metastatic rate (predominantly to the lungs, liver, brain, bones, and lymph nodes) directly correlates with the tumor grade. Overall, only 7% of sinonasal CSs develop metastases. Patients with mesenchymal CS in general have a 5-year survival rate ranging from 42% to 54.6% and a 10-year survival rate of 28%. Mesenchymal CS of the jaw bones (5- and 10-year survival rates of 82% and 56%, respectively) appears to have a more indolent course than axial skeletal or soft tissue mesenchymal CS.[304, 305]

On imaging, CS tends to occur at the cartilaginous junctions of the facial bones or in the cartilaginous nasal septum. Marginal bone erosion is typically present, and calcifications within the mass may or may not be seen. These tumors have fairly low T1-weighted and high T2-weighted signal intensities, and they enhance after contrast administration, either uniformly or nonuniformly. Without the presence of gross tumoral calcifications, the imaging appearance is not characteristic enough to establish a definitive diagnosis (Figs. 6-166 to 6-172). Rarely, a large, aggressive pituitary adenoma that extends into the nasal fossa may have similar imaging findings (Fig. 6-173).

With OS, there typically is a "sunburst" periosteal reaction, although this need not be present. Focal destruction is usually seen; however, dense sclerotic bone may be present, especially in the maxillary alveolus. Depending on the bone content of the tumor, the signal intensities can vary, usually being primarily a low T1-weighted and an intermediate T2-weighted signal intensity. Enhancement after contrast administration is present, although not usually to the degree seen in CS (Figs. 6-174 to 6-180).

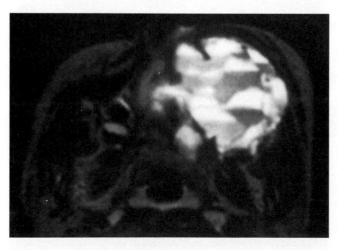

**FIGURE 6-158** Axial T2-weighted MR image shows multiple cystic components with fluid-fluid levels within a left maxillary sinus mass. This patient had an aneurysmal bone cyst. (Courtesy of Dr. Revel and Dr. Vanel.)

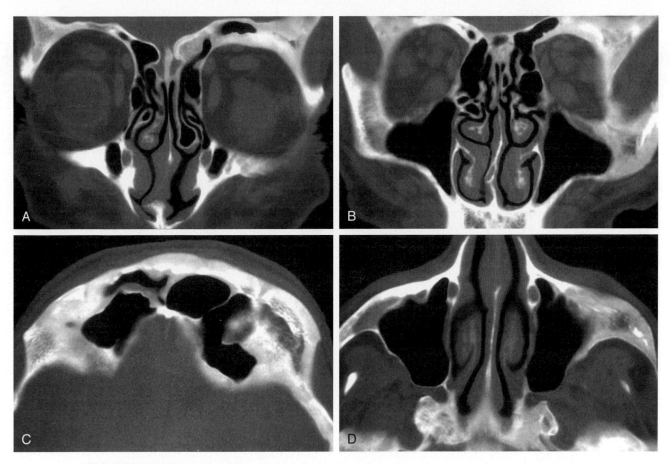

**FIGURE 6-160** Coronal (**A** and **B**) and axial (**C** and **D**) CT scans show the facial bones to be thickened, denser than normal, and with poorly defined trabeculae. Similar changes were present in the calvarium. This patient had Paget's disease.

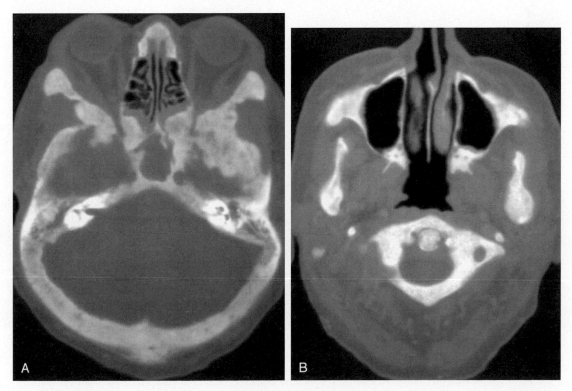

**FIGURE 6-161** Axial CT scans through the orbits (**A**) and the maxillary sinuses (**B**) show that the bones of the skull base, upper cervical vertebra, and face are thicker and denser than normal. The bones have a slightly irregular contour, and there is poor detail of the trabeculae. This patient had Paget's disease.

**FIGURE 6-162** Sagittal (**A**) and coronal (**B**) T1-weighted MR images show diffusely thickened bone in the facial region and the calvaria. The areas of high signal intensity in the calvaria correspond to regions of marrow, while the areas of low signal intensity correspond to regions of dense woven bone formation. The thickened calvaria has reduced the size of the intracranial compartment. The majority of the abnormal bone has a nonhomogeneous low to intermediate signal intensity. This patient had Paget's disease.

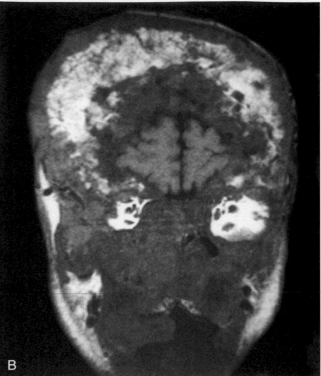

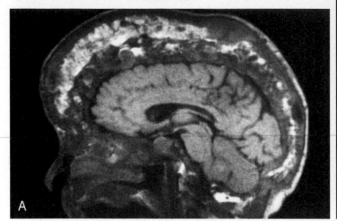

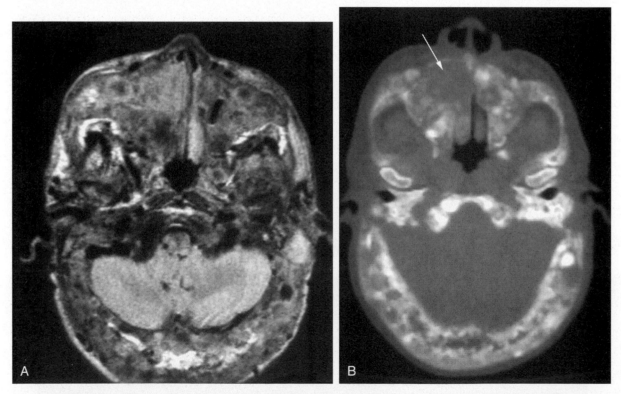

**FIGURE 6-163** Axial proton density MR image (**A**) and a corresponding axial CT scan (**B**) show marked thickening of the calvaria, with localized areas of dense woven bone. The expanded bone has virtually obliterated the maxillary sinuses. In **B** there is an area in the anterior medial right maxilla that is almost devoid of bone (*arrow*). This region, in retrospect, can be identified in **A**, but it is not as clearly evident. This patient had Paget's disease, and this localized area was an osteosarcoma.

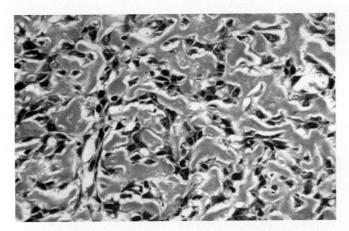

**FIGURE 6-164**  Osteogenic sarcoma: The malignant cells of this poorly differentiated OS are producing a lacelike osteoid stroma.

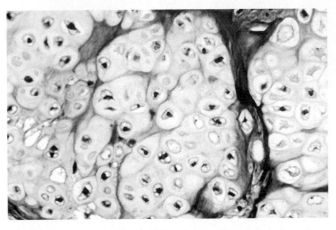

**FIGURE 6-165**  Chondrosarcoma grows in a lobulated fashion. These chondrocytes are atypical and crowded.

**FIGURE 6-166**  Axial (**A**) and coronal (**B**) CT scans show a destructive mass in the left ethmoid sinuses. The tumor has broken into the left orbit and the anterior cranial fossa. Gross, discrete calcifications are present within the mass. This patient had a chondrosarcoma.

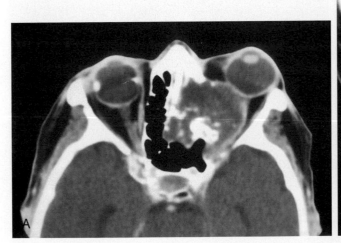

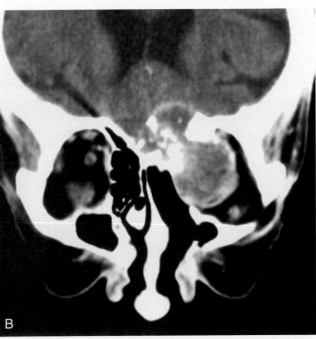

### Mesenchymal Chondrosarcoma

Mesenchymal CS is a rare variant of CS, representing approximately 10% of all CSs.[306] It can occur as an osseous (60% to 70%) or soft tissue (30% to 40%) neoplasm. Among 35 patients with mesenchymal CS seen at the Memorial Sloan-Kettering Cancer Center, 14% occurred in the head and neck, most commonly in the maxilla.[306] The craniospinal meninges and orbital soft tissues are the most common extraskeletal sites. These tumors also have been reported in the ethmoid sinuses. The majority of affected patients are 40 years old or younger (average, 26 years old). Mesenchymal CS is a bimorphic tumor composed of islands of well-differentiated hyaline cartilage juxtaposed to a small cell undifferentiated malignancy.

## ODONTOGENIC LESIONS AND TUMORS

Odontogenic and developmental cysts arise from the cystic expansion of epithelial remnants of various components of the dental apparatus or entrapped epithelium. They are generally uncommon entities and can be classified as either follicular cyst, periodontal cyst, odontogenic keratocyst, calcifying odontogenic cyst, nasopalatine cyst, median palatine cyst, and nasolabial cyst. The following discussion is limited to those jaw cysts that can present as maxillary or palatal lesions (also see Chapter 17).

### Jaw Cysts

#### Follicular Cyst

Follicular cysts (also referred to as dentigerous cysts) represents up to 24% of all odontogenic cysts. There is a pronounced predisposition for males and for African Americans. Most affected patients are diagnosed between the second and fourth decades of life. These cysts develop as

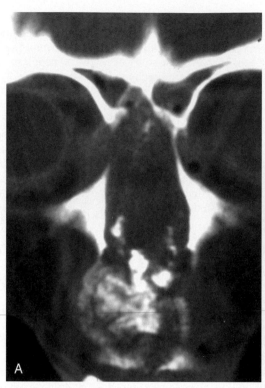

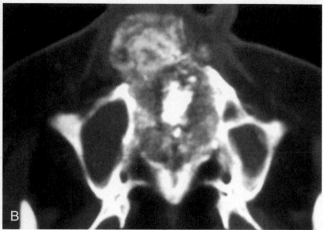

**FIGURE 6-167** Coronal (**A**) and axial (**B**) CT scans show a bulky mass arising in the hard palate and extending ventrally into the nose. There are innumerable calcifications spread throughout the tumor. This patient had a chondrosarcoma.

a result of fluid accumulation either around the tooth crown or within the enamel organ. They are invariably associated with impacted or unerupted teeth. The most commonly affected teeth are the mandibular third molars, maxillary canines, and third molars. Follicular cysts may also be associated with supernumerary teeth.[307]

Radiographically, one sees a well-circumscribed cyst that contains the crown of the tooth. As the cyst grows, it pulls the unerupted tooth with it. Small dentigerous cysts are unilocular. Large cysts may be multilocular, and the confined tooth may be displaced from its normal location. Resorption of adjacent teeth roots can occur.[308]

The dentigerous cyst must be distinguished radiographically from a normal dental follicle. If a dental follicle measures 2 cm or more, it is highly likely that the unerupted tooth will develop a dentigerous cyst. Similarly, a pericoronal space of 2.5 mm or more heralds an 80% likelihood that the unerupted tooth will become a dentigerous cyst.[309]

If the cyst erodes into the maxillary sinus, it may grow rapidly, remodeling the antral walls. Often the inferior maxillary sinus cortex is elevated over portions of the cyst. In the axial view, this can be detected by noting what appear to be two bony walls in the posterior sinus. Here the most posterior bone represents the true sinus wall, while the anterior bone represents the elevated sinus floor. If multiple dentigerous cysts are present, the patient should be examined for the basal cell nevus syndrome (see below). On MR imaging, the cyst fluid has intermediate signal intensity

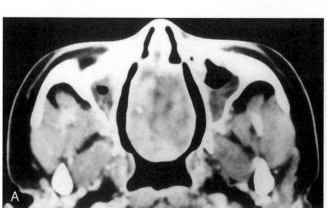

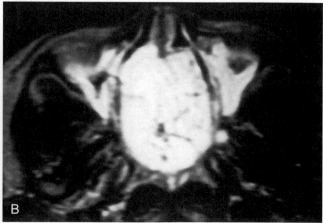

**FIGURE 6-168** Axial CT scan (**A**) and axial T2-weighted MR image (**B**) show a bulky mass arising from the nasal septum. Scattered calcifications are present within the mass. The lesion had an intermediate T1-weighted signal intensity. Obstructive inflammatory changes are present in the maxillary sinuses. This patient had a chondrosarcoma.

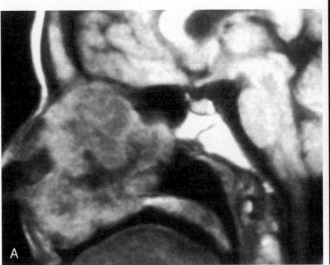
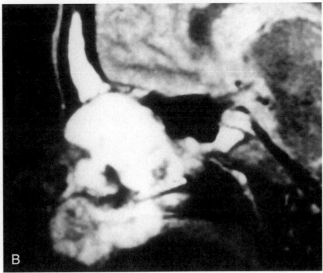

**FIGURE 6-169**    Sagittal T1-weighted (**A**) and T2-weighted (**B**) MR images show a slightly nonhomogeneous nasal septal mass that has a low to intermediate signal intensity in **A** and a high signal intensity in **B**. The frontal sinuses are obstructed by the tumor. This patient had a chondrosarcoma.

on T1-weighted images and high signal intensity on T2-weighted images; the displaced tooth gives a signal void on all imaging sequences. In this regard, the MR imaging appearance may be similar to that of an antral aspergilloma (Figs. 6-181 to 6-186).

Small dentigerous cysts are cured by curettage. Larger multiloculated cysts may require marsupialization. An ameloblastoma may arise within the wall of the dentigerous cyst. This mural or cystic ameloblastoma is often

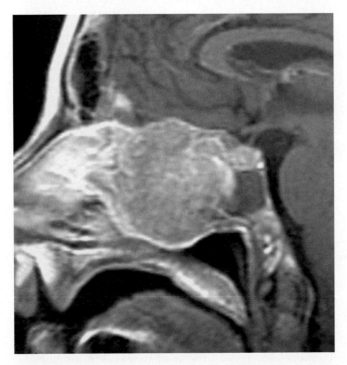

**FIGURE 6-170**    Sagittal T1-weighted, fat-suppressed, contrast-enhanced MR image shows an enhancing nasal septal mass that has extended into the sphenoid bone. A mucocele is present within the obstructed sphenoid sinus. This patient had a chondrosarcoma.

diagnosed only by the pathologist; the radiographic findings in such cases are those of a simple dentigerous cyst.[307, 309] There is a familial predisposition toward this transformation. The prognosis of a cystic ameloblastoma arising in a dentigerous cyst is excellent, as curettage is usually curative.

### Periodontal Cyst

Periodontal cysts are also referred to as periapical, radicular, apical periodontal, or dental cysts. They represent the most common jaw cyst and arise in erupted, infected carious teeth as sequelae to periapical granulomas. Maxillary teeth are most commonly involved. Maxillary periodontal cysts can erode into the maxillary sinus, remodeling the antral walls and elevating the inferior sinus cortex (Figs. 6-187 to 6-189).[309, 310]

The term *residual periodontal cyst (residual cyst)* refers to a periapical cyst developing after tooth extraction. Treatment of these cysts consists of simple enucleation.[306]

The lateral periodontal cyst (also referred to as a paradental cyst) is a noninflammatory developmental cyst that arises lateral to the tooth root. This cyst probably arises from proliferation of rests within the dental lamina. This cyst occurs most often in adults in the premolar and cuspid areas. Radiographically, there is an incidental multiloculated cyst along the lateral tooth root.

### Odontogenic Keratocyst

Odontogenic keratocysts (OKCs) can be subclassified as central (intraosseous), which are further subclassified as parakeratotic, orthokeratotic, or mixed, versus peripheral or mucosal. The central parakeratotic OKC (POKC) is most commonly encountered and is also referred to as a primordial cyst. POKC represents up to 16.5% of all jaw cysts and is most commonly seen in patients within the second and third decades of life. The mandible is affected two to four times more often than the maxilla, with a predilection for posterior jaws. Half of patients with POKC

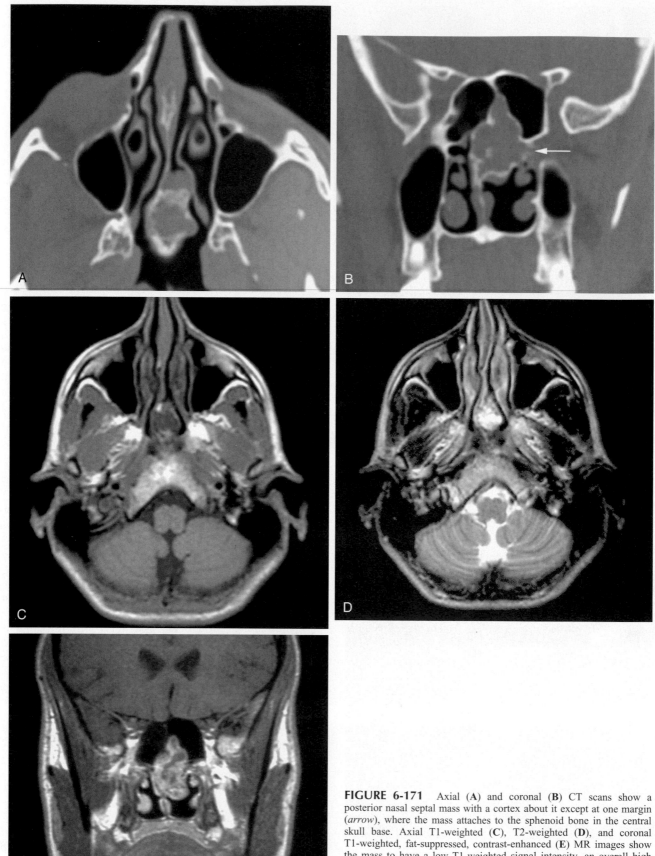

**FIGURE 6-171** Axial (**A**) and coronal (**B**) CT scans show a posterior nasal septal mass with a cortex about it except at one margin (*arrow*), where the mass attaches to the sphenoid bone in the central skull base. Axial T1-weighted (**C**), T2-weighted (**D**), and coronal T1-weighted, fat-suppressed, contrast-enhanced (**E**) MR images show the mass to have a low T1-weighted signal intensity, an overall high T2-weighted signal intensity, and nonhomogeneous, primarily peripheral enhancement. This patient had a low-grade chondrosarcoma.

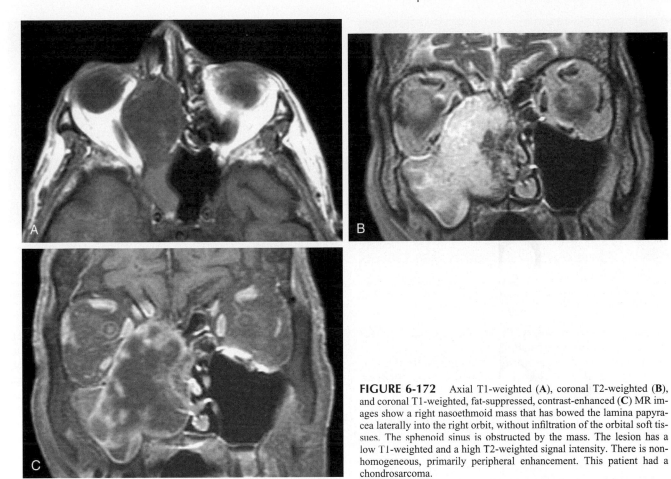

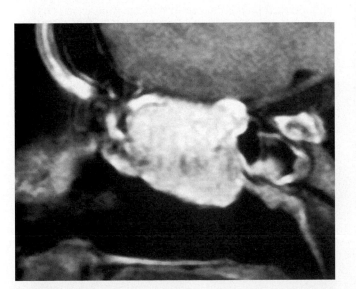

FIGURE 6-172  Axial T1-weighted (**A**), coronal T2-weighted (**B**), and coronal T1-weighted, fat-suppressed, contrast-enhanced (**C**) MR images show a right nasoethmoid mass that has bowed the lamina papyracea laterally into the right orbit, without infiltration of the orbital soft tissues. The sphenoid sinus is obstructed by the mass. The lesion has a low T1-weighted and a high T2-weighted signal intensity. There is nonhomogeneous, primarily peripheral enhancement. This patient had a chondrosarcoma.

FIGURE 6-173  Sagittal T1-weighted, fat-suppressed, contrast-enhanced MR image shows an enhancing mass that fills the nasal fossae and sphenoid sinuses. The tumor extends caudally into the roof of the nasopharynx. A small nodule of tumor projects above the sella turcica. This patient had an aggressive pituitary adenoma.

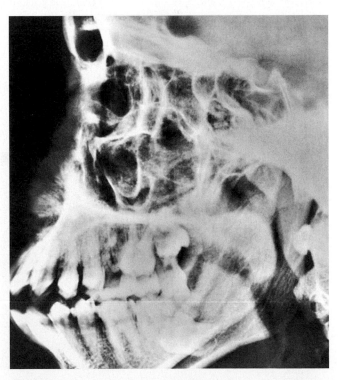

FIGURE 6-174  Lateral view shows an aggressive tumor of the maxilla that has caused a "sunburst" periosteal reaction anteriorly. This patient had an osteogenic sarcoma.

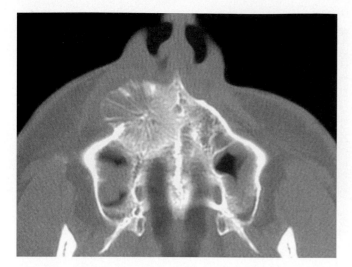

**FIGURE 6-175** Axial CT scan shows a destructive mass in the right anterior maxilla with a typical "sunburst"-type periosteal reaction. This patient had an osteogenic sarcoma.

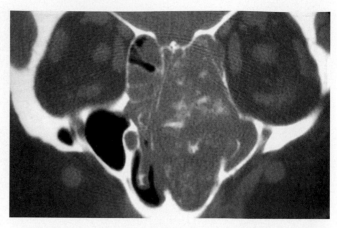

**FIGURE 6-176** Coronal CT scan shows a destructive mass in the nasal cavity and ethmoid sinuses, sphenoid sinuses, and right maxillary sinus. The tumor erodes the central skull base and the floor of the anterior cranial fossa. Within the mass are irregular areas of calcification or ossification. This appearance is highly suggestive of a sarcoma rather than a carcinoma. This patient had an osteogenic sarcoma.

complain of pain. Maxillary POKC can extend into the antrum, causing nasal obstruction.[307]

Historically, the term *primordial cyst* reflects the idea that these cysts were derived from degenerated stellate reticulum of the enamel organ prior to mineralization. However, these cysts are now believed to originate from dental lamina or its remnants or from extensions of basal cells from the overlying epithelium. Most are believed to develop from supernumerary teeth. When a rare cyst develops in place of a tooth, it is considered a replacement type of keratocyst.[307]

Radiographically, POKCs appear as unilocular or multilocular radiolucencies that may have a thin, reactive, sclerotic bony rim and smooth or scalloped margins or appear destructive, invading adjacent bone. Pathologically, these cysts are lined by stratified squamous epithelium, producing corrugated parakeratosis. The term *parakeratosis* refers to retained nuclei within the compact hyperkeratosis. The basal reserve cells reveal reverse palisading, which refers to the fact that the nuclei are oriented away from the basement membrane.

Multiple odontogenic keratocysts are associated with the nevoid basal cell carcinoma syndrome (Gorlin's syndrome). This condition is transmitted in an autosomal dominant fashion as a result of loss of a tumor suppressor gene on chromosome 9q22. Nevoid basal cell carcinoma syndrome is associated with the early development of multiple basal cell carcinomas, which can occur within preexisting sebaceous nevi, palmar and plantar pitting, and skeletal developmental abnormalities, as well as within the above-mentioned POKC. POKCs have also been associated with Marfan's syndrome. They are known for their aggressive potential for invasion and recurrence; up to 62.5% may recur. Simple POKC may be treated by enucleation, keeping the cyst intact. Multilocular or more destructive POKCs are better treated by en bloc resection.

Orthokeratosis is defined as compact keratin without retained nuclei. An orthokeratotic-type keratocyst (OOKC) represents 13% of OKCs. There is a male predisposition and no increased predominance in African Americans. OOKCs have a predilection for the mandible, but unlike POKCs, OOKCs are more likely to affect the anterior jaws. OOKCs are noteworthy in that they are generally unilocular.[307]

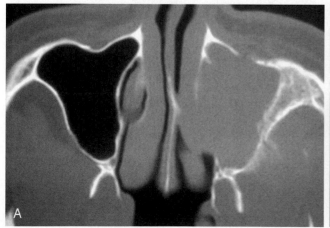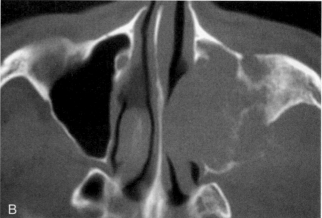

**FIGURE 6-177** Axial CT scans (**A** and **B**) show a mass in the left maxillary sinus, with destruction of portions of the anterior, medial, and posterior sinus walls. In addition, there is an aggressive periosteal reaction in the posterior sinus wall.

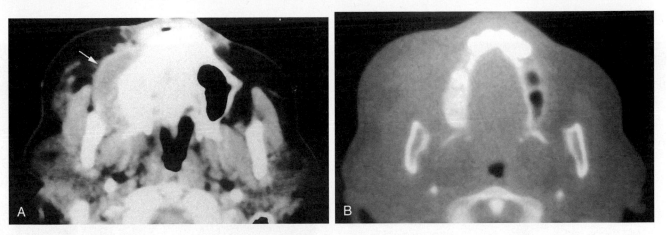

**FIGURE 6-178** Axial CT scans viewed at "soft-tissue" (**A**) and "bone" (**B**) window settings show a nonossified mass along the outer margin of the right maxillary alveolus (*arrow*). The alveolus in this area is minimally enlarged and very dense. This patient had an osteogenic sarcoma.

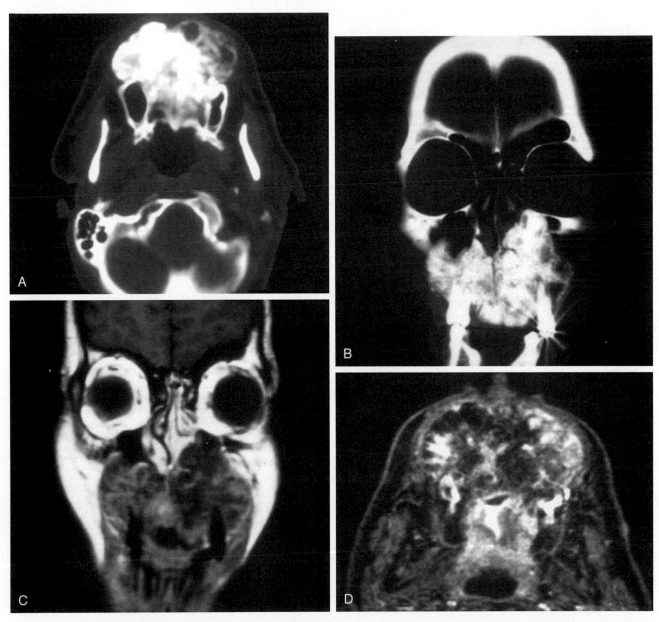

**FIGURE 6-179** Axial (**A**) and coronal (**B**) CT scans show a dense area of bony production in the hard palate. No intact cortex is identified in the region of the mass. Coronal T1-weighted (**C**) and axial T2-weighted (**D**) MR images show that this mass is quite nonhomogeneous. The areas of dense bone seen on the CT scan are for the most part of low signal intensity, but the lesion is not as clearly separated from the adjacent uninvolved maxilla and maxillary sinuses as it is on the CT scan. This patient had an osteogenic sarcoma.

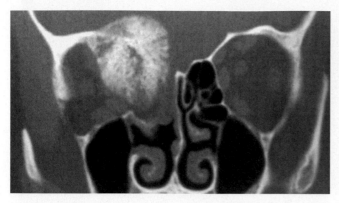

**FIGURE 6-180** Coronal CT scan on a patient who previously had a craniofacial resection for an osteogenic sarcoma shows a recurrent bony mass with aggressive periosteal production. This patient had a recurrent osteogenic sarcoma.

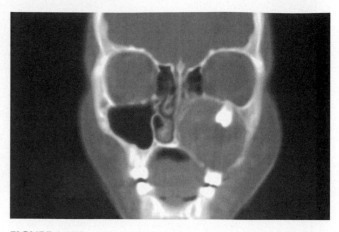

**FIGURE 6-182** Coronal CT scan shows an expansile mass in the left antrum. A molar tooth is present in the uppermost wall of the lesion. This patient had a dentigerous cyst.

Radiographically, one sees a unilocular radiolucent cyst. CT shows the bone morphology better than plain films; however, contrast-enhanced MR images provide the essential macroscopic detail, including focal wall enhancement and isointense intraluminal soft-tissue masses, which correlates with the histologic findings of focal inflammatory ulceration of the cyst lining, orthokeratosis, and cell debris. The cyst lining lacks the prominent corrugated proliferating basaloid reserve cells of POKC. Rather, these basal reserve cells are more flattened. The hyperkeratosis lacks retained nuclei, hence the classification "orthokeratosis." Curettage is curative. OOKCs are less aggressive than POKCs and recur infrequently.

### Calcifying Odontogenic Cyst

This cyst has a variety of names, including keratinizing ameloblastoma, keratinizing and calcifying ameloblastoma, melanotic ameloblastic odontoma calcifying cyst, cystic calcified odontogenic tumor, ghost cell tumor, and atypical adamantinoma.[307] The calcifying odontogenic cyst is an uncommon lesion, comprising only about 2% of all benign odontogenic lesions.[307] These cysts affect the maxilla and mandible equally. About 78% are intraosseous (central), and 22% are confined to the peripheral soft tissues. They are either unilocular or multilocular radiolucent cysts that frequently contain radiopaque material ranging from small flecks to large masses. The lesion can be well circumscribed or poorly demarcated. Radiographically, it resembles a calcifying epithelial odontogenic tumor, an odontoma, an ossifying fibroma, and fibrous dysplasia. The lining of a calcifying odontogenic cyst consists of ameloblastic epithelium and "ghost cells," which undergo dystrophic calcification. Treatment can be by curettage, enucleation, or conservative surgical excision; unlike the keratocyst, recurrences are unlikely.[310]

### Fissural Cyst

The term *fissural cyst* refers to a cystic expansion that had been attributed etiologically to entrapped epithelium within

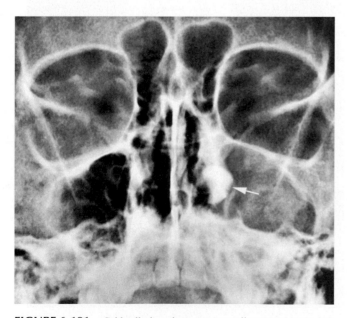

**FIGURE 6-181** Caldwell view shows an expansile process in the left maxillary sinus with a tooth in the medial antral wall (*arrows*). This patient had a dentigerous cyst.

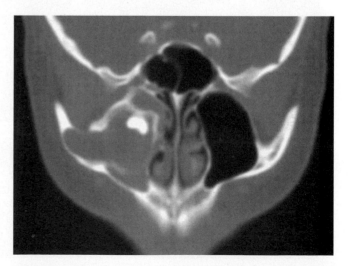

**FIGURE 6-183** Coronal CT scan shows an expansile right maxillary sinus mass with a tooth within the antrum. This patient had a dentigerous cyst.

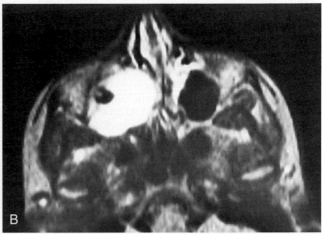

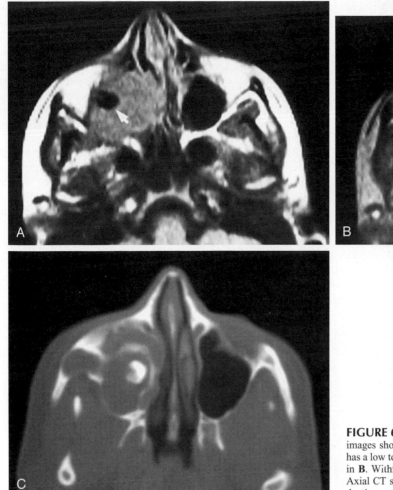

**FIGURE 6-184**   Axial proton density (**A**) and T2-weighted (**B**) MR images show an expansile mass in the right maxillary sinus. The mass has a low to intermediate signal intensity in **A** and a high signal intensity in **B**. Within the mass is an area of signal void (*arrow*) on all images. Axial CT scan (**C**) shows that this area was a tooth. This patient had a dentigerous cyst.

the fusion lines of the frontonasal and maxillary processes. However, it is apparent that these rare cysts may actually result from a variety of inflammatory as well as developmental etiologies. These cysts are classified as either globulomaxillary or median mandibular cysts.[307] Figure 6-190 is a diagrammatic overview of all of the cysts related to the maxillary alveolus and the palatal region.

The globulomaxillary cyst is found between the maxillary lateral incisor and canine teeth and represents less than 3% of all jaw cysts and 20% of maxillary cysts. Most occur in patients under 30 years of age. Radiographically, the globulomaxillary cyst appears as an inverted pear-shaped or ovoid cyst in the maxillary alveolus (Fig. 6-191). It often pushes apart the roots of the lateral incisor and canine teeth and can distort the lower anterior aspect of the maxillary sinus.[309]

Radiographically, the median mandibular cyst appears as a well-circumscribed radiolucency between the mandibular central incisors. The histologies of both cysts are nonspecific, and the diagnoses are confirmed radiographically.

### Developmental Cyst

Developmental cysts are the most commonly encountered nonodontogenic jaw cysts, representing 73% of these cysts.[307] They develop from entrapped ductal epithelium and may be classified anatomically as either nasopalatine

duct (also known as median anterior maxillary cysts), median palatal, or nasolabial cysts (Figs. 6-190, 6-192, and 6-193). Nasopalatine or median anterior maxillary cysts may be further subclassified as either incisive canal cyst (ICC) or palatine papilla cyst. The latter cyst is uncommon, derived from the incisor papilla soft tissue, and does not manifest itself radiographically. The ICC is thought to arise from remnants of the nasopalatine duct or as a result of degeneration of the contents of the incisive canal.[307] Patients with ICC present with a swelling of the anterior palate behind the central incisors.

Radiographically, ICC appears as a well-defined radiolucency above or between the root apices of the maxillary central incisors, exceeding 0.6 cm, that does not extend into the paranasal sinuses.[307] The cyst may be lined by either squamous or respiratory mucosa and may contain glandular or connective tissue remnants.

The median palatal cyst is an ICC that has extended posteriorly. Clinically, it appears as a midline palatine swelling that may also extend to the nasal floor. Radiographically, it appears as a midline palatal radiolucency. The histology is similar to that of ICC.

Lastly, the nasolabial (also referred to as nasoalveolar) cyst is thought to be derived from the nasolacrimal duct apparatus. Clinically, it appears as a small cystic mass in the upper lip, nasal vestibule, or nasal alae, obliterating the nasolabial fold. Nasolabial cysts are primarily soft-tissue based and therefore are rarely seen on plain films. If large, they may scallop the adjacent bone.

## Odontogenic Tumors

Odontogenic tumors arise from the dental apparatus, mimicking the various stages of odontogenesis; ameloblastoma, cementoma, odontoma, and fibromyxoma are the most common of these tumors, which can involve the paranasal sinuses (also see Chapter 17).

### Ameloblastoma (Including Unicystic Ameloblastoma)

Ameloblastoma represents only 1% of all pathologic lesions of the jaw and 18% of all odontogenic tumors.[307] Characteristically, this is a slowly growing solid and cystic tumor. Most affected patients are in the third and fourth decades of life. The ratio of mandibular to maxillary tumors is approximately 4:1, and the posterior mandible is the most common site. The majority of maxillary tumors (90%) involve the premolar-molar area. Noncentral ameloblastomas (those arising from peripheral, soft-tissue, nonosseous, or noncentral sites) are not considered in this discussion. An ameloblastoma presents as an enlarging, painless swelling, and large maxillary tumors can cause nasal obstruction. Other signs and symptoms include pain, bleeding, unhealed extraction sites, trismus, and neural involvement.[311, 312]

Radiographically, the ameloblastoma appears as a multiloculated, honeycombed lytic lesion devoid of mineralization. If the tumor extends into the antrum, the sinus will be clouded and the walls remodeled or destroyed. On CT, ameloblastomas have a nonenhancing, nonhomogeneous appearance, and on MR imaging they have nonhomogeneous mixed signal intensities. On T1-weighted images these tumors demonstrate intermediate signal intensity,

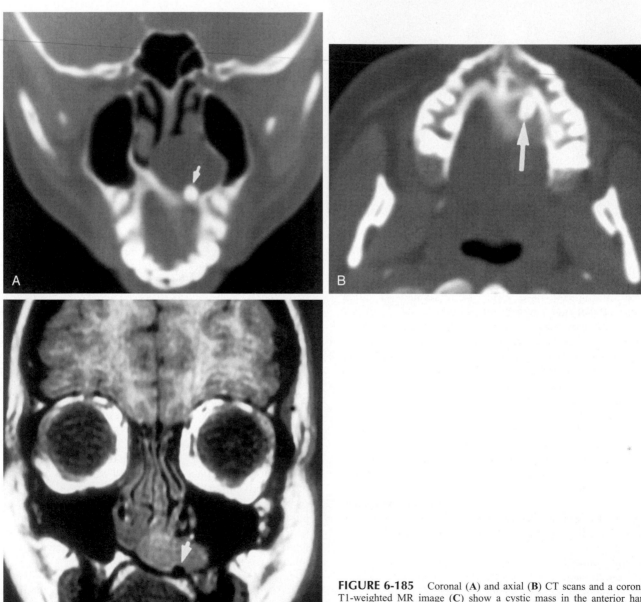

**FIGURE 6-185** Coronal (**A**) and axial (**B**) CT scans and a coronal T1-weighted MR image (**C**) show a cystic mass in the anterior hard palate (premaxilla). Within the cyst is a partially formed tooth (*arrow*). This patient had a dentigerous cyst of mesiodent tooth.

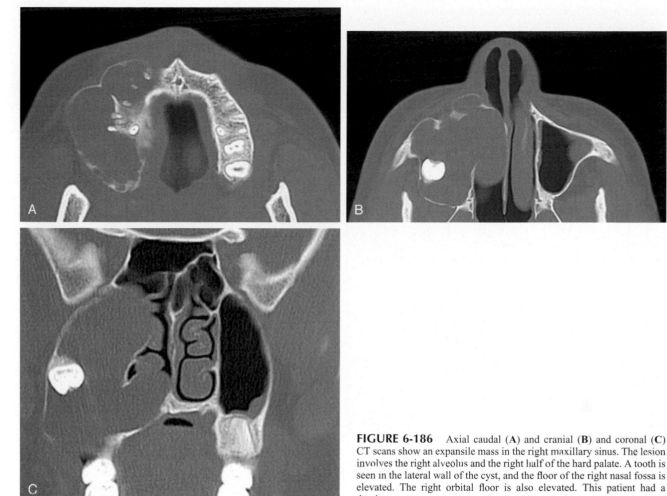

**FIGURE 6-186**   Axial caudal (**A**) and cranial (**B**) and coronal (**C**) CT scans show an expansile mass in the right maxillary sinus. The lesion involves the right alveolus and the right half of the hard palate. A tooth is seen in the lateral wall of the cyst, and the floor of the right nasal fossa is elevated. The right orbital floor is also elevated. This patient had a dentigerous cyst.

whereas on T2-weighted studies they have variable intermediate and high signal intensities (Figs. 6-194 and 6-195).

Histologically, the epithelial component is characterized by basaloid cells forming ribbons or lining the perimeter of nests and islands. These islands can contain spindled cells mimicking (and thus called) stellate reticulum. The epithelial component can also contain squamous cells or granular cells. The latter contain lysosomal granules and may represent a degenerative phenomenon.[307] The stromal component of ameloblastoma contains mature fibroblastic and myofibroblastic elements.

The clinical course of ameloblastomas is characterized by slow, destructive growth without metastatic capacity. The tendency toward recurrence is dependent upon tumor site, stage, and primary therapy. A low recurrence rate (15%) can be seen after complete resection with negative margins.[307] Conversely, curettage or enucleation can be associated with a much greater likelihood of local tumor recurrence. Maxillary ameloblastomas are more likely to present with cortical destruction and invasion of soft tissues than mandibular tumors, and hence are inherently more likely to recur after resection. Skull base invasion and intracerebral extension can thus lead to death. There are two rare malignant variants of ameloblastoma: malignant ameloblastoma and ameloblastoma carcinoma. Malignant ameloblas-

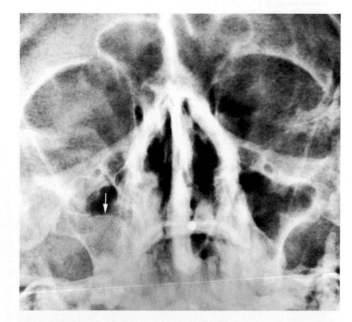

**FIGURE 6-187**   Waters view shows a mass in the lower right antrum that has elevated the inferior mucoperiosteal white line (*arrow*). This indicates that the mass arose in the alveolus below the sinus. This patient had a radicular cyst.

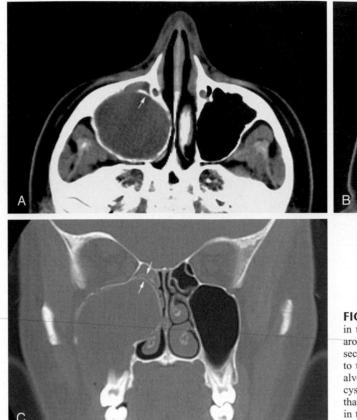

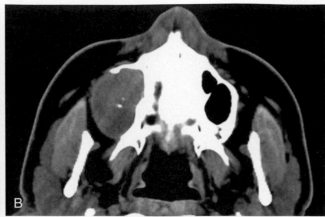

**FIGURE 6-188** Axial CT scans (**A** and **B**) show an expansile mass in the right maxillary sinus. In **A** there is an inner bony wall (*arrow*) around the watery contents of the mass. A small area of obstructed secretions is present within the remaining maxillary sinus cavity anterior to this inner bony rim. In **B** the mass is seen to involve the maxillary alveolus. No tooth is seen within the mass. This patient had a radicular cyst. Coronal CT scan (**C**) shows an expansile right maxillary sinus mass that involves the maxillary alveolus. A nondisplaced molar tooth is seen in the lower aspect of the mass. A double wall is seen along the upper margin of the mass (*arrows*). This patient had a radicular cyst.

toma is histologically benign, yet it metastasizes. This usually occurs after a long history of multiple unsuccessful surgical procedures or after radiation therapy. Most metastases occur in the lungs, pleura, and regional lymph nodes.[312]

Ameloblastic carcinoma is histologically malignant, and the metastases are less differentiated than the primary tumor.

Complete surgical resection is the treatment of choice for all ameloblastomas. Chemotherapy appears to be relatively ineffective against both the primary lesion and the metastases, and most lesions are not radiosensitive.[312]

Unicystic ameloblastoma deserves special mention. It represents 5% to 15% of all intraosseous ameloblastomas and occurs almost exclusively in the mandible.[307] This lesion appears radiologically as a unilocular mandibular cyst.

Histologically, one sees a unilocular simple or plexiform cyst lined by ameloblastomatous tissue (as described above). Unicystic ameloblastomas may be treated more conservatively than typical ameloblastomas, by curettage or enucleation, with a low recurrence rate.

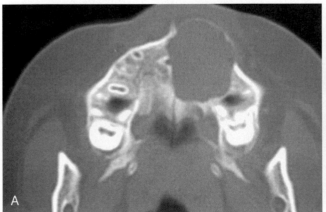

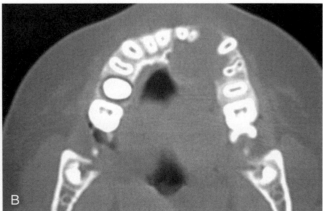

**FIGURE 6-189** Axial CT scans (**A** and **B**) show an expansile cystic mass in the left alveolus and hard palate. The cyst wall is seen in relationship to the left lateral incisor tooth. This patient had a radicular cyst.

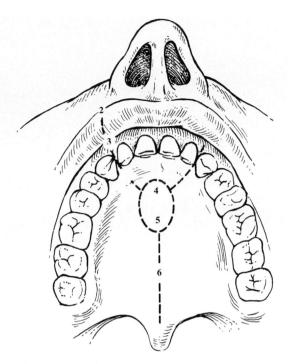

**FIGURE 6-190**   Diagram of distribution of fissural cyst. *1,* Nasolabial cyst; *2,* nasoalveolar cyst; *3,* globulomaxillary cyst; *4,* nasopalatine cyst; *5,* cyst of palatine papilla; and *6,* median palatal cyst.

### *Cementoblastoma*

Cementum-producing tumors can be classified as either benign cementoblastoma, gigantiform cementoma, periapical cemental dysplasia (previously discussed), and cemento-ossifying fibroma (previously discussed with fibroosseous jaw lesions). Cementoblastoma (also referred to as cementoma) is an uncommon neoplasm arising from the mesodermal periodontal ligament, which surrounds the tooth roots and contains cells able to produce cementum, bone, and fibrous tissue. Most patients are in their fourth decade of life or younger and present with a mandibular mass in the premolar-molar region. Because cementomas are attached to the tooth roots, tooth innervation can be disrupted and affected teeth can appear nonresponsive to vitality tests.[312]

Radiographically, these lesions appear as single or multiple well-defined radiopaque masses in continuity with the root apices of affected teeth. A zone of lucency, or "halo," surrounds each lesion (Figs. 6-196 to 6-198). The radiographic differential diagnosis is primarily hypercementosis, which refers to the excessive accumulation of cementum along the surface of the involved tooth root(s). Hypercementosis is associated with Paget's disease, periapical inflammation, and elongation of a tooth as a result of the loss of its antagonistic opposing tooth.[312]

Histologically, cementum appears as coalescing trabeculae of eosinophilic matrix with basophilic reversal lines. Numerous active cementoblasts can be seen in cementoblastomas. These tumors have limited growth potential and are usually cured by local excision.

The gigantiform cementoma (familial multiple cementoma, cemento-osseous dysplasia) is a rare lesion characterized by single or multiple nodular, irregular masses ranging from 1 to 10 cm in one or both jaws. Only the

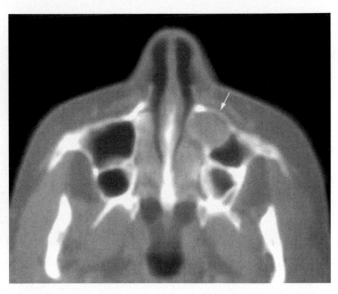

**FIGURE 6-191**   Axial CT scan shows an expansile soft-tissue mass (*arrow*) in the left anterior maxilla. The caudal aspect of the lesion extends down into the alveolus, separating the canine and lateral incisor teeth. This cyst has a thin rim of bone around its margin. This patient had a globulomaxillary cyst.

alveolar processes are affected, independent of the teeth. Radiographically, one sees expansion of the cortical plates with concomitant simple bone cysts. Serum alkaline phosphatase is not elevated, thus excluding Paget's disease.

Histologically, one sees solid sheets of acellular cementum and some proliferative areas. Clinically, this is a self-limiting process, and treatment depends on the clinical course. Osteomyelitis is the most common complication.

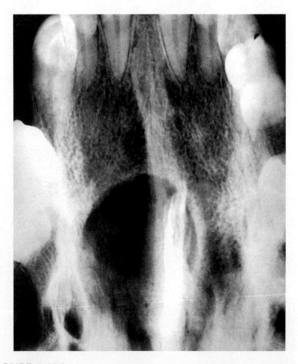

**FIGURE 6-192**   Intraoral occlusal film shows a well-demarcated cyst of the palate. This patient had a fissural cyst.

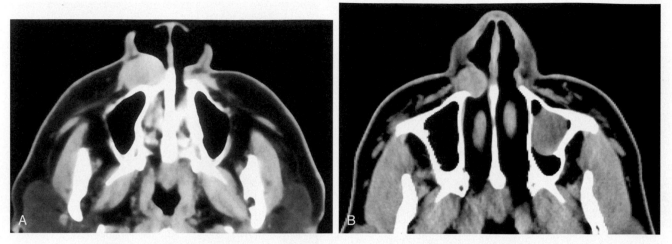

**FIGURE 6-193**   Axial CT scan (**A**) shows a soft-tissue density ovoid mass in the soft tissues of the right face deep to the lateral margin of the nose. The adjacent maxillary bone is uninvolved. In **B** a CT scan on another patient shows an ovoid mass in the lateral nostril region anterior to the medial maxilla. The bone is not involved. An incidental retention or polyp is present in the left antrum. Both of these patients had nasoalveolar cysts.

### Odontoma

Odontomas are tumors that produce both the epithelial and mesenchymal components of the dental apparatus with complete, mature differentiation. Enamel, dentin, cementum, and pulp production can be seen within these tumors. These lesions usually occur within the second decade of life, affecting both genders equally; 59% occur in the maxilla.[307]

Odontomas can be classified as either complex or compound; both occur with equal frequency. The complex odontoma has a haphazard arrangement of the elements. In compound odontomas the elements have a normal, more mature relationship to one another.[313]

Radiographically, the complex odontoma appears as an amorphous radiopacity. The compound odontoma has

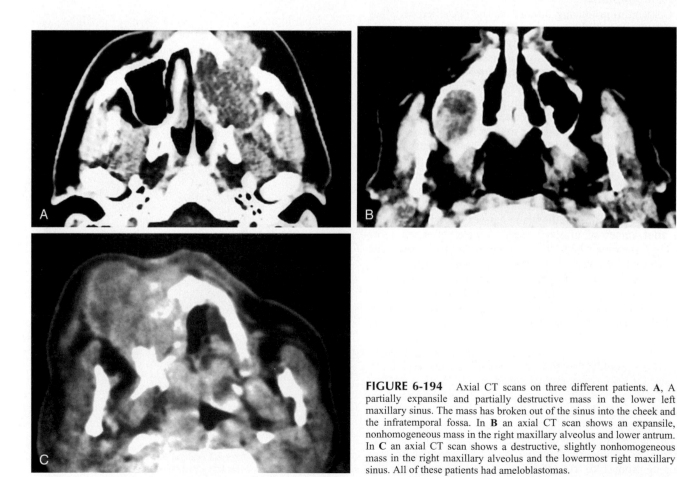

**FIGURE 6-194**   Axial CT scans on three different patients. **A**, A partially expansile and partially destructive mass in the lower left maxillary sinus. The mass has broken out of the sinus into the cheek and the infratemporal fossa. In **B** an axial CT scan shows an expansile, nonhomogeneous mass in the right maxillary alveolus and lower antrum. In **C** an axial CT scan shows a destructive, slightly nonhomogeneous mass in the right maxillary alveolus and the lowermost right maxillary sinus. All of these patients had ameloblastomas.

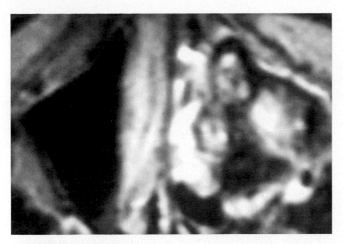

**FIGURE 6-195** Axial T2-weighted MR image shows a nonhomogeneous mass in the left maxillary sinus. The lesion has extended into the nasal fossa and the infratemporal fossa. This patient had an ameloblastoma. The imaging appearance is similar to that of a minor salivary gland tumor in this sinus.

anywhere from 3 to 2000 miniature teeth (or denticles), with single roots or no roots (Figs. 6-199 through 6-201). All odontomas are surrounded by a thin, radiolucent halo that represents the fibrous capsule. Radiographically, the differential diagnosis includes prior bone grafting.

Bone grafting to the maxillary floor can be performed for patients who require dental implants but have insufficient native bone to support them (Fig. 6-202). This imaging appearance should not be confused with that of an odontogenic tumor.

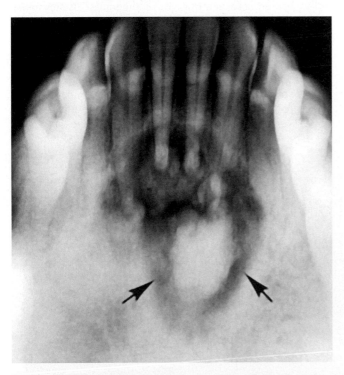

**FIGURE 6-196** Intraoral occlusal film shows a calcified palatal mass with a surrounding lucent zone (*arrows*). Note the small radiopaque densities surrounding the tooth roots (hypercementosis). This patient had a cementoma.

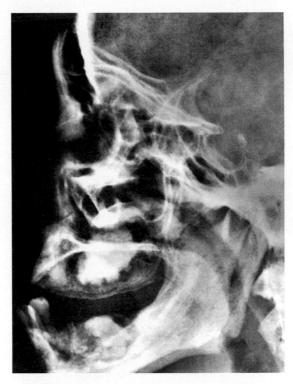

**FIGURE 6-197** Lateral view shows a calcified mass with a surrounding lucent zone in the maxillary alveolus and in the mandible. This patient had two cementomas.

Histologically, complex odontomas contain a disorganized array of dentin, cementum, enamel, and tooth pulp. In compound odontomas, one sees actual attempts at tooth formation. Treatment involves complete surgical excision; recurrences are rare.

### Calcifying Epithelial Odontogenic Tumor
The calcifying epithelial odontogenic tumor (Pindborg tumor) is a benign odontogenic neoplasm that constitutes

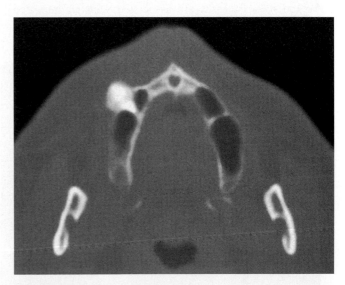

**FIGURE 6-198** Axial CT scan shows a dense osseous mass arising in the right maxillary alveolus. The lesion is localized to one area, and the remaining alveolus is normal. This patient had a cementoma.

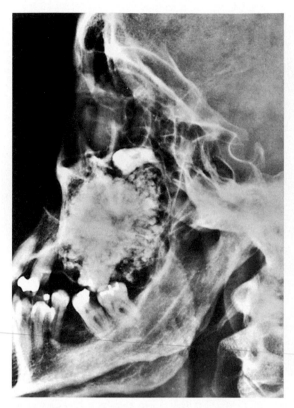

**FIGURE 6-199** Lateral view shows a large, expansile mass in the left maxillary alveolus and antrum. There are innumerable discrete, toothlike densities (denticles). This patient had a compound odontoma.

1% of this class of tumors. It usually occurs in patients in the fourth and fifth decades of life, although it has been reported in patients with an age range of 2 to 82 years.[307] These tumors are equally divided between males and females and occur twice as often in the mandible as in the maxilla. Most often the premolar teeth are affected. Although most tumors are asymptomatic and are discovered incidentally on dental radiographs, they also may cause jaw expansion. Between 35% and 45% of cases are associated with an impacted tooth.[307]

Pathologically, there are sheets of polyhedral or spindle cells, with sharply defined borders and prominent nuclei. The ultrastructure of the spindle cells has characteristics of myoepithelial cells. A capsule is variably present. Calcospherites composed of apatite crystals form laminations (Liesegang's rings) throughout the tumor. A variation of the tumor is a clear cell type, whose cells contain glycogen.[307]

Radiographically, most of these tumors are initially radiolucent, multilocular lesions with indistinct margins. The calcifications generally appear later and may be extensive or may not be seen on plain films, being too small. On CT and MR imaging these tumors are usually partially expansile, bulky maxillary sinus lesions with areas of calcification (Fig. 6-203). The differential diagnosis includes ameloblastoma, odontogenic myxoma, central GCG, follicular cyst, and OKC.

Metastatic renal cell carcinoma may at first be included in the differential diagnosis when there is a prominent clear cell population, but the presence of sheets of epidermoid-appearing cells in the Pindborg tumor helps eliminate this possibility.[307] A malignant variant with the capacity for metastasis has been described. This tumor revealed marked nuclear and cellular hyperchromatism, giant cells, and abnormal mitoses.[307]

Treatment of the Pindborg tumor varies from curettage for small lesions to en bloc resection for larger lesions. If not completely removed, these tumors will recur.

## HAMARTOMAS, TERATOMAS, AND TERATOCARCINOMAS

The term *hamartoma* refers to an abnormal, oncologically benign proliferation of indigenous tissues. The sinonasal tract is the most common site for head and neck hamartomas, usually in the area of the nasal septum. Histologically, one sees benign disorganized epithelium, salivary glands, muscle, and cartilaginous and vascular tissues.[314, 315]

An epithelial variant, respiratory epithelial adenomatoid hamartoma, has been reported. Clinically, these neoplasms appear similar to inflammatory polyps, but are more

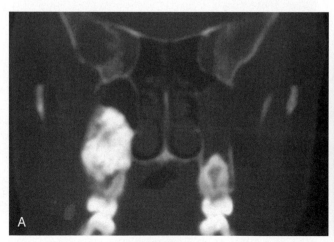
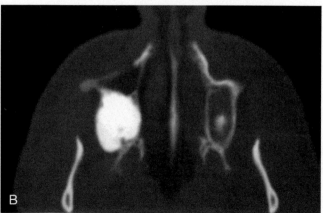

**FIGURE 6-200** Coronal (**A**) and axial (**B**) CT scans show a very dense nodular mass arising from the right maxillary alveolus and extending into the right antrum. This patient had a complex odontoma.

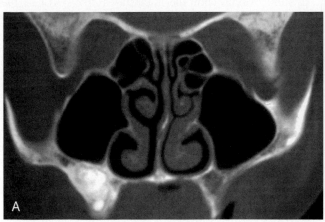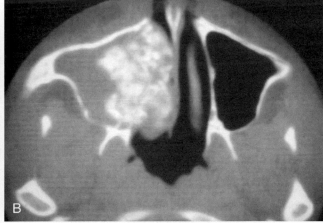

**FIGURE 6-201**   Coronal CT scan (**A**) shows a very dense nodular mass in the right maxillary alveolus. Axial CT scan (**B**) on another patient shows a mass in the right maxillary sinus with numerous discrete radiodensities. Obstructed secretions are present laterally in the sinus. Both of these patients had a complex odontoma.

indurated and occur at sites atypical for inflammatory polyps (posterior nasal septum). These differ from conventional sinonasal hamartomas in that there is a prominent glandular proliferation mimicking inverted Schneiderian papillomas or intestinal-type adenocarcinomas.

The term *teratoma* refers to a neoplasm-producing tissue that recapitulates all three germ layers (ectodermal, mesodermal, and endodermal). Teratomas may be histologically mature and oncologically benign, such as a dermoid cyst. A "hairy polyp" is essentially a polypoid, epithelium-lined dermoid of the nasopharynx that is seen in the pediatric population. It may be considered a benign teratoma; however, others believe it to be choristomatous since, unlike dermoids, it has limited growth potential.[316] Teratomas may also be histologically immature while being oncologically benign, or they may harbor malignant components and have aggressive biologic potential. As a general rule, pediatric head and neck teratomas tend to be oncologically benign, whereas adult teratomas tend to be histologically and thus oncologically malignant.[317] An epignathus, or "fetus-in-fetus" (unequal conjoined twins in which the smaller, incomplete one [the parasite] is attached to the larger twin [the autosite] at the jaw), is an extreme example of a neonatal teratoma originating from the jaw and presenting as a massive, protruding oral neoplasm. Other neonatal teratomas can originate from the soft tissues of the thyroid and cervical region. While these tumors are grotesquely manifest and can cause fatal upper airway obstruction, they are usually oncologically benign. Thus, prenatal surgical intervention can convert an otherwise moribund situation. Sinonasal teratomas (teratocarcinoma, malignant teratoma, teratocarcinosarcoma) have been reported predominantly in the adult population, with a male predominance.[314] The presenting symptoms are those associated with a sinonasal mass. Radiographically and grossly, these tumors are heterogeneous, with solid and cystic components. Histologically, one sees a mixture of immature, benign teratomatous tissue (e.g., epithelial, mesenchymal, differentiated cartilaginous) and a histologically malignant component that is usually carcinomatous but may be of any derivation. Sinonasal teratomas are

associated with a high mortality rate, despite multimodality treatment.

## METASTATIC DISEASE TO THE SINONASAL CAVITIES

Metastasis from primary tumors below the clavicles to the sinonasal cavities is infrequent. Only about 100 have been reported, the most common of which is metastatic renal cell carcinoma (RCC). Tumors found in the sinonasal cavities precede the diagnosis of the primary tumor in 8% of patients.[13] Next in frequency are tumors of the lung and breast; these are followed considerably less frequently by tumors of the testis, prostate, and gastrointestinal tract.[13, 318, 319] Soft-tissue sinonasal metastasis from esophageal carcinoma, initially mimicking acute sinusitis, has been rarely reported.[320]

The average age of patients with metastatic renal cell tumors to the sinonasal cavities is the sixth decade of life,

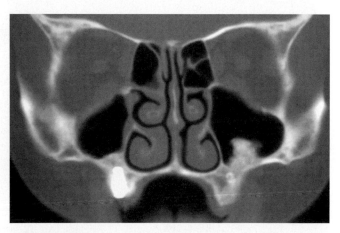

**FIGURE 6-202**   Coronal CT scan shows a dental implant in the right maxillary alveolus. In the floor of the left antrum, there is a bony prominence that represents transplanted bone placed to support a future left-sided dental implant.

similar to that of patients with breast carcinoma metastases. Bronchogenic and gastrointestinal tract metastases generally appear in the fifth decade of life.

Symptoms of metastases are nonspecific, except for the renal cell lesions, which commonly cause epistaxis.[321] Generally, metastatic neoplasia to the sinonasal tract is associated with a poor prognosis. However, isolated metastatic RCC to the sinonasal tract, in the absence of disease dissemination, may be associated with a good survival after resection.[322, 323]

We have recently seen a patient with histologically confirmed metastatic RCC to the sinonasal tract in the radiologic absence of a primary renal neoplasm. This metastasis presumably occurs with a regressed primary RCC, since spontaneous regression of primary or metastatic RCC can occur as a rare phenomenon (Fig. 6-204).[324, 325]

Squamous and basal cell carcinomas of facial and scalp skin may metastasize to the central skull base, usually along neurogenic pathways. These metastases can occur despite negative specimen margins of the resected primary skin tumor. In these cases, the most accurate prognostic finding is perineural tumor invasion in the primary lesion.[326–328] In rare instances, skin melanomas metastasize to the sinonasal

cavities. Along with the metastases from RCCs, these lesions are the most vascular metastases and often manifest with epistaxis.

Thyroid carcinoma metastatic to the paranasal sinuses is rare.[329–334] The patient may have symptoms related to the distant metastasis rather than the primary tumor. Such metastases in differentiated thyroid carcinoma portend a poor prognosis.

A case of an endometrial carcinoma metastatic to the paranasal sinuses has also been reported, as has a rare case of metastatic choriocarcinoma to the nasal cavity from testicular teratoma in a patient who presented with intractable epistaxis.[335, 336]

On CT, metastases from lung, breast, distal genitourinary tract, and gastrointestinal tract tumors are aggressive, bone-destroying soft-tissue masses that enhance minimally, if at all. The metastases are usually indistinguishable from a primary sinonasal SCC. By comparison, metastases from primary RCCs and melanomas are enhancing masses that may remodel the sinonasal walls as well as destroy them. Prostate carcinoma is one of the few primary tumors that may give a purely blastic metastasis to the facial bones and skull. Although a

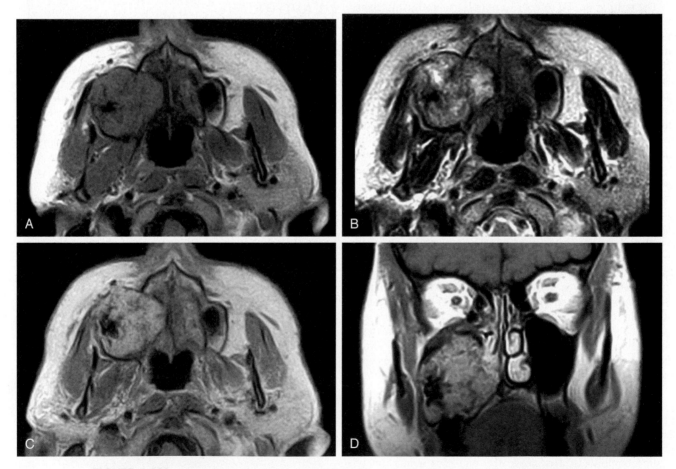

**FIGURE 6-203**  Axial T1-weighted (**A**), T2-weighted (**B**), and axial (**C**) and coronal (**D**) T1-weighted, contrast-enhanced MR images show a soft tissue mass in the right maxillary sinus with a low T1-weighted signal intensity and a nonhomogeneous T2-weighted signal intensity. The mass enhances slightly. There are areas of signal void within the lower lateral aspect of the mass on all sequences that were calcifications. This patient had a calcifying epithelial odontogenic tumor.

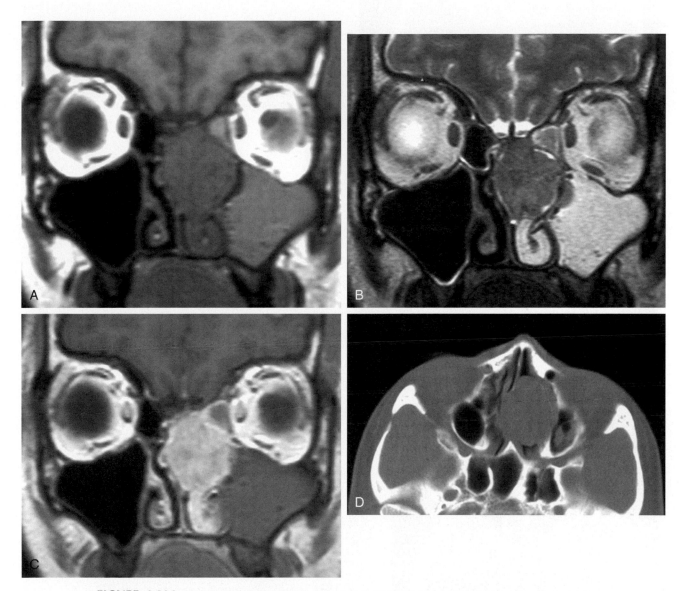

**FIGURE 6-204**   Coronal T1-weighted (**A**), T2-weighted (**B**), and T1-weighted, fat-suppressed, contrast-enhanced (**C**) MR images and an axial CT scan (**D**) show a spherical noninvasive mass in the upper left nasal fossa. The mass obstructs the remaining left ethmoid cells and the left maxillary sinus. The mass has a low T1- and T2-weighted signal intensity, and it enhances. The spherical shape suggests that this is either a minor salivary gland tumor or a lesion such as a schwannoma. This was a clear cell tumor metastatic from renal cell carcinoma.

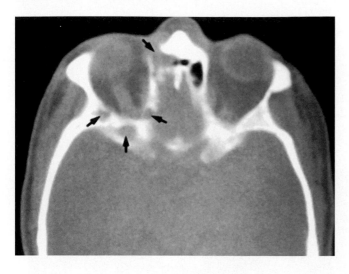

**FIGURE 6-205** Axial CT scan shows multiple discrete areas of lytic bone destruction (*arrows*). This patient had metastatic lung carcinoma.

soft-tissue mass may occur, often only a sclerotic, slightly thickened bone with an abnormal, irregular trabecular pattern is seen. On CT this pure bone disease can be overlooked unless wide windows are used to evaluate the bone.

The most important radiographic indication of metastasis is the presence of more than one lesion, particularly because sinonasal tumors usually do not erode multiple areas of bone. Rather, contiguous sites of bone erosion spread from an area of initial involvement. Thus, two areas of bone erosion with intervening normal bone suggest metastatic disease. However, a solitary destructive lesion may always represent a metastasis and the imaging appearance is nonspecific, often overlapping with that of other lesions that arise within the central skull base and sella (Figs. 6-205 to 6-214).

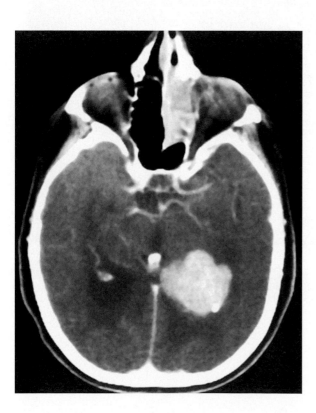

**FIGURE 6-206** Axial contrast-enhanced CT scan shows an enhancing mass in the left ethmoid sinuses and nasal cavity and a second mass in the occipital horn. This patient had metastatic melanoma.

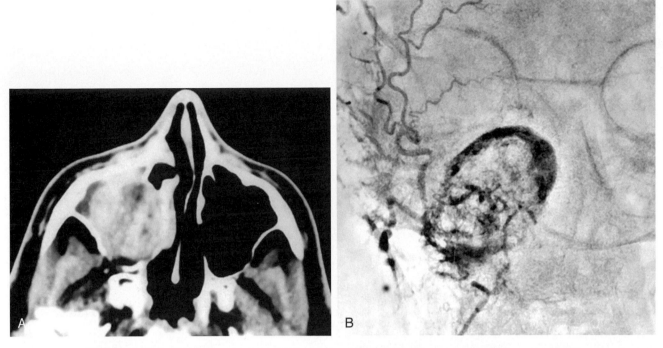

**FIGURE 6-207**   Axial contrast-enhanced CT scan (**A**) and coronal subtraction angiogram (**B**) show an expansile enhancing and vascular mass in the right maxillary sinus. This patient had metastatic hypernephroma.

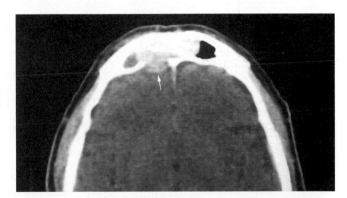

**FIGURE 6-208**   Axial contrast CT scan shows an enhancing frontal sinus mass that has eroded the posterior sinus table (*arrow*). This patient had metastatic hypernephroma.

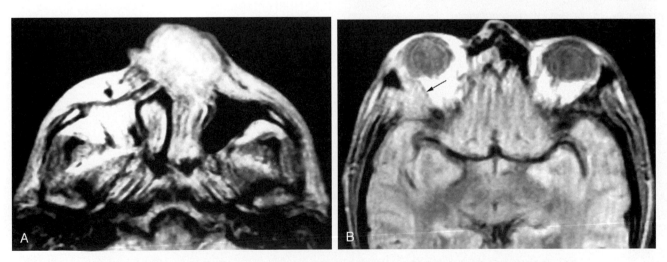

**FIGURE 6-209**   Axial proton density MR images through the level of the lower nasal fossa (**A**) and the orbits (**B**) show two distinct masses: one in the nose and one in the right lateral orbital wall (*arrow*). Both masses are homogeneous and of an intermediate to high signal intensity. This patient had metastatic lung carcinoma.

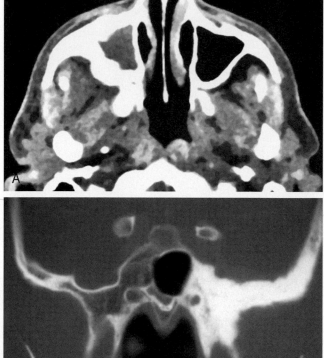

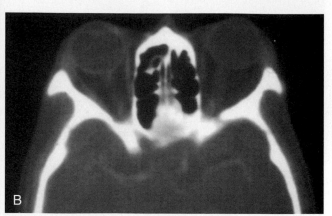

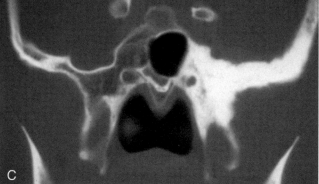

**FIGURE 6-210**   Axial CT scan (**A**) shows thickened, sclerotic bone in the right maxilla, zygoma, and lateral pterygoid plate. The right antrum is obstructed. Axial CT scan (**B**) on another patient shows thickened, sclerotic bone in the posterior left ethmoid and sphenoid regions. Both of these patients had metastatic prostate carcinoma. Coronal CT scan (**C**) shows thickened, sclerotic bone in the left sphenoid bone. On the narrow windows, some dural enhancement was present above this bone. This patient had a meningioma. In most cases, this should not be confused with metastatic prostate cancer.

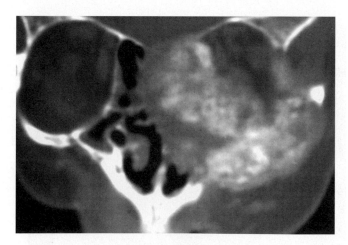

**FIGURE 6-211**   Coronal CT scan shows diffuse, irregular tumoral calcifications in the left face invading the ethmoid, anterior cranial fossa floor, nasal fossa, orbit, maxillary sinus, and cheek. This patient had metastatic sarcoma with calcium deposition.

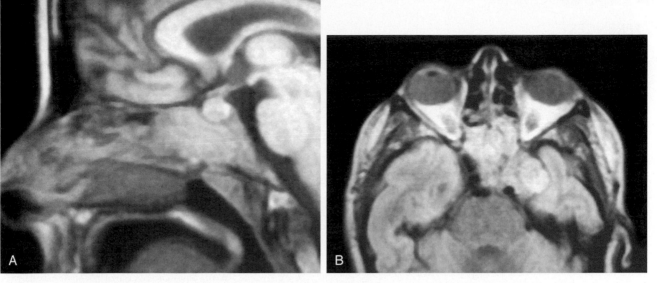

**FIGURE 6-212**    Sagittal (**A**) and axial (**B**) T1-weighted MR images show an intermediate signal intensity mass in the sphenoid sinus and clivus with invasion of the left temporal lobe. This patient had a rare metastatic pheochromocytoma.

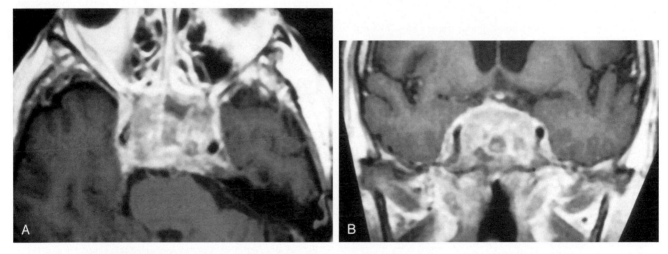

**FIGURE 6-213**    Axial (**A**) and coronal (**B**) T1-weighted, fat-suppressed, contrast-enhanced MR images show an enhancing mass in the sphenoid sinus, sella turcica, and both cavernous sinuses. This patient had metastatic prostate carcinoma.

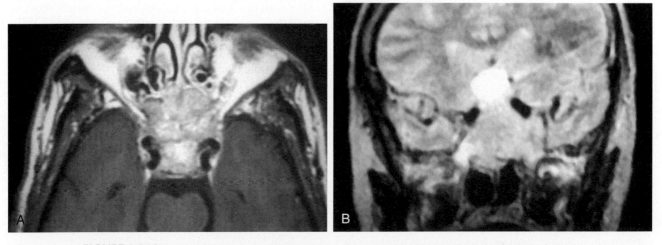

**FIGURE 6-214**    Axial (**A**) and coronal (**B**) T1-weighted, fat-suppressed, contrast-enhanced MR images show an enhancing mass in the sphenoid sinus extending into both cavernous sinuses and into the suprasellar region. This patient had an aggressive pituitary adenoma.

# REFERENCES

1. Batsakis J, ed. Tumor of the Head and Neck: Clinical and Pathological Considerations. 2nd ed. Baltimore: Williams and Wilkins, 1979;177–187.
2. Muir C, Weland L. Upper aerodigestive tract cancers. Cancer (Suppl) 1995;75:147–153.
3. Harrison D. The management of malignant tumors of the nasal sinuses. Otolaryngol Clin North Am 1971;4:159–177.
4. Harrison D. Problems in surgical management of neoplasms arising in the paranasal sinuses. J Laryngol 1976;90:69–74.
5. Jeans W, Gilani S, Bullimore J. The effect of CT scanning on staging of tumours of the paranasal sinuses. Clin Radiol 1982;33:173–179.
6. Nishijima W, Takooda S, Tokita N, et al. Analysis of distant metastases in squamous cell carcinoma of the head and neck and lesions above the clavicles at autopsy. Arch Otolaryngol Head Neck Surg 1993;119:65–68.
7. Elkeslassy A, Meder JF, Lafitte F, Rezeai K, Fredy D. [Imaging of non-osseous malignant tumors of the anterior skull base. Preoperative evaluation]. Neurochirurgie 1997;43:68–75.
8. Lloyd G, Lund V, Phelps PD, et al. Magnetic resonance imaging in the evaluation of nose and paranasal sinus disease. Br J Radiol 1987;60:957–968.
9. Som P, Shapiro M, Biller H, Sasaki C, Lawson W. Sinonasal tumors and inflammatory tissues: differentiation with MR imaging. Radiology 1988;167:803–808.
10. Dubois P, Schultz J, Perrin R, Dastur K. Tomography in expansile lesions of the nasal and paranasal sinuses. Radiology 1977;125:149–158.
11. Som P, Shugar J. The significance of bone expansion associated with the diagnosis of malignant tumors of the paranasal sinuses. Radiology 1980;136:97–100.
12. Som P, Shugar J. When to question the diagnosis of anaplastic carcinoma. Mt Sinai J Med 1981;48:230–235.
13. Barnes L, Verbin R, Gnepp D. Diseases of the nose, paranasal sinuses and nasopharynx. In: Barnes L, ed. Surgical Pathology of the Head and Neck. Vol 1. New York: Marcel Dekker, 1985;403–451.
14. Hyams V. Papillomas of the nasal cavity and paranasal sinuses: a clinicopathologic study of 315 cases. Ann Otol Rhinol Laryngol 1971;80:192–206.
15. Lasser A, Rothfeld P, Shapiro R. Epithelial papilloma and squamous cell carcinoma of the nasal cavity and paranasal sinuses: a clinicopathologic study. Cancer 1976;38:2503–2510.
16. Vrabec D. The inverted schneiderian papilloma: a clinical and pathological study. Laryngoscope 1975;85:186–220.
17. Brandwein M, Steinberg B, Thung S. HPV 6/11 and 16/18 in Schneiderian inverted papillomas. Cancer 1989;63:1708–1713.
18. McLachlin C, Kandel R, Colgan T. Prevalence of HPV in sinonasal papillomas. A study using PCR and in-situ hybridization. Mod Pathol 1992;5:406–409.
19. Norris H. Papillary lesions of the nasal cavity and paranasal sinuses. I Exophytic (squamous) papillomas: a study of 28 cases. Laryngoscope 1962;72:1784–1797.
20. Shohet JA, Duncavage JA. Management of the frontal sinus with inverted papilloma. Otolaryngol Head Neck Surg 1996;114:649–652.
21. Lund V, LLoyd G. Radiological changes associated with inverted papillomas of the nose and paranasal sinuses. Br J Radiol 1984;57:455–461.
22. Sukenik M, Casiano R. Endoscopic medial maxillectomy for inverted papillomas of the paranasal sinuses: value of the intraoperative examination. Laryngoscope 2000;110:39–42.
23. Momose K, Weber A, Goodman M. Radiological aspects on inverted papilloma. Radiology 1980;134:73–79.
24. Yousem D, Fellows S, Kennedy D, et al. Inverted papilloma: evaluation with MR imaging. Radiology 1992;185:501–505.
25. Woodruff W, Vrabec D. Inverted papilloma of the nasal vault and paranasal sinuses: spectrum of CT findings. AJR 1994;162:419–423.
26. Som P, Lidov M. The significance of sinonasal radiodensities: ossification, calcification, or residual bone? AJNR 1994;15:917–922.
27. Dammann F, Pereira P, Laniado M, et al. Inverted papilloma of the nasal cavity and the paranasal sinuses: using CT for primary diagnosis and follow-up. AJR 1999;172:543–548.
28. Slootweg P, Richardson M. Squamous cell carcinoma of the upper aerodigestive system. In: Gnepp D, ed. Diagnostic Surgical Pathology of the Head and Neck. Philadelphia: WB Saunders, 2001;19–78.
29. Barton R. Nickel carcinogenesis of the respiratory tract. J Otolaryngol 1977;6:412–422.
30. Perzin K, Lefkowitch J, Hui R. Bilateral nasal squamous carcinoma arising in papillomatosis: report of a case developing after chemotherapy for leukemia. Cancer 1981;48:2375–2382.
31. Weimert T, Batsakis J, Rice D. Carcinoma of the nasal septum. J Laryngol Otol 1978;92:209–213.
32. Baredes S, Cho H, Som M. Total maxillectomy. In: Blitzer A, Lawson W, Friedman W, eds. Surgery of the Paranasal Sinuses. Philadelphia: WB Saunders, 1985;204–216.
33. Harrison D. Critical look at the classification of maxillary sinus carcinoma. Ann Otol 1978;87:3–9.
34. Fleming I, Cooper J, Henson D, et al. American Joint Committee on Cancer Staging Manual. 5th ed. Philadelphia: Lippincott Raven, 1997.
35. Chaudhry A, Gorlin R, Mosser D. Carcinoma of the antrum: a clinical and histopathologic study. Oral Surg Oral Med Oral Pathol 1960;13:269–281.
36. Larsson L, Martensson G. Maxillary antral cancers. JAMA 1972;219:342–345.
37. Som M. Surgical management of carcinomas of the maxilla. Arch Otolaryngol 1974;99:270–273.
38. St. Pierre S, Baker S. Squamous cell carcinoma of the maxillary sinus: analysis of 66 cases. Head Neck Surg 1983;5:508–513.
39. Chowdhury AD, Ijaz T, el-Sayed S. Frontal sinus carcinoma: a case report and review of the literature. Australas Radiol 1997;41:380–382.
40. Kocak A, Erten SF, Mizrak B, et al. Unusual presentation of a sinonasal carcinoma mimicking an aneurysm rupture. Childs Nerv Syst 1998;14:338–342.
41. Ogura J, Schenck N. Unusual nasal tumors: problems in diagnosis and treatment. Otolaryngol Clin North Am 1973;6:813–837.
42. Conley J, ed. Concepts in Head and Neck Surgery. Stuttgart: Georg Thieme Verlag, 1970.
43. Phillips CD, Futterer SF, Lipper MH, Levine PA. Sinonasal undifferentiated carcinoma: CT and MR imaging of an uncommon neoplasm of the nasal cavity. Radiology 1997;202:477–480.
44. Som PM, Silvers AR, Catalano PJ, et al. Adenosquamous carcinoma of the facial bones, skull base, and calvaria: CT and MR manifestations. AJNR 1997;18:173–175.
45. Acheson E, Gowdell R, Jolles B. Nasal cancer in the Northamptonshire boot and shoe industry. Br Med J 1970;1:385–393.
46. Hadfield E. A study of adenocarcinoma of the paranasal sinuses in woodworkers in the furniture industry. Ann R Coll Surg Engl 1970;46:301–319.
47. Franquemont D, Fechner R, Mills S. Histologic classification of sinonasal intestinal-type adenocarcinoma. Am J Surg Pathol 1991;15:368–375.
48. Barnes L. Intestinal-type adenocarcinoma of nasal cavity and paranasal sinuses. Am J Surg Pathol 1986;10:192–202.
49. Batsakis J, ed. Tumor of the Head and Neck: Clinical and Pathological Considerations. 2nd ed. Baltimore: Williams and Wilkins, 1979;76–99.
50. Klintenberg C, Olofsson J, Hellquist H, et al. Adenocarcinoma of the ethmoid sinuses: a review of 38 cases with special reference to wood dust exposure. Cancer 1984;31:482–488.
51. Spiro R, Koss L, Hajdu S, et al. Tumors of minor salivary origin: a clinicopathologic study of 492 cases. Cancer 1973;31:117–129.
52. Yamamoto Y, Saka T, Makimoto K, et al. Histological changes during progression of adenoid cystic carcinoma. J Laryngol Otol 1992;106:1016–1020.
53. Goepfert H, Luna MA, Lindberg RD, White AK. Malignant salivary gland tumors of the paranasal sinuses and nasal cavity. Arch Otolaryngol 1983;109:662–668.
54. Tran L, Sidrys J, Horton D, et al. Malignant salivary gland tumors of the paranasal sinuses and nasal cavity. The UCLA experience. Am J Clin Oncol 1989;12:387–392.
55. Conley J, Dingman D. Adenoid cystic carcinoma in the head and neck (cylindroma). Arch Otolaryngol 1974;100:81–90.
56. Compagno J, Wong R. Intranasal mixed tumors (pleomorphic adenomas): a clinicopathologic study of 40 cases. Am J Clin Pathol 1977;68:213–218.
57. Suzuki K, Moribe K, Baba S. A rare case of pleomorphic adenoma of nasal cavity in Japan. Nippon Jibiinkoka Gakkai Kaiho 1990;93:740–745.
58. Freeman S, Kennedy K, Parker G, et al. Metastasizing pleomorphic adenoma of the nasal septum. Arch Otolaryngol Head Neck Surg 1990;116:1331–1333.

59. Sigal R, Monnet O, de Baere T, et al. Adenoid cystic carcinoma of the head and neck: evaluation with MR imaging and clinical-pathologic correlation in 27 patients. Radiology 1992;184:95–101.

60. Jin XL, Ding CN, Chu Q. Epithelial-myoepithelial carcinoma arising in the nasal cavity: a case report and review of literature. Pathology 1999;31:148–151.

61. Alarcos A, Matesanz A, Alarcos E. A glomus tumor of the nasal fossa and ethmoid sinus. Acta Otorrinolaringol 1992;34:291–295.

62. Staehler H. Paraganglioma of the nasal cavity. Laryngol Rhinol Otol 1985;64:399–402.

63. Sharma HS, Madhavan M, Othman NH, et al. Malignant paraganglioma of frontoethmoidal region. Auris Nasus Larynx 1999;26:487–493.

64. Shimono T, Hayakawa K, Yamaoka T, et al. Case report: glomus tumour of the nasal cavity and paranasal sinuses. Neuroradiology 1998;40:527–529.

65. Barnes L, Verbin R, Gnepp D. Diseases of the nose, paranasal sinuses and nasopharynx. In: Barnes L, ed. Surgical Pathology of the Head and Neck. Vol 1. New York: Marcel Dekker, 1985;659–724.

66. Elkon D, Hightower S, Lim M, et al. Esthesioneuroblastoma. Cancer 1979;44:1087–1094.

67. Kadish S, Goodman M, Wine C. Olfactory neuroblastoma: a clinical analysis of 17 cases. Cancer 1976;37:1571–1576.

68. Miyamoto R, Gleich L, Biddinger P, Gluckman J. Esthesioneuroblastoma and sinonasal undifferentiated carcinoma: impact of histological grading and clinical staging on survival and prognosis. Laryngoscope 2000;110:1262–1265.

69. Som P, Lawson W, Biller H, et al. Ethmoid sinus disease: CT evaluation in 400 cases. Part III: Cranio-facial resection. Radiology 1986 Jun; 159(3):605–609.

70. Morita A, Ebersold M, Olsen K. Esthesioneuroblastoma: prognosis and management. Neurosurgery 1993;32:706–715.

71. Levine P, Gallagher R, Cantrell R. Esthesioneuroblastoma: reflections of a 21-year experience. Laryngoscope 1999;109:1539–1543.

72. Dulgurov P, Calcaterra T. Esthesioneuroblastoma: the UCLA experience 1970–1990. Laryngoscope 1992;102:843–849.

73. Mack E, Prados M, Wilson C. Late manifestations of esthesioneuroblastoma in the central nervous system: report of two cases. Neurosurgery 1992;30:93–97.

74. Regenbogen V, Zinreich S, Kim K. Hyperostotic esthesioneuroblastoma: CT and MR findings. JCAT 1988;12:52–56.

75. Derdeyn C, Moran C, Wippold FI. MRI of esthesioneuroblastoma. JCAT 1994;18:16–21.

76. Som P, Lidov M, Brandwein M, et al. Sinonasal esthesioneuroblastoma with intracranial extension: marginal tumor cysts as a diagnostic MR finding. AJNR 1994;15:1259–1262.

77. Silva E, Butler J, MacKay B, Goepfert H. Neuroblastomas and neuroendocrine carcinomas of the nasal cavity: a proposed new classification. Cancer 1982;50:2388–2405.

78. Frierson H, Mills S, Fechner R, et al. Sinonasal undifferentiated carcinoma: an aggressive neoplasm derived from Schneiderian epithelium and distinct from olfactory neuroblastoma. Am J Pathol 1986;10:771–779.

79. Gallo O, Graziana P, Fini-Storchi O. Undifferentiated carcinoma of the nose and paranasal sinuses: an immunohistochemical and clinical study. ENT J 1993;72:588–595.

80. Freedman H, DeSanto L, Devine K, et al. Malignant melanoma of the nasal cavity and paranasal sinuses. Arch Otolaryngol 1973;97:322–325.

81. Batskis J, Sciubba J. Pathology. In: Blitzer A, Lawson W, Friedman W, eds. Surgery of the Paranasal Sinuses. Philadelphia: WB Saunders, 1985;74–113.

82. Brandwein M, Rothstein A, Lawson W, et al. Sinonasal melanoma—a clinicopathologic study of 25 cases and literature meta-analysis. Arch Otolaryngol Head Neck Surg 1997;123:290–296.

83. Welkosky H, Sorger K, Knuth A, et al. Malignant melanoma of the mucus sinuses of the upper aerodigestive tract. Clinical, histological and immunohistological characteristics. Laryngorhinootologie 1991;70:302–306.

84. Franquemont D, Mills S. Sinonasal malignant melanoma: a clinicopathologic and immunohistological study of 14 cases. Am J Clin Pathol 1991;96:689–697.

85. Jayaraj SM, Hern JD, Mochloulis G, Porter GC. Malignant melanoma arising in the frontal sinuses. J Laryngol Otol 1997;111:376–378.

86. Stowens D, Lin T. Melanotic progonoma of the brain. Hum Pathol 1974;5:105–113.

87. Kapadia S, Frisman D, Hitchcock C, et al. Melanotic neuroectodermal tumor of infancy. Clinicopathological, immunohistochemical, and flow cytometric study. Am J Surg Pathol 1993;17:566–573.

88. Huvos AG, ed. Bone Tumors: Diagnosis, Treatment, and Prognosis. 2nd ed. Philadelphia: WB Saunders, 1991;525.

89. Kapadia S. Tumor and tumor-like lesions of the soft tissue. In: Barnes L, ed. Surgical Pathology of the Head and Neck. Vol 2. 2nd ed. New York: Marcel Dekker, 2000;787–888.

90. Howard D, Daniels H. Ewing's sarcoma of the nose. Ear Nose Throat J 1993;72:277–279.

91. Lane S, Ironside J. Extra-skeletal Ewing's sarcoma of the nasal fossa. J Laryngol Otol 1990;104:570–573.

92. Klein E, Anzil A, Mezzacappa P, et al. Sinonasal primitive neuroectodermal tumor arising in a long-term survivor of heritable unilateral retinoblastoma. Cancer 1992;70:423–431.

93. Saw D, Chan J, Jagirdar J. Sinonasal small cell neoplasm developing after radiation therapy for retinoblastoma: an immunohistologic, ultrastructural and cytogenetic study. Hum Pathol 1992;23:896–899.

94. Klein E, Anzil A, Mezzacappa P. Sinonasal primitive neuroectodermal tumor arising in a long-term survivor of heritable unilateral retinoblastoma. Cancer 1992;70:423–431.

95. Chowdry K, Manoukian J, Rochon L. Extracranial primitive neuroectodermal tumor of the head and neck. Arch Otolaryngol Head Neck Surg 1990;116:475–478.

96. Schmidt D, Herrmann C, Jurgens H. Malignant peripheral neuroectodermal tumor and its necessary distinction from Ewing's sarcoma. A report from Kiel Pediatric Tumor Registry. Cancer 1991;68:2251–2259.

97. Hillstrom R, Zarbo R, Jacobs J. Nerve sheath tumors of the paranasal sinuses: electron microscopy and histopathologic diagnosis. Otolaryngol Head Neck Surg 1990;102:257–263.

98. Donnelly M, Saler M, Blayney A. Neurogenic sarcoma of the sinonasal tract. J Laryngol Otol 1992;105:186–190.

99. Som P, Biller H, Lawson W. An approach to parapharyngeal space masses: an updated protocol based upon 104 cases. Radiology 1984;153:149–156.

100. Sharma R, Tyagi I, Banerjee D, Pandey R. Nasoethmoid schwannoma with intracranial extension. Case report and review of literature. Neurosurg Rev 1998;21:58–61.

101. Fujiyoshi F, Kajiya Y, Nakajo M. CT and MR imaging of nasoethmoid schwannoma with intracranial extension [letter]. AJR 1997;169:1754–1755.

102. Hunt J, Pugh D. Skeletal lesions in neurofibromatosis. Radiology 1961;76:1–19.

103. Oberman H, Sullenger G. Neurogenous tumors of the head and neck. Cancer 1967;20:1992–2001.

104. D'Agostino A, Soule E, Miller R. Sarcomas of the peripheral nerves and somatic soft tissues associated with multiple neurofibromatosis (von Recklinghausen's disease). Cancer 1963;16:1015–1027.

105. Hellquist H, Lundgren J. Neurogenic sarcoma of the sinonasal tract. J Laryngol Otol 1991;105:186–190.

106. Guccion J, Enzinger F. Malignant schwannoma associated with von Recklinghausen's neurofibromatosis. Virchows Arch 1979;383:43–57.

107. Cadotte M. Malignant granular cell myoblastoma. Cancer 1974;33:1417–1422.

108. Farr H, Gray GJ, Vrana M. Extracranial meningioma. J Surg Oncol 1973;5:411–420.

109. Lopez D, Silvers D, Helwig E. Cutaneous meningioma: a clinicopathologic study. Cancer 1974;34:728–744.

110. Taxy J. Meningioma of the paranasal sinuses: a report of two cases. Am J Surg Pathol 1990;14:82–86.

111. Brunori A, Scarano P, Colacecchi R, Chiappetta F. A case of primary meningioma of the frontal sinus. Neurochirurgie 1999;45:307–311.

112. Bertrand B, Devars F, Aouadi A, et al. [Primitive extracranial meningioma: a case report of intratemporal and naso sinusal localization]. J Otolaryngol 1996;25:182–187.

113. Som P, Sacher M, Strenger S, et al. "Benign" metastasizing meningioma. AJNR 1987;8:127–130.

114. Chakrabarty A, Mitchell P, Bridges LR. Craniopharyngioma invading the nasal and paranasal spaces, and presenting as nasal obstruction. Br J Neurosurg 1998;12:361–363.

115. Jiang RS, Wu CY, Jan YJ, Hsu CY. Primary ethmoid sinus craniopharyngioma: a case report. J Laryngol Otol 1998;112:403–405.

116. Barnes L, Verbin R, Gnepp D. Diseases of the nose, paranasal sinuses and nasopharynx. In: Barnes L, ed. Surgical Pathology of the Head and Neck. Vol 2. New York: Marcel Dekker, 1985;912–1044.

117. Shugar J, Som P, Krespi Y. Primary chordoma of the maxillary sinus. Laryngoscope 1980;90:1825–1830.

118. Miro JL, Videgain G, Petrenas E, et al. Chordoma of the ethmoidal sinus. A case report. Acta Otorrinolaringol Esp 1998;49:66–69.

119. Wright D. Nasopharyngeal and cervical chordoma: some aspects of their development and treatment. J Laryngol 1967;81:1337–1355.

120. De las Casas L, Singh H, Halliday B, et al. Myxoid chondrosarcoma of the sphenoid sinus and chondromyxoid fibroma of the iliac bone: cytomorphologic findings of two distinct and uncommon myxoid lesions. Diagn Cytopathol 2000;22:383–389.

121. Rosenberg A, Nielsen G, Keel S, et al. Chondrosarcoma of the base of skull: a clinicopathologic study of 200 cases with emphasis on its distinction from chordoma. Am J Surg Pathol 1999;23:1370–1378.

122. Zacay G, Eyal A, Shacked I, et al. Chordoma of the cervical spine. Ann Otol Rhinol Laryngol 2000;109:438–440.

123. Hug E, Loredo L, Slater J, et al. Proton radiation therapy for chordomas and chondrosarcomas of the skull base. J Neurosurg 1999;91:432–439.

124. Yuh W, Flickinger F, Barloon T. MR imaging of unusual chordomas. JCAT 1985;12:30–35.

125. Fischbein NJ, Kaplan MJ, Holliday RA, Dillon WP. Recurrence of clival chordoma along the surgical pathway. AJNR 2000;21:578–583.

126. Pe'er J, Ilsar M. Ectopic lacrimal gland under the nasal mucosa. Am J Ophthalmol 1982;94:418–419.

127. Furukawa M, Takeuchi S, Umeda R. Ectopic tonsillar tissue in the nasal septum. Auris Nasus Larynx 1983;10:37–41.

128. Downs B, Shores C, Drake A. Choristoma of the nasopharynx. Otolaryngol Head Neck Surg 2000;123:523.

129. Esteban F, Ruiz-Avila I, Vilchez R, et al. Ectopic pituitary adenoma in the sphenoid causing Nelson's syndrome. J Laryngol Otol 1997;111:565–567.

130. McGurk M, Goepel J, Hancock B. Extranodal lymphoma of head and neck: a review of 49 consecutive cases. Clin Radiol 1985;36:455–458.

131. Fellbaum C, Hansmann M, Lennert K. Malignant lymphomas of the nasal and paranasal sinuses. Virch Arch A Pathol Anat Histopathol 1989;414:399–405.

132. Cleary K, Batsakis J. Sinonasal lymphomas. Ann Otol Rhinol Laryngol 1994 Nov;103:911–914.

133. Quraishi M, Bessell E, Clark D, et al. Non-Hodgkin's lymphoma of the sinonasal tract. Laryngoscope 2000;110:1489–1492.

134. Rodriguez J, Romaguera J, Manning J, et al. Nasal-type T/NK lymphomas: a clinicopathologic study of 13 cases. Leuk Lymphoma 2000;39:139–144.

135. Cuadra-Garcia I, Proulx G, Wu C, et al. Sinonasal lymphoma: a clinicopathologic analysis of 58 cases from the Massachusetts General Hospital. Am J Surg Pathol 1999;23:1356–1369.

136. Vidal R, Devaney K, Ferlito A, et al. Sinonasal malignant lymphomas: a distinct clinicopathological category. Ann Otol Rhinol Laryngol 1999;108:411–419.

137. van de Rijn M, Bhargava V, Molina-Kirsch H, et al. Extranodal head and neck lymphomas in Guatemala: high frequency of Epstein-Barr virus–associated sinonasal lymphomas. Hum Pathol 1997;28:834–839.

138. Pomilla P, Morris A, Jaworek A. Sinonasal non-Hodgkin's lymphoma in patients infected with human immunodeficiency virus: report of three cases and review. Clin Infect Dis 1995;21:137–149.

139. Strickler J, Meneses M, Habermann T, et al. Polymorphic reticulosis: a reappraisal. Hum Pathol 1994;25:659–665.

140. Arber D, Weiss L, Albujar P. Nasal lymphoma in Peru: high incidence of T-cell immunophenotype and Epstein-Barr virus infection. Am J Surg Pathol 1993;17:392–399.

141. Weiss L, Gaffey M, Chen Y, Frierson HJ. Frequency of Epstein-Barr viral DNA in "Western" sinonasal and Waldeyer's ring non-Hodgkin's lymphomas. Pathol Annu 1992;16:156–162.

142. Han J, Seo E, Kwon H, et al. Nasal angiocentric lymphoma with hemophagocytic syndrome. Korean J Intern Med 1999;14:41–46.

143. King AD, Lei KI, Ahuja AT, et al. MR imaging of nasal T-cell/natural killer cell lymphoma. AJR 2000;174:209–211.

144. Ooi GC, Chim CS, Liang R, et al. Nasal T-cell/natural killer cell lymphoma: CT and MR imaging features of a new clinicopathologic entity. AJR 2000;174:1141–1145.

145. Harnsberger H, Bragg D, Osborn A. Non-Hodgkin's lymphoma of the head and neck: CT evaluation of nodal and extranodal sites. AJNR 1983;8:673–679.

146. Kondo M, Hashimoto T, Shiga H. Computed tomography of sinonasal non-Hodgkin's lymphoma. JCAT 1984;8:216–219.

147. Duncavage J, Campbell B, Hanson G. Diagnosis of malignant lymphomas of the nasal cavity, paranasal sinuses and nasopharynx. Laryngoscope 1983;93:1276–1280.

148. Marsot-Dupuch K, Raveau V, Aoun N. Lethal midline granuloma: impact of imaging studies on the investigation and management of destructive midfacial disease in 13 patients. Neuroradiology 1992;34:155–161.

149. Borges A, Fink J, Villablanca P, et al. Midline destructive lesions of the sinonasal tract: simplified terminology based on histopathologic criteria. AJNR 2000;21:331–336.

150. Barnes L, Verbin R, Gnepp D. Diseases of the nose, paranasal sinuses and nasopharynx. In: Barnes L, ed. Surgical Pathology of the Head and Neck. Vol 2. New York: Marcel Dekker, 1985;1045–1209.

151. Uyesugi W, Watabe J, Petermann G. Orbital and facial granulocytic sarcoma (chloroma): a case report. Pediatr Radiol 2000;30:276–278.

152. Bassichis B, McClay J, Wiatrak B. Chloroma of the masseteric muscle. Int J Pediatr 2000;9:57–61.

153. Pomeranz S, Hawkins H, Towbin R, et al. Granulocytic sarcoma (chloroma): CT manifestations. Radiology 1985;155:167–170.

154. Castro E, Lewis J, Strong E. Plasmacytoma of paranasal sinuses and nasal cavity. Arch Otolaryngol 1973;97:326–329.

155. Fu Y-S, Perzin K. Nonepithelial tumors of the nasal cavity, paranasal sinuses and nasopharynx: a clinicopathologic study—IX plasmacytomas. Cancer 1978;42:2399–2406.

156. Bachmeyer C, Levy V, Carteret M, et al. Sphenoid sinus localization of multiple myeloma revealing evolution from benign gammopathy. Head Neck 1997;4:347–350.

157. Kondo M, Hashimoto S, Inuyama Y. Extramedullary plasmacytoma of the sinonasal cavities: CT evaluation. JCAT 1986;10:841–844.

158. Soo G, Chan A, Lam D, et al. Extramedullary nasal plasmacytoma—an unusual clinical entity. Ear Nose Throat J 1996;75:171–173.

159. Willman C, Busque L, Griffith B, et al. Langerhan's-cell histiocytosis (histiocytosis X), a clonal proliferative disease. N Engl J Med 1994;331:154–160.

160. Devaney K, Putzi M, Ferlito A, Rinaldo A. Head and neck Langerhan's cell histiocytosis. Ann Otol Rhinol Laryngol 1997;106:526–532.

161. Lieberman P, Jones C, Steinman R. Langerhans cell (eosinophilic) granulomatosis. A clinicopathologic study encompassing 50 years. Am J Surg Pathol 1996;20:519–552.

162. Alessi DM, Maceri D. Histiocytosis x in the head and neck in a pediatric population. Arch Otolaryngol Head Neck Surg. 1992;118:945–948.

163. Hussain SS, Simpson RD, McCormick D, Johnstone CI. Langerhan's cell histiocytosis in the sphenoid sinus: a case of diabetes insipidus. J Laryngol Otol 1989;103:877–879.

164. Stromberg JS, Wang AM, Huang TE, et al. Langerhan's cell histiocytosis involving the sphenoid sinus and superior orbital fissure. AJNR 1995;16:964–967.

165. Jaffe H, Lichtenstein L. Eosinophilic granuloma of bone; condition affecting one, several or many bones, but apparently limited to skeleton, and representing mildest clinical expression of peculiar inflammatory histiocytosis also underlying Siwe disease and Schuller-Christian disease. Arch Pathol 1944;37:99–118.

166. Ide F, Iwase T, Saito I. Immunohistochemical and ultrastructural analysis of the proliferating cells in histiocytosis X. Cancer 1984;53:917–921.

167. De Schepper A, Ramon F, Van Marck E. MR imaging of eosinophilic granuloma: report of 11 cases. Skeletal Radiol 1993;22:163–166.

168. Goodnight JW, Wang MB, Sercarz JA, et al. Extranodal Rosai-Dorfman disease of the head and neck. Laryngoscope 1996;106:253–256.

169. Gregor RT, Ninnin D. Rosai-Dorfman disease of the paranasal sinuses. J Laryngol Otol 1994;108:152–155.

170. Ku P, Tong M, Leung C, et al. Nasal manifestation of extranodal Rosai-Dorfman disease—diagnosis and management. J Laryngol Otol 1999;113:275–280.

171. Innocenzi D, Silipo V, Giombini S, et al. Sinus histiocytosis with massive lymphadenopathy (Rosai-Dorfman disease): case report with nodal and diffuse muco-cutaneous involvement. J Cutan Pathol 1998;25:563–567.

172. Smithson L, Lipper M, Hall JJ. Paranasal sinus involvement in thalassemia major: CT demonstration. AJNR 1987;8:564–565.

173. Olivieri N. The beta-thalassemias. N Engl J Med 1999;341: 99–109.

174. Tunaci M, Tunaci A, Engin G, et al. Imaging features of thalassemia. Eur Radiol 1999;9:1804–1809.

175. Apostol JV, Frazell E. Juvenile nasopharyngeal angiofibroma. Cancer 1965;18:869–878.

176. Som P, Cohen B, Sacher M. The angiomatous polyp and the angiofibroma: two different lesions. Radiology 1982;144:329–334.

177. Som P, Shugar J, Cohen B. The nonspecificity of the antral bowing sign in maxillary sinus pathology. JCAT 1981;5:350–352.

178. Bryan R, Sessions R, Horowitz B. Radiographic management of juvenile angiofibromas. AJNR 1981;2:157–166.

179. Som P, Lanzieri C, Sacher M. Extracranial tumor vascularity: determination by dynamic CT scanning. II The unit approach. Radiology 1985;154:407–412.

180. Herman P, Lot G, Chapot R, et al. Long-term follow-up of juvenile nasopharyngeal angiofibromas: analysis of recurrences. Laryngoscope 1999;109:140–147.

181. Lloyd G, Howard D, Phelps P, Cheesman A. Juvenile angiofibroma: the lessons of 20 years of modern imaging. J Laryngol Otol 1999;113:127–134.

182. Murray A, Falconer M, McGarry GW. Excision of nasopharyngeal angiofibroma facilitated by intra-operative 3D-image guidance. J Laryngol Otol 2000;114:311–313.

183. Fitzpatrick P, Briant D, Berman J. The nasopharyngeal angiofibroma. Arch Otolaryngol 1980;106:234–236.

184. Batsakis J, et al. Tumors of the Head and Neck: Clinical and Pathological Considerations. 2nd ed. Baltimore: Williams and Wilkins, 1979;139–143.

185. Barnes L, Verbin R, Gnepp D. Diseases of the nose, paranasal sinuses and nasopharynx. In: Barnes L, ed. Surgical Pathology of the Head and Neck. Vol 1. New York: Marcel Dekker, 1985;725–880.

186. Enziger F, Weiss S. Soft Tissue Tumors. 3rd ed. St Louis: CV Mosby, 1995.

187. Barnes L. Tumor and tumor-like lesions of the soft tissue. In: Barnes L, ed. Surgical Pathology of the Head and Neck. Vol 2. 2nd ed. New York: Marcel Dekker, 2000;991–993.

188. Kurien M, Nair S, Thomas S. Angiosarcoma of the nasal cavity and maxillary antrum. J Laryngol Otol 1989;103:874–876.

189. Solomons N, Stearns M. Haemangiosarcoma of the maxillary antrum. J Laryngol Otol 1990;104:831–834.

190. Kimura Y, Tanaka S, Furuka M. Angiosarcoma of the nasal cavity. J Laryngol Otol 1992;106:368–369.

191. Dorfman H, Steiner G, Jaffe H. Vascular tumors of bone. Hum Pathol 1971;2:349–375.

192. Joachims H, Cohen Y. Hemangioendothelioma of mastoid bone. Laryngoscope 1974;84:454–458.

193. Enzinger F, Smith B. Hemangiopericytoma: an analysis of 106 cases. Hum Pathol 1976;7:61–82.

194. El-Naggar A, Batsakis J, Garcia G, et al. Sinonasal hemangiopericytomas: clinicopathologic and DNA content study. Arch Otolaryngol Head Neck Surg 1992;118:134–137.

195. Hekkenberg RJ, Davidson J, Kapusta L, et al. Hemangiopericytoma of the sinonasal tract. J Otolaryngol 1997;26:277–280.

196. Catalano PJ, Brandwein M, Shah DK, et al. Sinonasal hemangiopericytomas: a clinicopathologic and immunohistochemical study of seven cases. Head Neck 1996;18:42–53.

197. Kauffaman S, Stout A. Hemangiopericytoma in children. Cancer 1960;13:695–710.

198. Herve S, Abd Alsamad I, Beautru R, et al. Management of sinonasal hemangiopericytomas. Rhinology 1999;37:153–158.

199. Gnepp D, Chandler W, Hyams V. Primary Kaposi's sarcoma of the head and neck. Ann Int Med 1984;100:107–114.

200. Lothe F, Murray J. Kaposi's sarcoma: autopsy findings in the African. Acta Unio Int Contra Cancrum 1962;18:429–452.

201. Greenberg J, Fischl M, Berger J. Upper airway obstruction secondary to AIDS-related Kaposi's sarcoma. Chest 1985;88:638–640.

202. Levy F, Tansek K. AIDS-associated Kaposi's sarcoma of the larynx. J Ear Nose Throat 1990;69:177–183.

203. Fliss D, Parikh J, Freeman J. AIDS-related Kaposi's sarcoma of the sphenoid sinus. J Otolaryngol 1992;21:235–237.

204. Barnes L, Verbin R, Gnepp D. Diseases of the nose, paranasal sinuses and nasopharynx. In: Barnes L, ed. Surgical Pathology of the Head and Neck. Vol 2. New York: Marcel Dekker, 1985;1834–1836.

205. Landis S, Murray T, Bolden S, Wingo P. Cancer statistics. CA Cancer J Clin 1999;49:8–31.

206. National Cancer Institute. (March 26, 2002). Surveillance, Epidemiology, and End Results [On-line]. Available: www-seer.ims.nci.nih.gov.

207. Lawrence WJ, Donegan W, Natarajan N, et al. Adult soft tissue sarcomas. A pattern of care survey of the American College of Surgeons. Ann Surg 1987;205:349–359.

208. Enziger F, Weiss S. Soft Tissue Tumors. 2nd ed. St Louis: CV Mosby, 1988.

209. Fu Y-S, Perzin K. Nonepithelial tumors of the nasal cavity, paranasal sinuses and nasopharynx: a clinicopathologic study. Cancer 1974;33: 1289–1305.

210. Ardekian L, Samet N, Talmi Y, et al. Vascular leiomyoma of the nasal septum. Otolaryngol Head Neck Surg 1996;114:798–800.

211. Nall A, Stringer S, Baughman R. Vascular leiomyoma of the superior turbinate: first reported case. Head Neck 1997;19:63–67.

212. Murono S, Ohmura T, Sugimori S, Furukawa M. Vascular leiomyoma with abundant adipose cells of the nasal cavity. Am J Otolaryngol 1998;19:50–53.

213. Huang C, Chien C, Su C, Chen W. Leiomyoma of the inferior turbinates. J Otolaryngol 2000;29:55–56.

214. Lippert B, Godbersen G, Luttges J, Werner J. Leiomyosarcoma of the nasal cavity. Case report and literature review. ORL 1996;58:115–120.

215. Strasser M, Gleich L, Hakim S, Biddinger P. Pathologic quiz case 2. Nasal leiomyosarcoma, low grade. Arch Otolaryngol Head Neck Surg 1998;124:715, 717.

216. Harcourt J, Gallimore A. Leiomyoma of the paranasal sinuses. J Laryngol Otol 1993;107:740–741.

217. Kuruvilla A, Wenig B, Humphrey D, et al. Leiomyosarcoma of the sinonasal tract: a clinicopathologic study of nine cases. Arch Otolaryngol Head Neck Surg 1990;116:1278–1286.

218. Dropkin L, Tang C, Williams J. Leiomyosarcoma of the nasal cavity and paranasal sinuses. Ann Otol Rhinol Laryngol 1976;85: 399–403.

219. Barnes L. Tumor and tumor-like lesions of the soft tissue. In: Barnes L, ed. Surgical Pathology of the Head and Neck. Vol 2. 2nd ed. New York: Marcel Dekker, 2001;889–1048.

220. Kapadia S, Meis J, Frisman D, et al. Fetal rhabdomyoma of the head and neck: a clinicopathologic and immunophenotypic study of 24 cases. Hum Pathol 1993;24:754–765.

221. Kapadia S, Meis J, Frisman D, et al. Adult rhabdomyoma of the head and neck: a clinicopathologic and immunophenotypic study. Hum Pathol 1993;24:608–617.

222. Young JJ, Miller R. Incidence of malignant tumors in U.S. children. J Pediatr 1975;86:254–258.

223. Sercarz J, Mark R, Tran L, et al. Sarcomas of the nasal cavity and paranasal sinuses. Ann Otol Rhinol Laryngol 1994;103:699–704.

224. Callender T, Weber R, Janjan N, et al. Rhabdomyosarcoma of the nose and paranasal sinuses in adults and children. Otolaryngol Head Neck Surg 1995;112:252–257.

225. Lee J, Lee M, Lee B, et al. Rhabdomyosarcoma of the head and neck in adults: MR and CT findings. AJNR 1996;17:1923–1928.

226. Licameli G, Tunkel D, Westra W. Pathologic quiz case 2. Rhabdomyosarcoma (RMS), alveolar type, of the paranasal sinus. Arch Otolaryngol Head Neck Surg 1997;123:881–883.

227. Daya H, Chan H, Sirkin W, Forte V. Pediatric rhabdomyosarcoma of the head and neck: is there a place for surgical management? Arch Otolaryngol Head Neck Surg 2000;126:468–472.

228. Golledge J, Fisher C, Rhys-Evans P. Head and neck liposarcoma. Cancer 1995;76:1051–1058.

229. Dooms G, Hricak H, Sollitto R, et al. Lipomatous tumors and tumors with fatty component: MR imaging potential and comparison of MR and CT results. Radiology 1985;157:479–483.

230. Gnepp D, Henley J, Weiss S, Heffner D. Desmoid fibromatosis of the sinonasal tract and nasopharynx: a clinicopathologic study of 25 cases. Cancer 1996;78:2572–2579.

231. Heffner D, Gnepp D. Sinonasal fibrosarcomas, malignant schwannomas, and "Triton" tumors: a clinicopathologic study of 67 cases. Cancer 1992;70:1089–1101.

232. Bortnick E. Neoplasms of the nasal cavity. Otolaryngol Clin North Am 1973;6:801–812.

233. Frankenthaler R, Ayala A, Hartwick R, Goepfert H. Fibrosarcoma of the head and neck. Laryngoscope 1990;100:799–802.

234. Barnes L, Kanbour A. Malignant fibrous histiocytoma of the head and neck. A report of 12 cases. Arch Otolaryngol Head Neck Surg 1988;114:1149–1156.

235. Brookes G, Rose P. Malignant fibrous histiocytoma of the ethmoid sinus. J Laryngol Otol 1983;97:279–289.

236. Nemes Z, Thomazy V, Adany R, Muszbek L. Identification of histiocytic reticulum cells by immunohistochemical demonstration of Factor XIII (F-XIIIa) in human lymph nodes. J Pathol 1986;149:121–132.

237. Nemes Z. Differentiation markers in hemangiopericytoma. Cancer 1992;69:133–140.

238. Merrick R, Rhone D, Chilis T. Malignant fibrous histiocytoma of the maxillary sinus. Arch Otolaryngol 1980;106:365–367.

239. Dai J, Shi M, Li G. [Computed tomographic features of malignant fibrous histiocytoma]. Chung Hua Chung Liu Tsa Chih 1996;18:140–142.

240. Basak S, Mutlu C, Erkus M, et al. Benign fibrous histiocytoma of the nasal septum. Rhinology 1998;36:133–135.

241. Som P, Brandwein M, Maldjiian C. Inflammatory pseudotumor of the maxillary sinus: CT and MR findings in six cases. Am J Roentgenol 1994;163:689–692.

242. Batsakis J, El-Naggar A, Luna M, Goepfert H. Pathology consultation—"inflammatory pseudotumor": What is it? How does it behave? Laryngology 1995;104:329–331.

243. Takimoto T, Kathoh T, Ohmura TR. Inflammatory pseudotumor of the maxillary sinus mimicking malignancy. Rhinology 1990;28:123–127.

244. Coffin C, Watterson J, Priest J, Dehner L. Extrapulmonary inflammatory myofibroblastic tumor (inflammatory pseudotumor). A clinicopathologic and immunohistochemical study of 84 cases. Am J Surg Pathol 1995;19:859–872.

245. Hytiroglu P, Brandwein M, Strauchen J. Inflammatory pseudotumor of the parapharyngeal space: case report and review of the literature. Head Neck 1992;14:230–234.

246. Chan Y, Ma L, Young C, Lam K. Parapharyngeal inflammatory pseudotumor presenting as a fever of unknown origin in a 3 year old girl. Pediatr Pathol 1988;8:195–203.

247. Keen M, Conley J, McBride T. Pseudotumor of the pterygomaxillary space presenting as anesthesia of the mandibular nerve. Laryngoscope 1986;96:560–563.

248. Drucker C, Brodin A, Wolff A. Pathological quiz. Arch Otolaryngol 1989;115:998–1000.

249. Zukerberg L, Rosenberg A, Randolph G, et al. Solitary fibrous tumor of the nasal cavity and paranasal sinuses. Am J Surg Pathol 1991;15:126–130.

250. Kohmura T, Nakashima T, Hasegawa Y, Matsuura H. Solitary fibrous tumor of the paranasal sinuses. Eur Arch Otorhinolaryngol 1999;256:233–236.

251. Kessler A, Lapinsky J, Berenholz L, et al. Solitary fibrous tumor of the nasal cavity. Otolaryngol Head Neck Surg 1999;121:826–828.

252. Barnes L. Tumor and tumor-like lesions of the soft tissue. In: Barnes L, ed. Surgical Pathology of the Head and Neck. Vol 2. 2nd ed. New York: Marcel Dekker, 2001;948.

253. Shugar J, Som P, Meyers R, et al. Intramuscular head and neck myxoma: report of a case and review of the literature. Laryngoscope 1987;97:105–107.

254. Barnes L, Verbin R, Appel B, Peel R. Diseases of bones and joints. In: Barnes L, ed. Surgical Pathology of the Head and Neck. Vol 2. 2nd ed. New York: Marcel Dekker, 2000;1049–1232.

255. Hurwitz JJ, Fine N, Howarth DJ, DeAngelis D. Lacrimal obstruction due to a nasal osteoma. Can J Ophthalmol 1999;34:296–298.

256. Osguthorpe J, Hungerford G. Benign osteoblastoma of the maxillary sinus. Head Neck Surg 1983;6:605–609.

257. Attane F, Tannier C, Vayr R. Pneumocephalus complicating osteoma of the frontal sinus. Rev Neurol (Paris) 1996;152:279–282.

258. Marras LC, Kalaparambath TP, Black SE, Rowed DW. Severe tension pneumocephalus complicating frontal sinus osteoma. Can J Neurol Sci 1998;25:79–81.

259. Koivunen P, Lopponen H, Fors AP, Jokinen K. The growth rate of osteomas of the paranasal sinuses. Clin Otolaryngol 1997;22:111–114.

260. Evans H, Ayala A, Romsdahl M. Prognostic factors in chondrosarcoma of bone: a clinicopathologic analysis with emphasis on histologic grading. Cancer 1977;40:818–831.

261. Chaudhry A, Robinovitch M, Mitchell D, et al. Chondrogenic tumors of the jaws. Am J Surg 1961;102:403–411.

262. McCoy J, McConnel F. Chondrosarcoma of the nasal septum. Arch Otolaryngol 1981;107:125–127.

263. Gay I, Elidan J, Kopolovic J. Chondrosarcoma of the skull base. Ann Otol Rhinol Laryngol 1981;90:53–55.

264. Huvos AG, ed. Bone Tumors: Diagnosis, Treatment, and Prognosis. 2nd ed. Philadelphia: WB Saunders, 1991;68.

265. Som P, Bellot O, Blitzer A. Osteoblastoma of the ethmoid sinus: the fourth reported case. Arch Otolaryngol 1979;105:623–625.

266. Coscina W, Lee B. Concurrent osteoblastoma and aneurysmal bone cyst of the ethmoid sinus: case report. CT J Comput Tomogr 1985;9:347–350.

267. Lucas D, Unni K, McLeod R, et al. Osteoblastoma: clinicopathologic study of 306 cases. Hum Pathol 1994;25:117–134.

268. Engelbrecht V, Preis S, Hassler W, Lenard HG. CT and MRI of congenital sinonasal ossifying fibroma. Neuroradiology 1999;41:526–529.

269. Lawton MT, Heiserman JE, Coons SW, et al. Juvenile active ossifying fibroma. Report of four cases. J Neurosurg 1997;86:279–285.

270. Tobey JD, Loevner LA, Yousem DM, Lanza DC. Tension pneumocephalus: a complication of invasive ossifying fibroma of the paranasal sinuses. AJR 1996;166:711–713.

271. Barnes L, Verbin R, Appel B, Peel R. Tumor and tumor-like lesions of the soft tissue. In: Barnes L, ed. Surigcal Pathology of the Head and Neck. Vol 2. 2nd ed. New York: Marcel Dekker, 2000;1091–1095.

272. Dehner L. Fibro-osseous lesions of bone. In: Ackerman L, Spjut H, Abell M, eds. Bones and Joints. Vol Monograph No. 17. Baltimore: International Academy of Pathology, 1976;209–235.

273. Som P, Lidov M. The benign fibro-osseous lesion: its association with paranasal sinus mucoceles and its MR characteristics. JCAT 1992;16:871–876.

274. Sterling K, Stollman A, Sacher M. Ossifying fibroma of sphenoid bone with coexistent mucocele: CT and MRI. JCAT 1993;17:492–494.

275. Commins DJ, Tolley NS, Milford CA. Fibrous dysplasia and ossifying fibroma of the paranasal sinuses. J Laryngol Otol 1998;112:964–968.

276. Barnes L, Verbin R, Gnepp D. Diseases of the nose, paranasal sinuses and nasopharynx. In: Barnes L, ed. Surgical Pathology of the Head and Neck. Vol 1. New York: Mercel Dekker, 1985;883–1044.

277. Von Wowern N, Odont D. Cherubism: a 36-year long-term follow-up of 2 generations in different families and review of the literature. Oral Surg Oral Med Oral Pathol Oral Radiol Endod 2000;90:765–772.

278. Hitomi G, Nishide N, Mitsui K. Cherubism: diagnostic imaging and review of the literature in Japan. Oral Surg Oral Med Oral Pathol Oral Radiol Endod 1996;81:623–628.

279. Yamaguchi T, Dorfman H, Eisig S. Cherubism: clinicopathologic features. Skeletal Radiol 1999;28:350–353.

280. Huvos AG, ed. Bone Tumors: Diagnosis, Treatment, and Prognosis. 2nd ed. Philadelphia: WB Saunders, 1991;432–441.

281. Kujas M, Faillot T, Van Effenterre R, Poirier J. Bone giant cell tumour in neuropathological practice. A fifty year overview. Arch Anat Cytol Pathol 1999;47:7–12.

282. Auclair P, Cuenin P, Kratochvil F, et al. A clinical and histomorphologic comparison of the central giant cell granuloma and the giant cell tumor. Oral Surg Oral Med Oral Pathol 1988;66:197–208.

283. Stolovitzky J, Waldron C, McConnel F. Giant cell lesions of the maxilla and paranasal sinuses. Head Neck 1994;16:143–148.

284. Barnes L, Verbin R, Appel B, Verbin R. Tumor and tumor-like lesions of the soft tissue. In: Barnes L, ed. Surgical Pathology of the Head and Neck. Vol 2. 2nd ed. New York: Marcel Dekker, 2000;1156–1169.

285. Som P, Lawson W, Cohen B. Giant cell lesions of the facial bones. Radiology 1983;147:129–134.
286. Rhea J, Weber A. Giant cell granuloma of the sinuses. Radiology 1983;147:135–137.
287. Friedman W, Pervez N, Schwartz A. Brown tumor of the maxilla in secondary hyperparathyroidism. Arch Otolaryngol 1974;100:157–159.
288. Smith G, Ward P. Giant cell lesions of the facial skeleton. Arch Otolaryngol 1978;104:186–190.
289. Becelli R, Cerulli G, Gasparini G. Surgical and implantation reconstruction in a patient with giant-cell central reparative granuloma. J Craniofac Surg 1998;1:45–47.
290. Citardi MJ, Janjua T, Abrahams JJ, Sasaki CT. Orbitoethmoid aneurysmal bone cyst. Otolaryngol Head Neck Surg 1996;114:466–470.
291. Kaffe I, Naor H, Calderon S, Buchner A. Radiological and clinical features of aneurysmal bone cyst of the jaws. Dentomaxillofac Radiol 1999;28:167–172.
292. Som P, Schatz C, Flaum E, Lanman T. Aneurysmal bone cyst of the paranasal sinuses associated with fibrous dysplasia: CT and MR findings. JCAT 1991;15:513–515.
293. Baker H, Papsidero M, Batsakis J, Krause C. Aneurysmal bone cyst of the ethmoid. Head Neck Surg 1982;5:177–180.
294. Barnes L, Verbin R, Appel B, Peel R. Tumor and tumor-like lesions of the soft tissue. In: Barnes L, ed. Surgical Pathology of the Head and Neck. Vol 2. 2nd ed. New York: Marcel Dekker, 2001;1084.
295. Som P, Hermann G, Sacher M. Paget disease of the calvaria and facial bones with an osteosarcoma of the maxilla: CT and MR findings. JCAT 1987;11:887–890.
296. Epley KD, Lasky JB, Karesh JW. Osteosarcoma of the orbit associated with Paget disease. Ophthalmol Plast Reconstr Surg 1998;14:62–66.
297. Huvos AG, ed. Bone Tumors: Diagnosis, Treatment, and Prognosis. 2nd ed. Philadelphia: WB Saunders, 1991;87.
298. Huvos AG, ed. Bone Tumors: Diagnosis, Treatment, and Prognosis. 2nd ed. Philadelphia: WB Saunders, 1991;349.
299. Hyde G, Yarington CJ, Chu F. Head and neck manifestations of Maffucci's syndrome: chondrosarcoma of the nasal septum. Am J Otolaryngol 1995;16:272–275.
300. Saito K, Unni K, Wollan P, Lund BC. Chondrosarcoma of the jaw and facial bones. Cancer 1995;76:1550–1558.
301. Gadwal S, Fanburg-Smith J, Gannon F, Thompson L. Primary chondrosarcoma of the head and neck in pediatric patients: a clinicopathologic study of 14 cases with a review of the literature. Cancer 2000;88:2181–2188.
302. Rassekh C, Nuss D, Kapadia S, et al. Chondrosarcoma of the nasal septum: skull base imaging and clinicopathologic correlation. Otolaryngol Head Neck Surg 1996;115:29–37.
303. Huvos AG, ed. Bone Tumors: Diagnosis, Treatment, and Prognosis. 2nd ed. Philadelphia: WB Saunders, 1991;399.
304. Vencio E, Reeve C, Unni K, Nascimento A. Mesenchymal chondrosarcoma of the jaw bones: clinicopathologic study of 19 cases. Cancer 1998;82:2350–2355.
305. Lockhart R, Menard P, Martin J, et al. Mesenchymal chondrosarcoma of the jaws. Report of four cases. Int J Oral Maxillofac Surg 1998;27:358–362.
306. Huvos AG, ed. Bone Tumors: Diagnosis, Treatment, and Prognosis. 2nd ed. Philadelphia: WB Saunders, 1991;382.
307. Verbin R, Barnes L. Cysts and cyst-like lesions of the oral cavity, jaws, and neck. In: Barnes L, ed. Surgical Pathology of the Head and Neck. Vol. 3. 2nd ed. New York: Marcel Dekker, 2001;1437–1555.
308. Verbin R, Barnes L. Cysts and cyst-like lesions of the oral cavity, jaws and neck. In: Barnes L, ed. Surgical Pathology of the Head and Neck. Vol 2. New York: Marcel Dekker, 1985;1278–1281.
309. Stafne E, Gibilisco J. Oral Roentgenographic diagnosis. 4th ed. Philadelphia: WB Saunders, 1975;147–168.
310. Barnes L, Verbin R, Gnepp D. Diseases of the nose, paranasal sinuses and nasopharynx. In: Barnes L, ed. Surgical Pathology of the Head and Neck. Vol 2. New York: Marcel Dekker, 1985;1233–1329.
311. Batsakis J, ed. Tumor of the Head and Neck: Clinical and Pathological Considerations. 2nd ed. Baltimore: Williams and Wilkins, 1979;531–560.
312. Mehhlisch D, Dahlin D, Masson J. Ameloblastoma: a clinicopathologic report. J Oral Surg 1972;30:9–22.
313. Barnes L, Verbin R, Gnepp D. Diseases of the nose, paranasal sinuses and nasopharynx. In: Barnes L, ed. Surgical Pathology of the Head and Neck. Vol 2. New York: Marcel Dekker, 1985;1409.
314. Ferlito A, Rinaldo A. Developmental lesions of the head and neck. In: Barnes L, ed. Surgical Pathology of the Head and Neck. Vol 3. 2nd ed. New York: Marcel Dekker, 2000;1649–1671.
315. Heffner D. Problems in pediatric otorhinolaryngic pathology, III. Teratoid and neural tumors of the nose, sinonasal tract, and nasopharynx. Int J Pediatr Otorhinolaryngol 1983;6:1–21.
316. Heffner DK, Thompson LD, Schall DG, Anderson V. Pharyngeal dermoids ("hairy polyps") as accessory auricles. Ann Otol Rhinol Laryngol 1996;105:819–824.
317. Batsakis J, el-Naggar A, Luna M. Teratomas of the head and neck with emphasis on malignancy. Ann Otol Rhinol Laryngol 1995;104:496–500.
318. Som P, Norton K, Shugar J, et al. Metastatic hypernephroma to the head and neck. AJNR 1987;8:1103–1106.
319. Maschka DA, McCulloch TM, Nerad JA. Prostate cancer metastatic to the orbit [see comments]. Ann Otol Rhinol Laryngol 1996;105:70–71.
320. Aw CY, Hwang JS, Brett RH, Lu PK. Metastatic oesophageal carcinoma to the paranasal sinuses—a case report. Singapore Med J 1999;40:539–541.
321. Batsakis J, ed. Tumor of the Head and Neck: Clinical and Pathological Considerations. 2nd ed. Baltimore: Williams and Wilkins, 1979;240–250.
322. Bernstein J, Montgomery W, Balogh K. Metastatic tumors to the maxilla, nose and paranasal sinus. Laryngoscope 1966;76:621–650.
323. Gottlieb MD, Roland JT Jr. Paradoxical spread of renal cell carcinoma to the head and neck. Laryngoscope 1998;108:1301–1305.
324. Vogelzang N, Priest E, Borden L. Spontaneous regression of histologically proved pulmonary metastases from renal cell carcinoma: a case with 5-year follow up. J Urol 1992;148:1247–1248.
325. Kallmeyer J, Dittrich O. Spontaneous regression of metastases in a case of bilateral renal cell carcinoma. J Urol 1992;148:138–140.
326. Cottel WI. Perineural invasion by squamous-cell carcinoma. J Dermatol Surg Oncol 1982;8:589–600.
327. Goepfert H, Dichtel W, Medina J, et al. Perineural invasion in squamous cell skin carcinoma of the head and neck. Am J Surg 1984;148:542–547.
328. Hanke C, Wolf R, Hochman S, et al. Chemosurgical reports: perineural spread of basal cell carcinoma. J Dermatol Surg Oncol 1983;9:742–747.
329. Altman KW, Mirza N, Philippe L. Metastatic follicular thyroid carcinoma to the paranasal sinuses: a case report and review. J Laryngol Otol 1997;111:647–651.
330. Freeman JL, Gershon A, Liavaag PG, Walfish PG. Papillary thyroid carcinoma metastasizing to the sphenoid-ethmoid sinuses and skull base. Thyroid 1996;6:59–61.
331. Yamasoba T, Kikuchi S, Sugasawa M, et al. Occult follicular carcinoma metastasizing to the sinonasal tract. J Otorhinolaryngol Relat Spec 1994;56:239–243.
332. Mochimatsu I, Tsukuda M, Furukawa S, Sawaki S. Tumours metastasizing to the head and neck—a report of seven cases. J Laryngol Otol 1993;107:1171–1173.
333. Renner GJ, Davis WE, Templer JW. Metastasis of thyroid carcinoma to the paranasal sinuses. Otolaryngol Head Neck Surg 1984;92:233–237.
334. Cinberg JZ, Terrife D. Follicular adenocarcinoma of the thyroid in the maxillary sinus. Otolaryngol Head Neck Surg 1980;88:157–158.
335. Scott A, Raine M, Stansbie JM. Ethmoid metastasis of endometrial carcinoma causing mucocele of maxillary antrum. J Laryngol Otol 1998;112:283–285.
336. Tariq M, Gluckman P, Thebe P. Metastatic testicular teratoma of the nasal cavity: a rare cause of severe intractable epistaxis. J Laryngol Otol 1998;112:1078–1081.

# 7

# Facial Fractures and Postoperative Findings

## Peter M. Som and Margaret S. Brandwein

## SECTION ONE

# FACIAL FRACTURES

## INTRODUCTION

The paranasal sinuses develop within and are protected by the facial bones. The facial bones also surround and protect the orbits, nasal fossae, and mouth, they support the maxillary dentition, and they serve as attachments for the facial muscles. The facial skeleton can be considered as a honeycombed structure of varying thickness and form that develops strength along stress zones by forming buttressed arches. In general, the most superficial portion of the facial skeleton is physically the strongest and serves the additional function of protecting the more delicate central part of the face. The honeycombed construction of the middle third of the facial skeleton evolved to resist the vertical masticatory forces, and in this regard it provides excellent stability. However, external impact forces directed toward the mid-face can disrupt this central structure, and the fracture of even one buttress can weaken the entire lattice, causing it to collapse. Fortunately, such collapse is often prevented by the strength of these same facial buttresses and the additional support of the skull base.[1, 2]

## FACIAL BUTTRESSES

The facial skeleton can be analyzed in terms of the supporting buttresses that comprise its structure. There are two main sagittal buttresses on either side of the face. There is a medial buttress that extends from the anterior maxillary alveolus up the lateral wall of the pyriform aperture, which is the opening in the facial skeleton that defines the margins of the nasal fossae, and into the medial orbital wall. This nasomaxillary buttress is thus formed by the lower maxilla, the frontal process of the maxilla, the lacrimal bone, and the nasal process of the frontal bone. There is also a lateral buttress, the zygomaticomaxillary buttress, which is formed on either side by the lateral wall of the maxilla, the body of the zygoma, and the orbital process of the frontal bone in the lateral orbital wall. A third buttress has been suggested, the pterygomaxillary buttress, which extends from the posterior maxillary alveolus (tuberosity) cranially along the pterygoid plates to the skull base.

These buttresses have evolved as mechanical adaptations of the skull to masticatory forces, and the greatest occlusal forces are absorbed by the zygomaticomaxillary buttress, as evidenced by the thick cortical bone present in the lateral maxillary-zygomatic region when compared with the more fragile medial maxillary wall. In addition to these sagittal buttresses, some authors believe that there is also a median buttress formed by the nasal septum. Overall these craniocaudal buttresses are curved, and analysis suggests that they need reinforcement by axial struts. Thus these sagittal buttresses are interconnected by three axial (horizontal) struts that are formed by the floor of the anterior cranial fossa, the orbital floor and zygomatic arches, and the maxillary alveolus and hard palate. In addition, the skull base, which is oriented at approximately a 45° angle to the occlusal plane of the maxilla, acts as an additional axial buttress. Together these buttresses or struts form an interconnecting facial support system.

The facial skeleton can also be conceptualized as being formed by two coronal buttresses: an anterior plane formed by the vertical portion of the frontal bone (glabellar region), the orbital rims, the anterior maxilla, and the alveolus; and a posterior plane formed by the posterior wall of the maxilla and the pterygoid processes.[1, 3, 4]

Such analyses, first studied experimentally by Le Fort, have led to an understanding of the major lines of weakness in the midfacial skeleton, and these, in turn, have helped explain why certain fractures follow an overall predictable course. The efforts of Le Fort are recognized today by the Le Fort types I, II, and III fractures. The forces he used experimentally are similar to the low-velocity impact forces that occur today in fist fights and sporting events. However, at present there are also high-velocity impact injuries such as those that occur in high-speed vehicular accidents and with violence involving blunt devices or gunshot wounds. Despite the much greater order of magnitude of these impact forces, the same fracture lines are still encountered, albeit in various combinations other than those originally observed by Le Fort.[1, 2]

In addition to causing complicated facial fractures, such high-impact trauma rarely may be associated with cervical spine injury. In one study of 582 consecutive patients with facial fractures, 1.04% (6) were found to have a cervical spine injury, all of which were the result of a car accident.[5] Thus, the proper workup of a patient with severe facial fractures should also include evaluation of the cervical spine. In addition, imaging of these patients should include the brain and the carotid arteries for associated trauma.

## CLINICAL DIAGNOSIS AND TREATMENT

The diagnosis of facial fractures usually is accomplished by a combination of clinical and imaging examinations. The clinician is primarily concerned with the detection of malocclusion, abnormal mobility, and crepitation as signs of fracture. Often, deformity of the facial skeleton is initially concealed by overlying edema, hemorrhage, and soft-tissue injury. Any evidence of a palpable step-off at the orbital rim, diplopia, hypertelorism, midfacial elongation, cerebrospinal fluid (CSF) rhinorrhea, or flattening of the cheek further helps the clinician identify the type of fracture present. However, only after imaging studies can the fractures be completely identified and characterized. It is now recognized that the information gained from CT scans is of greater net value than that gained from a combination of routine radiographs and clinical examination. Thus imaging is essential for proper treatment planning in these cases.[1, 2, 6]

In many instances, clinicians wait several days after the trauma before reducing the fracture(s). This delay allows some of the soft-tissue injury to subside and may be necessary if the patient has other life-threatening injuries that require immediate attention (before the less critical facial fractures are addressed). However, if possible, a delay of more than 7 days is to be avoided, because after this time fibrous fixation of the fracture occurs and fracture reduction becomes more difficult, often requiring refracturing to attain normal positioning.

The basic principles of treating midfacial fractures are (1) reduction of the fractures and (2) fixation of the fractured bones to one another and to the skull. Absolute immobilization of the fractures is the main prerequisite for rapid and undisturbed healing because the main interferences with fracture healing are local mechanical factors. In the early phase of fracture healing, mobility can disturb the normal course of bone regeneration and lead to faulty differentiation of the callus.[1, 2, 7-9] Of primary clinical concern is the restoration of occlusion and facial form, because these provide a means of restoring the essential masticatory function. Midfacial restoration is accomplished by means of arch bars applied to the maxillary and mandibular teeth and then, after manipulation is held in good occlusion, by fixing the arch bars together with small rubber bands. Such fixation of the midface must be maintained until bony union and consolidation are achieved. If internal wire fixation is used, immobilization usually takes 6 to 8 weeks. Intermaxillary fixation alone requires 3 to 4 weeks to prevent further occlusal malalignment.[8, 9] However, today most internal fixation is accomplished by the use of microplates or miniplates and screws (Fig. 7-1).[8-10] With this technique, intermaxillary fixation is accomplished without a waiting interval. In addition, the growing use of microplate fixation has almost made obsolete the complex internal fixation schemes accomplished with wire sutures and wire suspensions (Fig. 7-2). External fixation for facial fractures using a halo frame with fixation bars is also less common due to the utilization of microplates.

Infections of the fracture line are among the most serious complications of facial fractures. Any fracture must be considered potentially infected if it traverses the alveolus, the walls of the nasal skeleton, or the paranasal sinuses or communicates with a soft-tissue wound. Such fractures are called *compound fractures,* and appropriate antibiotic therapy reduces the chances of infection in these fractures.[1, 2, 8, 9] With good treatment the risk of infection of a maxillary or midfacial fracture is only about 2%, and the risk of osteomyelitis is 0.5%. However, a treatment delay of 2 to 3 weeks raises the incidence of osteomyelitis to 1.3%.[8, 9] Similarly, posttraumatic sinusitis occurs in 7.25% to 9% of all the patients with midfacial fractures, and proper maintenance of sinus drainage must be a therapeutic consideration.[7]

It is not uncommon to encounter multiple bone fragments during open reduction of facial bone fractures. When these fragments are few and their size is large, there is no problem. However, multiple small, thin bone fragments are difficult to handle, making accurate reduction with interfragmentary wires problematic. This is frequently encountered in

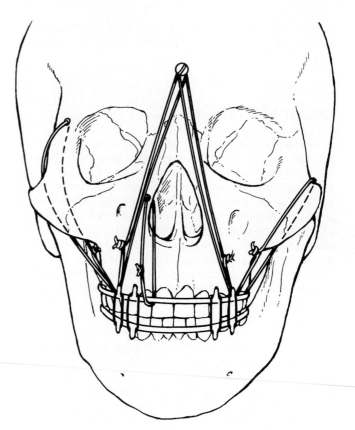

**FIGURE 7-2**  Frontal diagram of the different types of intraosseous wiring. The maxillary and mandibular teeth are fitted with arch bars, which are held together with rubber bands. With the patient in good occlusion, fixation can be achieved by frontomalar suspension, glabella (screw) suspension, pyriform aperture suspension, or circumzygomatic suspension.

fractures of the anterior maxillary wall, orbital floor, orbital roof, and frontal sinus. Therefore, many surgeons reconstruct the larger segments and discard the smaller segments. In one study, 10 patients who sustained facial fractures with multiple small, thin fragments were treated with tissue adhesive (*n*-butyl-2-cyanoacrylate). Postoperative three-dimensional (3D) CT scans demonstrated excellent reconstruction following this technique.[11]

Thus, the concepts of treating craniomaxillofacial fractures have changed over the last 15 years, and modern imaging techniques play a central part in establishing a proper diagnosis. In addition, advanced life support and intensive care medicine now allow for early primary fracture treatment. The former principles of minimal exposure of bone fragments using small incisions have been replaced by principles from reconstructive craniofacial surgery comprising extensive subperiosteal dissection, exposure of all fracture lines, open reduction, and rigid internal fixation. Missing bony structures are replaced primarily by autogenous bone grafts or the use of exogenous materials. By using these concepts, most late esthetic and functional sequelae of facial fractures can be dramatically reduced.[12]

The final goal in reconstructing the facial skeleton of trauma patients is to obtain good cosmetic and functional outcomes. To accomplish those goals, many surgeons believe that the key to repairing midfacial fractures is the correct placement of the zygomatic arch in relation to the cranial base and the midface. In this way the transverse,

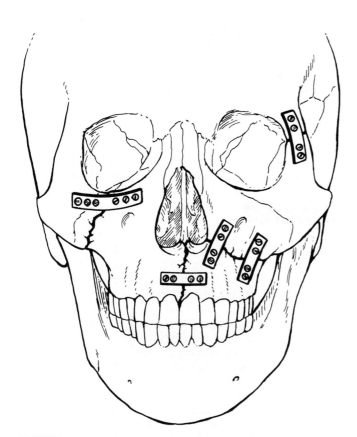

**FIGURE 7-1**  Frontal diagram of the use of microplates or miniplates in the fixation of midfacial fractures at typical fracture sites.

vertical, and sagittal diameters are regained in their correct spacial relationships.[13]

## IMAGING

CT is the modality of choice for the most complete evaluation of the facial skeleton and facial soft tissues.[14] Although contrast-enhanced CT scans can assess the brain and dural spaces, which so often have associated damage in the severe accidents that cause facial trauma, these structures are better evaluated with MR imaging.[15] The most useful diagnostic information is gained by utilizing both axial and coronal CT scans.[16, 17] That is, a single-plane CT study does not provide as detailed information as an orthogonal two-plane examination. Specialized sagittal or oblique plane studies, although helpful in specific cases, are generally considered optional.[8] These specialized reconstructions usually appear degraded when compared to the original acquisition plane images; however, with the use of multidetector CT units, such deficiency may be a thing of the past.

Helical CT provides a means of obtaining better-quality two-dimensional (2D) reconstructions in any plane and provides excellent 3D reconstructions. Although some detail is lost as part of the smoothing algorithm, the 3D images serve as an excellent communication tool with the surgeons.[18, 19] These 3D images usually allow clinicians to visualize the fracture segments and their relationship to one another better than on a series of 2D scans in any one plane. Although these 3D images have been shown to be of little value in the temporal bone, they have considerable value in the skull base and the facial skeleton, especially if surfaces are involved or fragments are displaced.[20] With the newer 3D software, the fracture segments can be manipulated on screen so that the clinician can evaluate a particular treatment approach or the results of a treatment plan. In addition, 3D models can now be constructed from the CT data, allowing hands-on preoperative planning in complex cases.[18] It has been shown that measurement of the skull and facial bone landmarks by 3D reconstruction is quantitatively accurate for surgical planning and treatment evaluation of craniofacial fractures.[21]

Because MR imaging does not visualize the bone directly, small yet unstable nondisplaced facial fractures may not be seen. Although MR imaging can be helpful in differentiating blood from inflammatory reactions and edema fluid, such a distinction is rarely of clinical importance. By 48 hours after the trauma, intrasinus blood has a high methemoglobin content. If MR imaging is performed at this time, the blood has a high T1-weighted signal intensity, while edema and infection have intermediate to low T1-weighted signal intensities.[22]

In addition to evaluating the facial bones, the skull base also must be carefully examined, as fractures of the anterior cranial fossa are found in 7.1% of central midfacial fractures, 14.7% of centrolateral midfacial fractures, and 1.1% of lateral midfacial fractures.[7] The midfacial area is formed by the paired maxillae, palatal bones, inferior turbinates, lacrimal bones, nasal bones, zygomas, and solitary vomer and ethmoid bones. Central midfacial fractures include all forms of fractures that occur between the root of the nose and the alveolar processes of the maxillae, without involvement of the zygomas. These fractures include the alveolar process fracture of the maxilla, with detachment of teeth; the transverse fracture just above the floor of the nasal cavity, with separation of the palate and alveolus (Le Fort I, or Guérin's, fracture); the median or paramedian sagittal fracture of the hard palate; the pyramidal fracture, with separation of the midface either with the nasal bones (Le Fort II and Wassmund II) or without the nasal bones (Wassmund I); and fractures of the nasal bones and the nasoethmoidal region.[7]

Lastly, it must be remembered that with minor trauma, no fracture may be present and yet there are reportable findings. Thus, intrasinus hemorrhage, subcutaneous edema, subcutaneous hematomas, and foreign bodies may be present (Fig. 7-3). These findings must be noted, as they serve to explain

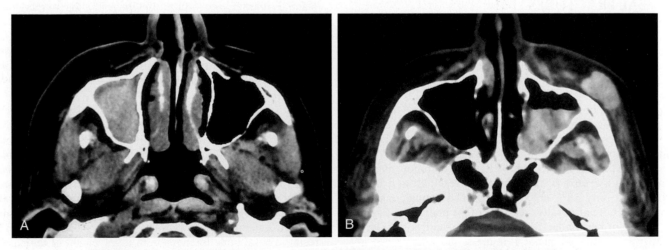

**FIGURE 7-3**   Axial CT scan (**A**) shows high-attenuation hemorrhage within the right maxillary sinus. There is slight fullness of the soft tissues in the right cheek area. This patient had received blunt trauma to the right face and presented with epistaxis. No fractures were present. Axial CT scan (**B**) on another patient shows high-attenuation fluid within the left maxillary sinus. There is also edema and a hematoma within the subcutaneous tissues of the left cheek. This patient was in the passenger seat during a low-velocity car accident and presented with a cheek deformity and epistaxis. No fractures were present.

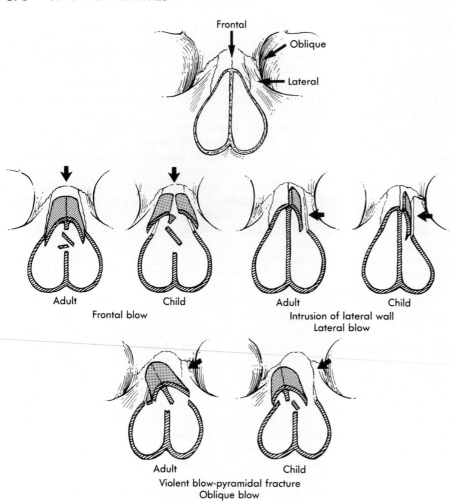

**FIGURE 7-4** Frontal diagram showing different common types of nasal fractures in children and adults that result from frontal, lateral, and oblique blows.

## NASAL FRACTURES

Nasal injuries are the most common fractures of the facial skeleton; about 50% of facial fractures are isolated fractures of the nasal pyramid.[10, 14] That is, nasal fractures can occur either as isolated fractures or in association with other facial injuries. A distinction should be made between fractures of the cartilaginous nasal structures and those of the nasal bones because they represent different types of injuries.[1, 2]

The extent of disruption of the nasal structure relates to the direction and degree of the force causing the injury (Fig. 7-4). The lateral impact injury is more common than the frontal injury; 66% of nasal fractures result from a lateral force, but only 13% are the result of a frontal impact.[23] Although not universally used, one of the main classification systems for nasal bone fractures divides the frontal injuries into three types. In plane 1 injuries, the injury does not extend dorsal to a plane that extends from the caudal tip of the nasal bones to the anterior nasal spine. The majority of the impact is absorbed by the lower nasal cartilages and the nasal tip. Separation and avulsion of the upper lateral nasal cartilages occur, and occasionally there is posterior disloca-

tion of the septal and alar cartilages. In plane 2 injuries, the external nose, the nasal septum, and the anterior nasal spine are all involved. There is splaying or flattening of the nasal bones; septal cartilage tears and overriding may occur. In plane 3 injuries, the orbital and possibly the intracranial structures are also involved. Typically there are comminuted nasal bone fractures, and fractures of the frontal processes of the maxillae, the lacrimal bones, and the ethmoid labyrinth. Severe nasal septal injuries can result in upward extension that may involve the cribriform plate and orbital roof.[23]

With weak lateral (oblique) impacts, plane 1 injuries result and involve only the ipsilateral nasal bone. Typically the lower nasal bone, the frontal process of the maxilla, and possibly the pyriform aperture margin are medially displaced. Lateral plane 2 injuries result from a greater force than plane 1 injuries. The fracture results in medial displacement of the ipsilateral nasal bone and lateral displacement of the contralateral nasal bone and nasal septum. Lateral plane 3 injuries are still more severe and result in nasal bone fractures with involvement of the nasal septum, the frontal process of the maxilla, and the lacrimal bone.[23]

In summary, the majority of nasal bone fractures involve the thinner, distal third of the nasal bones, and the nasoethmoid margin remains intact.[1, 2, 10] A lateral blow to

facial deformity and epistaxis that may clinically suggest a fracture.

the nose usually causes a simple cartilage depression or fracture of only the ipsilateral nasal bone (Fig. 7-5). However, an anteriorly placed nasal blow usually fractures both nasal bones at their lower ends, and because the force is absorbed by the nasal septum, the septum is also displaced and fractured.

With a greater force, the entire nasal pyramid, including the frontal processes of the maxillae, may become detached (Fig. 7-6).[10] When the nasal bones and septum are displaced posteriorly, a saddle nose deformity and splay-

ing of the nose result.[1, 2] In more severe fractures, traumatic hypertelorism and telecanthus may occur, and hemorrhage caused by rupture of the anterior or posterior ethmoidal arteries may be severe.

In adults, the internasal suture is solidly ossified so that the nasal bones function as a unit between the frontal processes of the maxilla. However, in children the internasal suture is not yet ossified, and the nasal bones are essentially hinged on each other while resting on the frontal processes of the maxillae. As a result, the frontal processes usually are

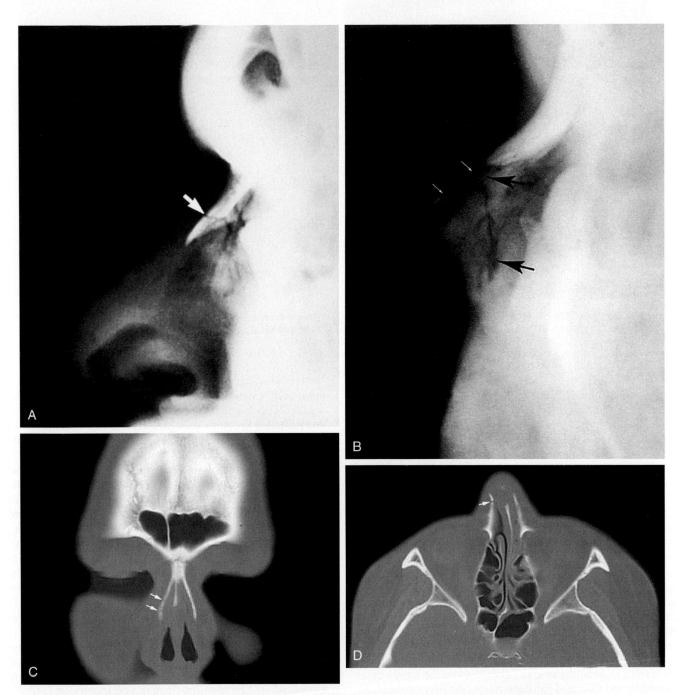

**FIGURE 7-5**    Lateral plain film (**A**) shows a nondisplaced fracture (*arrow*) extending from the midline nasal bones laterally. Lateral plain film (**B**) shows comminuted nasal bone fractures (*small arrows*) with extension into the frontal processes of the maxilla (*arrows*). Coronal (**C**) and axial (**D**) CT scans on another patient show minimally displaced right nasal fractures (*arrows*).

*Illustration continued on following page*

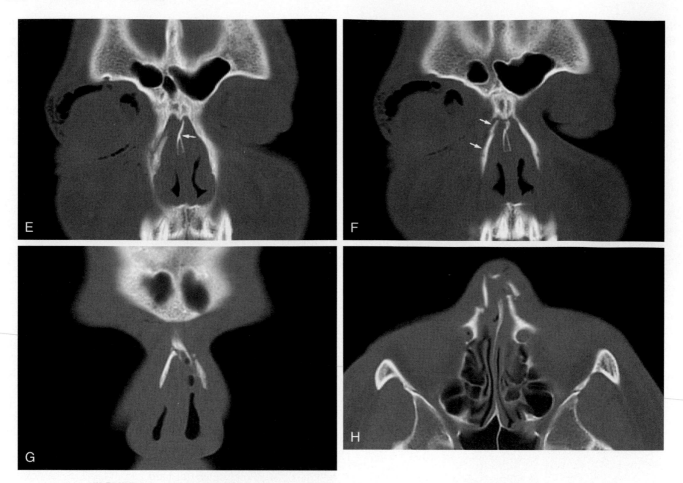

**FIGURE 7-5** *Continued.* Coronal CT scans (**E, F**) on a different patient show medially displaced comminuted fractures of the right nasal bone (*arrow* in **E**) and a displaced fracture of the anterior bony nasal septum (*arrows* in **F**). There is also orbital emphysema on the right side from an ethmoid fracture. Coronal (**G**) and axial (**H**) CT scans on yet another patient show comminuted fractures of the nasal bones and the right frontal process of the maxilla.

not fractured in childhood nasal injuries.[1, 2] In fact, it has been noted that in children there is a less prominent nasal projection (the nasal bone length is almost equal to the width), and there is increased elasticity and stability of the midface due to the presence of developing bone, the relative lack of sinus pneumatization, and the state of mixed dentition. There is also increased shielding of the facial skeletal structure due to the disproportionate amount of soft tissue relative to bone, and the small weight and size of the child decrease inertial impact forces.[23]

If the nose is struck from the side and near its base, the lateral cartilaginous walls may be displaced, and this type of injury is not identified radiographically. Further, edema and hemorrhage usually fill in the resulting surface depression and obscure clinical detection of the deformity. If these injuries and simple nasal fractures initially go undetected, especially if they occur in conjunction with more serious injuries, the inadequately treated nasal trauma may result in cosmetic deformity and functional impairment.[1, 2]

If the nasal trauma results in buckling of the nasal septal cartilage, the fractured cartilage fragments may overlap one another, thereby separating the perichondrium from the cartilage. This event allows a hematoma to develop in the space between the perichondrium and the cartilage, and this hematoma interferes with the cartilage's overlying muco-

periosteal vascular supply. Eventual cartilage necrosis occurs. If such a septal hematoma is not initially identified and treated, it becomes an organized hematoma that causes a firm, unyielding thickening of the septum and impaired breathing.

If a septal hematoma becomes infected after mucosal injury, a septal abscess develops, with fever, pain, septal swelling, eventual cartilage necrosis and resulting loss of nasal support and the development of a saddle nose deformity, and possible intracranial spread of the infection.[1, 2] To avoid these complications, it is essential to have careful clinical examination of the nasal septum and early evacuation of a septal hematoma. If imaging studies of the nose and nasal fossae are also performed, the radiologist should always direct attention to the nasal septum to identify any localized septal swelling or traumatic deviation (septal bone fracture and/or cartilage dislocation).[1, 2]

One study demonstrated that, based on clinical examination, 25% of patients required surgical reduction of a nasal fracture or dislocation despite a negative plain film examination.[24] In addition, there is a poor correlation (6.6% to 10%) between the plain film demonstration of a fracture and the need for surgical reduction.[23] In more severe injuries, a higher detection rate and better clinical correlation are achieved with the use of CT. Actual fracture of cartilage may not be imaged by any modality. However, in these cases, cartilage dislocation or a focal hematoma usually draws attention to the injury.

# CENTRAL MIDFACIAL FRACTURES

## Nasoorbital Fractures

The nasoorbital fracture most often results from a blow over the bridge of the nose. The force displaces the nasal pyramid posteriorly, fracturing the nasal bones, frontal processes of the maxillae, lacrimal bones, ethmoid sinuses, walls of the frontal sinuses, cribriform plate, and nasal septum. The ethmoid lamina usually fractures on itself in an accordion fashion, and this is best visualized on CT in the axial plane. Posttraumatic hypertelorism and telecanthus may result, as well as associated damage to the lacrimal apparatus and the medial canthal tendon (Fig. 7-7). Careful attention also should be given to any fractures involving the bones near the optic canal, as a surgical attempt to reduce the facial bone fractures may displace such an optic canal fracture and cause blindness.

In the floor of the anterior cranial fossa the dura is thin and firmly adherent to the bone. Thus the skull base and dura in the anterior cranial fossa function as a unit, and a fracture through this region invariably tears the dura. Dural tears provide a pathway for CSF rhinorrhea and the development of an intracranial pneumocele or infection (Fig. 7-8).[1, 2] In one series, motor vehicle accidents accounted for nearly 70% of these cases, and 63% of the patients had associated severe nonfacial injuries. In addition, 51% of the cases had central nervous system injury and 42% of the patients had CSF leakage. Telecanthus was present in 12% of the cases.[25, 26] Thus, if a fracture in the region of the nasion is identified on imaging, a careful search should always be made for any associated intracranial traumatic complications.

## Isolated Maxillary/Palatal Fractures

Alveolar fractures are the most common isolated maxillary fractures. An upward blow to the mandible can thrust the mandible into the maxilla and push the maxillary teeth upward and outward. This movement, in turn, fractures the alveolus. Because of the strong soft-tissue support over the alveolus, these isolated fractures rarely are displaced. The involved teeth often are displaced or devitalized, and such alveolar fractures in children may damage the tooth germs.[7] Partial fractures of the maxilla can result from a blow delivered by a narrow object directly over the anterior maxillary wall. The fractures usually involve the anterior and lateral antral walls and extend toward the pyriform aperture and down into the maxillary alveolus (Figs. 7-9 to 7-12).

Sagittal fractures of the palate result from either an axial or an oblique blow to the chin or a direct blow to the upper jaw. The fracture passes through the weakest portion of the palatine process of the maxilla, which is in a sagittal plane just off of the midline. The midline itself is reinforced by the vomer, whereas the lateral hard palate is supported by the alveolus. In more violent trauma a sagittal midline fracture can occur, and comminuted palatal fractures are associated with other central or centrolateral facial fractures.[7]

## Le Fort I Fractures

The Le Fort I (Guérin's) fracture results from a blow delivered over the upper lip region and is characterized by detachment, at a level just above the floor of the nasal cavity, of the upper jaw with the tooth-bearing segments from the caudal portions of the maxillary sinuses and the lower nasal septum. The fracture extends through the lower nasal septum, the lower walls of the maxillary sinuses, and the lower pterygoid plates. Thus the fracture segment includes the entire palate, maxillary alveolus and teeth, and portions of the pterygoid plates. This "floating palate" is displaced posteriorly, resulting in malocclusion and hemorrhaging into the antra (Figs. 7-13 and 7-14).[7]

The presence of upper arch dentures can modify the fracture patterns occurring in midfacial trauma. In a group of such patients with predominantly Le Fort I fractures, an atypical fracture path was noted, with a vertical fracture passing from the main Le Fort I fracture to the inferior orbital rim. Full upper arch dentures generally protected the upper alveolus from fracture but, where there was discontinuity of the prosthesis, alveolar fractures mirrored the edge of the denture as it crossed the alveolus. Thus the clinician should be alerted to the possibility of unusual maxillary fractures in denture wearers.[27]

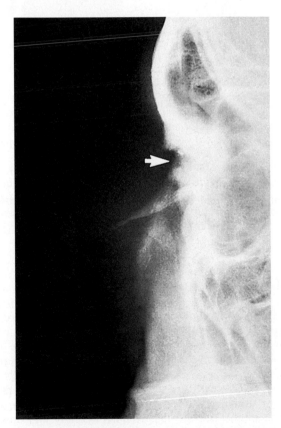

**FIGURE 7-6**   Lateral plain film shows a nasal fracture through the frontonasal suture (*arrow*) with posterior displacement of the nasal bones.

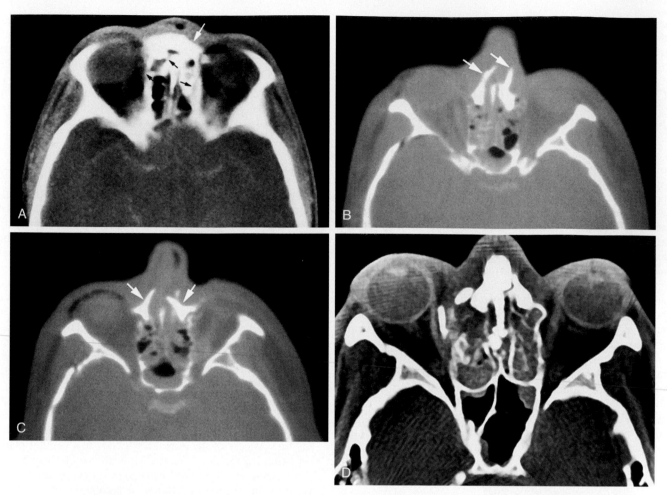

**FIGURE 7-7**   Axial CT scan (**A**) shows a nasoorbital fracture with posterior displacement of the region of the nasion (*white arrow*) and fractures through the fovea ethmoidalis (*small arrows*). Axial CT scan (**B**) shows a nasoorbital fracture with posterior displacement and rotation to the left side of both nasal bones and the frontal processes of each maxilla (*arrows*). There are also fractures of the ethmoids with some hypertelorism. Axial CT scan (**C**) shows a nasoorbital fracture with posterior and medial displacement of both nasal bones and each frontal process of the maxilla. There are also multiple fractures of the ethmoid complex and some hypertelorism. Axial CT scan (**D**) shows a nasoorbital fracture with posterior displacement of the nasal bones and fractures and hypertelorism of the ethmoid complex.

## Le Fort II Fractures

A strong, broad blow over the central facial region causes a pyramidal fracture, one of the most severe midfacial fractures. The high, central midface fracture (Le Fort II) is characterized by a fracture line that extends through the root of the nose, then runs bilaterally to involve the lacrimal bones and medial orbital walls. On each side the fracture line then turns anteriorly along the floor of the orbit near the infraorbital canal and extends down the zygomaticomaxillary suture and the anterior wall of the maxilla; posteriorly the fracture goes down across the infratemporal surface of the maxilla and finally extends through the lower pterygoid plates. This creates a pyramid-shaped central facial fracture segment. The deep central midface (Wassmund I) fracture spares the nasal bones and extends from the lateral edges of the pyriform aperture back across to the lacrimal bones and into the medial orbital walls. From this point the fracture is the same as the Le Fort II (Figs. 7-15 and 7-16).[7] In the Le Fort II and Wassmund I

fractures the zygomatic bones remain attached to the cranium. The pyramid-shaped fracture segment (the central midface) is posteriorly displaced, resulting in a "dishface" deformity, malocclusion, and hemorrhage. Anesthesia or paresthesia of one or both of the infraorbital nerves occurs in 78.9% of the cases.[10]

## Le Fort III Fractures

Centrolateral midfacial fractures are characterized by separation of the entire facial skeleton from the skull base. Such a craniofacial dysjunction has a fracture line that extends through the root of the nose, then runs bilaterally across the lacrimal bones and medial orbital walls, to continue posterolaterally across the floor of each orbit to the inferior orbital fissure. At this point on each side, one portion of the fracture line extends laterally and upward across the lateral orbital wall to end near the zygomatico-frontal sutures. A second fracture line extends from the

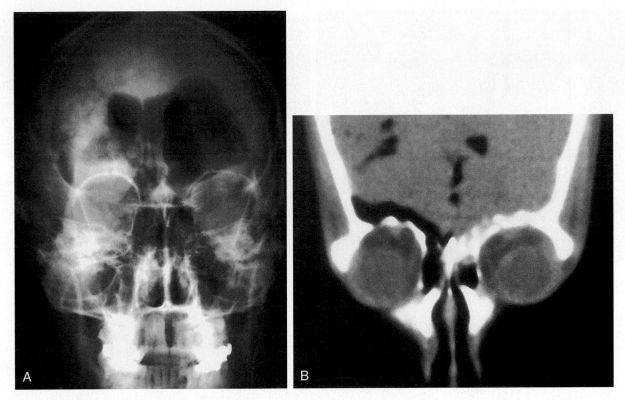

**FIGURE 7-8**   The Caldwell view (**A**) shows massive intracranial air in a patient who had a nasoorbital fracture. Coronal CT scan (**B**) shows intracranial air in another patient with a nasoorbital fracture.

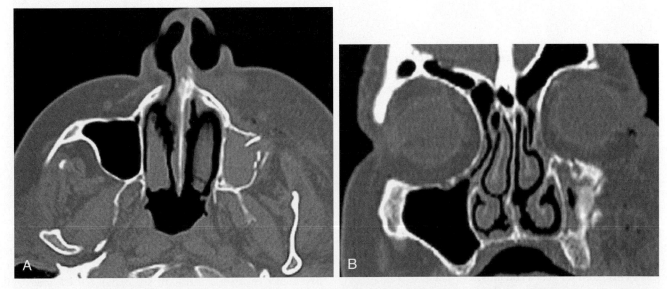

**FIGURE 7-9**   Axial (**A**) and Coronal (**B**) CT scans show a comminuted fracture of the anterolateral left antral wall. This type of fracture usually is the result of a blow from a narrow object.

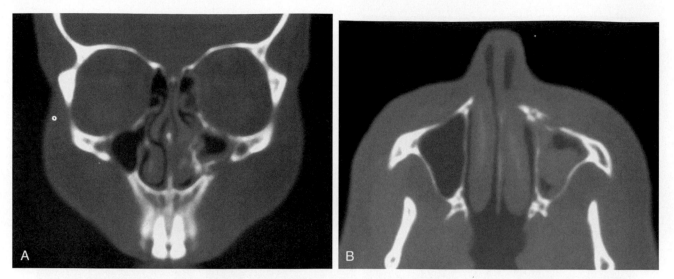

**FIGURE 7-10** Coronal (**A**) and axial (**B**) CT scans show comminuted fractures involving the left anteromedial maxilla.

orbital floor down across the back of each maxilla to the lower portion of the pterygoid plates. The zygomatic arches also are fractured, thereby completing the separation of the facial skeleton from the skull base. Such a fracture is called a Le Fort III or Wassmund IV fracture (Figs. 7-17 to 7-19). The same fracture without inclusion of the nasal bones is called a Wassmund III fracture (Fig. 7-17B), and the fracture line extends from each side of the pyriform aperture up to the lacrimal bones. The fracture then continues as a Le Fort III fracture. The distinguishing feature between the Le Fort III fracture and the Le Fort II fracture is the inclusion in the Le Fort III fractured segment of the zygomas and lateral orbital walls. These patients have a dishface deformity, CSF rhinorrhea, hemorrhage, damage to the lacrimal apparatus, and malocclusion. The infraorbital nerves are involved in 69.3% of cases.[10]

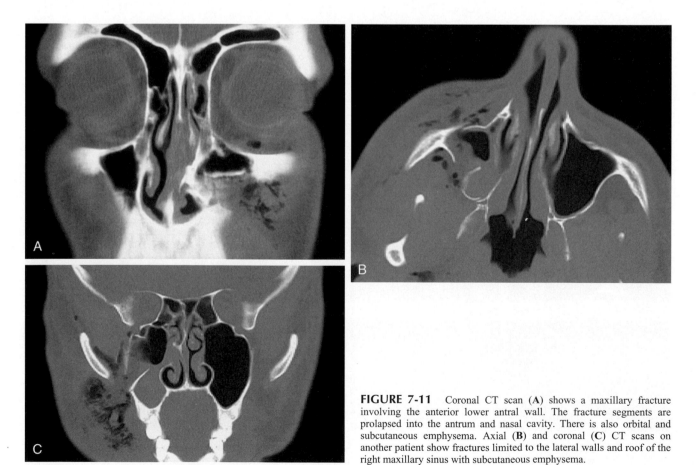

**FIGURE 7-11** Coronal CT scan (**A**) shows a maxillary fracture involving the anterior lower antral wall. The fracture segments are prolapsed into the antrum and nasal cavity. There is also orbital and subcutaneous emphysema. Axial (**B**) and coronal (**C**) CT scans on another patient show fractures limited to the lateral walls and roof of the right maxillary sinus with subcutaneous emphysema.

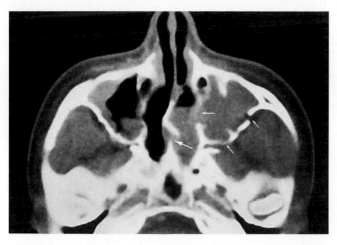

**FIGURE 7-12**   Axial CT scan shows fractures of the left maxillary sinus's posterolateral and medial walls (*small arrows*) and a fracture of the nasal septum (*large arrow*).

## LATERAL MIDFACIAL FRACTURES

Lateral midfacial fractures include the zygomatic fractures (trimalar, or tripod), zygomatic arch fractures, zygomaticomaxillary fractures, zygomaticomandibular fractures, and fractures of the floor of the orbit (blow-out fractures).

## Trimalar (Zygomatic) Fractures

Zygomatic fractures are the second most common facial fractures after nasal bone trauma. The fracture line in a

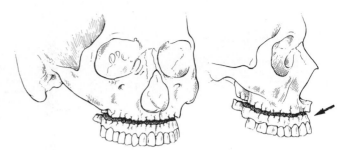

**FIGURE 7-13**   Diagram of a Le Fort I fracture, which results in a "floating" palate.

zygomatic fracture extends from the lateral orbital wall (zygomaticofrontal suture and the zygomaticosphenoid suture) to the inferior orbital fissure, then across the orbital floor near the infraorbital canal, down the anterior maxilla near the zygomaticomaxillary suture, and up the posterior maxillary wall back to the inferior orbital fissure. There is also a fracture through the weakest part of the zygomatic arch, which is about 1.5 cm dorsal to the zygomaticotemporal suture. The infraorbital nerve is impaired in 94.2% of the cases.[10] These fractures are usually and traditionally referred to as trimalar or tripod fractures because these are fractures through the three bony connections of the zygoma. That is, there are fractures (1) through the lateral orbital wall, (2) separating the zygoma and maxilla, and (3) through the zygomatic arch. Rarely these fractures have been referred to as quadramalar fractures, because the fractures extend through four suture lines (zygomaticofrontal, zygomaticosphenoid, zygomaticotemporal, and zygomaticomaxillary). Nonetheless, the more common term is trimalar fracture, recognizing that there is one fracture line through the

**FIGURE 7-14**   Coronal (**A**) and lateral (**B**) multidirectional tomograms show a Le Fort I fracture (*curved arrows*) and its extension through the pterygoid plates (*arrows*).

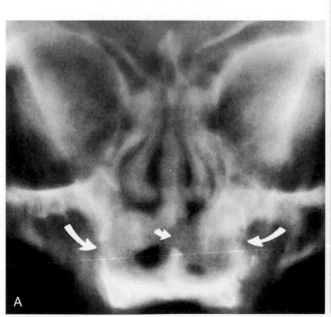

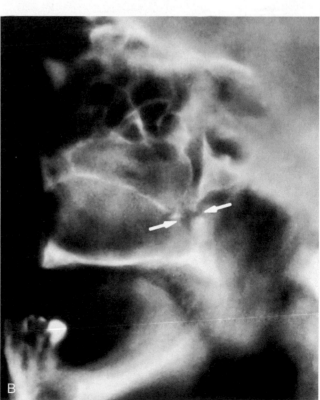

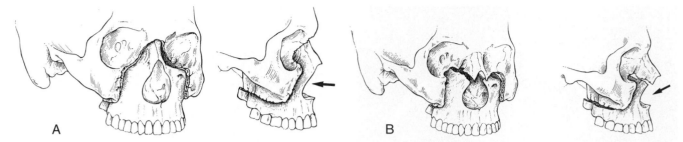

**FIGURE 7-15** Diagram (**A**) of a Le Fort II fracture. The midfacial fracture segment is pyramidal in shape, and these fractures are often called *pyramidal fractures*. Diagram (**B**) of a Wassmund I fracture. This is the same type of fracture as Le Fort II, except that the nasal bones are spared.

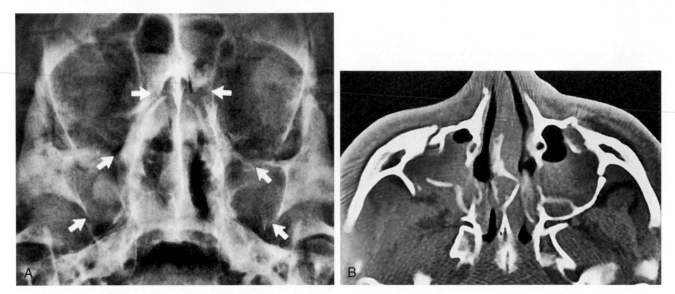

**FIGURE 7-16** Waters view (**A**) shows a Le Fort II fracture (*arrows*) that creates a pyramid-shaped fracture segment. Axial CT scan (**B**) shows a Le Fort II fracture. The midface fracture segment is clearly seen, and the zygomas are uninvolved. On more caudal scans the pterygoid plates were fractured, and on more cranial scans the ethmoid sinuses and orbital floors were fractured.

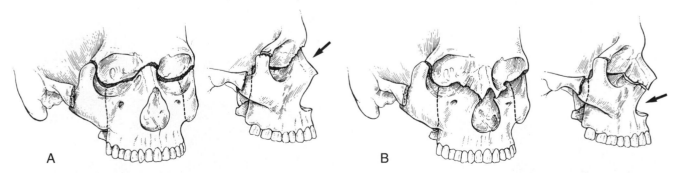

**FIGURE 7-17** Diagram (**A**) of a Le Fort III fracture. There is separation of the viscerocranium and the facial bones. The dotted fracture lines extend down the posterior maxillary sinus walls. The fracture involves the lateral orbital walls and the zygomatic arches. Diagram (**B**) of a Wassmund III fracture. This fracture is similar to the Le Fort III fracture, except that the nasal bones are not involved. The dotted fracture lines extend down the posterior maxillary sinus walls.

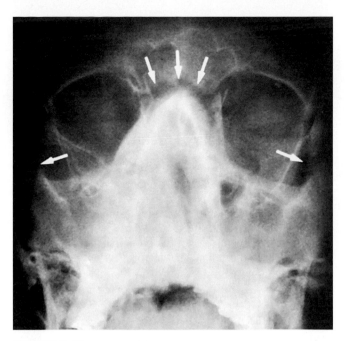

**FIGURE 7-18**   Waters view shows a Le Fort III fracture (*arrows*). Hemorrhage is present in both antra.

**Table 7-1**
**TYPE, FREQUENCY, AND POSTREDUCTION STABILITY OF ZYGOMATIC FRACTURES**

| Fracture Type | Frequency | Postreduction Stability (%) |
|---|---|---|
| Nondisplaced | 11 | 100 |
| Isolated arch | 16 | 93 |
| Rotation around vertical axis | 12 | |
| Medial | 3.5 | 57 |
| Lateral | 8.5 | 88 |
| Rotation around horizontal axis | 6 | |
| Medial | 10 | |
| Lateral | 5 | 50 |
| Displacement without rotation | 31 | |
| Medial | 11.5 | 39 |
| Lateral | 1 | 0 |
| Posterior | 12 | 92 |
| Inferior | 6.5 | 0 |
| Isolated rim | 9.5 | 47 |
| Complex | 14.5 | 0 |

lateral orbital wall that actually goes through two suture lines (zygomaticofrontal and zygomaticosphenoid).

In one study, as many as one-third of all patients who suffered comminuted malar fractures had an ocular disorder, but only 16.7% of patients with a blow-out fracture had ocular problems. Decreased visual acuity was the primary problem accompanying the majority of significant eye injuries.[28–30]

Several classifications of lateral midface fractures have been proposed.[31] Each considers the displacement of the zygoma as it relates to the clinical severity of the fracture and how the malar position may be used to plan treatment. Zygomatic fractures account for 49% to 53% of the midface fractures, and in one study 69% of midfacial fractures involved the zygomatic complex, either alone or in combination with other midface fractures.[7, 31] The reports vary considerably as to the frequency of the different malar fracture positions. One of the more complete classifications, including the fracture type, frequency, and postreduction stability, is shown in Table 7-1.

Before the use of miniplates and microplates, this type of classification allowed the clinician to better predict the postoperative stability of the fracture and thus influence the degree of fixation needed (Figs. 7-20 to 7-25). When the malar eminence is rotated in more than one axis or displaced in more than one direction, the primary rotation and displacement are usually used to classify the fracture. However, these complex cases point out the limitation of any of these classification systems. In the present era, the use of miniplates and microplates is common, and there is little

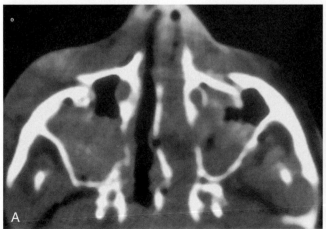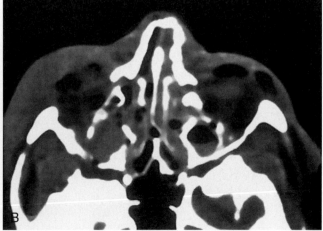

**FIGURE 7-19**   Axial CT scans show a Le Fort III fracture. The more caudal aspects of the fracture (**A**) are similar to those of a Le Fort II fracture. However, the more cranial fractures (**B**) separate the facial bones from the cranium.

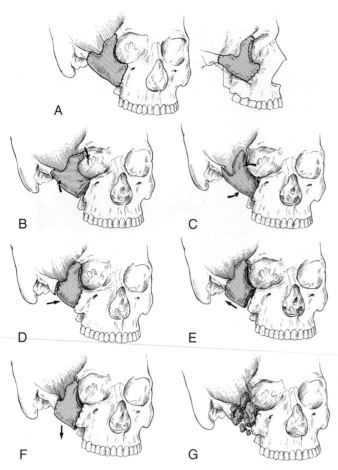

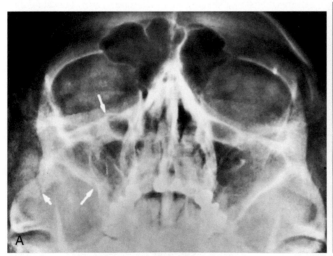

reliance on a classification system to determine the treatment type. It is used by the few surgeons who believe that not all zygomatic fractures need fixation after reduction. It is generally believed that the primary cause of movement of a reduced but nonfixed malar fracture is the masseter muscle's pulling force on the zygoma.[32]

## Zygomaticomaxillary Fractures

Zygomaticomaxillary fractures differ from trimalar fractures in that the former fractures include a maxillary segment. Thus, a zygomaticomaxillary fracture involves the orbital floor, extends down the anterior maxilla (often more medially than in a typical trimalar fracture) near the infraorbital foramen, runs to the premolar region, and then extends across the palate to the maxillary tuberosity and lower pterygoid plates.

## Zygomaticomandibular Fractures

Zygomaticomandibular fractures differ from zygomatic fractures only by the additional fracture of the mandibular condyle, coronoid process, or both.

## Zygomatic Arch Fractures

When there are isolated fractures of the zygomatic arch, there usually are at least three discrete fracture lines, creating two fracture segments. These pieces are displaced medially and downward, reflecting the direction of the impact force. The fracture pieces may impinge on the temporalis muscle or coronoid process of the mandible and interfere with movement of the lower jaw (Figs. 7-26 and 7-27). Trismus is reported in 45% of zygomatic arch fractures and in about 33% of all zygomatic fractures.

**FIGURE 7-20**    Diagram (**A**) of a nondisplaced trimalar zygomatic fracture. Diagram (**B**) of a zygomatic fracture with clockwise (medial) rotation around a horizontal axis (anterior to posterior) through the zygoma. Diagram (**C**) of a zygomatic fracture with counterclockwise (lateral) rotation around a horizontal axis (anterior to posterior) through the zygoma. Diagram (**D**) of a zygomatic fracture with pure medial displacement. Diagram (**E**) of a zygomatic fracture with pure posterior displacement. Diagram (**F**) of a zygomatic fracture with pure inferior displacement. Diagram (**G**) of a zygomatic comminuted (complex) fracture.

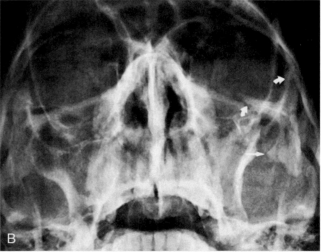

**FIGURE 7-21**    Waters view (**A**) shows a nondisplaced right zygomatic fracture. The fractures through the maxilla and the zygomatic arch are seen (*arrows*). However, the zygomaticofrontal fracture is not visualized because there was only a slight diastasis at this point. Waters view (**B**) shows a left zygomatic fracture that is laterally displaced (*arrow*) and slightly clockwise rotated (*curved arrows*).

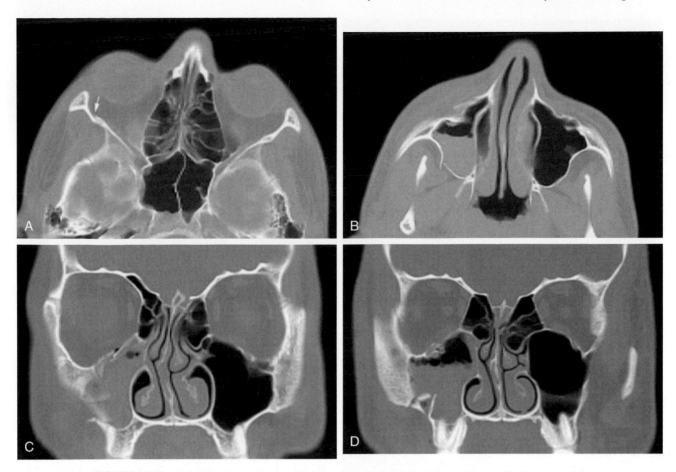

**FIGURE 7-22**    Axial images through the orbit (**A**) and the maxilla (**B**) and coronal images (**C, D**) show a right trimalar fracture. The right frontosphenoid fracture is minimally displaced (*arrow* in **A**), and the zygoma is inferiorly and posteriorly displaced. Hemorrhage is present in the right antrum, and a small amount of orbital emphysema is present.

## Blow-out and Blow-in Orbital Wall Fractures

Fractures of the orbital floor may occur as either simple or comminuted fractures in conjunction with midfacial fractures, with atypical periorbital fractures (orbital roof), or as isolated blow-out fractures.

The term *orbital blow-out fracture* describes the injury that results from a blow to the orbit by an object that is too large to enter the orbit (fist, baseball, etc.). The force of the blow is absorbed by the orbital rim and is transmitted to the thinner orbital floor, which shatters, usually in the middle third near the infraorbital canal (presumably the floor is

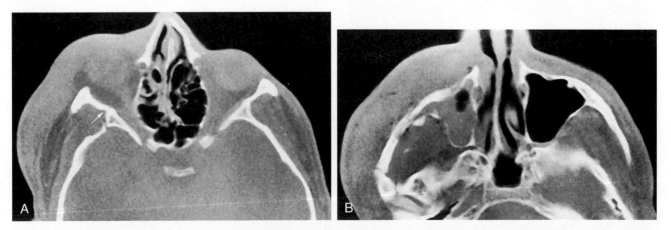

**FIGURE 7-23**    Axial CT scans through the orbit (**A**) and the zygomatic arch (**B**) show a right zygomatic fracture with posterior displacement and clockwise (medial) rotation of the zygoma. The site of the zygomatico-frontosphenoid fracture is also seen (*arrow* in **A**).

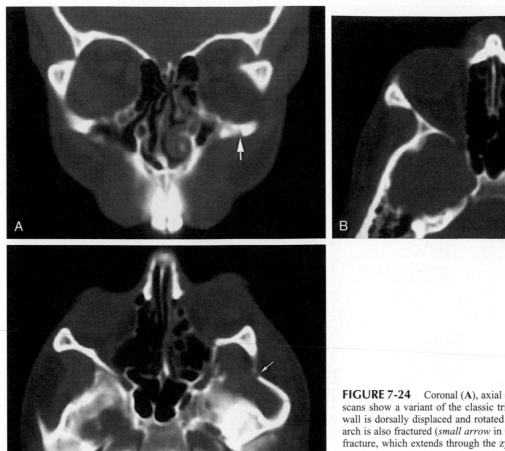

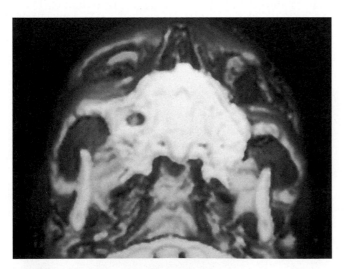

**FIGURE 7-24**  Coronal (**A**), axial (**B**), and more caudal axial (**C**) CT scans show a variant of the classic trimalar fracture. The lateral orbital wall is dorsally displaced and rotated counterclockwise. The zygomatic arch is also fractured (*small arrow* in **C**). Rather than the more common fracture, which extends through the zygomaticomaxillary suture region, this fracture extends through the lateral zygoma or lower lateral orbital wall (*large arrow* in **A**).

**FIGURE 7-25**  Three-dimensional reconstruction on a patient with a left trimalar fracture. The zygoma is posteriorly displaced compared with the normal right side. The white area in the center of the picture is the hard palate seen en face. Most of the mandible was removed from the computerized picture.

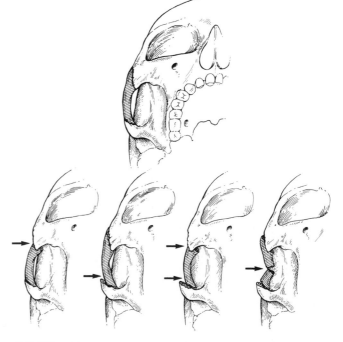

**FIGURE 7-26**  Diagram of different types of isolated zygomatic arch fractures. The last type may impinge medially on the coronoid process of the mandible.

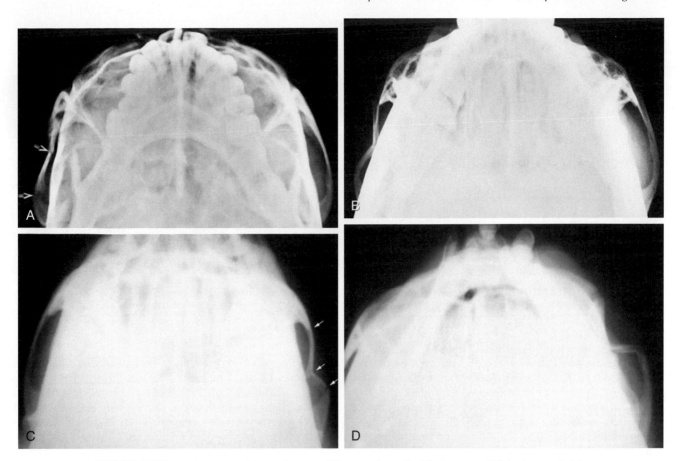

**FIGURE 7-27**   Underpenetrated base views on different patients. In (**A**) there are slightly depressed right zygomatic arch fractures (*arrows*). In (**B**) there is a solitary right depressed zygomatic arch segment. In order to create this type of depression, there must be at least three fractures. In (**C**) a left zygomatic arch depressed fracture similar to that seen in (**B**) is present, and the actual three fractures (*arrows*) are more clearly seen. In (**D**), there is a more severely depressed left zygomatic arch fracture that impinges on the coronoid process of the mandible and locked mandibular motion.

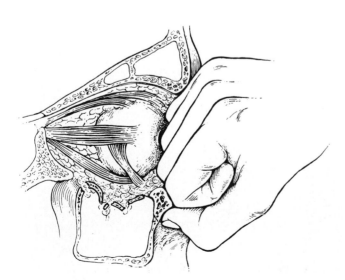

**FIGURE 7-28**   Diagram of blow-out fracture. The impacting object is larger than the orbital rim diameter. The blow fractures the orbital floor and pushes the eye back. The eye then displaces the fractured floor into the maxillary sinus.

weakened by the presence of the infraorbital canal, which is often also dehiscent). As the eye is pushed back into the conical orbital apex, it increases intraorbital pressure and this "blows out" the fractured floor into the maxillary sinus. Usually the orbital rim is not fractured (pure blow-out fracture) and the globe remains undamaged. Less commonly the inferior orbital rim also is fractured; this is referred to as an impure blow-out fracture. Blow-out fractures represent only 3% to 5% of all midface fractures (Figs. 7-28 to 7-34).[33]

Herniation of orbital fat, inferior rectus muscle, and inferior oblique muscle can occur with occasional muscle entrapment in the fracture line, resulting in diplopia on upward gaze. However, diplopia is the most frequent complaint in all patients with blow-out fractures and may occur solely because of periorbital edema and hemorrhage, which exert pressure on the globe. This type of diplopia resolves in several days, whereas entrapment diplopia remains. If the cause of diplopia is in doubt, a traction test can be performed on the inferior muscles. Rarely a depression fracture of the orbital roof or superior orbital rim can impinge on the upper globe, prohibiting upward gaze and clinically mimicking an inferior muscle entrapment (Fig. 7-35). Imaging studies clarify this situation. In these

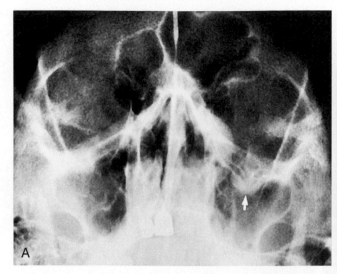
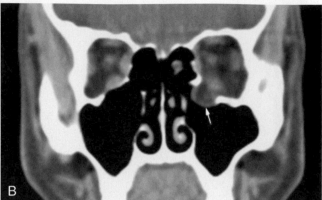

**FIGURE 7-29**    Waters view (**A**) shows polypoid soft-tissue mass in the roof of the left antrum (*arrow*). This was a blow-out fracture of the orbital floor. Coronal CT scan (**B**) shows a blow-out fracture of the left orbital floor. The herniated soft tissues (*arrow*) mimic an antral polyp on plain films.

latter cases, communication with the base of the anterior cranial fossa can lead to CSF leakage into the orbit or herniation of meninges or brain through the fracture line.

Rarely the orbital floor fracture segments can herniate upward into the orbit, impinging on the inferior orbital muscles or the globe. This unusual occurrence has been called a blow-in fracture, and on imaging it must be clearly identified so that the clinician can reposition this fractured bone. Laceration of the globe can rarely occur.[10, 34]

Despite the fact that many reports have indicated that the middle third of the orbital floor is the weakest portion of the orbit, the thin lamina papyracea of the medial wall should theoretically be the weakest area. In one study of clinically suspected orbital blow-out fractures evaluated with CT scans, the most common fracture was an isolated medial wall fracture (55%), followed by medial and inferior wall fractures (27%). The most common facial fracture associated with a medial wall fracture was a nasal fracture (51%), not an inferior wall fracture (33%). This suggests that the force causing a nasal fracture is an important causative factor in creating a pure medial wall fracture. Of patients with medial wall fractures, 25% had diplopia and 40% had enophthalmos.[35]

In another article analyzing 2741 patients with facial fractures, 273 patients (9.9%) were identified with 304 medial orbital wall fractures. The male-to-female ratio was 5:1, and most injuries involved the left orbit. Most fractures were caused by fist fights, but more complex injuries were noted secondary to car accidents and falls. The fractures were divided into types based on the location and severity of

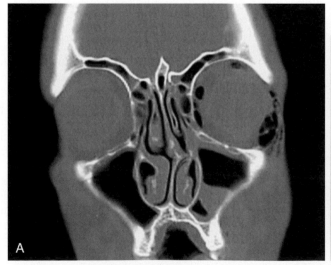
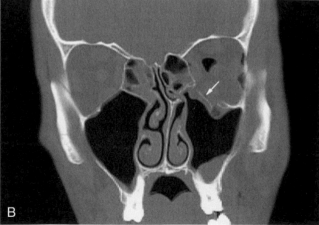

**FIGURE 7-30**    Coronal CT scans. In (**A**) there is an intact orbital rim anteriorly. In (**B**) there is an orbital floor fracture (*arrow*) in the midfloor just posterior to the orbital rim. This was a pure blow-out fracture. The fracture is just medial to the infraorbital canal, and this patient had hypesthesia in the cheek. Secretions are seen in both ethmoid sinuses, and hemorrhage occurred in the left antrum. There is also subcutaneous and orbital emphysema.

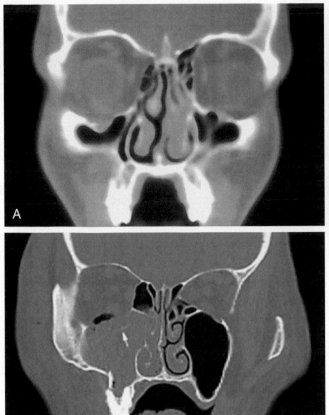

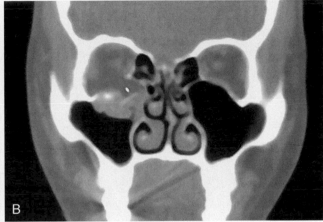

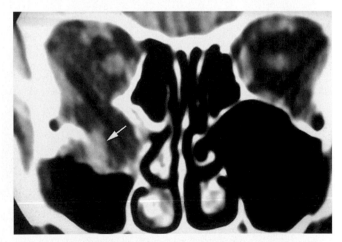

**FIGURE 7-31**   Coronal CT scans. In (**A**) there is a small, depressed blow-out fracture of the right orbital floor. In (**B**) there is a comminuted right orbital floor fracture that also involves the lower medial orbital wall. A large, depressed bone fragment is seen in the antrum. In (**C**), there is hemorrhage within the right antrum and nasal fossa. There is a depressed, comminuted fracture (*arrow*) of the orbital floor. There is also orbital emphysema and another fracture of the lower antral wall.

the injury. Type I fractures were confined to the medial orbital wall. Type II fractures involved the medial orbital wall and continuous orbital floor. Type III fractures involved the medial orbital wall and orbital floor and malar fractures. Type IV fractures involved the medial orbital wall and complex midfacial injuries. Although visual loss (2%), diplopia (41%), and enophthalmos (12%) were seen, diplopia and enophthalmos were commonly observed with type II injuries. Imaging studies showed that about 52% of

the fractures were associated with prolapse of orbital fat, but only 43% could be diagnosed on plain films.[36]

Thus, fractures of the medial orbital wall can occur either as isolated fractures or in conjunction with orbital floor fractures or more complex fractures. Traditionally, such medial wall fractures were considered to accompany nearly 50% of orbital floor fractures, but as discussed, the incidence may be far greater. Often the ethmoid fracture is poorly visualized on plain films, with only some clouding of the

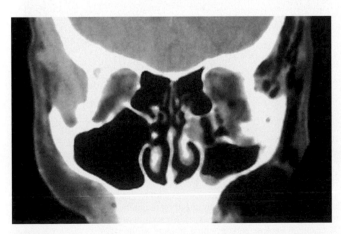

**FIGURE 7-32**   Coronal CT scan shows a moderately large blow-out fracture in the floor and medial wall of the left orbit. Orbital emphysema is also present.

**FIGURE 7-33**   Coronal CT scan shows a large right orbital floor blow-out fracture. The inferior rectus muscle (*arrow*) is depressed into the fracture. This muscle was entrapped on the lateral fracture margin.

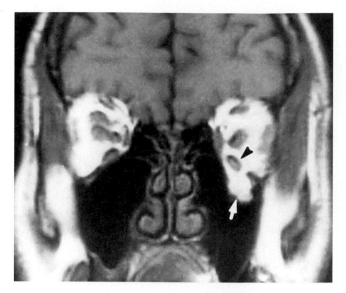

**FIGURE 7-34**    Coronal T1-weighted MR image shows a left blow-out fracture. Fat has herniated into the left antrum (*arrow*), and there is minimal depression of the inferior rectus muscle (*arrowhead*).

ethmoid cells being evident. Even on CT scans, if there is no bone displacement, the actual fractures may not be identified. However, on CT, fat that has herniated into the fractured ethmoid complex is well visualized (Figs. 7-36 to 7-41). Herniated fat can also be identified on MR imaging, although small fracture segments may not be identified. Muscle entrapment in these fractures is rare.[37] The only imaging differential diagnosis is a congenital dehiscence of the lamina papyracea (actually, a hypoplasia of the ethmoid complex). In congenital dehiscence, on CT and MR imaging, portions of the lamina papyracea are either not visualized or are medially bowed and orbital fat lies in the ethmoid complex. However, unlike in trauma cases, the margins of the defect are smooth and there is no history of trauma.

Medial wall fractures can also be inferred by the presence of orbital emphysema. Such orbital air most commonly comes from an ethmoid sinus fracture and rarely results from an isolated maxillary fracture. The infrequent occurrence of orbital emphysema with orbital floor blow-out fractures is attributed to the rapid sealing of the fracture by edema, hemorrhage, and periorbital herniation of orbital fat

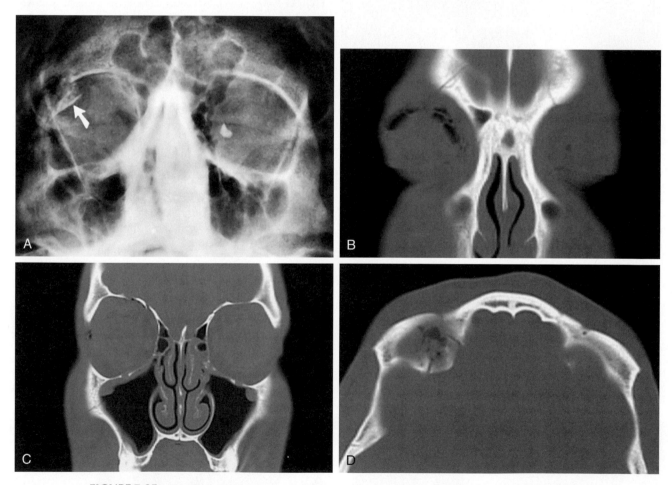

**FIGURE 7-35**    Waters view (**A**) shows a depressed orbital roof fracture (*arrow*) that impinged on the globe and clinically mimicked a blow-out fracture of the orbital floor with entrapment. A foreign body is also seen in the left eye. Coronal anterior (**B**) and posterior (**C**) and axial (**D**) CT scans on another patient with a fracture of the right frontal bone and orbital roof. There is minimal displacement of the right orbital roof fracture, as well as orbital emphysema and a small amount of extradural air. There is also a similar nondisplaced left frontal and orbital roof fracture.

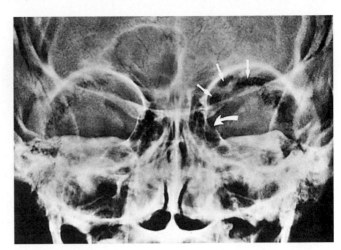

**FIGURE 7-36**    Caldwell view shows orbital emphysema (*three arrows*) and a defect in the left lamina papyracea (*curved arrow*). This was a medial wall blow-out fracture.

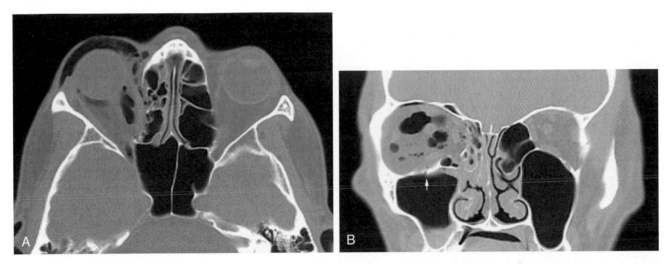

**FIGURE 7-37**    Axial (**A**) and coronal (**B**) CT scans show a comminuted right medial wall blow-out fracture with extensive orbital emphysema. There is also a right orbital floor fracture (*arrow* in **B**). Hemorrhage is present in the right ethmoid sinuses.

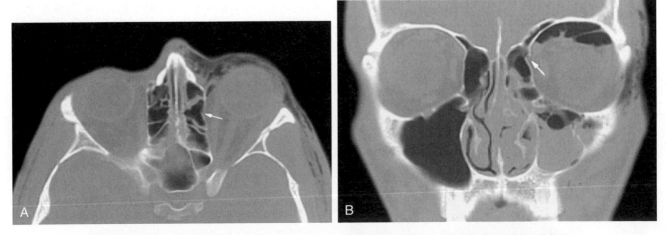

**FIGURE 7-38**    Axial (**A**) and coronal (**B**) CT scans show left orbital emphysema. In (**A**), the medial wall fracture is not as well seen (*arrow*) as it is in (**B**) (*arrow*). Minimal hemorrhage is present in the left ethmoid sinuses. Hemorrhage and secretions are present in the left maxillary sinus.

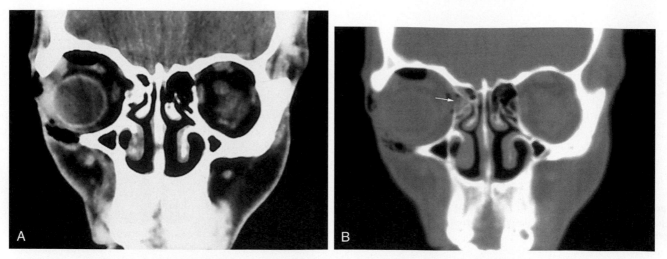

**FIGURE 7-39**   Coronal CT scans at soft-tissue (**A**) and bone (**B**) settings show a medial wall right blow-out fracture (*arrow* in **B**). There is also orbital emphysema. Note how much more difficult it is to detect the findings in (**A**).

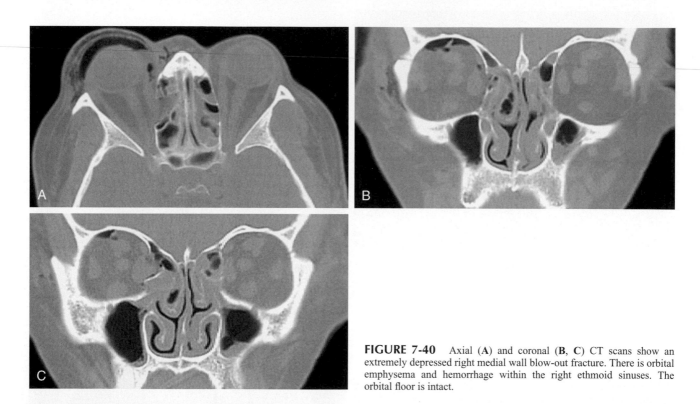

**FIGURE 7-40**   Axial (**A**) and coronal (**B, C**) CT scans show an extremely depressed right medial wall blow-out fracture. There is orbital emphysema and hemorrhage within the right ethmoid sinuses. The orbital floor is intact.

**FIGURE 7-41**   Axial CT scan shows a left medial wall blow-out fracture with a large herniation of orbital fat into the fracture site. This is the type of fracture that can result in chronic enophthalmos.

and muscle. Orbital emphysema develops after an ethmoid fracture when nose blowing by the patient increases intranasal pressure, which in turn raises the intrasinus pressure and forces air into the orbit. In most patients, refraining from nose blowing allows the fracture line to seal and the orbital air to resorb.[10]

Rarely, air can enter the orbit from a complex fracture involving the frontal or sphenoid sinuses. However, these cases are associated with severe facial trauma, and the source of the air becomes evident on imaging studies. Even more rarely, pneumomediastinum can occur following a blow-out fracture.[38]

The two clinical indications for immediate surgery on an orbital blow-out fracture are definite muscle entrapment and acute enophthalmos. In the most dramatic case, the globe is almost completely displaced into the maxillary sinus and there are reports of complete globe herniation into a fractured maxillary sinus.[39–41] However, milder and more common degrees of acute enophthalmos may take several days to confirm clinically because of the presence of periorbital edema and hemorrhage.

The development of chronic enophthalmos is also to be avoided, because it leads to cosmetic deformity and in some cases diplopia. Chronic enophthalmos develops when too much orbital fat has herniated from the orbit. Although initially the increased orbital volume clinically goes unnoticed because of compensatory intraorbital edema, the subsequent loss of edema, scarring, and lipogranulation of the herniated tissues eventually cause sufficient volume loss that the globe recedes. The patients who are at greatest risk are those who have sizable herniations of fat into one sinus (maxillary or ethmoid) or moderate herniations into both medial wall and orbital floor fractures. The imager must draw the clinician's attention to any such cases that may have the potential to develop chronic enophthalmos, even in the absence of acute enophthalmos or muscle entrapment.

Alloplasts are often used to reconstruct the orbital floor where they have been effective in the long-term reconstruction of this orbital margin. However, such products rarely work effectively in the long-term attempted repair of the medial orbital wall, as invariably there is movement of the alloplast. The products most often used include Teflon, Silastic, and Marlex mesh, all of which have the benefit of not being absorbed.[42] However, these alloplasts have the disadvantages of extrusion and infection. They can be identified on CT, which is a useful modality to detect early displacement of the graft.

On plain films, soft-tissue swelling over the inferior orbital rim, antral opacification with or without an air-fluid level, and subcutaneous emphysema in the cheek are often the only indirect signs of a blow-out fracture. An actual depressed or displaced orbital floor bone fragment may not be seen. Occasionally a soft-tissue polypoid density can be visualized in the antral roof. This may represent the site of the blow-out fracture filled with orbital contents and hemorrhage or it may represent an unrelated antral cyst or polyp. Only on coronal CT or MR imaging can the actual fracture and herniated tissue be clearly seen. A completely displaced piece of bone, a trapdoor fracture, or a hinged fracture can then be identified, as can the typical "teardrop" herniation of orbital contents. On CT the orbital fat may be of a higher attenuation than expected because of hemorrhage; in some cases an antral air-blood level may be present.[22] On MR imaging, the high T1-weighted signal intensity of the orbital fat and any hemorrhage can be well seen; however, a small bone fracture segment may not be identified.

Supraorbital roof fractures are uncommon, and the incidence has been reported to be between 1% and 5%. In one study of 621 patients with facial fractures, 9.3% had supraorbital roof fractures. The average age of these patients was 31 years, and the predominant mechanism of injury was from motor vehicle accidents. Sixty-nine percent of the patients had associated skull fractures and 54% had frontal sinus fractures. Dural tears were present in 14 patients, traumatic encephalocele in 3, proptosis in 6, pulsatile proptosis in 3, orbital apex syndrome in 1, persistent CSF leak in 3, and meningitis in 5. A majority of the patients had associated intracranial bleeds.[43]

## FRONTAL SINUS FRACTURES

Frontal sinus fractures are the result of either direct trauma or an extension of a calvarial fracture into the sinus. Of all the fractures involving the frontal sinuses, 67% are limited to the anterior table, 28% involve both the anterior and posterior sinus walls, and only 5% are limited to the posterior sinus table.[44] Most commonly a linear fracture occurs in the anterior sinus wall. This fracture tears the mucosa and produces hemorrhage, edema, and sinus opacification. The fracture line may extend downward, often involving the superomedial orbital rim (Figs. 7-42 to 7-48).

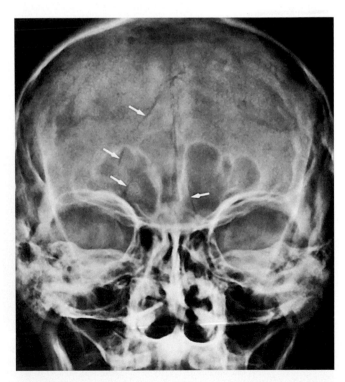

**FIGURE 7-42**   Caldwell view shows a comminuted fracture of the frontal bone (*arrows*) that extends into the frontal sinus.

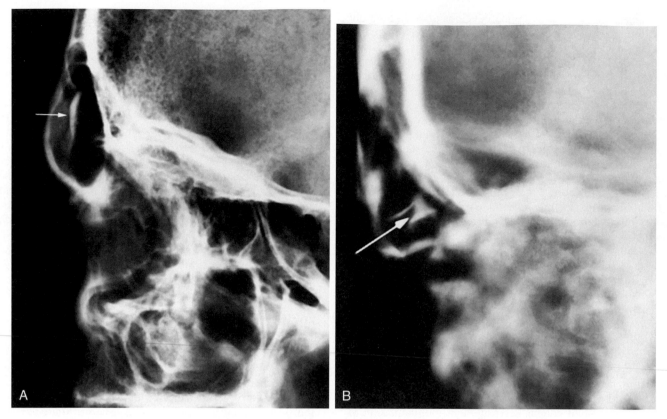

**FIGURE 7-43**   Lateral plain film (**A**) shows a depressed anterior frontal sinus wall fracture (*arrow*). Lateral tomogram film (**B**) shows a depressed fracture (*arrow*) of the anterior wall and floor of the frontal sinus.

Comminuted fractures of the anterior wall also occur and frequently reflect the size and shape of the object causing the fracture. On plain film Caldwell and Waters views, only a vague density may appear in the frontal sinus. However, on a lateral view, bone fragments may be identified within the sinus. Axial CT most clearly confirms the presence of such depressed fractures, which often are clinically unobserved because the forehead soft-tissue depression is filled by edema and hemorrhage.[45]

Complex fractures of both the anterior and posterior frontal sinus tables usually are associated with other midfacial fractures. Isolated fractures of the posterior sinus wall are rare. They occur either as an extension of a skull base fracture or as an extension of a calvarial fracture.[46–49] Any fracture involving the posterior frontal sinus wall opens communication with the dural spaces, and CSF leakage into the sinus and intracranial infection or a pneumocele can develop. Rarely, orbital emphysema or CSF leakage into the orbit can result from frontal sinus fractures. In one study of CT scans on patients with suspected intracranial posttrau-

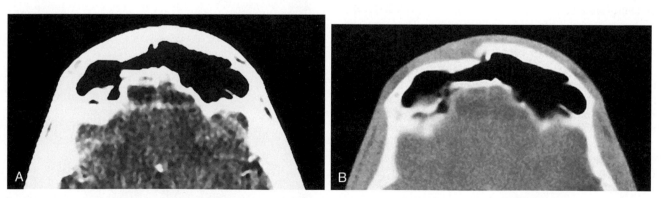

**FIGURE 7-44**   Axial CT scans seen at narrow window settings (**A**) and wide window settings (**B**). In (**A**) there is no obvious depression of the forehead, nor is there an obvious fracture of the right anterior frontal sinus table. In (**B**) the fracture is clearly seen. There was no soft-tissue depression in the forehead because the defect was filled with hemorrhage and edema fluid.

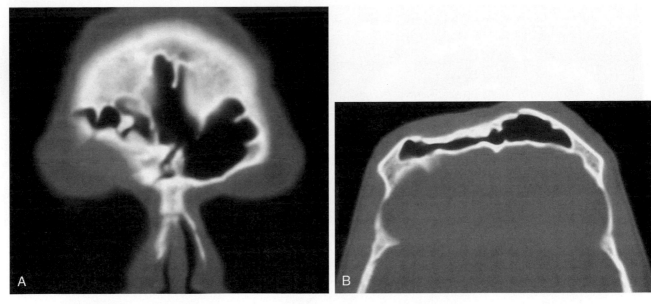

**FIGURE 7-45**   Coronal (**A**) and axial (**B**) CT scans show a depressed comminuted fracture of the right anterior frontal sinus table that also involves the right orbital roof.

matic injuries, 90% of the patients had a frontal sinus fracture identified on the initial CT scan. Complex fractures involving the anterior and posterior walls accounted for 65% of the cases, and isolated anterior wall (24%) or posterior wall (11%) fractures were less common.[45] This study reflects the severity of the trauma that led to both the fractures and the intracranial damage. In fact, it has been determined that it takes two to three times the force to fracture the frontal sinus than it does to fracture the zygoma, maxilla, or mandible.[50]

In general, nondisplaced frontal sinus fractures are treated conservatively. Uncomplicated anterior table fractures with cosmetic deformity are treated by fragment reduction and stabilization, usually with microplates or miniplates. Nasofrontal duct obstruction is usually managed by sinus obliteration. Finally, comminuted, displaced anterior and posterior table fractures, especially those associated with persistent CSF leakage, are often treated by frontal sinus cranialization.[47]

## SPHENOID SINUS FRACTURES

Fractures of the sphenoid sinus seldom occur, but when they do, they are associated with severe cranial trauma and basilar skull fractures. Often, these patients are recumbent due to the associated intracranial injuries. In these cases, sphenoid opacification or a sphenoid sinus air-fluid level may indicate intrasinus hemorrhage, leakage of CSF directly into the sinus from a sphenoid sinus fracture, CSF drainage into the sinus via the nasopharynx from a temporal bone fracture in a patient with an intact tympanic membrane, poor sinus drainage due to supine position, and edema around indwelling nasogastric or orotracheal tubes. Rarely, milder trauma to the midfacial region may extend back into the

sphenoid sinus. If the fracture injures the adjacent internal carotid arteries or cavernous sinuses, these events may be life-threatening.

## PEDIATRIC FACIAL FRACTURES

When compared with the adult skeleton, the pediatric facial bones behave differently with regard to fracture patterns, healing, and treatment. The inherent elasticity of the facial bones in a young patient is advantageous in trauma because the bone yields more easily and does not fracture as readily as it does in an adult.[1] When a fracture does occur, the thick, elastic periosteum usually prevents bone displacement and a green-stick fracture results. In addition, fractures heal faster in children than in adults, so the period of immobilization is shorter. However, if treatment is delayed, the fragments may become fixed, making fracture reduction more difficult. Malocclusions in the primary dentition that are not completely corrected may be spontaneously compensated for by the secondary dentition or may be treated by orthodontic therapy.[1]

Although children have many advantages in terms of healing, they are at a disadvantage with regard to dentition. In 30% to 50% of pediatric facial fractures, the tooth germs lie in the fracture. These teeth fall out during healing or have delayed development and deformities that do not manifest clinically until the permanent teeth erupt. Facial fractures also can damage the bony growth centers and result in osseous hypoplasia, functional abnormalities, and cosmetic deformities. Some clinicians believe that the child's parents should be informed of these potential problems at the time of the initial injury.

Children generally have too few teeth for fixation splints,

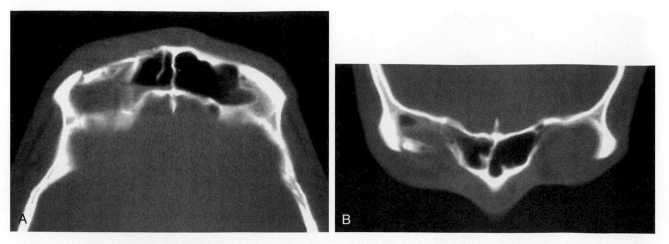

**FIGURE 7-46**  Axial (**A**) and coronal (**B**) CT scans show a fracture involving the right orbital roof and the lower anterior frontal sinus table.

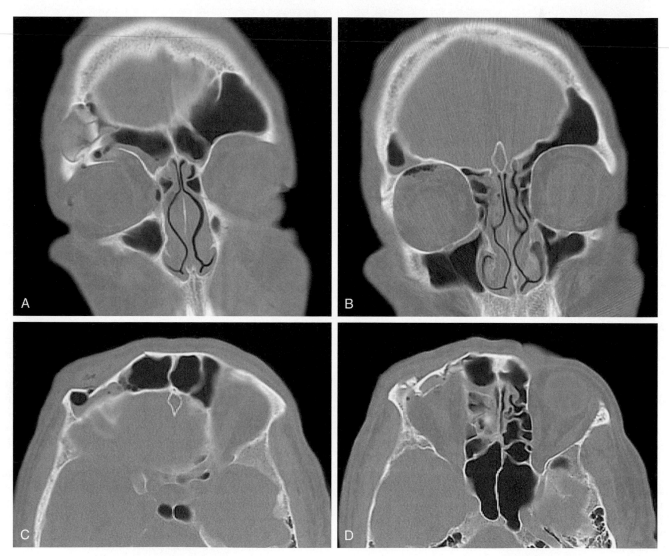

**FIGURE 7-47**  Coronal anterior (**A**) and posterior (**B**) CT scans and axial cranial (**C**) and caudal (**D**) CT scans show a comminuted right frontal sinus fracture that involves the anterior table and the roof of the orbit. A fracture segment impinges on the upper globe and prevents upward gaze. Orbital emphysema is also present.

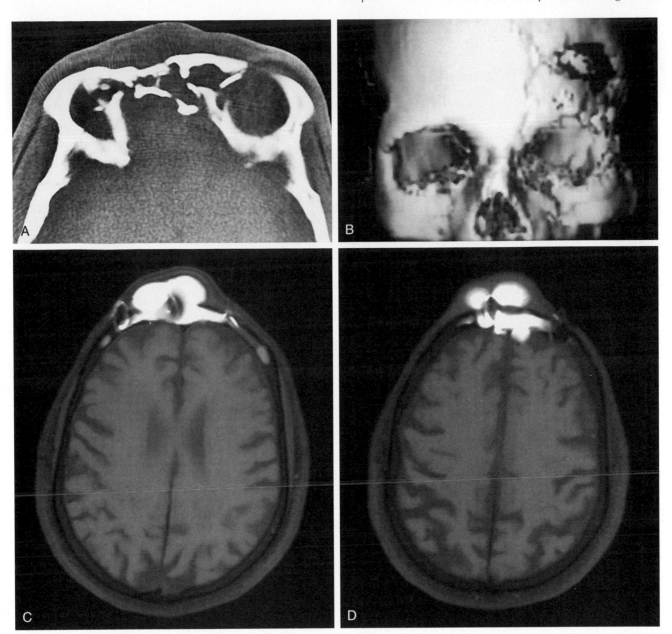

**FIGURE 7-48**   Axial CT scan (**A**) shows a comminuted midfacial fracture that involves the orbital roof bilaterally, as well as the anterior and posterior frontal sinus walls. Coronal 3D reconstructed image (**B**) on a different patient shows a markedly depressed left frontal bone fracture that involved the lateral margin of the left frontal sinus. As in Figure 7-42, frontal bone fractures often may involve the frontal sinuses. Axial T1-weighted, fat-suppressed MR images (**C, D**) on a patient who had prior frontal sinus trauma and an osteoplastic flap repair and then reinjured the frontal sinus. Hemorrhage has occurred within the flap fat, expanding it through the anterior and posterior fracture defects.   *Illustration continued on following page*

and treatment plans must be modified from those used in adult patients. No wire ligatures can be placed in children under 2 years of age. After this age, it may be possible to fix interdental wires and arch bars if the primary teeth have not been damaged by caries and their crowns have an adequately retentive form. However, with the appearance of interdental spaces caused by eruption of the secondary teeth, the possibility of fixing dental splints becomes less likely. Similarly, erupted permanent teeth can accept such ligatures only after their greatest convexity has passed the gingival margin. This period lasts from about the fifth to the eighth years of life.[1]

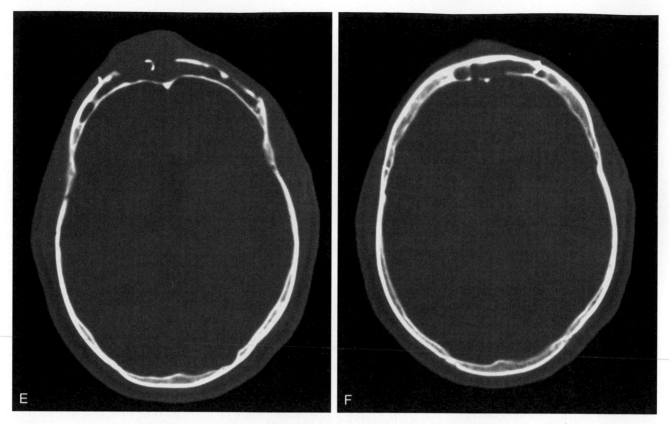

**FIGURE 7-48**    *Continued.* Corresponding axial CT scans (**E, F**) show the bone defects.

## SECTION TWO

# POSTOPERATIVE SINONASAL CAVITIES

## IMAGING EVALUATIONS

The proper imaging evaluation of the postoperative patient requires the radiologist to be knowledgeable about a number of facts, some of which are often obscure at the time of performing and then interpreting the imaging examination. Ideally, the radiologist should know what operation was performed, when it was done, and what disease prompted it. Familiarity with the various surgical procedures enables the radiologist to determine which bone(s), if any, can be expected to be removed, what soft-tissue defects may be created, and what soft tissue or foreign material is usually placed to repair the surgical defect. This knowledge is essential for proper imaging interpretation and should help prevent the misdiagnosis of a surgical defect as a site of bone erosion or a muscle-fascia graft as a tumor recurrence.

The interval between the surgery and the time of imaging helps the radiologist determine the type of soft-tissue reaction to expect. For recent surgery, the primary healing reaction is active inflammation with edema and possible hemorrhage. However, if the surgery was performed months

to years ago, the primary expected healing reaction is mature granulation tissue or vascularized scar with varying degrees of fibrosis. In some patients, a reactive bony sclerosis may occur after those procedures that denude mucosa. Such a reaction requires time to develop and produce sufficient bone thickening to possibly reduce the sinus cavity size. This is a reactive process to the surgery and, although it may appear the same on imaging as the sclerosis associated with chronic inflammation, there is no evidence of active disease or pain in the majority of these patients. However, in some patients, recurrent sinusitis can coexist with the reactive postoperative changes. In these cases, one cannot know whether the bone changes are attributable to the active inflammation, the postoperative reaction, or both.

Knowledge of the disease process that initially prompted the surgery allows the radiologist to anticipate the types of imaging changes to expect. Thus, if the initial disease was chronic infection, one may commonly expect recurrent sinus mucosal thickening, reactive bone sclerosis and thickening, and possible nasal polyposis. If the initial disease was a granulomatous process, one may expect sinus mucosal thickening, nasal mucosal changes, septal erosions, and bone erosions intermixed with areas of reactive bone. If the initial disease was a tumor, the concern will be to characterize any nodular or localized soft-tissue disease, differentiate recurrent tumor from infection, and observe the presence of progressive bone erosion or soft-tissue extension to areas not normally involved by the surgery.

The best and most efficacious way to interpret a

postoperative imaging study, especially on a patient with a malignancy, is to compare it with a prior examination. Initially, this is best accomplished by comparing a follow-up study to a baseline postoperative CT or MR examination. This baseline scan is important for the imaging monitoring of a patient after surgery because it provides an anatomic reference with which all future examinations can be compared. If this baseline study is obtained too close to the time of surgery, the imaging findings are dominated by changes of hemorrhage and edema and thus may give a false impression of what the eventual stable postoperative appearance will be. However, if one waits too long after surgery, recurrent disease may be present. The best compromise appears to be a postoperative waiting period of 6 to 8 weeks. This time allows most of the hemorrhage and edema to resolve, whereas few if any tumors (or chronic inflammatory diseases) will recur within this period.[51, 52]

Although the baseline study is less important in patients with inflammatory disease, it still provides a reference standard against which future imaging studies can be compared, and a few physicians routinely obtain such a study for future comparison.

On subsequent follow-up CT or MR examinations, any progressive soft-tissue resolution can be interpreted as a further reduction of any postoperative edema and inflammation. However, the appearance of any new soft-tissue changes, or sites of bone erosion, must be considered recurrent disease until proven otherwise. Patients who have been operated on for inflammatory disease usually do not need periodic follow-up scans and are only imaged if symptoms reappear. By comparison, those patients who have been operated on for tumors should have scheduled periodic follow-up scans if early tumor recurrences are to be diagnosed. The time interval between these examinations usually is 4 to 6 months for the first 2 or 3 postoperative years and then 6 to 12 months for the next 2 to 3 years.[51, 52]

Plain films do not allow detailed evaluation of the postoperative patient because of the overall survey nature of these studies and the unique anatomy of the paranasal sinuses, where focal soft-tissue disease is best assessed by its relationship to the adjacent bone (which may now be resected) and sinus cavity air (which may be obscured by fibrosis or disease). Thus CT and MR imaging are the examinations of choice in monitoring the course of postoperative patients. CT allows the detailed evaluation of bone and a fairly accurate assessment of the soft tissues, provided that both axial and coronal views are available. The use of contrast is desirable because it provides some distinction between inflammatory tissue, tumor, and scar.

MR imaging offers the possibility of further differentiating recurrent tumors from sites of active infection. However, even when contrast is used, the distinction between vascularized scar and tumor may be impossible and early bone erosions may go undetected.[53] Tumor invasion into marrow-containing bone is, however, usually detected earlier on MR imaging than on CT.

Ultimately the examination of choice depends on the surgical procedure and the disease. In general, recurrent inflammatory disease is best followed on CT. The appearance of mucosal thickening is easily identified, and interval changes can be assessed by comparison to a previous CT study.

The radiologist is presented with more serious diagnostic problems when following a patient with a tumor, as the distinction between inflammatory disease, scar, and tumor is of critical importance. On CT, inflammatory secretions and reactions tend to have lower attenuation than most sinonasal tumors. On contrast-enhanced CT, active inflammatory changes tend to enhance more than most tumors. However, variations in this pattern commonly exist, and in many cases vascularized scar tissue cannot be confidently differentiated from either inflammation or tumor.

On MR imaging, inflammatory tissues usually have a low to intermediate T1-weighted and a high T2-weighted signal intensity. As mentioned in Chapter 6, about 95% of sinonasal tumors have intermediate signal intensity on all imaging sequences. Thus, in most cases, a good distinction can be made between tumor and adjacent inflammation.[54] On contrast-enhanced MR imaging, inflammatory tissues enhance intensely, and they tend to follow the contour of the sinus cavity wall fairly smoothly. Tumors, on the other hand, usually enhance only moderately and have a distinctly nodular configuration. As mentioned, the vascularized scar tissue that often develops in the postoperative sinonasal cavities has the identical imaging characteristics as tumor on both CT and MR imaging. Ultimately the distinction between these tissues is made either by comparing the imaging findings on serial studies or by biopsy of any suspicious regions. In general, MR imaging is the preferred modality to follow patients with sinonasal tumors. Newer approaches to detect early tumor recurrence include the use of MR spectroscopy and PET scanning. These topics are discussed in Chapter 45.

# OPERATIVE PROCEDURES

## NASAL SURGERY

Although surgery on the nose is primarily cosmetic, posttraumatic airway reconstruction accounts for many procedures. Surgery confined to the nasal or septal cartilages rarely leaves an imaging identification. However, during a rhinoplasty, use of the saw, chisel, and file to remove bone leaves a slight irregularity along the midline contour of the nasal bones. This is best seen on lateral plain films of the nose (Fig. 7-49). The nasal bones are also purposely fractured in cases of nasal bone "hump" removal. Once this bony mound has been removed, the resulting broad nasal base is cosmetically too wide. Because of this, the lateral nasal walls are fractured and turned inward, re-creating a thin midline nasal contour. Such iatrogenic fractures may mimic a recent traumatic fracture, and only the patient's history may resolve any confusion. After 6 to 12 months, the sharp edges of all nasal fractures become smooth, and the fracture lines are less sharply identified. Old fractures also can prove confusing when evaluating recent nasal trauma.

In more severe nasal injuries in which the nasal bones have been crushed, cartilage or rib implants may be used to reconstruct a normal nasal contour. These implants give a unique radiographic appearance that, once identified, indicates to the imager that reconstructive surgery was performed (Figs. 7-50 to 7-52).

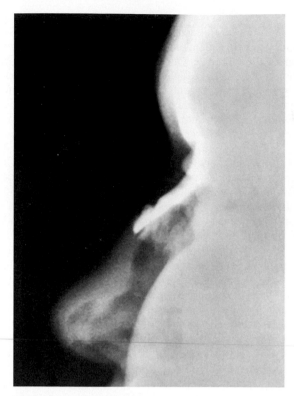

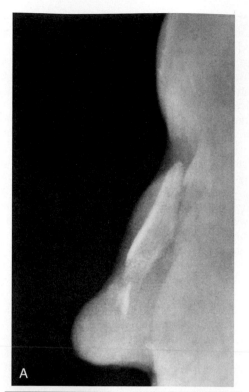

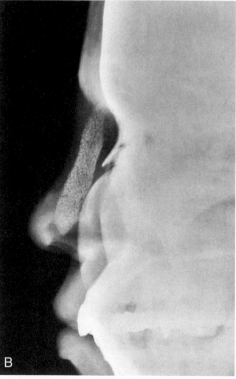

**FIGURE 7-49** Lateral plain film shows a patient who has had a prior rhinoplasty. The irregularity of the nasal bone contour is postsurgical in etiology.

The topics of endoscopic sinonasal surgery and the post-operative complications associated with this surgery are covered in Chapters 3 and 4. The following discussion concerns those more classic, nonendoscopic operations.

## FRONTAL SINUS SURGERY

### Trephination

Statistically, most frontal sinus disease stems from infection and can be classified as acute or chronic. In acute infections, especially if an air-fluid level is found on plain films or imaging, factors such as the time to diagnosis and the patient's immediate response to treatment determine whether a trephination (essentially an incision and drainage) procedure should be performed. The operation consists of drilling a small hole 0.5 to 1 cm to the side of the midline, usually near the upper edge of the eyebrow. After the sinus is entered and drained (the sinus mucosa is not stripped), a drainage tube or cannula is placed in the sinus for 8 to 14 days, after which it is removed to prevent a foreign body reaction in the sinus mucosa.[55] Most often the surgeon determines, by means of a Caldwell view, the sinus size and the presence of any sinus loculations. Care must be taken so that the drill does not enter either the orbit below, the anterior cranial fossa through the posterior sinus wall, or, for a small sinus, the calvarium outside of the sinus margin. The surgical defect is poorly visualized on coronal and axial CT unless the scans happen to pass directly through the site (Fig. 7-53). If the scan is performed while the drain is in place, the drain can be followed to its exit point from the sinus.

**FIGURE 7-50** Lateral plain film (**A**) shows a patient with a rib nasal graft replacing badly fractured nasal bones. Lateral plain film (**B**) shows a patient with a partially calcified cartilage graft replacing crushed nasal bones.

In patients with chronic inflammatory disease, two types of procedures can be performed: those that do not obliterate the sinus cavity and the more commonly performed procedures that obliterate the sinus cavity. Although not commonly performed today, there are mainly three frontal sinus

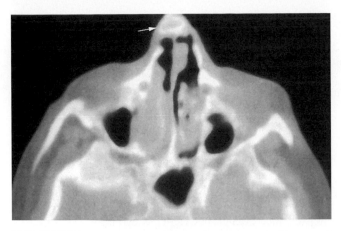

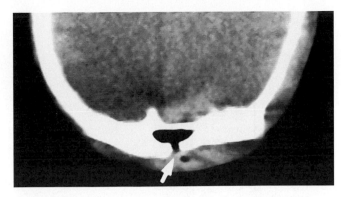

**FIGURE 7-53**   Coronal CT scan shows a frontal sinus that was trephined because of an acute unresponsive sinusitis. The site of the trephination is seen as a hole in the anterior sinus wall (*arrow*).

**FIGURE 7-51**   Axial CT scan shows a rib (*arrow*) used in a nasal reconstruction. There is unrelated inflammatory disease in the nasal cavities.

nonobliterative procedures: the Lynch, Killian, and Riedel procedures. For the most part, these operations have been replaced by endoscopic approaches or, for large sinuses, the obliterative osteoplastic flap procedure.

## Lynch Procedure

The Lynch procedure is utilized primarily for disease in the ethmoid sinuses and supraorbital ethmoid cells. However, it also provides good entrance into a small to moderate-sized frontal sinus. The Lynch incision is buried in the creases and concavity of the lateral nose and the superomedial orbital margin. The frontal sinus is entered from below and behind the orbital rim, and the region of the nasofrontal duct is exposed by a lateral (external) ethmoidectomy. The diseased frontal sinus and ethmoid mucosa are removed, and a tube is placed in the nasofrontal duct to promote sinus drainage through a reconstructed duct. This tube remains in place for 6 to 8 weeks and then is removed intranasally (Figs. 7-54 to 7-56).

If the frontal sinus is too large for all of its diseased mucosa to be effectively removed by the standard Lynch procedure, an extended Lynch incision can be used, extending the incision more laterally over the orbit. Alternatively, in past years, a larger bony defect was made in the anterior frontal sinus wall, using either the Killian or Riedel procedure.

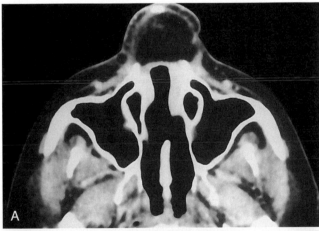

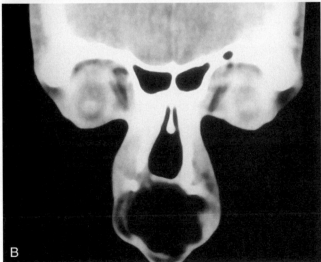

**FIGURE 7-52**   Axial (**A**) and coronal (**B**) CT scans show a free flap reconstruction of the lower nose after a rhinectomy. The bulk of the graft is fatty.

## Killian Procedure

In a moderately large frontal sinus the Killian procedure can be used. Via two bony defects, this approach creates a larger entrance into the frontal sinus than can be obtained with an extended Lynch procedure. In the Killian approach the first bony defect is created above the orbital rim in the anterior frontal sinus wall, and the second defect is created below and behind the orbital rim in the frontal sinus floor (via a standard Lynch incision). The intact superior orbital rim partially prevents the overlying soft tissues of the forehead from collapsing into the sinus, and when compared with the Riedel procedure, the resulting cosmetic deformity is minimized (Fig. 7-57). However, the soft tissues of the forehead region do partially prolapse into the sinus cavity and create a noticeable cosmetic deformity, which is well

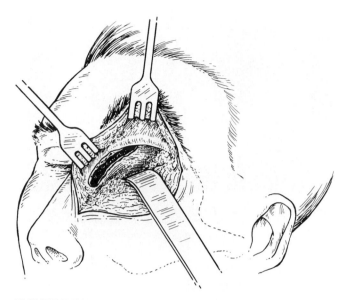

**FIGURE 7-54** Diagram of a Lynch procedure. The ethmoid sinuses, supraorbital ethmoid cells, and small frontal sinuses can be approached by this procedure. The incision is buried in the creases of the lateral nose and the superomedial orbital rim.

seen on axial scans. As in the Lynch procedure, the nasofrontal duct is reconstructed through an external ethmoidectomy.

## Riedel Procedure

For the reliable removal of diseased sinus mucosa in a large frontal sinus, the Riedel procedure can be used. In this approach the two surgical defects created in the Killian procedure are joined into one large defect, which includes the superior orbital rim (Fig. 7-58). At the completion of the procedure the soft tissues of the forehead are laid on the posterior frontal sinus wall, which has been denuded of its mucosa. This effectively obliterates the upper sinus cavity but creates a cosmetically undesirable soft-tissue defect in the forehead. The nasofrontal duct is reconstructed as in the Lynch procedure.[55, 56]

Because of the cosmetic deformities associated with these procedures, particularly the latter two techniques, and because the nasofrontal duct becomes obstructed postoperatively in about 50% of these patients, the cosmetically less deforming obliterative osteoplastic flap procedure has gained great popularity, especially in the moderate to large frontal sinuses in which mucosa cannot be removed by a Lynch approach.

## Osteoplastic Flap Procedure

The osteoplastic flap incision is either a curved coronal scalp incision that is hidden in the scalp hair or a brow incision that extends between the eyebrows, crossing the intervening skin crease near the root of the nose or nasion. Once the periosteum over the frontal bone is exposed, a template made from a Caldwell view is used to trace the frontal sinus contour on the bone and periosteum. This template should come from a film taken on a dedicated head unit such as the Franklin head unit, which has a magnification factor of only 3.4% (compared with 10.3% on a standard 40-inch posteroanterior Caldwell film).[57] The template is made by cutting out on this film the sinus contour and the contour of the upper orbits. The resulting template is then gas sterilized. The orbital contours can be used to localize the template on the patient, and then the sinus outline is traced on the patient's exposed frontal bone with its intact periosteum.

The periosteum is incised on all except its inferior margin, and the frontal sinus contour is drilled into the anterior frontal sinus table. The drill line is beveled medially and downward into the sinus to help ensure that the frontal sinus and not the anterior cranial fossa is entered. The inferior margin of this anterior wall is not drilled but is fractured from side to side, elevated, and turned downward off of the sinus, with its overlying periosteum intact. This technique yields a viable bone flap. The sinus mucosa is then drilled out, and the sinus cavity is obliterated with fat or muscle, usually taken from the abdominal wall. The anterior sinus wall is then replaced, the periosteum sutured, and the skin closed, leaving literally no cosmetic deformity (Fig. 7-59).

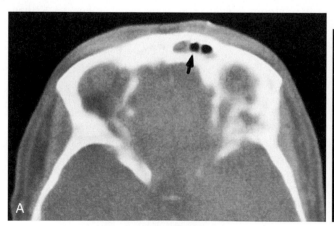
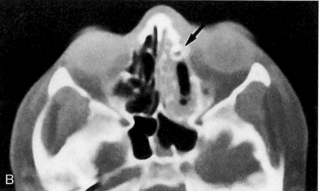

**FIGURE 7-55** Axial CT scan (**A**) shows an air-filled tube (*arrow*) in the left frontal sinus. The sinus is partially filled with secretions. Axial CT scan (**B**) through the ethmoid sinuses shows the drainage tube (*arrow*) extending down into the nose. There has been an external ethmoidectomy, and the anterior lamina papyracea has been removed. The left ethmoid cavity and the left sphenoid sinus have inflammatory changes.

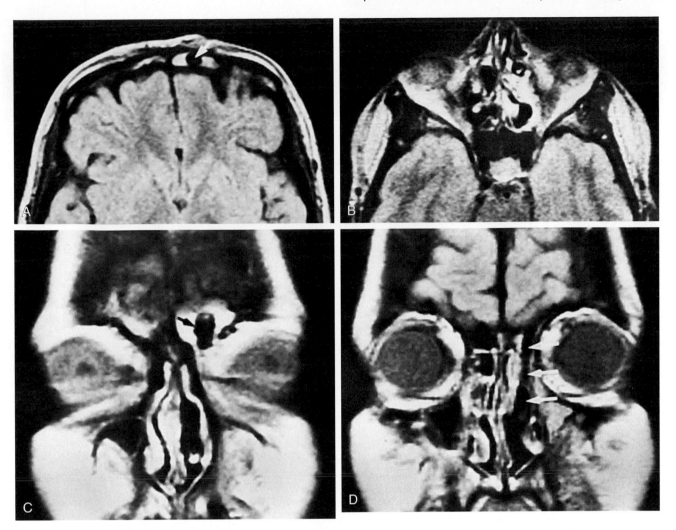

**FIGURE 7-56**   Axial proton density MR images (**A**, **B**) show a drainage tube in the left frontal sinus (**A**) (*arrow*) and sinus secretions. In (**B**), the drainage tube can barely be seen in the left ethmoid sinuses (*arrow*), and inflammatory changes are present as well. On the MR images, it is almost impossible to appreciate that an external ethmoidectomy has been performed. Coronal proton density MR images (**C**, **D**) show the tube in the left frontal sinus (*black arrow*) and the drainage tube extending through the ethmoid sinuses into the nasal fossa (*arrows*).

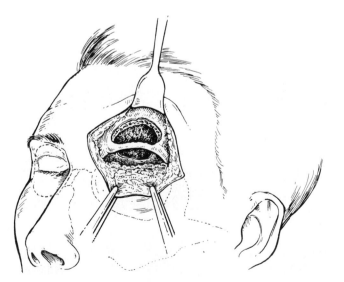

**FIGURE 7-57**   Diagram of a Killian procedure in which the superior orbital rim remains intact. Because of the forehead deformity, this procedure has for the most part been abandoned.

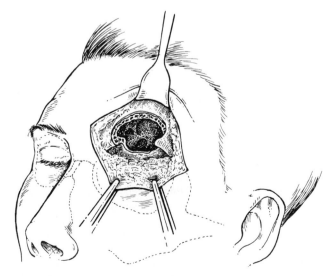

**FIGURE 7-58**   Diagram of a Riedel procedure in which the superior orbital rim has been removed. Because this operation causes a large deformity of the forehead, it has been almost entirely abandoned.

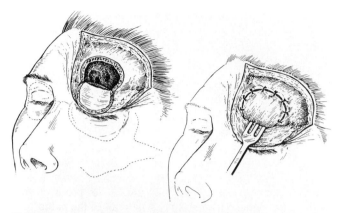

**FIGURE 7-59**  Diagram of an osteoplastic flap procedure. The anterior sinus wall is flipped down, with the inferior periosteum left intact. After the sinus mucosa and disease are removed, the sinus is obliterated with fat and then the flap is replaced. This procedure leaves almost no cosmetic deformity.

The fat progressively and gradually undergoes fibrosis, usually until the fibrosis represents one-third to one-half the volume of the obliterating material. More extensive fibrosis of the fat does not appear to occur normally. Throughout this fibrosing process, no volume loss occurs so that the sinus remains obliterated.

Infection of the bone flap or the operative margins, with or without associated osteomyelitis, and infection of the obliterating fat are the two most significant complications of the osteoplastic flap procedure. If the infection cannot be controlled with antibiotic treatment, reoperation is necessary. This often necessitates the removal of the anterior sinus wall bone flap, with some resulting inward prolapse of the forehead soft tissues. A plastic reconstruction can then be performed at a later date once the infection is cured.

If the osteoplastic flap procedure was performed to obliterate a mucocele that thinned or destroyed a portion of the posterior or anterior sinus tables, these defects will also be visualized on subsequent imaging studies. On plain films the osteoplastic bone flap is identified by a variably thin zone of lower density at its margins. This zone represents the bone that was drilled out of the frontal table during surgery (Figs. 7-60 and 7-61). In a few cases the flap fit may be so good as to make visualization of the surgical margin almost impossible on Caldwell or Waters views. However, a lateral view clearly shows the beveled surgical defect. In fact, if a history of prior surgery is not obtained, this defect may be misinterpreted as an anterior frontal table fracture (Fig. 7-62). If the sinus margin was altered before surgery, it will remain so after surgery. Thus the mucoperiosteal white line may be absent or replaced by a thick zone of sclerosis, and the sinus contour may be remodeled. Although this appearance can be confusing and suggests that whatever caused these changes is still present in the sinus, these sinus alterations merely reflect whatever process originally necessitated the surgery. The fat used to obliterate the sinus usually causes the sinus to have a hazy soft-tissue density on plain film, suggesting sinusitis. The surgical bony margins should be sharp and of a normal texture even though the bone flap does not fit precisely against the adjacent frontal bone. An air-fluid level indicates reinfection of the sinus, a serious complication.

On CT the bone flap may go unnoticed if only narrow window images are available. At wide window settings the bone flap should have a normal texture (Fig. 7-63). How-

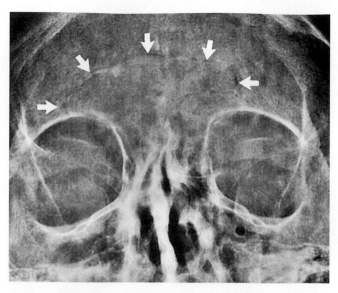

**FIGURE 7-60**  Waters view shows a patient after bilateral osteoplastic flap surgery. The flap margins can barely be identified (*arrows*).

ever, the edges of the flap and the adjacent frontal bone occasionally have a ragged, irregular appearance that reflects the beveling surgical procedure. Without any associated clinical or soft-tissue changes of infection, this irregular bone should not elicit a diagnosis of osteomyelitis. Frank osteomyelitis appears as areas of bone demineralization, erosion, or sequestration accompanied by swelling and cellulitis of the overlying forehead soft tissues. There usually is also evidence of infection in the underlying fat (Fig. 7-64).

The bone flap should be in a normal alignment with the adjacent frontal bone contour, that is, the flap should not be either depressed into the sinus or elevated over the adjacent frontal bone. When the flap is elevated, infection of the underlying obliterating fat must be considered. The obliter-

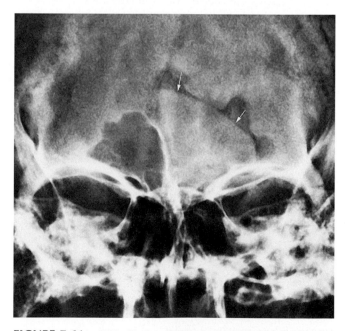

**FIGURE 7-61**  Caldwell view shows a patient after left osteoplastic flap surgery. The margins of the flap are well seen (*arrows*). The space between the flap and the calvarium is a normal postoperative finding resulting from the bone removal that occurs during surgery.

ated sinus is best examined at both narrow and wide windows. The entire sinus cavity should be airless and filled with fat that has randomly scattered strands of soft-tissue-dense fibrous tissue. Whenever a focal mass of soft-tissue density is seen within the fat or whenever more than half of the fat content is of fibrous density, the imager should raise the possibility of infection (Figs. 7-64, 7-66, and 7-68 to 7-70). This type of infection is usually associated with elevation of the flap secondary to swelling of the fibrous fatty material (Figs. 7-65, 7-69, and 7-70). In these cases the intracranial compartment should also be examined for evidence of spread of the infection.

Occasionally the osteoplastic bone flap fractures during surgery; however, as long as the overlying periosteum remains intact, the fracture pieces usually remain viable. The imager should verify that the bony pieces have a normal texture, that there are no sites of osteomyelitis, and that the bone fragments are not elevated. In rare instances after many years, some calcification can occur in the obliterating fat; this should be considered a normal postoperative variant.

On MR imaging the signal intensities in the normal postosteoplastic flap sinus reflect the obliterating fat. Thus there is a high T1-weighted and an intermediate T2-weighted signal intensity (Fig. 7-71). Although infection in the fat will produce a high T2-weighted signal intensity, occasionally areas of high T2-weighted signal intensity are seen in noninfected sinuses (Fig. 7-72). The precise cause of this is unclear. Thus, the mere presence of a high T2-weighted signal intensity within the obliterating fat should not warrant a diagnosis of postoperative infection. Infection should be considered if there is high T2-weighted signal intensity in the obliterating fat, elevation of the bony flap, and evidence of swelling and inflammation in the surrounding forehead soft tissues.

## ETHMOID SINUS SURGERY

Although today the ethmoid sinuses are most often approached endoscopically, traditionally the ethmoid complex can be partially resected via three major approaches: the external, the internal (intranasal), and the transmaxillary (transantral) (Fig. 7-73). These procedures are performed for inflammatory disease, and the aim is to progressively remove the disease from each cell until all of the pathologic material is extirpated. The primary areas of complication are entrance into the floor of the anterior cranial fossa and damage to the orbital contents.[51, 52, 57]

### External Ethmoidectomy

The external approach provides the best overall access and visualization of the ethmoid cells. After a Lynch incision, the periorbita is elevated and the surface of the lamina papyracea is viewed to identify prior fractures and any areas of dehiscence or erosion. The anterior and posterior ethmoidal canals are exposed. A line connecting these canals lies just below the floor of the anterior cranial fossa, and if the surgeon stays caudal to this line, entrance into the anterior cranial fossa should not occur. The surgical field can be enlarged to the frontal sinus, supraorbital cells, orbit, anterior sphenoid sinus, or base of the skull; the nasofrontal duct is best opened with this approach. In an external ethmoidectomy, the anterior cells are first entered through the lamina papyracea, and then the posterior cells are progressively opened as needed. As a Lynch incision must be made, this external approach has a scar hidden in the crease of the medial orbital margin.

### Internal Ethmoidectomy

The internal ethmoidectomy is an intranasal approach and usually includes resection of the middle turbinate to provide better access to the ethmoid and sphenoid cells. The ethmoid complex is usually entered via the bulla ethmoidalis; the anterior cells are resected and then the more posterior cells are opened. Although in experienced hands the lamina papyracea is not violated in this procedure, dehiscence of the lamina papyracea or a prior external ethmoidectomy is a contributing factor to inadvertant entrance into the orbit. The internal ethmoidectomy approach is used for isolated ethmoid sinus disease, for biopsies in patients who do not have coexistent antral disease, and in patients who do not wish to have an external incision.

### Transantral Ethmoidectomy

The transantral approach is used when the antral cavity has coexistent sinusitis or when the intranasal approach is not possible for anatomic or technical reasons. The antrum is entered using a Caldwell-Luc approach,

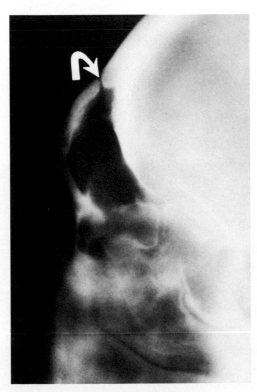

**FIGURE 7-62**  Lateral multidirectional tomogram shows a patient's status after an osteoplastic flap procedure. The surgical margin of the flap (*arrow*) is seen and may simulate a fracture.

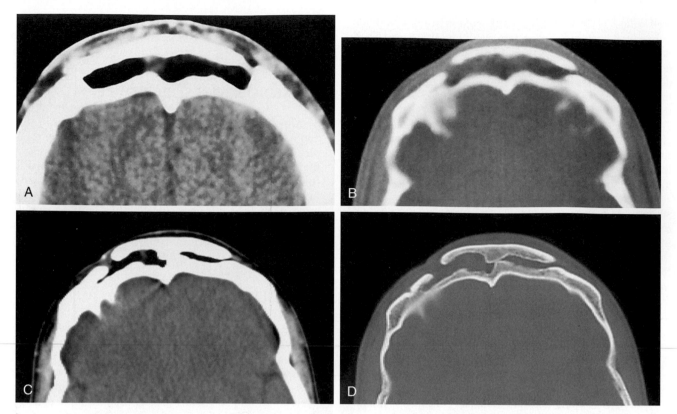

**FIGURE 7-63** Axial CT scans at narrow (**A**) and wide (**B**) window settings. The patient has had an osteoplastic flap procedure. The sinus is filled with fat, and the flap is clearly seen in a good position. In (**A**), the presence of the flap can be easily overlooked. Axial CT scans at narrow (**C**) and wide (**D**) window settings on another patient who has also had an osteoplastic flap procedure. The sinus is filled with fat; however, the bone flap appears elevated. This is secondary to abutting of the residual sinus septum on the flap bone and the posterior sinus wall. This will be the new normal frontal sinus appearance for this patient and demonstrates why baseline postoperative scans should be obtained.

and the medial, upper maxillary sinus wall (ethmoidomaxillary plate) is taken down so that the ethmoid cells can be entered. The ethmoid cells are then progressively resected.

In all of these ethmoidectomy procedures, the surgeon is essentially blindly cutting through the most inaccessible ethmoid septa, those located at the cranial and posterior margins of the ethmoid complex. Even when the surgeon believes that the resection extended back into the sphenoid sinus, CT often shows that the most posterior ethmoid cells and the sphenoid sinus remain untouched. Because entrance into the anterior cranial fossa is to be avoided, most surgeons favor caution and many of the most cranial ethmoid cells also remain intact. These remaining cells point out the difficulty of intraoperatively estimating one's precise anatomic position. Because disease can recur in these remaining cells, postoperative scans should be obtained if the patient's symptoms persist or recur (Figs. 7-74 to 7-84).[51, 52]

Because of the relatively small, boxlike anatomy of the ethmoid complex, postoperative hemorrhage can fill some unresected cells, and on occasion, rather than resorb, the blood becomes fibrosed or even ossified. Such en bloc fibrosis does not often occur after surgery in the other paranasal sinuses, but it is fairly common in the ethmoid complex. The imaging differentiation of recurrent disease from fibrosis can be difficult, as the attenuation values frequently are not sufficiently different to establish a

definitive diagnosis. In general on CT, recurrent inflammation enhances and the fibrosis does not.

Uncommonly, a dense fibrous scar develops within the postoperative ethmoid bed. This usually has low T1-weighted and T2-weighted signal intensity and thus can be distinguished from active infection on the T2-weighted

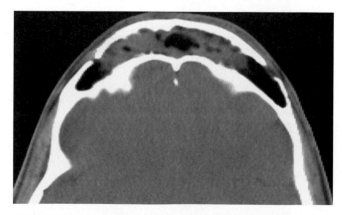

**FIGURE 7-64** Axial CT scan shows an osteoplastic flap. Although over half of the fat has soft tissue rather than fat attenuation, the bone flap is in a good position and there are no inflammatory changes in the overlying soft tissues. This is a normal imaging variant of this procedure.

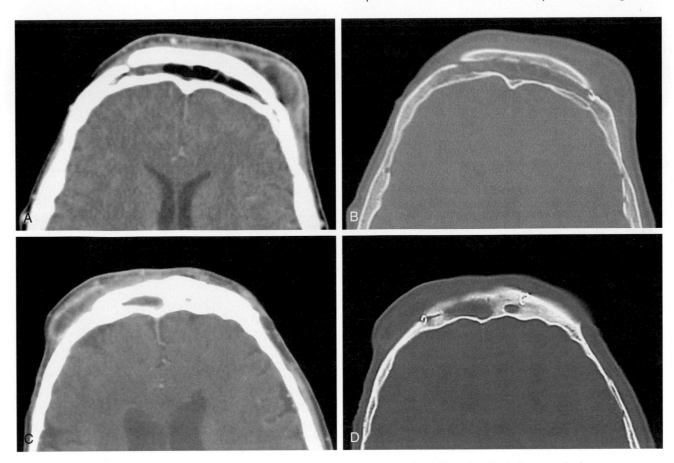

**FIGURE 7-65**     Axial CT scans at narrow (**A**) and wide (**B**) window settings. The patient has had an osteoplastic flap procedure. Despite the presence of primarily fat attenuation within the sinus, the right side of the bone flap is elevated, there is an abscess at the left margin of the flap, and there is swelling of the forehead soft tissues. This was an infected flap. Axial CT scans at narrow (**C**) and wide (**D**) window settings on another patient. In (**C**), an abscess is seen in the forehead soft tissues. Although it lies at the right margin of an osteoplastic flap, the bony flap cannot be seen clearly. In (**D**), the bony flap is clearly seen. This was an early abscess, developing after local head trauma to the region. The flap is otherwise normal on imaging.

scans. The denuded ethmoid bone may also develop a hyperostotic reaction that produces variable amounts of bone. In some cases, a localized osteoma-like bone develops; in other cases, the entire postoperative cavity may be obliterated by the bone that often mimics the appearance of fibrous dysplasia. This type of bone reaction also occurs in

the maxillary sinus and to a lesser degree in the sphenoid sinus. It is rare that this reactive bone develops in the postoperative frontal sinus.

In addition to noting how extensive is the removal of the ethmoid septae, the imager should anticipate (1) an absent anterior third to half of the lamina papyracea from an

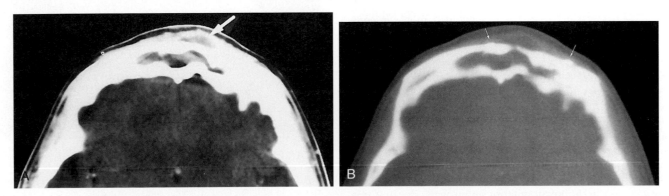

**FIGURE 7-66**     Axial CT scans at soft tissue (**A**) and bone (**B**) window settings show a patient who had a left osteoplastic flap. The small wire sutures stabilizing the flap can barely be seen in (**B**) (*small arrows*). There is erosion of the midanterior bone flap, and an abscess is present in the forehead (*arrow* in **A**). The fat used to obliterate the sinus is also dense, reflecting infection.

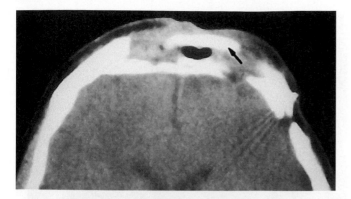

**FIGURE 7-67** Axial CT scan shows an infected osteoplastic flap. There is swelling of the overlying forehead soft tissues, and the bone flap (*arrow*) has been partially eroded. In addition, just behind the flap there is air, which should not be present in an obliterated sinus. The defect in the left posterior sinus table was related to the surgery.

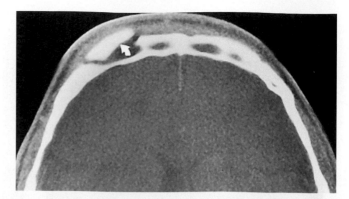

**FIGURE 7-68** Axial contrast CT scan shows a patient's status after a right osteoplastic flap procedure. Although the obliterating fat is only slightly denser than expected, there is elevation and rotation of the bone flap (*arrow*) and swelling of the forehead soft tissues. This was an infected flap.

external approach, (2) an absent medial ethmoid wall and probably an absent middle turbinate from an internal approach, and (3) a Caldwell-Luc defect in the lower anterior antral wall, absent bone in the upper medial antral wall, and possibly an absent middle turbinate from a transantral approach. Any residual soft tissues in the remaining ethmoid cells should be clearly noted by the imager for future reference.

If a postethmoidectomy cavity becomes obstructed after mucosal reepithelialization, a postoperative mucocele may develop (Fig. 7-85). This mucocele usually does not grow like a typical ethmoid mucocele, which tends to expand laterally into the orbit. Rather, this postoperative mucocele takes the course of least resistance and expands within the enlarged postoperative ethmoid cavity. It is only after the entire ethmoid cavity is filled that the mucocele bulges into the orbit. On imaging, characteristically there is a collection of entrapped secretions within the postoperative ethmoid.[58]

## MAXILLARY SINUS SURGERY

Today the most common diagnostic and therapeutic procedures performed on the antrum and the osteomeatal complex are endoscopic. However, intranasal antrostomy and the Caldwell-Luc operation are still performed. The endoscopic techniques and their postoperative appearances are discussed in Chapters 3 and 4.

### Intranasal Antrostomy and the Caldwell-Luc Procedure

In an intranasal antrostomy the membranous and bony lateral nasal wall of the inferior meatus is partially resected in an attempt to create better gravity drainage for the sinus. In the Caldwell-Luc procedure, in addition to the intranasal antrostomy, the maxillary sinus is entered via the canine fossa region in the lower anterior antral wall. Because this entrance scar is intraoral, there is no facial scarring (Fig. 7-86). Once the sinus is entered, the diseased mucosa is removed. Initially the anterior wall bony defect is closed by

a hematoma that eventually undergoes fibrosis (Figs. 7-87 to 7-90). However, this hematoma can uncommonly become infected, and in rare instances an oroantral fistula may be created. If this complication occurs, it is usually within the first or second postoperative week.

Via the Caldwell-Luc approach, the bone of the posterior sinus wall can also be removed to provide access for internal maxillary artery ligation or to expose the pterygopalatine fossa, vidian nerve, and pterygopalatine ganglion.[55] In such cases, a bony defect in the upper medial and posterior antral wall also can be seen on imaging.

In some patients, synechiae develop between the posterior maxillary sinus wall and the margins of the canine fossa/Caldwell-Luc defect in the anterior sinus wall. Such synechiae may form the basis for the development of a membrane that extends across the sinus between the anterior and posterior walls. Once formed, this membrane may obstruct the drainage of the lateral portion of the maxillary sinus and lead to the appearance of a postoperative antral

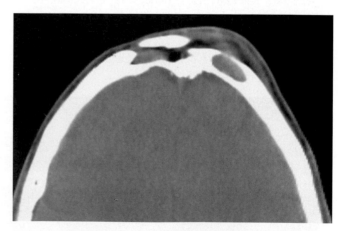

**FIGURE 7-69** Axial CT scan of a patient who had a right osteoplastic flap procedure. There is an ovoid soft tissue density within the right sinus. The bone flap is elevated, and there is thickening of the forehead soft tissues. In addition, the left frontal sinus is opacified, and there is a soft tissue mass in the overlying forehead with thinning of the intervening anterior frontal sinus bone. This patient had a recurrent mucopyocele in the right frontal sinus. There was a mucocele in the nonoperated left frontal sinus.

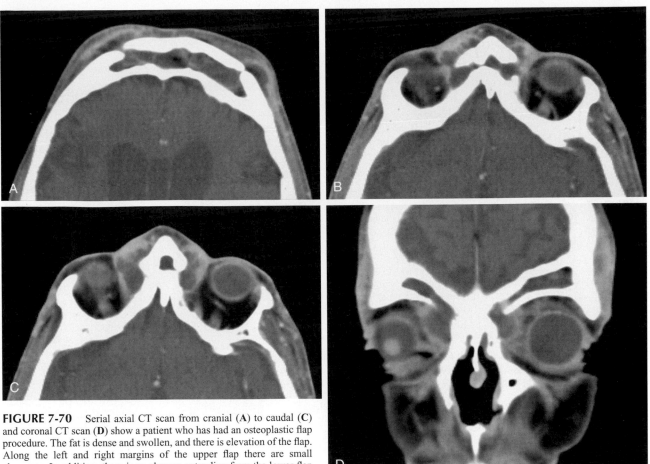

**FIGURE 7-70**   Serial axial CT scan from cranial (**A**) to caudal (**C**) and coronal CT scan (**D**) show a patient who has had an osteoplastic flap procedure. The fat is dense and swollen, and there is elevation of the flap. Along the left and right margins of the upper flap there are small abscesses. In addition, there is an abscess extending from the lower flap margin into the upper medial aspect of each orbit. There is unrelated ventricular dilatation.

**FIGURE 7-71**   Sagittal T1-weighted (**A**) and axial proton density (**B**) MR images show high signal intensity material (fat) within the obliterated sinus. The bone flap, which is often hard to identify on MR images, is in a good position.

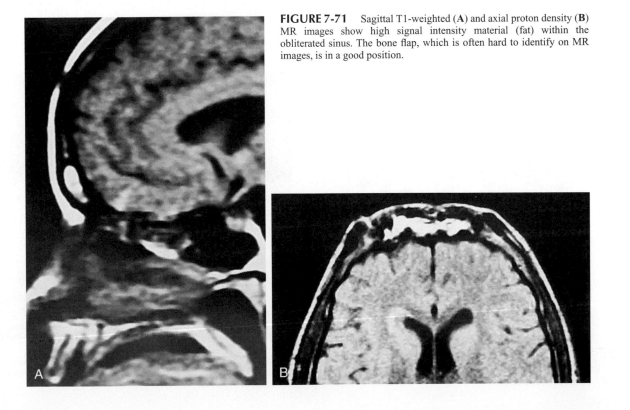

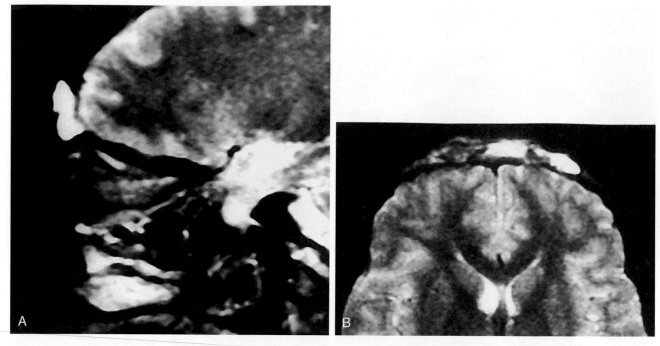

**FIGURE 7-72**    Sagittal (**A**) and axial (**B**) T2-weighted MR images on a patient who has had an osteoplastic flap procedure. The right side of the obliterated sinus has a normal fat signal intensity. However, the middle and left regions of the sinus have high signal intensity. This usually indicates the presence of infection, but this patient was asymptomatic. Such high T2-weighted signal intensity may be a normal postoperative MR finding. There is no elevation of the bone flap, and there are no inflammatory changes in the forehead soft tissues.

mucocele. In these cases, the medial postoperative sinus cavity remains aerated, while the lateral sinus cavity first becomes obstructed and then, as a mucocele develops, expanded. The imaging appearance of a laterally expanded mucoid mass in such a sinus signifies the presence of a postoperative mucocele (Figs. 7-91 and 7-92). Less often, postoperative antral mucoceles can occur in the maxillary recesses in the tuberosity and in the hard palate.

As previously mentioned, once the sinus mucosa has been stripped from the sinus wall, a bony reaction may be elicited that results in reactive bone formation, thickening of the sinus wall, and reduction or obliteration of the sinus cavity. Such a reaction is an expected consequence of the procedure and should not necessarily signify to the radiologist that active infection is present (Figs. 7-88 and 7-89).[59]

Optic nerve compression and decreased visual acuity in

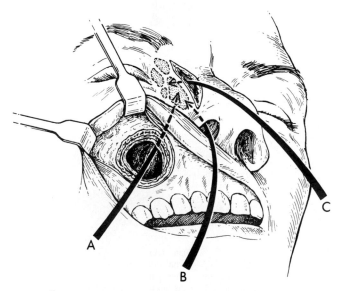

**FIGURE 7-73**    Diagram of the three major surgical approaches to the ethmoid sinuses. (**A**) Transmaxillary or transantral. (**B**) Internal or intranasal. (**C**) External (Lynch).

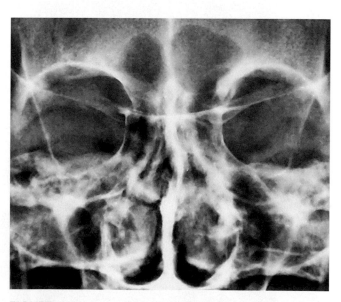

**FIGURE 7-74**    Caldwell view shows clouding of the left ethmoid sinuses. This appearance suggests infection. However, in this patient it was due to fibrosis after an ethmoidectomy.

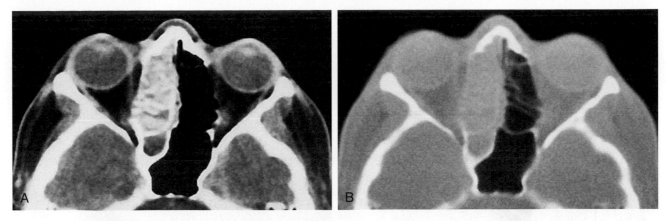

**FIGURE 7-75**   Axial CT scans at narrow (**A**) and wide (**B**) window settings show inflammatory disease in the right ethmoid and sphenoid sinuses. In (**A**), there appears to have been a left sphenoethmoidectomy, as the septations are not seen. However, in (**B**), the left ethmoid septa and the anterior sphenoid sinus wall are intact, indicating that no surgery was performed. In order to avoid such mistakes, these cases should always be viewed at wide window settings.

patients with thyroid ophthalmopathy may be treated by surgical decompression of the orbit. The procedures most commonly employed are a lateral orbitotomy (Krönlein's procedure); an antral (orbital floor) decompression using a Caldwell-Luc approach; an ethmoid decompression using an external ethmoidectomy approach; and an orbital roof decompression accomplished via a craniotomy. Of these operations, the greatest degree of decompression from a single procedure is obtained from the orbital floor approach. However, this procedure must be performed bilaterally so that the visual axes are not made asymmetric, resulting in diplopia and cosmetic deformity. The lateral and ethmoid decompressions can be combined with antral decompressions to achieve maximal relief of exophthalmos and a decrease in intraorbital pressure. The orbital roof approach provides relatively little decompression, and because it is a

*Text continued on page 420*

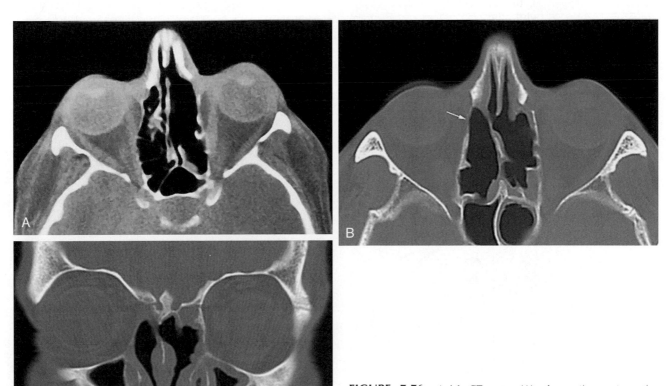

**FIGURE 7-76**   Axial CT scan (**A**) shows the postoperative appearance of a complete left internal ethmoidectomy. Axial (**B**) and coronal (**C**) CT scans show another patient who has had bilateral ethmoidectomies. On the left side, the lamina papyracea is intact and the operation was an internal ethmoidectomy. On the right side, the anterior lamina papyracea is not seen (*arrow* in **B**). This is a result of an external ethmoidectomy.

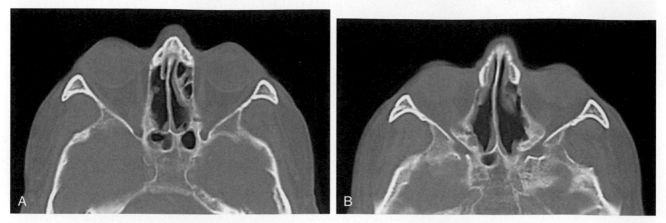

**FIGURE 7-77**     Axial CT scans at cranial (**A**) and caudal (**B**) levels of the ethmoid complex on a patient who has had bilateral internal ethmoidectomies. On the right side, almost all of the cells were removed. On the left side, the uppermost anterior cells remain. This appearance is typical of this operation, and the location of any remaining cells should be noted in the imaging reports of these cases.

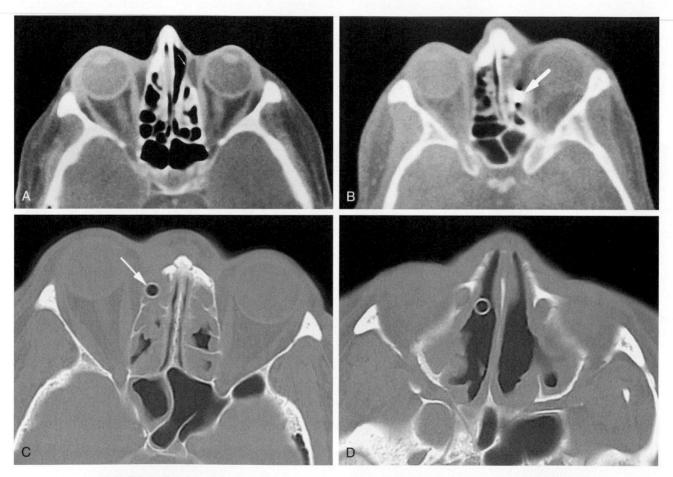

**FIGURE 7-78**     Axial CT scan (**A**) shows the postoperative appearance of a left external ethmoidectomy. The anterior lamina papyracea has been surgically removed and is replaced by fibrosis (*arrow*). Axial CT scan (**B**) shows a patient's status after a left external ethmoidectomy. The surgical clip (*arrow*) is used to control bleeding from the ethmoidal vessels. The soft tissue in the anterior ethmoid cavity was fibrosis and granulation tissue in this asymptomatic patient. Axial CT scans (**C, D**) on another patient show that a Lynch procedure was performed on the right side, and the drainage tube extends from the frontal sinus down through the ethmoid (*arrow* in **C**) sinus into the right nasal fossa (**D**).

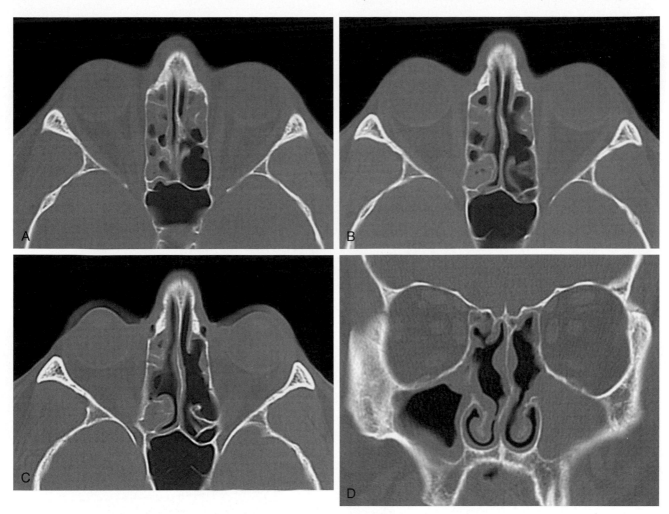

**FIGURE 7-79**   Serial axial CT scans from cranial (**A**) to caudal (**C**) and a coronal CT scan (**D**) on this patient who has had bilateral internal ethmoidectomies. The most superior cells remain anteriorly on both sides. The upper middle and posterior cells are also still present on the right side. Inflammatory disease is present in these remaining cells. Typically, the upper and posterior cells are not removed in internal ethmoidectomies because the surgeon does not want to enter the anterior cranial fossa inadvertently. The middle turbinates were removed at surgery, and inflammatory disease is present in both maxillary sinuses.

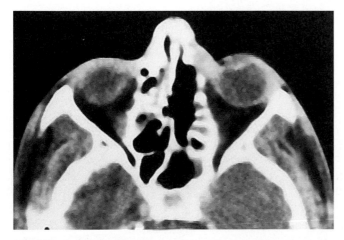

**FIGURE 7-80**   Axial CT scan shows the appearance of a left ethmoidectomy. Several of the posterior and more cranial ethmoid septa are still seen. This is a common finding, and these areas may be sites of residual disease.

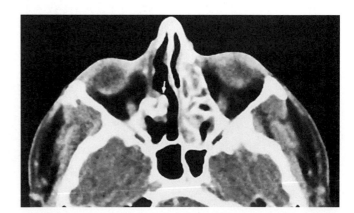

**FIGURE 7-81**   Axial CT scan shows a patient who has had a right ethmoidectomy. There is a focal area of bone production within the postoperative cavity (*arrow*). This represents reactive bone in response to surgery occurring in residual septae. It has no pathologic significance.

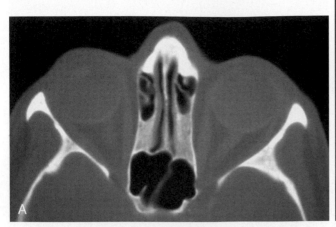

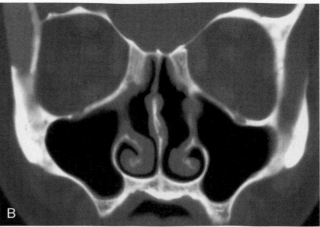

**FIGURE 7-82** Axial (**A**) and coronal (**B**) CT scans on a patient who has had bilateral internal ethmoidectomies. "Ground glass"–appearing bone is present in the upper posterior and middle postoperative cavities, partially obliterating the postoperative ethmoid cavities. This is a normal postoperative bony reactive change and should not be misinterpreted as an abnormality.

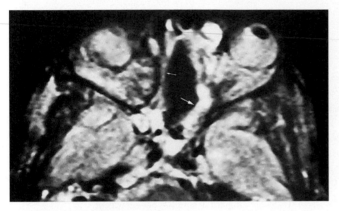

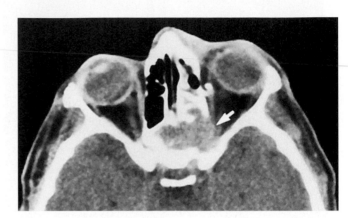

**FIGURE 7-83** Axial T2-weighted MR image shows the appearance of prior complete bilateral internal ethmoidectomies. Part of the postoperative cavity is lined with fibrotic tissue (*small arrow*), and other areas have inflammatory tissue with a high T2-weighted signal intensity (*large arrow*).

**FIGURE 7-84** Axial CT scan shows a destructive mass in the left posterior sphenoethmoid region (*arrow*). This patient had a limited left ethmoidectomy for suspected infectious disease. No preoperative scan was obtained. It was only when postoperative left eye signs developed that a scan was obtained. This patient had both infection and a squamous cell carcinoma.

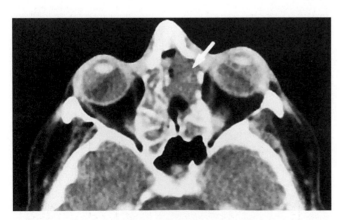

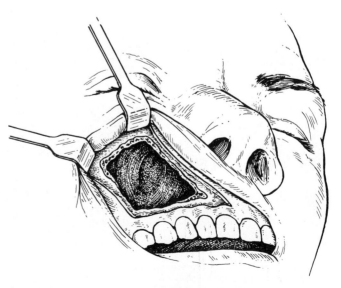

**FIGURE 7-85** Axial CT scan shows the appearance of a left ethmoidectomy that has an accumulation of mucoid material within the postoperative cavity (*arrow*). Rather than extending into the left orbit as a typical ethmoid mucocele, the postoperative mucocele tends to fill the post-ethmoidectomy cavity first.

**FIGURE 7-86** Diagram of the Caldwell-Luc approach. The maxillary sinus is entered anteriorly under the lip via the canine fossa. The hole in the sinus can be variable in size.

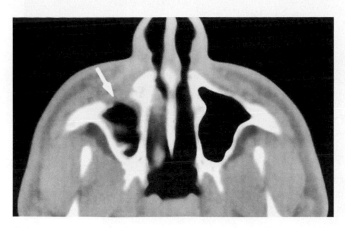

**FIGURE 7-87**   Axial CT scan shows the anterior sinus wall Caldwell-Luc defect (*arrow*). The soft tissues in the sinus were senechia.

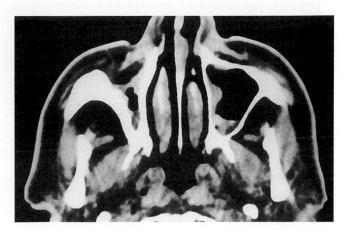

**FIGURE 7-88**   Axial CT scan shows a patient after a right Caldwell-Luc procedure. Fat from the cheek has partially prolapsed into the defect, and some inflammatory mucosal thickening is present bilaterally.

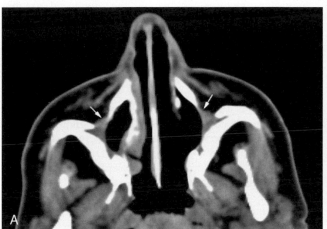

**FIGURE 7-89**   Axial CT scans seen at narrow (**A**) and wide (**B**) window settings on a patient after bilateral Caldwell-Luc procedures. The thickening of the posterolateral sinus bony walls is a reaction to the denuding of the sinus mucosa during the procedure and is an expected postoperative finding. Note the fibrous tissue that closes off the anterior sinus wall defect (*arrows* in **A**).

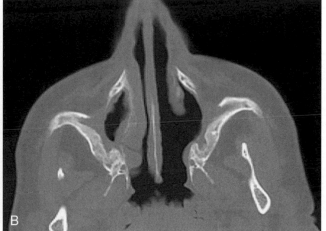

**FIGURE 7-90**   Coronal CT scan shows the Caldwell-Luc defect in the anterior left maxillary sinus wall (*arrow*) and inflammatory mucosal thickening in both antra.

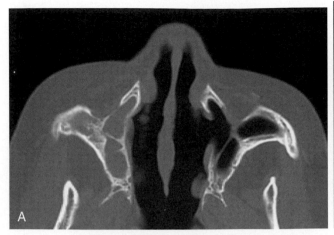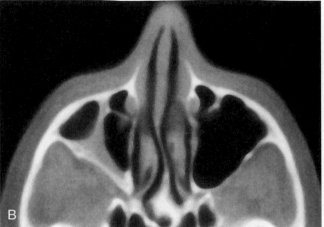

**FIGURE 7-91**    Axial CT scan (**A**) on a patient who has had bilateral Caldwell-Luc procedures. On the right side, the defect is fibrosed over and the sinus cavity is opacified. On the left side, fibrous strands extend from the surgical defect to the posterior sinus wall. Axial CT scan (**B**) on a patient after a right Caldwell-Luc procedure. On this more cranial scan through the antrum, a septum has formed between the anterior and posterior sinus walls. If this septum completely obstructs the lateral portion of the sinus, a postoperative mucocele will develop.

more extensive surgical approach, it is reserved for the most severe cases.

On sectional imaging, the absence of the lateral portion of the orbital wall may at first elude detection, the imager's attention being drawn by pronounced proptosis with muscle enlargement. However, careful evaluation of the bony orbital walls will show that a Krönlein procedure was performed (Figs. 7-93 and 7-94). The ethmoid decompression has the same appearance as an external ethmoidectomy, and it is the orbital muscle findings of thyroid ophthalmopathy that suggest the diagnosis (Figs. 7-93 to 7-95). The antral decompression reveals prolapse of the orbital fat and inferior muscles into the upper maxillary sinuses. Without a history, on axial scans this operation may present a confusing picture, often mimicking unusual antral disease. However, coronal scans reveal that most of the orbital floor bone is missing, a finding that differentiates this postoperative appearance from the rare event of bilateral orbital floor blow-out fractures, in which the displaced fracture's segments can be identified (Figs. 7-94 and 7-96).

## SPHENOID SINUS SURGERY

The sphenoid sinuses can be approached through the anterior sinus wall for biopsy, to improve sinus drainage, or to remove inflammatory tissue. The sphenoid sinusotomy opens the anterior wall of the sinus and creates a wide-open cavity that leads into the nasopharynx (Fig. 7-97). The sinus can be reached by intranasal, transseptal, transmaxillary, or transethmoidal approaches.

In the transnasal approach, portions of the posterior middle turbinate, the superior turbinate, and some of the posterior ethmoid cells are removed to gain exposure. In the transseptal approach, portions of the cartilaginous and bony nasal septum (vomer) are removed. The transmaxillary

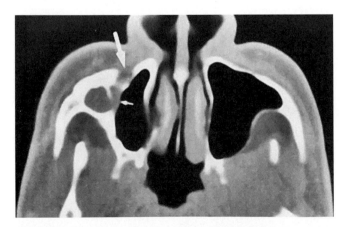

**FIGURE 7-92**    Axial CT scan shows an anterior Caldwell-Luc defect in the right maxillary sinus wall (*large arrow*). There is an expansile mass in the lateral portion of the right antrum (*small arrow*). This patient had a postoperative antral mucocele.

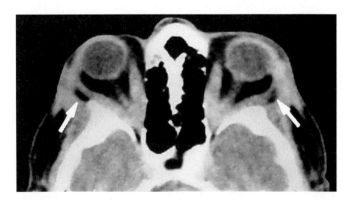

**FIGURE 7-93**    Axial CT scan shows a patient with the changes of thyroid ophthalmopathy. All of the extraocular muscle bellies are enlarged, and there is tapering at the tendon insertions. There is also bilateral proptosis. The lateral orbital walls (*arrows*) have been surgically removed, making the proptosis appear even greater than it is. This patient has had bilateral lateral orbitotomies (Krönlein's approaches).

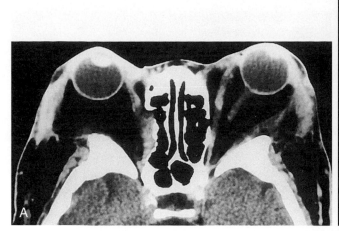
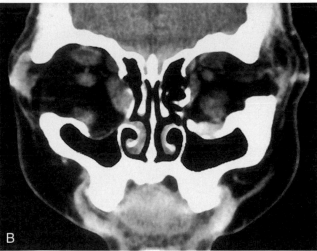

**FIGURE 7-94**   Axial (**A**) and coronal (**B**) CT scans show a patient with bilateral thyroid ophthalmopathy and bilateral Krönlein's and orbital floor decompression procedures. A medial right ethmoid decompression was also performed.

approach is an extension of a Caldwell-Luc procedure in which a transmaxillary ethmoidectomy is extended to include the anterior sphenoid sinus wall. The transethmoidal approach is simply a posterior extension of an external ethmoidectomy procedure. Thus, depending on the approach used, in addition to a widened ostium or an absence of one or both anterior sphenoid sinus walls, the respective surgical defects just described should be observed on images.[55, 56]

When a sphenoid sinusotomy is performed, care must be taken to avoid trauma to the carotid artery. In 17% of patients the bony wall separating the sinus and artery is so thin that it provides little if any protection from trauma, and carotid artery damage may lead to a posttraumatic aneurysm or a carotid-cavernous fistula.[60, 61] Similarly, damage can occur to the cavernous sinus and to the vidian, maxillary, and optic nerves in those patients who have these nerves running within the sinus (see Chapters 2 and 3).

A transsphenoidal hypophysectomy can be performed as an extension of a sphenoid sinusotomy. Once the sphenoid

sinus cavity is surgically exposed, portions of the anterior wall and the floor of the sella turcica can be removed and the pituitary fossa entered from below. Muscle, fat, cartilage, or bone may be used to seal the surgical defect. On sectional imaging, in addition to the site of surgical bone removal, sclerotic thickening of the remaining portions of the anterior wall and the floor of the sella turcica may be observed. Some postoperative prolapse of sellar contents, including fat, into the sphenoid sinus can occur, and without benefit of the surgical history, the imaging picture can simulate that of a large pituitary tumor with extension into the sphenoid sinus.

In the preoperative evaluation of patients being considered for a transsphenoidal hypophysectomy, the imager must direct special attention to the thickness of the bone forming the anterior wall of the sella turcica. In nearly 99% of patients, the sphenoid sinus development extends back to within 1 mm of the anterior wall or under the sellar floor. However, in the 1% of patients in whom a thick margin of bone remains between the sinus and sella, the transsphenoi-

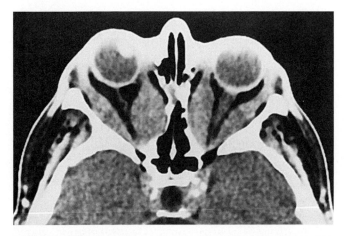

**FIGURE 7-95**   Axial CT scan shows large muscle bellies in the extraocular muscles with tapering at the anterior tendon insertions. The ethmoid complexes have been collapsed by a decompression. This patient had thyroid ophthalmopathy.

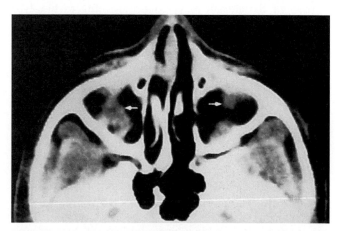

**FIGURE 7-96**   Axial CT scan through the upper maxillary sinuses shows the inferior rectus muscles (*arrows*) and orbital fat in the upper antra. The orbital floors have been surgically removed. This patient had thyroid ophthalmopathy and bilateral orbital floor decompressions.

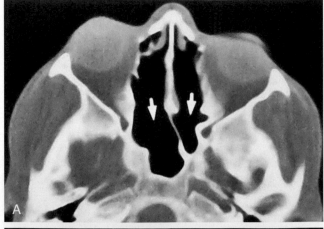

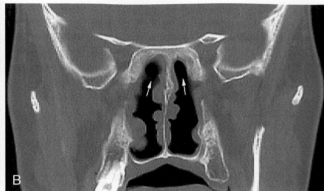

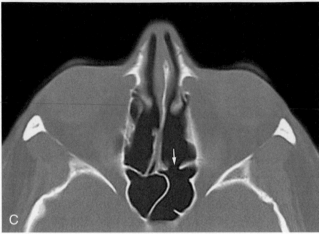

**FIGURE 7-97**    Axial CT scan (**A**) shows a patient with bilateral ethmoidectomies and sphenoid sinusotomies. The anterior sphenoid sinus walls have been removed (*arrows*). Coronal CT scan (**B**) on another patient who has had bilateral sphenoid sinusotomies. Note that the lower anterior sinus walls (*arrows*) have been removed. An axial CT scan (**C**) on another patient shows that bilateral internal ethmoidectomies and a left sphenoid sinusotomy (*arrow*) have been performed.

dal approach is not desirable; instead, an intracranial approach is used often.[31]

## SURGERY FOR SINUS MALIGNANCY

The type of tumor-curative operation performed on the maxillary sinus varies, depending upon the precise location of the primary neoplasm. Thus a tumor affecting the lower portion of the antrum may require an infrastructure-type partial maxillectomy, while a nasal tumor may require a medial maxillectomy. More extensive tumor necessitates a total maxillectomy with or without removal of the pterygoid plates and adjacent structures. A partial or total ethmoidectomy is often combined with a maxillectomy for complete tumor extirpation.

### Medial Maxillectomy

For localized nasal tumors that only involve a portion of the medial antral wall, a partial or medial maxillectomy is performed, usually in association with a partial ethmoidectomy and a resection of the nasal tumor. If the lower antral wall is involved, portions of the adjacent hard palate and maxillary alveolus may also be included in the resection (Fig. 7-98). Thus, in a partial maxillectomy, the medial antral wall, the inferior turbinate, often the middle turbinate, the lower ethmoid cells, and, if appropriate, portions of the hard palate and alveolus are removed. The lateral portion of the antrum and its mucosa remain intact.

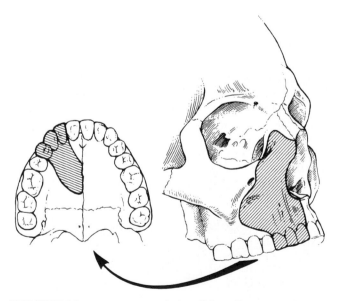

**FIGURE 7-98**    Diagram of a typical medial maxillectomy resection. A portion of the palate is removed if needed to obtain a tumor-free margin. The medial antral wall and inferior turbinate are also included in the resection.

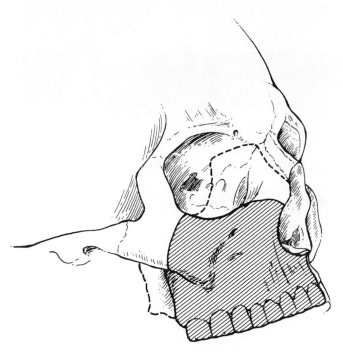

**FIGURE 7-99**  Diagram of a typical total maxillectomy resection. Variable portions of the zygoma and pterygoid plates may be included in the resection. Similarly, the orbital floor may be taken in its entirety, and an ethmoid resection (*dotted line*) may also be included to obtain a tumor-free margin.

## Total Maxillectomy

For more extensive tumors, a total maxillectomy is performed (Fig. 7-99). In addition to resection of the maxilla, there is some variation as to what is included in the resection. Such surgery may include the body of the zygoma, the ipsilateral hard palate and alveolus, the inferior turbinate, and often the pterygoid plates and portions of the ethmoid sinuses.[62, 63] Modifications are made to fit the specific tumor location. Thus the orbital floor may be left in place or it may be included along with an orbital exenteration. The latter is performed when there is gross tumor extension into the orbit.

Erosion of the bones lining the orbit may necessitate an orbital exenteration, and the degree of orbital involvement must be noted by the imager in order to aid the clinician in planning surgery. Gross orbital invasion almost always requires an orbital exenteration. However, erosion of bone, without gross penetration of the periorbita, may or may not necessitate an orbital exenteration. To some degree, this depends on the particular philosophy of the clinician and the tumor histology.

Today, there is a tendency not to exenterate an orbit for minimal disease, especially if the periorbita remains intact. This is a less aggressive approach than that of several decades ago, when exenteration was almost always performed. This is due in part to better chemo/radiation treatments and in part to a change in philosophy based on statistics noting tumor recurrences.

For squamous cell carcinoma, the initial involvement of any orbital bone must be considered when surgery is performed, even if preoperative chemo/radiation has shrunk the tumor away from the orbit. Failure to do so usually results in an orbital margin recurrence. With other tumors such as olfactory neuroblastomas, initial involvement of the orbital wall need not result in an exenteration. If there is a good preoperative tumor response to chemo/radiation and the orbit becomes grossly free of tumor, in most cases tumor resection without an exenteration may be curative.

After the bone is resected, the postmaxillectomy cavity can be lined with a split-thickness skin graft to create an immediate epithelial surface, or a muscle graft can be placed to fill the cavity. If the orbital floor was removed, various synthetic grafts can be placed to help support the orbital contents. Similarly, bone and prosthetic material can be placed to support the anterior and lateral facial structure, and prostheses can be placed to fill the surgical defects created in the hard palate and alveolus. These foreign substances can cause imaging problems either because they may degrade the image quality or because, in the case of some plastics and musculofascial grafts, on MR imaging they may simulate normal bone and go undetected. Eye prostheses also may cause degradation artifacts on scans.

As mentioned, there is a tendency today to obliterate the postoperative maxillectomy cavity created, with or without an ethmoidectomy, by using a rotated myocutaneous graft. Such a graft brings muscle, fat, and soft tissues into an area in which they normally are not present, and recognition of such a graft will obviate difficulties in interpreting postoperative CT and MR images.

The sinus cavity in a partial maxillectomy patient is lined by normal mucosa. The defect after a total maxillectomy can be lined either by a split-thickness skin graft or a myocutaneous graft. In any case, after a 6- to 8-week postoperative interval, nearly all of the operative-related edema and hemorrhage will have subsided and a baseline scan should be performed. This scan maps the patient's new anatomy and establishes the contour and thickness of the postoperative mucosal surfaces. The normal postoperative mucosa is smooth and moderately thin. Any localized area of soft-tissue nodularity or mucosal-submucosal thickening must be suspected of representing recurrent tumor until proven otherwise. If such an area develops that was not noted on the baseline scan, the imager should direct the clinician specifically to this site for biopsy (Figs. 7-100 to 7-109). This approach has led to more positive biopsy specimens than are obtained from clinical assessment alone. The routine postoperative imaging follow-up of patients has also led to identification of small, early recurrences that were overlooked on routine clinical follow-up.[62]

## EXTENSIVE NASOETHMOID SURGERY

The lateral rhinotomy provides access to the entire nasal cavity and the maxillary, ethmoid, and sphenoid sinuses. Modifications and extensions of this approach can be used to include access to the frontal sinuses. The typical incision extends from just below the medial end of one eyebrow, caudally between the nasal dorsum and medial canthus of the eye, down the nasofacial crease, and along the nasal alar rim. The incision is then extended down the upper lip if necessary. The nose is turned to the side, thereby exposing the pyriform aperture. This procedure gives access to the entire lateral nasal wall and nasal septum. Usually removed

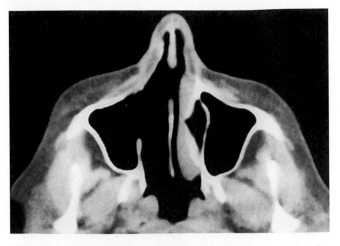

**FIGURE 7-100** Axial CT scan shows the normal appearance after partial right maxillectomy. The medial antral wall has been removed, and the soft tissues in and around the antrum should be smooth.

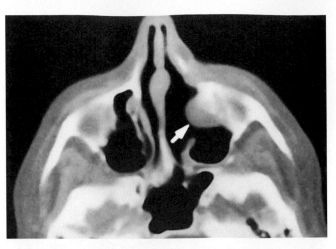

**FIGURE 7-101** Axial CT scan on a patient after partial left maxillectomy with a smooth nodular mass (*arrow*) in the antrum. Although this could be an inflammatory mass, tumor should be suspected until proven otherwise. This patient had tumor recurrence.

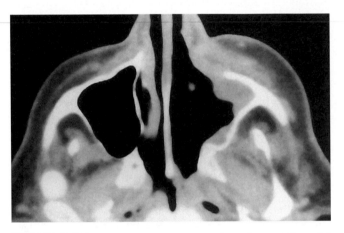

**FIGURE 7-102** Axial CT scan on a patient after a left medial maxillectomy. There is a nodular fullness in the soft tissues filling the postoperative cavity. This smooth nodule was a retention cyst and not recurrent tumor.

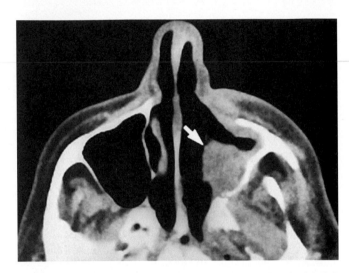

**FIGURE 7-103** Axial CT scan on a patient after partial left maxillectomy with irregularly nodular tumor recurrence (*arrow*) in the antrum. The smooth soft tissues lining the anterior left antrum were scar tissue.

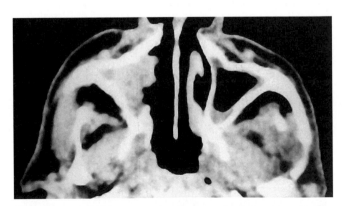

**FIGURE 7-104** Axial CT scan on a patient after right medial maxillectomy. The soft tissues within the right sinus have a nodular contour and suggest recurrent tumor. Inflammatory disease is present in the left antrum. This patient had recurrent inverted papilloma.

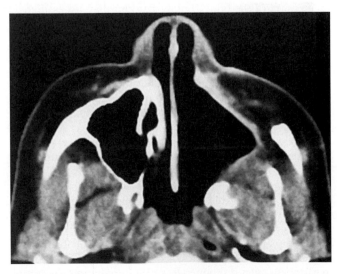

**FIGURE 7-105** Axial CT scan on a patient who has had a total left maxillectomy. The postoperative cavity is smoothly lined with thin soft tissue from a split-thickness skin graft. This is the normal appearance of a total maxillectomy. The pterygoid plates were not resected in this patient.

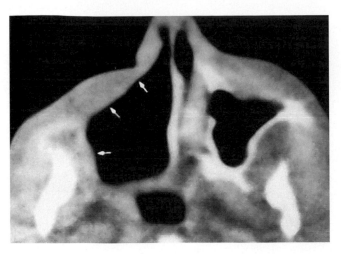

**FIGURE 7-106** Axial CT scan shows the normal postoperative appearance of a right total maxillectomy. The postoperative cavity is smoothly lined (*arrows*). The pterygoid plates were resected in this patient.

at surgery are the medial antral wall, the ethmoid cells, and the inferior and middle turbinates. The anterior sphenoid wall can be resected via this procedure, and the operation can be extended to include the entire nasal septum and contralateral nasal cavity structures, resulting in a total rhinotomy. In general, the operation of choice for a unilateral nasal tumor is a medial maxillectomy with a lateral rhinotomy and ethmoidectomy. Despite the extent of the resection, the cosmetic and functional results are excellent. Regarding patient follow-up, as with the postmaxillectomy patient, the same general imaging rules apply, namely, one must suspect tumor at sites of soft-tissue nodularity and mucosal thickening (Figs. 7-110 to 7-113).

## CRANIOFACIAL RESECTION

This large operation is reserved for patients with tumors of the superior nasal cavity, ethmoid sinuses, frontal sinuses, anterior sphenoid sinuses, and orbits. The operation essentially combines a frontal craniotomy with a resection of the

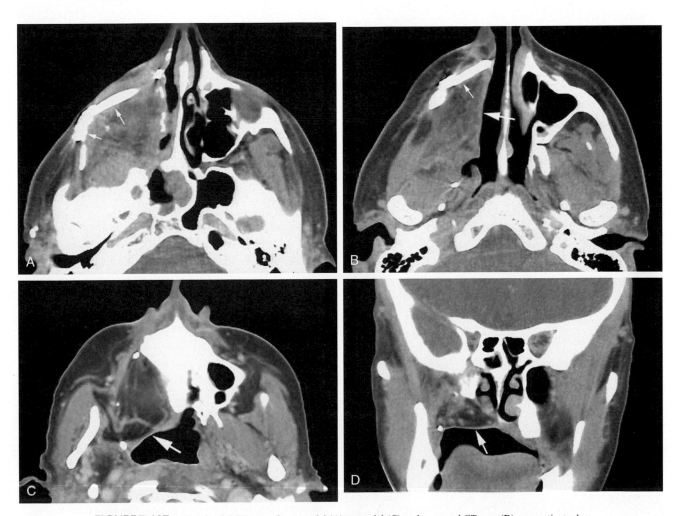

**FIGURE 7-107**   Serial axial CT scans from cranial (**A**) to caudal (**C**) and a coronal CT scan (**D**) on a patient who has had a right total maxillectomy with a graft reconstruction. Plated bone (*small arrows*) is present superficially to give a better contour to the cheek. The fat of the graft fills most of the postoperative cavity and forms the right side of the reconstructed palate. Notice that the free margins of the graft (*large arrows*) are smooth, with a thin mucosal lining. This is the expected normal postoperative appearance for such an operation.

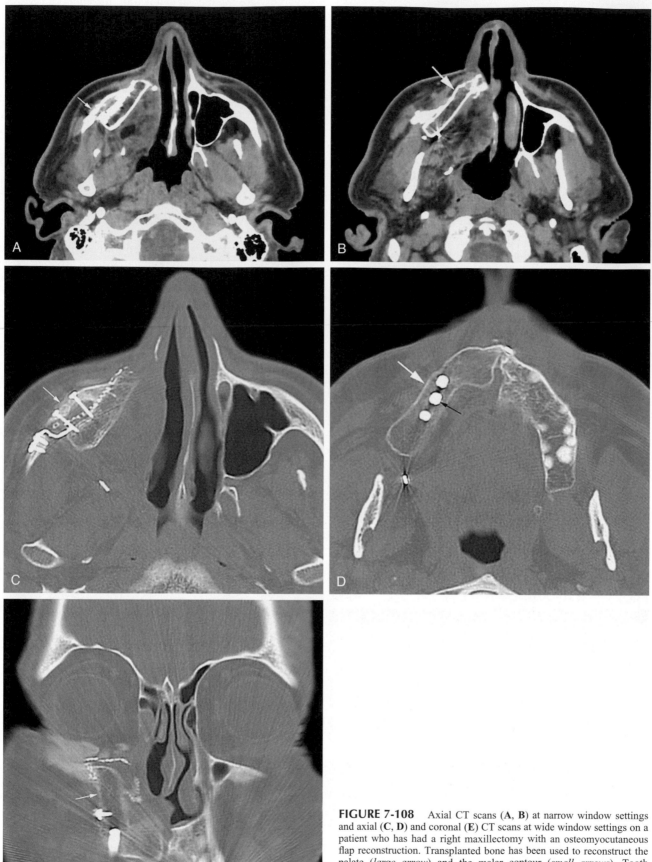

**FIGURE 7-108** Axial CT scans (**A**, **B**) at narrow window settings and axial (**C**, **D**) and coronal (**E**) CT scans at wide window settings on a patient who has had a right maxillectomy with an osteomyocutaneous flap reconstruction. Transplanted bone has been used to reconstruct the palate (*large arrow*) and the malar contour (*small arrows*). Tooth implants (*black arrows*) were then placed in the reconstructed palate/alveolar region.

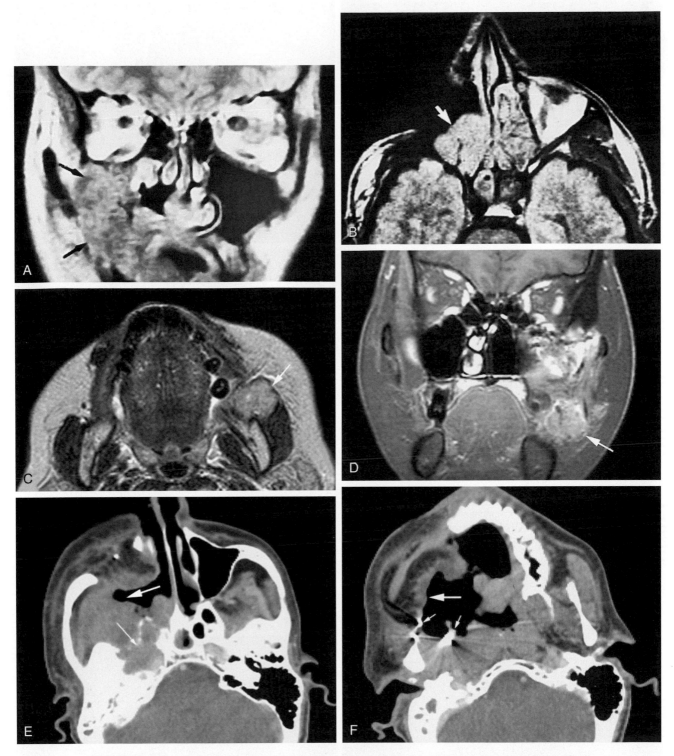

**FIGURE 7-109**   Coronal proton density MR image (**A**) shows a large right recurrent tumor with an intermediate signal intensity (*arrows*) in a patient who has had a total right maxillectomy. Axial proton density MR image (**B**) shows a patient who has had a total right orbital exenteration and a total maxillectomy. Tumor recurrence is seen in the right orbital apex (*arrow*). Axial FSE T2-weighted (**C**) and coronal T1-weighted, fat-suppressed, contrast-enhanced MR image (**D**) on a different patient who has had a left maxillectomy with a graft reconstruction. A tumor nodule is seen at the lower lateral margin of the graft (*arrows*). This was not clinically evident and points out the value of surveillance imaging. Axial CT scans (**E, F**) on another patient who has had a right total maxillectomy with a flap reconstruction. Tumor is present along the upper margin of the flap, eroding the skull base (*thin arrow*). Tumor fills the flap, and the medial side of the flap has become necrotic and ulcerated (*large arrow*). In (**F**), surgical clips that were within the flap are now exposed (*small arrows*) at the necrotic surface of the flap.

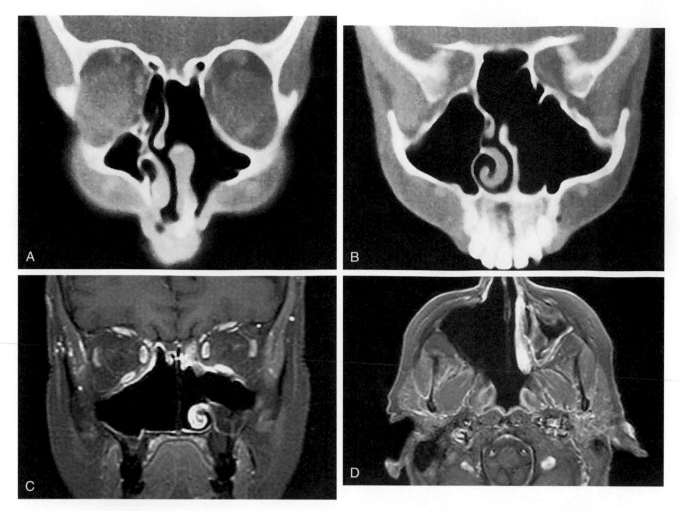

**FIGURE 7-110**  Coronal CT scan through the anterior antrum (**A**) and posterior antrum and sphenoid sinus (**B**) in a patient who has had a left lateral rhinotomy. There has been a left ethmoidectomy and a medial maxillectomy. The upper nasal septum has also been removed. This is the typical appearance of this operative procedure. Coronal (**C**) and axial (**D**) T1-weighted, fat-suppressed, contrast-enhanced MR images of another patient who has had a lateral rhinotomy including a right total maxillectomy and ethmoidectomy and a left medial antrostomy and a partial ethmoidectomy. Note the absence of any focal enhancing nodules.

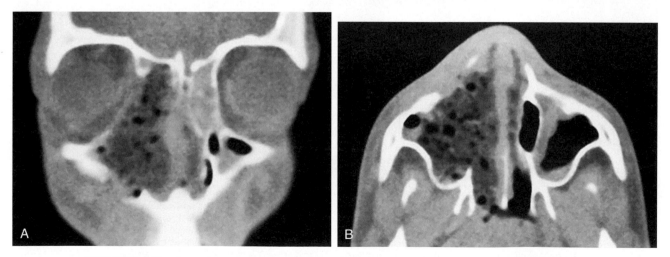

**FIGURE 7-111**  Coronal (**A**) and axial (**B**) CT scans show a patient who has had a right lateral rhinotomy. The postoperative cavity is filled with packing.

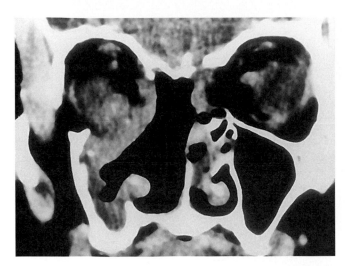

**FIGURE 7-112**   Coronal CT scan on a patient after an extended right lateral rhinotomy. The floor and medial wall of the right orbit have been removed. Although the thickened soft tissues along the orbital margin could be either scar or recurrent tumor, the smooth margin suggests that tumor is not present. The best way to evaluate this disease is to compare this scan with a previous study. Biopsy may be necessary. No tumor was present in this patient.

midportion of the floor of the anterior cranial fossa and an extended lateral rhinotomy. The surgery is often performed by a skull-base team comprised of a neurosurgeon and an otolaryngologist. Initially, one of several types of frontal or bifrontal craniotomies is performed, the frontal lobes are elevated, and any tumor extension into the brain is resected. The bone and dura in the floor of the anterior cranial fossa are then incised. The typical resection includes the posterior wall of the frontal sinuses, the cribriform plate, the fovea ethmoidalis on each side, and as much of the medial orbital roof as is necessary to obtain a margin around the tumor. The posterior incision runs along the posterior roof of the sphenoid sinus, and it can extend back to the tuberculum sella. An extended lateral rhinotomy is then performed, and the resection includes one or both ethmoid sinuses (includ-

ing the corresponding medial orbital wall), the nasal septum, and if necessary a portion of the medial maxilla. Once the entire specimen is free, the surgeons proceed with an en bloc extirpation. An anterior dural flap and a temporalis free musculofascial graft are used to close and support the cranial floor defect, and the lateral rhinotomy is closed separately (Fig. 7-114).[51, 64, 65]

Postoperative CT scans contain several areas that may cause diagnostic difficulties. First, the anterior dura adjacent to the frontal osteotomy becomes thickened and enhances on contrast studies. This appearance may persist indefinitely and relates to a low-grade reactive process that obliterates the dural spaces (Fig. 7-115). Second, the musculofascial flap that supports the central region of the floor of the anterior cranial fossa can bulge slightly downward into the upper postoperative nasoethmoid cavity (Figs. 7-116 and 7-117). This can simulate a tumor mass on axial CT scans and MR images, but usually can be identified as representing the graft region on coronal studies. This is especially true during the period before the free flap becomes completely fibrosed, usually between 2 and 8 months after the surgery. Although the CT appearance is not effectively altered once the flap is completely fibrosed, the MR imaging findings are changed. The initial intermediate T1-weighted and high T2-weighted signal intensities are gradually replaced by low signal intensities or signal voids on all imaging sequences. This change corresponds to replacement of the graft by scar. The thickness of the fibrosed graft may occasionally be sufficiently similar to that of the remaining bony floor of the adjacent anterior cranial fossa that on coronal MR images the radiologist may not detect that bone has been removed (Fig. 7-118). Only the altered contour of the bony floor of the anterior cranial fossa (absent the crista galli and fovea ethmoidalis) may signify that the surgery included the bone in this region. Such bone defects are seen easily on coronal CT. There are slight variations in the imaging appearance of patients who have had craniofacial procedures, primarily reflecting variations in the surgical approach (Figs. 7-119 and 7-120).

Any nodularity along the cranial or nasal margin of the graft or postoperative sinonasal cavity must be suspected of

*Text continued on page 435*

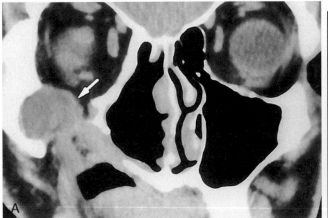
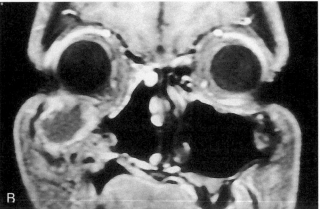

**FIGURE 7-113**   Coronal CT (**A**) and coronal T1-weighted, contrast-enhanced, fat-suppressed MR (**B**) image show a patient's status after an extended right lateral rhinotomy. No nodularity is present within the postoperative cavity. However, there is a mass (*arrow* in **A**) in the right zygomatic recess of the right antrum, which has broken into the floor of the right orbit. The lesion has surrounding mucosal enhancement, but the secretions within it do not enhance. This patient had a postoperative mucocele.

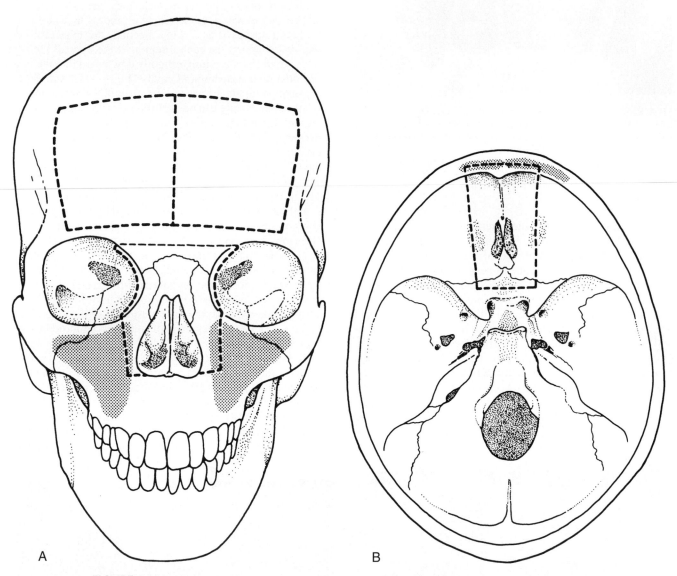

A                                              B

**FIGURE 7-114**    Diagrams of the skull in the frontal view (**A**) and the axial view (**B**) as seen from above with the calvarium removed. The osteotomies typically performed in the craniofacial procedure (*dashed lines*) are outlined.

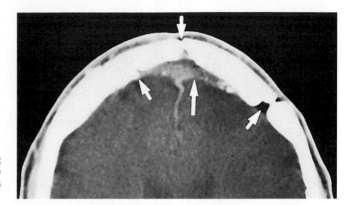

**FIGURE 7-115**   Axial contrast-enhanced CT scan shows dural thickening and enhancement (*large arrow*) that normally is seen as a postoperative finding in a patient who has had a craniofacial resection. The osteotomy sites in the frontal bones (*small arrows*) are also seen.

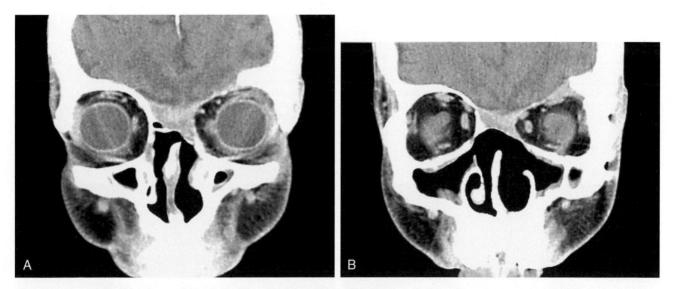

**FIGURE 7-116**   Coronal CT scans through the anterior (**A**) and posterior (**B**) ethmoid sinus levels in a patient who has had a craniofacial procedure. The ethmoid bones including the medial wall of the left orbit, the medial wall of the left antrum, and most of the roof of the left orbit were removed. Note the smooth margins of the intracranial portion of the flap and the sinonasal and orbital margins. Any focal nodule or mass should raise suspicion of a tumor recurrence.

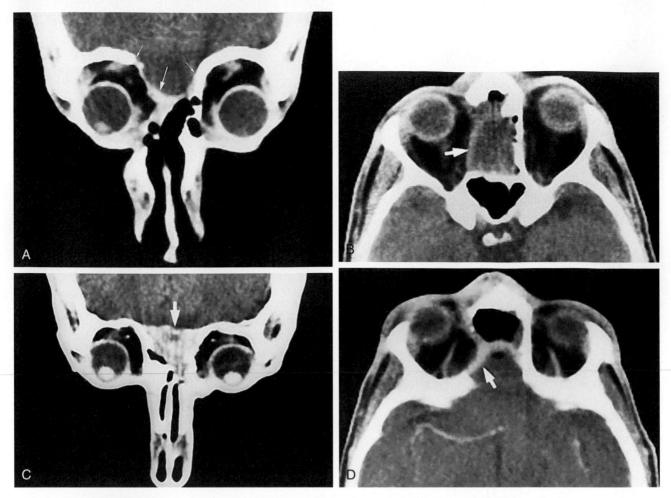

**FIGURE 7-117** Coronal contrast-enhanced CT scan (**A**) on a patient who has had a craniofacial procedure. There is enhancement of the muscle fascial graft (*large arrow*) between the margins of the bony resection (*small arrows*). The intracranial and sinonasal contours of the graft are smooth. Axial CT scan (**B**) shows a soft-tissue mass (*arrow*) in the postoperative upper nasoethmoid cavity. This is the fascial-muscle graft of an osteoplastic flap as it prolapses slightly below the level of the anterior skull base. Any confusion regarding this "pseudomass" can be resolved with a coronal study. Coronal contrast-enhanced CT scan (**C**) on a patient who has had a craniofacial resection. The fascial-muscle graft and adjacent dura enhance (*arrow*), filling the surgical defect in the floor of the anterior cranial fossa. The graft hangs down into the postoperative nasoethmoid cavity. Axial contrast-enhanced CT scan (**D**) shows enhancement of dura and granulation tissue (*arrow*) partially below the level of the fascial-muscle graft in a patient who has had a craniofacial resection. The air anteriorly is actually in the upper postoperative nasoethmoid cavity.

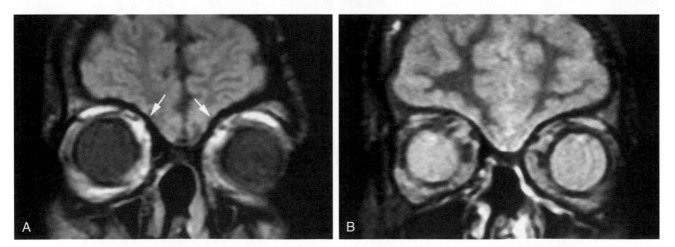

**FIGURE 7-118** Coronal T1-weighted (**A**) and proton density (**B**) MR images on a patient who has had a craniofacial resection. The graft has fibrosed, giving it signal void on all sequences. Because the graft has about the same thickness as the adjacent bone (*arrows* in **A**) in the remaining floor of the anterior cranial fossa, no obvious defect is seen. The imaging key to identifying that this surgery was performed is the absent normal contour of the crista galli and fovea ethmoidalis. Note that the cranial and sinonasal margins of the graft site are smooth.

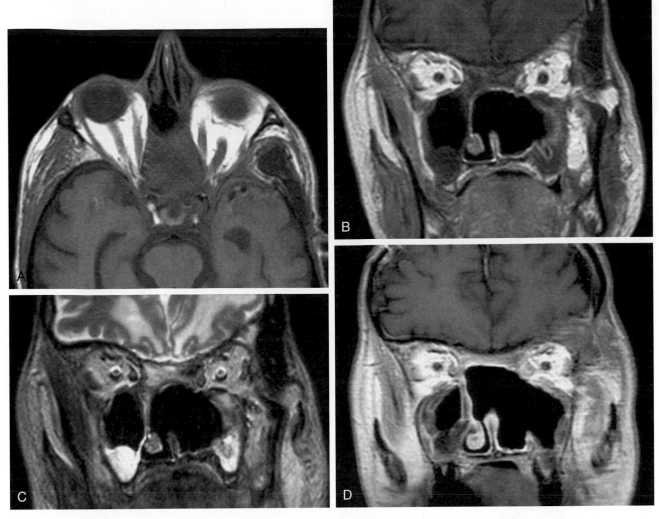

**FIGURE 7-119** Axial T1-weighted (**A**) and coronal T1-weighted (**B**), T2-weighted (**C**), and T1-weighted, fat-suppressed, contrast-enhanced (**D**) MR images on a patient who has had a craniofacial procedure. In (**A**) a "pseudomass" is seen in the midline upper nasoethmoid region. This is the flap as it hangs down into the upper sinonasal cavity. This is confirmed on the coronal images, where smooth margins are seen along the intracranial, sinonasal, and orbital margins. Incidental inflammatory disease is present in the right maxillary sinus. This is the normal postoperative appearance of a patient who has had a craniofacial procedure.

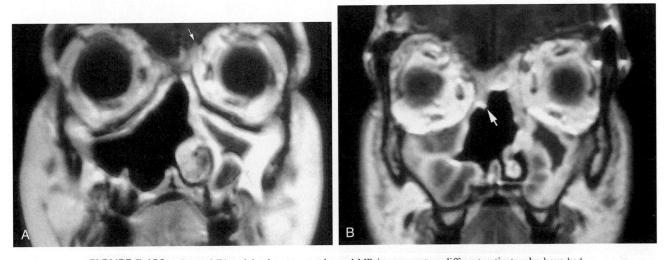

**FIGURE 7-120** Coronal T1-weighted, contrast-enhanced MR images on two different patients who have had craniofacial procedures. In (**A**) the mucosa lining the postoperative nasal cavity and the right maxillectomy cavity is smooth and normal. There is a sinusitis with entrapped secretions in the left antrum. The graft in the floor of the anterior cranial fossa enhances minimally, and if one is not careful, one may overlook the extent of the removed bone, especially in the skull base. A focal area of nodularity is seen (*arrow*) along the intracranial margin near the left attachment of the graft to the bone. This remained stable in appearance over several postoperative years. In this patient, this was a postoperative variant, and it points out the value of obtaining baseline postoperative images. In (**B**) the intracranial margin is smooth, but there is a focal nodule along the right sinonasal margin (*arrow*). Although this area is easily accessible to clinical observation, it was also present on the baseline scan and remained unchanged. There is also bilateral antral inflammatory disease.

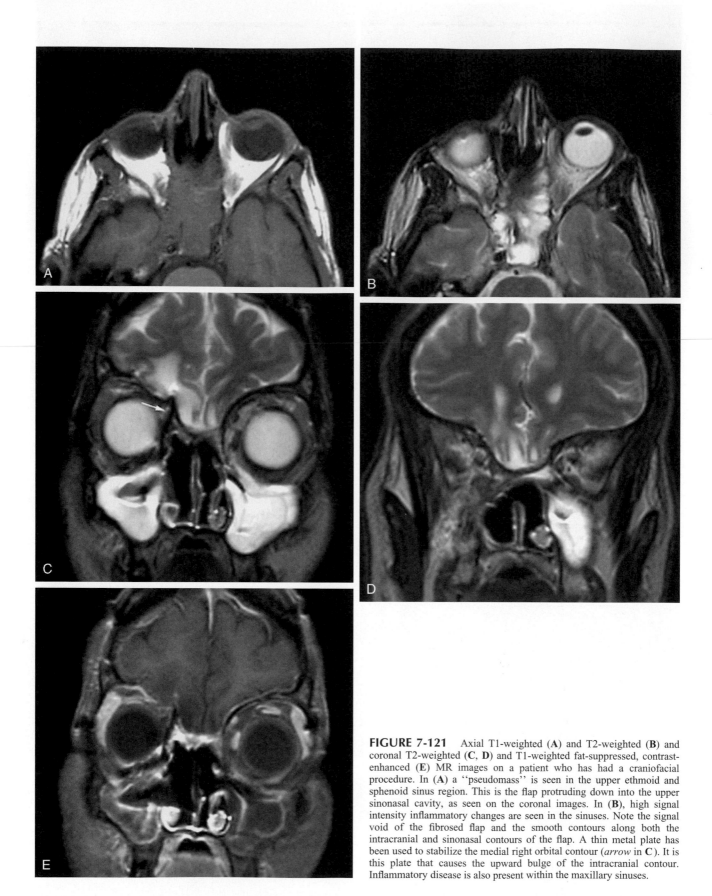

**FIGURE 7-121**    Axial T1-weighted (**A**) and T2-weighted (**B**) and coronal T2-weighted (**C, D**) and T1-weighted fat-suppressed, contrast-enhanced (**E**) MR images on a patient who has had a craniofacial procedure. In (**A**) a ''pseudomass'' is seen in the upper ethmoid and sphenoid sinus region. This is the flap protruding down into the upper sinonasal cavity, as seen on the coronal images. In (**B**), high signal intensity inflammatory changes are seen in the sinuses. Note the signal void of the fibrosed flap and the smooth contours along both the intracranial and sinonasal contours of the flap. A thin metal plate has been used to stabilize the medial right orbital contour (*arrow* in **C**). It is this plate that causes the upward bulge of the intracranial contour. Inflammatory disease is also present within the maxillary sinuses.

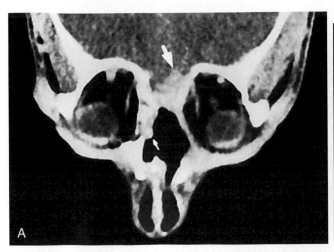

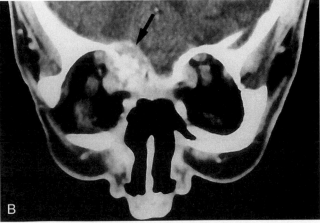

**FIGURE 7-122**    Coronal contrast-enhanced CT scan (**A**) on patient who has had a craniofacial resection. The upper fascial-muscle graft contour is nodular (*arrow*). This should raise the suspicion of early tumor recurrence. This patient had recurrent tumor. Coronal CT scan (**B**) on a patient who has had a craniofacial resection. There is a soft-tissue mass (*arrow*) along the graft margin in the floor of the anterior cranial fossa. The mass has also invaded the right orbit. This patient had recurrent adenocarcinoma.

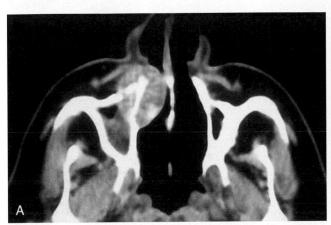

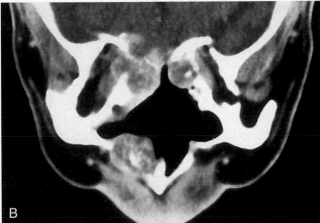

**FIGURE 7-123**    Axial (**A**) and coronal (**B**) CT scans on a patient who has had a craniofacial procedure. There are tumor nodules along the upper sinonasal cavity, in the right orbit, and along the right intracranial graft margin. There is also tumor in the right anterior maxilla. Speckled calcifications are seen within each tumor nodule. This patient had recurrent adenocarcinoma.

representing tumor. Progressive thickening of the graft or an upward convexity along the cranial margin of the graft are possible signs of tumor recurrence. Unfortunately, a vascularized scar tissue develops postoperatively that has imaging findings similar to those of recurrent tumor on both CT and MR imaging, with or without contrast. However, this tissue will not progressively grow on serial imaging studies. Thus, tumor recurrence in these patients is best detected by a change in the mucosal or graft surface contour or thickness.[51] Occasionally, inflammatory disease including abscess formation may be seen after surgery. However, in these cases, the clinical presentation usually suggests the diagnosis (Figs. 7-121 to 7-124).

Although technically large graft replacements of the facial area can be performed, the cure rate of such major surgery is often disappointing. Tumor recurrences can occur either deep within the graft or adjacent to the surgical bed (Figs. 7-125 and 7-126).

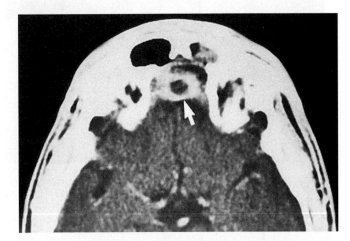

**FIGURE 7-124**    Axial contrast-enhanced CT scan shows a ring-enhancing mass (*arrow*) just cranial to the fascial-muscle graft in a patient who has had a craniofacial resection. This patient had a postoperative abscess.

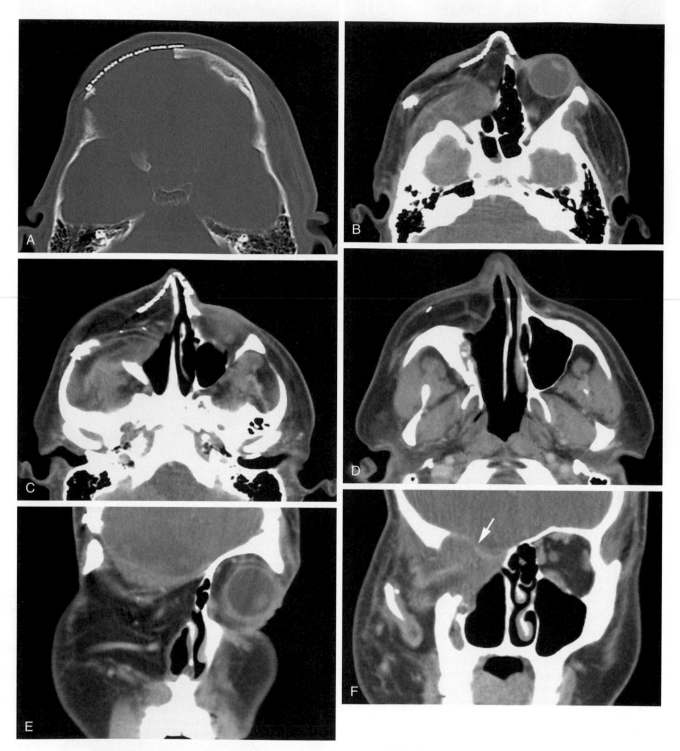

**FIGURE 7-125**    Serial axial CT scans from cranial (**A**) to caudal (**D**) and coronal CT scans from anterior (**E**) to posterior (**F**) on a patient who has had a craniofacial procedure, with a myocutaneous graft replacing the right orbit and face. Metal plates have been used to form a nasal contour. Although soft-tissue attenuation is seen near the cranial margin of the craniofacial graft, the intracranial margin (*arrow*) is smooth, as is the sinonasal margin. No recurrence is present.

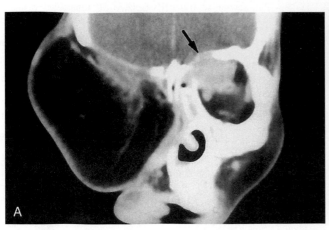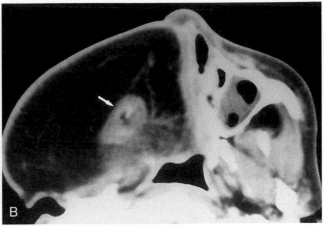

**FIGURE 7-126**  Coronal (**A**) and axial (**B**) CT scans on a patient who has had multiple recurrences of a rhabdomyosarcoma after chemotherapy, irradiation, and numerous operations. Finally, a large myocutaneous graft was used to replace her entire right facial region. The bulk of this graft makes clinical detection of a recurrence within it extremely difficult. Imaging shows the muscle (*arrow* in **B**) within the graft and no evidence of tumor recurrence. However, tumor has now recurred on the left side of the craniofacial graft and in the upper left orbit (*large arrow* in **A**).

# REFERENCES

1. Stanley RB Jr, Nowak GM. Midfacial fractures: importance of angle of impact to horizontal craniofacial buttresses. Otolaryngol Head Neck Surg 1985;93:186–192.
2. Stanley RB Jr. Use of intraoperative computed tomography during repair of orbitozygomatic fractures. Arch Facial Plast Surg 1999;1: 19–24.
3. Gentry LR, Manor WF, Turski PA, Strother CM. High-resolution CT analysis of facial struts in trauma: 1. Normal anatomy. AJR 1983;140:523–532.
4. Gentry LR, Manor WF, Turski PA, Strother CM. High-resolution CT analysis of facial struts in trauma: 2. Osseous and soft-tissue complications. AJR 1983;140:533–541.
5. Beirne JC, Butler PE, Brady FA. Cervical spine injuries in patients with facial fractures: a 1-year prospective study. Int J Oral Maxillofac Surg 1995;24:26–29.
6. Manson PN, Iliff N. Management of blow-out fractures of the orbital floor. II. Early repair for selected injuries. Surv Ophthalmol 1991;35:280–292.
7. Schwenzer N. [Corrective operations following primary surgical management of facial cleft patients]. Fortschr Kieferorthop 1986;47:540–546.
8. Kreipke DL, Moss JJ, Franco JM, et al. Computed tomography and thin-section tomography in facial trauma. AJR 1984;142:1041–1045.
9. Kreipke DL, Lingeman RE. Cross-sectional imaging (CT, NMR) of branchial cysts: report of three cases. J Comput Assist Tomogr 1984;8:114–116.
10. Rowe NL. Maxillofacial injuries—current trends and techniques. Injury 1985;16:513–525.
11. Kim DB, Sacapano M, Hardesty RA. Facial fractures in children. West J Med 1997;167:100.
12. Schierle HP, Hausamen JE. [Modern principles in treatment of complex injuries of the facial bones]. Unfallchirurg 1997;100:330–337.
13. Becelli R, Renzi G, Frati R, Iannetti G. [Maxillofacial fractures in children]. Minerva Pediatr 1998;50:121–126.
14. Manson PN, Markowitz B, Mirvis S, et al. Toward CT-based facial fracture treatment. Plast Reconstr Surg 1990;85:202–212; discussion 213–214.
15. Brant-Zawadzki MN, Minagi H, Federle MP, Rowe LD. High resolution CT with image reformation in maxillofacial pathology. AJR 1982;138:477–483.
16. Zilkha A. Computed tomography in facial trauma. Radiology 1982;144:545–548.
17. Zilkha A. Multiplanar reconstruction in computed tomography of the orbit. Comput Radiol 1982;6:57–62.
18. Lill W, Solar P, Ulm C, et al. Reproducibility of three-dimensional CT-assisted model production in the maxillofacial area. Br J Oral Maxillofac Surg 1992;30:233–236.
19. Carls FR, Schuknecht B, Sailer HF. Value of three-dimensional computed tomography in craniomaxillofacial surgery. J Craniofac Surg 1994;5:282–288.
20. Bruning R, Quade R, Keppler V, Reiser M. [3-D CT reconstruction of fractures of the skull base and the facial skeleton]. Rofo Fortschr Geb Rontgenstr Neuen Bildgeb Verfahr 1994;160:113–117.
21. Cavalcanti MG, Haller JW, Vannier MW. Three-dimensional computed tomography landmark measurement in craniofacial surgical planning: experimental validation in vitro. J Oral Maxillofac Surg 1999;57:690–694.
22. Zimmerman R, Bilaniuk L, Hackney D, et al. Paranasal sinus hemorrhage: evaluation with MR imaging. Radiology 1987;162:499–503.
23. Arden RL, Crumley RL. Cartilage grafts in open rhinoplasty. Facial Plast Surg 1993;9:285–294.
24. Clayton MI, Lesser TH. The role of radiography in the management of nasal fractures. J Laryngol Otol 1986;100:797–801.
25. Stranc MF. The pattern of lacrimal injuries in naso-ethmoid fractures. Br J Plast Surg 1970;23:339–346.
26. Stranc MF. Primary treatment of naso-ethmoid injuries with increased intercanthal distance. Br J Plast Surg 1970;23:8–25.
27. Cooter RD, Dunaway DJ, David DJ. The influence of maxillary dentures on mid-facial fracture patterns. Br J Plast Surg 1996;49:379–382.
28. al-Qurainy IA, Titterington DM, Dutton GN, et al. Midfacial fractures and the eye: the development of a system for detecting patients at risk of eye injury. Br J Oral Maxillofac Surg 1991;29:363–367.
29. al-Qurainy IA, Stassen LF, Dutton GN, et al. Diplopia following midfacial fractures. Br J Oral Maxillofac Surg 1991;29:302–307.
30. al-Qurainy IA, Stassen LF, Dutton GN, et al. The characteristics of midfacial fractures and the association with ocular injury: a prospective study. Br J Oral Maxillofac Surg 1991;29:291–301.
31. Yanagisawa E, Smith H. Normal radiographic anatomy of the paranasal sinuses. Otolaryngol Clin North Am 1973;6:429–457.
32. Ellis E 3rd, Ghali GE. Lag screw fixation of mandibular angle fractures. J Oral Maxillofac Surg 1991;49:234–243.
33. Smith PH. Blow out fracture of the floor of the orbit. Aust NZ J Surg 1967;36:319–322.
34. Gruss JS, Hurwitz JJ. Isolated blow-in fracture of the lateral orbit causing globe rupture. Ophthalmol Plast Reconstr Surg 1990;6:221–224.

35. Burm JS, Chung CH, Oh SJ. Pure orbital blowout fracture: new concepts and importance of medial orbital blowout fracture. Plast Reconstr Surg 1999;103:1839–1849.

36. Nolasco FP, Mathog RH. Medial orbital wall fractures: classification and clinical profile. Otolaryngol Head Neck Surg 1995;112:549–556.

37. Coker NJ, Brooks BS, El Gammal T. Computed tomography of orbital medial wall fractures. Head Neck Surg 1983;5:383–389.

38. Almog Y, Mayron Y, Weiss J, et al. Pneumomediastinum following blowout fracture of the medial orbital wall: a case report. Ophthalmol Plast Reconstr Surg 1993;9:289–291.

39. Berkowitz RA, Putterman AM, Patel DB. Prolapse of the globe into the maxillary sinus after orbital floor fracture. Am J Ophthalmol 1981;91:253–257.

40. Raghav B, Vashisht S, Keshav BR, Berry M. The missing eyeball—CT evaluation (a case report). Ind J Ophthalmol 1991;39: 188–189.

41. Pelton RW, Rainey AM, Lee AG. Traumatic subluxation of the globe into the maxillary sinus. AJNR 1998;19:1450–1451.

42. Lee FY, Hazan EJ, Gebhardt MC, Mankin HJ. Experimental model for allograft incorporation and allograft fracture repair. J Orthop Res 2000;18:303–306.

43. Martello JY, Vasconez HC. Supraorbital roof fractures: a formidable entity with which to contend. Ann Plast Surg 1997;38:223–227.

44. Shockley WW, Stucker FJ Jr, Gage-White L, Antony SO. Frontal sinus fractures: some problems and some solutions. Laryngoscope 1988;98:18–22.

45. Olson EM, Wright DL, Hoffman HT, et al. Frontal sinus fractures: evaluation of CT scans in 132 patients. AJNR 1992;13:897–902.

46. Whelan MA, Reede DL, Meisler W, Bergeron RT. CT of the base of the skull. Radiol Clin North Am 1984;22:177–217.

47. Rohrich RJ, Hollier LH. Management of frontal sinus fractures. Changing concepts. Clin Plast Surg 1992;19:219–232.

48. Rohrich RJ, Hollier LH, Watumull D. Optimizing the management of orbitozygomatic fractures. Clin Plast Surg 1992;19:149–165.

49. Rohrich RJ, Shewmake KB. Evolving concepts of craniomaxillofacial fracture management. Clin Plast Surg 1992;19:1–10.

50. Nahum AM. The biomechanics of facial bone fracture. Laryngoscope 1975;85:140–156.

51. Som PM, Lawson W, Biller HF, et al. Ethmoid sinus disease: CT evaluation in 400 cases. Part III. Craniofacial resection. Radiology 1986;159:605–609.

52. Som PM, Lawson W, Biller HF, Lanzieri CF. Ethmoid sinus disease: CT evaluation in 400 cases. Part II. Postoperative findings. Radiology 1986;159:599–604.

53. Som PM, Urken ML, Biller H, Lidov M. Imaging the postoperative neck. Radiology 1993;187:593–603.

54. Som P, Shapiro M, Biller H, et al. Sinonasal tumors and inflammatory tissues: differentiation with MR imaging. Radiology 1988;167: 803–808.

55. Naumann H, Buckingham R. Head and Neck Surgery: Indications, Techniques, Pitfalls. Vol. 1. Philadelphia: WB Saunders, 1980; 173–462.

56. Ballantyne J, Harrison D. Operative Surgery: Nose and Throat. London: Butterworth, 1986;1–177.

57. Urken M, Som P, Lawson W, et al. The abnormally large frontal sinus. Part I: a practical method for its determination based upon an analysis of 100 normal patients. Laryngoscope 1987;97:602–605.

58. Som P, Shugar J. The CT classification of ethmoid mucoceles. J Comput Assist Tomogr 1980;4:199–203.

59. Unger JM, Dennison BF, Duncavage JA, Toohill RJ. The radiological appearance of the post-Caldwell-Luc maxillary sinus. Clin Radiol 1986;37:77–81.

60. Johnson D, Hopkins R, Hanafee W. The unprotected parasphenoidal carotid artery studied by high resolution computed tomography. Radiology 1985;155:137–141.

61. Pedersen R, Troost B, Schramm V. Carotid-cavernous sinus fistula after external ethmoid-sphenoid surgery. Arch Otolaryngol 1981;107:307–309.

62. Som P, Shugar J, Biller H. The early detection of antral malignancy in the post maxillectomy patient. Radiology 1982;143: 509–512.

63. Baredes S, Cho H, Som M. Total maxillectomy. In: Blitzer A, Lawson W, Friedman W, eds. Surgery of the Paranasal Sinuses. Philadelphia: WB Saunders, 1985;204–216.

64. Lund V, Howard D, Lloyd G. CT evaluation of paranasal sinus tumors for craniofacial resection. Br J Radiol 1983;56:439–446.

65. Nuss D, Janecka I. Surgery of the anterior and middle cranial base. In: Cummings C, Fredrickson J, Harker L, et al, eds. Otolaryngology—Head and Neck Surgery. Vol 4. St. Louis: CV Mosby, 1993; 3300–3337.

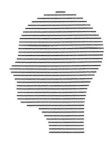

# Orbit and Visual Pathways

# 8

# The Eye

*Mahmood F. Mafee*

# EMBRYOLOGY OF THE EYE

The globe is formed from the neuroectoderm of the forebrain, the surface ectoderm from the head, the mesoderm lying between these layers, and neural crest cells.[1] The neural tube ectoderm (neuroectoderm) gives rise to the retina, the fibers of the optic nerve, and the smooth muscles (the sphincter and dilator papillae) of the iris.[1] The surface ectoderm on the side of the head forms the corneal and conjunctival epithelium, the lens, and the lacrimal and tarsal glands.[1, 2] Although the mesenchymal cells are derived from mesenchyme, neural crest cells also migrate into this mesenchyme, and it is from this combined mesenchyme that the corneal stroma, the sclera, the choroid, the iris, the ciliary musculature, part of the vitreous body, and the cells lining the anterior chamber are formed.[2]

The rudimentary eyes appear as two neuroectodermally lined hollow diverticula (grooves) extending from the lateral aspects of the forebrain (diencephalon) (Fig. 8-1). It is in the third week of gestation (22 days) that these diverticulae appear, one on either side of the neural groove. These are the optic pits, and they deepen to form the optic vesicles, which can be identified in the 4 mm embryo (less than 4 weeks of gestation)[3] (Fig. 8-1). The diverticula grow out laterally, and their ends come into close apposition with the overlying surface ectoderm. The apposition of the outer wall of each optic vesicle to the overlying surface epithelium is essential for the transmission of inductive messages that stimulate the surface ectoderm to form a small area overlying the optic vesicle that thickens and forms the lens placode. As the process of lens induction proceeds, the outer surface of the optic vesicle flattens and then becomes concave toward

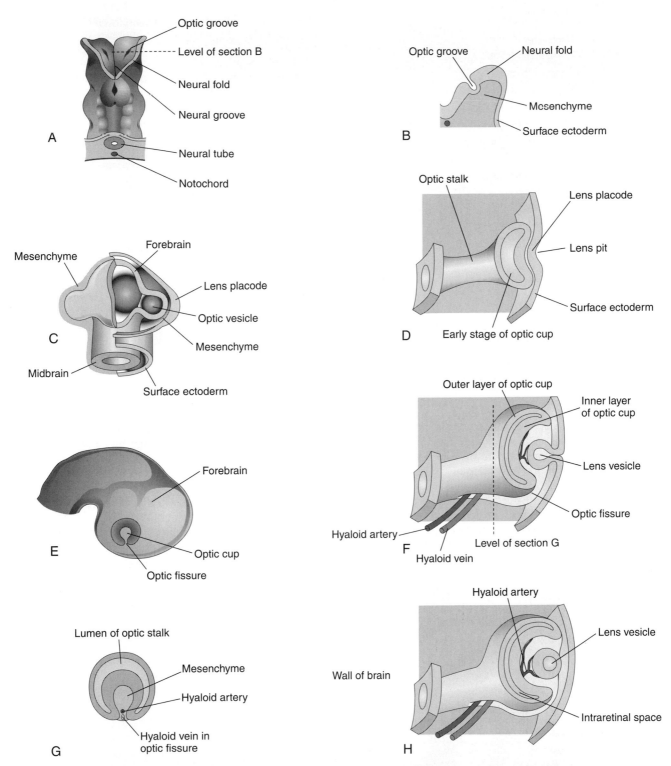

**FIGURE 8-1**   Drawings showing early eye development. **A,** Optic sulci or grooves are seen in the cranial end of an embryo at about 22 days of gestation. The neural folds have not yet fused to form the primary forebrain vesicles. **B,** Transverse section of a neural fold showing the optic sulcus. **C,** Schematic drawing of an embryo at about 28 days of gestation shows the covering layers of mesenchyme and surface ectoderm. **D, F,** and **H,** Schematic sections of the developing eye showing the successive stages in the development of the optic cup and lens vesicle. **E,** Lateral view of the brain of an embryo at about 32 days of gestation showing the external appearance of the optic cup. **G,** Transverse section of the optic stalk showing the optic fissure and its contents. Note that the edges of the fissure are growing together, thereby completing the optic cup and enclosing the central artery and vein of the retina in the optic stalk and cup. (From Moore KL, Persaud TVN. The Developing Human: Clinically Oriented Embryology 6th ed. Philadelphia, Pa: Saunders, 1998; 493.)

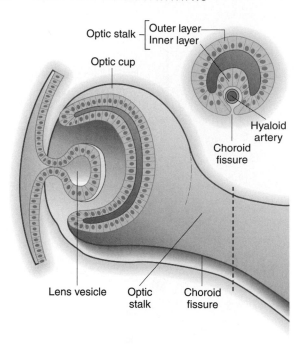

**FIGURE 8-2** Drawing of the optic cup and stalk showing the choroid fissure containing the hyaloid artery. The cross section (top) is through the level of the dashed line. (From Carlson BM. Human Embryology and Developmental Biology, 2nd ed. St. Louis, Mo: Mosby, 1994; 265.)

the surface of the embryo. This results in the transformation of the distal end of the optic vesicle into the double-layered optic cup. The proximal portion of each optic vesicle becomes constricted to form the optic stalk[1-6] (Figs. 8-1 and 8-2). The lens placode invaginates and sinks below the surface ectoderm to become the lens pit, and its edges come together and fuse to enclose a hollow lens vesicle[1-6] (Figs. 8-2 and 8-3). By the fifth week, the lens vesicle loses contact

with the surface ectoderm and lies within the mouth of the optic cup, the edges of which form the future pupil[1-7] (Figs. 8-1 and 8-3). The lens vesicle initiates a new series of inductive reactions by acting on the overlying surface ectoderm to begin development of the cornea.

In the 5 mm embryo, the invagination is not limited to the outer wall of the optic vesicle, but also involves its caudal surface and extends in the form of a groove for some distance along the optic stalk[2] (Figs. 8-1 and 8-2). Thus, for a time, a wide hiatus, the optic fissure or choroidal fissure (embryonic fissure), exists in the inferior edge of the optic cup.[1,2] The embryonic fissure remains open for some distance along the optic stalk at the inferior and slightly nasal aspect of the optic cup (Figs. 8-1 and 8-2). Through the embryonic fissure, the mesenchyme extends into the optic stalk and cup, carrying the hyaloid artery with it to the posterior surface of the lens[1-3] (Fig. 8-3). The hyaloid artery, a branch of the ophthalmic artery, supplies the inner layer of the optic cup, the lens vesicle, and the mesenchyme in the optic cup (Figs. 8-4 and 8-5). The hyaloid vein drains blood from these structures. Later, as growth proceeds, the edges of this fissure become narrowed, and by the seventh week of embryonic development the fissure closes, forming a narrow tube, the optic canal, inside the optic stalks. Failure of the choroidal fissure to close completely results in a coloboma (a notched defect) formation, which may include the iris, ciliary body, choroid, retina, or optic nerve.

The retina develops from the optic cup (Figs. 8-2 and 8-3). For purposes of description, the retina may be divided into two developmental layers, the pigment layer and the neural layer. Its two layers are at first equipotential and mutually interchangeable. The pigment layer is formed from the outer thinner layer of the optic cup. It is a single layer of cells that becomes columnar in shape, and pigment granules develop within the cytoplasm of these cells. The neural layer is formed from the inner layer of the optic cup.[1-6] It is

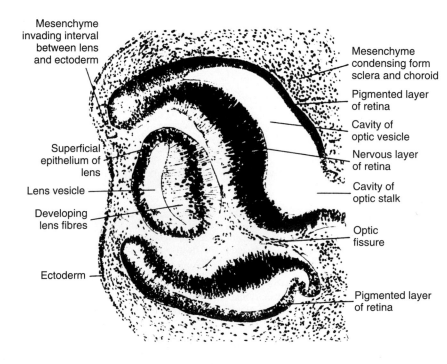

**FIGURE 8-3** A lateral section through the developing eye of a human embryo 13.2 mm long. (From Bannister LH, Berry MM, Collins P, Dyson M, et al. (eds). Gray's Anatomy, 38th ed. Edinburgh: Churchill Livingstone, 1999; 259.)

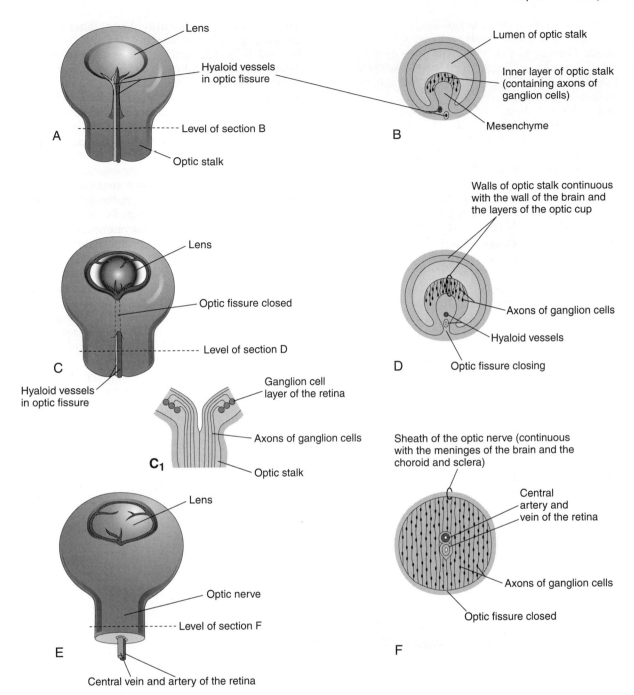

**FIGURE 8-4**   Diagrams showing the closure of the optic fissure and the formation of the optic nerve. **A, C,** and **E,** Views of the inferior surface of the optic cup and stalk showing progressive stages in the closure of the optic fissure. **C₁,** Schematic drawing of a longitudinal section of a part of the optic cup and stalk showing axons and ganglion cells of the retina growing through the optic stalk to the brain. **B, D,** and **F,** Transverse sections of the optic stalk showing successive stages in the closure of the optic fissure and the formation of the optic nerve. (From Moore KL, Persaud TVN. The Developing Human: Clinically Oriented Embryology 6th ed. Philadelphia, Pa: Saunders, 1998; 495.)

important to realize that in the region of the cup that overlaps the lens, the inner layer is not differentiated into neural elements. This anterior one-fifth of the inner layer persists as a layer of columnar epithelium, which, together with the corresponding part of the pigmented epithelium of the outer layer, extend forward onto the posterior surface of the developing ciliary body and iris to form the double epithelium of the ciliary body and iris.[1,2] The posterior four-fifths of the inner layer of the optic cup undergoes cellular proliferation, forming an outer nuclear zone and an inner marginal zone devoid of nuclei (Fig. 8-3). Later, at the 12 mm stage, the cells of the nuclear zone invade the marginal zone, so that at the 17 mm stage, the neural part of the retina consists of an inner and an outer neuroblastic layer.[2] The inner neuroblastic layer of the retina forms the ganglion cells, the amacrine cells, and the somata of the sustentacular fibers of Müller.[1, 2, 8, 9] The outer neuroblastic layer of the retina gives rise to the horizontal cells, the nuclei of the bipolar rod and cone nerve cells, and probably the rod and cone cells as well (Fig. 8-6).[1, 2]

By the eighth month of fetal life, all the layers of the retina can be recognized[1, 2] (Fig. 8-7). Thus, the inner layer of the optic cup may be divided into a small nonneural portion near the edge of the cup and a large photosensitive portion, the two being separated by a wavy line, the ora serrata. It is interesting to remember that the cavity of the optic vesicle is continuous through the optic stalk (optic canal) with the cavity of the diencephalon (i.e., the part that forms the third ventricle) (Figs. 8-1 and 8-2). Early in development, the outermost layer of cells of the nuclear zone have cilia, which are continuous with the ciliated ependymal cells of the third ventricle.[2] Later, during the seventh week of development, the cilia of the cells of the nuclear zone disappear and are believed to be replaced by the outer segments of the rods and cones during the fourth month of gestation.[2]

## Optic Nerves, Macular Area, and Fovea Centralis

The deepest part of the optic (embryonic) fissure is at the center of the floor of the optic cup[1] (Figs. 8-1 and 8-2). In this region, which later is the site of the optic disc, the inner (neural) cell layer of the cup is continuous with the corresponding invaginated cell layer of the optic stalk (Fig. 8-3). As a result, the developing nerve fibers of the ganglion cells can pass directly into the wall of the stalk to become the optic nerve.[1] At the 7.5 mm embryonic stage, the area in the optic cup where the optic nerve head will develop can be identified.[5] It is referred to as the primitive epithelial papilla and is located at the superior end of the embryonic fissure.[10] Once the axons pass through the primitive epithelial papilla, it is referred to as the optic nerve head.[5, 10, 11]

The macular area first develops as a localized increase of superimposed nuclei in the ganglion cell layer, lateral to the optic disc, just after midterm. During the seventh month there is a peripheral displacement of the ganglion cells, leaving a central shallow depression, the fovea centralis. The foveal cones decrease in width in their inner segments, but

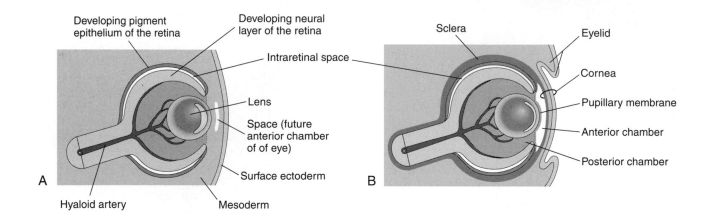

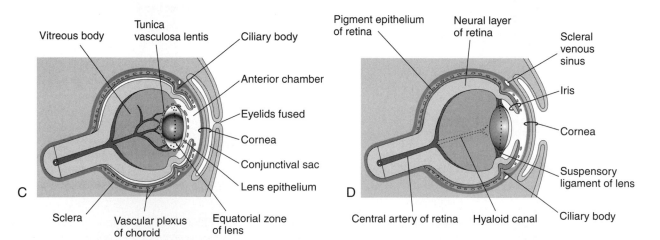

**FIGURE 8-5**    Drawings of sagittal sections of the eye showing successive developmental stages of the lens, retina, iris, and cornea. **A**, 5 weeks; **B**, 6 weeks; **C**, 20 weeks; **D**, newborn. Note that the layers of the optic cup fuse to form the retinal pigment epithelium and neural retina and extend anteriorly as the double epithelium of the ciliary body and its iris. The retina and optic nerve are formed from the optic cup and stalk (outgrowths of the brain). At birth the eye is about three quarters of its adult size. Most successive growth occurs during the first year of life. (From Moore KL, Persaud TVN. The Developing Human: Clinically Oriented Embryology 6th ed. Philadelphia, Pa: Saunders, 1998; 498.)

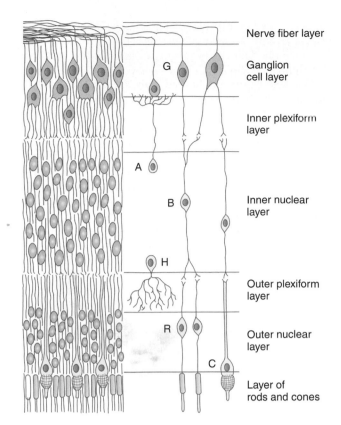

Nerve fiber layer

Ganglion cell layer

Inner plexiform layer

Inner nuclear layer

Outer plexiform layer

Outer nuclear layer

Layer of rods and cones

**FIGURE 8-6**   Drawing of the tissue and cellular organization of the neural retina of the human fetus. **A**, Amacrine cell; **B**, bipolar cell; **C**, cone, **G**, ganglion cell; **H**, horizontal cell. **R**, Rod. (From Carlson BM. Human Embryology and Developmental Biology, 2nd ed. St. Louis, Mo: Mosby, 1994; 271.)

their outer segments are elongated. This permits an increase in foveal cone density.[2] At birth, the ganglion cells have been reduced to a single layer in the fovea, and by 4 months of age, the cone nuclei in the center of the fovea have no

ganglion cells covering them. The reason for the newborn's imperfect central fixation is that the cones do not fully develop until several months after birth.[2]

The ganglion cells of the retina develop axons that converge to a point where the optic stalk leaves the posterior surface of the optic cup (Fig. 8-3). This site will later become the optic disc.[1-3, 9] The axons now pass among the cells that form the inner layer of the stalk. Gradually, the inner layer encroaches on the cavity of the stalk until the inner and outer layers fuse. The cells of the optic stalk form neuroglia-supporting cells to the axons, and the cavity of the stalk disappears. The stalk, together with the optic axons, forms the optic nerve. The surrounding mesenchyme condenses and later differentiates into the meninges, which form a sheath for the optic nerve. The axons of the optic nerve begin to develop their myelin sheaths just before birth, but the process of myelination continues for some time after birth.[1-3] After the eyes have been exposed to light for about 10 weeks, myelination is complete. The hyaloid artery and vein become the central artery and vein of the retina, running for a distance within and along the optic nerve.[1, 2]

## Lens

As described, the rudimentary lens is first seen as a thickening of the surface ectoderm, the lens placodes, at 22 days of gestation; it overlies the optic vesicle (Figs. 8-1 and 8-2). The lens placode invaginates and sinks below the surface ectoderm to form the lens vesicle, which is overlapped by the margin of the optic cup and becomes separated from the overlying ectoderm by mesenchyme.[1, 2] The cells forming the posterior wall of the lens vesicle rapidly elongate and form transparent lens fibers known as the primary lens fibers (Fig. 8-3). At the cellular level, the relatively unspecialized lens epithelial cells undergo a

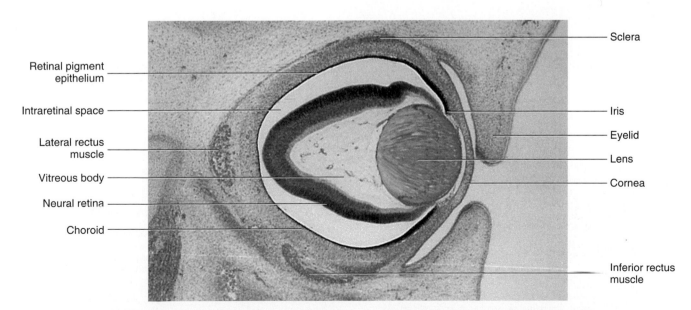

Retinal pigment epithelium

Intraretinal space

Lateral rectus muscle

Vitreous body

Neural retina

Choroid

Sclera

Iris

Eyelid

Lens

Cornea

Inferior rectus muscle

**FIGURE 8-7**   Sagittal section of the eye of an embryo at about 56 days of gestation. Note the developing neural retina and the retinal pigment epithelium. The intraretinal space normally disappears as these two layers of the retina fuse. (From Moore KL, Persaud TVN, Shiotak: Color Atlas of Clinical Embryology. Philadelphia, WB Saunders, 1994.)

profound transformation into transparent, elongated cells that contain large quantities of crystallin proteins, the primarily proteins being α, β, and γ.[12] With the increase in length of these cells, the cavity of the lens vesicle gradually becomes obliterated.[2] The primary lens fibers become attached to the apical surface of the anterior lens epithelium.[2] All additional lens fibers are formed by the division of the anterior epithelial cells at the equatorial zone or rim of the lens (Figs. 8-8 and 8-9). These are known as the secondary lens fibers, and new secondary lens fibers are formed throughout life.

By the second month of gestation, the lens is invested by a vascular mesenchymal condensation termed the *vascular capsule of the lens*, the ventral part of which, covering the lens, is named the pupillary membrane. The blood vessels supplying the dorsal part of this capsule are derived from the hyaloid artery, and those for the ventral part are derived from the anterior ciliary arteries.[1,2] By the sixth month, all the vessels of the capsule are atrophied except the hyaloid artery, which becomes occluded during the eighth month of gestation.[1,2] With the loss of its blood vessels the vascular capsule of the lens disappears (Fig. 8-4, 8-5), but sometimes the pupillary membrane persists at birth, giving rise to the condition termed *congenital atresia of the pupil*.[1,2] In the fetus the lens grows rapidly because it is supplied by the hyaloid artery, which forms a plexus on the posterior surface of the lens capsule. By the time the infant is born, the anteroposterior diameter of the lens is nearly that of an adult. Its equatorial diameter is about two-thirds of that reached in the adult.[2]

The lens capsule is formed from the mesenchyme that surrounds the lens. As mentioned, in the earliest stages of development, it receives an abundant arterial supply from the hyaloid artery as the tunica vasculosa lentis. Later, this blood supply regresses, and it disappears before birth. In the 40 mm human embryo, the layers of the retina, developing lens, pupillary membrane, cornea, conjunctival sac, anterior and posterior aqueous chambers, the developing vitreous body, the condensing circumoptic mesenchyme, and the fused eyelids are recognized (Fig. 8-7).[1]

Throughout most of its life, the lens is under the influence of the retina. Thus, following induction of the lens, chemical secretions from the retina accumulate in the vitreous humor behind the lens and appear to stimulate the formation of lens fibers.[12]

## The Ciliary Body and Suspensory Ligaments of the Lens

The mesenchyme, situated at the edge of the optic cup, differentiates into the connective tissue of the ciliary body,

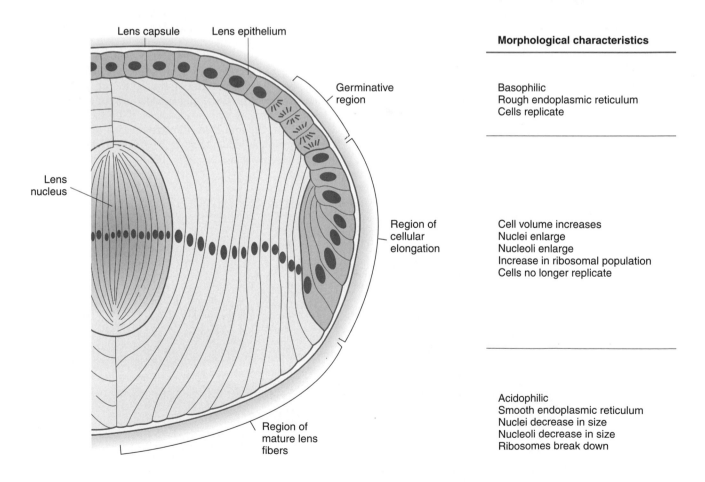

**FIGURE 8-8** Drawing of the organization of the vertebrate lens. As the lens grows, epithelial cells from the germinative region stop dividing, elongate, and differentiate into lens cells that produce lens crystallin proteins. (Papaconstantinou J. Molecular aspects of lens cell differentiation. Science 156:338–346, 1967.)

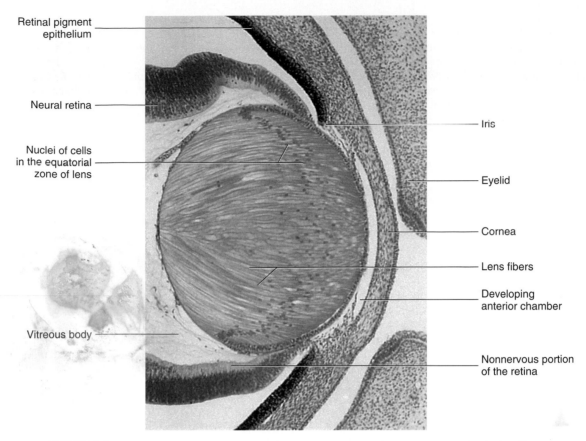

Retinal pigment epithelium

Neural retina

Nuclei of cells in the equatorial zone of lens

Vitreous body

Iris

Eyelid

Cornea

Lens fibers

Developing anterior chamber

Nonnervous portion of the retina

**FIGURE 8-9**   Higher magnification of a portion of the developing eye seen in Figure 8-7. Note that the lens fibers have elongated and obliterated the cavity of the lens vesicle. The inner layer of the optic cup has thickened to form the neural retina, and the outer layer is heavily pigmented (retinal pigment epithelium). (From Moore KL, Persaud TVN, Shiotak: Color Atlas of Clinical Embryology. Philadelphia, WB Saunders, 1994.)

the smooth muscle fibers of the ciliary muscle, and the suspensory ligaments of the lens. The two layers of neuroectoderm (the outer pigment layer and the anterior one-fifth of the inner layer) forming the edge of the optic cup grow onto the posterior surface of the ciliary muscle, forming the two epithelial layers covering the ciliary body.[2] The fibers of the ciliary muscles are derived from the mesoderm, but those of the sphincter and dilator pupillae are of ectodermal origin, being developed from the cells of the pupillary part of the optic cup (Fig. 8-10).[1, 2]

## The Iris and the Aqueous Chamber

The mesenchyme, situated on the anterior surface of the lens, condenses to form the pupillary membrane. The two layers of neuroectoderm (the pigment layer of the retina and the neural layer of the retina) forming the growing edge of the optic cup, having covered the ciliary muscle, now extend onto the posterior surface of the pupillary membrane. These structures fuse to become the iris.[2] The sphincter and dilator muscles of the pupil are derived from the pigment cells of the neuroectoderm. The mesenchyme forms the connective tissue and blood vessels of the iris. Pigment cells derived from the neuroectoderm penetrate the sphincter muscle and enter the connective tissue. The opening in the central part of the iris becomes the pupil. The pupillary membrane begins

to separate from the iris, and at about the eighth month of gestation, the pupillary membrane starts to degenerate and eventually disappears.[2]

The anterior (aqueous) chamber of the eye appears as a cleft in the mesenchyme between the surface ectoderm and the developing iris.[1, 2] The posterior chamber develops as a slit in the mesenchyme posterior to the developing iris and anterior to the developing lens (Fig. 8-5). The mesenchyme superficial to the cleft forms the substantia propria of the cornea. The mesenchyme deep to the cleft forms the mesenchymal stroma of the iris and the pupillary membrane (Fig. 8-10).[1] When the pupillary membrane disappears, the anterior and posterior chambers of the eye communicate with each other through a circumferential scleral venous sinus (sinus venosus sclerae, canal of Schlemm).[1] This sinus (canal) is the outflow site of aqueous humor from the anterior chamber of the eye to the venous system. Temporally, the anterior and posterior chambers communicate when the pupillary membrane disappears and the pupil is formed.[1]

## The Vitreous

The vitreous body develops between the developing lens and the optic cup. The primitive or primary vitreous body consists of a network of delicate cytoplasmic processes that are derived partly from the ectodermal cells of the developing lens and partly from the neuroectoderm of the retinal layer of the optic cup. The mesenchyme that enters the cup through the choroidal (embryonic or optic) fissure and around the equator of the lens becomes intimately united with this reticular tissue and also contributes to the formation of the vitreous body, which is therefore derived partly from the ectoderm and partly from the mesoderm.[1, 2] It contains many vascular elements, including the vasa hyaloidea propria, which join the primitive vitreous. At this stage, the primitive vitreous is supplied by the hyaloid artery and its branches. The definitive or secondary vitreous arises between the primitive vitreous and the retina. It is at first a homogeneous gel, which rapidly increases in volume and pushes the primitive vitreous anteriorly behind the iris. Hyalocytes, derived from the mesenchyme around the hyaloid vessels, now migrate into the secondary vitreous. Later the hyaloid vessels atrophy and disappear, leaving the acellular hyaloid canal.[2] The hyaloid artery becomes occluded during the eighth month of intrauterine life.[2] Prior to this, during the fourth month, the hyaloid artery gives off retinal branches, and its proximal part persists in the adult as the central artery of the retina.[2] The hyaloid canal, which carries the artery through the vitreous during development of the primitive (primary) vitreous, persists after the vessel has become occluded.[1, 13–15]

## The Choroid

Outside the optic cup, there is a layer of mesenchymal cells that are primarily of neural crest origin. As a result of induction from the pigmented epithelium of the retina, these mesenchymal cells differentiate into structures that provide the vascular and mechanical support of the eye.[12] The innermost cells of this mesenchymal layer become the highly vascular choroid, and the anterior part of the choroid is eventually modified to form the ciliary body and ciliary processes.

## The Sclera

The sclera is also derived from the mesenchyme surrounding the optic cup, outside the choroid. This mesenchyme forms a densely collagenous covering, the sclera, which is continuous with the cornea. It first forms near the future insertion of the rectus muscle.[1]

## The Cornea

The formation of the cornea is the last in the series of inductive events in the formation of the eye. Corneal development is induced by the lens and the optic cup.[1] The corneal epithelium is formed from the surface ectoderm and the mesothelium of the anterior chamber from the mesenchyme[2] (Figs. 8-5, 8-9). The substantia propria and the endothelium covering the posterior surface of the cornea are formed from mesenchyme.[1] Bowman's membrane, which lies immediately beneath the basal lamina of the corneal epithelium, is formed from mesenchyme.[1] Descemet's membrane, which is the basement membrane of the endothelial cells, is synthesized by the endothelial cells

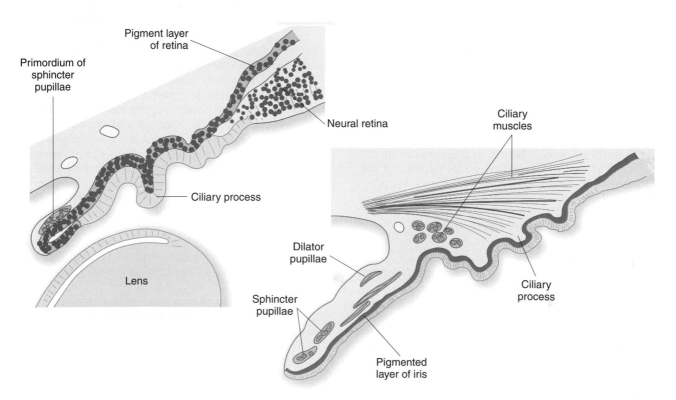

**FIGURE 8-10**  Drawing of two stages (earlier on the left) in the development of the iris and ciliary body, including the sphincter and dilator pupillae muscles. (From Carlson BM. Human Embryology and Developmental Biology, 2nd ed. St. Louis, Mo: Mosby, 1994; 274.)

formed from mesenchyme.[1] Listed from outside to inside, the layers that form the mature cornea are the outer epithelium, Bowman's membrane, the secondary stroma, Descemet's membrane, and the corneal endothelium.

## Vascular System

The development of the vascular system of the eye is a complex process that involves the appearance of vessels to meet the nutritional needs of the developing eye and subsequent regression of those same vessels.[3] In the early embryo, the internal carotid artery supplies a fine capillary plexus to the dorsal aspect of the optic cup (dorsal ophthalmic artery). Soon afterward, a second branch of the internal carotid artery is given off to supply the medial aspect of the optic cup.[3] This branch is called the ventral ophthalmic artery and is anastomosed with the dorsal ophthalmic artery.[3] The hyaloid artery is a branch of the dorsal ophthalmic artery that passes through the embryonic fissure into the optic cup. Simultaneously, the orbital tissues are supplied by the stapedial artery, a branch of the internal carotid artery.[3] The hyaloid artery extends toward and around the lens vesicle and projects a vascular meshwork across the lens to form the tunica vasculosa lentis.[3] During the sixth week of gestation, the primitive dorsal ophthalmic artery is transformed into the definitive ophthalmic artery, and the ventral ophthalmic artery regresses and transforms into the posterior nasal ciliary artery.[3] The ophthalmic artery's branches become the central retinal artery, the temporal long posterior ciliary artery, and the short posterior ciliary artery.[3] In the third trimester, the hyaloid system begins to regress and the tunica vasculosa lentis becomes thin and atrophic, and eventually disappears.[3–5] Remnants of this system may sometimes be seen in the adult as a persistent pupillary membrane.[6] The hyaloid artery is no longer patent and loses its connection to the disc in the eighth month of intrauterine life (Figs. 8-4 and 8-5). Occasionally, a connective bud may remain attached to the disc as Bergmeister's papilla.[3]

## IMAGING TECHNIQUES

Computed tomography (CT) provided a major imaging advance over conventional radiography and multidirectional tomography in examining the eye. However, the development of magnetic resonance (MR) imaging has proven to be an even greater breakthrough in diagnostic medical imaging and biomedical research.[16–20] This section discusses CT and MR imaging of the normal globe and the features of ocular pathology, with particular emphasis on the potential of MR imaging in the practice of ophthalmology.

## MR Imaging

The success of MR imaging depends on the cooperation of the patient and, in the case of infants and children, appropriate sedation. The procedure should be carefully explained to the patient and the family or accompanying persons, especially to the person who will stay in the MR scanner room with the patient. For sedation, oral chloral hydrate (75 to 100 mg/kg body weight) usually affords satisfactory sedation in children up to 2 to 4 years of age. When this proves inadequate, intramuscular diphenhydramine (Benadryl, a one-time dose of 1 mg/kg) or midazolam (Versed, 0.05 to 0.08 mg/kg) for children 5 to 8 years of age can be added.[7] Other children may need intravenous medication or general anesthesia, and there may be variations among institutions regarding the doses and medications used. Because of the importance of monitoring sedated patients, sedation procedures should be performed by a trained, dedicated MR imaging nurse. The patient should be monitored during MR imaging using pulse oximetry, allowing evaluation of the arterial oxygen saturation. When general anesthesia is required, anesthesiologists use MR-compatible monitoring and ventilation equipment.

The majority of MR imaging studies described in this section were performed on a 1.5-T Signa unit (General Electric, Milwaukee) with 3 or 5 mm thick sections, with no gap or a 0, 0.6 to 1.5 mm interslice gap. A complete MR evaluation of the eye should consist of high-resolution axial, coronal, and sagittal images of the eye and surrounding structures. The globe can be successfully evaluated with the standard head coil. The field of view, however, should be maintained between 12 and 16 cm and in plane resolution of $256 \times 192$, $256 \times 256$, or $512 \times 256$. Orbital surface coils are used to improve the spatial resolution of MR images.[21] If they are available, they should be used primarily for lesions limited to the globe and for smaller lesions that may not be detected by a head coil. For intraocular lesions that have invaded the optic nerve and retrobulbar space, a head coil is preferred. The use of contrast-enhanced MR imaging of the orbit and brain, using a head coil, is recommended for the evaluation of children with suspected retinoblastoma and, in particular, for patients with possible subarachnoid seeding of retinoblastoma and those with bilateral disease. This technique allows early detection of optic nerve involvement, orbital spread, or asymptomatic pineoblastoma and suprasellar tumors.[21] Although the examination should always be tailored to the problems of the individual patient, in general for ocular lesions the routine MR imaging examination consists of both T1- and T2-weighted images and precontrast and postcontrast T1-weighted images with and without fat suppression. The suggested head coil or surface coil protocol for ocular MR imaging is as follows:

*Axial View*
   TR 2000–3000 ms, TE 30/80–120 ms
   $256 \times 192$, 3 mm slice thickness, 0.5 mm skip
   Field of view (FOV) $16 \times 16$ cm, 2 number of excitation (NEX), no phase wrap (NP)
   This may be replaced by a fast spin echo, single echo, T2-weighted, fat suppression acquisition technique

*Precontrast Axial View*
   TR 500 ms, TE 20 ms
   $256 \times 192$, 3 mm slice thickness, 0.5 mm skip
   FOV 14–16, 2 or 3 NEX, NP

*Postcontrast Axial and Coronal Views*
   TR 500 ms, TE 20 ms
   $256 \times 192$, 2 or 3 mm slice thickness, 0.5 mm skip
   FOV 14–16, 3 NEX, NP

*Postcontrast Fat Suppression Axial View*
TR 500 ms, TE 20 ms
256 × 192, 3 mm slice thickness, 0.5 mm skip
FOV 14–16, 3 NEX, NP

An additional postcontrast, fat suppression, T1-weighted sagittal view may be obtained according to the findings in the axial or coronal sections.

*Postcontrast Axial View of the Orbit and Head Using a Head Coil*
TR 500 ms, TE 20 ms
256 × 192, 5-mm slice thickness, 1.5-mm skip
FOV 22–24 cm, 1 NEX

Because motion artifact is more pronounced on images obtained with a surface coil due to the inherent sensitivity of the coil, a lesion is sometimes seen better on images obtained with a head coil.[21] With the surface coil, a 3 mm section thickness is used to reduce the problem of partial volume averaging. The thin section has the disadvantage of generating less signal (a small volume), and this may result in a decreased amount of T2-weighted information in later echoes, particularly in rapidly decaying T2-weighted signals. For these reasons, at times a uveal melanoma may be better seen on T2-weighted images obtained with a head coil rather than with a surface coil. This is extremely important because the hypointensity of melanotic tissues in T2-weighted images is an important diagnostic feature of these lesions.[19, 21] Despite the difficulties encountered with inhomogeneity in the face and orbit, fat suppression MR techniques are most often utilized. Fat suppression pulse sequences are important for the detection of intraocular (small) lesions and for the evaluation of extraocular extension of eye tumors and inflammation. Fat suppression is also useful in the T2-weighted acquisitions of the optic nerve and optic pathway.

## CT Technique

The CT protocol for intraocular lesions includes 1.5 to 3 mm axial sections of the globe. For all foreign bodies and lesions at 6 o'clock and 12 o'clock, additional direct 3 to 5 mm coronal sections are obtained. Additional 1.5, 3, or 5 mm axial sections (depending on the size of the lesion) of the orbit are obtained following administration of iodinated contrast material (meglumine diatrizoate, 1 ml per pound of body weight). In cases of suspected retinoblastoma and uveal melanoma, additional 5 to 10 mm axial sections of the head are obtained to investigate the possibility of an intracranial abnormality. The major application of CT for ocular lesions is the detection of foreign bodies and intraocular calcification. For intraocular tumors and other intraocular pathology, MR imaging is the preferred initial study.

## MR Imaging and Evaluation of Intraocular Foreign Bodies

Despite the many advantages of MR imaging, it may not be indicated as a primary modality in the evaluation of the traumatized eyes harboring a possible intraocular foreign body. This cautionary advice is based on the possibility of additional damage to the injured eye by ferromagnetic foreign bodies that are induced to move during the imaging process. A study conducted in vitro and in vivo (rabbit) experiments to examine the effects of MR imaging (1.5 Tesla Units) on intraocular foreign bodies showed that diamagnetic and paramagnetic foreign bodies were imaged without artifacts and without movement during the imaging process, and ferromagnetic foreign bodies produced large amounts of artifact that prevented meaningful images.[22] All ferromagnetic foreign bodies moved during in vitro imaging. During in vivo imaging, three of four ferromagnetic foreign bodies moved, producing substantial retinal injury. It was concluded that MR imaging is contraindicated in the patient with a traumatized eye and a suspected ferromagnetic foreign body. For those patients with a remote history of a traumatic foreign body, or in metal workers or other high-risk individuals, high-resolution 1.5 mm or thinner CT scans of the orbits and 5 to 10 mm thick CT scans of the head are recommended to rule out the possibility of foreign bodies. Patients with stapedectomy (metallic) or other metallic prostheses that have proved to be safe for 1.5T MR unit should be carefully screened for MR study using a 3T or higher field. Not enough data are available to demonstrate that these devices may not move at field strengths higher than 1.5T.

## MR Imaging Artifacts

Motion artifacts may result in marked degradation of MR images. It is important to tell patients to close their eyes during the examination. Artifacts may occur as a result of tattooing of eyelids with iron oxide and even from the external application of eye cosmetics (Fig. 8-11). The artifacts arising from tattooing or related to eye cosmetics usually appear as distortion of the skin contours in the location of the iron oxide. There also may be distortion of the shape of the globe and multiple artifacts consisting of hyperintense areas around the contour of the eyelids.

## NORMAL OCULAR ANATOMY

### Ocular Structures

The eyeball (eye or globe) is made up of the segments of two spheres of different sizes placed one in front of the other. The anterior, smaller segment is transparent (cornea) and forms about one-sixth of the eyeball. The posterior, larger segment is opaque (sclera) and forms about five-sixths of the eyeball.[23] The anterior pole of the eyeball is the center of curvature of the transparent segment, or cornea. The posterior pole is the center of the posterior curvature of the eyeball, and it is located slightly temporal to the optic nerve. The geometric or optic axis is a line connecting the two poles. The equator lies midway between the two poles. Because the fovea centralis is temporal and slightly inferior to the posterior pole, the visual axis and the optic axis do not coincide.[24]

The eye consists of three primary layers (Fig. 8-11): (1) the sclera, or outer layer, which is composed primarily of

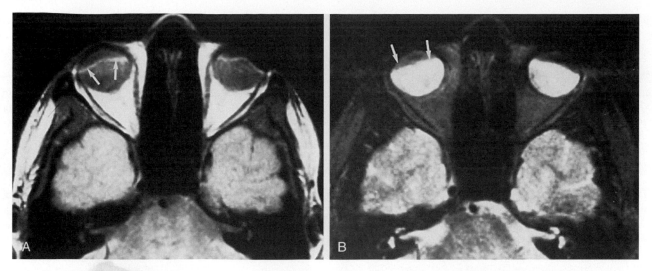

**FIGURE 8-11**    Axial PW (**A**) and T2-weighted (**B**) MR images show makeup artifacts (*arrows*).

collagen-elastic tissue; (2) the uvea, or middle layer, which is richly vascular and contains pigmented tissue consisting of three components: the choroid, ciliary body, and iris; and (3) the retina, or inner layer, which is the neural, sensory stratum of the eye.

## Tenon's Capsule

The fascial sheath of the eyeball, also called the fascia bulbi or Tenon's capsule, is a thin membrane that envelops the eyeball and separates it from the central orbital fat. It thus forms a socket for the eyeball.[23] Tenon's capsule blends with the sclera just behind the corneoscleral junction and fuses with the bulbar conjunctiva. Tenon's capsule is perforated behind by the optic nerve and its sheath, the ciliary nerves and vessels. The capsule fuses with and extends to the sheath of the optic nerve and the sclera around the entrance of the optic nerve.[25] Septa of fibrous tissue are attached to the outer surface of Tenon's capsule, and near the equator it is perforated by the vortex (vorticose) veins (draining veins of the choroid and sclera).[25] The inner surface of Tenon's capsule is smooth and shiny and is separated from the outer surface of the sclera by the episcleral (Tenon's) space.[25] This is a potential space that is traversed by fibers of loose connective (areolar) tissue, which extend between the fascia and the sclera.[26] The episcleral space starts anteriorly, at the bulbar conjunctiva near the sclerocorneal junction, and extends to the optic nerve, where it firmly attaches to the nerve and then is continuous with the subdural and subarachnoid spaces about the nerve.[26] The tendons of all extrinsic ocular muscles pierce the capsule to reach the sclera. At the site of perforation, the fascial sheath is reflected back along the tendons of these muscles to form on each a tubular sleeve.[23] The connection between the muscle fibers and the sheath is especially strong at the point where the two fuse.[25, 26] For this reason, the muscles retain their attachment to the capsule and do not retract extensively after enucleation (tenotomy).[25, 26] The superior oblique muscle sleeve extends as far as the trochlea. The inferior oblique muscle sleeve

extends to the origin of the muscle on the floor of the orbit.[23] The tubular sleeves for the four recti muscles have important expansions. Those for the medial and lateral recti are strong and are attached to the lacrimal and zygomatic bones. Because these expansions may limit the actions of these muscles on the eyeball, they are called medial and lateral check ligaments.[23] Thinner and less distinct expansions extend from the superior rectus tendon to that of the levator palpebrae superior, and from the inferior rectus to the inferior tarsal plate. The inferior part of the fascial sheath of the eyeball is thickened and is continuous medially and laterally with the medial and lateral check ligaments.[23] This hammock-like arrangement of the fascial sheath constitutes what is known as the suspensory ligament of Lockwood.[23] This thickened area receives contributions from the fascia of the inferior rectus and inferior oblique muscles as they cross each other below the eyeball. The close relationship between the suspensory ligament of Lockwood and the tendons of the inferior oblique and inferior rectus muscles makes operations on these muscles very difficult and the results unpredictable.[23] The suspensory ligament is strong enough to provide the eyeball with adequate support in case of maxillectomy. Inflammatory and intraocular neoplastic processes are the most common lesions to involve Tenon's space. In posterior scleritis, episcleritis, Tenon's fasciitis, and pseudotumor, an inflammatory effusion produces a characteristic circular or semicircular distention of Tenon's capsule (Fig. 8-12). Retinoblastomas (Fig. 8-13) and melanomas (Fig. 8-14) also may invade Tenon's space.[21]

## Sclera

The sclera is the globe's outer white leathery coat. It extends from the limbus at the margin of the cornea to the optic nerve, where it becomes continuous with the dural sheath.[27] The external side of the sclera lies against Tenon's capsule. The internal surface of the sclera blends with the suprachoroidal tissues.[27] Posteriorly the sclera is perforated by the vortex veins, the long posterior ciliary arteries and nerves, and the short posterior ciliary arteries and nerves.

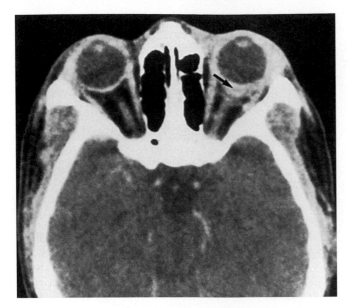

**FIGURE 8-12** Pseudotumor. Axial CT scan shows fluid (*arrow*) and inflammatory infiltration in Tenon's space.

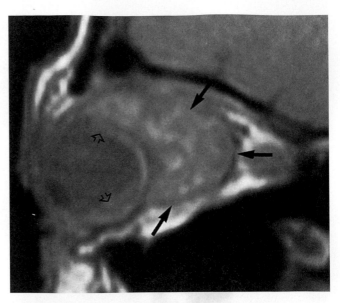

**FIGURE 8-14** Uveal melanoma with extension into Tenon's capsule. Sagittal PW MR image shows a large, well-capsulated retrobulbar mass (*arrows*) in this patient with uveal melanoma (not seen in this section). Note the subretinal fluid (*open arrows*). Surgery confirmed the intraocular tumor and massive extension into Tenon's capsule.

The sclera is composed predominantly of extracellular bundles of collagen. The sclera forms the posterior five-sixths of the eyeball and is opaque. In the adult the sclera is 1 mm thick posteriorly, thinning at the equator to 0.6 mm. It is thinnest, 0.3 mm, immediately posterior to the

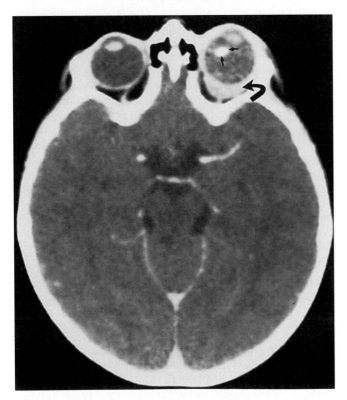

**FIGURE 8-13** Axial CT scan shows retinoblastoma with extension into Tenon's capsule. A mass with focal calcification (*arrows*) fills the entire left globe and extends into Tenon's space (*curved arrow*). (From Mafee MF et al. Malignant uveal melenoma and similar lesions studied by CT. Radiology 1985;156:403–408.)

tendinous insertions of the recti muscles.[23] At the corneoscleral junction the sclera is 0.8 mm thick. The medial rectus muscle inserts 5.5 mm posterior to the limbus; the inferior rectus 6.5 mm; the lateral rectus 6.9 mm; and the superior rectus 7.7 mm.[23] The insertions of the superior oblique and inferior oblique muscles are posterior to the scleral equator. The sclera is perforated posteriorly about 3 mm medial and 1 mm above the posterior pole by the optic nerve. The site of this perforation is referred to as the posterior scleral foramen.[23] Here the sclera is fused with the dural and arachnoid sheaths of the optic nerve. The lamina cribrosa is where the optic nerve fibers pierce the sclera. One of the openings in the lamina is larger than the rest and transmits the central retinal artery and vein. Since the lamina cribrosa is relatively a weak point, it can be made to bulge outward by a rise in intraocular pressure, producing a cupped disc. The sclera is pierced anteriorly at the insertion of the recti muscles by the branches of anterior ciliary arteries. Each rectus muscle has two anterior ciliary arteries, with the exception of the lateral rectus muscle, which only has one.[23]

The sclera is pierced about 4 mm posterior to the equator of the eye by the vortex veins (four or five). The posterior scleral apertures are numerous and are located around the optic nerve. They transmit the long and short ciliary nerves and vessels.[23] Anteriorly, the sclera is continuous with the cornea. Just posterior to the corneoscleral junction, and lying within the sclera, is a circularly running canal called the sinus venous sclerae or the canal of Schlemm. The sclera may be divided, for purpose of description, into three layers: (1) the episclera, (2) the scleral stroma, and (3) the lamina fusca.[23] The episclera is the outermost layer and consists of loose connective tissue. It is connected to Tenon's capsule by fine strands of tissue. Anteriorly, the episclera has a rich blood supply from the anterior ciliary arteries, which form a plexus that extends between the extrinsic muscle insertions and the corneoscleral junction. These vessels lie deep to the conjunctiva and normally are nonconspicuous. However, in the presence of inflammatory disease they become very red and congested. The scleral stroma consists of dense fibrous tissue intermingled with fine elastic fibers. The lamina fusca is the innermost layer of the sclera. It is separated from the external surface of the choroid by a potential space, the suprachoroidal (perichoroidal) space. Connecting the lamina fusca with the choroid are fine collagen fibers that provide a weak attachment between the sclera and the choroid.[23]

### Blood Supply and Nerve Supply of the Sclera

The sclera is a relatively avascular structure. However, anterior to the insertions of the recti muscles, the branches of the anterior ciliary arteries form a dense episcleral plexus. This plexus exists beneath the conjunctiva and is normally inconspicuous; however, in the presence of inflammation involving the cornea, iris, and ciliary body, marked vasodilatation may occur. This pronounced vasodilatation is known as a ciliary flush.[23] This rich blood supply to the anterior episclera results in rapid healing of surgical incisions.[23] The posterior sclera receives small branches from the long and short posterior ciliary arteries. The sclera is innervated by the ciliary nerves that arise from branches of the trigeminal nerve.

## Cornea

Microscopically, the cornea consists of five layers. From front to back, they are (1) the corneal epithelium, (2) Bowman's layer (membrane), (3) the substantia propria, (4) Descemet's membrane, and (5) the corneal endothelium. Bowman's layer is acellular and consists of interwoven collagen fibers embedded in intercellular substances. It ends abruptly at the limbus. The substantia propria forms 90% of the corneal thickness. It is transparent and consists of many lamellae of collagen fibers that run parallel to the surface.[23] Descemet's membrane is the basement membrane of the endothelium. It is thicker than the endothelium. The corneal epithelium is stratified and consists of five layers of cells. The corneal endothelium consists of a single layer of flattened cells.[23]

### Blood Supply and Nerve Supply of the Cornea

The cornea is avascular and devoid of lymphatic drainage. It is nourished by diffusion from the aqueous humor and from the capillaries of the sclera and conjunctiva that end at its edge. The cornea is innervated by the ophthalmic division of the trigeminal nerve, mainly through the long ciliary nerves.[23]

## Uvea (Choroid, Ciliary Body, and Iris)

The uveal tract lies between the sclera and the retina (Fig. 8-15). The choroid is the section of the uveal tract that lies between the sclera and the retinal pigment epithelium, the outer layer of the retina (Fig. 8-15). It forms a membrane of predominantly vascular tissue extending from the optic nerve to the ora serrata (Fig. 8-15), beyond which it continues as the ciliary body.[23, 27] Its thickness varies from approximately 0.22 mm at the posterior pole to 0.10 mm

near the ora, at the optic nerve, where it forms part of the optic nerve canal, and at the point of internal penetration of the vortex veins. Its inner surface is smooth and firmly attached to the retinal pigment epithelium; its outer surface is roughened. It is firmly attached to the sclera in the region of the optic nerve and where the posterior ciliary arteries and ciliary nerve enter the eye. It is also tethered to the sclera where the vortex veins leave the eyeball.[23] This accounts for the characteristic shape of choroidal detachment, which shows valleys at the site of the vortex veins.[28] The choroid can be divided into four layers, which are, extending from internally to externally, Bruch's membrane, the choriocapillaris, the stroma, and the suprachoroidea.[23, 28]

### Bruch's Membrane

Bruch's membrane (2 to 4 μm thick) is a tough, acellular, amorphous, bilamellar structure situated between the retina and the rest of the choroid.[29] Microscopically, Bruch's membrane consists of five layers: the basement membrane of the retinal pigment epithelium, the inner collagenous zone, a meshwork of elastic fibers, the outer collagenous zone, and the basement membrane of the choriocapillaris.[23, 30] The function of Bruch's membrane is not exactly known, although it is believed to play a role in the passage of tissue fluid from the choriocapillaris to the retina.[23] When a choroidal tumor breaks through Bruch's membrane, it results in a characteristic mushroom-shaped growth configuration (Fig. 8-16).

### Choriocapillaris

The choriocapillaris is the capillary layer of the choroid, lying immediately external to Bruch's membrane. The capillaries are drained by the vortex veins. The choriocapillaris is a visceral type of vasculature containing wide-bore

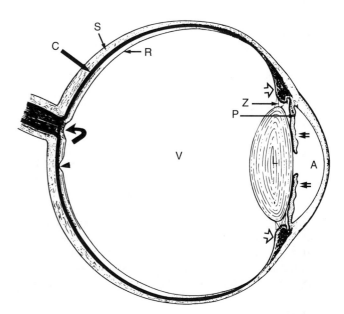

**FIGURE 8-15** Ocular coats and chambers. The three ocular coats consist of the sclera (*S*), middle layer: uvea (*black layer*), consisting of choroid (*C*), ciliary body (*hollow arrows*), and iris (*double black arrows*); the inner layer: the retina (*R*). Note the optic nerve disc (*curved arrow*), fovea (*arrowhead*), vitreous chamber (*V*), lens (*L*), zonule fibers (*Z*), posterior chamber (*P*), and anterior chamber (*A*).

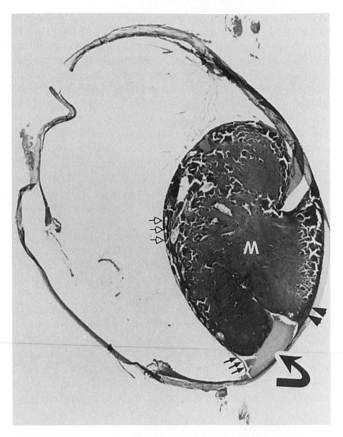

**FIGURE 8-16**  Uveal melanoma. Tissue section shows a mushroom-shaped uveal melanoma (*M*) arising from the choroid (*arrowheads*) and breaking through Bruch's membrane (*curved arrows*). The retina (*open arrows*) is elevated to the top of the tumor and is detached (*arrows*) at the slope of the tumor. (From Mafee MF et al. Malignant uveal melanoma and similar lesions studied by CT. Radiology 1985;156:403–408.)

capillaries with fenestrations in the vessels. These openings are covered by diaphragms, which permit the relatively free exchange of material between the choriocapillaris and the surrounding tissues.[31] By contrast, the retinal capillaries show no fenestrations and present a strong barrier to the interchange of material from capillary to retinal tissue.[27] It should be noted that the density of the capillaries is greatest and the bore is widest at the macula.

### Choroidal Stroma

The choroidal stroma lies external to the choriocapillaris and consists of blood vessels, nerves, fibroblasts, a collection of immunologic cells, macrophages, lymphocytes, mast cells, plasma cells, and loose collagenous supporting tissue containing melanocytes. The blood vessels of the stroma are branches of the short posterior ciliary arteries and extend anteriorly. The veins are much larger and converge to join four or five vortex (vorticose) veins that drain into the ophthalmic veins.

### Suprachoroidea

The suprachoroidea, also called the perichoroidal/suprachoroidal space, is a potential space, approximately 30 μm thick, that lies between the stroma and the sclera.[27] Running across this space are thin pigmented sheets of connective tissue called the suprachoroid lamina.[23] Running

in the suprachoroidal space are the long and short posterior ciliary arteries and nerves. At the optic nerve the choroid becomes continuous with the pia and arachnoid.[23]

### Blood Supply of the Choroid

The choroid receives its blood supply mainly from the posterior ciliary arteries. A number of recurrent branches arise from the anterior ciliary arteries. All of these arteries are branches of the ophthalmic artery. The four or five vortex (vorticose) veins drain the choroid into the ophthalmic veins.

### Function

The most important functions of the uvea are to provide a vascular supply to the eye and to regulate the ocular temperature.[20] The choroid is also responsible for nourishing the pigment epithelium and the outer one-third of the retina.[27] The fenestrations in its capillaries permit proteins and other larger molecules to diffuse through Bruch's membrane, and the selectivity of passage of these materials anterior to Bruch's membrane depends on the retinal pigment epithelium.[27] It is also thought that changes in the blood flow in the choroidal blood vessels may produce heat exchange from the retina.[23] The pigment cells in the choroid absorb excess light, preventing reflection.[23]

### Nerve Supply of the Choroid

The choroid is innervated by the long and short ciliary nerves. The long ciliary nerves are branches of the nasociliary nerve, a branch of the ophthalmic division of the trigeminal nerve. They carry sensory nerve and sympathetic fibers. The short ciliary nerves arise from the ciliary ganglion and carry sympathetic and parasympathetic fibers.[23]

## Ciliary Body

The ciliary body is continuous posteriorly with the choroid and anteriorly with the peripheral margin of the iris (Fig. 8-15). Considered as a whole, the ciliary body is a complete ring that runs around the inside of the anterior sclera. It is about 6 mm wide and extends forward to the scleral spur (a projecting ridge of scleral tissue along the internal scleral sulcus) and backward to the ora serrata of the retina.[23] On cross section the ciliary body is triangular, with its small base facing the anterior chamber of the eye and its anterior outer angle facing the scleral spur. Its apex extends posteriorly and laterally to become continuous with the choroid.[23] The anterior surface or base is ridged or plicated and is called the pars plicata. The posterior surface is smooth and flat and is called the pars plana. It is the pars plicata that surrounds the periphery of the iris and gives rise to the ciliary processes. The fibers of the zonule of the lens attach to the surface of the pars plicata (Fig. 8-15). The posterior margin of the pars plana has a scalloped edge that fits into and corresponds with the tooth-like edge of the ora serrata. Surgically, the pars plana is an important anatomic structure. Because of its relative avascularity and its position anterior to the retina, incisions through the sclera and choroid into the vitreous should be made at this point to avoid hemorrhagic complications and retinal detachments.

The ciliary body is made up of (1) the ciliary epithelium, (2) the ciliary stroma, and (3) the ciliary muscle. The epithelium consists of two layers of cuboidal cells that cover the inner surface of the ciliary body.[23] Embryologically, they represent the two layers of the optic cup. The inner layer of cubical cuboidal cells is nonpigmented and constitutes the anterior continuation of the nervous layer of the retina. These cells also line the anterior chamber.[23] The deeper outer layer consists of cuboidal cells that are packed with melanin pigment and constitutes the anterior continuation of the pigmented layer of the retina.[23] These cells rest against the stroma of the ciliary body. The structures of the two layers of ciliary epithelium on electron microscopy appear to suggest that both layers are involved in producing aqueous humor.[23] The ciliary stroma consists of loose connective tissue, rich in blood vessels and melanocytes, containing the embedded ciliary muscle. The ciliary muscle consists of smooth muscle fibers. It is innervated by the postganglionic parasympathetic fibers derived from the oculomotor nerve. The nerve fibers reach the muscle via the short ciliary nerves.

## Iris

The iris is a thin, contractile, pigmented diaphragm with a central aperture, the pupil (Fig. 8-15). It is suspended in the aqueous humor between the cornea and the lens. The periphery of the iris that is attached to the anterior surface of the ciliary body is called the ciliary margin or root of the iris.[23, 32] The iris divides the space between the lens and the cornea into an anterior and a posterior chamber. The aqueous humor, formed by the ciliary processes in the posterior chamber, circulates through the pupil into the anterior chamber and exits into the sinus venosus (canal of Schlemm) at the iridocorneal angle.[23, 32] The iris consists of a stroma and two epithelial layers located posteriorly and derived from the neural ectoderm. The stroma consists of highly vascular connective tissue containing melanocytes. The stroma also contains nerve fibers, the smooth muscle of the sphincter pupillae, and the myoepithelial cells of the dilator pupillae.[23] The nerve supply of the sphincter pupillae is from the parasympathetic postganglionic fibers in the short ciliary nerves. They are derived from the oculomotor nerve. The dilator pupillae muscle is a thin layer of myoepithelium.[23] The myoepithelial cells are derived from the anterior layer of the iris pigment epithelium that covers the posterior surface of the iris.[23] The arterial blood supply of the iris is from the major arterial circle located in the stroma of the ciliary body. The major arterial circle is formed from the two long posterior ciliary arteries and the seven anterior ciliary arteries.[23]

## Retina

The retina is the internal layer of the eyeball. It is a thin, transparent membrane having a purplish-red color in living subjects. The external surface of the retina is in contact with the choroid and the internal surface with the vitreous body. Posteriorly the retina is continuous with the optic nerve. The optic nerve and the inner layer of the eye represent an anteriorly protruding portion of the brain. Grossly the retina has two layers: (1) the inner layer, which is the sensory retina, that is, photoreceptors, and the first- and second-order neurons (ganglion cells) and neuroglial elements of the retina (Müller's cells, or sustentacular gliocytes); and (2) the outer layer, which is the retinal pigment epithelium (RPE), consisting of a single lamina of cells whose nuclei are adjacent to the basal lamina (Bruch's membrane) of the choroid.[20, 32]

The retina is very thin, measuring 0.056 mm near the disc and 0.1 mm anteriorly at the ora serrata.[32, 33] It is much thinner at the optic disc and thinnest at the fovea of the macula. The retina consists of a single-layer outer RPE and an inner neurosensory layer, which are both derived from neuroectoderm. The sensory retina extends forward from the optic nerve to a point just posterior to the ciliary body. Here the nervous tissues of the retina end and its anterior edge forms a crenated wavy ring called the ora serrata (Fig. 8-15). The anterior, nonreceptive part of the retina at the ora serrata becomes continuous with the pigmented and nonpigmented columnar cell layers of the ciliary body and its processes. At the iris, both layers of cells continue on its posterior surface, and they both become pigmented. The macula, the center of the retina, lies 3.5 mm temporal to the margin of the optic nerve (Fig. 8-15). The retina is attached tightly at the margin of the optic disc and at its anterior termination at the ora serrata. It is also firmly attached to the vitreous but loosely to the RPE, and it is nourished by the choroid and the RPE.[27] The macula lutea is the retinal area for the most distinct vision.[23] The optic disc is pierced by the central retinal artery and vein. At the disc there is a complete absence of rods and cones. Thus, it is insensitive to light and is referred to as the blind spot. On ophthalmoscopic examination the optic disc is paler than the surrounding retina. The RPE cells contain numerous round or ovoid melanin granules. The cells have numerous functions, including the absorption of light, participation in the turnover of the outer segments of the photoreceptors, and the formation of rhodopsin and iodopsin by storing and releasing vitamin A, which is a precursor of the photosensitive pigment.[23, 33] The RPE cells are joined to each other by tight junctions. This arrangement forms a barrier (blood retinal barrier) that limits the flow of ions and prevents diffusion of large toxic molecules from the choroid capillaries to the photoreceptors of the retina. In oculocutaneous and ocular albinism, there is a lack of melanin pigment in the pigment cells of the retina and the uvea.[23, 33] The neural retina consists of three main groups of neurons: (1) the photoreceptors (cone and rod cells), (2) the bipolar cells, and (3) the ganglion cells. Its also possesses other important neurons, the horizontal cells and the amacrine cells, that modulate their activity.[23, 33] Supporting cells (Müller cells) are also present. The photoreceptors are similar to other sensory receptors elsewhere in the body. The bipolar cells are similar to the neurons in the posterior root ganglia and form the first-order neurons. The ganglion cells are similar to the relay neurons found in the spinal cord and brainstem and form the second-order neurons.[23] The axons of the ganglion cells form the optic nerve, and its fibers become myelinated after they have passed through the lamina cribrosa. The myelin sheaths of these axons are formed from oligodendrocytes rather than Schwann cells. The nerve cells of the lateral geniculate body form the third-order neurons, and their axons terminate in the visual cortex. Thus, the number of neurons involved in conducting light impulses from the retina to the visual cortex is the same as that found in other sensory pathways.[23] Based on light microscopic findings, the retina is said to be composed of 10 layers. These are, from peripheral (farthest away from the center of the eye) to central, (1) the pigment epithelium, (2) the rods and cones, (3) the external limiting membrane, (4) the outer nuclear layer, (5) the outer plexiform layer, (6) the inner nuclear layer, (7) the inner plexiform layer, (8) the ganglion cells, (9) the nerve fiber layer, and (10) the internal limiting membrane. The outer nuclear layer consists of the nuclei of the rod and cone cells. The outer plexiform layer is made up of the synapses between the terminal processes of the rod and cone cells, the bipolar cells, and the horizontal cells. The inner nuclear layer consists of the nuclei of the bipolar cells, the horizontal cells, the amacrine cells, and the Müller cells. The inner plexiform layer is made up of synaptic connections between the bipolar, amacrine, and ganglion cells. The ganglion cell layer consists of the nuclei of the ganglion cells. The nerve fiber layer consists of the axons of the ganglion cells that are converging toward the optic disc. The external and internal limiting membranes are formed by the cell processes of the supporting Müller cells.[23, 33] There are two types of photoreceptors, the rods (110 to 125 million) and the cones (6.3 to 6.8 million).[23] The cones are responsible for vision in dim light. The rods are absent at the fovea. The cones, by contrast, are most dense at the fovea. There are approximately 1 million ganglion cells in each retina and about 100 photoreceptor cells per ganglion cell. The rod cells contain rhodopsin. The cone cells contain several photochemicals, similar in composition to rhodopsin, and are known as iodopsins.[23] The bipolar cells have a radial orientation. One or more dendrites of the bipolar cells pass outward to synapse with the photoreceptor cell terminals. The single axon is directed inward to synapse with ganglion and amacrine cells. The ganglion cells resemble cells found in nervous ganglia. They are situated in the inner part of the retina. The ganglion cells are the second type of neurons in the visual pathway. Most of them are small (midget ganglion cells), but a small number are large.[23] They are absent at the fovea. The ganglion cells are multipolar cells, and their dendrites synapse with the axons of bipolar and amacrine cells. The axons of ganglion cells converge at the exit of the optic nerve at the optic disc. After piercing the lamina, the nerve fibers become myelinated. In some individuals, the ganglion cell axons are partially myelinated; such areas are non-seeing and will produce a blind spot.[23] In addition to rod and cone cells, bipolar cells, and ganglion cells, there are two types of neurons in the retina called horizontal and amacrine cells. The horizontal cells are located close to the terminal expansion of the rods and cones. The horizontal cells respond to the neurotransmitter liberated by the rods and cones following excitation by light.[23] It is believed that the horizontal cells integrate visual stimuli. The amacrine cells are situated close to the ganglion cells. These cells are stimulated by the bipolar cells, which in turn excite the ganglion cells.[23]

The retinal supporting cells are similar to the neuroglial cells. One of them runs radially and is called the Müller cell. These cells fill in most of the space of the neural retina not occupied by the neurons. Other glial-like cells, called retinal astrocytes, perivascular glial cells, and microglial cells, have also been described.[23]

The macula lutea is an oval, yellowish area at the center of the posterior part of the retina. It measures about 4.5 mm in diameter and lies about 3 mm to the lateral side of the optic disc. Its yellow coloration is caused by a yellow carotenoid pigment, xanthophyll, which is present in the retina layers from the outer nuclear layer inward. The fovea centralis is a depression in the center of the macula lutea. It measures about 1.5 mm in diameter. The depression is made by the peripheral displacement of the nerve cells and fibers of the inner layers of the retina, leaving only the photoreceptors in the center. This greater light accessibility explains why this central depression has the most distinct vision. There are no blood vessels overlying the fovea and no rod cells in the floor of the fovea. It is here that the highest concentration of cones exists. The optic disc measures about 1.5 mm in diameter. A rise in CSF pressure causes the optic disc to bulge into the eyeball. It is believed that the pressure on the optic nerve impedes the axoplasmin flow of its fibers, and this causes the optic disc to swell.

### Blood Supply of the Retina

The blood supply of the retina is from two sources. (1) The outer lamina, including the rods and cones and outer nuclear layer, is supplied by the choroidal capillaries; the vessels do not enter these laminae, but tissue fluid exudes between these cells. (2) The inner laminae are supplied by the central retinal artery. The retinal arteries are anastomotic end arteries, and there are no arteriovenous anastomoses. The retina depends on both of these circulations, neither of which alone is sufficient.[23] The central retinal artery is the first branch of the ophthalmic artery,[23, 33] measuring about 0.3 mm in diameter, and runs forward adherent to the dural sheath of the optic nerve. It enters the inferior and medial side of the optic nerve about 12 mm posterior to the eyeball. The artery is surrounded by a sympathetic plexus and accompanied by the central vein. It pierces the lamina cribrosa to enter the eyeball. At this location the posterior ciliary arteries form an anastomotic circle in the sclera around the optic nerve. Small branches from this circle penetrate the choroid to supply the optic disc and the adjacent retina. Small anastomoses occur between the branches of the posterior ciliary arteries and the central retinal artery (cilioretinal artery). The central vein of the retina leaves the eyeball through the lamina cribrosa. The vein crosses the subarachnoid space and drains directly into the cavernous sinus or the superior ophthalmic vein. The retina has no lymphatic vessels.

## Vitreous

The vitreous body occupies the space between the lens and retina and represents about two thirds of the volume of the eye or approximately 4 ml.[34, 35] All but 1% to 2% of the vitreous is water, which is bound with a fibrillar collagen meshwork of soluble proteins, some salts, and hyaluronic acid.[20, 23, 34, 35] It possesses a network of fine collagen fibrils that form a scaffolding.[23] The vitreous is the largest and simplest connective tissue present as a single structure in the human body.[32] Any insult to the vitreous body may result in

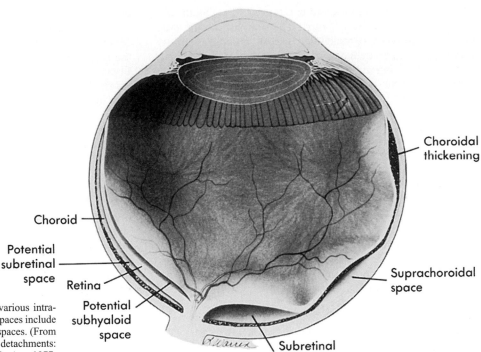

**FIGURE 8-17**   Diagram demonstrates various intra-ocular potential spaces. Principal potential spaces include subretinal, suprachoroidal, and subhyaloid spaces. (From Mafee MF et al. Retinal and choroidal detachments: role of MRI and CT. Radiol Clin North Am 1977; 25:487–507.)

a fibroproliferative reaction (such as proliferative vitreoret-inopathy), which can subsequently result in a tractional retinal detachment.[20] The vitreous body has been said to be bounded by membranes, such as the anterior and posterior hyaloid membranes.[23] Anteriorly the vitreous body has a saucer-shaped depression for the lens called the hyaloid fossa.[23] The vitreous body is attached to the sensory retina, especially at the ora serrata and the margin of the optic disc.[23] It is also attached to the ciliary epithelium in the region of the pars plana.[23] The attachment of the vitreous to the lens along the periphery of the hyaloid fossa is firm in young people and weakens with age.

Within the vitreous, the hyaloid (Cloquet's) canal (channel) runs forward from the optic disc to the posterior pole of the lens. During fetal life this channel contains the hyaloid artery, a branch of the central artery of the retina. In developing eyes it nourishes the lens. The hyaloid artery disappears about 6 weeks before birth, and the canal becomes filled with liquid.[23] The vitreous body transmits light, supports the posterior surface of the lens, and assists in holding the sensory retina against the RPE.

## INTRAOCULAR POTENTIAL SPACES

There are basically three potential spaces in the eye that can accumulate fluid, resulting in detachment of the various coats of the globe (Fig. 8-17)[20, 32, 36, 37]: (1) the posterior hyaloid space, the potential space between the base of the hyaloid (posterior hyaloid membrane) and the sensory retina (Fig. 8-17). Separation of the posterior hyaloid membrane from the sensory retina is referred to as posterior hyaloid detachment[35] (see Fig. 8-17); (2) the subretinal space, the potential space between the sensory retina and the RPE.

Separation of the sensory retina from the retinal pigment epithelium is referred to as retinal detachment (Fig. 8-17); and (3) the suprachoroidal space, the potential space between choroid and the sclera. The RPE and Bruch's membrane are tightly adherent to the choroid and become separated only when both layers are torn. However, the choroid is loosely attached to the sclera and can be separated, resulting in choroidal detachment (Fig. 8-17). The hyaloid fossa (patellar fossa) on the anterior surface of the vitreous for the lens is also a potential space called the retrolenticular space. Exudates and hemorrhage can accumulate in this space in some pathologic conditions.[23] Another potential space is the episcleral or Tenon's space, which was described earlier.

## NORMAL IMAGING OF OCULAR ANATOMY

Regarding the anatomy and pathology of the globe, MR imaging is a modality that provides both excellent contrast for ocular imaging and good sensitivity for detecting gross as well as incipient pathology.[20, 21, 23, 37, 38] The globe is unique in that it contains both the most (vitreous) and least (lens) water-laden soft tissues in the body.[37, 38] Since the MR appearance of the vitreous and lens is a function of the interaction between tissue protein and water and because of the wide variation in water content of the eye's various tissues, the eye is an ideal organ for an MR imaging study (Fig. 8-18). The vitreous water content is 98% to 99%, that of the cornea is 80%, and that of the lens is 65% to 69%; these differences produce different water proton relaxation times for each of these tissues.[19, 32, 38]

The vitreous represents about two thirds of the volume of the eye, or approximately 4 ml.[29] The vitreous humor is a gel-like transparent extracellular matrix composed of a meshwork of 0.2% collagen fibrils interspersed with 0.2% hyaluronic acid, polymers, water (98% to 99%), and a small amount of soluble proteins.[17, 32, 38] In a number of ocular disease states and as part of the aging process, the vitreous can degenerate to a liquid state devoid of collagen.[18, 32, 39] The vitreous is both viscous and gel-like, and has characteristics associated with both the hyaluronic acid and collagen components, respectively. In a manner similar to that of synovial fluid, the vitreous serves as somewhat of a biologic shock absorber.[39] Because the vitreous is a gel composed of long, fixed collagen fibrils bathed only with dilute dissolved proteins, just a fraction of its water content is in contact with macromolecules.[38] Consequently, the bulk of the water in the vitreous relaxes on MR imaging as pure water, with only a small protein–water interaction.[19, 38] Thus the vitreous has T1 and T2 relaxation times that are longer than those of most tissues but are shorter than those of water (Fig. 8-18).

## LENS

The lens is made up of three parts: (1) an elastic capsule, (2) a lens epithelium, which is confined to the anterior surface of the lens, and (3) the lens fibers. The capsule envelops the entire lens. The lens epithelium is cuboidal and lies beneath the capsule. It is found only on the anterior surface of the lens. The lens fibers constitute the main mass of the lens. The fibers are formed by the multiplication and differentiation of the lens epithelial cells at the equator. The lens is held in position by a series of delicate fibers known as the suspensory ligament of the lens, or zonule. The zonule fibers arise from the epithelium of the ciliary process.

The lens is approximately 9 mm in diameter and 4 to 4.5 mm thick. Anterior to the lens are the iris and the aqueous humor; posteriorly, the lens is bordered by the vitreous humor (Fig. 8-15). The zonular fibers (zonules of Zinn) are inserted on the outermost surface of the equatorial lens capsule and extend to the ciliary body (Fig. 8-15). Chemically, the lens is 66% water, making the lens the least hydrated organ of the body.[23] The remainder of the lens is composed of protein forming a liquid crystal. On MR imaging the normal lens is characteristically darker than the surrounding fluid-laden tissue on T2-weighted pulse sequences, predominately because of the dominance of its ultrashort T2 relaxation time (Fig. 8-18).[38] The lens nucleus has both a lower water content and a shorter T2 relaxation time than the cortex.

MR imaging provides precise information regarding other ocular structures as well. The anterior chamber is crescent-shaped, is just anterior to the lens, and is almost isointense to the vitreous humor on both short and long TR images (Fig. 8-18A and 8-18B).[32, 38] The ciliary body may be seen on T2-weighted MR images as a hypointense area running from the edge of the lens to the wall of the globe (Fig. 8-19). Differentiation by MR imaging of individual layers of the sclera, choroid, and retina is impossible in the normal eye.[18, 19, 32]

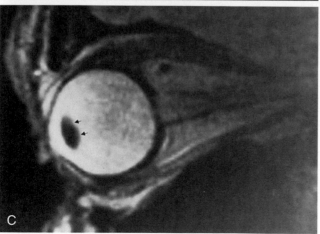

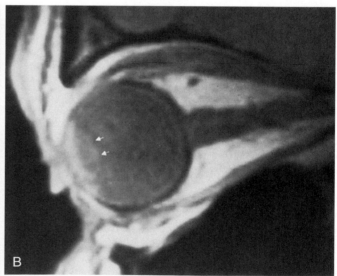

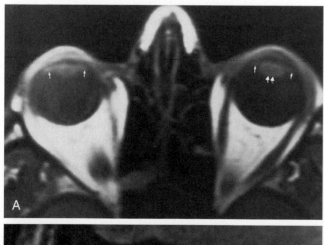

**FIGURE 8-18** Axial (**A**) T1-weighted and sagittal (**B**) PW and (**C**) T2-weighted MR images show the cornea, anterior chamber, lens, and vitreous chamber. The three ocular coats may not be distinguished as distinct individual layers. The lens capsule (*double arrows*) appears hyperintense relative to its nucleus in T1-weighted and PW images. The ciliary body and lens zonules appear slightly hyperintense in T1-weighted images (*arrows* in **A**) and usually hypointense in T2-weighted images. The lens nucleus appears hypointense on the T2-weighted scan.

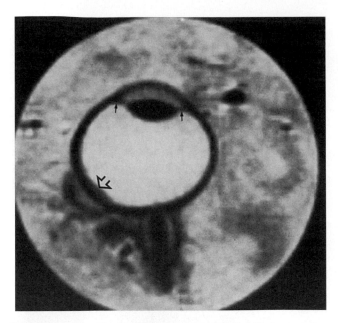

**FIGURE 8-19** Uveal melanoma. T2-weighted MR image of an enucleated eye shows a hypointense posterior uveal melanoma (*hollow arrow*). Note the hypointensity of the lens and the hyperintensity of the vitreous humor. The ciliary body and lens zonules appear hypointense (*arrow*).

The anterior chamber is a small cavity (3 mm anteroposteriorly) lying behind the cornea and in front of the iris (Fig. 8-15). The chamber contains aqueous humor. Its volume is about 0.2 ml. The aqueous fluid nourishes the corneal epithelium and the lens.[27] The iris, which is the most anterior extension of the uveal tract, lies at the anterior surface of the lens (Fig. 8-15). The ciliary body, which is just posterior to the iris, is responsible for producing aqueous fluid, which drains from the eyeball through the trabecular meshwork at the angle formed by the joining of the root of the iris, the anterior margin of the ciliary body, and the corneoscleral junction.[27] The ciliary body divides the globe into two compartments (segments)—the anterior segment and the posterior segment. The anterior and posterior chambers belong to the anterior segment. The anterior chamber is anterior to the iris and posterior to the cornea (Fig. 8-15). It is filled with aqueous humor. Its volume is about 0.2 ml. It measures about 3 mm anteroposteriorly in its central portion.[23] The posterior chamber is a small stilt-like cavity posterior to the iris and anterior to the lens. Its volume is about 0.6 ml. It is filled with aqueous fluid and communicates with the anterior chamber through the pupil. The posterior chamber is bounded anteriorly by the iris, peripherally by the ciliary processes, and posteriorly by the lens and the zonule (Fig. 8-15).

## OCULAR PATHOLOGY

## Congenital Anomalies

### Anophthalmia

Anophthalmia denotes the complete absence of an eye due to a developmental defect and is extremely rare.[40] More commonly, a small cystic remnant is seen and the term *clinical anophthalmia* is used. Bilateral cases suggest an early teratogenic event related to failure of the optic pit to develop.[40] In true anophthalmia, there is absence of neuroectodermal tissue within the orbit. Those structures not derived from neuroectoderm such as extraocular muscles, eyelids, conjunctiva, lacrimal apparatus, and bony orbit are present; however, the orbit is diminished in size, and orbital soft tissues including the optic nerve and extraocular muscles are rather hypoplastic. In true anophthalmia, in addition to absence of the globes, the optic nerves and the optic chiasm may be absent. The optic tracts may be rudimentary, and the lateral geniculate nuclei may be gliotic.[41] On CT and MR imaging there may be either rudimentary tissue or no globe present. At times, dystropic calcification may be present within the rudimentary tissue. The extraocular muscles, lacrimal glands, and eyelids are present.

### Microphthalmia

Microphthalmia refers to a congenital underdevelopment of or acquired diminution in the size of the globe (Fig. 8-20). Congenital microphthalmia (microphthalmos) is a continuation of a spectrum that begins with anophthalmia. Microphthalmos is defined as an eye that has an axial length less than 21 mm in an adult or less than 19 mm in a 1-year-old child.[40] Microphthalmia can occur as an isolated disorder or may be associated with other ocular, craniofacial anomalies (Hallerman-Streiff syndrome) or systemic abnormalities such as MIDS (microphthalmos, dermal aplasia, and sclerocornea).[40] Other causes of microphthalmia include the congenital rubella syndrome, persistent hyperplastic primary vitreous (PHPV), and retinopathy of prematurity (ROP). Bilateral microphthalmia and cataract may be seen in Lowe's syndrome (oculocerebral renal disease).[41] Microphthalmia results from an insult to the embryo after the outgrowth of the optic vesicle. If the insult occurs before complete invagination of the optic vesicle, an orbital cyst may result. This condition is referred to as microphthalmos with *cyst*. It can present as a progressive swelling from birth. The cyst may course along the optic nerve, with free communication with the intraocular contents.

In some cases in which a baby is born with a unilateral small orbit and no visible eye, a small microphthalmic globe is present in the orbital soft tissues. All such children have hypoplastic orbits. CT and MR imaging in congenital microphthalmia demonstrate a small globe as well as a small, poorly developed orbit. In older patients microphthalmia may occur as the result of trauma, surgery, inflammation, radiation, or other processes, which result in disorganization of the eye (phthisis bulbi). In these patients, CT and MR imaging demonstrate a small, shrunken globe, often with extensive intraocular calcification or ossification (Fig. 8-21). The principal conditions with which microphthalmia may be associated are listed in Table 8-1.

### Macrophthalmia
#### Buphthalmos and Megalophthalmos

Macrophthalmia, or enlargement of the globe, is seen in patients with axial myopia, congenital glaucoma (buphthalmos), Sturge-Weber syndrome, and neurofibromatosis. As many as 50% of patients with lid and facial involvement in neurofibromatosis exhibit glaucoma on the affected side. Up to 30% of patients with Sturge-Weber syndrome have glaucoma, and nearly two thirds of these patients develop buphthalmos.[24] The hallmark of all forms of glaucoma in infants and young children is ocular enlargement (Fig. 8-22), which occurs because the immature and growing collagen that constitutes the cornea and sclera in the young eye still responds to increased intraocular pressure by stretching.[40] All parts of the globe may stretch in response to the elevated intraocular pressure until 3 to 4 years of age, and glaucoma-related axial myopia may be seen until the early teenage years.[40] Buphthalmos, the most extreme form of macrophthalmia, consists of elevated intraocular pressure and an enlarged globe, as well as an enlarged cornea. Megalocornea is characterized by bilateral anterior segment enlargement with a corneal horizontal diameter of more than 12 mm at birth and more than 13 mm after 2 years of age. Megalocornea may be present without other ocular abnormalities. Megalophthalmos is an enlarged cornea in an overall enlarged eye that does not have glaucoma. There is an increased ocular axial length, often more than 30 mm. The condition is most likely autosomal recessive, and its findings are similar to those of X-linked megalocornea.[40] The most common cause of macrophthalmia is axial elongation of the eye associated with high myopia.[41] The normal adult eye has an axial length of about 24 mm. Using CT data, the axial length and width of the globe have been

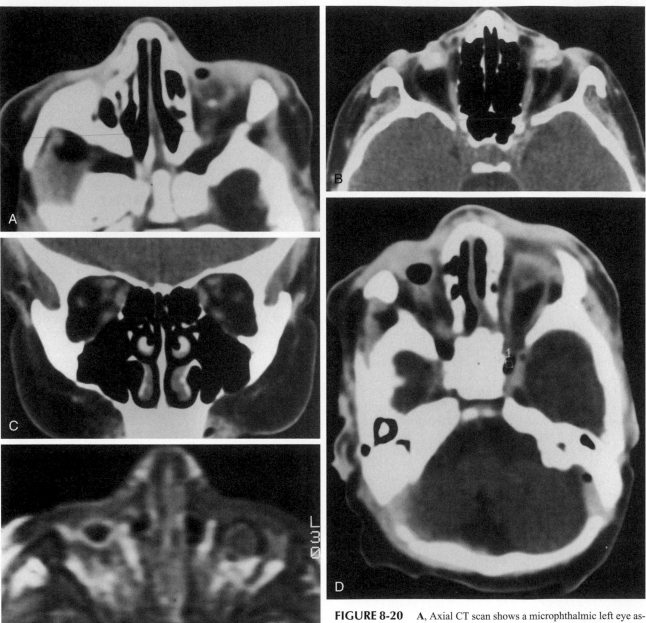

**FIGURE 8-20** **A**, Axial CT scan shows a microphthalmic left eye associated with a small calcification. **B**, Axial CT scan in another patient shows bilateral microphthalmia with marked calcifications. **C**, Coronal CT scan of the same patient in **B** showing normal development of the extraocular muscle but hypoplastic optic nerves. **D**, Axial CT scan shows bilateral microphthalmia. There is an air pocket in the remnant of the right dysplastic globe. **E**, Axial PW (2000/30, TR/TE) image (same patient as in **D**), showing a dysplastic right eye and a microphthalmic left eye.

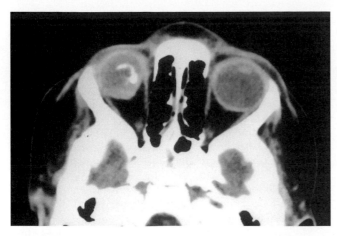

**FIGURE 8-21**   Phthisis bulbi: Axial CT scan shows a dense right eye with irregular calcification. This child with acquired immune deficiency syndrome developed cytomegalovirus chorioretinitis, resulting in a disorganized eye with associated dystrophic calcification.

published.[42] In addition to ocular elongation, CT and MR imaging may demonstrate thinning of the posterior scleral-uveal rim.

### Staphyloma

Staphyloma refers to thinning and stretching (ectasia) of the scleral-uveal coats of the eyeball. Progressive myopia (megamyope) results in posterior staphyloma. The progressively myopic eye expands in all of its posterior dimensions, and the formation of an equatorial staphyloma with scleral dehiscences is not uncommon,[40] especially in the superotemporal quadrant. As the scleral shell expands, the retina and choroid stretch and thin to accommodate the area they cover. Staphyloma has also been reported in glaucoma, scleritis, necrotizing infection after surgery or radiation therapy, and with trauma. Anterior staphyloma also may occur as a result of inflammatory or infectious corneal thinning.[40]

**Table 8-1**
**MICROPHTHALMIC EYE, ISOLATED AND ASSOCIATED WITH SOME SYNDROMES**

Isolated microphthalmia

Microphthmos with orbital cyst

Persistent hyperplastic primary vitreous

Retinopathy of prematurity

Congenital rubella syndrome

Congenital toxoplasmosis

Congenital syphilis

Posttraumatic

Postinflammation (herpes, cytomegalovirus)

Postradiation therapy

Hallerman-Streipp syndrome

MIDS syndrome

Lowe's syndrome

Norrie's syndrome

Warburg's syndrome

Meckel's syndrome

Other craniofacial and systemic syndromes

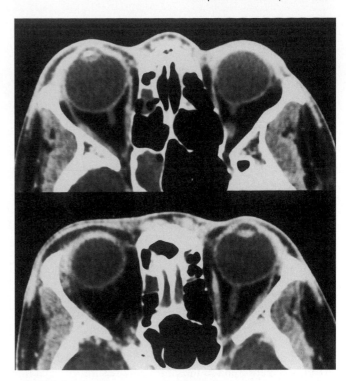

**FIGURE 8-22**   Glaucoma and enlarged eye. Axial CT scans shows moderate enlargement of the right globe (top). This child presented with eye pain and was found to have cataracts, anterior uveitis of unknown etiology, and glaucoma on the right side. Note the irregularity of the right lens as well as a shallow right anterior chamber (bottom).

### Cryptophthalmos

Cryptophthalmos consists of partial or complete failure of development of the eyelids (eyebrow, palpebral fissure, eyelashes, and conjunctiva). It may be unilateral or bilateral. It may be associated with a skin-like cornea, an incompletely developed anterior segment, or a rudimentary cyst-like globe. Cryptophthalmos may be associated with systemic anomalies such as syndactyly and genitourinary anomalies.

### Coloboma and Morning Glory Anomaly

A coloboma (Greek, a mutilation) is a notch, gap, hole, or fissure that is congenital or acquired and in which a tissue or portion of a tissue is lacking. Ocular coloboma may involve the iris, lens, ciliary body, retina, choroid, optic nerve, or sclera.[43] Three types of optic nerve colobomas occur: (1) isolated coloboma of the optic nerve, (2) retinochoroidal coloboma, and (3) Fuchs' coloboma.[44-46] In a typical coloboma, the cleft appears in the inferonasal quadrant of the globe and results from the failure of the embryonic fissure to close.[44-46] Fuchs' coloboma (tilted disc syndrome, nasal fundus ectasia syndrome) is a form of coloboma in which there is a congenital, inferiorly tilted optic disc in conjunction with an inferonasal crescent or conus along the border of the disc in the direction of the tilt.[45, 46] Myopia and astigmatism accompany these changes.[45, 46] Ophthalmoscopically, optic nerve coloboma characteristically shows enlargement of the papillary areas, with partial or total excavation of the disc (Fig. 8-23A). The embryonic derivation of the ocular structures was discussed previously in this chapter. A study of this embryology is important to understand the origin of optic nerve colobomas. Isolated

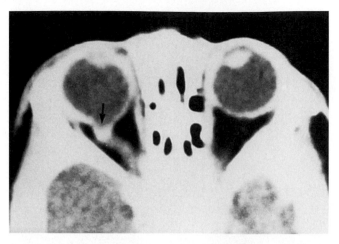

**FIGURE 8-23** Typical coloboma of the optic disc. Axial CT scan shows a large posterior global defect (*arrow*) with optic disc excavation on the right side. The defect appears to be surrounded by an enhancing, deformed sclera and seems to have a direct connection with the vitreous body. (From Mafee MF et al. CT of optic nerve colobomas, morning glory anomaly, and colobomatous cyst. Radiol Clin North Am 1987; 25:693–699.)

optic nerve colobomas arise from failure of closure of only the most superior end of the embryonic fissure.[45–47] Failure of closure of other parts of the embryonic fissure causes iridic, lenticular, ciliary body, and retinochoroidal colobomas.[48] The visual acuity in eyes with optic nerve colobomas is variable and may range from normal to abnormal light perception. Both nonrhegmatogenous and rhegmatogenous (tear of the retina) retinal detachments have been well described in association with optic nerve coloboma.[45, 48] Optic nerve colobomas have been observed in association with ocular abnormalities, including congenital optic pit,

cyst of the optic nerve sheath, posterior lenticonus, and remnant of the hyaloid artery.[45, 46] These colobomas also have been associated with nonocular abnormalities including cardiac defects, dysplastic ears, facial palsy, and transsphenoidal encephalocele.[49] A coloboma can form in normal-sized eyes as well as microphthalmic eyes. In a small percentage of microphthalmic eyes with coloboma, a defect in the sclera allows an extraocular herniation of the intraocular neural ectoderm to form an orbital cyst with a tunnel-like connection to the globe.[43] The relative sizes of the microphthalmic eye and colobomatous cyst, and the direction of cyst growth, are quite variable (Figs. 8-24 and 8-25). Colobomatous cysts have been associated with a number of systemic syndromes, chromosomal anomalies, and familial cases (Table 8-2).[43]

Morning glory disc is an anomaly that was first characterized by Kindler in 1970.[50] He described a unilateral congenital anomaly of the optic nerve head in 10 patients. Because of the similarity in appearance between the nerve head and a morning glory flower, he referred to the anomaly as the morning glory syndrome. Ophthalmoscopically, the disc is enlarged and excavated and has a central core of white tissue. The disc is surrounded by an elevated annulus of light and also by variable pigmented subretinal tissue.

### Diagnostic Imaging

The CT and MR appearance of optic disc coloboma includes a posterior global defect with optic disc excavation (Fig. 8-23). The imaging appearance of the morning glory anomaly is characteristic and corresponds to its clinical appearance as a large funnel-shaped disc (Fig. 8-24). The colobomatous cyst associated with coloboma of the optic nerve head can be readily identified on CT and MR imaging (Figs. 8-25 and 8-26).

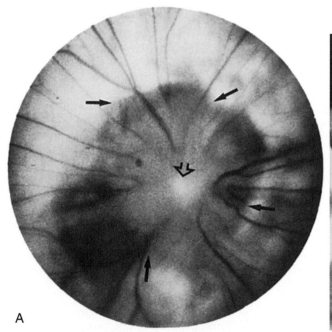

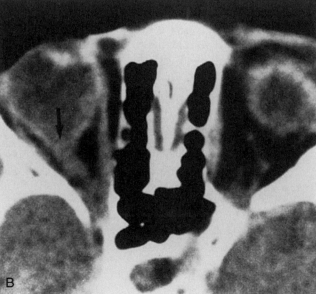

**FIGURE 8-24** Morning glory anomaly. **A**, Disc is enlarged (*solid arrows*) and has a central core of white glial tissue (*open arrows*). **B**, Axial CT scan shows a funnel-shaped deformity of the posterior globe (*arrow*). (From Mafee MF et al. CT of optic nerve colobomas, morning glory anomaly, and colobomatous cyst. Radiol Clin North Am 1987;25:693–699.)

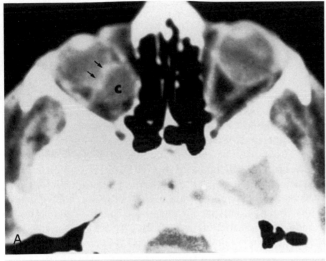

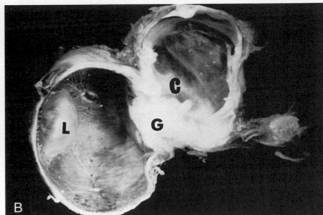

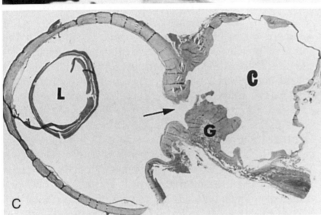

**FIGURE 8-25** Colobomatous cyst. **A**, Axial CT scan shows bilateral microphthalmia and a large cyst (*C*) separated from the right globe by a band of enhancement (*arrows*), which is related to abnormal gliotic tissue. **B**, Anatomic section of an enucleated right eye. Note the small eye, large colobomatous defect, abnormal white tissues, gliotic tissues (*G*), and large cyst (*C*). Note the lens (*L*) and the optic nerve. **C**, Histologic section of an eye shows a large retinochoroidal coloboma (*arrow*), gliotic tissue (*G*), cyst (*C*), and lens (*L*). (From Mafee MF et al. CT of optic nerve colobomas, morning glory anomaly, and colobomatous cyst. Radiol Clin North Am 1987;25:693–699.)

**Table 8-2**
**COLOBOMATOUS CYSTS ASSOCIATED WITH SYSTEMIC SYNDROMES**

Oculocerebrocutaneous syndrome (Dellman's syndrome)
Focal dermal hypoplasia (Goltz's syndrome)
Brachio-oculofacial syndrome
CHARGE association
VATER association
Aicardi's syndrome
Proboscis lateralis
Lenz's syndrome
Meckle's syndrome
Warburg's syndrome
Triploidy
Trisomy 13
Trisomy 18
Cat-eye syndrome
4p depletion

Source: Adopted from Kaufman LM, Villablanca PJ, Mafee MF. Diagnostic imaging of cystic lesions in the child's orbit. Radiol Clin North Am 1998;36:1149–1163.

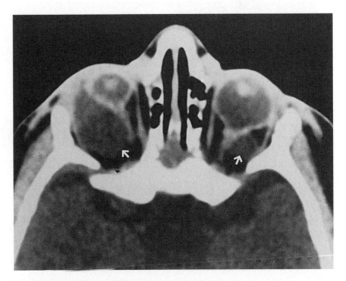

**FIGURE 8-26** Colobomatous cyst. Axial CT scan shows microphthalmic eyes with large cysts (*arrows*).

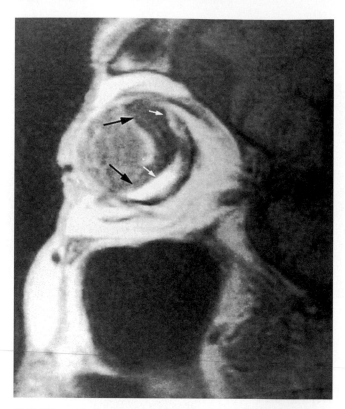

**FIGURE 8-27** Posterior hyaloid detachment and retinal detachment in a patient with complicated macular degeneration. Sagittal T1-weighted MR image shows two semilunar regions; the posterior region (*white arrows*) is caused by chronic subretinal hemorrhage, and the anterior region (*black arrows*) is caused by posterior hyaloid detachment. Surgery confirmed these findings.

## OCULAR DETACHMENTS

### Posterior Hyaloid Detachment

Posterior hyaloid detachment usually occurs in adults over the age of 50 years but may occur in children with persistent hypertrophic primary vitreous (PHPV).[37, 39, 40] In the older population, the vitreous tends to undergo degeneration and liquefaction. This process may lead to posterior vitreous detachment and predispose to retinal detachment.[23] Posterior hyaloid detachment in adults may be associated with macular degeneration (Fig. 8-27).

The posterior hyaloid membrane is very thin and is invisible on MR imaging or CT, but it can be made visible when blood or other fluid fills the posterior hyaloid space, causing thickening of this membrane (Fig. 8-27). Fluid in the retrohyaloid space is seen on CT and MR imaging as a layered abnormality that shifts its location in the lateral decubitus position (Figs. 8-28 and 8-29). The retrohyaloid-layered fluid is shifted in the decubitus position because it is not within the substance of the vitreous (Fig. 8-28B). Hemorrhage within the vitreous mixes with the vitreous humor, which is a gel-like extracellular material and therefore does not show intragel layering. Fluid in the retrohyaloid space and the subretinal space may not be differentiated from each other on CT and MR imaging.[36]

### Retinal Detachment

Retinal detachment occurs when the sensory retina is separated from the retinal pigment epithelium. The retinal pigment epithelium has a barrier function that, once damaged, allows fluid to leak into the potential subretinal space.[20, 36] Retinal detachment resulting from a hole (or tear) in the retina is referred to as rhegmatogenous retinal

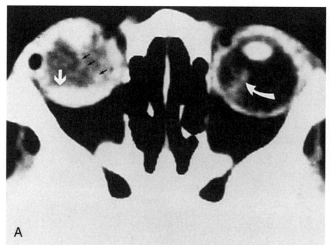
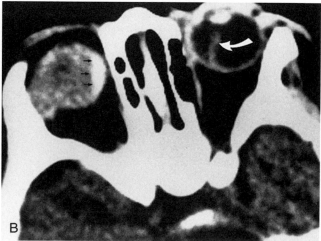

**FIGURE 8-28** Posterior hyaloid detachment and congenital nonattached retina. Axial CT scans obtained without contrast in the supine position (**A**) and the decubitus position (**B**) show gravitational layering fluid (*white arrow* in **A**), which is related to hemorrhage in the subhyaloid space. Fluid shifts more freely in the subhyaloid space than in the subretinal space (*black arrows* in **B**). Note the congenitally nonattached retina of the left eye (*curved arrows*). Increased density, as well as retrolental soft tissue of the right eye (*black arrows* in **A**), are related to PHPV. (From Mafee MF et al. CT in the evaluation of patients with persistent hyperplastic primary vitreous [PHPV]. Radiology 1982;145:713–717.)

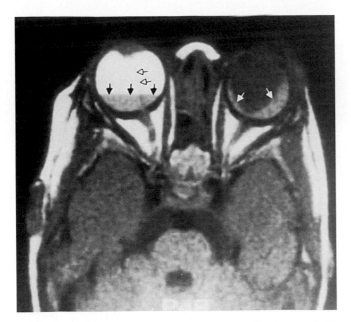

**FIGURE 8-29**  Posterior hyaloid and retinal detachment. Axial T1-weighted MR image shows the fluid-fluid level (*black arrows*) in the right vitreous chamber. This is thought to be caused by chronic (hyperintense) and acute (hypointense) hemorrhage in the subhyaloid or subretinal space. Note the detached leaves of the retina of the left eye (*white arrows*). The patient was diagnosed as having Warburg's syndrome. (From Mafee MF et al. Persistent hyperplastic primary vitreous [PHPV]: role of CT and MRI. Radiol Clin North Am 1987;25:683–692.)

detachment. The sensory retina is part of the central nervous system, so if there is a tear, the sensory retina cannot heal. By contrast, retinal pigment epithelium has healing potential. In laser treatment for retinal detachment, the energy of the laser beam is absorbed by RPE at the retinal detachment, and the resultant heat heals and closes the tear. Fluid in the subretinal space can be detected by CT and MR imaging (Fig. 8-30). Rhegmatogeneous retinal detachments are rare in the pediatric population. The majority of retinal detachments in children are nonrhegmatogenous and are secondary

to other ocular diseases (Fig. 8-31). Retinal detachment usually is the result of retraction caused by a mass, a fibroproliferative disease in the vitreous such as vitreoretinopathy of prematurity or vitreoretinopathy of diabetes mellitus, or accompanying an inflammatory process such as the larval granuloma of toxocara endophthalmitis.[20, 36] Retinal detachment also may occur because of retinal vascular leakage, which is seen in patients with Coats' disease, a primary vascular anomaly of the retina characterized by telangiectasia. The telangiectatic vessels leak serum and lipid, resulting in accumulation of a lipoproteinaceous exudate in the subretinal space (Fig. 8-32). Retinal detachment is sometimes the result of subretinal hemorrhage and occurs following trauma, senile macular degeneration, or persistent hyperplastic primary vitreous. Any choroidal lesions can cause retinal detachment (Figs. 8-33 and 8-34). In an axial CT or MR imaging scan taken below or above the lens, the retinal detachment appears as a homogeneous increased density (Fig. 8-32A). Although the retina is very thin and is beyond the limits of resolution of CT and MR scanners, it may be shown when outlined by the significant contrast difference between the density or intensity of the subretinal effusion on one side and the vitreous cavity on the other side (Fig. 8-35). The appearance of the retinal detachment varies with the amount of exudation (Figs. 8-32 to 8-37) and organization of the subretinal materials. In a section taken at the level of the optic disc, retinal detachment is seen with a characteristic indentation at the optic disc (Figs. 8-36 and 8-37). When total retinal detachment is present and the entire vitreous cavity is ablated, the leaves of the detached retina may not be clearly detected (Fig. 8-38). Retinal detachment is seen on coronal MR imaging as a characteristic folding membrane (Fig. 8-39). The subretinal fluid of an exudative retinal detachment is rich in protein, giving higher CT numbers and stronger MR signal intensities (on T1-weighted MR images) than those seen in the subretinal fluid (transudate) of a rhegmatogenous detachment. A rhematogeneous retinal detachment is produced by a retinal tear and subsequent ingress of vitreous fluid into the subretinal space.[20, 36] In many cases of shallow retinal detachment, the

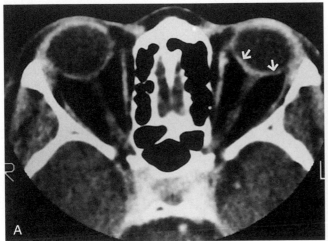

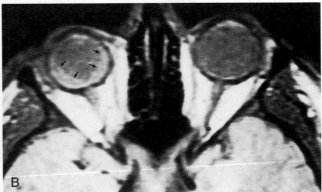

**FIGURE 8-30**  Retinal detachment. **A,** Axial CT scan shows a dependent image of increased density (*arrows*) of the left eye caused by retinal detachment. **B,** Axial PW MR image shows a dependent hyperintense image (*arrows*) of the right vitreous chamber caused by a subretinal exudate.

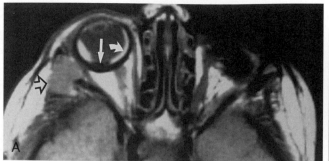

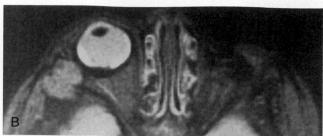

**FIGURE 8-31**    Exudative retinal detachment and regressed retinoblastoma after radiation therapy. **A**, Axial PW and **B**, T2-weighted MR images. **A** and **B** show a mass (*white arrow*) and a hyperintense subretinal exudate (*curved arrows*). The mass is hypointense in PW and T2-weighted MR images because of calcification. Note the destructive lesion (*open arrow*), presumably a sarcoma, that developed in the field of radiation therapy. The left eye has been enucleated in this patient, who had bilateral Rb.

MR image and in particular the CT scan may not show the detached retina. In these patients, ultrasonography is superior to MR imaging and CT. Retinal detachment is characteristically seen on CT or MR imaging as a V-shaped abnormality, with its apex at the optic disc and its extremities toward the ciliary body (Figs. 8-36 and 8-37). This appearance of retinal detachment may be confused

with the appearance of choroidal detachment. However, choroidal detachment, in the region of the optic disc and macula, involves detachment of the choroid that is restricted by the anchoring effect of the vortex veins, short posterior ciliary arteries, and nerves. This restriction usually results in a characteristic appearance of the leaves of the detached choroid, which, unlike the detached

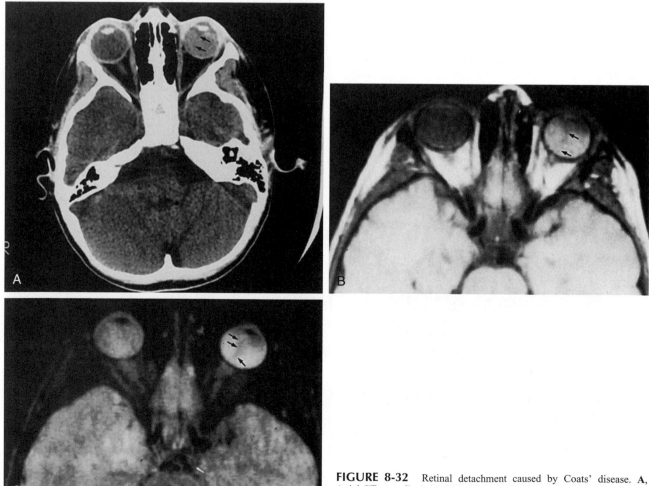

**FIGURE 8-32**    Retinal detachment caused by Coats' disease. **A**, Axial CT scan. **B**, Axial PW and **C**, Axial T2-weighted MR images. All images show total retinal detachment (*arrows*).

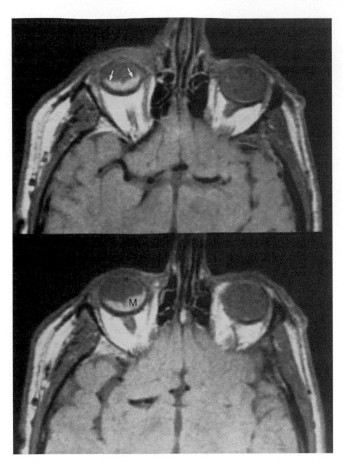

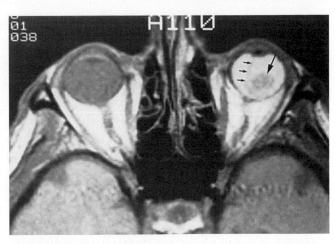

FIGURE 8-34  Total retinal detachment. Axial PW MR image shows a mass (*arrow*) with total retinal detachment (*arrows*). The subretinal exudate is hyperintense.

usually involved, producing scleritis or chorioretinitis, respectively. Inflammation of the choroid can damage the retinal pigment epithelial cells. Such damage causes breakdown of the ocular blood barrier, with subsequent outpouring of proteinaceous fluid (exudate) into the subretinal space, producing an exudative retinal detachment.[20] The sensory retina subsequently detaches. Interestingly, neoplastic diseases of the choroid may produce similar changes in the retinal pigment epithelium; however, these changes usually occur in a more advanced stage of the disease (Figs. 8-33 and 8-34).

Malignant melanomas and choroidal hemangiomas are the most common choroidal neoplasms producing retinal detachment in adults (Figs. 8-33 and 8-34).[19, 36] These tumors produce various degrees of subretinal fluid accumulation, depending on the size and location of the tumor (Figs. 8-33 and 8-34). These tumors produce shifting fluid when the retinal detachment approaches at least one quarter of the circumference of the eye.[20] The subretinal exudate

FIGURE 8-33  Retinal detachment caused by uveal melanoma. Axial PW MR images shows a mass (*M*) and exudative retinal detachment (*arrows*).

retinal leaves, do not extend to the region of the optic disc (Fig. 8-40).[20, 36]

Inflammatory diseases of the uvea are seldom limited to this vascularized layer of the eye. The sclera and retina are

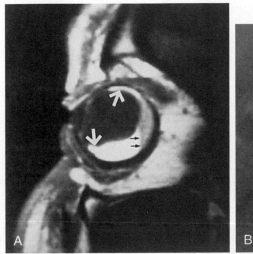

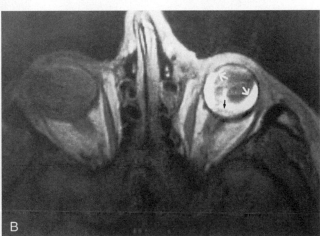

FIGURE 8-35  Retinal detachment. **A,** Sagittal T1-weighted sagittal MR image shows the leaves of a detached retina (*white arrows*). Subretinal fluid is hyperintense because of either exudate or chronic hemorrhage. Note the layered fluid (*black arrows*) caused by recent hemorrhage. **B,** Axial PW axial MR image shows leaves of a detached retina (*white arrows*) and layered recent hemorrhage (*black arrow*).

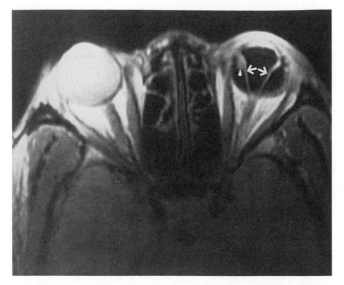

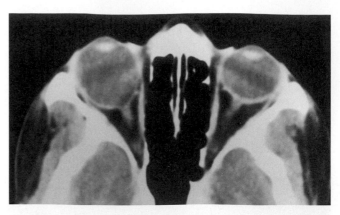

**FIGURE 8-38**   Axial myopia and staphyloma. Axial CT scan shows marked enlargement of the right globe associated with thinning of the sclera and bulging of the posterior globe including the peripapillary region.

**FIGURE 8-36**   Total retinal detachment. Axial T2-weighted MR image shows a detached retina (*arrows*) with the characteristic V-shaped configuration with the apex at the optic disc. Hypointensity of the left globe is caused by injection of silicone oil into the vitreous, which also has escaped into the subretinal space. The arrowhead points to residual subretinal fluid not replaced by silicone oil. (From Mafee MF et al. Retinal and choroidal detachments: role of MRI and CT. Radiol Clin North Am 1977;25:487–507.)

## Choroidal Detachment, Choroidal Effusion, and Ocular Hypotony

Choroidal detachment is caused by the accumulation of fluid (serous choroidal detachment) or blood (hemorrhagic choroidal detachment) in the potential suprachoroidal space.[20, 51–54] Serous choroidal detachment (Fig. 8-40) frequently occurs after intraocular surgery, penetrating ocular trauma, or inflammatory choroidal disorders.[52] Hemorrhagic choroidal detachment often occurs after a contusion, after a penetrating injury, or as a complication of intraocular surgery. Such detachment significantly influences the prognosis of the involved eye.[52] In these cases, ophthalmoscopic visualization of the fundus may be precluded by hyphema (blood in the anterior chamber) or vitreous hemorrhage. Ultrasound, although useful, has

often has a high density on CT and high signal intensity on MR imaging. MR imaging is superior to CT in differentiating choroidal lesions and suprachoroidal fluid from retinal lesions and subretinal fluid. Ultrasonography is superior to MR imaging and CT in the evaluation of retinal detachment.[20]

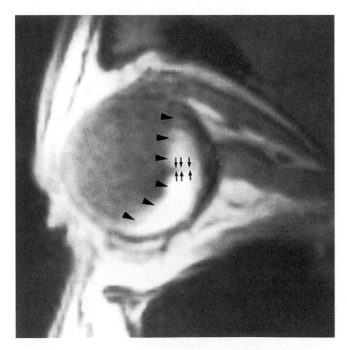

**FIGURE 8-37**   Retinal detachment. Sagittal PW MR image shows a detached retina (*arrowheads*) with characteristic folding of the retinal leaves (*arrows*) toward the optic disc.

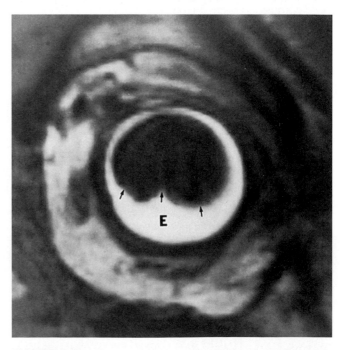

**FIGURE 8-39**   Retinal detachment. T1-weighted coronal MR image shows the characteristic appearance of retinal folds (*arrows*) and a hyperintense subretinal exudate (*E*).

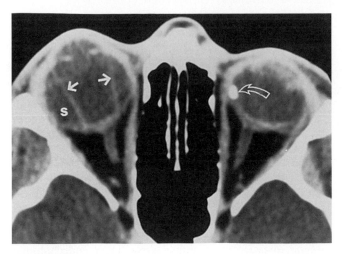

**FIGURE 8-40**   Serous choroidal detachment. Axial CT scan shows two prominent linear images (*solid arrows*) in the right eye. Because of the anchoring effect of posterior ciliary arteries and nerves, detached leaves of choroid usually do not appear to converge at the disc, unlike retinal leaves in retinal detachment. The suprachoroidal space (*S*) is isodense with vitreous, indicating serous choroidal detachment. The enlarged right globe results from known congenital glaucoma. Note the postsurgical changes in the left eye and the scleral-encircling silicone band (*curved arrow*). (From Mafee MF et al. Malignant uveal melanoma and simulating lesions: MRI evaluation. Radiology 1986;160:773–780.)

certain shortcomings in examining the traumatized eyes in the presence of an opaque medium. Contact B-scan ultrasound can expel the intraocular contents, is not tolerated by a patient with a painful eye, and increases the risk of inflammation.[54, 55] A-scan ultrasound, though less traumatic, is not often used because it is time-consuming and its interpretation requires experience. If air or gas is present in the vitreous cavity, the ultrasound postoperative evaluation of choroidal detachment is difficult. CT is best suited for the evaluation of a lacerated globe. If there is no suspicion of a ferromagnetic foreign body, MR imaging may be used.

Ocular hypotony is the essential underlying cause of serous choroidal detachment.[52] Ocular hypotony may be the result of inflammatory diseases (uveitis, scleritis), accidental perforation of the eyeball, ocular surgery, or intensive glaucoma therapy.[52–55] The pressure within the suprachoroidal space is determined by the intraocular pressure, the intracapillary blood pressure, and the oncotic pressure exerted by the plasma protein colloids.[51] The capillaries of the choriocapillaris differ from those of other capillary beds in the body because the choriocapillaris is a visceral type of vasculature with fenestrations in the vessels.[27, 31] These openings are covered by diaphragms, which permit the relatively free exchange of material between the choriocapillaris and the surrounding tissues.[27] Ocular hypotony causes increased permeability of the choroidal capillaries. This increased permeability leads to the transudation of fluid from the choroidal vasculature into the uveal tissue and causes diffuse swelling of the entire choroid (choroidal effusion). As the edema of the choroid increases, fluid accumulates in the potential suprachoroidal space, resulting in serous or exudative choroidal detachment.[51, 52, 54, 56] Choroidal effusion, like choroidal hematoma, may be preceded by surgery or other types of trauma to the eye.[57, 58] In fact, choroidal effusion may be a common, albeit

transient, occurrence after intraocular surgery.[59] Other causes of choroidal effusion include inflammatory disorders of the eyeball, myxedema, photocoagulation, retinal cryopexy, Vogt-Koyanagi-Harada syndrome, and the uveal effusion syndrome.[59, 60] Clinically the choroidal detachment appears as a smooth gray-brown elevation of the choroid extending from the ciliary body to the posterior segment.[52, 54] Even when the ocular media are clear in pigmented eyes, it is difficult with ophthalmoscopy to differentiate between a serous and a hemorrhagic choroidal detachment.[52, 54] The appearance of serous choroidal detachment on CT has been described.[52] It appears as a semilunar or ring-shaped area of variable attenuation. The degree of attenuation depends on the cause but is generally greater with inflammatory disorders of the eyeball. Inflammatory diseases of the choroid (uveitis) seldom appear as a localized mounding of the choroid; however, they generally produce a diffuse thickening with no localized area of mounding unless there is a choroidal abscess.[20]

Hemorrhagic choroidal detachments appear as either a low or high mound-like area of high density on CT, which can be quite large and irregular (Fig. 8-41). In a fresh hemorrhagic choroidal detachment, the choroid and hemorrhage in the potential suprachoroidal space are isodense. However, in a patient with chronic choroidal hematoma or a serosanguineous choroidal detachment, it may be possible to separate choroid and suprachoroidal fluid accumulation (Fig. 8-42).[52]

MR imaging, with its direct multiplanar imaging ability, is an excellent method for evaluating the eye in patients with choroidal detachment, particularly if ultrasound or CT, in conjunction with the clinical examination, has not provided sufficient information. MR imaging shows a choroidal hematoma as a focal, well-demarcated, lenticular mass in the wall of the eyeball (Fig. 8-43). This characteristic configuration usually does not change as the hematoma ages.[53] However, a decrease in the size of the choroidal hematoma may be observed. Multiple lesions occasionally may be seen (Fig. 8-43). The signal intensity of the choroidal hematoma depends on its age. Within the first 48 hours or so, the hematoma is isointense to slightly hypointense relative to

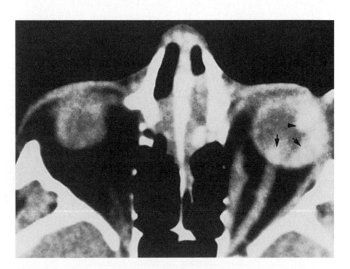

**FIGURE 8-41**   Acute choroidal hemorrhage (detachment). Axial CT scan shows choroidal hematomas (*arrows*).

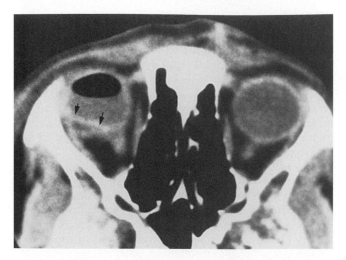

**FIGURE 8-42** Choroidal detachment. Axial CT scan shows detached choroid (*arrows*). Note the air in the right vitreous caused by air-fluid exchange from a detached choroid.

the normal vitreous body on T1-weighted and proton density MR images (Fig. 8-43A) but is markedly hypointense on T2-weighted images (Fig. 8-43B). After 5 days, its signal intensity characteristics are different, being relatively hyperintense on T1-weighted and proton density images (Fig. 8-44A) and only slightly hypointense on T2-weighted images (Fig. 8-44B).[20, 52, 53] At this stage, the choroidal hematoma may be confused with a choroidal melanoma.[53] The hematoma usually continues to increase in signal intensity on T1-weighted, proton density, and T2-weighted images (Fig. 8-44) and usually becomes markedly hyperintense by 2 weeks on all MR sequences (Figs. 8-44 and 8-45).[20, 52, 53]

Serous choroidal detachment (Figs. 8-46 and 8-47) and choroidal effusion (Figs. 8-48 and 8-49) have a different appearance on CT and MR imaging from choroidal hematoma (Figs. 8-41 and 8-43). Serous choroidal detach-

ment is caused by a nonhemorrhagic accumulation of fluid in the suprachoroidal potential space. The choroidal detachment appears as a smooth elevation of the choroid (Figs. 8-46 and 8-47), the fluid in the suprachoroidal space is often hypodense on CT (Fig. 8-46), and its MR appearance is that of an exudate (Fig. 8-47). A choroidal effusion usually is seen as a crescentic or ring-shaped lesion on both CT and MR imaging (Figs. 8-48 and 8-49).[20, 52, 53] It does not resemble the lenticular appearance of a hematoma. Inflammatory choroidal effusions usually appear as increased signal intensity on all MR images (Figs. 8-48 and 8-49). This high signal intensity is thought to be due to the high protein content of the effusion fluid.[53] Posttraumatic effusions, although also demonstrating increased signal on T1-weighted and T2-weighted images, are not as hyperintense as the inflammatory effusions.[53] At times it may be difficult to differentiate retinal detachment and choroidal detachment, since the distinction of choroidal effusion from subretinal effusion is not always clear.[20, 53, 54] Shifting of subretinal fluid occurs rather rapidly, whereas shifting of suprachoroidal fluid occurs slowly.[20] Therefore, rapidly shifting fluid within the wall of the eye, demonstrated on CT or MR imaging, favors the diagnosis of retinal detachment.

## Ocular Inflammatory Disorders

The eye may be affected by either known systemic or idiopathic ocular inflammatory processes. A host of infectious diseases may affect the glove. Viral diseases include herpes simplex, rubella, rubeola, mumps, variola, varicella, cytomegalovirus (Fig. 8-50), and infectious mononucleosis. Bacterial diseases include syphilis, brucellosis, tuberculosis, and leprosy. Fungal infections, particularly candidiasis, may also involve the globes in diabetic and immunocompromised patients.[41] Chronic inflammatory processes may cause calcification of the sclera, choroid and

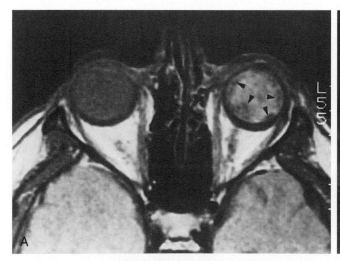
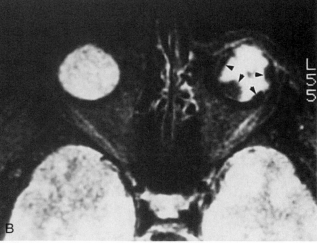

**FIGURE 8-43** Acute choroidal hemorrhage (detachment). **A,** Axial PW and **B,** T2-weighted MR images. Scans show choroidal hematomas (*arrowheads*). The increased intensity of the left globe is probably caused by protein leaking into the vitreous as a result of an impaired retinal-blood barrier. (From Mafee MF et al. Retinal and choroidal detachments: role of MRI and CT. Radiol Clin North Am 1977;25:487–507.)

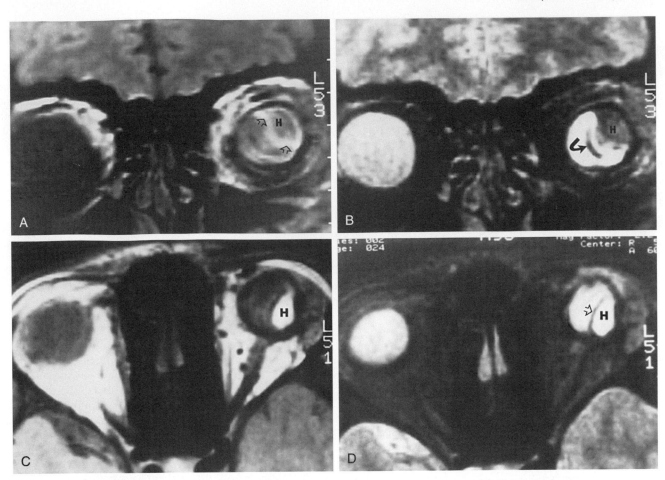

**FIGURE 8-44**   Subacute and chronic hemorrhagic choroidal detachment. **A,** Coronal PW MR image shows choroidal hematoma (*H*) as an area of mixed signal intensity. The peripheral part of the hematoma is hyperintense (*arrows*). **B,** Coronal T2-weighted MR image shows a choroidal hematoma (*H*) as a hypointense area. The curved image (*curved arrow*) is thought to be caused by residual intravitreal silicone oil. **C,** Axial PW and **D,** T2-weighted MR images. Scans obtained about 9 days after the scans in **A** and **B** show that the hematoma is markedly hyperintense.

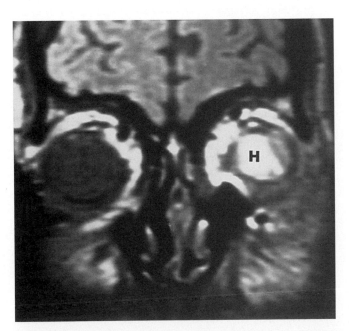

**FIGURE 8-45**   Chronic hemorrhagic choroidal detachment. Coronal PW MR image shows a hyperintense choroidal hematoma (*H*).

lens. Extensive disease may result in irregular calcific intraocular masses and a small, deformed globe (phthisis bulbi) (Fig. 8-21).

## Other Inflammatory Conditions

### Lymphoid Hyperplasia

Lymphoid hyperplasia of the uvea may cause thickening of the posterior wall of the globe, a finding that can simulate melanoma, uveitis, and posterior scleritis (see Fig. 8-12). Lymphoma and leukemic infiltration of the globe may also simulate uveitis.

### Papilledema

Increased intracranial pressure may result in papilledema with elevation of the optic discs. On CT and MR scans, elevation and bulging of the optic disc into the posterior aspect of the globe is observed (Fig. 8-51). The diameter of the optic nerve sheath complex may be increased. On postcontrast T1-weighted MR imaging scans, there may be increased enhancement of the optic discs (Fig. 8-51).

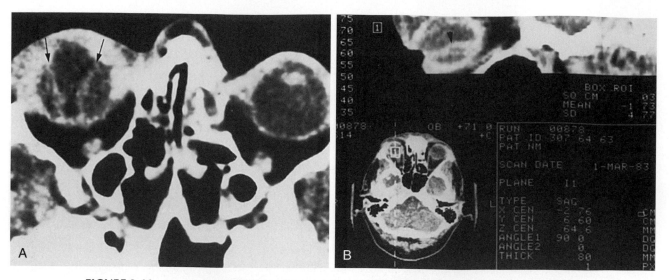

**FIGURE 8-46** Serous choroidal detachment. **A,** Axial CT scan. **B,** Reformatted sagittal CT image. Scans show detached choroid (*arrows* and *arrowhead*). The suprachoroidal space is isodense to vitreous compatible with serous fluid.

### Episcleritis

Episcleritis is a relatively common idiopathic inflammation of the thin layer of tissue lying between the conjunctiva and the sclera. It may be unilateral (66%) or bilateral. In some cases, episcleritis is associated with deeper inflammation (scleritis). Episcleritis is usually self-limited and resolves within 1 to 2 weeks. Imaging evaluation is not indicated in episcleritis.

### Scleritis

Scleritis can occur either as an idiopathic condition or in association with systemic diseases.[41] The process may be unilateral or bilateral. Patients with anterior scleritis

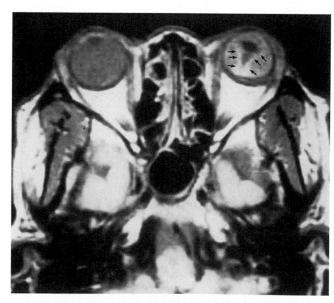

**FIGURE 8-47** Serous choroidal detachment. Axial PW MR image shows a kissing choroidal detachment. Suprachoroidal fluid is slightly hyperintense compared with that of the normal right vitreous. The detached choroid (*arrows*) appears thick, and its hyperintensity is caused by accumulation of fluid in its interstitium.

present with pain, erythema, photophobia, and tenderness.[41, 61] Scleritis may be caused by collagen-vascular disorders, granulomatous diseases, metabolic disorders, infections, and trauma. The sclera is basically an avascular structure deriving its blood supply from the choroidal episcleral plexus.[62] Scleritis may be bacterial, fungal, or viral in origin.[62] It may be caused by metabolic disease (gout) or by a group of autoimmune disorders, including rheumatoid arthritis, polyarthritis nodosa, lupus erythematosus, Wegener's granulomatosis, and relapsing polychondritis.[41, 61] Inflammatory bowel disease, especially Crohn's disease, can be associated with scleritis. Sarcoidosis and Cogan's syndrome also can be associated with scleritis. In most cases of posterior scleritis, however, no underlying cause is found.[61] Scleritis is classified as anterior or posterior scleritis. Scleritis may be acute or chronic. Posterior scleritis results in thickening of the sclera and choroid.[61, 62] There may be associated thickening of Tenon's capsule, as well as secondary serous or exudative retinal detachment (Fig. 8-52).[61, 62] Histopathologically, posterior scleritis is classified into two forms: (1) nodular and (2) diffuse. Nodular posterior scleritis is a focal or zonal necrotizing granulomatous inflammation surrounding a discrete sequestrum of scleral collagen.[61, 62] This type can mimic uveal melanoma (Fig. 8-53). Diffuse posterior scleritis appears as diffuse thickening of the uveoscleral coat, with some degree of contrast enhancement on both CT and MR scans.[61, 62] Fluid between the sclera and Tenon's capsule often causes choroidal detachment, which can be detected by CT and MR imaging or ultrasonography. Perforation of the sclera may be seen in necrotizing scleromalacia, a rare disease usually associated with severe rheumatoid arthritis.[41] At times, in addition to posterior scleritis, other features in support of a diagnosis of pseudotumor may be present on CT and MR scans. These findings suggest that several entities (posterior scleritis, scleritis, sclerotenonitis, periscleritis, and orbital pseudotumor) represent a continuum of the same disease.[62]

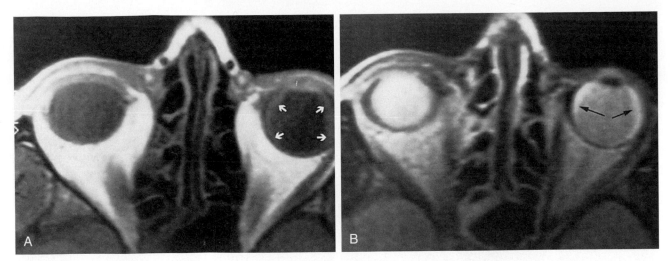

**FIGURE 8-48**   Choroidal detachment. **A**, Axial PW and **B**, T2-weighted MR images. Scans show the choroidal effusion of the left eye as a ring-shaped area of increased signal intensity (*arrows*).

## Uveitis

Uveitis is an inflammatory process of the intraocular contents, often prominently involving the uveal tract.[41] The etiology of uveitis is often unknown. Many patients appear to have a perturbation of lymphocytic control mechanisms.[41] Intraocular lymphoma can mimic posterior uveitis, pars planitis, or pars plana endophthalmitis; the last condition is an idiopathic form of uveitis. Uveitis may be caused by a specific organism such as *Toxoplasma* or cytomegalovirus. Ocular tuberculosis results from endogenous spread of systemic disease (Fig. 8-54). Toxoplasmosis is a common cause of posterior chorioretinitis. In congenital toxoplasmosis, the fetus is infected in utero and the infection is arrested by the time of diagnosis. Many of these children have cerebral toxoplasmosis and the detection of CNS calcifications by CT helps to establish the etiology.[41] In the adult form of ocular toxoplasmosis, associated CNS involvement is much less common.

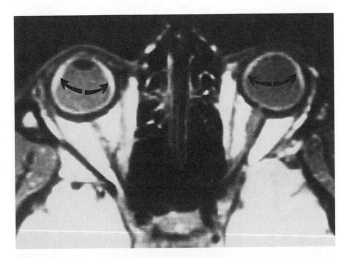

**FIGURE 8-49**   Bilateral choroidal effusion. Axial PW MR image shows bilateral ring-shaped areas of increased signal intensity (*arrows*). This MR appearance may be difficult to differentiate from that of retinal detachment. (From Mafee MF et al. Choroidal hematoma and effusion: evaluation with MRI. Radiology 1988;168:781–786.)

## Parasitic Infections

Larval granulomatosis usually affects children between 2 and 8 years of age. The process causes uveitis resulting from ingestion of the eggs of the nematode *Toxocara canis* or *T. cati* (Fig. 8-55).[41] Three clinical patterns occur: (1) a unilateral localized granuloma that may mimic retinoblastoma, (2) endophthalmitis, and (3) pars plana disease.[41]

## Intraocular Calcifications

Deposition of calcium in ocular tissues is a complex process, the pathophysiology of which depends on the specific site of calcification. Intraocular calcifications may be metastatic (hypercalcemic states) or dystrophic, and arise in association with diverse degenerative ocular conditions (neoplasia, inflammation, congenital dysplasias, and senescent or traumatic degeneration).[41, 63] Calcifications in neoplasms may be a result of tumor necrosis. Such neoplasms include retinoblastoma and astrocytic hamartomas seen in tuberous sclerosis or neurofibromatosis Type I. Fifty percent of patients with tuberous sclerosis may develop retinal hamartomas, which often calcify. Ocular calcification or ossification may also occur in congenital vascular lesions such as Sturge-Weber syndrome and Von Hippel-Lindau disease.[41] Scleral calcification has been reported in patients with linear sebaceous nevus syndrome.[41] The association of the nevus sebaceous syndrome of Jadassohn with seizures, mental deficiency, and ocular abnormalities has been reported.[41] The ocular anomalies may include coloboma of the iris and choroid, conjunctival lipodermoids, horizontal and rotational nystagmus, and vascularization of the cornea.[41] Chronic posttraumatic degeneration is probably the most common cause of dystrophic intraocular calcification. Choroidal osteoma, episcleral choristoma, and optic disc drusen are other causes of intraocular calcification.[41] Retinopathy of prematurity also may cause delayed unilateral or bilateral ocular calcification.[63] Scleral calcification may be seen in elderly people at or anterior to the sites of insertion of the horizontal extraocular muscles.[63] *Phthisis bulbi* refers to calcification or ossification within a shrunken or atrophic globe. It may be the result of any ocular insult with subsequent degeneration. It is most commonly a result

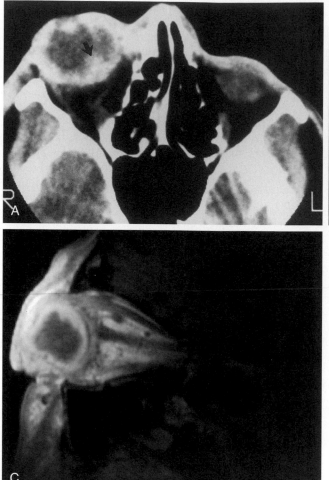

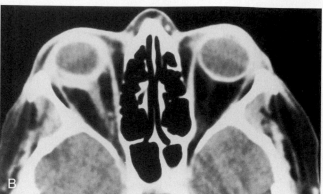

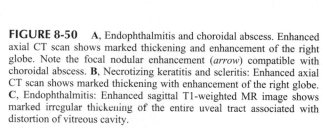

**FIGURE 8-50** **A,** Endophthalmitis and choroidal abscess. Enhanced axial CT scan shows marked thickening and enhancement of the right globe. Note the focal nodular enhancement (*arrow*) compatible with choroidal abscess. **B,** Necrotizing keratitis and scleritis: Enhanced axial CT scan shows marked thickening with enhancement of the right globe. **C,** Endophthalmitis: Enhanced sagittal T1-weighted MR image shows marked irregular thickening of the entire uveal tract associated with distortion of vitreous cavity.

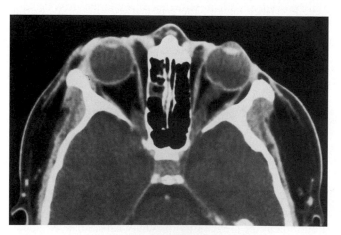

**FIGURE 8-51** Optic papilledema. Axial CT scan shows bulging of the left optic disc in this patient with bilateral papilledema. There was bilateral optic disc enhancement on enhanced T1-weighted MR images.

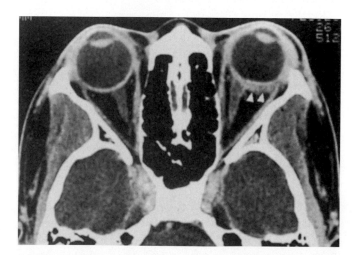

**FIGURE 8-52** Posterior scleritis. Enhanced axial CT scan shows thickening with enhancement of the posterior scleral-uveal coat (*arrowheads*). (Courtesy of M.F. Mafee, MD, FACR, Chicago.)

of trauma or infection.[63] Table 8-3 lists the most frequent causes of intraocular calcifications.[63]

## LEUKOKORIA

Leukokoria is a white, pink-white, or yellow-white pupillary reflex (cat's eye). It is a sign that results from any intraocular abnormality that reflects the incident light back through the pupil toward the observer. This reflection of light is the result of a white or light-colored intraocular mass, membrane, retinal detachment, or a retinal storage disease.[40, 64] Leukokoria is dependent on the size, location, and pigmentation of the intraocular pathology. When examining a child with leukokoria, the major diagnostic considerations are retinoblastoma, persistent hyperplastic primary vitreous (PHPV), retinopathy of prematurity (ROP), congenital cataract, Coats' disease, toxocariasis, total retinal detachment, and a variety of other nonspecific diseases.

Leukokoria is the most common presenting sign of retinoblastoma, the highly malignant primary retinal cancer. Howard and Ellsworth studied 500 consecutive patients in whom the diagnostic possibility of retinoblastoma was raised.[65] Of these 500 patients, diagnoses other than retinoblastoma were made in 265 cases (53%). Out of 27 different conditions, the most common was PHPV, followed by ROP, posterior cataract, coloboma of the choroid or optic disc, uveitis, and larval granulomatosis. Identification of the cause of the leukokoria is critical to ensure prompt recognition and appropriate treatment, and diagnostic accuracy is particularly important because retinoblastoma is one of the few human cancers for which definitive treatment is carried out without a confirmed histopathologic diagnosis.[21] Common ocular and orbital disorders in children are listed in Table 8-4.

## RETINOBLASTOMA

Retinoblastoma (Rb) is the most common intraocular tumor of childhood. It is a highly malignant primary retinal tumor that arises from neuroectodermal cells (nuclear layer of the retina) that are destined to become retinal photoreceptors.[66, 67] The manner of intraocular and extraocular extension, patterns of metastasis and recurrence, ocular complications, and associated malignancies make the diagnosis of retinoblastoma one of the most challenging problems of pediatric ophthalmology and radiology. To ensure appropriate therapy, retinoblastoma must be differentiated from a host of benign lesions that stimulate it (Table 8-5). This diagnosis must be established rapidly to permit maximum ocular salvage and to minimize tumor-associated mortality.[64, 68] When the disease extends beyond the eye, mortality approaches 100%.[68] With earlier diagnosis, the 5-year survival rate with tumors limited to the globe is greater than 90%.[32, 69] The classification of retinoblastomas has been established in regard to expected results of therapy. Group I includes tumors with a very favorable prognosis. These are either solitary tumors or multiple tumors less than four disc diameters in size at or behind the equator. Useful vision in the treated eye is attained in 90% of these patients and overall in about 75% of eyes that are not enucleated.[69] In group II the prognosis is also favorable, including patients with one or several tumors measuring between 4 and 10 disc diameters. In group III the tumors are anterior to the equator or there is a solitary tumor larger than 10 disc diameters. In these cases the prognosis is guarded. Group IV includes tumors that are multiple and extend up to the ora serrata. Group V includes those tumors that involve half of the retina or tumors that also have vitreous seeds. Groups IV and V have unfavorable prognoses.[21, 32]

Virchow was the first to postulate that retinoblastoma is of glial origin. He used the term *glioma of the retina* to describe the tumor.[32] Bailey and Cushing divided Rb into two types: (1) medulloblastoma and (2) neuroepithelioma. It is now well known that retinoblastoma is derived from primitive embryonal retinal cells (either photoreceptor or neuronal retinal cells).[70] This tumor can be undifferentiated or well-differentiated and can display evidence of photoreceptor differentiation in the form of Flexner-Wintersteiner rosettes and fleurettes.[66, 67, 71, 72] The tumor is composed of small round or ovoid cells with scant cytoplasm and relatively large nuclei. There is marked variability in the histologic features of retinoblastoma. Some tumors display

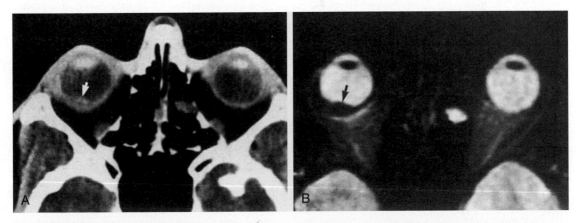

**FIGURE 8-53**   Posterior nodular scleritis. **A**, Axial CT scan shows a mass-like lesion (*arrow*). **B**, Axial T2-weighted MR image. The lesion (*arrow*) appears hypointense, simulating a choroidal melanoma. It was barely recognized on T1-weighted images (not shown). The patient improved and his symptoms resolved following a short course of steroid therapy. (Courtesy of M.F. Mafee, MD, FACR, Chicago.)

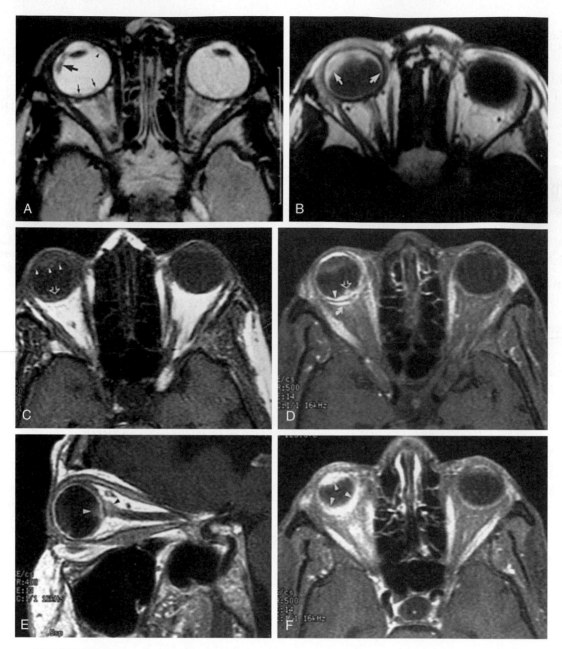

**FIGURE 8-54** (1) Granulomatous uveitis. **A**, Axial T2-weighted (2800/95, TR/TE) MR image shows hypointense lesions (*arrows*). **B**, Axial enhanced, T1-weighted (400/15, TR/TE) MR image shows marked enhancement of the entire uveal tract (*arrow*). Rb is unlikely because the lesion appears to have arisen within the uvea rather than the retina. (2) Ocular sarcoidosis panuveitis. **C**, Unenhanced axial T2-weighted (500/13, TR/TE) MR image shows nodular thickening of the posterior aspect of the right globe (*arrow*) and thickening of the anterior segment (*arrowheads*) of the right globe. **D**, Enhanced axial fat-suppressed, T1-weighted (500/13, TR/TE) MR image shows nodular enhancement of the posterior aspect of the right globe (*arrowhead* and *open arrow*) related to granulomatous involvement of the choroids. Note the enhancement of the anterior segment of the right globe and the abnormal enhancement of Tenon's capsule (*curved arrow*). **E**, Enhanced sagittal T1-weighted (400/13, TR/TE) MR image shows granuloma at the optic disc (*white arrowhead*) as well as involvement of the optic nerve (*black arrowhead*). **F**, Enhanced axial fat-suppressed, T1-weighted (500/14, TR/TE) MR image shows enhancement of the markedly thickened uveal tract (*arrowheads*).

significant necrosis and prominent foci of calcification. A few tumors show areas of glial differentiation.[67, 71] The occurrence of a second cancer arising outside the treatment radiation field was pointed out by Jensen and Miller[73] and Abramson, Ellsworth, Kitchin, and Tung.[74] Abramson et al.[74] demonstrated that patients with heritable retinoblas-toma are highly susceptible to the development of other nonocular cancers, usually osteogenic sarcomas, and other neoplasms at sites of irradiation. The worldwide incidence of retinoblastoma has been reported to be 1 in 18,000 to 30,000 live births.[75] Although the tumor is congenital in origin, it usually is not recognized at birth.[32] However,

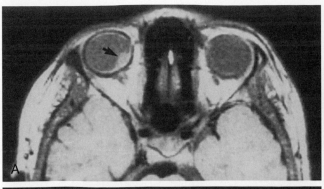

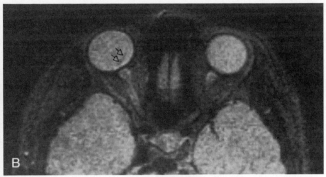

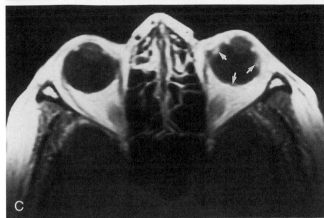

**FIGURE 8-55** Ocular toxocariasis. **A**, Axial PW and **B**, T2-weighted MR images. Scans show a hyperintense mass (*black arrow*) with associated minimum subretinal effusion. The mass remains hyperintense on the T2-weighted MR image, unlike Rb, which is almost always hypointense in T2-weighted scans. Note the ill-defined image of hypointensity (*open arrows*), which may represent scar tissue. Clinical and ophthalmologic findings were most compatible with granuloma of *Toxocara canis*. (From Mafee MF et al. Retinoblastoma and simulating lesions: role of CT and MRI. Radiol Clin North Am 1987;25:667–682.) **C**, Toxocariasis. Postcontrast axial T1-weighted MR image shows multiple abscesses in this 54-year-old woman with a positive ELISA test for *T. canis*.

**Table 8-3**
**CAUSES AND SITES OF CALCIUM DEPOSITION IN INTRAOCULAR TISSUE**

| Site of Calcification | Description | Causes |
|---|---|---|
| Cornea | Basement membrane of corneal epithelium, Bowman's membrane, anterior stromal lamellae | Chronic iridocyclitis |
| Sclera | Focal, near insertion of rectus muscles | Idiopathic sclerochoroidal calcification<br>Hypercalcemia*<br>Rheumatoid arthritis*<br>Microphthalmic with cyst*<br>Metastatic calcification*<br>Linear sebaceous nevus syndrome |
| Lens | Focal or diffuse, in the subcapsular or equatorial region (especially in hypermature cataracts) | Any condition that causes hypermature cataract |
| Ciliary body | Focal | Trauma<br>Medulloepithelioma (teratoid)*<br>Myopia |
| Choroid/RPE | Focal or diffuse (from RPE metaplasia or choroid osteoma) | Trauma<br>Uveitis, *Toxocara* granuloma*<br>Sturge-Weber syndrome*<br>Choroidal osteoma* |
| Retina | Focal, scattered or diffuse | Retinoblastoma<br>Drusen<br>Phthisis bulbi<br>Subretinal membrane<br>Periretinal membrane<br>PHPV*<br>ROP*<br>Coats' disease*<br>Astrocytoma*<br>CMV retinitis*<br>Tuberous sclerosis*<br>Von Hippel-Lindau disease*<br>Chronic organized retinal detachment<br>Medulloepithelioma* |
| Optic nerve | Focal, near the surface of the optic nerve | Drusen<br>Astrocytoma*<br>Optic nerve sheath dural idiopathic calcification* |

*Uncommon causes.
*RPE*, retinal pigment epithelium; *PHPV*, persistent hyperplastic primary vitreous; *ROP*, retinopathy of prematurity; *CMV*, cytomegalovirus.
Source: Yan X, Edward DP, Mafee MF. Ocular calcification: radiologic–pathologic correlation and literature review. Int J Neuroradiol 1998;4:81–96.

**Table 8-4**
**COMMON OCULAR AND ORBITAL DISORDERS OF CHILDREN**

Retinoblastoma—most common malignant ocular cancer in children

Persistent hyperplastic primary vitreous

Retinopathy of prematurity

Coats' disease

Microphthalmos with or without orbital cyst

Ocular trauma

Ocular inflammation, including granulomatous conditions

*Toxocara* larval granulomatosis

Orbital cellulitis—most common cause of proptosis in children

Dermoid and epidermoid cysts—most common orbital masses

Capillary hemangioma and lymphangioma—most common vascular masses

Optic nerve glioma—most common optic nerve tumor in children

Rhabdomyosarcoma—most common primary malignant orbital tumor in children

Leukemia

Pseudotumor

Neurofibroma

Metastatic neuroblastoma—most common metastatic cancer of the orbit in children

Subperiosteal hematoma

ocular involvement and metastasis may be present at birth.[62] In the United States, the average age of the child at diagnosis is 13 months.[76] In other countries, the disease is often not detected until the fourth year of life, when it is usually far advanced.[77] Over 90% of all diagnoses are made in children younger than 5 years of age. The sex distribution is equal, and there is no preference for either the right or the left eye.[78] Retinoblastoma results when an individual retinal cell has inactivation or loss of both alleles of the Rb1 gene on chromosome 13q14.[79–83] Transformation of the retinal cell occurs only if the genetic events occur during the age of vulnerability, usually when the patient is less than 3 years old. Retinoblastoma occurs in two distinct patterns: (1) a nonfamilial sporadic form and (2) a familial, hereditary form that appears at the clinical level to be autosomal dominant.[21] In both forms, the biology of the retinoblastoma tumor is identical. In nonfamilial retinoblastoma, an individual somatic retinal cell undergoes two sequential genetic events resulting in the loss or inactivation of both Rb1 alleles. All of the patients with nonfamilial retinoblastoma have unilateral solitary tumors. In the familial form, the patient's first loss or inactivation of an Rb1 allele occurs during gametogenesis at the germ cell level (either an inherited or a new mutation), so that every cell in the patient has only one working Rb1 allele. Retinoblastoma results if one of the patient's ''primed'' retinal cells has loss or inactivation of the second Rb1 allele (statistically, a 90% chance). With familial retinoblastoma, 85% of the cases are bilateral and 15% are unilateral.[21] Overall, approximately one third of the patients with retinoblastoma have bilateral disease.[19, 78, 84]

A parent with bilateral retinoblastoma has about a 50% chance of passing retinoblastoma on to one child.[78] Some affected children have been found to have an associated

deletion of the long arm of chromosome 13 involving band 13q14.[81, 82] The association between retinoblastoma and deletion of the q14 band of chromosome 13j (13q14) has been convincingly documented.[81–83, 85] Esterase D, an electrophoretically polymorphic human enzyme, has also been mapped to chromosomal band 13q14.[86] In several families with hereditary retinoblastoma with no apparent chromosomal deletion, the gene for retinoblastoma has been shown to be closely linked to that for esterase D and assigned to chromosome band 13q14.[86, 87] Compilation of data from recent studies suggests an approximately 7% incidence of 13q chromosomal deletion in patients with retinoblastoma.[88, 89] Only a few of the patients with retinoblastoma have a sufficiently large chromosomal deletion to produce systemic dysmorphic features such as microcephaly, genital malformations, ear abnormalities, mental retardation, and toe and finger abnormalities.[89] Karyotype analysis of these children with congenital dysmorphic features may allow detection of chromosome 13 deletion involving band 13q14, prompting ophthalmic examination and therefore allowing early diagnosis of retinoblastoma.[89] Patients with familial Rb are highly susceptible to the development of other nonocular cancers, usually osteogenic sarcoma, as well as other neoplasms at the site of external beam irradiation (see Fig. 8-31).[32] A second neoplasm may also arise outside the field of radiation.[32] Of 688 patients who survived therapeutic external beam irradiation for retinoblastoma, 89 developed second tumors, 62 in the field of radiation and 27 outside of the field.[32, 74] Of 23 patients who received no radiation, five developed second tumors, either osteosarcoma or soft tissue

**Table 8-5**
**INTRAOCULAR MASS AND MASS-LIKE LESIONS SIMULATING RETINOBLASTOMA**

| | |
|---|---|
| Coats' disease | Uveitis |
| Toxocariasis | Vitreous hemorrhage |
| Medulloepithelioma | Endophthalmitis |
| Retinal astrocytoma | Organized vitreous |
| Combined hamartoma of retinal pigment epithelium and retina | Retinal detachments |
| Choroidal osteoma | Persistent hyperplastic primary vitreous |
| Incontinetia pigmenti | Retinopathy of prematurity |
| Juvenile xanthogranuloma | X-linked retinoschisis |
| Mesoectodermal leiomyoma | Retinal dysplasia |
| Papillitis | Syndrome |
| Optic nerve head drusen | Norrie's disease |
| Retinal gliosis | Developmental retinal cyst |
| Myelinated nerve fibers | Falciform fold |
| Chorioretinal coloboma | Familial exudative vitreoretinopathy |
| Optic disc coloboma | Trauma |
| Walker-Warburg morning glory disc | Myopia |
| Von Hippel-Landau retinal angiomatosis | Stickler's syndrome |
| Choroidal hemangioma | Congenital cataract |
| Subretinal neovascular membrane | Congenital glaucoma |
| Vitreous opacities | Myiasis |

sarcoma.[74] The incidence of second tumors is 20% 10 years after initial diagnosis, 50% at 20 years, and 90% at 30 years.[32, 65, 74]

## Trilateral Retinoblastoma

The occurrence of ectopic retinoblastoma in the pineal body or in a parasellar region (*trilateral retinoblastoma*) has been reported by Jakobiec et al.[90] and Bader et al.[91, 92] The association of retinoblastoma with pinealoblastoma suggests that these tumors may be related.[93] In addition to having a common neuroectodermal origin, it is well known that in lower vertebrates the pineal gland has photoreceptor functions (similar to those seen in their retinas) and endocrine functions.[93] The development of an ectopic midline neuroblastic tumor in a patient with bilateral retinoblastoma probably represents an additional focus of a multicentric malignancy rather than a second primary tumor or metastatic disease.[91] It is also well known that the histologic appearance of retinoblastomas and pinealoblastomas may not be distinguished from each other.[90] It is postulated that, because of their similar origin, the same mutations may be cancerogenic for both retinoblasts and pinealoblasts. The failure of pineoblastomas to develop in all patients with heritable retinoblastoma may be due to a smaller cell population in the pineal gland or to other unrecognized factors.[94]

## Tetralateral Retinoblastoma

Trilateral retinoblastoma is the syndrome of bilateral retinoblastoma with a solitary midline intracranial tumor in the pineal gland, suprasellar region, or parasellar region.[70] El-Nagger et al.[95] reported an 11-month-old infant with bilateral and two distinct partially calcified intracranial tumors: a large mass in the area of the pineal gland and a second tumor in the suprasellar region. On biopsy, the pineal mass was compatible with a neuroblastic tumor (pinealoblastoma). The authors coined the term *tetralateral retinoblastoma* for this case of two distinct midline intracranial neuroblastic tumors associated with bilateral Rb.

## Clinical Diagnosis

Retinoblastoma accounts for about 1% of all deaths from childhood cancer in the United States.[96] The diagnosis of retinoblastoma usually can be made by an ophthalmoscopic examination. However, the detection and clinical differentiation of retinoblastoma from a host of benign simulating lesions may be difficult.[35, 82–99] The most common sign associated with retinoblastoma is leukokoria, which is present in 60% of patients (Fig. 8-56).[21, 32, 78] Strabismus (deviation of the eye) is the second most common sign. Pain caused by secondary glaucoma, often with heterochromia (different-colored irides), is the next most common symptom and sign, which leads to ophthalmologic evaluation. The ophthalmologic recognition of retinoblastoma is quite reliable. Small lesions are seen as gray-white intraretinal foci. Because of the difference in color from the surrounding retina and choroid, retinoblastomas can be seen when they are as small as 0.02 mm.[71] Other characteristic ophthalmoscopic findings include tumor calcification and vitreous seeding. As tumors grow in size, they often assume a convex configuration and produce three growth patterns: (1) In endophytic retinoblastoma, the tumor projects anteriorly, breaks through the internal limiting membrane of the retina, and grows into the vitreous. (2) In exophytic retinoblastoma, the tumor arises intraretinally and subsequently grows into the subretinal space, causing elevation of the retina.[64, 86] With continued tumor growth, there is an associated exudation and, rarely, a subretinal hemorrhage, which progressively cause retinal detachment; ophthalmoscopically, the exophytic tumors can simulate a traumatic retinal detachment. (3) In diffuse retinoblastoma, the tumor grows along the retina, appearing as a placoid mass. This diffuse form presents a perplexing diagnostic difficulty because of its atypical ophthalmoscopic feature (which simulates inflammatory or hemorrhagic conditions), its characteristic lack of calcification, and its occurrence usually outside of the typical age group.[64] All three growth forms, but especially the exophytic and diffuse infiltrating forms, may result in a tractional or exudative retinal detachment. Vitreous seeding of the tumor is more common in the endophytic and diffuse forms. Thus retinoblastoma may present as (1) a retinal or subretinal mass, with or without an associated retinal detachment or vitreous opacity; (2) a retinal detachment, with little indication of its etiology; (3) an opaque vitreous, with a limited view of the retinal structures and few clues to the etiology of the vitreous changes; or (4) some combination of the above forms.[64]

## Diagnostic Imaging

Although ophthalmoscopic recognition of retinoblastoma is often reliable, imaging modalities should be used on all patients suspected of harboring a retinoblastoma to determine the presence of gross or subtle retrobulbar spread, intracranial metastasis, and the presence of a second tumor. In addition, imaging techniques may allow differentiation of retinoblastoma from lesions such as PHPV, Coats' disease, ROP, toxocariasis, retinal detachment, organized subretinal hemorrhage, organized vitreous, endophthalmitis, retinal dysplasia, retinal astrocytoma (hamartoma), retinal gliosis, myelinated nerve fibers, choroidal hemangioma, coloboma, morning glory anomaly, congenital cataract, choroidal osteoma, drusen of the optic nerve head, and other so-called pseudogliomas and leukokorias. These lesions may have a clinical appearance similar to that of retinoblastoma (Table 8-6). Ultrasonography, CT, and MR are the most useful imaging techniques in the evaluation of these lesions. The tumor and calcification can be diagnosed by ultrasonography; however, the accuracy of ultrasonography for this condition is only 80%.[88] Diagnosis of tumor extension to the medial and lateral aspects of the orbit and extraocular extension are particularly limited with ultrasound.

High-resolution, thin-section (1.5 mm) CT can detect tumor and calcification within it with a high degree of accuracy.[24, 32, 84, 100] More than 90% of retinoblastomas show evidence of calcification on CT.[100] Calcification may be small and single, large and single, multiple and punctate

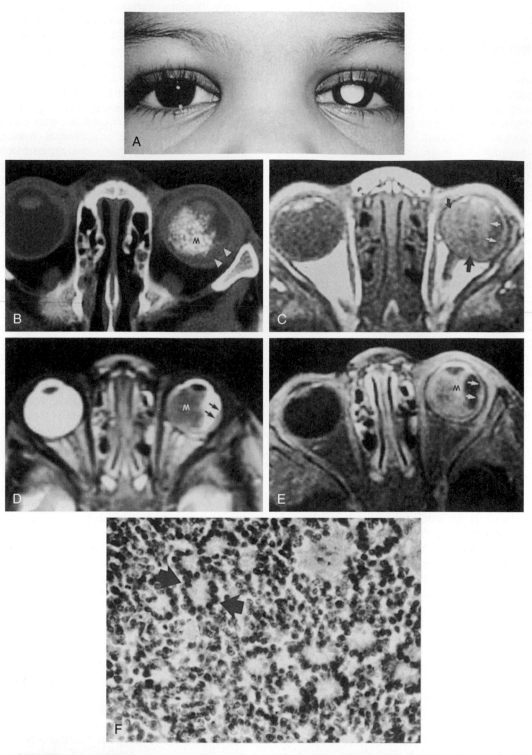

**FIGURE 8-56**    Retinoblastoma. **A,** Leukokoric left eye (whitish papillary reflex). **B,** Axial CT scan shows a large calcified intraocular mass (*M*). Note the noncalcified component (*arrowhead*). **C,** Axial T1-weighted (500/15, TR/TE) MR image shows a relatively hyperintense infiltrative mass (*arrows*). **D,** Axial T2-weighted (2000/102) MR image shows a hypointense infiltrative mass (*M*). Note the extension along the temporal aspect of the globe (*arrows*). **E,** Axial enhanced, fat-suppressed, T1-weighted (400/15, TR/TE) MR image shows moderate enhancement (*arrows*) of the mass (*M*). Note the enhancement along the temporal aspect of the globe (*arrows*). **F,** Histopathologic examination reveals well-differentiated retinoblastoma with numerous Flexner-Winterstein rosettes (*arrows*).

**Table 8-6**
**CT AND MR IMAGING DIFFERENTIAL DIAGNOSIS**
**OF CHOROIDAL OSTEOMA**

Choroidal hemangioma

Amelanotic choroidal nevus or melanoma

Regressed retinoblastoma

Metastatic carcinoma to choroid (prostate)

Idiopathic or dystrophic sclerochoroidal calcification

Posttraumatic or postinflammatory ocular calcification

Bone formation in phthisical eyes

Neurilemoma or neurofibroma of choroid

Intraocular foreign body

Calcification related to macular degeneration

Peripapillary choroidal calcification in chronic retinal detachment

(Fig. 8-56), or a few fine-speckled foci.[84] The DNA released from necrotic cells in retinoblastoma has a propensity to form a DNA–calcium complex. It is the frequent presence of this calcified complex that allows the intraocular tumor to be identified by fundoscopic, ultrasonic, and CT imaging.[32, 84, 100–102] In the extraocular component of retinoblastoma, calcification is rarely present.[84] The presence of intraocular calcification in children under 3 years of age (98% of cases present prior to age 6 months) is highly suggestive of retinoblastoma because none of the simulating lesions, except microphthalmos and colobomatous cyst, contain calcification.[32, 84] Retinoblastoma in a microphthalmic eye is extremely rare. In children over 3 years of age, some of the simulating lesions, including retinal astrocytoma, ROP, toxocariasis, and optic nerve head drusen can produce calcification.[32, 84] The diffuse infiltrating form of retinoblastoma is rare and may have no calcification (Fig. 8-57).[40, 86]

A retinal astrocytoma (astrocytic hamartoma) may initially appear like a retinoblastoma,[32, 76, 84] and the retinal astrocytoma may be present before any of the neurologic or dermatologic manifestations of tuberous sclerosis appear.[84] The CT appearance of these myelinated nerve fibers may also be similar to that of retinoblastoma.[84]

## MR Imaging

MR imaging has been used to evaluate retinoblastoma and other simulating lesions.[84, 96, 99, 103–105] In the diagnosis of retinoblastoma, MR imaging is not as specific as CT (Fig. 8-56) because of its lack of sensitivity in detecting calcification. However, the MR imaging appearance of retinoblastoma may be specific enough to differentiate retinoblastoma from simulating lesions (Fig. 8-57).[105] Retinoblastomas appear slightly or moderately hyperintense in relation to normal vitreous on T1-weighted (Fig. 8-56) and proton density images. On T2-weighted images, they appear as areas of markedly (Fig. 8-56) to moderately low signal intensity. Tumors elevated 3 to 4 mm in height may not be definitely identified on MR imaging,[84, 105] and lesions less than 2 to 3 mm in height are not confidently recognized by present MR imaging technology. Calcifications on MR imaging may be seen as varied degrees of hypointensity in

all pulse sequences (Fig. 8-56). In contrast to CT scanning, which is highly specific for calcification, MR imaging may be nonspecific. In many cases a calcification may not be recognized on MR imaging (Fig. 8-58). Thus, in the diagnosis of retinoblastoma, CT is more specific because of its superior sensitivity for detecting calcifications. Calcifications as small as 2 mm can be reliably detected by CT.[105] MR imaging, however, has better contrast resolution than CT, and MR imaging provides more information for differentiation of leukokoric eyes.[21, 105] The use of paramagnetic gadolinium contrast material has improved the sensitivity of MR imaging. Retinoblastomas show moderate to marked enhancement on postcontrast MR images (Figs. 8-56 and 8-57).

In a study of 27 patients with leukokoria, MR in all retinoblastomas (17 cases) showed a mass.[105] These masses had relatively short T1 and short T2 relaxation times. All retinoblastomas were seen as mildly to moderately hyperintense lesions on T1-weighted and proton density MR imaging (Figs. 8-56 to 8-58), and this appearance was very similar to that of uveal melanoma. None of the patients with PHPV, ROP, Coats' disease, or toxocariasis demonstrated MR imaging characteristics similar to those of retinoblastomas.[105]

Of the various imaging modalities, MR imaging has become the most useful in evaluating the challenging retinoblastoma patient.[21, 32] Ultrasound is limited by the presence of complex intraocular interfaces when vitreous opacities, retinal masses, subretinal fluid, and retinal detachments are present. As stated, CT is valuable in demonstrating calcification, but both ultrasound and CT are of lesser value in showing local spread of retinoblastoma (Fig. 8-59) or in distinguishing retinoblastoma from stimulating lesions. In the study of eyes with suspected retinoblastoma, our protocol includes plain CT (1.5 to 3 mm thick sections) of the eyes and MR imaging of the eyes and brain, because optic nerve (Fig. 8-59), extracranial (Figs. 8-60 and 8-61) and intracranial involvement (Figs. 8-62 and 8-63) may be better evaluated by MR imaging than by CT scanning. Both techniques can detect the intra- and extraocular lesions; however, MR imaging provides more information about the differentiation of other pathologic intraocular conditions that cause leukokoria, as well as other lesions such as medulloepithelioma and mesoectodermal leiomyoma.[21, 32] Patients with familial retinoblastoma are highly susceptible to the development of other nonocular cancers, usually osteogenic sarcoma as well as other neoplasms at the site of external beam radiation (see Fig. 8-31). Second neoplasms may also arise outside the field of radiation.[21, 32]

## Intraocular Mass and Mass-Like Lesions Simulating Retinoblastoma

There are other pediatric intraocular disorders that may clinically simulate retinoblastoma by presenting as a retinal or subretinal mass or mass-like lesion, retinal detachment, or a vitreous opacity.[21, 32] Further taxing the clinician's skills, (1) many of these other intraocular masses or mass-like lesions may secondarily result in retinal detachment or vitreous opacity, (2) the vitreous opacity disorders may secondarily result in a retinal detachment, (3) retinal detachments may undergo organization and contracture so as to resemble an intraocular mass, and (4) secondary cataracts may prevent direct viewing of the primary intraocular condition.

In a study of 500 consecutive patients with leukokoria in whom the diagnostic possibility of retinoblastoma was raised, diagnoses other than retinoblastoma were made in 265 cases.[65] The most common causes of leukokoria include retinoblastoma, PHPV, ROP, Coats' disease, posterior cataract, coloboma of the choroid or optic disc, uveitis, larval granulomatosis, and a variety of other processes (see Table 8-5).[21]

## PERSISTENT HYPERPLASTIC PRIMARY VITREOUS

PHPV is a condition that needs to be differentiated from retinoblastoma. Clinically, this condition is characterized by a unilateral leukokoria in a microphthalmic eye of a full-term baby. Rarely, PHPV may be bilateral. It is caused by the failure of the embryonic hyaloid vascular system to regress normally. The basic lesion is caused by a persistence of various portions of the primary vitreous and tunica vasculosa lentis, with hyperplasia and extensive proliferation of the associated embryonic connective tissue. In a study by Howard and Ellsworth,[65] of 500 children with leukokoria, PHPV accounted for 51 of the 265 non-Rb

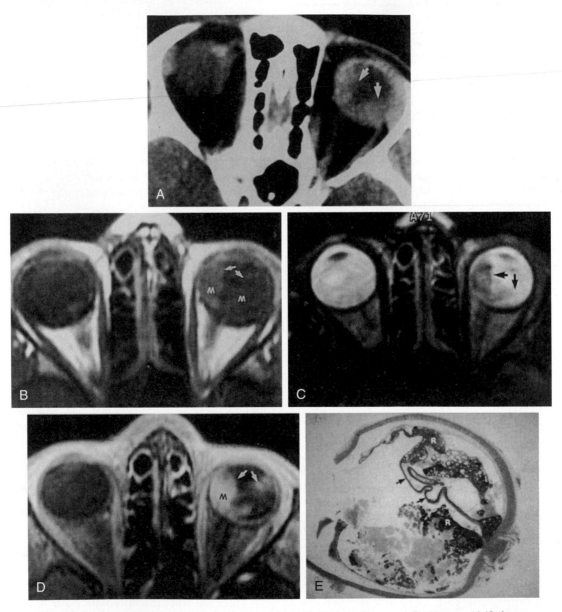

**FIGURE 8-57**   Diffuse infiltrating retinoblastoma. **A**, Axial CT scan shows an infiltrative noncalcified mass (*arrows*). **B**, Axial T1-weighted MR image shows a slightly hyperintense infiltrative exophytic mass (*MR*) under a detached retina (*arrows*). **C**, Axial T2-weighted MR image shows a hypointense infiltrative mass (*arrows*). **D**, Axial enhanced, fat-suppressed, T1-weighted MR image shows moderate enhancement of the tumor (*M*) under the associated retinal detachment (*arrows*). **E**, Photomicrograph of an enucleated eye showing diffuse retinoblastoma (*R*) with a detached retina (*arrows*) and no calcification.

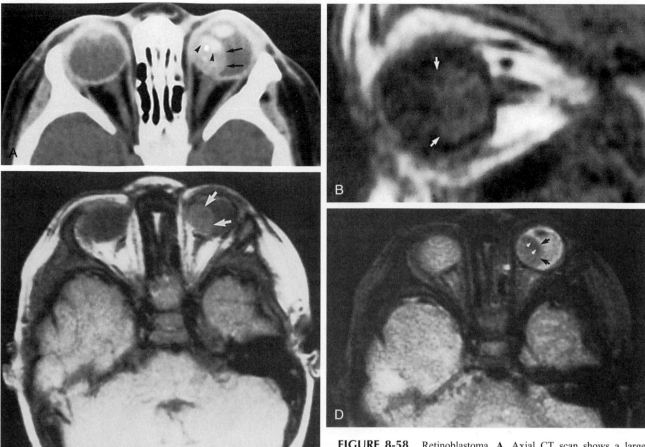

**FIGURE 8-58**   Retinoblastoma. **A**, Axial CT scan shows a large mass (*arrows*) with areas of calcification (*arrowheads*). **B**, T1-weighted sagittal MR image shows slight hyperintensity of the lesion (*arrows*). **C**, Axial PW MR image shows a moderately hyperintense mass (*arrows*). **D**, Axial T2-weighted MR image shows a hypointense mass (*arrows*). (From Mafee MF et al. MRI versus CT of leukokoric eyes and use of in vitro proton magnetic resonance spectroscopy of retinoblastoma. Ophthalmology 1989;96:965–976.)

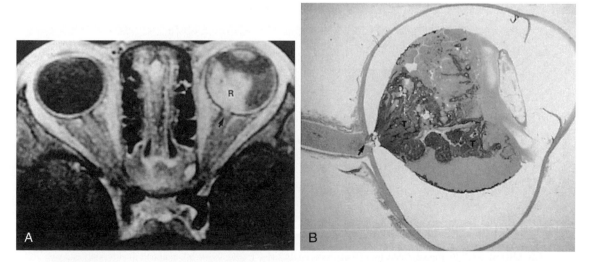

**FIGURE 8-59**   Retinoblastoma with optic nerve involvement. **A**, Enhanced, fat-suppressed, axial T1-weighted MR image shows marked enhancement of a retinoblastoma (*R*) with extension into the optic nerve (*arrow*). **B**, Photomicrograph of an enucleated eye showing the tumor (*T*) as well as extension into the optic nerve head (*arrow*). (Courtesy of D. Ainbinder, MD, Tacoma, WA.)

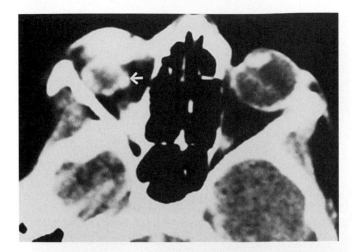

**FIGURE 8-60** Recurrent retinoblastoma. Axial CT scan shows recurrent disease (*arrow*) after enucleation. Note the right false eye. (Courtesy of Dr. G. Schullman.)

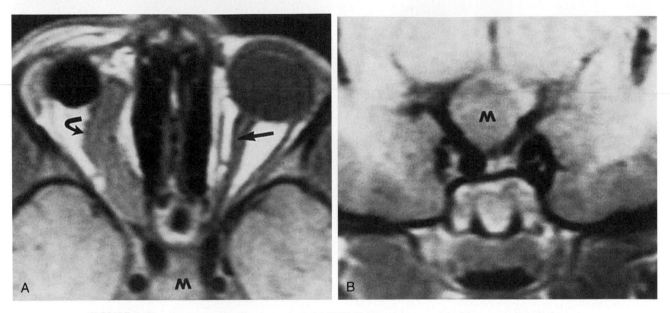

**FIGURE 8-61** Recurrent retinoblastoma. **A**, Axial PW MR image shows a right false eye and marked tumor along the right optic nerve (*curved arrow*). Note the normal left optic nerve (*arrow*) and the tumor mass (*M*) in the sellar region. **B**, Coronal PW MR image shows a marked tumor mass (*M*) in the sellar and suprasellar region.

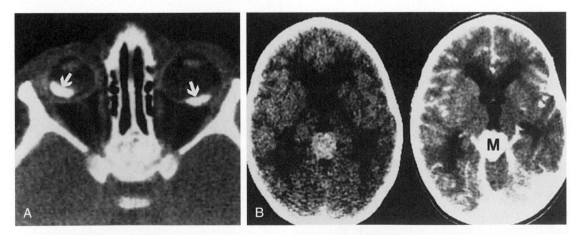

**FIGURE 8-62** Presumed trilateral retinoblastoma. **A**, Axial CT scan shows bilateral calcified retinoblastomas (*arrows*). **B**, Axial CT scans with and without contrast enhancement show a large mass (*M*) in the region of the pineal gland with associated moderate hydrocephalus. This presumed pinealoma (retinoblastoma?) developed 2 years after external irradiation to both eyes through lateral ports. (From Mafee MF et al. Retinoblastoma and simulating lesions: role of CT and MRI. Radiol Clin North Am 1987;25:667–682.)

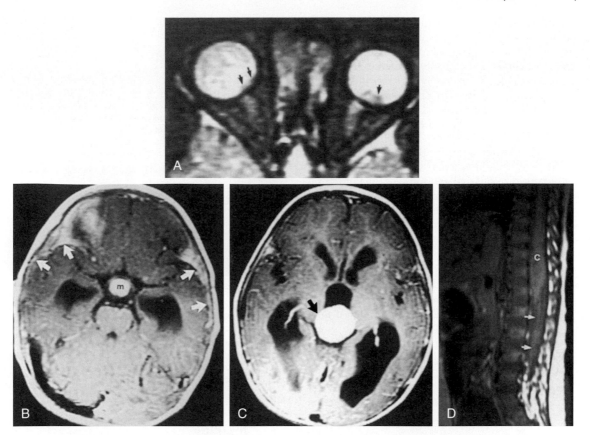

**FIGURE 8-63**   Tetralateral retinoblastoma. **A,** Axial T2-weighted MR image shows bilateral retinoblastoma (*arrows*). **B,** Enhanced axial T1-weighted MR image shows a markedly enhancing suprasellar mass (*m*). Note the subarachnoid spread of the tumor, seen as leptomeningeal enhancement along the sylvian fissures (*arrows*). **C,** Enhanced axial T1-weighted MR image shows marked enhancement of a pinealoblastoma (*arrow*). **D,** Enhanced sagittal T1-weighted MR image obtained a few months later shows diffuse distal spinal cord (*C*) and subarachnoid metastases (*arrows*).

cases. The authors concluded that except for retinoblastoma, PHPV is the most frequent cause of leukokoria in childhood. The nosology of PHPV is extremely complex.[105–107] The ocular malformation can reflect either an isolated congenital defect or a manifestation of more extensive ocular or systemic involvement. The term *persistent hyperplastic primary vitreous* therefore is a marked oversimplification that has no etiologic precision and only the grossest prognostic implications.[108] The embryonic intraocular vascular system may be divided into two components: an anterior system in the region of the iris and a posterior (retrolental) component within the vitreous. The anterior system is composed of the pupillary membrane, which is formed by small vascular buds that grow inwardly to vascularize the iris mesoderm anterior to the lens.[29] The posterior system includes the main hyaloid artery, vasa hyaloidea propria, and tunica vasculosa lentis.[29, 35] The first vessels to undergo regression are the vasa hyaloidea propria, followed by the tunica vasculosa lentis and eventually the main hyaloid artery.[29, 35, 108] During the first month of gestation, the space between the lens and the retina contains the primary vitreous. It consists of two parts: mesodermally derived tissue, including the hyaloid vessel and its branches, and a fibrillar meshwork that is of ectodermal origin.[109] In the second month of embryonic development, collagen fibers and a ground substance or gel component consisting of hyaluronic acid are produced. They form the secondary vitreous and begin to replace the vascular elements of the primary vitreous. By the fourteenth week, the secondary vitreous begins to fill the vitreous cavity.[109] By the fifth to sixth month of development, the cavity of the eye is filled primarily with the secondary vitreous that represents the adult vitreous. The primary vitreous is thus reduced to a small central space, Cloquet's canal, which runs in an S-shaped course between the optic nerve head and the posterior surface of the lens.[35, 36]

## Clinical Diagnosis

Diagnosis of PHPV often is made difficult by its extremely broad array of clinical manifestations, etiologic heterogeneity, and frequently opaque ocular media.[106, 108, 110] Complete inspection of the interior of the eye may be precluded not only by cataract but also by vitreous hemorrhage or by opaque retrolental fibrovascular tissue. This condition usually manifests clinically as unilateral leukokoria in a microphthalmic eye. At birth the lens is clear, with a white to pinkish fibrovascular mass behind it; later, the lens usually becomes swollen and cataractous.[111] In the natural course of untreated PHPV, the eye often develops glaucoma and eventually buphthalmos or phthisis, sometimes leading to loss of the globe.[111] The clinical presentation of PHPV is variable. Its main features include a unilateral (rarely bilateral) presentation, usually with leukokoria, microphthalmos, lens opacity, retinal detachment, and vitreous hemorrhage. In severe forms, elongated ciliary processes, elongated radial iris vessels, a shallow anterior chamber, and phthisis may occur. The diagnosis of the different types or causes of PHPV can sometimes be inferred from the family and birth histories, as well as from the details of the clinical examination.[108] Direct visualization of remnants of the fetal hyaloid vascular system offers the best evidence. However, direct visualization by ophthalmoscopy or microscopy is sometimes impossible because of the opaque media. In these circumstances, indirect visualization by CT and MR imaging can be diagnostically useful.[35, 108] The CT findings of PHPV were first reported by Mafee and Goldberg and their colleagues.[35, 108] Maximum information was derived from the use of CT following intravenous contrast administration and repeated scanning in the lateral decubitus position.[35] The CT findings include (1) microphthalmos, which is usually detectable, although it may be minimal or absent, and other deformities in the globe configuration, which may have been undetectable by physical examination or ultrasonography;[108] (2) calcification is absent within or around the globe; (3) generalized increased density of the entire vitreous chamber may be visible (Fig. 8-64), although minimally affected patients may show normal attenuation values in the vitreous chambers; (4) enhancement of abnormal intravitreal tissue may be seen after intravenous administration of a contrast medium; (5) tubular, cylindrical, triangular, or other discrete intravitreal densities suggest the persistence of fetal tissue in Cloquet's canal or congenital nonattachment of the retina (Fig. 8-65); (6) decubitus positioning may show a gravitational effect on a fluid level within the vitreous chamber (see Fig. 8-28), reflecting the presence of serosanguineous fluid in either the subhyaloid or subretinal space; and (7) the lens may be small and irregular, and the anterior chamber may be shallow.

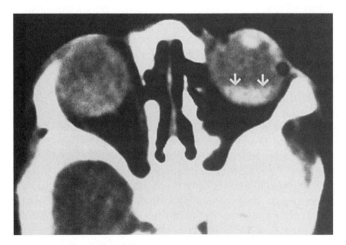

**FIGURE 8-64** PHPV. Axial CT scan shows an increase in the density of both vitreous chambers, with gravitational layering of high-density fluid in the left eye (*arrows*). The high-density fluid is most likely caused by blood in the subhyaloid space.

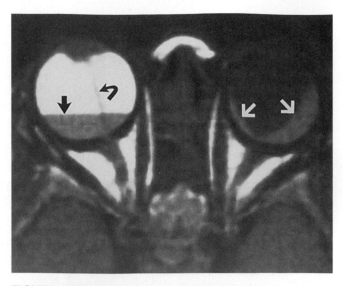

**FIGURE 8-65** PHPV. This 5-month-old girl was diagnosed as having Warburg's syndrome (congenital oculocerebral disorder). Axial T1-weighted MR image shows hyperintense subretinal fluid in the left eye with a detached retina (*arrows*). Note the fluid-fluid level in the right vitreous (*solid arrow*). This is thought to be caused by chronic (hyperintense) and acute (hypointense) hemorrhage in the subhyaloid or subretinal space. Note the tubular image (*curved arrow*), which suggests a congenital nonattached retina or Cloquet's canal.

## MR Imaging

The MR appearance of the different types of PHPV may be different. Early experience with MR imaging in patients with PHPV has revealed marked hyperintensity of the vitreous chamber on T1-weighted, proton density, and T2-weighted images.[36] The MR appearance of eyes with ROP may be identical to that of eyes with PHPV. The appearance of retinal detachment in PHPV has two forms: (1) retinal elevation into the vitreous from the optic nerve, resembling acquired forms of retinal detachment (Fig. 8-65), and (2) retinal elevation from a point in the wall of the eye that was eccentric to the optic nerve, suggesting a falciform fold or congenital nonattachment of the retina.[106, 108] Contrast-enhanced CT or MR imaging may demonstrate an enhanced retrolental mass (Fig. 8-66), and there may be increased enhancement in the anterior segment of the involved eye (Fig. 8-66). PHPV is often associated with severe malformations of the optic nerve and retina.[108] The ocular malformation usually reflects a manifestation of more extensive disease including Norrie's disease, Warburg's syndrome, primary vitreoretinal dysplasia, and other congenital defects. Nonetheless, the clinical or imaging detection of PHPV alerts the clinician to the appropriate diagnostic and prognostic possibilities. CT and MR imaging certainly are not indicated if the diagnosis and management of PHPV can be determined easily by conventional techniques. On the other hand, any procedure such as CT or MR imaging that aids the complex diagnostic and therapeutic decision-making that is often required for such affected children should be considered clinically useful and employed in these selected circumstances. In a CT study by Goldberg and Mafee[108] of eight children referred with several diagnoses, including Rb, congenital cataract, and microphthalmos, after collation of data from clinical examinations under anesthesia and from CT scanning, although PHPV was not the initial diagnosis in any case, it proved to be the most acceptable diagnosis for all patients. MR imaging provides even more information in the diagnosis of PHPV because no patient with PHPV has the hypointensity of the vitreous chamber that is characteristic of retinoblastoma (Figs. 8-56 and 8-57). However, on CT, differentiation of a retinoblastoma from PHPV is not always easy.

## RETINAL DYSPLASIA

Retinal dysplasia includes a group of disorders, such as Norrie's disease and Walker-Warburg's syndrome, in which abnormal proliferation and folding of the developing outer retina leads to congenital retinal detachment.[21] PHPV is manifested with more severe malformation in diseases such as Norrie's disease, Warburg's syndrome, and retinal dysplasia.

## Norrie's Disease

Norrie's disease, or congenital progressive oculoacousticocerebral degeneration, is a rare X-linked recessive syndrome consisting of retinal malformation, deafness, and mental retardation or deterioration.[112] In 1927, Norrie described seven cases in two families with the same hereditary blindness.[113] In 1961, Warburg described the entity with other congenital eye diseases, coined the eponym *Norrie's disease*,[114] and later added the features of hearing loss and mental retardation. Warburg also described the disorder as *congenital progressive oculoacousticocerebral degeneration*.[115] Warburg established that Norrie's disease has an X-linked recessive pattern of inheritance, affects only males, and has ophthalmologically unaffected female carriers.[116] The affected males can exhibit ocular changes, including partial or complete retinal detachment; vitreoretinal hemorrhage, which can be present in the early neonatal

period;[112] a retrolental mass; cataract; glaucoma; optic nerve atrophy; choroidal hypercellularity; and phthisis bulbi, which after varying periods of time lead to bilateral blindness.[112] Other findings include progressive high-tone sensorineural hearing loss,[116, 117] congenital nystagmus,[112] mild to severe mental retardation, and psychotic symptoms.[112, 116, 117]

The pathogenesis of Norrie's disease is unknown. Warburg[116] postulated that the basic lesion is a genetically determined biochemical defect that causes primary arrest in the development of the embryonic neuroectodermal structures of the retina, with consequent changes within the primary and secondary vitreous. Neuroectodermal changes also occur in the cerebral cortex.

Histopathologically, in the early stage the condition is characterized by absence of retinal ganglion cells and absence of normal nerve fiber layer structures in the retina.[118] In the more advanced stages of the disease, most authors have been impressed with the similarity between Norrie's disease and Coats' disease.[119] However, Apple, Fishman, and Goldberg[118] believed that in the earlier stages it is possible to differentiate Norrie's and Coats' diseases. Associated changes in Norrie's disease that may be present include optic nerve atrophy, atrophy of visual pathways, incomplete stratification of the brain cortex, and abnormalities of the brain.[115]

### Diagnostic Imaging

The CT findings in Norrie's disease were first reported by Mafee and Goldberg.[35, 108] These included bilaterally dense vitreous chambers (Fig. 8-67A), a retrolental mass, retinal detachment, microphthalmia,[36] optic nerve atrophy, a shallow anterior chamber, and a small, highly dense lens.[36] There was no evidence of intraocular or extraocular calcification, nor was there any evidence of gravitational layering of intravitreal fluid. The MR imaging findings of Norrie's disease include bilateral hyperintense vitreous caused by chronic vitreous or subretinal hemorrhage (Fig. 8-67B,C); persistence of the primary vitreous may be present, the optic nerves may be hypoplastic, and there may be associated developmental anomalies of the brain (Fig. 8-67D).

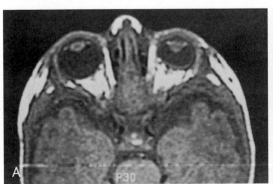
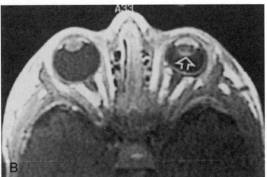

**FIGURE 8-66**  PHPV. Axial Precontrast (**A**) and postcontrast (**B**) T1-weighted (450/15, TR/TE) MR images show a microphthalmic left eye. Note the abnormal signal of the left lens, the retrolental enhancing mass (*arrow*), and the increased enhancement in the left anterior chamber related to elongated ciliary processes, possibly caused by leaking vessels.

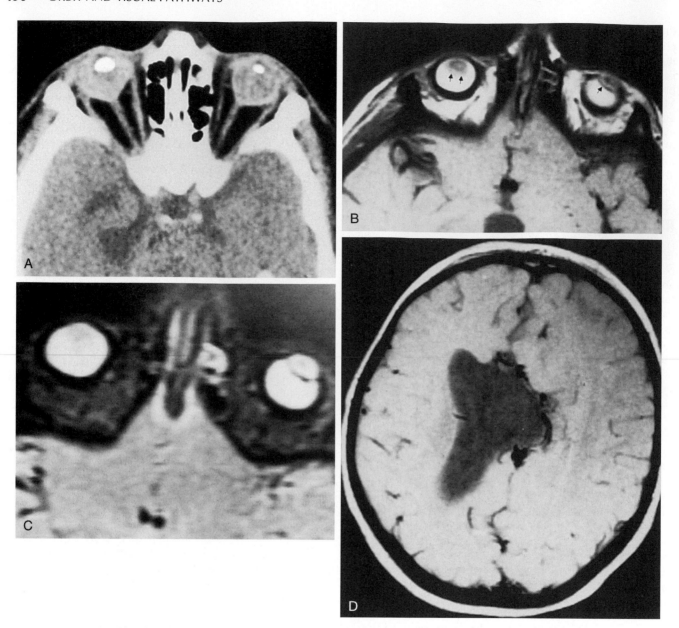

**FIGURE 8-67**   Norrie's disease with bilateral PHPV. **A,** Axial CT scan shows bilateral dense vitreous chambers and small eyes. The left lens is smaller than the right lens, and both are rather peculiar in shape. **B,** Axial PW MR image shows marked hyperintensity of both globes. **C,** Axial T2-weighted MR image shows hyperintensity of both globes. These changes are caused by proteinaceous fluid or chronic hemorrhage in the subhyaloid or subretinal space or within the vitreous chamber. Note the abnormal tissue in the retrolental regions (*arrows*), better seen in **B** than in **C**. These changes may be difficult to differentiate from ROP. **D,** Axial PW MR image shows a developmental anomaly of the lateral ventricles, a cavum septum pellucidum, and flattening of some of the cortical gyri (lissencephaly). (**A** to **C** from Mafee MF et al. Persistent hyperplastic primary vitreous (PHPV): role of CT and MRI. Radiol Clin North Am 1987;25:683–692.)

## Warburg's Syndrome

Complex syndromes with congenital malformations of the central nervous system, microphthalmia, and congenital unilateral or bilateral retinal nonattachment have been described in a number of disorders such as Meckel's syndrome, a disorder with malformations of the central nervous system, including encephalocele, cleft palate, polydactyly, cysts of the liver and kidneys, genital malformations, and microphthalmia.[120]

In 1971, Warburg suggested that such patients might suffer from a nosologically distinct syndrome.[121] She described an autosomal recessive disorder consisting of profound mental retardation with death in infancy, hydrocephaly, microphthalmia, and congenital nonattachment of the retina.[121] Subsequent postmortem studies confirmed these clinical observations and noted the coexistence of lissencephaly in these patients.[122, 123]

In 1978 the syndrome was redescribed and the mnemonic HARDTE was coined to point out the following characteristic features: hydrocephaly, agyria, and retinal dysplasia (detachment), with or without encephalocele.[124] The

HARDTE, or Warburg's syndrome, is a congenital oculocerebral disorder caused by a genetic defect that simultaneously affects ocular and cerebral embryogenesis and specifically involves the retina and the brain.[125] The syndrome emphasizes the developmental and morphologic similarities between the cerebral cortex and the retina. The syndrome is characterized by congenital bilateral leukokoria.

The ophthalmic findings associated with this syndrome include microphthalmos and retinal dysplasia with congenital retinal nonattachment.[115, 126] Associated anomalies may include vitreous hemorrhage, a large intravitreal vessel, opaque retrolental tissue, persistent hyperplastic primary vitreous, and a hypoplastic optic disc.[125] The lens may have a pear-shaped configuration because of a posterior bulge (posterior lenticonus).[125] Postmortem studies of the brain attest to the poor growth of the cerebral hemisphere, with disorganization and dysgenesis of the cerebral and cerebellar gray and white matter.[122, 123, 125]

### Clinical Diagnosis

Microphthalmia and hydrocephaly may be seen in children with congenital toxoplasmosis, rubella syndrome, congenital syphilis, and herpes and cytomegalovirus (CMV) infections. In toxoplasmosis, there may be characteristic chorioretinal scars and a positive serologic test. The presence of significant serum antibody titers against rubella, CMV, herpes virus, and syphilis should serve to distinguish Warburg's syndrome from these simulating disease entities.[32]

### Diagnostic Imaging

The CT and MR imaging findings in the eyes of patients with Warburg's syndrome include bilateral retinal detachment (Fig. 8-68A), subretinal hemorrhage, vitreous hemorrhage, and gravitational intravitreal fluid (Fig. 8-68B). Persistence of the primary vitreous also may be present.[125] The congenital nonattached retina or the totally detached retina exhibits a characteristic narrow funnel shape or a triangular intravitreal mass adjacent to Cloquet's canal (see Figs. 8-28 and 8-65).

## Retinopathy of Prematurity

In contrast to PHPV, ROP (retrolental fibroplasia, retinal fibroplasia) is seen in premature low-birth-weight infants. ROP is usually bilateral and fairly symmetric. The essential feature of ROP appears to be prematurity. The smaller the infant, the greater the risk of developing this disease. ROP usually develops as a response to prolonged exposure to supplemental oxygen therapy. It is possible that excessive oxygen plays only a participating role in the development of ROP. Eller et al.[127] noted that 14 patients had an associated persistent hyaloid vascular system. A massive persistent hyaloid vascular system was found in seven of their patients. The authors concluded that ROP may be related to a combination of developmental and environmental factors that prevent normal retinal vasculogenesis outside the womb.

### Ophthalmoscopic Picture

In ROP, proliferation of abnormal peripheral retinal vessels occurs, with subsequent hemorrhage and cicatrization, which may organize and contract, leading to tractional retinal detachment in the advanced stages. The detachment may be partial or total, anterior or posterior, or in an open or closed funnel configuration. The ophthalmoscopic findings of ROP have been divided into active, regressive, and cicatricial phases. The initial active phase is characterized by arteriolar narrowing caused by a spastic response of the vessels to hyperoxia.[128] The vessels then start to dilate and become tortuous. A subsequent sign is the presence of fine, delicate neovascularization in the periphery, changes that are most marked in the temporal periphery because this is the region where the retinal vascularization develops last. Commonly, as long as premature infants are under oxygen therapy, there is no vascular dilatation or tortuosity, which

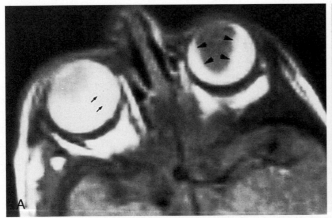
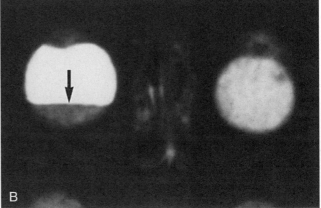

**FIGURE 8-68**   Warburg's syndrome. **A,** Axial T1-weighted MR image shows subretinal effusion with a detached retina (*arrows*) of the left eye. Hyperintensity of the right globe is caused by chronic hemorrhage in the subhyaloid or subretinal space. Note the congenitally nonattached retina or Cloquet's canal and the abnormal retrolental soft tissue. **B,** Axial T1-weighted MR image obtained 4 months later reveals progression of disease in both eyes with a fluid-fluid level (*arrow*) caused by chronic (hyperintense) and acute (hypointense) hemorrhage in the subhyaloid or subretinal space.

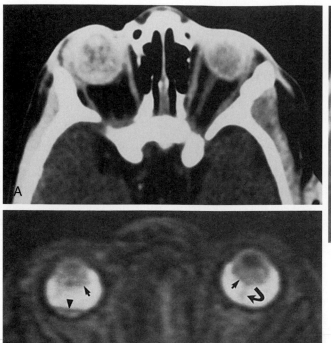

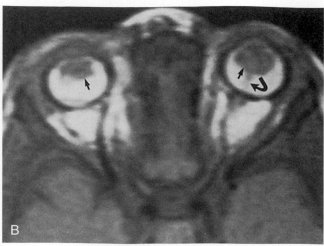

**FIGURE 8-69**   ROP. **A,** Axial CT scan shows increased density of the globes and left microphthalmos. **B,** Axial PW MR image shows hyperintensity of both globes, presumably caused by subretinal hemorrhage. Note the retrolental abnormal tissues (*arrows*) and detached retina (*curved arrow*). **C,** Axial T2-weighted MR image shows hyperintensity of the globes and abnormal retrolental soft tissues (*arrows*). Note the detached retina (*curved arrow*) and the layered acute hemorrhage in the right subretinal space (*arrowhead*).

occurs 24 to 48 hours after the infants are removed rapidly from the oxygen incubator.[129] Gradually, strands containing new vessels pass into the vitreous from the retina. There may be vitreous hemorrhage, which may be massive, and the retina may become partially or completely detached.[129]

### Regressive Phase

A characteristic of the disease is that during the early stage, there is a tendency to regress spontaneously, with disappearance of the neovascularization and even of a general detachment of the retina.[129] The detached retina, however, may not always become reattached. About 85% to 90% of cases show spontaneous regression.[129]

### Cicatricial Phase

Finally, a dense membrane or a gray-white vascularized mass will be left as permanent evidence of the active phase. The lens always remains clear. The retina is detached, with associated retinal scars. The growth of the eye is often inhibited, with microphthalmos as the final outcome.

### Diagnostic Imaging

The early stage of ROP may have no specific CT and MR imaging findings except that the eyes may be microphthalmic. In more advanced cases, the CT and MR differential diagnosis between ROP (Fig. 8-69) and PHPV, retinoblastoma, endophthalitis, or a number of pathologic conditions wherein retinal detachment is a common feature may be difficult.[36, 84, 126, 129] The history of incubator

treatment, birth weight, bilaterality, and the ophthalmoscopic, ultrasound, and CT findings are usually sufficient to establish the diagnosis. Calcification is rare in ROP. However, in the more advanced stage, calcification may be present. In the most advanced cases of ROP, both eyes are microphthalmic, with very shallow anterior chambers. Calcification in a microphthalmic eye is less indicative of retinoblastoma, although rarely retinoblastoma has been reported in microphthalmic eyes with or without ROP or PHPV. ROP may on occasion present as unilateral leukokoria. However, in the majority of cases, ROP presents as bilateral but often markedly asymmetric disease.[110] A persistent hyaloid vascular system may be an associated finding in patients with ROP, and the recognition of a massive persistent hyaloid vascular system on clinical examination, MR imaging, CT, or ultrasound is of prognostic importance.[127] In these cases, the surgical dissection of the retrolental membrane in the presence of a persistent hyaloid vascular system is more difficult because these vessels tend to bleed, and the retrolental membrane is tightly adherent to the detached retina.[127]

## Coats' Disease

Coats' disease (primary retinal telangiectasis) is a primary vascular anomaly of the retina characterized by idiopathic retinal telangiectatic and aneurysmal retinal vessels, with progressive deposition of intraretinal and subretinal exudates that leads to massive exudative retinal detachment (exudative retinopathy).[27, 130, 131] The condition occurs more frequently in juvenile males than in females. However, it is also seen in adults, in whom it is almost always unilateral.[27, 130, 132, 133] The formation of retinal telangiectasia, and the breakdown in the blood-retinal barrier with leakage of a lipoproteinaceous exudate at the telangiectasis, are the essential underlying causes of the pathologic changes that occur in Coats' disease.[27] The primary cause for the telangiectasis, and for the leakage of serum and lipid and eventual closure of the retinal vessels in the area of the telangiectasis, is unknown.[27] The degree of lipoproteinaceous subretinal exudation in Coats' disease appears to be proportional to the extent of the retinal telangiectasis.[134] The spectrum of pathologic changes in Coats' disease includes intraretinal or subretinal exudation, hemorrhages, lipid and fibrin deposition, phagocytic proliferation (ghost cells), and, ultimately, glial and fibrous tissue organization of the retina.[27] The vascular anomaly of Coats' disease, although present at birth, usually does not cause symptoms until the retina detaches and central vision is lost.[135]

### Clinical Presentation and Diagnosis

Coats' disease usually occurs in young boys, with the onset of symptoms in most patients occurring before age 20. Although the incidence peaks between 6 and 8 years,[134] cases have been reported in patients ranging from 4 months old to the seventh decade.[134] The modes of presentation include leukokoria, strabismus, a failed school screening test, or painful glaucoma secondary to angle closure. Although the cause of Coats' disease remains unknown, there are isolated reports associating the disease with fasciocapsulohumeral muscular dystrophy, Turner's syndrome, Senior-Loken syndrome (familial renal-retinal dystrophy), the ichthyosis hystrix variant of epidermal nevus syndrome, inversion on chromosome 3, and a deletion of chromosome 13.[134] The ophthalmoscopic findings in Coats' disease vary with the stage of disease. In the early stages, the telangiectasis can be observed. In the later stages, when the retina is filled with and detached by a mass of cholesterol exudate (total bullous exudative retinal detachment), the telangiectasis can be seen only on fluorescein angiography.[27] In the early stage of the disease, while the retinal disease is not too extensive and the retinal detachment is shallow, photocoagulation, cryotherapy, or both usually obliterate the telangiectatic vessels and reduce or eliminate the exudative retinal detachment.[134] When there is extensive retinal telangiectasis and a total bullous exudative retinal detachment, cryotherapy and photocoagulation may not be sufficient to obliterate the leaking vessels. Such eyes commonly progress to secondary angle closure or iris neovascularization, becoming blind and painful as a result of acute congestive (neovascular) glaucoma.[134, 135]

### Diagnostic Imaging

The ophthalmoscopic and biomicroscopic features of eyes with advanced Coats' disease may closely resemble findings in eyes with exophytic retinoblastoma and leukokoria.[136] It is important to distinguish retinoblastoma from Coats' disease. Many eyes with advanced Coats' disease are enucleated because retinoblastoma cannot be excluded.[135] In a study of 62 eyes satisfying the histologic diagnostic criteria of Coats' disease submitted to the Armed Forces Institute of Pathology, Chang, McLean, and Merritt[131] found that 52 (79%) were enucleated, with the diagnosis of retinoblastoma or to rule out retinoblastoma. Coats' disease is almost always unilateral, and it usually appears in boys slightly older (4 to 8 years) than those who have retinoblastoma.[21, 32] Many diagnostic techniques, including ultrasound, CT, and MR imaging, are available that help the ophthalmologist to diagnose clinical conditions, and CT and MR imaging have been shown to be extremely valuable in the diagnosis of Coats' disease.[84, 105, 134]

The CT and MR imaging findings in Coats' disease vary with the stage of the disease. In the early stages, both techniques may yield little information. In the later stages, retinal detachment accounts for all the pathologic findings in CT and MR imaging. Sherman, McLean, and Brallier[137] reported two children with Coats' disease. They concluded that CT could not differentiate between Coats' disease and unilateral noncalcifying retinoblastoma. Haik et al. reported the CT findings in 14 patients with Coats' disease; total retinal detachment (Fig. 8-70A) was routinely seen in advanced disease.[99] Calcification is not a feature of Coats' disease; however, in advanced Coats' disease, in up to one fifth of all cases, there is a fibrous submacular nodule that occasionally is calcified or ossified.[134] These nodules might represent exuberant proliferation and metaplasia of the retinal pigment epithelium (RPE).[134] MR imaging is superior to CT in differentiating Coats' disease from retinoblastomas and other leukokoric eyes.[105, 134] The subretinal exudation of Coats' disease is usually seen as hyperintense on T1-weighted, proton density, and T2-weighted MR images (Fig. 8-70B,C). In retinoblastomas, MR characteristically shows a mass that can be easily differentiated from an associated subretinal exudate. The retinoblastoma is relatively hyperintense on T1-weighted and proton density images (Figs. 8-56 and 8-57) and becomes hypointense on T2-weighted images (Figs. 8-56 and 8-57). The subretinal fluid of an associated retinal detachment is seen as various degrees of hyperintensity in all pulse sequences. Although Coats' disease can produce a subretinal mass resembling retinoblastoma, the mass in Coats' disease is caused by cholesterol, organized hemorrhage, and fibrosis, and therefore its signal is presumed to be inhomogeneous in character. The MR findings in patients with Coats' disease are compatible with retinal detachment without the presence of an intraocular mass (Fig. 8-71). In Coats' disease the detached retina may show enhancement following intravenous injection of Gd-DTPA contrast (Fig. 8-71D). The enhancement is due to idiopathic intraretinal telangiectasia and microaneurysms, the underlying pathology of Coats' disease. The MR findings in some of these patients in the early stages of the disease are normal.

In general, if an ophthalmologist suspects advanced Coats' disease but is uncertain about the correct clinical diagnosis and is unable to rule out retinoblastoma conclusively, a diagnostic imaging study should be requested.[135] When a patient presents with what appears to be a retinoblastoma with total retinal detachment, there are basically three diagnoses to consider: PHPV, Coats' disease, and ROP. In the appropriate clinical setting, the MR imaging and CT findings of Coats' disease should help establish a correct diagnosis.[21, 32, 134]

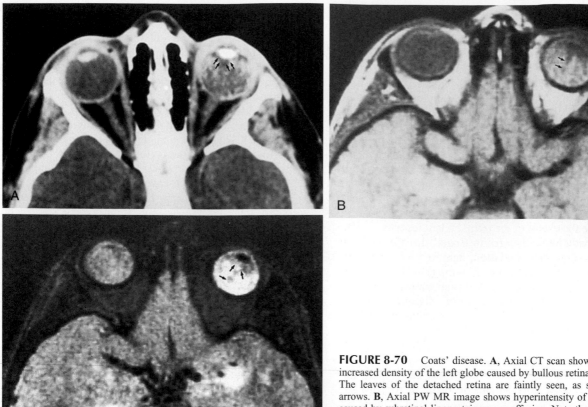

FIGURE 8-70   Coats' disease. **A,** Axial CT scan shows generalized increased density of the left globe caused by bullous retinal detachment. The leaves of the detached retina are faintly seen, as shown by the arrows. **B,** Axial PW MR image shows hyperintensity of the left globe caused by subretinal lipoproteinaceous effusion. Note the leaves of the detached retina (*arrows*). **C,** Axial T2-weighted MR image shows the detached retina (*arrows*).

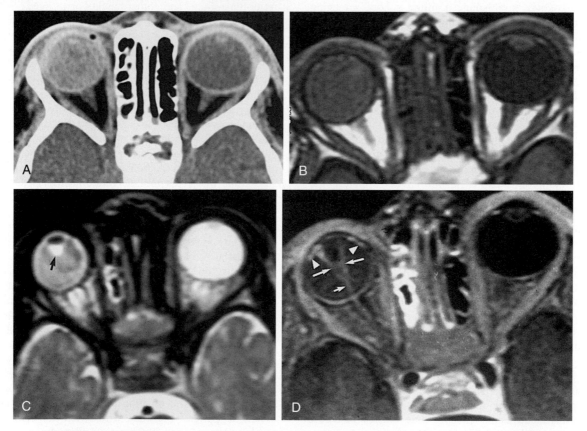

FIGURE 8-71   **A,** Axial CT scan shows the diffuse increased density of the right globe caused by total retinal detachment. A retinoblastoma cannot be excluded. **B,** Nonenhanced axial T1-weighted MR image shows slightly increased intensity of the right globe caused by total exudative retinal detachment. **C,** Axial T2-weighted MR image shows mixed signal intensities caused by a lipoproteinaceous exudate. The collapsed remaining part of the vitreous (*arrow*) appears hyperintense. **D,** Axial fat-suppressed, contrast-enhanced, T2-weighted MR image shows enhancement of the thickened, detached sensory retina (*arrows*). Note the enhancement of the peripheral retina (*arrowheads*) characteristically seen in Coats' disease, consistent with enhancement of telangiectatic vessels seen in **F** and **G**. A retinoblastoma can now be excluded.

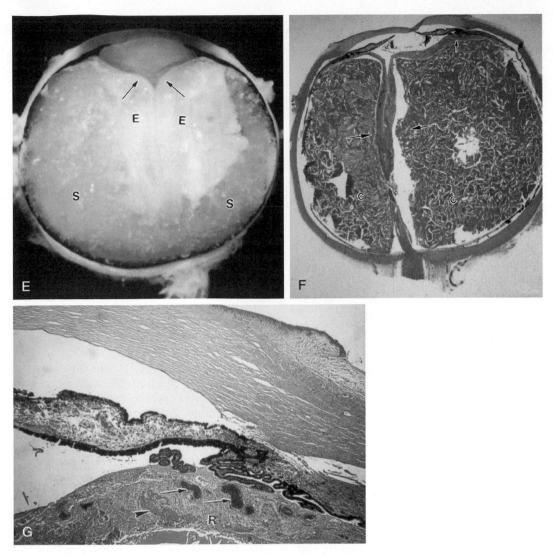

**FIGURE 8-71**   *Continued.* **E**, Gross photomicrograph of the eye. Note the large exudative detachment, with retinal elevation touching the posterior lens surface. The peripheral retina is markedly thickened (*arrows*). Areas of thick subretinal exudate (*E*) and cholesterol crystals are seen in the subretinal space (*S*). **F**, Photomicrograph of the eye. Note the bullous retinal detachment (*long arrows*) with peripheral telangiectatic vessels (*short arrow*). The subretinal space contains an eosinophilic exudate with cholesterol crystals (*C*). **G**, Peripheral detached retina (*R*) behind the iris showing telangiectatic blood vessels (*arrows*) and an intraretinal (*arrowhead*) and subretinal exudate. (Hematoxylin-eosin; original magnification × 10.)

## Ocular Toxocariasis (Sclerosing Endophthalmitis)

Ocular toxocariasis is a chorioretinitis caused by an inflammatory response to the nematode *Toxocara canis*.[21] Infected puppies excrete worm ova that may survive in soil for years. The granuloma of *T. canis* is actually an eosinophilic abscess that contains the second-stage larva of *Toxocara* within it.[21] The infection results from ingestion of the ova (eggs) in contaminated soil. In these patients the death of the larva results in a wide spectrum of intraocular inflammatory reactions,[138–140] the more severe of which has the characteristic pathologic appearance of sclerosing endophthalmitis.[139, 140] Ocular toxocariasis is usually unilateral and is seen in older children. Clinically, it may present as endophthalmitis with vitreous haze from a profound inflammatory response or as posterior or peripheral retinal

granuloma.[32] The granuloma appears a white, elevated lesion in the retina and may have associated adherent vitreous bands, vitreous traction, tractional retinal detachment, and dragging of the retina and optic disc.[32] In most but not all instances, the anterior segment is uninvolved, and a funnel-shaped retinal detachment is typically associated with an organized vitreous.[138] The histologic changes of the globe are characterized by an infiltration with lymphocytes, plasma cells, eosinophils, and giant cells. Retinal, subretinal, and vitreous hemorrhages may frequently occur. Remnants of the secondary larval stage of *T. canis* are often difficult to find. In 46 cases originally reported by Wilder,[139] larvae were present in 24. However, in the remaining 22 cases, larvae were not identified. In many cases, the diagnosis of ocular nematode infection is based presumptively on the characteristic histopathologic features of sclerosing endophthalmitis. A diagnostic enzyme-linked immunosorbent assay

(ELISA) for *Toxocara* is now available. In addition, analysis of vitreous fluid by ELISA testing reveals eosinophils. Eosinophilia may not be seen in peripheral blood.[64]

### Diagnostic Imaging

Margo et al.[138] reported the CT findings in three cases of histopathologically proven sclerosing endophthalmitis. These findings consisted of a homogeneous intravitreal density that corresponded to a detached retina, an organized vitreous, and an inflammatory subretinal exudate. These investigators concluded that the findings are similar to those seen in Coats' disease and noncalcified retinoblastoma. Three cases of toxocariasis in young adults appeared on CT as a localized or diffuse ill-defined mass with no significant enhancement (Fig. 8-72). Clinical examination in these patients frequently shows vitreous, retinal, or choroidal signs of previous inflammation.[78] This inflammatory process (chronic abscess) is seen on CT as an irregularity of the uveoscleral coat with a diffuse or locally thickened, slightly enhanced uveoscleral coat (Fig. 8-72). This CT appearance usually favors a diagnosis of toxocariasis or another granulomatous disease of the globe and is due to diffuse inflammatory infiltration of the choroid and sclera (Fig. 8-72).[84]

In the appropriate clinical setting, the CT findings of the granuloma of *T. canis* should be relied on to establish a presumptive diagnosis.[84] MR imaging has been reported to have the ability to detect the site of the larval granuloma.[99] The MR images of a patient with a presumptive diagnosis of toxocariasis are shown in Figure 8-55A,B. In general, the proteinaceous subretinal exudate produced by the inflammatory response to the larval infiltration is seen as variably hyperintense on T1-weighted, proton density, and T2-weighted images. These MR imaging characteristics were found in two patients with suspected toxocariasis. Further studies are needed to establish the spectrum of MR imaging characteristics of this relatively uncommon ocular disease. The postcontrast MR imaging appearance of multiple *Toxocara* abscesses in a patient with a positive ELISA test is

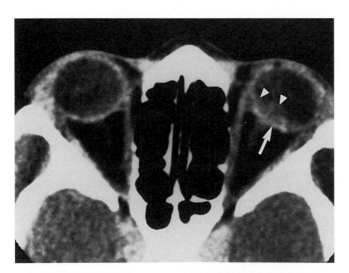

**FIGURE 8-72**  Ocular toxocariasis. Axial CT scan shows an irregular, moderately enhancing mass (*arrowheads*) with irregularity of the uveoscleral coat (*arrow*).

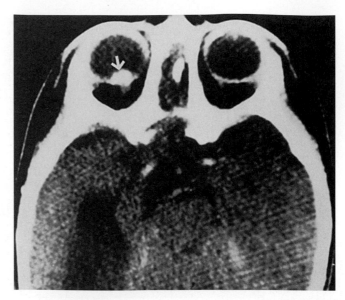

**FIGURE 8-73**  Astrocytic hamartoma. Axial CT scan shows a mass (*arrow*) in the posterior aspect of the right eye.

shown in Figure 8-55C. It should be noted that at times it may be very difficult to differentiate the MR imaging and CT appearances of chronic retinal detachment and organized vitreous from *Toxocara* granuloma, Coats' disease, and even ROP, PHPV, and noncalcified retinoblastoma.[84]

## Ocular Astrocytic Hamartoma (Retinal Astrocytoma)

Although retinoblastoma is the major life-threatening cause of leukokoria in children, a host of other simulating conditions (pseudogliomas) can cause diagnostic confusion.[21, 32, 138] In some cases of leukokoria, it is exceedingly difficult to exclude the possibility of retinoblastoma without having to resort to enucleation.[138] Retinal astrocytoma is a benign yellow-white rare retinal tumor that occurs in association with tuberous sclerosis or neurofibromatosis or in isolation.[141] Early retinal astrocytoma (astrocytic hamartoma) may look exactly like early retinoblastoma and may be present before any neurologic or dermatologic manifestations of tuberous sclerosis appear.[32, 78] These tumors may appear in the retina or in the optic nerve. The usual appearance is that of a single nodule or multiple nodules elevated 1 or 2 mm above the surface of the retina. At this stage, CT and MR imaging cannot visualize the lesions. Tumors elevated more than 3 mm can be demonstrated on CT and MR imaging. The CT appearance of astrocytic hamartomas is similar to that of retinoblastoma (Fig. 8-73). If typical features of tuberous sclerosis are not present, the differentiation between astrocytic hamartomas and other ocular lesions may be very difficult. The CT appearance of myelinated nerve fibers in astrocytic hamartomas also may be similar to that of retinoblastoma (Fig. 8-74). In several patients with known tuberous sclerosis and clinical evidence of retinal nodules (dots), because of the small size of the lesions the ocular nodules were not seen on MR imaging.

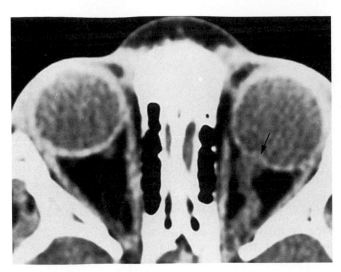

**FIGURE 8-74**   Myelinated nerve fiber (retinal gliosis). Axial CT scan shows a tortuous left optic nerve and soft tissue density at the optic disc (*arrow*). (From Mafee MF et al. Retinoblastoma and simulating lesions: role of CT and MRI. Radiol Clin North Am 1987;25:667–682.)

## Combined Hamartoma of the Retinal Pigment Epithelium and Retina

Combined hamartoma of the retinal pigment epithelium and retina is a rare congenital ocular tumor, and patients present with painless loss of vision.[21] This benign proliferation of mature cells involving the retinal pigment epithelium, retina, and vitreous leads to an elevated lesion in the posterior pole or optic disc and occurs with varying pigmentation. The less pigmented lesions simulate retinoblastoma clinically.[21]

## Incontinentia Pigmenti

Incontinentia pigmenti is a disorder associated with abnormalities of the skin, eye, and skeletal system.[21] The disease is inherited in an X-linked dominant pattern, although sporadic cases may occur. This condition is lethal in boys. Infants with this condition exhibit pigmentary skin abnormalities including erythematous skin with linear bullae at birth.[21] Ocular involvement is bilateral but often asymmetric. Retinal vascular abnormalities, pigmentary changes, and proliferation of retinal pigment epithelium lead to an intraocular nodular mass (pseudoglioma) that is usually seen in the first year of life. Peripheral fibrovascular proliferation may lead to tractional retinal detachment.[21]

## Juvenile Xanthogranuloma

Juvenile xanthogranuloma (non-Langerhans' cell histiocytosis) is a benign cutaneous disorder affecting the skin and eye.[21] The cutaneous lesions are yellow-orange granulomatous nodules composed of histiocytes. This condition usually affects the iris and ciliary body,[142–144] but lesions in the choroid, retina, or optic nerve have also been reported.[143] Juvenile xanthogranuloma has also been noted to present as a solitary orbital granulomatous mass (Fig. 8-75). Infiltration of the iris can cause spontaneous hyphema, glaucoma, and uveitis.

## Glioneuroma

Glioneuroma is an exceedingly rare neoplasm that arises from neuroepithelial cells that compromise the anterior margin of the embryonic optic cup.[145] The lesion usually appears at birth or in early childhood but is occasionally diagnosed in adulthood.[145] The tumor appears as a yellow or pink mass in the iris. Histopathologically, the ganglioneuroma is composed of an admixture of glial cells and neurons.[145]

## Papillitis

Papillitis, inflammation of the optic nerve head, has multiple causes including ischemia, infections, and autoim-

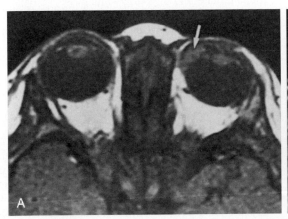
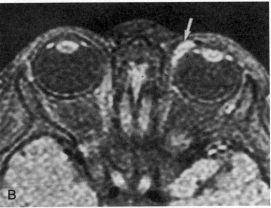

**FIGURE 8-75**   Juvenile xanthogranuloma. Precontrast axial T1-weighted (500/23, TR/TE) (**A**) and postcontrast T1-weighted (533/23, TR/TE) (**B**) MR images show an infiltrative enhancing mass involving the left eye (*arrow*). (Courtesy of A. Hidayat, MD, Washington, DC.)

mune diseases. If the inflammatory process is severe, the optic disc can be massively enlarged and hemorrhagic so as to resemble Rb.[21]

## Optic Nerve Head Drusen

Optic nerve head drusen is a benign, usually bilateral cause of pseudopapilledema and is occasionally inherited as an autosomal dominant condition.[146, 147] Disc drusen or hyaline bodies are spherical, acellular, laminated concretions from an unknown source, often partially calcified and possibly related to accumulation of axoplasmic derivatives of degenerating retinal nerve fibers.[146, 147] Drusen are buried within the substance of the nerve head, usually anterior to the lamina cribrosa. They are covered by axonal and glial tissue, together with the vascular supply of the nerve head. Therefore, drusen of the optic nerve head are recognizable because of characteristic distortion in the shape of the nerve head. Drusen of the optic nerve head are usually bilateral. Clinically, the term *drusen* is more frequently applied to the very common multiple small, round, discrete punctate subretinal nodules (drusen of the pigmented retinal epithelium) at the posterior pole. From the standpoint of pathology, drusen of the optic disc should not be confused with drusen of the pigmented retinal epithelium, which are deposits of basement membrane material between the pigment epithelium of the retina and Bruch's membrane. Bruch's membrane is a tough, acellular, amorphous, bilamellar structure situated between the outer layer of the retina, that is, the RPE, and the choroid. Microscopically, Bruch's membrane consists of five layers: (1) basement membrane of the RPE, (2) inner collagenous zone, (3) elastic layer, (4) outer collagenous zone, and (5) basement membrane of the choriocapillaris. RPE drusen are extracellular deposits that lie between the basement membrane of the RPE and the inner collagenous zone of Bruch's membrane. It has been suggested that apoptosis, a process by which cells cast off part of their cytoplasm, may lead to formation of drusen.[63, 146, 147] The RPE drusen are believed to develop by the shedding of basal cytoplasm of RPE through its basement membrane. Over time, RPE and optic disc drusen change their size, shape, and consistency and may become calcified.[63, 146, 147] Drusen contain sialic acid, cerebrosides, calcium, carbohydrate, mucopolysaccharides, and iron. Optic disc drusen may vary in size (from 59 to 750 mm in diameter) and number; often, smaller drusen appear to coalesce to form larger aggregates. Once their calcified component is more than 1 to 1.5 mm, they should be recognized on thin-section (1 to 1.5 mm) CT scans.[146] RPE drusen are not large enough to be visible on CT scans.

Although optic disc drusen are rarely seen in early childhood, most drusen are believed to be present at birth.[146, 147] They become more apparent in later life as they enlarge and approach the disc surface, becoming ophthalmologically visible as hyaline or colloid bodies.[146] Drusen are rarely detected by CT scanning in early childhood. In order to suggest the diagnosis in early childhood, the CT scans should be carefully evaluated, as the optic disc drusen is not calcified enough at this age. Careful evaluation of the optic disc may reveal a small area that is slightly more dense than the rest of the disc. Some children and adults with drusen of

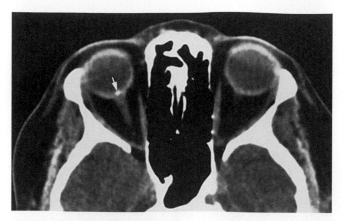

**FIGURE 8-76** Optic nerve head drusen. Axial CT scan shows increased density at the optic disc (*arrow*).

the optic disc may undergo a number of diagnostic studies, including cranial CT and MR imaging, to exclude an intracranial process. Optic disc drusen have been reported in 20 to 24 per 1000 patients at autopsy and are bilateral in 73% of cases.[146, 147] When drusen are located well beneath the surface of the disc, they may blur the disc margin and may lead to misdiagnosis of papilledema. Clinically, drusen are usually asymptomatic, but arcuate field defects (arcuate scotomas) or peripheral field constrictions may be present. These field defects are usually not apparent until adulthood, which further emphasizes the slowly progressive nature of drusen. There also appears to be an association between drusen of the optic disc and retinal hemorrhages.[146] Clinical findings in optic disc drusen range from a small, subtle elevation of the disc to a large, globular yellow-white mass containing calcified concretions.[21] On CT drusen appear as discrete, rounded, high-density or calcified bodies that are confined to the optic disc surface and are found at any level within the prelaminar zone of the optic nerve (Fig. 8-76). Optic nerve drusen are difficult to visualize by MR imaging.

## Choroidal Osteoma

Choroidal osteoma is a benign tumor that is typically found unilaterally in young white girls.[21, 63] Histopathologic evaluation reveals mature bone with marrow spaces containing loose fibrovascular tissue.[63] Choroidal osteoma originally was classified as a choristoma (a benign congenital tumor composed of normal tissue elements that do not normally occur at that site), but currently it is regarded by some as an acquired benign choroidal neoplasm of unknown etiology.[145]

### Clinical Diagnosis

Patients with choroidal osteoma present with painless progressive loss of vision over several months or years or abrupt recent blurring of central vision. Some lesions are detected initially on routine eye examination.[145] The tumor appears as a yellow-white or orange-red choroidal mass, depending on the amount of depigmentation or hyperplasia of the overlying retinal pigment epithelial layer. This calcified lesion is found in the macula or in the juxtapapillary region extending toward the macula.[21] Small vessels can be seen on the surface of the osteoma. Choroidal osteoma involves one eye only in 70% to 80% of cases and both eyes in 20% to 30%.[145] If the lesion involves the macular choroid, visual acuity can be impaired because of degeneration of the overlying RPE and the neurosensory retina.[145] In other cases, a choroidal neovascular membrane arises from the inner surface of the lesion and produces a serous or serosanguineous macular retinal detachment that results in loss of vision.[145]

### Imaging Diagnosis

Ultrasound and CT are useful in detecting choroidal osteoma. On a CT scan, choroidal osteomas appear as a plate-like calcified thickening of the posterior ocular wall, typically in the juxtapapillary region; unlike drusen, calcification typically does not involve the center of the optic disc (Fig. 8-77).

### Differential Diagnosis

The most important lesions in the differential diagnosis of choroidal osteoma are listed in Table 8-6.

## Retinal Gliosis

Retinal and optic nerve astrocytes are analogous to fibroblasts in the body.[21] *Retinal gliosis* refers to reactive proliferation and hypertrophy of astrocytes in the retina, especially occurring in response to injury. Gliotic tissue growth may appear mass-like or may cause tractional retinal detachment.

## Myelinated Nerve Fibers

Oligodendrocytes and myelin are not usually present in the human retina.[21] Approximately 1% of eyes have myelinated nerve fibers within the retina, however, usually in a peripapillary distribution. This myelination results in a slightly elevated white retinal plaque and, if extensive, can

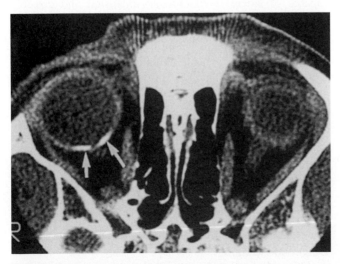

**FIGURE 8-77**   Choroidal osteoma. Axial CT scan shows a peripapillary calcified mass (*arrows*) compatible with choroidal osteoma.

produce leukokoria. The CT appearance of myelinated nerve fibers may be similar to that of noncalcified retinoblastoma (see Fig. 8-74).

## X-Linked Retinoschisis

X-linked retinoschisis is a congenital disorder in which there is splitting of the retina within the nerve fiber layer. This causes the inner layers of the retina to be elevated, or the schisis may result in retinal holes, eventually leading to a full-thickness retinal tear and detachment. The CT and MR imaging appearance of X-linked retinoschisis is nonspecific and compatible with retinal detachment.[21]

## Retinal Detachment

Retinoblastoma may produce a retinal detachment, which in turn can obscure from view the underlying tumor. Therefore, a retinal detachment resulting from any other etiology can simulate Rb.[21, 32] Rhegmatogenous retinal detachments arise from full-thickness retinal breaks that occur secondarily from retinal atrophy, deterioration, trauma, or vitreous traction. The retinal break allows passage of liquified vitreous into the subretinal space,[21] subsequently causing retinal detachment. Predisposing conditions include trauma, high myopia, Stickler's syndrome, congenital cataract surgery, congenital glaucoma, and myiasis.[21] Nonrhegmatogenous retinal detachments result from traction on the surface of the retina or from exudation under or within the retina, as seen in conditions such as familial exudative vitreoretinopathy, falciform fold, or retinal cyst.[21]

## Subretinal Neovascular Membranes

Subretinal neovascular membrane is an acquired abnormality in which growth of new blood vessels from the choriocapillaris occurs beneath the neurosensory retina, usually in response to some retinal injury. These new vessels may hemorrhage or leak, leading to serous retinal detachment. The lesion may organize, resulting in a gliotic, elevated retinal scar and retinal traction.[21]

## Vitreous Opacities

Any disease, such as uveitis (see Fig. 8-38), vitreous hemorrhage, endophthalmitis, or organized vitreous, associated with cells in the vitreous can simulate retinoblastoma with vitreous seeding.[21, 32] These vitreous cells or opacities often obscure the view of the retina, causing more difficulty for the clinician in differentiating the etiology of the vitreous cells.

## Von Hippel-Lindau Retinal Angiomatosis

Von Hippel-Lindau retinal angiomatosis is an autosomal dominant disorder characterized by retinal capillary hemangiomas.[21] Ophthalmoscopic examination of the fundus reveals a red-orange mass lesion with tortuous feeder and draining vessels.[21] The lesion is usually located in the midperipheral retina and may be associated with exudates and retinal detachment. Aside from ocular conditions, these patients may develop cerebellar hemangioblastoma, optic nerve or optic chiasm hemangioblastoma, renal cell carcinoma, pheochromocytoma, cysts in the kidney or pancreas, and endolymphatic sac tumors.[21]

## Choroidal Hemangioma

Choroidal hemangiomas are congenital vascular hamartomas of the choroid that are typically seen in middle-aged individuals. Normal retinal vessels overlie the mass. Choroidal hemangioma in children can simulate retinoblastoma.[21] The CT and MR imaging characteristics of choroidal hemangioma are described elsewhere in this chapter.

## Malignant Uveal Melanoma

The uvea (choroid, ciliary body, and iris) is derived from both the mesoderm and the neuroectoderm and may harbor tumors from both of these origins. Because it is the most highly vascular portion of the eyeball, the uvea provides a suitable substrate for tumor cells. Most primary and metastatic ocular neoplasms involve the choroid, and the most common tumor is malignant melanoma.[148] Malignant melanomas of the uvea are unusual in blacks, with the white/black patient ratio being about 15:1.[149] Those melanomas involving the ciliary body and choroid are thought to originate from preexisting nevi.[148] The neoplasm has a capacity to metastasize hematogenously. Its favored metastatic site is the liver. The incidence of malignant melanoma of the choroid has been estimated to be 5.2 to 7.5 cases per million per year.[150] The incidence of uveal melanoma increases with age. Less than 2% of tumors are seen in patients below 20 years of age.[62] Congenital melanosis, ocular melanocytosis, oculodermal melanocytosis, and uveal nevi are predisposing lesions that precede the development of uveal melanoma.[62]

Callender's classification of melanotic lesions, which is based on cellular features, offers the best indication of the prognosis.[151, 152] The spindle-A tumors, which are composed of spindle cells with elongated nuclei, characteristically lacking nucleoli, have the best prognosis. The next best prognoses involve the spindle-B tumors, whose cells have the same shape as spindle-A lesions but are slightly larger and have a nucleus containing a prominent nucleolus. The next worst prognosis concerns the epithelioid-cell tumors, which are composed of larger, more pleomorphic cells than the spindle-cell tumors. Finally, there are mixed-cell tumors composed of both spindle and epithelioid cells.[148, 152] Some of the tumors may be amelanotic, especially the spindle-cell tumors.

### Clinical Diagnosis

An iris melanoma is seen as a visible spot on the iris or as a discoloration of the iris in one eye. The typical ciliary body melanoma appears as a highly elevated, nodular, dark brown

lesion in the peripheral fundus.[153] The typical choroidal melanoma appears as a dark brown solid tumor and has a biconvex, lenticular cross-sectional shape.[153] The tumor initially grows flat within the choroid, later elevates Bruch's membrane, and finally ruptures through it so that the melanoma assumes a characteristic mushroom shape, growing toward the vitreous cavity. The retina over the surface of the tumor becomes elevated and detached (solid retinal detachment). This detachment gradually extends as a serous detachment over the slopes of the tumor.

Ophthalmoscopically, the lesion is seen as a circumscribed mass of varied pigmentation along with a solid retinal detachment, and the retinal vessels over the surface of the mass are elevated. The retina usually is attached to the mass and does not float easily, as seen in rhegmatogenous retinal detachments. In some cases, the subretinal fluid extends only around the base of the lesion; in others, it accumulates to the extent that the retina is extensively or even totally detached.[153] In some cases, the subretinal fluid is bloody, almost exclusively in eyes that have tumor eruption through Bruch's membrane.[153]

If the tumor is not treated, it may cause secondary glaucoma and eventually break through the eye into the retrobulbar region. Metastases occur primarily to the liver. Management of clinically suspected choroidal melanomas has been the subject of some controversy in recent years. Enucleation has been a standard treatment for more than a century.[154] However, enucleation has not been proven to prevent metastasis. Furthermore, Zimmerman, McLean, and Foster have hypothesized a potentially harmful effect from intraoperative dissemination of tumor cells.[155] The controversy over the efficacy of enucleation remains unresolved.[156]

In general, relatively small choroidal melanomas measuring less than 10 mm in diameter and 3 mm in thickness have a relatively favorable prognosis, with a 10% to 15% incidence of death in 5 years.[157] Biologic aggressiveness has been judged by a clinically visible increase in the size of the tumor. Clinically stable choroidal melanomas are managed with longitudinal observations by clinical examination, echography, CT, and MR imaging, and no treatment. Nevertheless, visibly stationary melanomas have been capable of extensive extraocular extension and possibly even distant metastasis.[158, 159] Furthermore, it has been suggested that tumor cell dissemination may occur early in the course of the disease, with distant metastasis appearing many years later.[160] Thus the clinical management of even small and relatively stable choroidal melanomas warrants careful consideration and the use of all reasonable clinical aids.[156] If there is evidence of tumor growth, enucleation, or local excision, other modes of therapy such as photocoagulation and radiation therapy are indicated.[157, 161] Some advocate early enucleation of all melanomas to prevent metastasis.[160] Metastatic sites of primary uveal melanoma include liver, lung, bone, kidney, and brain in order of decreasing frequency, and a thorough search for metastasis is important to save the patient an unnecessary enucleation.[156]

### Diagnostic Imaging

Although uveal melanomas can be accurately diagnosed by ophthalmoscopy, fluorescein angiography, or ultrasonog-

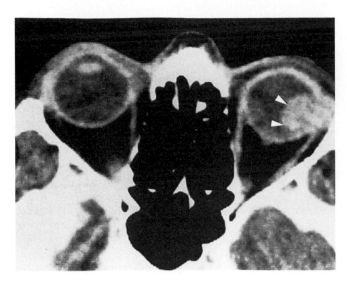

**FIGURE 8-78**  Malignant melanoma of the choroid. Axial CT scan shows a mushroom-shaped mass with increased density in the temporal quadrant of the left globe (*arrowheads*). (From Mafee MF et al. Malignant uveal melanoma and similar lesions studied by CT. Radiology 1985;156: 403–408.)

raphy, misdiagnosis continues to occur, particularly when opaque media preclude direct visualization.[137, 162–164] CT has proven to be a highly accurate method for demonstrating uveal melanoma, and dynamic CT can provide information about the vascularity and perfusion of intraocular lesions and can help distinguish uveal melanomas from other lesions such as choroidal hemangiomas. Most uveal melanomas are seen on CT as an elevated, hyperdense, sharply marginated lenticular or mushroom-shaped lesion (Figs. 8-78 and 8-79A).

MR imaging has been used to diagnose intraocular lesions.[21, 32, 165] On T1-weighted and proton density images, uveal melanomas are seen as areas of moderately high signal (greater signal intensity than in the vitreous) (Fig. 8-79B top). On T2-weighted images, melanomas are seen as areas of moderately low signal (lesser intensity than in the vitreous) (Fig. 8-79B bottom). These MR characteristics of uveal melanomas are very similar to those of retinoblastomas (Fig. 8-80). Associated retinal detachment is better visualized by MR imaging than by CT (Fig. 8-81). Exudative retinal detachment is usually depicted on MR imaging as a dependent area of moderate to very high signal intensity in T1-weighted, proton density, and T2-weighted images (Figs. 8-79 and 8-81), and total retinal detachment may be present. Chronic retinal detachment and hemorrhagic subretinal fluid have varied MR imaging appearances. Most uveal melanomas appear as a well-defined solid mass (Figs. 8-82 and 8-83). However, atypical features of ocular melanoma may be present. When necrotic or hemorrhagic foci are present within the uveal melanoma, the inhomogeneity present within the tumor can be problematic (Fig. 8-82). Some melanomas may be seen better on T1-weighted images (Fig. 8-82); discoid or ring melanomas may be difficult to detect if they are flat. Additionally, an organized subretinal exudate, with or without associated hemorrhage, may have MR characteristics similar to those of a uveal melanoma (Fig. 8-84). Tumor invasion of the sclera, optic disc, Tenon's capsule, and the extraocular orbit can be easily detected by MR imaging (Fig. 8-85). Paramagnetic contrast material is very useful in the diagnosis of uveal melanomas, in particular for evaluation of the optic nerve, as well as retrobulbar extension of ocular tumors (Fig. 8-86). Uveal melanomas demonstrate moderate enhancement on postgadolinium T1-weighted MR images. On fat suppression, the T1-weighted MR images demonstrate marked expansion of gray scale with apparently increased signal intensity of the extraocular muscles and lacrimal gland (Fig. 8-86C). Therefore, one should look carefully for extraocular tumor extension adjacent to the area of contact of extraocular muscles with the globe. Fat-suppressed T1-weighted MR images are prone to artifacts related

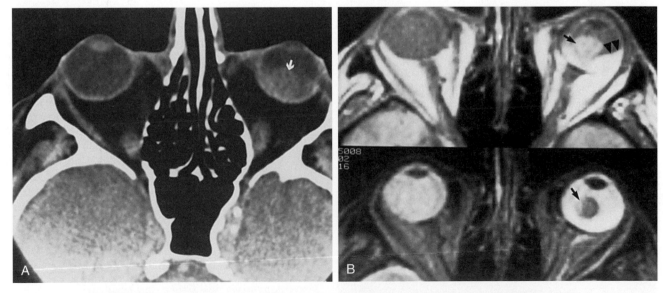

**FIGURE 8-79**  Malignant melanoma of the choroid. **A,** Axial CT scan shows a mass (*arrow*). **B,** Axial PW MR image (top) and T2-weighted MR image (bottom) show a mass (*arrow*) and exudative retinal detachment (*arrowheads*). Retinal detachment is distinguished better on MR imaging than on CT.

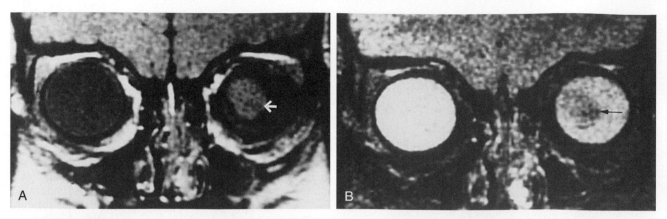

**FIGURE 8-80**    Retinoblastoma. **A,** Coronal PW and **B,** T2-weighted MR images. Scans show retinoblastoma (*arrows*). (From Mafee MF et al. Retinoblastoma and simulating lesions: role of CT and MRI. Radiol Clin North Am 1987;25:667–682.)

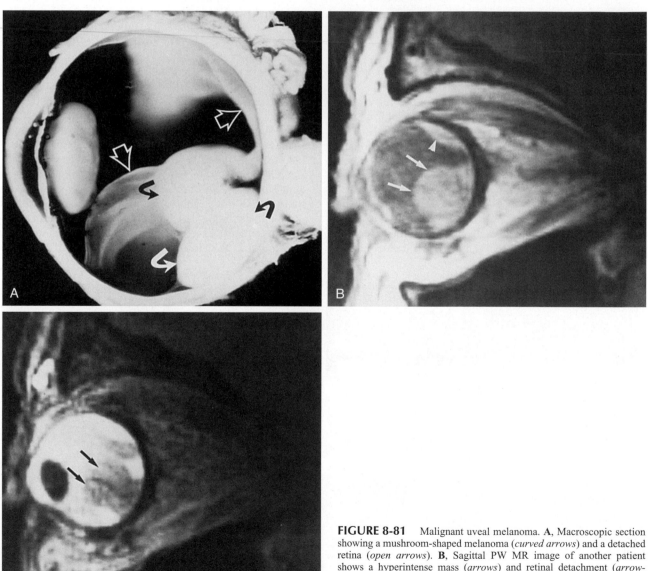

**FIGURE 8-81**    Malignant uveal melanoma. **A,** Macroscopic section showing a mushroom-shaped melanoma (*curved arrows*) and a detached retina (*open arrows*). **B,** Sagittal PW MR image of another patient shows a hyperintense mass (*arrows*) and retinal detachment (*arrowhead*). **C,** Sagittal T2-weighted MR image shows a mushroom-shaped hypointense melanoma (*arrows*). The subretinal effusion remains hyperintense.

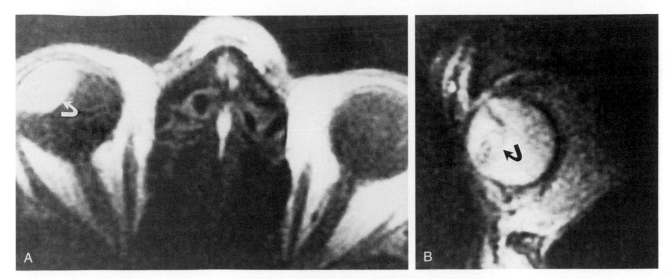

**FIGURE 8-82**   Malignant uveal melanoma. **A,** Axial T1-weighted MR image shows a hyperintense mass (*arrow*). **B,** Sagittal T2-weighted MR image shows the mixed signal appearance of the lesion (*arrow*). The anterior portion is hyperintense because of necrosis or hemorrhage.

to dental fillings or other foreign bodies around the orbit (Fig. 8-87).

Choroidal lesions elevated more than 3 mm are usually well visualized on MR imaging. Any lesion less than 3 mm is better studied with ultrasound.[21, 32] The MR imaging characteristics of melanotic lesions are believed to be related to the paramagnetic properties of melanin.[166–168] Damadian et al. reported that, unlike other tumors, melanomas have short T1 relaxation times, which the authors attributed to paramagnetic proton relaxation by stable radicals in melanin.[166] Electron spin-resonance studies have shown that melanin produces a stable free radical signal under all

known conditions, and these stable radicals cause proton relaxation enhancement that shortens both T1 and T2 relaxation time values.[167] However, a recent study[169] has shown that with the use of synthetic models, the content of free radicals in melanin ($10^{18}$ spins per gram or one free radical per 3000 subunits), at the average concentration of melanin estimated within melanoma tissue (15 mg/ml), is too low to affect substantially the tissue TI relaxation time.[169]

It has been shown that melanin has a high affinity and binding capacity for metal ions,[169] and natural melanin contains a wide variety of bound metals in vivo (iron,

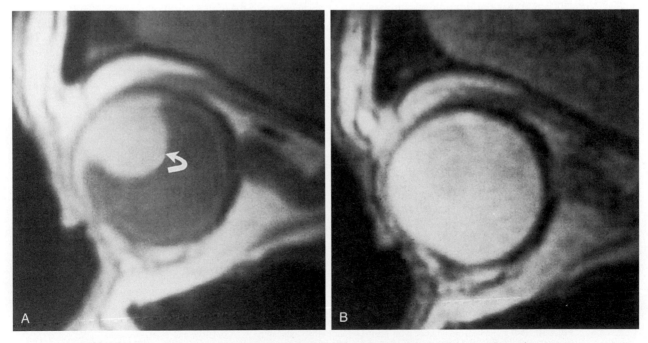

**FIGURE 8-83**   Malignant uveal melanoma. **A,** Sagittal PW and **B,** T2-weighted MR images. Scans show a mass (*arrow*), which is better seen in the PW MR image. The lesion remains slightly hypointense on the T2-weighted MR image.

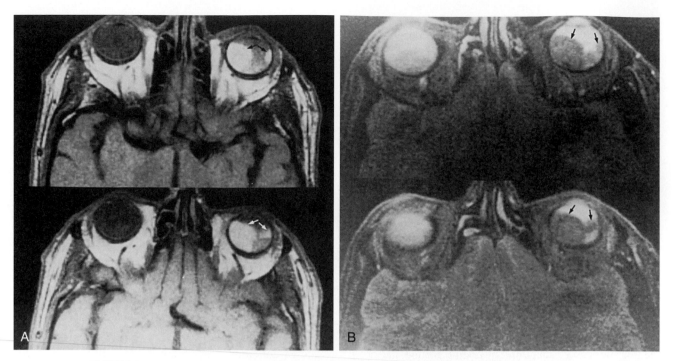

**FIGURE 8-84**   Malignant uveal melanoma and postradiation retinal detachment simulating recurrent tumor. **A,** Axial PW MR images show hyperintense masses (*arrows*). **B,** Axial T2-weighted MR images show hypointense masses. The eye was enucleated, and masses were found to be caused by highly proteinaceous, organized subretinal fluid with some degree of hemorrhage as well. The uveal melanoma was seen as a small, partially necrotic lesion. The MR imaging appearance of these subretinal changes is identical to the MR imaging characteristics of melanotic lesions. Therefore, caution must be exercised in MR imaging interpretation of intraocular lesions. When highly proteinaceous lesions are present, such as in this case or in the case of mucin-producing metastatic adenocarcinoma, MR imaging may not differentiate them from uveal melanomas.

copper, manganese, and zinc).[62] This indicates that melanin may have a cytoprotective function as an intracellular scavenger of free metals. The work of Enochs and associates[169] revealed that it is the binding of paramagnetic metals (paramagnetic metal scavenging) that is responsible for the high signal intensities of melanomas on T1-weighted MR images. Uveal melanomas therefore are unique in that both T1 and T2 relaxation values are relative shortened.

Hence, on T1-weighted images, the lesion should be relatively hyperintense, the opposite of that predicted for T2-weighted images, and these signal intensities have been observed in the overwhelming majority of uveal melanomas. At times, uveal melanomas may have mixed or high signal intensity on T2-weighted scans (Fig. 8-83). The MR imaging diagnosis of uveal melanomas is greatly enhanced by the use of gadolinium contrast material. Uveal melano-

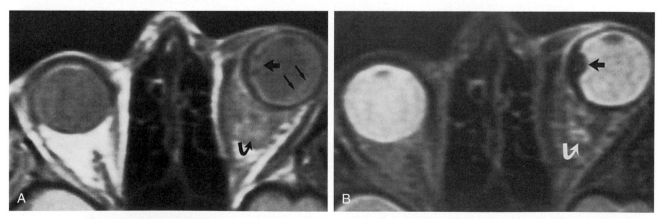

**FIGURE 8-85**   Uveal melanoma with massive retrobulbar extension. **A,** Axial PW and **B,** T2-weighted MR images. Scans show uveal melanoma (*large arrow*), subretinal fluid (*small arrows*), and massive extraocular tumor extension (*curved arrow*).

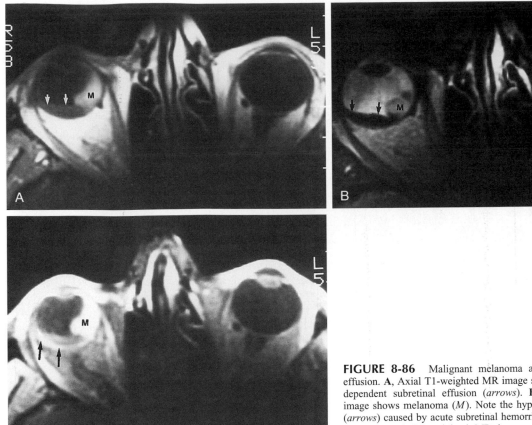

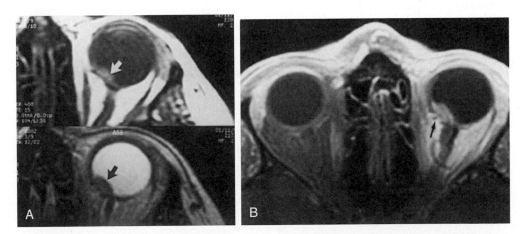

**FIGURE 8-86** Malignant melanoma and hemorrhagic subretinal effusion. **A,** Axial T1-weighted MR image shows melanoma (*M*) and a dependent subretinal effusion (*arrows*). **B,** Axial T2-weighted MR image shows melanoma (*M*). Note the hypointense subretinal effusion (*arrows*) caused by acute subretinal hemorrhage. **C,** Axial postcontrast, fat-suppressed, T1-weighted MR image shows melanoma (*M*) and enhancement of the thickened uvea (*arrows*).

mas show moderate enhancement (Figs. 8-86 and 8-87), and ocular and extraocular invasion can be easily detected on postcontrast, fat-suppressed, T1-weighted scans. Extension into the orbit of a primary ocular melanoma is not common. The size of the extraocular extension is independent of the size of the ocular tumor (Fig. 8-85).

### Differential Diagnosis

A number of benign and malignant lesions of the eye may be confused with malignant uveal melanomas. These conditions include metastatic tumors (Fig. 8-88), choroidal detachment, choroidal nevi, choroidal hemangioma, choroidal cyst, neurofibroma and schwannoma of the uvea,

**FIGURE 8-87** Malignant uveal melanoma. **A,** Axial T1-weighted (top) and T2 weighted (bottom) MR images showing a choroidal melanoma (*arrows*). **B,** Enhanced, fat-suppressed, T1-weighted MR image showing moderate tumor enhancement. Note the irregularity of the scleral and tumor nodule (*arrow*) caused by scleral invasion and retrobulbar extension, confirmed on histologic examination. The hyperintensity of the retrobulbar fat on the left in this image is due to dental metallic filling, causing a problem in suppressing the fat. (Courtesy of M.F. Mafee, MD, FACR, Chicago.)

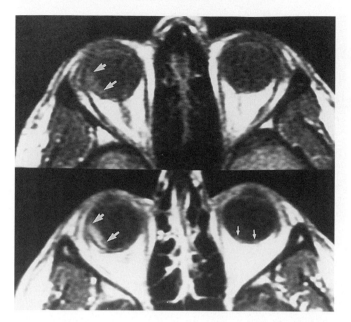

**FIGURE 8-88** Uveal metastasis. Axial precontrast (top) and postcontrast (bottom) T1-weighted MR images show bilateral choroidal metastases (*arrows*).

leiomyoma, choroidal lymphoma (Fig. 8-89), adenoma of the ciliary body, medulloepithelioma, retinal detachment, and disciform degeneration of the macula.[19, 170, 171] The most important lesions in the differential diagnosis of iris melanomas and choroidal and ciliary body melanomas are listed in Tables 8-7 and 8-8.

## Melanocytoma

Melanocytoma is a deeply pigmented benign tumor that usually occurs at the optic disc but may also arise anywhere in the uvea. Iris melanocytomas are rare and have a predisposition to release pigment into the anterior chambers, which causes a secondary open-angle glaucoma. Approxi-

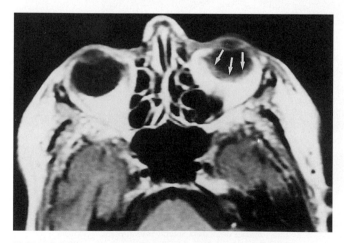

**FIGURE 8-89** Choroidal lymphoma. Axial postcontrast T1-weighted MR image shows an irregular, infiltrative, moderately enhancing mass (*arrows*) involving the left globe. The appearance cannot be differentiated from that of uveal metastasis.

**Table 8-7**
**DIFFERENTIAL DIAGNOSIS OF IRIS MELANOMAS**

Nevus of the iris

Medulloepithelioma

Metastasis

Juvenile xanthogranuloma

Adenoma and adenocarcinoma of the ciliary epithelium

Cyst of the iris

Inflammatory granuloma

Leiomyoma of the iris and ciliary body

Choristoma, teratoma

mately 50% of melanocytomas develop in blacks, whereas the incidence of malignant uveal melanoma in blacks is less than 1%.[150] The MR imaging appearance of melanocytoma is similar to that of malignant uveal melanoma (Fig. 8-90). Melanocytomas are special types of uveal nevus. Melanocytoma of the optic disc usually is composed entirely of maximally pigmented, polyhedral nevus cells (magnocellular nevus cells).[40] Clinically, the lesion is a dark tumor that involves the substance of the optic disc. The melanocytomas appear homogeneously very hypointense on T2-weighted MR images (Fig. 8-90). Primary malignant melanoma of the optic nerve head is an exceedingly rare tumor.[172] Most melanomas of the optic nerve head are related to extension of a peripapillary choroidal melanoma.[173] The tumors are found to involve the choroid adjacent to the optic disc. Figure 8-91 shows a clinicopathologically proved primary malignant melanoma of the optic disc without choroidal involvement. The clinical appearance simulated that of a melanocytoma so precisely that the proper diagnosis was delayed. MR imaging demonstrated a discoid mass with

**Table 8-8**
**DIFFERENTIAL DIAGNOSIS OF CHOROIDAL AND CILIARY BODY MELANOMAS**

Choroidal nevus including ocular melanocytosis

Melanocytoma of optic disc

Melanocytoma of choroid

Metastasis (often bilateral)

Choroidal hemangioma

Choroidal osteoma

Inflammatory granuloma of the uvea (tuberculosis, sarcoidosis)

Nodular posterior scleritis

Localized choroidal-suprachoroidal hematoma

Localized subretinal or subpigment epithelial hematoma (senile macular degeneration)

Medulloepithelioma

Choroidal lymphoma (almost always bilateral)

Primary ocular adenoma and adenocarcinoma

Hemangiopericytoma (ciliary body)

Leukemic infiltration of the uvea

Pseudotumor of the uvea

Massive gliosis of the retina

Astrocytoma of the retina

Uveal neurilemoma/neurofibroma

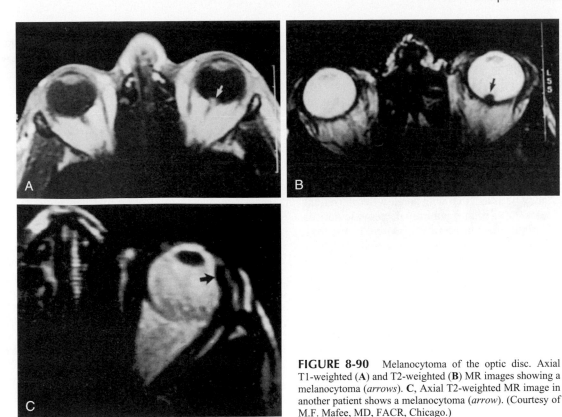

**FIGURE 8-90**   Melanocytoma of the optic disc. Axial T1-weighted (**A**) and T2-weighted (**B**) MR images showing a melanocytoma (*arrows*). **C**, Axial T2-weighted MR image in another patient shows a melanocytoma (*arrow*). (Courtesy of M.F. Mafee, MD, FACR, Chicago.)

involvement of the optic nerve (Fig. 8-91), and the patient underwent enucleation of the right eye. Even though 17 mm of nerve was obtained, tumor was present at the point of surgical resection. Later, the patient underwent right frontotemporal craniotomy to remove the remainder of the optic nerve to the chiasm.

## Uveal Metastasis

Uveal metastasis can be confused with uveal melanoma both clinically and on imaging. Metastatic lesions

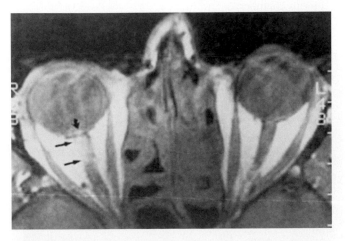

**FIGURE 8-91**   Melanoma of the optic nerve with optic nerve involvement. Enhanced, fat-suppressed, proton density MR image shows an optic nerve head lesion (*curved arrow*) with marked extension into the optic nerve (*arrows*). (Courtesy of M.F. Mafee, MD, FACR, Chicago.)

of the uvea extend chiefly in the plane of the choroid, usually with relatively little increase in thickness. Unlike uveal melanomas, which tend to form a protuberant mass, metastatic lesions have a mottled appearance and a diffuse outline, causing relatively little increase in their thickness.[62] The malignant cells (emboli) obtain access to the eye via the bloodstream by means of the short posterior ciliary arteries, and this may be the reason that the majority of metastases occur in the posterior half of the eye. The most common source of secondary carcinoma within the eye is from the breast or lung. Tumor metastasis may occur in both the retina and the choroid, both eyes being affected in about one-third of the cases. Unlike uveal metastasis, bilateral uveal melanomas are rare. Metastatic carcinoma of the pancreas and stomach also have been reported in the retina.[62] On CT, uveal metastasis may be difficult to differentiate from uveal melanoma.[19, 62, 174] MR imaging has been shown to be superior to CT in differentiating uveal metastasis from uveal melanoma.[19] However, uveal metastases may have signal characteristics similar to those of uveal melanomas (Fig. 8-92). Metastatic lesions of the choroid may lead rapidly to prominent and widespread detachment of the retina. In these patients, the mottled appearance and diffuse outline of the lesion may be rather different from those of uveal melanoma. Gd-DTPA has increased the sensitivity of MR for detection of uveal metastasis (Fig. 8-89). A mucin-producing metastatic lesion (adenocarcinoma) may also simulate a uveal melanoma because the proteinaceous fluid tends to decrease the T1 and T2 relaxation times of the lesion. We have seen metastatic carcinoid as well as hypernephroma that were indistinguishable from other uveal metastasis on MR imaging.

## Uveal Nevus

Uveal nevi are congenital lesions, usually recognized late in the first decade of life and most frequently located in the posterior one third of the choroid.[40] Most choroidal nevi are less than 5 mm in basal diameter and less than 1 mm in thickness, but occasionally lesions of this type attain a basal diameter of 10 mm or more and a thickness of 3 mm or more.[40] They appear clinically as a flat or minimally elevated slate-gray choroidal mass with slightly indistinct margins. The color of these lesions depends largely on the composition of cell types within the nevus. Occasionally, choroidal nevi may be associated with shallow serous retinal detachment, with or without subretinal neovascularization.[168, 175, 176] If the macula becomes involved, this may cause visual field defects with decreased vision.[176] Under such circumstances, a choroidal nevus may simulate a choroidal melanoma both ophthalmoscopically and angiographically. The choroidal nevus is one of the most commonly misdiagnosed lesions to be enucleated under the misdiagnosis of malignant melanoma.[163, 164, 170] It is sometimes extremely difficult to differentiate these two lesions, with long-term follow-up being the only possible solution.[176] Most of the important lesions in the differential diagnosis of uveal nevi include melanoma of the iris, ciliary body, and choroid, metastatic carcinoma to the uvea, inflammatory granuloma, leiomyoma of the iris and ciliary body, juvenile xanthogranuloma of the iris and ciliary body, circumscribed choroidal hemangioma, choroidal osteoma, choroidal neurilemoma, subretinal or suprachoroidal hematoma, and foreign body in the iris.

### Diagnostic Imaging

CT and MR imaging studies of several patients in whom uveal nevus was considered the likely ophthalmoscopic diagnosis showed that many lesions could not be visualized because of their small size, with most uveal nevi being less than 2 mm. In two uveal nevi seen on CT and MR imaging, the appearance was identical to that of uveal melanoma. Both of these patients underwent internal eye wall resection of the lesions, and a histopathologic study led to a diagnosis of choroidal nevus. It should be emphasized that CT and MR imaging are unable to differentiate uveal nevi from uveal melanomas. Internal eye wall resection may provide an alternative approach for suspicious lesions near the posterior pole, and this procedure has the advantage of preserving the globe.

## Choroidal and Retinal Hemangiomas

Choroidal hemangiomas are seen usually in association with Sturge-Weber disease (encephalotrigeminal syndrome). Retinal angiomas (angiomatosis retinae), on the other hand, are seen in patients with von Hippel-Lindau disease. The diagnosis of choroidal hemangiomas on clinical grounds presents some difficulty. In the majority of cases, the lesion is discovered in the course of a pathologic examination, and in cases where an ophthalmoscopic examination had been performed, the tumor was concealed by the detachment of the retina.[177] The diagnosis of angiomatosis retinae of von Hippel-Lindau disease, by contrast, is chiefly dependent on the ophthalmoscopic appearance of the lesion. Sturge-Weber disease and von Hippel-Lindau disease belong to the general class of disorders referred to as phakomatoses. The major syndromes include neurofibromatosis, tuberous sclerosis (Bourneville's disease), encephalotrigeminal syndrome (Sturge-Weber disease), cerebelloretinal hemangioblastomatosis (von Hippel-Lindau disease), and ataxia-telangiectasia (Louis-Bar disease).

Sturge-Weber disease consists of capillary or cavernous hemangiomas that have a cutaneous distribution along the trigeminal nerve and of a predominantly venous hemangioma of the leptomeninges.[177, 178] The intracranial or cutaneous lesions may occur separately. The most familiar manifestation takes the form of the port-wine stain, or capillary nevus of the face, varying in its extent and sometimes being limited to the skin of the eyelids and conjunctiva. The eye changes are usually ipsilateral to the changes elsewhere, may be bilateral, and may be found without any surface angiomas. The ophthalmic changes consist of an angioma of the choroid, buphthalmos, or chronic glaucoma with atrophy and cupping of the optic nerve.[62, 177] The glaucoma may be explained by the angiomatous changes in the ciliary body or the angle of the anterior chamber.

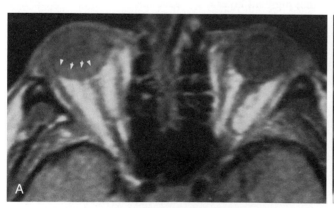
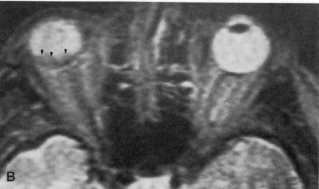

**FIGURE 8-92**  Choroidal metastasis. **A,** Axial PW MR image shows a hyperintense lesion (*arrows*) consistent with an ophthalmoscopic finding of choroidal metastasis. Note the irregularity of the lesion's surface. **B,** The lesion remained slightly hyperintense in this axial T2-weighted MR image.

Choroidal hemangiomas are congenital vascular hamartomas that are typically seen in middle-aged to elderly individuals, although they can be seen in children. Two different forms have been reported: (1) a circumscribed or solitary type not associated with other abnormalities and (2) a diffuse angiomatosis often associated with facial nevus flammeus or variations of Sturge-Weber syndrome.[62]

### Clinical Features

Uveal hemangiomas are classified histologically into three descriptive categories: (1) cavernous, (2) capillary, and (3) mixed type. Regardless of their histologic classification, these lesions follow two major growth patterns: (1) the solitary circumscribed choroidal form and (2) the diffuse form associated with Sturge-Weber syndrome. Solitary choroidal hemangioma is confined to the choroid, shows distinct margins, and characteristically lies posterior to the equator of the globe.[62, 177] It is typically seen as a focal reddish orange choroidal tumor located in the juxtapapillary or macular regions of the fundus. In contrast, the hemangioma associated with Sturge-Weber syndrome is a diffuse process that may involve the choroid, ciliary body, iris, and occasionally other nonuveal tissues such as the episclera, conjunctiva, and limbus.

### Diagnostic Imaging

Although uveal hemangiomas can be diagnosed by ophthalmoscopy, fluorescein angiography, or ultrasound, the clinical diagnosis may be difficult.[62, 177] In recent years, increased awareness of the various lesions of the uvea that may mimic melanoma (pseudomelanomas), combined with CT and MR imaging, has greatly decreased the frequency of erroneous diagnosis, so fewer eyes with choroidal hemangioma are enucleated.[62] A choroidal hemangioma is seen on plain CT as an ill-defined mass (Fig. 8-93A) that demonstrates marked enhancement with contrast infusion (Fig. 8-93B,C) and on dynamic CT (Fig. 8-93D). In some cases, the choroidal angioma may be concealed by the detachment of the retina (Fig. 8-93C). On MR imaging, a choroidal hemangioma may be seen as a hypointense area on T1-weighted (Fig. 8-93E) and T2-weighted images (Fig. 8-93F). Some choroidal hemangiomas are seen as a moderately intense area on T1-weighted, proton density, and T2-weighted images (Figs. 8-94 and 8-95). Whenever a choroidal hemangioma cannot be definitely differentiated from a uveal melanoma by MR imaging, contrast-enhanced CT is recommended using a combination of infusion-bolus (Fig. 8-93B) or dynamic CT techniques (Fig. 8-93D).[19, 36] Alternatively, gadolinium MR imaging may differentiate these entities (Fig. 8-95). The diagnosis of angiomatosis retinae of von Hippel-Lindau disease is chiefly dependent on the ophthalmoscopic appearance of the lesion. Because of the small size of the lesion (1.5 to 2 mm), retinal angiomas usually are not identified on MR imaging.

### Angiomatosis Retinae and Von Hippel-Lindau Disease

*Angiomatosis retinae* and *von Hippel-Lindau disease* are interchangeable names for phakoma of the retinal angioma.[27] This syndrome consists of a vascular malformation of the retina and cerebellum. The retinal lesion usually has the characteristics of a malformation, and the cerebellar lesion consists of a slowly growing cystic hemangioblastoma(s). The cerebellar lesions may be multiple and associated with one or more spinal hemangioblastomas. Von Hippel described the ocular changes in 1895 and the clinical and pathologic changes in 1911. In 1926, Lindau described the frequent occurrence of von Hippel's ocular findings in patients with hemangioblastoma in the cerebellum, medulla, and spinal cord, with angiomas or cysts of the pancreas, liver, kidney, adrenals, epididymis, or ovaries.[27] This combination has been recognized as von Hippel-Lindau disease. Not all patients have a retinal lesion, the von Hippel part of the disease. Both eyes are affected in about 50% of cases, and 25% of the patients with retinal angioma manifest systemic involvement.[27, 40] Retinal angiomas are present at birth as hamartomatous collections of small nests of angioblastic and astroglial rest cells, but it is not until the second or third decade of life that an angioma grows sufficiently large to be clinically detected.[27] Among the conditions that must be considered in the differential diagnosis of angiomatosis retinae of von Hippel-Lindau disease are Eales' disease, Coats' disease, multiple retinal aneurysms (Leber's disease), and capillary angiectasis of the retina.[27, 40] Eales' disease, or retinal periphlebitis, occurs in young men (15 to 35 years old) and is characterized by vessel sheathing of the retina and vitreous hemorrhage. The retinal veins show sheathing with exudates, hemorrhage, and vasoproliferation.[40] There are also recurrent vitreous hemorrhages from affected veins.

## Choroidal Hemorrhage and Choroidal Detachment

In discussing the differential diagnosis of uveal melanoma, choroidal hemorrhage and choroidal detachment must be considered because they may be easily mistaken for a choroidal tumor. A massive choroidal hemorrhage that has failed to rupture the lamina of Bruch may simulate the ophthalmoscopic, CT, and MR imaging appearance of a choroidal tumor because it forms a round, even globular, dark brown prominence that is opaque to transillumination (Figs. 8-96 and 8-97). The covering of the pigmented choroid, if the hemorrhage is in the suprachoroidal space, and of the retinal pigment layer may cause the hemorrhage's color to be even darker than that of the majority of melanomas. Such hemorrhage may become encapsulated and subsequently absorbed, leaving behind a more- or less-dense membrane. Choroidal effusion (uveal effusion) is another pathologic entity that can be confused with a ring melanoma.[53, 54] The CT and MR imaging appearances of choroidal hemorrhage (Figs. 8-41 and 8-97), choroidal detachment (Figs. 8-40, 8-46, and 8-47), uveal effusion (Fig. 8-48), were discussed earlier in this chapter.

## Choroidal Cyst

Choroidal cysts are very rare. However, they can be mistaken for a choroidal tumor. They may be bilateral, and they may cause retinal detachment. The cyst may be successfully treated by the removal of its fluid content.

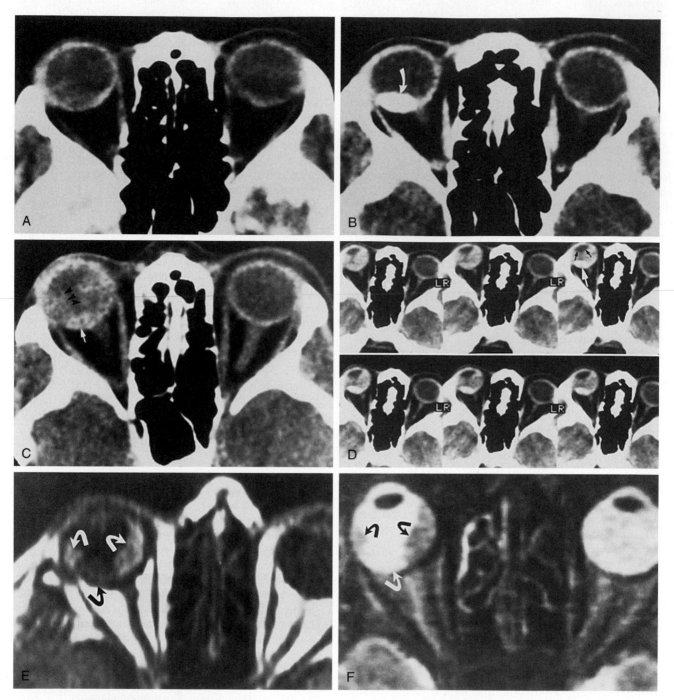

**FIGURE 8-93** Choroidal hemangioma. **A**, Noncontrast axial CT scan shows a faint lesion of the right globe. **B**, Contrast axial CT scan obtained with rapid injection of contrast shows marked enhancement of a hemangioma (*arrow*). This patient later developed total retinal detachment. **C**, Routine axial contrast enhancement shows a mass (*arrow*) and retinal detachment (*arrowheads*). **D**, Dynamic CT scans show a hemangioma (*white arrow*), differentiating it from total retinal detachment (*black arrows*). **E**, Axial T1-weighted MR image shows hemangioma (*black arrow*) and chronic subretinal effusion (*white arrows*). **F**, Axial T2-weighted MR image shows the hemangioma as a hyperintense image (*white arrow*) and chronic subretinal effusion as a hypointense image (*black arrows*). The hypointensity of the subretinal effusion is thought to be caused by highly organized proteinaceous fluid. (From Mafee MF et al. Malignant uveal melanoma and simulating lesions: MRI evaluation. Radiology 1986;160:773–780.)

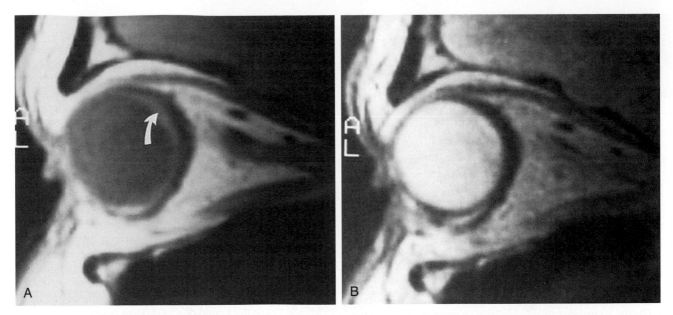

**FIGURE 8-94**  Choroidal hemangioma. **A,** Sagittal PW MR image shows a hyperintense mass (*arrow*). **B,** Sagittal T2-weighted MR image shows that the mass remains hyperintense. Ophthalmoscopic findings were most compatible with hemangioma. This MR imaging appearance may be difficult to differentiate from retinal detachment. Combined clinical and MR imaging findings should help the clinician make the right diagnosis.

## Other Tumors of the Uvea

### Ocular Lymphoma

Primary non-Hodgkin's lymphoma involving the eye is a rare condition. Modern immunohistochemical analysis shows that primary lymphomas of the retina and central nervous system (CNS) are usually large B-cell lymphomas.[40] The number of primary lymphomas of the retina and CNS has increased because of patients with acquired immune deficiency syndrome (AIDS) and other causes of immunodeficiency.[40] In contrast to primary ocular lymphoma, secondary ocular involvement by a systemic malignant lymphoma manifests itself mainly as a uveal tumor. Most often, the disease presents initially with signs of uveitis. Primary lymphoma of the eye is typically bilateral. Primary lymphoma of the retina can masquerade as a corticosteroid-resistant chronic uveitis.[40] Extensive infiltration of the retina and optic nerve head may lead to coagulative necrosis. Many atypical presentations of intraocular lymphoma have been reported, including a hemorrhagic retinal vasculitis that mimics a viral retinitis.[40] A secondary glaucoma may be present. The most important differential diagnosis includes the majority of cases of granulomatous uveitis, particularly ones that involve the retina, such as toxoplasmosis.[40] Ocular lymphoma can be mistaken for choroidal tumor.[62] On MR imaging, ocular

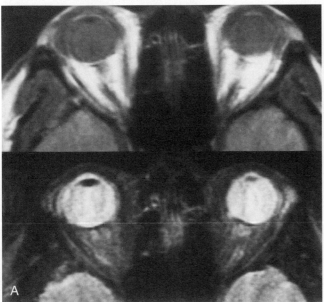

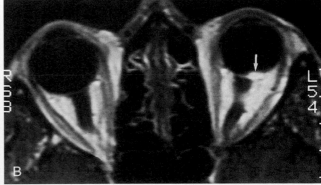

**FIGURE 8-95**  Choroidal hemangioma. **A,** Axial proton (top) and T2-weighted (bottom) MR images show no obvious intraocular mass. **B,** Axial postcontrast T1-weighted MR image shows intense enhancement of a left ocular hemangioma (*arrow*).

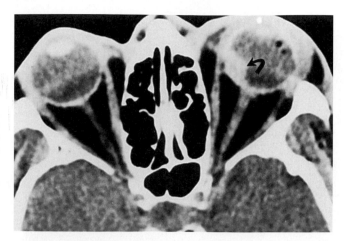

**FIGURE 8-96** Acute choroidal hematoma. Axial CT scan shows a hyperdense mass (*arrow*) related to traumatic choroidal hematoma. Note the air bubbles in the left globe.

lymphoma may have signal characteristics similar to those of uveal melanomas (Fig. 8-98). They are often bilateral (Fig. 8-98). Bilateral melanomas are extremely rare.

### Ocular Leukemia

Leukemic intraocular infiltration may involve the uvea, retina, optic disc, or vitreous. This is an uncommon ophthalmic disorder and unfortunately has a poor prognosis.[40] Leukemic intraocular infiltrates can present in one eye or both eyes. On MR imaging, leukemic infiltrates may have signal characteristics similar to those of uveal melanomas, metastasis, and intraocular inflammation (microbial and nonmicrobial).

### Primary Ocular Schwannoma (Neurilemoma)

Primary ocular schwannoma is an extremely rare lesion that can cause diagnostic confusion with uveal melanoma. This benign neoplasm arises from the Schwann cells of the peripheral nerves in the uvea or sclera.[40] Primary ocular schwannoma occurs either in patients who have neurofibromatosis Type I or in patients who do not have this condition. It usually occurs as an amelanotic mass in the choroid or

ciliary body that is indistinguishable clinically, by fluorescein angiography, and by ocular ultrasonography from a uveal melanoma.[40] The tumor consists of an encapsulated proliferation of amelanotic Schwann cells. Tumor cells exhibit positive immunoreactivity to S-100 protein but negative immunoreactivity to HMB-45 (melanoma-specific antigen) and muscle-specific markers (muscle-specific action).[40] The CT and MR imaging appearance of primary ocular schwannoma cannot be distinguished from that of uveal melanoma.[62] Primary intraocular neurofibroma is an extremely uncommon lesion that occurs in patients with neurofibromatosis Type I, although it has been reported in patients who have no manifestations of this syndrome.[40] The tumor is composed of an admixture of Schwann cells, fibroblasts, connective tissue, and neural axons and is usually nonencapsulated. The tumor typically arises in the choroid or ciliary body as an amelanotic mass that is indistinguishable from an amelanotic uveal melanoma by clinical examination and on imaging studies. At times in patients with neurofibromatosis Type I, the entire choroid may become thickened due to diffuse neurofibroma.

### Leiomyoma

Smooth muscle tumors of the ciliary body are extremely rare and must be distinguished from other spindle-cell tumors, especially the more common amelanotic spindle-cell melanoma.[179, 180] Electron microscopic examination is necessary to prove the smooth muscle origin of these tumors.[179] Pathologically, leiomyoma consists of amelanotic spindle-shaped cells of benign appearance. Immunohistochemical staining shows positive immunoreactivity to muscle markers (muscle-specific action and smooth muscle action).[180] Jakobiec et al.[180] reported two benign tumors of the ciliary body (one in a 37-year-old woman and another in a 20-year-old woman), which were diagnosed as neurogenic tumors by light microscopy but which on electron microscopic examination were found to be composed of smooth

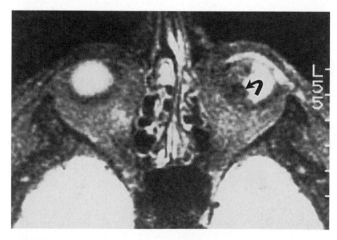

**FIGURE 8-97** Acute choroidal hematoma. Axial T2-weighted MR image shows hypointense fresh choroidal hematoma (*arrow*).

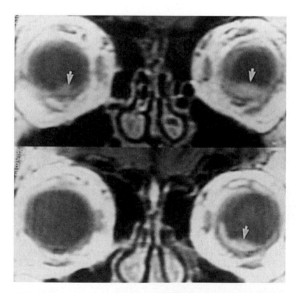

**FIGURE 8-98** Uveal lymphoma. Enhanced T2-weighted MR images showing bilateral, intraocular, irregular enhanced masses (*arrows*). (Courtesy of M.F. Mafee, MD, FACR, Chicago.)

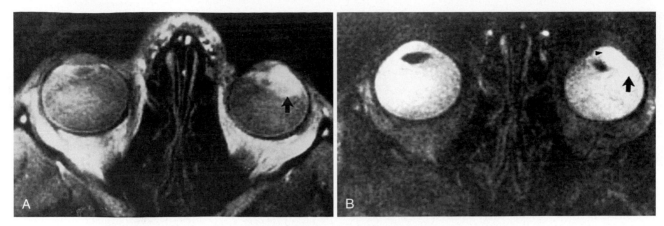

**FIGURE 8-99**    Leiomyoma of the ciliary body. **A,** Axial PW MR image shows a large, hyperintense mass (*arrow*). **B,** Axial T2-weighted MR image shows that the lesion remains hyperintense (*arrow*). Note the extension into the anterior chamber (*arrowhead*). (From Mafee MF et al. Retinoblastoma and simulating lesions: role of CT and MRI. Radiol Clin North Am 1987;25:667–682.)

muscle cells with unusual morphologic features. The authors concluded that myogenic and neurogenic characteristics reside in the neural crest origin smooth muscle of the ciliary body (mesectoderm) and that these tumors constitute a new nosologic entity of myogenic neoplasia. They coined the term *mesectodermal leiomyoma of the ciliary body* because the cells of the neural crest that contribute to the formation of bone, cartilage, connective tissue, and smooth muscle in the region of the head and neck have been called mesectoderm.[180] The MR appearance of a mesectodermal leiomyoma of the ciliary body has been reported.[84, 105] The lesion appeared as a well-defined noninfiltrative mass that demonstrated hyperintensity on T1-weighted, proton density, and T2-weighted images (Fig. 8-99). The CT and MR imaging appearance of ocular leiomyoma cannot be confidently distinguished from that of uveal melanoma and uveal neurogenic tumors.

## Ocular Adenoma and Adenocarcinoma

Ocular adenoma and adenocarcinoma may arise from the pigment epithelium of the iris, ciliary body, or retina. Adenomas and adenocarcinomas of the ciliary epithelia appear as solid nodular lesions in the ciliary body region.[40] Those that arise from the pigmented ciliary epithelium are darkly melanotic, whereas those that arise from the nonpigmented ciliary epithelium are amelanotic. Ocular adenoma and primary adenocarcinoma are extremely rare tumors and may not be differentiated from ocular melanoma by CT and MR imaging.

## Medulloepithelioma

Medulloepithelioma, or dictyoma, is a rare primary intraocular neoplasm derived from neuroectoderm, which characteristically arises from the primitive nonpigmented epithelium of the ciliary body.[40] Medulloepithelioma is usually seen in young children, although it can be seen in adults.[170, 181] Histologically, the tumor resembles embry-

onic retina and neural tissue.[181] This tumor has been divided into teratoid and nonteratoid types. The nonteratoid type (diktyoma) is a pure proliferation of cells of the medullary epithelium.[62] The teratoid type is distinguished by the additional presence of heteroplastic elements, particularly cartilage, skeletal muscle, and brain tissue.[62] Although most medulloepitheliomas are cytologically malignant, distant metastasis is uncommon.[62] From its point of origin on the ciliary body, the tumor may spread forward along the surface of the iris or backward along the surface of the retina.[62]

Medulloepithelioma generally occurs in the first decade of life as a nonpigmented ciliary body mass. In children, medulloepithelioma should be considered in the differential diagnosis of retinoblastoma, nematoid granuloma, and juvenile xanthogranuloma. In adults, this tumor may simulate amelanotic uveal melanoma and leiomyoma on ciliary body ophthalmoscopic evaluation, fluorescein angiography, ultrasonography, and CT (Fig. 8-100).[36] On MR imaging, medulloepithelioma appears similar to retinoblastoma and uveal melanoma.

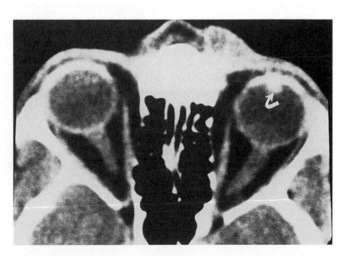

**FIGURE 8-100**    Medulloepithelioma. Axial CT scan shows a hyperdense mass (*arrow*).

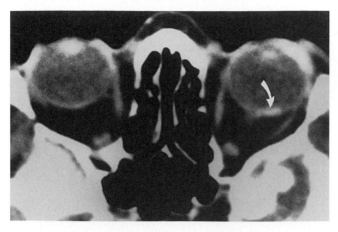

**FIGURE 8-101** Senile macular degeneration. Axial PW MR image shows a hyperintense mass (*arrow*) compatible with discoid macular degeneration. The lesion remained mixed in signal intensity on a T2-weighted image with a small, ill-defined area that appeared hypointense.

## Retinal Detachment in the Differential Diagnosis of Uveal Melanoma

The ophthalmoscopic appearance of a smooth globular outline of an elevated retina, characteristic of most cases of malignant uveal melanoma, on occasion may be caused by a simple retinal detachment. However, in practically all cases of simple retinal detachment, there is a retinal hole. On MR imaging, the appearance of a simple retinal detachment is characteristic, and provided that a mass is elevated more than 3 mm, the absence or presence of the mass can be readily assessed (Fig. 8-33). However, chronically organized or hemorrhagic subretinal fluid may have MR characteristics identical to those of uveal melanomas (Fig. 8-84).

## Senile Macular Degeneration

Macular degeneration in the elderly is a leading cause of legal blindness. Arteriosclerosis of the choriocapillaries,

dysfunction of the pigment epithelial cells, and loss of neuroepithelial cells are the fundamental causes of the macular degeneration syndrome in the elderly.[27] The earliest change at the macula is hyalinization and thickening of Bruch's membrane. Later, ingrowth of choroidal neovascularization into the subpigment epithelial space occurs, and eventually this results in detachment of the pigment epithelium. The serous fluid that accumulates in the subpigment space eventually finds its way into the subretinal space. One of the serious possible complications is hemorrhage, which is limited at first to the subpigment epithelial space but later extends into the subretinal space, eventually forming an organized fibrous scar, with consequent loss of almost all function of the involved macular.[27] The process of senile macular degeneration may be associated with liquefaction of the vitreous, which may cause posterior hyaloid detachment. The CT appearance of senile macular degeneration may be similar to that of uveal melanoma (Fig. 8-101). However, there may be more iodinated contrast enhancement in macular degeneration than in uveal melanomas. The MR imaging appearance of macular degeneration varies, depending on the stage of the disease. The lesion may show hyperintensity on all pulse sequences because of fluid in the subretinal space (Fig. 8-102), or there may be varied MR characteristics if there is associated hemorrhage and other complications (Fig. 8-102).

## Ocular Trauma

Ocular trauma can be categorized as blunt or penetrating. Either mechanism can cause corneal tear, scleral rupture, lens dislocation, hemorrhage, retinal detachment, or choroidal detachment. Because of the pressure changes and radial distortions of the globe, blunt trauma may actually cause more damage to the eye than a small projectile passing through the globe.[182] There are imaging findings that may suggest many of the ocular injuries, but most are clinically obvious on clinical examination, and imaging is not usually ordered to assess these problems primarily. Ultrasound may

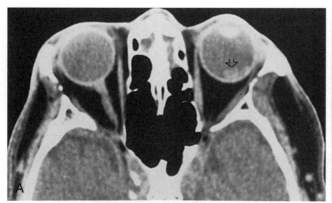
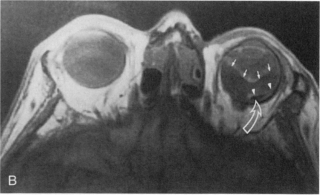

**FIGURE 8-102** Senile macular degeneration associated with complications. **A,** Axial CT scan shows a mass (*arrow*) and a dependent image probably caused by effusion in the subretinal space. **B,** Axial T1-weighted MR image shows the characteristic posterior hyaloid detachment (*arrows*). Unlike retinal detachment, a detached posterior hyaloid membrane does not extend toward the optic disc. Note the detached retina (*arrowheads*) and the hypointense image (*curved arrow*) related to scar tissue in the subretinal and retinal regions. Surgery confirmed these findings. Notice that information obtained by MR imaging is far superior to that obtained by CT.

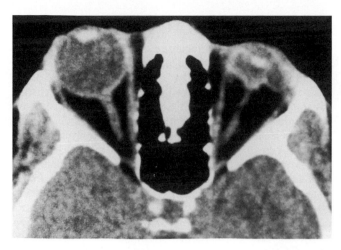

**FIGURE 8-103**   Ocular rupture. Axial CT scan shows deformity of the left eye with uveoscleral infolding due to ocular hypotony related to a rupture.

be used as part of an assessment, but the study is difficult to perform in the traumatized eye and is contraindicated in an open globe injury. Usually the most immediate concern for imaging is the possible presence of a foreign body, and the type of possible foreign body will determine the imaging modality used.

Intraocular foreign bodies (IOFBs) constitute a large percentage of ocular traumas, and advanced diagnostic and surgical techniques are required to manage them successfully.[183] Factors that influence the prognosis of IOFBs include the size, type of material, location, trajectory, reactivity, inflammatory response, degree and type of tissue damage, and length of time since the injury.

Patients presenting with ocular trauma are always examined for the presence of retained IOFBs. Indirect ophthalmoscopy, standard x-rays including the soft tissue (bone free) technique, CT, ultrasound, and, rarely, MR imaging are used to locate the foreign body. Localization of IOFBs is most often accomplished by CT, and this modality has proven valuable not only in detecting of IOFBs, but also

in detecting ocular rupture (Fig. 8-103) and choroidal hematoma (Figs. 8-104 and 8-105).[52] Ultrasound is useful to examine the relationship of IOFBs to soft tissue pathology such as retinal detachment.[183]

The advent of endovitreal microsurgery has allowed a spectrum of treatment possibilities to be offered to the patient with a severely injured eye as well as for the removal of IOFBs. Therefore, a detailed diagnostic imaging study is vital to evaluate these patients properly. Of all ocular perforations, IOFBs occur in about 40%.[184] DeJuan et al.,[185] who reported a series of 453 cases seen at the Wilmer Eye Institute, found ocular perforations to be caused by projectiles (41%), lacerations (37%), and blunt trauma (22%). Of the 35 cases of IOFB studied by Coleman et al.,[183] 30 (86%) were due to metallic IOFBs; the remaining 5 (14%) consisted of three glass fragments and two concrete particles. Twenty-five of the metallic IOFBs proved to be magnetic. This means that magnetic IOFBs constitute 71% of all IOFBs and 83% of all metallic IOFBs. Three foreign bodies (8.5%) were due to BB guns. The high compressive and concussive forces seen in BB injuries are usually regarded as the reason for the poor prognosis.[183] The natural course of a retained IOFB varies widely. Small IOFBs may be completely resorbed,[186] and the IOFB may become encapsulated. Sederosis bulbi may develop in an eye with a retained iron-containing IOFB. The siderotic changes may stabilize or regress[187]; the foreign body may lose its magnetic properties or become radiolucent on x-ray.[187] Patients with a clinical diagnosis of siderosis bulbi may develop iris heterochromia, papillary mydriasis, cataract formation, retinal pigmentary degeneration, and occasionally optic disc hyperemia.[187] The diagnosis of IOFB is often made ophthalmoscopically or by slit-lamp examination. Gonioscopy will detect a foreign body in the anterior chamber angle. The removal of an IOFB should be strongly entertained in an eye with siderosis if a diminished electroretinographic response is noted or in an eye with a mobile foreign body in the vitreous or a nonencapsulated foreign body in the retina. Because up to 90% of IOFBs are magnetic,[183] the use of magnets has long been advocated for their removal. The magnets used in ophthalmic surgery

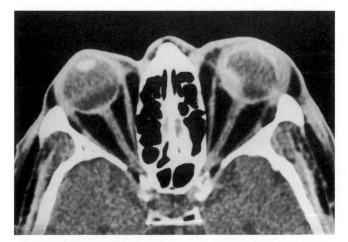

**FIGURE 8-104**   Ocular trauma and choroidal hematoma. Axial CT scan shows a hyperdense left choroidal hematoma. This can be confused with a choroidal melanoma.

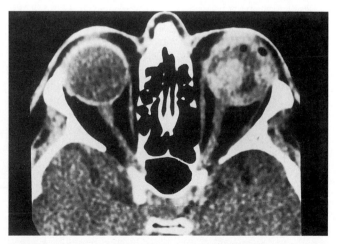

**FIGURE 8-105**   Choroidal hematoma following ocular surgery. Axial CT scan shows multiple choroidal hematomas of various sizes involving the left eye.

are of two general types: electromagnets and rare earth magnets.

Nonmagnetic IOFBs and even ferromagnetic foreign bodies are currently extracted in conjunction with posterior vitrectomy, endocoagulation, and removal of the foreign body by a forceps or other instrument. Retinal breaks may result from IOFBs. A retinal break encountered during vitrectomy generally is treated with retinopexy, often followed by fluid gas exchange and sometimes scleral buckling. Amber et al.[188] suggested that retinopexy may be avoided for retinochoroidal injury from a posteriorly situated metallic IOFB when there is no associated retinal detachment. The avoidance of retinopexy and fluid gas exchange may decrease the risk of retinal detachment and periretinal macular fibrosis.[188] Intraocular gas is known to cause breakdown of the blood-retina barrier, a situation that is significant in the stimulation of proliferative vitreoretinopathy.[188] Retained IOFBs are associated with endophthalmitis in approximately 7 to 13% of cases.[189] The use of intravitreal antibiotics in high-risk injuries and the possible use of vitrectomy surgery may reduce the incidence and severity of endophthalmitis.[189] Mieler et al.,[189] based on their experience, recommended prompt evaluation and surgical removal of acute retained IOFBs.

The optimal CT evaluation of intraocular pathology may consist of contiguous 1.5 mm axial sections parallel to the canthomeatal line. Thin sections are particularly valuable when evaluating small foreign bodies. Coronal and sagittal orbital reconstructions are helpful in confirming the intraocular location of a foreign body, especially when it is peripherally located. Direct coronal scanning is the best means of evaluating suspected foreign bodies at the 6 or 12 o'clock position in the globe. Plastic IOFBs are better demonstrated at a narrow window width, as described for intraorbital wood fragments.[190, 191] The plastics have a wide range of CT attenuation values (−125 to +364).[192] Most of the plastics are polyethylene, polystyrene, and polystyrene mixtures, which are inexpensive plastics often found in cheap disposable products such as fireworks.

CT scanning may fail to detect retained nonmetallic foreign bodies, especially when they are composed of organic material such as plastic[193, 194] or wood.[195] Ultrasound has the disadvantage of being technically difficult to perform; usually it is contraindicated in an open globe, and it does a poor job of identifying IOFBs when more than one is present.[193] MR imaging is contraindicated in the presence of a metallic foreign body.[193] Lobue et al.[193] performed CT and MR imaging on 10 enucleated eyes with wood, glass, and plastic foreign bodies. MR imaging detected all eight of the IOFBs compared to seven of eight found by CT. The authors noted that in three cases utilizing CT and involving wood or radiolucent plastic foreign bodies, confusion existed regarding whether a foreign body or merely an air bubble was detected. The authors stated that if a CT scan is normal and has ruled out a metallic IOFB, MR imaging may be useful in detecting and localizing a small nonmetallic foreign body. Williamson et al.[196] inserted a variety of magnetic and nonmagnetic IOFBs in 15 eyes. MR imaging (performed with a low-field MR unit) was accurate in locating 11 of the 15 foreign bodies that were nonmagnetic. The two foreign bodies not detected were located in the suprachoroidal space, suggesting that as with CT scanning, foreign bodies

located near the sclera are hard to detect. Small steel foreign bodies produced artifact obscuring all intraocular details. Using a low-field MR unit caused no intraocular injuries and was considered safe by these authors. However, higher field strength MR imaging units have been demonstrated to apply torque to ferromagnetic foreign bodies, which are then capable in both animals[195] and humans[197] of causing intraocular damage. In general, MR imaging is contraindicated in traumatized eyes with suspected ferromagnetic foreign bodies. For those patients with a remote history of traumatic foreign body to the eye or in those people with jobs in a high risk field such as metal lathe work, a high-resolution 1.5 mm thick CT scan of the orbits and a 5 to 10 mm thick CT study of the head are recommended to rule out the possibility of foreign bodies.[198] An MR imaging study may be recommended after CT has ruled out the presence of a magnetic (metallic) foreign body.

Lagouros and associates[195] conducted in vitro and in vivo experiments to study MR imaging of IOFBs. Diamagnetic and paramagnetic foreign bodies were imaged without artifact and without movement during the imaging process, while ferromagnetic foreign bodies, as expected, produced large amounts of artifact that prevented meaningful imaging. All ferromagnetic foreign bodies moved during in vitro imaging. During in vivo imaging, three of four ferromagnetic foreign bodies moved, producing substantial retinal injury.

In general, all substances are influenced by a magnetic field, and their behavior in it is determined by their magnetic susceptibility according to the following equation:

$$X = \frac{\text{Intensity of Magnetization}}{\text{Magnetic Force}^{199}}$$

If $X$ is negative, the substance is said to be diamagnetic; if $X$ is positive, the substance is considered paramagnetic. In diamagnetic materials, the molecular currents (caused by electrons revolving in their orbit around their parent nuclei) in one direction are equal to those in the other direction. In the absence of an external field, the molecules of these substances have no net magnetic moment.[195] Paramagnetism occurs when the molecules of a substance have a permanent magnetic movement. A magnetic field acts on a molecule by aligning it with the external field and adding the molecular field to the external field. When an insulated wire is wound around a ring of any substance and an electrical current is passed through this system, a magnetic field is generated. With paramagnetic substances, this field is greater than that of the current in the winding alone. This field is 100 to 1000 times greater in a subclass of paramagnetic substances known as ferromagnetic substances. At room temperature, iron, nickel, cobalt, and gadolinium are the only ferromagnetic elements.[195] Alloys containing these elements also may be ferromagnetic.

The CT appearance of various plastics has been described by Henrikson and associates.[192] The authors concluded that plastics may not be readily apparent on a CT scan when they are small and in the negative CT number range (<−30 HU). Lagouros and associates[195] were able to image polystyrene with MR imaging, which had a CT density of −35 HU in the study by Henrikson et al.[192] It would seem that all plastics, being relatively hydrogen poor, have a signal void on MR images, especially when they are in a relatively hydrogen-rich vitreous.[195]

The detection of an intraorbital wooden foreign body is difficult, particularly in cases of apparently minor trauma.[200–204] Orbital x-rays rarely detect wooden fragments.[203] CT has been shown to detect intraorbital wood associated with metallic paint[205] or a granuloma.[206] Wooden orbital foreign bodies are seen on CT scans as a site of low density; they often are mistaken for air or partial volume averaging of orbital fat. Both experimental[207] and clinical[208] studies have shown that CT has little value in detecting dry wood alone. Tate and Cupples[207] found that the high-resolution CT scanner could not detect small pieces of wood. Myllyla et al.[208] reported that CT scanning did not detect intraorbital wood in their two patients. They noted that the CT density of wood ranged from −618 to +23 HU. Orbital ultrasound also has some limitation in detecting intraorbital wood.[209] Intraorbital wooden foreign bodies are seen on MR imaging as an area of low signal intensity on T1-weighted, proton density, and T2-weighted images. They are particularly well delineated in T1-weighted MR images.[200] The usefulness of MR imaging in detecting orbital wooden foreign bodies was first reported by Green et al.[200] The authors recommended that MR imaging be done in all cases where orbital penetration by a wooden foreign body is suspected and the CT scan has not shown a foreign body. The possibility of an IOFB should be suspected in any patient sustaining minor lid trauma, especially when there is a history of injury caused by a pointed object. Second, if orbital fat is seen on direct physical examination, indicating violation of the orbital septum, an IOFB must be excluded. If standard x-rays and CT scans reveal a radiolucent focus anywhere within the orbit, particularly in a linear configuration, within the setting of orbital trauma, there should be a high index of suspicion for an organic foreign body.[210]

### Globe Injury

The globe can be torn by penetrating injury or by blunt trauma. A projectile can perforate the globe or simple compression of the globe can cause tears in weak areas.[182] Pressure waves transmitted through the globe contribute to injury to the retina and choroid. In blunt trauma, the globe is usually compressed posteriorly, diminishing the anterior-to-posterior dimension. When this happens there is transient radial expansion at the equator followed by rebound in all directions.[182] This rapid variation in shape can tear the globe wall at various weak points. There can be vitreous extrusion and collapse of the globe. The sclera will fold inward, giving a wrinkled grape or "crenated" globe appearance (Figs. 8-106 to 8-108). More minor injuries can cause loss of pressure limited to the vitreous compartment or the aqueous chamber, and the aqueous chamber may appear less voluminous than normal (Fig. 8-109). There may slight distortion of the vitreous chamber. With slight loss of tone, the lens may appear to move slightly anteriorly or posteriorly, depending on the chamber involved.[211] In some cases, air is demonstrated in the globe and hemorrhage into the vitreous can be present. Of note, the globe may be normal in appearance; thus, imaging is not relied upon for exclusion of open globe injury or perforation of the globe.[212]

Hemorrhage into the eye is appreciated as increased density on CT. A hyphema, blood in the anterior chamber, may not be identifiable because the volume is small. Larger hemorrhages into the vitreous are more obvious. Hemorrhage may be seen as an isolated phenomenon or associated with wall rupture. Small foci of hemorrhage may mimic a foreign body. Retinal or choroidal detachments can be immediate or delayed. The retina can be torn by the acute injury, with hemorrhage pushing the retina away from the wall of the globe and into the vitreous compartment. Alternatively, injury to the vitreous can cause a fibrotic reaction, and subsequent retraction of scar can cause a delayed tractional detachment. Retinal and choroidal detachments were discussed earlier in this chapter.

The lens itself can be dislocated (Fig. 8-110; see also 8-106 and 8-107). With penetrating injury, the lens can be pushed directly into the vitreous cavity. In blunt trauma, the rapid changes in the shape of the globe can disrupt the zonule and suspensory fibers, destroying the supporting structure of the lens. In addition, the lens can be dislocated completely or can be dislocated along one margin if only a partial disruption occurs. The normal lens is a liquid crystal

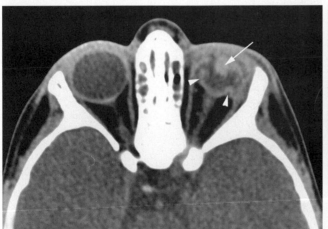
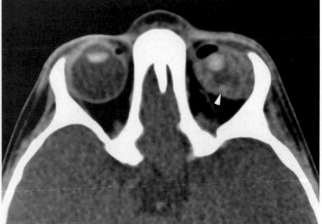

**FIGURE 8-106**  Perforation and collapse of the globe. Axial CT scans show infolding (*arrowheads*) of the posterior aspect of the globe, and the lens (*arrow*) is partially displaced.

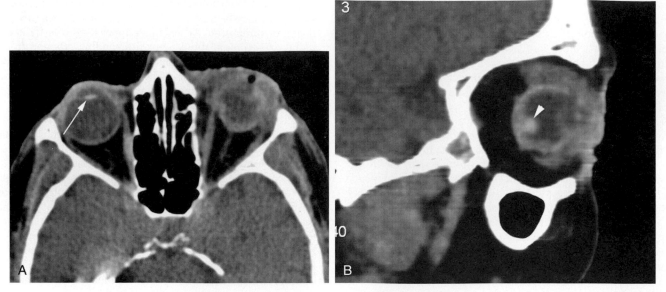

**FIGURE 8-107**   Perforated globe with loss of tone and lens displacement on the left side. Intraocular lens implant, right side. **A**, Axial CT scan shows the intraocular lens (*arrow*) on the right side. Note that the left globe has lost tone and has partially collapsed, with infolding of the posterior sclera. **B**, Sagittal reconstruction shows the displacement of the lens (*arrowhead*) into the posterior aspect of the vitreous compartment.

structure with an extremely high protein content, and therefore is visible as a high density on CT contrasted against the vitreous. Any deviation from its normal position should suggest the possibility of zonular rupture with complete or partial dislocation. Patients with Marfan's syndrome are particularly prone to dislocations of the lens. Dislocations can be bilateral and can occur with minor trauma.

The lens capsule can be perforated. Fluid then moves into the lens, diluting the normally high protein (Fig. 8-111). On CT, the density decreases.[213–215] This decreased density represents early cataract formation. Later calcification can occur.

Avulsions of the extraocular muscles can give the appearance of a shorter, fatter muscle displaced or contracted posteriorly into the orbit. Because the sheath of the muscle may remain intact, a linear structure may remain, connecting the enlarged muscle belly to the globe. The optic nerve can also be torn or avulsed from the posterior globe.

### Postsurgical Changes

Many surgical interventions result in a change in the appearance of the globe that is detectable on CT or MR imaging. Most of these findings relate to surgery for detached retina or cataracts.

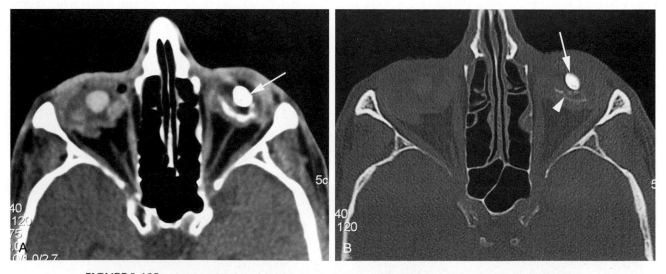

**FIGURE 8-108**   Acute perforation of the globe on the right side. Phthisis bulbi and calcified lens on the left side. Axial CT scans at narrow (**A**) and wide (**B**) window settings. There is inward buckling of the sclera of the right globe after acute trauma. There is calcification along the wall of the globe on the left, with a calcified lens (*arrow*) from a previous insult.

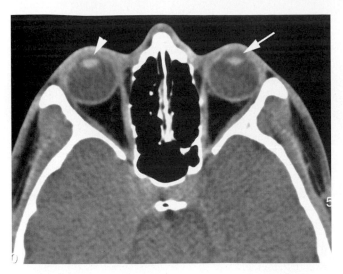

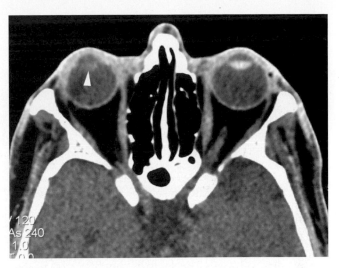

**FIGURE 8-109** Perforation of the cornea. Axial CT scan shows perforation of the cornea with hypotony of the aqueous chamber. The fluid space between the cornea and the lens on the right side (*arrowhead*) is diminished compared to the left. A normal aqueous chamber is seen on the left side (*arrow*).

**FIGURE 8-111** Axial CT. Acute perforation of the lens capsule. The abnormal lens (*arrowhead*) has low density due to the influx of fluid diluting the normally high protein of the lens. Compare with the opposite side.

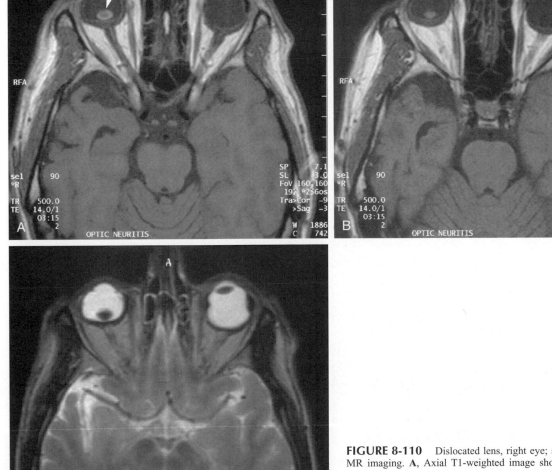

**FIGURE 8-110** Dislocated lens, right eye; scleral buckle, left eye. MR imaging. **A**, Axial T1-weighted image shows the dislocated lens (*arrow*) posteriorly positioned in the right globe. **B**, Axial T1-weighted axial image. On the left side, the low-signal areas (*arrowheads*) on the medial and lateral aspect of the globe represent the scleral buckle. **C**, Axial T2-weighted image shows the dislocated lens on the right and the scleral buckle (low signal) on the left.

Scleral buckle or banding, a procedure done for a detached retina, produces a very typical appearance.[216, 217] A plastic or composite band is placed completely around the equator of the globe, passing close to the insertion points of the rectus muscles (Fig. 8-112; see also Fig. 8-110). The inward "squeeze" decreases the likelihood that the retina will pull away from the wall of the globe once the retina has been reattached or reapproximated to its normal position. Most scleral buckles are made of silicone or hydrogel, are dense on CT, and have low signal intensity on MR imaging.[217] A silicone sponge can give the appearance of air and thus can be of low density on CT. The appearance of some materials can be variable, particularly on MR imaging, but the characteristic position of the buckle circling the globe usually makes the banding obvious. The inward "girdling" or bowing of the wall of the globe is also usually appreciable on imaging.

After the detached retina is repositioned against the wall of the globe, a laser or cryoprobe is used to fuse the retina to the more peripheral layers. The ophthalmologist may place a gas or fluid into the vitreous chamber to push the retina outward and tamponade the retina against the wall of the globe. Silicone oil, fluorosilicone oil, perfluorocarbon liquid, saline, and various other substances including expanding gases have been used for such tamponade retinopexy procedures. The appearance varies with the materials used.[217–220] Many materials are dense on CT and variable on MR imaging (Fig. 8-113). Some materials can be confused with diffuse hemorrhage if the history of previous surgery is not given. Silicone, for example, is dense on CT and has high signal intensity on T1-weighted images and low signal intensity on T2-weighted images.[221]

Probably the most common postsurgical change seen at imaging is the artificial intraocular lens (IOL) placed after cataract extraction. The lens is surgically removed via an incision in the sclera or a phacoemulsification is performed. In phacoemulsification, an instrument or probe is inserted into the lens, and ultrasound is used to disrupt and liquify the inner structure of the lens

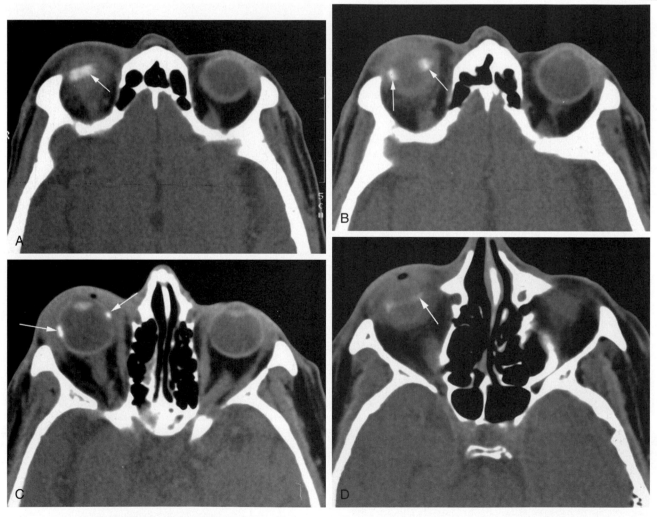

**FIGURE 8-112**   Scleral buckle in retinal detachment. **A** to **D**, Axial CT images showing the linear radial density encircling the globe (*arrows*). Note that if followed on all images, the radiodensity makes a complete ring around the globe.

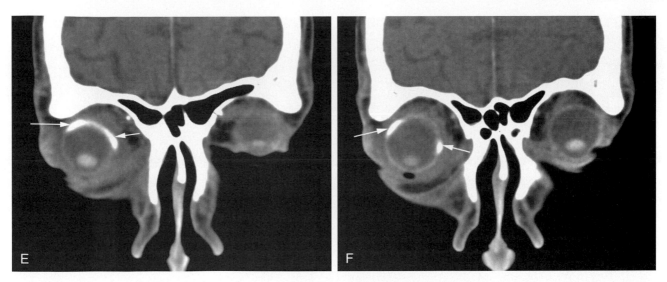

**FIGURE 8-112**   *Continued.* **E** and **F**, Coronal images show the encircling band (*arrowheads*).

including the cataract. The contents are then removed by suction. After either procedure, an IOL is then usually inserted.

With CT, rather than the biconvex structure characteristic of a normal lens, an IOL implant is typically seen as a thin, radiodense line (Fig. 8-107). A similar linear structure frequently can be appreciated on MR imaging. IOLs are commonly seen incidentally in patients undergoing imaging for nonorbital problems.

Finally, various drainage shunts and filters can be placed as decompression procedures in patients with glaucoma (Fig. 8-114), and the aqueous humor may collect in a reservoir-like "bleb" beneath the conjunctiva. Such a collection may be visible along the margin of the globe, usually close to the limbus.

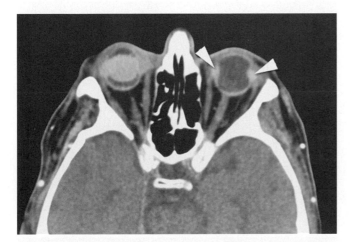

**FIGURE 8-113**   Silicone tamponade for retinal detachment of the right eye. Axial CT scan shows the radiodensity of the silicone in the globe. As with the normal lens, though radiodense on CT, the silicone is transparent to visible light. Note the scleral buckle (*arrowheads*) on the left side.

### Anophthalmic Socket and Orbital Implant

CT and MR imaging play an important role in the examination of the anophthalmic socket and the orbital implant.[222] There are two types of orbital implants: (1) spherical orbital implants, used following enucleation, and (2) reconstructive orbital implants, including plates, sheets, and fixation screws, which are used to repair nonsurgical and surgical trauma.[222] The spherical orbital implant is sutured within the intraconal space (Fig. 8-115). The layered closure includes the rectus muscles, Tenon's capsule, and the conjunctiva. An external custom-fit ocular prosthesis is then worn on the ocular surface (Fig. 8-115). Spherical orbital implants can be made of nonporous materials, such as silicone and polymethylmethacrylate, or of porous materials, such as porous polyethylene or hydroxyapatite (Fig. 8-116). Postenucleation imaging requests frequently involve such concerns as porous spherical orbital implant vascularization (Fig. 8-117), migration, exposure, orbital tumor recurrence, and associated craniofacial abnormalities.[222] Gadolinium-enhanced MR imaging has proven to be very valuable in determining the vascularization of hydroxyapatite implants following enucleation (Fig. 8-117).[223, 224] Based upon the extent of relative MR imaging enhancement within the implant, surgeons determine the appropriate time to integrate the spherical orbital implant surgically with an overlying external ocular prosthesis.[222–224] Integration involves drilling a hole through the overlying soft tissues into the spherical orbital implant and placing an integrational peg.[222] The peg, which is positioned inside the conjunctiva-lined hole is coupled with the external ocular prosthesis to improve motility.[222] A sufficient blood supply to the orbital implant must be present to support a conjunctival lining of the drilled interface.[222] Motility coupling pegs for porous polyethylene orbital implants recently have been introduced, and surgeons may request an MR study prior to placement of a peg.[225] MR documentation of fibrovascular ingrowth has broad clinical importance, and the rate of fibrovascular ingrowth is both patient and surgical technique dependent.[222]

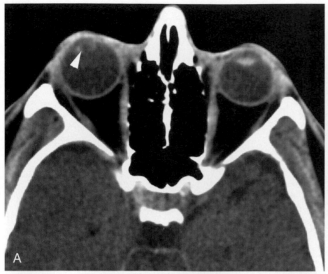

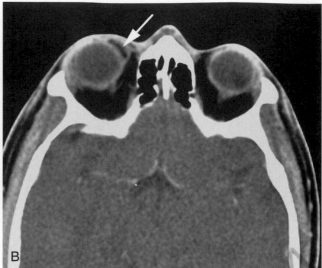

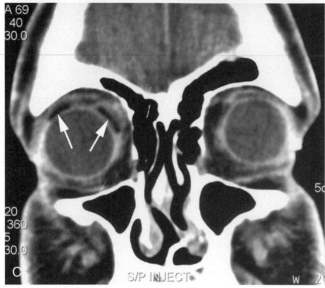

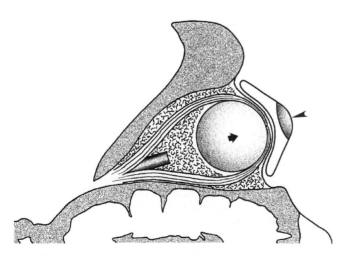

**FIGURE 8-114** Aqueous shunt. Axial CT scans show a shunt implant placed into the right aqueous chamber (*arrowhead* in **A**). A small bleb of aqueous (*arrows* in **B** and **C**) collects beneath the conjunctiva. The patient has undergone phakoemulsification on the right. No IOL was inserted.

**FIGURE 8-115** Enucleation with placement of an orbital implant. The orbital implant is sutured within the intraconal space (*arrow*). The layered closure includes the rectus muscles, Tenon's capsule, and the conjunctiva. A custom-fit ocular prosthesis is worn on the ocular surface (*arrowhead*).

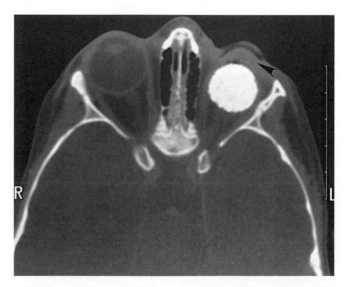

**FIGURE 8-116** Enucleation with placement of an unwrapped hydroxyapatite orbital implant. Axial CT scan shows the coarse surface of the hydroxyapatite implant and the position of the overlying prosthesis (*arrowhead*).

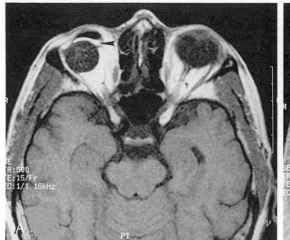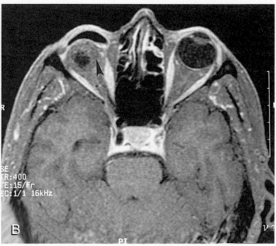

**FIGURE 8-117**   Enucleation with a porous polyethylene implant and an overlying dermis fat graft. **A**, Axial T1-weighted MR image shows the hyperintense signal of the dermis fat graft (*arrowhead*) anterior to the orbital implant and posterior to the ocular prosthesis. **B**, Axial T1-weighted, gadolinium-enhanced, fat-suppressed MR image shows the hyperintense signal of the rectus muscles consistent with a favorable blood supply. The hyperintense signal of the periphery of the orbital implant is consistent with early vascularization of the porous implant (*arrowhead*).

# REFERENCES

1. Warwick R, Williams PL. Gray's Anatomy, 35th British ed. Philadelphia: WB Saunders, 1973;145–147.
2. Snell RS, Lemp MA (eds). Clinical Anatomy of the Eye. Boston: Blackwell Scientific, 1989;1–15.
3. Mann IC. Developmental Abnormalities of the Eye, 2nd ed. Philadelphia: JB Lippincott, 1957;74–78.
4. Mann IC. On the development of the fissure and associated regions in the eye of the chick and some observations of the mammal. J Anat 1921;55:113–118.
5. Mann IC. The Development of the Human Eye. New York: Grune & Stratton, 1969.
6. Yanoff M, Duke JS, eds. Ophthalmology. Philadelphia: CV Mosby, 1999;3.1–3.6.
7. Mafee MF, Jampol LM, Langer BC, Tso M. Computed tomography of optic nerve colobomas, morning glory anomaly, and colobomatous cyst. Radiol Clin North Am 1987;25:693–699.
8. Driell D, Provis JM, Billson FA. Early differentiation of ganglion, amacrine, bipolar and Müeller cells in the developing fovea of the human retina. J Comp Neurol 1990;291:203–219.
9. Hollenberg J, Spira AW. Human retinal development. Ultrastructure of the outer retina. Am J Anat 1973;137:357–386.
10. Mann IC. On the morphology of certain developmental structures associated with the upper end of the choroidal fissure. Br J Ophthalmal 1922;6:145–163.
11. Brown G, Tasman W (eds). Congenital Anomalies of the Optic Disc. New York: Grune & Stratton, 1983;97–191.
12. Carlson BM. Human Embryology and Developmental Biology. St. Louis: CV Mosby, 1994;252–268.
13. Jack RL. Regression of the hyaloid vascular system: an ultrastructural analysis. Am J Ophthalmal 1972;74:261–271.
14. Renz BE, Vygantas CM. Hyaloid vascular remnants in human neonates. Ann Ophthalmal 1977;9:179–184.
15. Mafee MF, Goldberg MF, Valvassori GE, et al. Computed tomography in the evaluation of patients with persistent hyperplastic primary vitreous (PHPV) Radiology 1982;145:713–717.
16. Aguayo JB, Glaser B, Mildvan A, et al. Study of vitrous liquifaction by NMR spectroscopy and imaging. Invest Ophthalmol Vis Sci 1985;26:692–697.
17. Wehrli FW, Shimakawa A, Gullberg GT, et al. Time of flight MR flow imaging. Selective saturation recovery with gradient refocusing. Radiology 1986;160:781–785.
18. Mafee MF, Peyman GA, Grisolano JE, et al. Malignant uveal melanoma and simulating lesions: MR imaging evaluation. Radiology 1986;160:773–780.
19. Mafee MF, Puklin J, Barany M, et al. MRI and in vivo proton spectroscopy of the lesions of the globe. Semin Ultrasound CT MR 1988;9:59–71.
20. Mafee MF, Peyman GA. Retinal and choroidal detachments: role of MRI and CT. Radiol Clin North Am 1987;25:487–507.
21. Kaufman LM, Mafee MF, Song CD. Retinoblastoma and simulating lesion: role of CT, MR imaging and use of GD-DTPA contrast enhancement. Radiol Clin North Am 1998;36:1101–1117.
22. Lagouros PA, Langer BG, Peyman GA, et al. Magnetic resonance imaging and intraocular foreign bodies. Arch Ophthalmol 1987;105:551–553.
23. Snell RS, Lemp MA (eds). Clinical Anatomy of the Eye. Boston: Blackwell Scientific, 1989.
24. Zion VM. Phakomatoses. In: Tasman W, Jaeger EA, eds. Duane's Clinical Ophthalmology, Vol 5. Chapter 36:1–12.
25. Reeh MF, Wobij JL, Wirtschafter JD. Ophthalmic Anatomy: A Manual with Some Clinical Applications. San Francisco: American Academy of Ophthalmology, 1981;11–54.
26. Mafee MF, Putterman A, Valvassori GE, et al. Orbital space-occupying lesions: role of computed tomography and magnetic resonance imaging. An analysis of 145 cases. Radiol Clin North Am 1987;25:529–559.
27. Siegelman J, Jakobiec FA, Eisner G, eds. Retinal Diseases: Pathogenesis, Laser Therapy and Surgery. Boston: Little, Brown, 1984;1–66.
28. Rutmin U. Fundus appearance in normal eye. I. The choroid. Am J Ophthalmol 1967;64:821–857.
29. Anderson H, Apple D. Anatomy and embryology of the eye. In: Peyman GA, Sanders DR, Goldberg MF, eds. Principles and Practice of Ophthalmology, Vol 1. Philadelphia: WB Saunders, 1980;3–68.
30. Nakaizumi Y. The ultrastructure of Bruch's membrane. II. Eyes with a tapetum. Arch Ophthalmol 1964;72:388–394.
31. Wudka E, Leopold IM. Experimental studies of the choroidal blood vessels. Arch Ophthalmol 1956;55:857–885.
32. Mafee MF. Magnetic resonance imaging: Ocular anatomy and pathology. In: Newton TH, Bilanuik LT, eds. Modern Neuroradiology, Vol 4. Radiology of the Eye and Orbit. New York: Clavadel Press/Raven Press, 1990;2.1–3.45.
33. Warwick R, Williams PL, eds. Gray's Anatomy, 35th British ed. Philadelphia: WB Saunders, 1973.
34. Balaz EA. Physiology of the vitreous body. In: Schepens CL, ed. Importance of the Vitreous Body in Retinal Surgery with Special Emphasis on Reoperations. St. Louis: CV Mosby, 1960;29–48.
35. Mafee MF, Goldberg MF, Valvassori GE, et al. Computed tomography in the evaluation of patients with persistent hyperplastic primary vitreous (PHPV). Radiology 1982;145:713–714.

36. Mafee MF, Goldberg MF. CT and MR imaging for diagnosis of persistent hyperplastic primary vitreous (PHPV). Radiol Clin North Am 1987;25:683–692.

37. Aguayo JB, Blackband SJ, Schoeniger J, et al. Nuclear magnetic resonance imaging for a single cell. Nature 1986;322:190–191.

38. Penning DJ, et al. MRI imaging of enucleated human eye at 1.5 Tesla. J Comput Assist Tomogr 1986;10:55.

39. Balaz EA. The molecular biology of the vitreous. In: McPhearson A, ed. New and Controversial Aspects of Retinal Detachment. New York: Harper & Row, 1968;3–15.

40. Yanoff M, Duker JS. Ophthalmology. Philadelphia: CV Mosby, 1999.

41. Char DH, Unsold R. Computed tomography: ocular and orbital pathology. In: Newton TH, Bilanuik LT, eds. Modern Neuroradiology, Vol 4. Radiology of the Eye and Orbit. New York: Clavadel Press/Raven Press, 1990;9.1–9.64.

42. Mafee MF, Pruzansky S, Corrales MM, et al. CT in the evaluation of the orbit and the bony interorbital distance. AJNR 1986;7:265–269.

43. Kaufman LM, Villablanca PJ, Mafee MF. Diagnostic imaging of cystic lesions in the child's orbit. Radiol Clin North Am 1998;36:1149–1163.

44. Lyle DJ. Coloboma of the optic nerve. Am J Ophthalmol 1932;15:347–349.

45. Brown G, Tasman W, eds. Congenital Anomalies of the Optic Disc. New York: Grune & Stratton, 1983;97–191.

46. Mafee MF, Jampol LM, Langer BG, et al. Computed tomography of optic nerve colobomas, morning glory anomaly, and colobomatous cyst. Radiol Clin North Am 1987;25:693–699.

47. Mann I. Developmental Abnormalities of the Eye, 2nd ed. Philadelphia: JB Lippincott, 1957;74–78.

48. Savell J, Cook JR. Optic nerve colobomas of autosomal dominant heredity. Arch Ophthalmol 1976;94:395–400.

49. Pollock JA, Newton TH, Hoyt WF. Transsphenoidal and transethmoidal encephaloceles. Radiology 1968;90:442–453.

50. Kindler P. Morning glory syndrome: unusual congenital optic disc anomaly. Am J Ophthalmol 1970;69:376–384.

51. Capper SA, Leopold IH. Mechanism of serous choroidal detachment. Arch Ophthalmol 1956;55:101–113.

52. Mafee MF, Peyman GA. Choroidal detachment and ocular hypotony: CT evaluation. Radiology 1984;153:697–703.

53. Mafee MF, Linder B, Peyman GA, et al. Choroidal hematoma and effusion: evaluation with MR imaging. Radiology 1988;168:781–786.

54. Peyman GA, Mafee MF, Schulman JA. Computed tomography in choroidal detachment. Ophthalmology 1984;91:156–162.

55. Iijima Y, Asanagi K. A new B-scan ultrasonographic technique for observing ciliary body detachment. Am J Ophthalmol 1983;95:498–501.

56. Wing GL, Schepens CL, Trempe CL, et al. Serous choroidal detachment and the thickened choroid sign detected by ultrasonography. Am J Ophthalmol 1982;84:499–505.

57. Archer DB, Canavan YM. Contusional eye injuries: retinal and choroidal lesions. Aust J Ophthalmol 1983;11:251–264.

58. Gole GA. Massive choroidal hemorrhage as a complication of krypton red laser photocoagulation for disciform degeneration. Aust N Z J Ophthalmol 1985;13:37–38.

59. Maumenee AE, Schwartz MF. Acute intraoperative choroidal effusion. Am J Ophthalmol 1985;100:147–154.

60. Schepens CL, Brockhurst RJ. Uveal effusion. I. Clinical picture. Arch Ophthalmol 1963;70:189–201.

61. Chaques VJ, Lam S, Tessler HH, Mafee MF. Computed tomography and magnetic resonance imaging in the diagnosis of posterior scleritis. Ann Ophthalmol 1993;25:89–94.

62. Mafee MF. Uveal melanoma, choroidal hemangioma, and simulating lesions: role of MR imaging. Radiol Clin North Am 1998;36:1083–1099.

63. Yan X, Edward DP, Mafee MF. Ocular calcification radiologic–pathologic correlation and literature review. Int J Neuroradiol 1998;4:81–96.

64. Weiter JJ, Ernest JT. Anatomy of the choroidal vasculature. Am J Ophthalmol 1974;78:583–590.

65. Howard GM, Ellsworth RM. Differential diagnosis of retinoblastoma: a statistical survey of 500 children. I. Relative frequency of the lesions which stimulate retinoblastoma. Am J Ophthalmol 1965;60:610–618.

66. Popoff NA, Ellsworth RM. The fine structure of retinoblastoma: in vivo and in vitro observations. Lab Invest 1971;25:389–402.

67. Tso MO. Clues to the cells of origin of retinoblastoma. Int Ophthalmol Clin 1980;20(2):191–210.

68. Kodilyne HC. Retinoblastoma in Nigeria: problems in treatment. Am J Ophthalmol 1967;63:467–481.

69. Abramson DH, Ellsworth RM, Tretter P, et al. Treatment of bilateral groups I through III retinoblastoma with bilateral radiation. Arch Ophthalmol 1981;99:1761–1762.

70. Kyritsis AP, Tsokos M, Triche TJ, et al. Retinoblastoma: origin from a primitive neuroectodermal cell? Nature 1984;307:471–473.

71. Tso MOM, Fine BS, Zimmerman LE. The nature of retinoblastoma. I. Photoreceptor differentiation: a clinical and histopathologic study. Am J Ophthalmol 1970;69:339–349.

72. Tso MOM, Zimmerman LE, Fine BS, et al. A cause of radioresistance in retinoblastoma: photoreceptor differentiation. Trans Am Acad Ophthalmol Otolaryngol 1970;74:959–969.

73. Jenson RD, Miller RW. Retinoblastoma: epidemiologic characteristics. N Engl J Med 1971;285:307–311.

74. Abramson DH, Ellsworth RM, Kitchin DF, Tung G. Second nonocular tumors in retinoblastoma survivors. Ophthalmology 1984;91:1351–1355.

75. Pendergrass TW, Davis S. Incidence of retinoblastoma in the United States. Arch Ophthalmol 1980;98:1204–1210.

76. Ellsworth RM. The management of retinoblastoma. Trans Am Ophthalmol Soc 1969;67:462–534.

77. Lennox EL, Draper GJ, Sanders BM. Retinoblastoma: a study of natural history and prognosis of 268 cases. Br Med J 1975;3:731–734.

78. Abramson DH. Retinoblastoma: diagnosis and management. Cancer J Clin 1982;32:130–140.

79. Kundson AG. Retinoblastoma: a prototype heredity neoplasm. Semin Oncol 1978;5:57–60.

80. Kundson AG Jr. Mutation and cancer: a statistical study of retinoblastoma. Proc Natl Acad Sci USA 1971;68:820–823.

81. Lele KP, Penrose LS, Stallard HE. Chromosome deletion in a case of retinoblastoma. Ann Hum Genet 1963;27:171–174.

82. Kundson AG Jr, Meadows AT, Nichols WW, et al. Chromosomal deletion and retinoblastoma. N Engl J Med 1976;295:1120–1123.

83. Yunis JJ, Ramsey N. Retinoblastoma and subband deletion chromosome 13. Am J Dis Child 1978;132:161–163.

84. Mafee MF, Goldberg MF, Greenwald MJ, et al. Retinoblastoma and simulating lesions: role of CT and MR imaging. Radiol Clin North Am 1987;25:667–681.

85. Cavenee WX, Murphree AL, Shul MM, et al. Prediction of familial predisposition to retinoblastoma. N Engl J Med 1986;314:1201–1207.

86. Sparkes RS, Sparkes MC, Wilson MG, et al. Regional assignment of genes for human esterase D and retinoblastoma to chromosome band 13q14. Science 1980;208:1042–1044.

87. Sparkes RS, Murphree AL, Lingua RW, et al. Gene for hereditary retinoblastoma assigned to human chromosome 13 by linkage to esterase D. Science 1983;219:971–973.

88. Motegi T. High rate of detection of 13q-14 deletion mosaicism among retinoblastoma patients (using more extensive methods). Hum Genet 1982;61:95–97.

89. Seidman DJ, Shields JA, Augsburger JJ, et al. Early diagnosis of retinoblastoma based on dysmorphic features and karyotype analysis. Ophthalmology 1987;94:663–666.

90. Jakobiec FA, Tso MOM, Zimmerman LE, et al. Retinoblastoma and intracranial malignancies. Cancer 1977;39:2048–2058.

91. Bader JL, Miller RW, Meadows AT, et al. Trilateral retinoblastoma. Lancet 1980;2:582–583.

92. Bader JL, Meadows AT, Zimmerman LE, et al. Bilateral retinoblastoma with ectopic intracranial retinoblastoma: trilateral retinoblastoma. Cancer Genet Cytogenet 1982;5:203–213.

93. Judisch GF, Patil SR. Concurrent heritable retinoblastoma, pinealoma and trisomy X. Arch Ophthalmol 1981;99:1767–1769.

94. Stefanko SZ, Manschot WA. Pinealoblastoma with retinoblastomas differentiation. Brain 1979;102:321–332.

95. El-Naggar S, Kaufman LM, Chapman LI, Miller MT, Mafee MF. Tetralateral retinoblastoma. Ann Ophthalmol 1995;27(6):360–363.

96. Schulman JA, Peyman GA, Mafee MF, et al. The use of magnetic resonance imaging in the evaluation of retinoblastoma. J Pediatr Ophthalmol Strabismus 1986;23:144–147.

97. Robertson DM, Campbell RJ. Analysis of misdiagnosed retinoblastoma in a series of 726 enucleated eyes. Mod Probl Ophthalmol 1977;18:156–159.
98. Char DH. Current concepts in retinoblastoma. Ann Ophthalmol 1980;12:792–804.
99. Haik BG, Saint Louis L, Smith ME, et al. Magnetic resonance imaging in the evaluation of leukokoria. Ophthalmology 1985;92:1143–1152.
100. Char DH, Hedges TR, Norman D. Retinoblastoma: CT diagnosis. Ophthalmology 1984;91:1347–1350.
101. Goldberg BB, Kotler MN, Ziskin MD. Diagnostic Uses of Ultrasound. New York: Grune & Stratton, 1975;100.
102. Danziger A, Price MI. CT findings in retinoblastoma. AJR 1979;133:695–702.
103. Daniel AF, Shurin SB, Bardenstein DS. Trilateral retinoblastoma: two variations. AJNR 1995;16:166–170.
104. Provenzale JM, Weber AL, Klintworth GK, et al. Radiologic–pathologic correlation. Bilateral retinoblastoma with coexistent pinealoblastoma (trilateral retinoblastoma). AJNR 1995;16:157–165.
105. Mafee MF, Goldberg MF, Cohen SB, et al. Magnetic resonance imaging versus computed tomography of leukokoric eyes and use of in vitro proton magnetic resonance spectroscopy of retinoblastoma. Ophthalmology 1989;96(7):965–976.
106. Warburg M. Retinal malformations: aetiological heterogeneity and morphological similarity in congenital retinal non-attachment and falsiform folds. Trans Ophthalmol Soc UK 1979;99:272–283.
107. Ohba N, Watanabe S, Fujita S. Primary vitreoretinal dysplasia transmitted as an autosomal recessive disorder. Br J Ophthalmol 1981;65:631–635.
108. Goldberg MF, Mafee MF. Computed tomography for diagnosis of persistent hyperplastic primary vitreous (PHPV). Ophthalmology 1983;90:442–451.
109. Peyman GA, Sanders DR. Vitreous and vitreous surgery. In: Peyman GA, Sanders DR, Goldberg MF, eds. Principles and Practice of Ophthalmology, Vol. 2. Philadelphia: WB Saunders, 1980;1327–1401.
110. Katz NNK, Margo CE, Dorwart RH. Computed tomography with histopathologic correlation in children with leucocoria. J Pediatr Ophthalmol Strabismus 1984;21:50–56.
111. Caudhill JW, Streeten BW, Tso MOM. Phacoanaphylactoid in persistent hyperplastic primary vitreous. Ophthalmology 1985;92:1153–1158.
112. Liberfarb RM, Eavey RD, DeLong GR, et al. Norrie's disease: a study of two families. Ophthalmology 1985;92:1445–1451.
113. Norrie G. Causes of blindness in children: twenty-five years experience of Danish institutes for the blind. Acta Ophthalmol 1927;5:357–386.
114. Warburg M. Norrie's disease: a new hereditary bilateral pseudotumour of the retina. Acta Ophthalmol 1961;39:757–772.
115. Warburg M. Norrie's disease (atrofia bulborum hereditaria): a report of eleven cases of hereditary bilateral pseudotumour of the retina, complicated by deafness and mental deficiency. Acta Ophthalmol 1963;41:134–146.
116. Warburg M. Norrie's disease: a congenital progressive oculo-ocoustico cerebral degeneration. Acta Ophthalmol 1966(suppl 89);1–47.
117. Holmes LB. Norrie's disease: an X-linked syndrome of retinal malformation, mental retardation, and deafness. J Pediatr 1971;79:89–92.
118. Apple DJ, Fishman GA, Goldberg MF. Ocular histopathology of Norrie's disease. Am J Ophthalmol 1974;78:196–203.
119. Blodi FC, Hunter WS. Norrie's disease in North America. Doc Ophthalmol 1969;26:434–450.
120. Mecke S, Passarge E. Encephalocele, polycystic kidneys and polydactyly as an autosomal recessive trait simulating certain other disorders: the Meckel syndrome. Ann Genet 1971;14:97–103.
121. Warburg M. The heterogeneity of microphthalmia in the mentally retarded. Birth Defects 1971;7:136–154.
122. Chemke J, Czernobilsky B, Mundel G, et al. A familial syndrome of central nervous system and ocular malformation. Clin Genet 1975;7:1–7.
123. Chan CC, Egbert PR, Herrick MK, et al. Oculocerebral malformations: a reappraisal of Walker's "lissencephaly." Arch Neurol 1980;37:104–108.
124. Pagon RA, Chandler JW, Collie MR, et al. Hydrocephalus, agyria, retinal dysplasia, encephalocele (HARDTE) syndrome: an autosomal recessive condition. Birth Defects 1978;14(6B):233–241.
125. Levine RA, Gray DL, Gould N, et al. Warburg syndrome. Ophthalmology 1983;90:1600–1603.
126. Warburg M. Hydrocephaly, congenital retinal nonattachment, and congenital falciform fold. Am J Ophthalmol 1978;85:88–94.
127. Eller AW, Jabbour NM, Hirose T, et al. Retinopathy of prematurity: the association of a persistent hyaloid artery. Ophthalmology 1987;94:444–448.
128. Ashton N, Ward B, Sperpell G. Role of oxygen in the genesis of retrolental fibroplasia: a preliminary report. Br J Ophthalmol 1953;37:513–520.
129. Michaelson IC. Retrolental fibroplasia. In: Michaelson IC, ed. Textbook of the Fundus of the Eye. Edinburgh: Churchill Livingstone, 1980;303–315.
130. Coats G. Forms of retinal disease with massive exudation. R Lond Ophthalmol Hosp Rep 1908;17:440–525.
131. Chang M, McLean IW, Merritt JC. Coats' disease: a study of 62 histologically confirmed cases. J Pediatr Ophthalmol Strabismus 1984;21:163–168.
132. Reese AB. Telangiectasis of the retina and Coats' disease. Am J Ophthalmol 1956;42:1–8.
133. Woods AC, Duke JR. Coats' disease. I. Review of the literature, diagnostic criteria, clinical findings, and plasma lipid studies. Br J Ophthalmol 1963;47:385–412.
134. Edward DP, Mafee MF, Valenzuela EG, Weiss RA. Coats' disease and persistent hyperplastic primary vitreous: Role of MRI and CT. Radiol Clin North Am 1988;36:1119–1131.
135. Silodor SW, Augsburger JJ, Shields JA, et al. Natural history and management of advanced Coats' disease. Ophthalmic Surg 1988;19:89–93.
136. Shields JA. Diagnosis and Management of Intraocular Tumors. St. Louis: CV Mosby, 1983;497–533.
137. Sherman JL, McLean IW, Brallier DR. Coats' disease. CT pathologic correlation in two cases. Radiology 1983;146:77–78.
138. Margo CE, Katz NN, Wertz FD, et al. Sclerosing endophthalmitis in children: computed tomography with histopathologic correlation. Pediatr Ophthalmol Strabismus 1983;20:180–184.
139. Wilder HC. Nematode endophthalmitis. Trans Am Acad Ophthalmol Otolaryngol 1950;55:99–104.
140. Zinkham WM. Visceral larva migrans: a review and reassessment indicating two forms of clinical expression, visceral and ocular. Am J Dis Child 1978;132:627–633.
141. Reesner FH, Aaberg TM, VanHorn DL. Astrocytic hamartoma of the retina not associated with tuberous sclerosis. Am J Ophthalmol 1978;86:688–698.
142. Zimmerman LE. Ocular lesions of juvenile xanthogranuloma. Trans Am Acad Ophthalmol Otolaryngal 1965;69:412.
143. Wertz FD, Zimmerman LE, McKeown CA, et al. Juvenile xanthogranuloma of the optic nerve, disk, retina, choroid. Ophthalmology 1982;89:1331–1335.
144. Shields CL, Shields JA, Buchanon HW. Solitary orbital involvement in juvenile xanthogranuloma. Arch Ophthalmol 1990;108:1587.
145. Augsburger JJ, Guthoff R. Benign intraocular tumors. In: Yanoff M, Duker JS, eds. Ophthalmology. St. Louis: CV Mosby, 1999;9.9.1–9.14.2.
146. Mafee MF. Calcifications of the eye. Head and Neck Disorders (Fourth Series) test and syllabus. Reston, Va: American College of Radiology, 1992;70–116.
147. Friedman AM, Henkind P, Gartner S. Drusen of the optic disk: a histopathological study. Trans Ophthalmol Soc UK 1975;95:4–9.
148. McMahon RT. Anatomy, congenital anomalies, and tumors. In: Peyman CA, Sanders DR, Goldberg MF, eds. Principles and Practice of Ophthalmology. Philadelphia: WB Saunders, 1980;1491–1553.
149. Yanoff M, Fine BS. Ocular Pathology. A Text and Atlas. Hagerstown, Md: Harper & Row, 1975;831.
150. Depotter P, Shields JA, Shields CL, eds. MRI of the Eye and Orbit. Philadelphia: JB Lippincott, 1995;35–92.
151. Callender GR. Malignant melanotic tumors of the eye: a study of histologic types in III cases. Trans Am Acad Ophthalmol Otolaryngol 1931;36:131–142.
152. McLean JW, Foster WU, Zimmerman LE. Prognostic factors in small malignant melanomas of choroidal and ciliary body. Arch Ophthalmol 1977;95:148–158.
153. Augsburger JJ, Damato BE, Bornfeld N. Malignant intraocular tumors. In: Yanoff M, Duker JS, eds. Ophthalmology. St. Louis: CV Mosby, 1999;9.3.1–9.8.4.

154. Donders PC. Malignant melanoma of the choroid. Trans Ophthalmol Soc UK 1973;93:745–751.

155. Zimmerman LE, McLean IW, Foster WD. Does enucleation of the eye containing a malignant melanoma prevent or accelerate the dissemination of tumor cells? Br J Ophthalmol 1978;62: 420–425.

156. Duffin RM, Straatsma BR, Foos RY, et al. Small malignant melanoma of the choroid with extraocular extension. Arch Ophthalmol 1981;99:1827–1830.

157. Char DH. The management of small choroidal melanomas. Surv Ophthalmol 1978;22:377–387.

158. Canny CLB, Shields JA, Kay ML. Clinically stationary choroidal melanoma with extraocular extension. Arch Ophthalmol 1978;96: 436–439.

159. Ruiz RS. Early treatment in malignant melanomas of the choroid. In: Brockhurst RJ, Boruchoff SA, Hutchinson BR, et al, eds. Controversy in Ophthalmology. Philadelphia: WB Saunders, 1977; 604–610.

160. Manschot WA, VanPeperzeel HA. Choroidal melanoma: enucleation or observation? A new approach. Arch Ophthalmol 1980;98:71–77.

161. Peyman GA, Juarez CP, Diamond DG, et al. Ten years' experience with eye wall resection for uveal melanomas. Ophthalmology 1984;91:1720–1725.

162. Mauriello JA Jr, Zimmerman LE, Rothstein TB. Intrachoroidal hemorrhage mistaken for malignant melanoma. Ann Ophthalmol 1983;15:282–284.

163. Ferry AP. Lesions mistaken for malignant melanoma of the posterior uvea: a clinicopathologic analysis of 100 cases with ophthalmoscopically visible lesions. Arch Ophthalmol 1964;72S:463–469.

164. Shields JA, Zimmerman LE. Lesions simulating malignant melanoma of the posterior uvea. Arch Ophthalmol 1973;89:466–471.

165. Peyster RG, Augsburger JJ, Shields JA, et al. Intraocular tumors: evaluation with MR imaging. Radiology 1988;68:773–779.

166. Damadian R, Zaner K, Hor D, et al. Human tumors by NMR. Physiol Chem Phys 1973;5:381–402.

167. Gomori JM, Grossman RI, Shields JA, et al. Choroidal melanomas: correlation of NMR spectroscopy and MR imaging. Radiology 1986;158:443–445.

168. Mafee MF, Peyman GA, McKusick MA. Malignant uveal melanoma and similar lesions studied by computed tomography. Radiology 1985;156:403–408.

169. Enochs SW, Petherick P, Bogdanova A, et al: Paramagnetic metal scavenging by melanin: MR imaging. Radiology 1997;204:417–423.

170. Zimmerman LE. Problems in the diagnosis of malignant melanomas of the choroid and ciliary body. Am J Ophthalmol 1973;75:919–929.

171. Depotter P, Shields JA, Shields JA, Shields CL. Computed tomography and magnetic resonance imaging of intraocular lesions. Ophthalmol Clin North Am 1994;7:333–346.

172. Erzurum SA, Jampol LM, Territo C, O'Grady R. Primary malignant melanoma of the optic nerve simulating a melanocytoma. Arch Ophthalmol 1992;110:684–686.

173. Deveer JA. Juxtapapillary malignant melanoma of the choroid and so-called malignant melanoma of the optic disk. Arch Ophthalmol 1973;51;147–751.

174. Mafee MF, Peyman GA, Peace JH, et al. Magnetic resonance imaging in the evaluation and differentiation of uveal melanoma. Ophthalmology 1987;94:341–348.

175. Naumann G, Yanoff M, Zimmerman LE. Histogenesis of malignant melanomas of the uvea: histopathologic characteristics of nevi of the choroid and ciliary body. Arch Ophthalmol.1966;76:784–796.

176. Gonder JR, Augsburger JJ, McCarthy FF, et al. Visual loss associated with choroidal nevi. Ophthalmology 1982;89:961–965.

177. Mafee MF, Ainbinder DJ, Hidayat AA, Friedman S: MRI and CT in the evaluation of choroidal hemangioma. Int J Neuroradiol 1995;1:67–77.

178. Adams RD, DeLong GR. Developmental and other congenital abnormalities of the nervous system. In: Harrison TR. Harrison's Principles of Internal Medicine. New York: McGraw-Hill, 1974; 1849–1863.

179. Meyer SI, Fine BS, Font RI, et al. Leiomyoma of the ciliary body: electron microscopic verification. Am J Ophthalmol 1968;66:1061–1068.

180. Jakobiec FA, Font RL, Tso MOM, et al. Mesectodermal leiomyoma of the ciliary body: a tumor of presumed neural crest origin. Cancer 1977;2102–2113.

181. Apt L, Heller MD, Moskovitz M, et al. Dictyoma (embryonal medulloepithelioma): recent review and case report. J Pediatr Ophthalmol 1973;10:30–38.

182. Pieramici DJ, Parver LM: A mechanistic approach to ocular trauma. Ophthalmol Clin North Am 1995;8(4):569–587.

183. Coleman DF, Lucas BC, Rondeau MJ, et al. Management of intraocular foreign bodies. Ophthalmology 1987;94:1647–1653.

184. Benson WE, Machemer R. Severe perforating injuries treated with pars plana vitrectomy. Am J Ophthalmol 1976;81:728–732.

185. de Juan E Jr, Stemberg P Jr, Michels RG. Penetrating ocular injuries: types of injuries and visual results. Ophthalmology 1983;90:1318–1322.

186. Begle HL. Perforating injuries of the eye by small steel fragments. Am J Ophthalmol 1929;12:970–977.

187. Scott RS, Weigeist TA. Management of siderosis bulbi due to a retained iron containing intraocular foreign body. Ophthalmology 1990;97:375–379.

188. Ambler JS, Sanford F, Meyers M. Management of intraretinal metallic foreign bodies without retinopexy in the absence of retinal detachment. Ophthalmology 1991;39:391–394.

189. Mieler WF, Ellis MK, Williams DF, et al. Retained intraocular foreign bodies and endophthalmitis. Ophthalmology 1990;97:1532–1538.

190. Grove AS. Orbital trauma and computed tomography. Ophthalmology 1980;403–411.

191. Grove AS Jr. Orbital trauma evaluation by computed tomography. Comput Tomogr 1979;3:267–278.

192. Henrickson GC, Mafee MF, Flanders AE, Kriz RJ, Peyman GA, et al. CT evaluation of plastic intraocular foreign bodies. AJNR 1987;8: 378–379.

193. Lobue TD, Deutsch TA, Lobick J. et al. Detection and localization of nonmetallic intraocular foreign bodies by magnetic resonance imaging. Arch Ophthalmol 1988;106:260–261.

194. Duker JS, Fisher DH. Occult plastic intraocular foreign body. Ophthalmic Surg 1989;20:169–170.

195. Lagouras PA, Langer BG, Peyman GA, et al. Magnetic resonance imaging and intraocular foreign bodies. Arch Ophthalmol 1987;105: 551–553.

196. Williamson THE, Smith FW, Forrester JV. Magnetic resonance imaging of intraocular foreign bodies. Br J Ophthalmol 1989;73: 555–558.

197. Kelly WN, Paglen PG, Pearson JA, et al. Ferromagnetism of intraocular foreign body causes unilateral blindness after MR study. AJNR 1986;7:243–245.

198. Zheutlin JD, Thompson JT, Shofner RS. The safety of magnetic resonance imaging with intraorbital metallic objects after retinal reattachment or trauma (letter). Am J Ophthalmol 1987;103:831.

199. Sears FW, Zenansky MW (eds). University Physics, ed 4. Reading, MA: Addison-Wesley, 1970.

200. Green BF, Kraft SP, Carter KD, et al. Intraorbital wood: detection by magnetic resonance imaging. Ophthalmology 1990;97:608–611.

201. Ferguson EC III. Deep, wooden foreign bodies of the orbit: a report of two cases. Trans Am Acad Ophthalmol Otolaryngol 1970;74: 778–787.

202. Macrae JA. Diagnosis and management of a wooden orbital foreign body: case report. Br J Ophthalmol 1979;848–851.

203. Brock L, Tanenbaum HL. Retention of wooden foreign bodies in the orbit. Can J Ophthalmol 1980;15:70–72.

204. Reshef DS, Ossoinnig KC, Nerad JA. Diagnosis and intraoperative localization of a deep orbital organic foreign body. Orbit 1987;6:3–15.

205. Weisman RA, Savino PJ, Schut L, et al. Computed tomography in penetrating wounds of the orbit with retained bodies. Arch Otolaryngol 1983;109:265–268.

206. Grove AS Jr. Computed tomography in the management of orbital trauma. Ophthalmology 1982;89:433–440.

207. Tate E, Cupples H. Detection of orbital foreign bodies with computed tomography: current limits. AJR 1981;137:493–495.

208. Myllyla V, Pyhtinen J, Pajvansalo M, et al. CT detection and location of intraorbital foreign bodies: experiments with wood and glass. ROFO 1987;146:639–643.

209. Coleman DJ. Reliability of ocular and orbital diagnosis with B-scan ultrasound orbital diagnosis. Am J Ophthalmol 1972;74:704–718.

210. Macrae JA. Diagnosis and management of a wooden orbital foreign body: case report. Br J Ophthalmol 1979;63:848–851.

211. Weissman JL, Beatty R, Hirsch WL, Curtin HD. Enlarged anterior chamber: CT finding of a ruptured globe. AJNR 1995;16(4 Suppl):936–938.
212. Joseph DP, Pieramici DJ, Beauchamp NJ Jr. Computed tomography in the diagnosis and prognosis of open-globe injuries. Ophthalmology 2000;107(10):1899–1906.
213. Segev Y, Goldstein M, Lazar M, Reider-Groswasser I. CT appearance of a traumatic cataract. AJNR 1995;16(5):1174–1175.
214. Boorstein JM, Titelbaum DS, Patel Y, Wong KT, Grossman RI. CT diagnosis of unsuspected traumatic cataracts in patients with complicated eye injuries: significance of attenuation value of the lens. AJR 1995;164(1):181–184.
215. Almog Y, Reider-Groswasser I, Goldstein M, Lazar M, Segev Y, Geyer O. ''The disappearing lens'': failure of CT to image the lens in traumatic intumescent cataract. J Comput Assist Tomogr 1999;23(3):354–356.
216. Bressler EL, Weinberg PE, Zaret CR. Silicone encircling bands for retinal detachment: CT appearance. J Comput Assist Tomogr 1984;8(5):960–962.
217. Girardot C, Hazebroucq VG, Fery-Lemonnier E, et al. MR imaging and CT of surgical materials currently used in ophthalmology: in vitro and in vivo studies. Radiology 1994;191(2):433–439.
218. Herrick RC, Hayman LA, Maturi RK, Diaz-Marchan PJ, Tang RA, Lambert HM. Optimal imaging protocol after intraocular silicone oil tamponade. AJNR 1998;19(1):101–108.
219. Manfre L, Fabbri G, Avitabile T, Biondi P, Reibaldi A, Pero G. MRI and intraocular tamponade media. Neuroradiology 1993;35(5):359–361.
220. Yoshida A, Cheng HM, Kwong KK, Ogasawara H, Garrido L, McMeel JW. Magnetic resonance imaging of intraocular tamponades. Ophthalmic Surg 1991;22(5):287–291.
221. Mathews VP, Elster AD, Barker PB, Buff BL, Haller JA, Greven CM. Intraocular silicone oil: in vitro and in vivo MR and CT characteristics. AJNR 1994;15(2):343–347.
222. Ainbinder DJ, Haik BG, Mazzoli RA. Anophthalmic socket and orbital implants: role of CT and MR imaging. Radiol Clin North Am 1998;36:1133–1147.
223. DePotter P, Shields CL, Shields JA, et al. Role of magnetic resonance imaging in the evaluation of the hydroxyapatite orbital implant. Ophthalmology 1992;99:824.
224. Shields CL, Shields JA, DePotter P. Hydroxyapatite orbital implant after enucleation: experience with initial 100 consecutive cases. Arch Ophthalmol 1992;110:333.
225. Rubin PA, Green JP, Keur C, et al. Medpur motility coupling post: primary placement in humans. Am Soc Ophthal Plast Reconstr Surg 28th Annual Symposium, 1997.

# 9

# Orbit: Embryology, Anatomy, and Pathology

*Mahmood F. Mafee*

# EMBRYOLOGY OF THE ORBIT

## The Orbit

The orbital bones develop from the mesenchyme that encircles the optic vesicle (see also the discussion of embryology in Chapter 8).[1,2] The medial wall forms from the lateral nasal process. The lateral wall and inferior wall develop from the maxillary process. The superior wall forms from the mesenchymal capsule of the forebrain. The posterior orbit is formed by the bones of the base of the skull.[2] The bones of the orbit form as membranous bone, except for the ethmoid, which is enchondral in origin.[1,2] It is interesting to note that early in development, the eye develops at a faster rate than the orbit, so that in the sixth month of fetal life the anterior half of the eye projects beyond the orbital opening. The eye increases rapidly in size during the first years of life. The rate of growth then slows but increases again at puberty. The cornea, which is relatively large at birth, reaches adult size by the time the child is 2 years old.[2] Pigmentation of the iris stroma occurs during the first years after birth.[2] The lens grows rapidly after birth and continues to grow throughout life. At birth the eye is hypermetropic (hyperopic or farsighted). Later, as the anteroposterior axis of the eye increases in length, this condition is corrected. A further increase in the anteroposterior axis could cause myopia, but generally this is prevented by the simultaneous flattening of the lens as growth proceeds.[2]

## Extraocular Muscles

The extraocular muscles of the eye are formed from the mesenchyme in the region of the developing eye (preotic myotomes).[1] Originally represented as a single mass of mesenchyme, they later separate into distinct muscles, first at their insertions and later still at their origins. The levator palpebrae superioris is formed last, splitting off from the mesenchyme that forms the superior rectus muscle. During their development, the extraocular muscles become associated with the third, fourth, and sixth cranial nerves.[1]

## The Eyelids

The eyelids develop as folds of surface ectoderm above and below the developing cornea (Figs. 9-1 and 9-2). As they grow, they become united with each other at about the third month of gestation.[1] The lids remain fused until about the fifth month of gestation, when they start to separate. Separation of the eyelids is completed by the seventh month of intrauterine life.[1] While the lids are fused, a closed space, the conjunctival sac, exists in front of the cornea. The mesenchymal core of the lids forms the connective tissue and tarsal plates. The mesenchyme of the second pharyngeal arch invades the eyelids to form the orbicularis oculi muscle supplied by the seventh cranial nerve. The cilia develop as epithelial buds from the surface ectoderm. The ciliary glands of Moll and Zeis grow out from the ciliary follicles. The tarsal glands (meibomian glands) develop as columns of ectodermal cells from the lid margins.[1] The epithelium of the cornea and conjunctiva is of ectodermal origin, as are the eyelashes and the lining cells of the tarsal and other glands opening onto the margins of the eyelids.[2]

## The Lacrimal Gland

The lacrimal gland forms as a series of ectodermal buds that grow superolaterally from the superior conjunctival

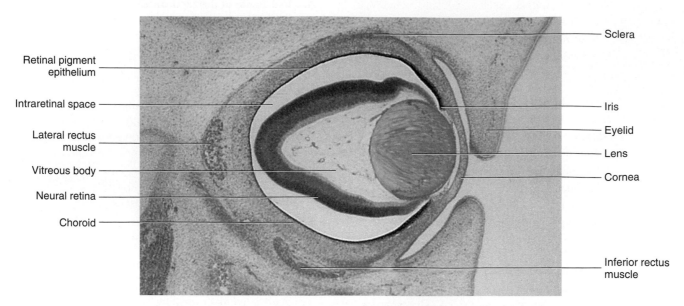

Sclera

Retinal pigment
epithelium

Intraretinal space

Lateral rectus
muscle

Vitreous body

Neural retina

Choroid

Iris

Eyelid

Lens

Cornea

Inferior rectus
muscle

**FIGURE 9-1**   Photomicrograph of a sagittal section of the eye of an embryo (×50) at Carnegie stage 23, about 56 days. Observe the developing neural retina and the retinal pigment epithelium. The intraretinal space normally disappears as these two layers of the retina fuse. (From Moore KL, Persaud TVN, Shiota K: *Color Atlas of Clinical Embryology*. Philadelphia, WB Saunders, 1994.)

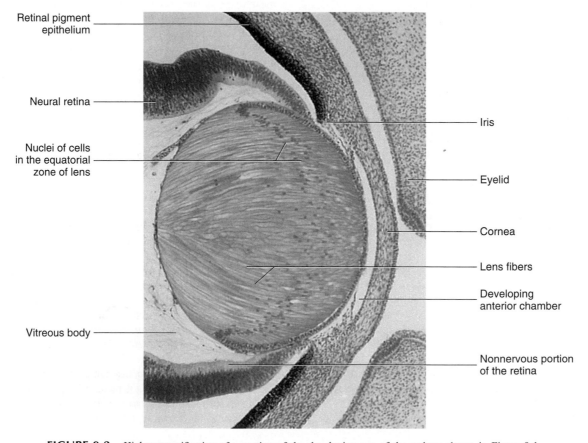

Retinal pigment
epithelium

Neural retina

Nuclei of cells
in the equatorial
zone of lens

Vitreous body

Iris

Eyelid

Cornea

Lens fibers

Developing
anterior chamber

Nonnervous portion
of the retina

**FIGURE 9-2**   Higher magnification of a portion of the developing eye of the embryo shown in Figure 9-1. Observe that the lens fibers have elongated and obliterated the cavity of the lens vesicle. Note that the inner layer of the optic cup has thickened greatly to form the neural retina and that the outer layer is heavily pigmented (retinal pigment epithelium). (From Moore KL, Persaud TVN, Shiota K: *Color Atlas of Clinical Embryology*. Philadelphia, WB Saunders, 1994.)

fornix into the underlying mesenchyme.[1] These buds are arranged in two groups, one forming the gland proper and the other its palpebral process.[2] These buds later canalize, forming the secretory units and multiple ducts of the gland. The gland becomes divided into orbital and palpebral parts with the development of the levator palpebral superioris. Tears are usually not produced until 1 to 3 months after birth.

## The Lacrimal Sac and Nasolacrimal Duct

The lacrimal sac and nasolacrimal duct initially develop as a solid cord of ectodermal cells in the nasomaxillary groove between the lateral nasal elevation and the maxillary process of the developing face.[1, 2] Later, this solid cord of cells sinks into the mesenchyme, and during the third month of embryonic life, the central cells of the cord break down and the cord becomes canalized to form the nasolacrimal duct. The superior end becomes dilated to form the lacrimal sac. Incomplete canalization, particularly in the lower end of the system, is common, even in full-term infants. Further cellular proliferation results in the formation of the inferior, superior, and common lacrimal ducts. The lacrimal canaliculi (superior and inferior) arise as buds from the upper part of the cord of cells and secondarily establish openings (puncta lacrimalia) on the margins of the lids.[2]

## INTRODUCTION TO THE ORBIT

The orbits are two recesses that contain the globes, extraocular muscles, blood vessels, nerves (cranial nerves II, III, IV, V, VI and the sympathetic and parasympathetic nerves), adipose and connective tissues, and most of the lacrimal apparatus. The orbit is bordered by the periosteum of seven bones (frontal, sphenoid, ethmoid, lacrimal, maxilla, zygoma, and palatine), and it is separated from the globe by Tenon's capsule.[1, 3, 4] Anteriorly are the orbital septum and the lids. The orbital cavity is pyramidal in shape, with its apex directed posteromedially and its base, the orbital opening, directed anterolaterally. Its bony walls separate it from the anterior cranial fossa superiorly; the ethmoid air cells, sphenoid sinus, and nasal cavity medially; the maxillary sinus inferiorly; and the lateral face and temporal fossa laterally and posteriorly. The volume of the orbit in adult is about 30 cc. The orbital entrance averages about 35 mm in height and 45 mm in width, and the maximum width occurs about 1 cm behind the anterior orbital margin.[5, 6] In adults, the depth of the orbit varies from 40 to 45 mm from the orbital entrance to the orbital apex.

## BONY ORBIT

Each orbit presents a roof, floor, medial wall, lateral wall, base (or orbital opening), and apex (Figs. 9-3 and 9-4). The orbital ventral margin or rim forms a quadrilateral spiral. The superior margin is formed by the frontal bone, which is interrupted medially by the supraorbital notch or foramen that transmits the supraorbital blood vessels and the supraorbital nerve, a branch of the ophthalmic division of the trigeminal nerve. The medial margin is formed by the frontal bone above and by the posterior lacrimal crest of the maxillary bone and the anterior lacrimal crest of the lacrimal bone below. The inferior margin is formed by the maxillary and zygomatic bones, while the lateral margin is formed by the zygomatic and frontal bones.

## Orbital Roof

The orbital roof is formed from the orbital plate of the frontal bone and most of the lesser wing of the sphenoid bone (Fig. 9-3). Anteromedially is the floor of the frontal sinus, and anterolaterally is the lacrimal fossa, in which lies the orbital part of the lacrimal gland. Posteriorly, at the junction of the roof and the medial wall, are the optic canal and optic foramen (Fig. 9-4), which establish communication between the orbit and the suprasellar cistern and cavernous sinuses. The optic canal contains the optic nerve, ophthalmic artery, and sympathetic fibers. Medially and anteriorly is the fovea (fossa) trochlearis, which is located approximately 4 mm from the superior orbital margin. From it is formed the trochlea or pulley of the superior oblique muscle. The trochlea is a curved plate of hyaline cartilage attached to the trochlear fossa. Calcification of the trochlea is common.

## Medial Orbital Wall

The medial wall is exceedingly thin, except at its most posterior part. This wall is formed by a small portion of the frontal process of the maxilla, the lacrimal bone, the ethmoid bone, and the body of the sphenoid (Figs. 9-3, 9-4). The medial wall slopes gently downward and laterally into the floor. Anteriorly is the lacrimal groove for the lacrimal sac. The groove communicates below with the nasal cavity through the nasolacrimal canal, which is about 1 cm long

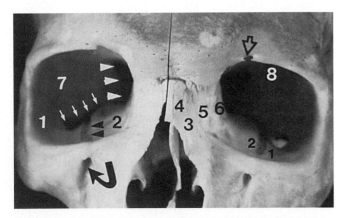

**FIGURE 9-3**    Frontal view of orbits. *1*, Orbital process of zygomatic bone; *2*, orbital process of maxilla; *3*, frontonasal process of maxilla; *4*, nasal bone; *5*, lacrimal bone; *6*, orbital plate of ethmoid bone (lamina papyracea); *7*, orbital surface of greater wing of sphenoid bone; *8*, orbital surface of frontal bone. Note supraorbital foramen (notch) (*hollow arrow*), superior orbital fissure (*white arrowheads*), inferior orbital fissure (*white arrows*), infraorbital groove (*black arrowheads*), and infraorbital foramen (*curved arrow*).

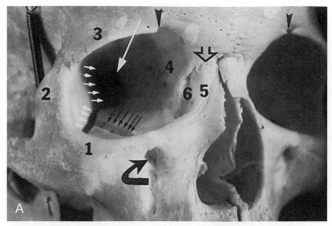

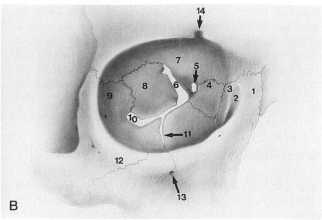

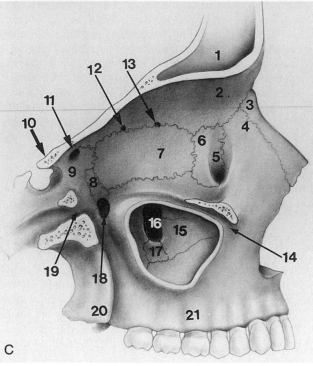

**FIGURE 9-4**  Frontal and slightly oblique view of orbits. **A**, *1*, Zygomatic bone; *2*, frontal process of zygomatic bone; *3*, zygomatic process of frontal bone; *4*, orbital plate of ethmoid bone (lamina papyracea); *5*, nasal bone; *6*, lacrimal bone and lacrimal fossa. Note frontonasal suture (*hollow arrow*), supraorbital notch foramen (*black arrowheads*), optic canal (*white long arrow*), superior orbital fissure (*white short arrows*), inferior orbital fissure (*white arrowheads*), infraorbital groove (*black arrows*), and infraorbital foramen (*curved arrow*). **B**, Schematic frontal drawing of bony orbit. *1*, Frontal process of maxilla; *2*, lacrimal groove; *3*, lacrimal bone; *4*, lamina papyracea; *5*, optic canal (foramen); *6*, superior orbital fissure; *7*, frontal bone; *8*, greater wing of the sphenoid; *9*, orbital plate of zygomatic bone; *10*, inferior orbital fissure; *11*, infraorbital groove; *12*, zygoma (malar bone); *13*, infraorbital foramen; *14*, supraorbital foramen. **C**, Schematic sagittal drawing of the orbital maxillary region. *1*, Frontal sinus; *2*, orbital plate of frontal bone; *3*, nasal bone; *4*, frontal process of maxilla; *5*, lacrimal groove; *6*, lacrimal bone; *7*, lamina papyracea; *8*, palatine bone; *9*, sphenoid bone; *10*, lesser wing of the sphenoid bone; *11*, optic canal; *12*, posterior ethmoid foramen; *13*, anterior ethmoid foramen; *14*, infraorbital canal (foramen); *15*, inferior concha; *16*, maxillary hiatus; *17*, palatine bone; *18*, sphenopalatine foramen opening into pterygopalatine fossa; *19*, vidian canal, opening into pterygopalatine fossa; *20*, pterygoid plate; *21*, alveolar process of maxilla.

and contains the nasolacrimal duct. The duct opens into the inferior meatus of the nasal cavity. Also in the medial wall are two canals for the anterior and posterior ethmoidal nerves and vessels. These canals are situated at the level of the floor of the anterior cranial fossa, as their lower margins are formed by the ethmoid bone and their upper margins are formed by the frontal bone. The anterior ethmoidal foramen is located at the frontal-ethmoidal suture and transmits the anterior ethmoidal vessels and nerve. The posterior ethmoidal foramen transmits the posterior ethmoidal vessels and nerve.[1,3–6] If an external ethmoidectomy is performed and the surgeons keep their bone incision caudal to a line between these canals, the incision will be into the ethmoid complex and not into the anterior cranial fossa.

## Orbital Floor

The inferior wall, or floor of the orbit, is relatively thin, and in most of its extent it is also the roof of the maxillary antrum or sinus (Figs. 9-3 and 9-4). The floor actually is made up of the orbital part of the maxilla, the orbital process of the zygomatic bone, and the orbital process of the palatine bone (Figs. 9-3 and 9-4). The orbital process of the palatine bone forms a small triangular area in the posteromedial corner of the orbital floor, where the floor meets the medial wall. The floor is not horizontal, but slants upward so that the posteromedial portion is higher than the flatter anterolateral portion.[1] Anteriorly, for about 1.0 to 1.5 cm, the floor is continuous with the lateral orbital wall. However, posterior to this area, the floor and lateral wall are separated by the inferior orbital fissure (Figs. 9-3 and 9-4). This fissure connects the orbit medially and posteriorly with the pterygopalatine fossa, and laterally and anteriorly with the retromaxillary and temporal fossae. The medial lip of the fissure is notched by the infraorbital groove, or fissure (Figs. 9-3 and 9-4), which passes forward in the orbital floor (usually in the middle third of the orbital floor), sinks into the orbital floor about 1 cm behind the orbital rim, and becomes the infraorbital canal that opens on the anterior face of the maxilla as the infraorbital foramen, about 1 cm below the inferior orbital rim (Figs. 9-3 and 9-4).[1] The groove, canal, and foramen transmit the infraorbital nerve, the continuation of the maxillary nerve ($V_2$).[1, 3–6] The inferior oblique muscle arises from the floor of the orbit just lateral to the opening of the nasolacrimal canal.[5, 6] It is the only extraocular muscle that does not originate from the orbital apex.

## Lateral Orbital Wall

The lateral wall of the orbit is the thickest wall, and it is formed by the orbital surface of the greater wing of the sphenoid bone behind and the orbital surface of the frontal process of the zygomatic bone in front (Figs. 9-3 and 9-4). The two bones meet at the sphenozygomatic suture. This aspect of the zygomatic bone presents the openings of two minute canals, one for the zygomaticofacial nerve and artery (near the junction of the floor and lateral walls) and the other for the zygomaticotemporal nerve and artery, which are slightly higher on this wall.[1, 5, 6] The lateral orbital tubercle, a small elevation of the orbital margin of the zygoma, lies approximately 11 mm below the frontal-zygomatic suture.

This important landmark is the site of attachment for (1) the check ligament of the lateral rectus muscle, (2) the suspensory ligament of the eyeball, (3) the lateral palpebral ligament, and (4) the aponeurosis of the levator palpebrae muscle.[5, 6]

## ORBITAL APEX

The apex of the orbit is basically formed by the optic canal and the superior orbital fissure.[1, 3] The optic canal and the superior and inferior orbital fissures allow various structures to enter and exit the orbit. The optic canal, having virtually no length at birth, becomes 4 mm long by 1 year of age and is up to 9 mm long in adults. The optic canal is directed forward, laterally (about 45° from the midsagittal plane), and somewhat downward (about 12° from the horizontal plane) and has orbital and intracranial openings (foramina). The configuration of the intracranial opening is oval, with its long axis in the horizontal plane. The configuration of the midportion of the optic canal is circular, and the configuration of the orbital opening is an oval with its long axis in the vertical plane. The optic canal is bounded medially by the body of the sphenoid bone (Figs. 9-5 and 9-6),

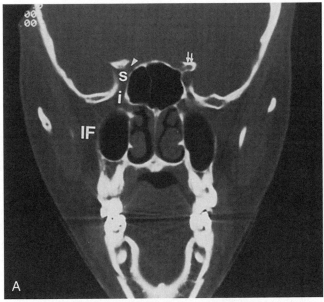

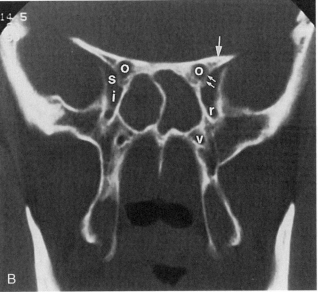

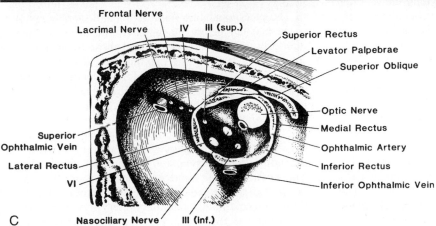

**FIGURE 9-5   A,** Coronal CT scan shows anterior clinoid (*arrows*); optic canal (*arrowhead*); superior orbital fissure (*S*); inferior orbital fissure (*i*); and lateral extension of interior orbital fissure into infratemporal fossa (*IF*). **B,** Coronal CT scan a few millimeters posterior to view in **A** shows anterior clinoid (*arrow*); optic canal (*o*); optic strut (*two small arrows*); superior orbital fissure (*s*); inferior orbital fissure (*i*); foramen rotundum (*r*); and pterygoid (*vidian*) canal (*v*). **C,** Frontal view of right orbital apex. The anulus of Zinn encircles the optic canal and the medial aspect of the superior orbital fissure. (**C** from Daniels DL, Pech P, Kay MC, et al. Orbital apex: correlative anatomic and CT study. AJNR 1985;6:705–710.)

Labels for Figure 9-5C:
Frontal Nerve
Lacrimal Nerve
IV
III (sup.)
Superior Rectus
Levator Palpebrae
Superior Oblique
Optic Nerve
Medial Rectus
Ophthalmic Artery
Inferior Rectus
Inferior Ophthalmic Vein
Superior Ophthalmic Vein
Lateral Rectus
VI
Nasociliary Nerve
III (inf.)

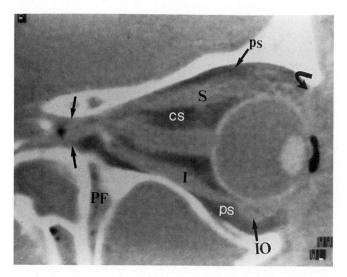

**FIGURE 9-6**   Orbital CT anatomy. Direct parasagittal CT scan of cadaver head shows peripheral orbital space (*ps*); central orbital (intraconal) space (*CS*); optic nerve; superior rectus muscle (*S*) and inferior rectus muscle (*I*); inferior oblique muscle (*IO*); orbital septum (*curved arrow*); and common tendon of Zinn (*arrows*). Periosteum (periorbita) lines bony orbit as orbital fascia and is loosely attached to bony orbit. Periosteum is united with dura mater and sheath of optic nerve at optic canal. Normally, periosteum cannot be differentiated from adjacent soft tissues. Periosteum is continuous with periosteum of the bones of the face and is also continuous with layer of dura at superior orbital fissure. Note continuity of periorbita with periosteum of pterygomaxillary fossa (*PF*). Infection or infiltrative process of pterygomaxillary fossa may invade orbital subperiosteal space (periorbita) or vice versa. (CT scan courtesy of FW Zonneveld.) (From Mafee MF et al. Orbital space-occupying lesions: role of CT and MRI: an analysis of 145 cases. Radiol Clin North Am 1987;25:529.)

superiorly by the superior root of the lesser wing of the sphenoid bone, and inferiorly and laterally by the inferior root (optic strut) of the lesser wing of the sphenoid bone.[4] Attached to the orbital wall surrounding the opening of the optic canal (and thus the optic nerve, ophthalmic artery, and sympathetic nerves) and extending around the lower aspect of the vertical portion of the superior orbital fissure (encircling cranial nerves III and VI) is the common tendinous ring (annulus) of Zinn, which gives origin to the inferior, medial, lateral, and superior rectus muscles (Fig. 9-6).[1] Usually the inferior ophthalmic vein is below the annulus of Zinn in the lower aspect of the superior orbital fissure. Above the annulus of Zinn and within the superior orbital fissure are the superior ophthalmic vein, the recurrent meningeal artery, the lacrimal nerve, the frontal nerve, and cranial nerve IV.

## Superior Orbital Fissure

Just inferolateral to the optic canal and separated from it by the optic strut is the superior orbital fissure, located between the greater and lesser wings of the sphenoid bone (Fig. 9-5). This fissure is approximately 22 mm long and is somewhat comma-shaped, with the bulbous or wider portion inferomedially and the thin portion superolaterally. The inferior part of the superior orbital fissure is divided from the superior part by the origin of the lateral rectus muscle.[1, 6]

Where the fissure begins to widen, its lower border is marked by a bony projection, often sharp in character, which gives attachment to the lateral part of the common tendinous ring of Zinn. The superior orbital fissure communicates with the middle cranial fossa and transmits the oculomotor, trochlear, and abducens nerves and the terminal branches of the ophthalmic nerve ($V_1$) and the ophthalmic veins. The lacrimal, frontal, and trochlear nerves traverse the narrow lateral part of the fissure, which also transmits the meningeal branch of the lacrimal artery and the occasional orbital branch of the middle meningeal artery. The trochlear nerve is situated more medially and lies just outside the common tendinous ring of Zinn.[1] The two divisions (superior and inferior) of the oculomotor nerve, the nasociliary nerve (a branch of the ophthalmic nerve), the abducens nerve, and the sympathetic plexus pass within the tendinous ring and therefore traverse the wider medial part of the fissure. They may be accompanied by the superior and inferior ophthalmic veins, but the superior ophthalmic vein may also accompany the trochlear nerve, and the inferior ophthalmic vein may pass through the medial end of the fissure below the ring.[1]

## Inferior Orbital Fissure

At the posterior aspect of the orbit, the inferior and lateral walls of the orbit are separated by the inferior orbital fissure (Figs. 9-3 to 9-5). The fissure lies just below the superior orbital fissure and is bounded above by the greater wing of the sphenoid, below by the maxilla and the orbital process of the palatine bone, and laterally by the zygomatic bone (the zygomaticomaxillary suture). The inferior orbital fissure extends obliquely as a gently curving continuation of the more medial pterygopalatine fossa (Figs. 9-6 and 9-7). The maxillary nerve is the most important structure traversing the inferior orbital fissure. The inferior orbital fissure also transmits the infraorbital vessels, the zygomatic nerve, and a few minute twigs from the pterygopalatine ganglion. Through the anterior part of the inferior orbital fissure, a vein passes to connect the inferior ophthalmic vein with the pterygoid plexus in the infratemporal fossa.[1] The inferior ophthalmic vein passes through its lower portion before entering the cavernous sinus.[6]

## Pterygopalatine Fossa

The pterygopalatine fossa is a small, narrow pyramidal space situated below the apex of the orbit and tapering inferiorly[7] (Fig. 9-6). It is bounded above by the body of the sphenoid, in front by the maxilla, behind by the pterygoid processes and the greater wing of the sphenoid, and medially by the palatine bone (Fig. 9-6). It communicates with the infratemporal fossa through the pterygomaxillary (retromaxillary) fissure. The five foramina that open into this fossa are (1) the foramen rotundum, (2) the pterygoid (vidian) canal, (3) the pharyngeal (palatovaginal) canal (Fig. 9-5B), (4) the sphenopalatine foramen, and (5) the pterygopalatine canal. The most important contents of the fossa are the maxillary nerve, the pterygopalatine (sphenopalatine) ganglion, and the terminal part of the maxillary artery. The maxillary nerve ($V_2$) runs from the inferior aspect of the cavernous sinus and exits the skull base through the foramen rotundum. The nerve then runs through the upper part of the pterygopalatine fossa, just above the pterygopalatine ganglion, and enters the inferior orbital fissure, passing forward and laterally to reach the posterior end of the infraorbital groove in the floor of the orbit. The nerve finally exits to the face through the infraorbital foramen.

Below and medial to the foramen rotundum, the pterygoid (vidian) canal (Fig. 9-5B) transmits the vidian nerve and vidian artery. The vidian nerve is formed by the joining of the superficial petrosal nerve (from the geniculate ganglion of the facial nerve containing parasympathetic and motor fibers) and the deep petrosal nerve, a branch from the sympathetic plexus on the internal carotid artery. The pterygoid nerve ends in the pterygopalatine ganglion.

The pharyngeal (palatovaginal) canal transmits the pharyngeal branch of the maxillary artery and the pharyngeal nerve, a branch of the pterygopalatine ganglion, to the roof of the pharynx. This nerve is distributed to the mucous membrane of the nasal part of the pharynx, behind the auditory tube.[1] The sphenopalatine foramen is on the medial wall of the pterygopalatine fossa. It is bounded above by the body of the sphenoid, in front by the orbital process of the palatine bone, behind by the sphenoidal process, and below by the upper border of the perpendicular plate of the palatine bone. It transmits the nasopalatine nerve and accompanying vessels from the pterygopalatine fossa to the nasal cavity.

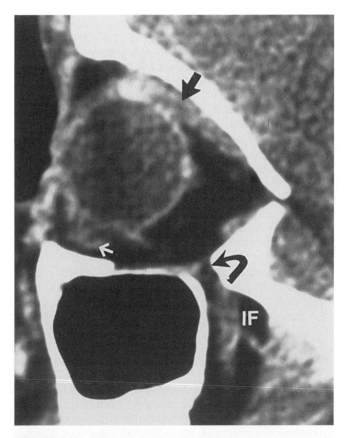

**FIGURE 9-7**    Direct parasagittal CT scan shows lateral extension of inferior orbital fissure (*curved arrow*) into infratemporal fossa (*IF*). Note inferior oblique muscle (*white arrow*) and superior rectus muscle (*black arrow*).

The pterygopalatine canal extends from the inferior margin of the pterygopalatine fossa, at the junction of the anterior and posterior walls, to the greater palatine canal opening in the palate. The greater palatine canal transmits the greater (anterior) and lesser (middle and posterior) palatine nerves and the palatine vessels. In general, the pterygopalatine ganglion supplies parasympathetic innervation to the pharynx, palate, nasal cavity, and lacrimal gland.[4] Thus, in summary, the pterygopalatine fossa communicates with five major anatomic regions: (1) the nasal cavity via the pterygopalatine (sphenopalatine) foramen, (2) the oral cavity via the pterygopalatine canals, (3) the infratemporal fossa via the pterygomaxillary (retromaxillary) fissure, (4) the orbit via the inferior orbital fissure, and (5) the middle cranial fossa via the foramen rotundum and the vidian canal.

## PERIORBITA

The periosteum of the bony orbit is known as the *periorbita* or the *orbital fascia*.[8] The periosteum is a specialized connective tissue structure that covers the bones. It consists of two strata: a superficial fibrous mantle and an active inner layer known as the *cambium*.[9] Duhamel is credited with the first scientific investigation of the osteogenic properties of the periosteum.[10] The periorbita (orbital fascia) is generally loosely adherent to the surrounding bones except at the anterior orbital margin, trochlear fossa, lacrimal crests, and margins of the fissures and canals.[1, 3, 4, 8] Anteriorly, it is continuous with the periosteum of the orbital margins (Figs. 9-6 to 9-8). Posteriorly, it is continuous with the dura of the optic nerve and the dura surrounding the superior orbital fissure. Thus, posteriorly located surgery or trauma may result in cerebrospinal fluid (CSF) leaks.[3] The dura matter is composed of a meningeal layer and a periosteal layer. These two layers are so closely bound together that they can be separated only with difficulty.[4, 7] After these layers pass through the optic foramen, however, they become separated. The meningeal layer continues as the sheath of the optic nerve, and the periosteal layer lines the bony orbit as the orbital fascia or periorbita. Numerous septae and fascial bands from various structures in the orbit are attached to the inner surface of this periosteum.[4] In front, the periorbita is fused with the orbital septum along the margins of the base (anterior rims) of the orbit.[5] The orbital septum is the continuation of the periosteum.[4, 8]

## ORBITAL SEPTUM AND EYELIDS

The orbital septum is a thin sheet of fibrous tissue that forms the fibrous layer of the eyelids and is attached to the margins of the bony orbit, where it is continuous with the periorbita. In the upper eyelid, it fuses with the levator aponeurosis. In the lower eyelid, the orbital septum fuses with the capsulopalpebral fascia (see below) approximately 3 to 5 mm below the inferior tarsal border. The fused capsulopalpebral fascia/orbital septum complex, along with a small contribution from the inferior tarsal smooth muscle, inserts on both the posterior and inferior tarsal surfaces, as well as on the tapered inferior border of the tarsus.[5] The

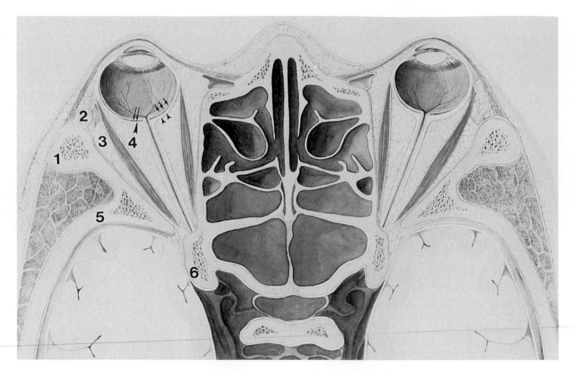

**FIGURE 9-8**    Diagram of the orbital-cranial region showing the zygomatic bone, (*1*); lacrimal gland, (*2*); peripheral orbital fatty reticulum, (*3*); central orbital fatty reticulum, (*4*); greater wing of the sphenoid, (*5*); lesser wing (anterior choroid) of the sphenoid, (*6*). Notice the retina (*three arrows*), choroid (*two arrows*), sclera (*arrowhead*), and Tenon capsule (*two arrowheads*).

palpebral portion of the orbicularis oculi muscle lies in front of the orbital septum (Fig. 9-8).[5] Moving from the skin inward toward the orbit, in general, each eyelid or palpebra consists of skin, subcutaneous areolar tissue, fibers of the orbicularis oculi, the tarsus and orbital septum, tarsal glands (meibomian), and conjunctiva. The conjunctiva is the transparent vascularized mucous membrane that covers the inner surfaces of the eyelids, and is reflected over the front part of the sclera and cornea.[1, 5] The line of reflection of the conjunctiva from the eyelids on the eyeball is called the *conjunctival fornix*. The palpebral conjunctiva is highly vascular, and its deeper part contains a considerable amount of lymphoid tissue, especially near the fornices. It is intimately adherent to the tarsi.[1] The ocular conjunctiva is loosely connected to the eyeball. On reaching the cornea, the ocular conjunctiva continues as the corneal epithelium.[1] The palpebral conjunctiva is covered by a nonkeratinized epithelium that contains the mucin-secreting goblet cells and the accessory lacrimal glands of Krause and Wolfring.[5] Secretions from these accessory glands form the major components of the lacrimal secretion, in contrast to the reflex tear secretion from the parasympathetically innervated main lacrimal gland.[5] Thus, anteriorly, the orbit can be considered as being closed by the orbital septum (Figs. 9-6, 9-8), which forms the fibrous layer of the eyelids. Within each eyelid, the orbital septum is thickened to form a tarsal plate. The levator palpebrae superioris has a broad anterior aponeurosis. Some of its fibers attach to the superior tarsal plate, while other terminal filaments interdigitate with the superior tarsal muscle (Müller's muscle), a smooth muscle that extends along the upper margin of the superior tarsal plate. As a result, some of the action of the levator palpebrae

superioris must extend through Müller's muscle before it affects the superior tarsal plate. In Horner's syndrome, the ptosis associated with that syndrome occurs because Müller's muscle is paralyzed and the upper eyelid cannot be elevated until this muscle has been passively stretched out to its full length by the action of the levator palpebrae superioris. This results in end-stage ptosis and minimal lid elevation after the complete contraction of the levator palpebrae superioris. A few fibers of the inferior rectus muscle are attached to the lower edge of the inferior tarsal plate.[5, 6] Posteriorly, each plate is covered by conjunctiva and has meibomian glands (modified sebaceous glands) embedded in its deep surface.

The tarsal plates consist of dense connective tissue and serve as the skeleton of the eyelids. They are attached to the orbital margin by the lateral and medial palpebral ligaments. The length (22 mm) and thickness (1 mm) of the upper and lower tarsal plates are similar.[6] The upper tarsus is more than twice as wide (11 mm) as the lower tarsus.[6] The tarsal (meibomian) glands are modified sweat glands, and their oily secretion passes through small orifices into the tear film.

## ORBICULARIS OCULI

The orbicularis oculi muscle is a flat, elliptical muscle that surrounds the orbital margin, extending onto the temporal region and cheek (orbital portion), onto the eyelids (palpebral portion), and behind the lacrimal sac (lacrimal portion) (Fig. 9-8). The palpebral portion of the orbicularis muscle consists of thin bundles of fibers that arise from the medial palpebral ligament (Fig. 9-8). The fibers sweep laterally and concentrically across the eyelids and in front of the orbital septum. At the lateral angle of the eye, the fibers interlace at the lateral palpebral raphe.

## TENON'S CAPSULE (FASCIA BULBI) AND TENON'S SPACE

Tenon's capsule is a fibroelastic membrane that envelops the eyeball from the optic nerve to the level of the ciliary muscle. Tenon's capsule is also called the *fascial sheath*, *fascia bulbi*, and *bulbar fascia* of the eyeball. This fibroelastic socket, which encloses the posterior four fifths of the eyeball, separates it from the central orbital fat (Figs. 9-6 and 9-8).[4, 8] Movement of the eyeball is facilitated by the fascia bulbi, which invests but does not adhere to the sclera. The bulbar fascia is discussed in Chapter 8.

## ORBITAL FATTY RETICULUM

Within the orbit, all structures are embedded in a fatty reticulum. The fibroelastic tissue that makes up the reticulum divides the fat into lobes and lobules.[4–8] The fatty reticulum is divided into (1) peripheral orbital fat, which is outside the muscle cone and its intermuscular membranes (Figs. 9-4, 9-6, and 9-8), and (2) central orbital fat, which is within the muscle cone (Figs. 9-6 and 9-8).

## EXTRAOCULAR MUSCLES

The six striated extraocular muscles, including the four recti and two oblique muscles, control eye movement (Figs. 9-6, 9-8). The rectus muscles arise from the annulus of Zinn, which is a funnel-shaped tendinous ring that encloses the optic foramen and the medial end of the superior orbital fissure, where it is continuous with the dural sheath of the optic nerve and periorbita.[3, 8–11] The annulus has an upper portion, called the *superior orbital tendon* or the *upper common tendon of Lockwood*, and a lower portion, called the *lower common tendon of Zinn*.[12] Because of this intimate relationship, apical disease frequently affects all of these structures simultaneously. In addition, surgical removal of optic nerve tumors must be done within the annulus, which is most safely entered superomedially after removing the orbital roof.[3] The inferior rectus muscle originates from the common tendon of Zinn below the optic foramen. It inserts into the inferior sclera 6.5 mm from the limbus. The superior rectus (the longest of the four recti) originates from the common tendon of Lockwood above the optic foramen and from the sheath of the optic nerve. It passes below the levator aponeurosis and inserts into the upper sclera 7.7 mm from the limbus. The medial rectus muscle (the thickest of the recti) arises from the upper tendon of Lockwood, the lower tendon of Zinn, and the sheath of the optic nerve and inserts 5.5 mm from the limbus.[11, 12] The lateral rectus originates from the lower common tendon of Zinn and the upper common tendon of Lockwood and inserts 6.9 mm from the limbus.[12] The superior oblique (longest and thinnest of the extraocular muscles) originates from the

periosteum of the body of the sphenoid bone, above and medial to the annulus of Zinn and the origin of the medial rectus.[11, 12] It passes anteriorly along the upper part of the medial orbital wall as a slender tendon and enters the trochlea, a fibrocartilaginous ring lined with a synovial-type sheath.[13] The tendon slides through the trochlea and then turns sharply posterolaterally and downward beneath the superior rectus muscle to insert in the lateral sclera, behind the equator of the eye. The inferior oblique muscle is the only extrinsic eye muscle that originates not from the orbital apex but from a shallow depression in the orbital plate of the maxilla at the anteromedial corner of the orbital floor just posterolateral to the orifice of the nasolacrimal duct. It passes under the inferior rectus and runs posteriorly, laterally, and superiorly before inserting into the inferolateral aspect of the globe.[14] All extraocular muscles are about 40 mm in length except for the 37 mm inferior oblique.[15] One important difference among these muscles is the ratio of tendinous tissue to muscle fibers. The inferior oblique muscle contains essentially no tendon, and the superior oblique has 20 mm of tendon.[15]

### Spiral of Tillaux

The four rectus muscles insert on the anterior portion of the globe in a configuration called the *spiral of Tillaux*.[6] The medial rectus muscle inserts closest to the limbus, and the superior rectus muscle inserts farthest from the limbus. The relationship between the muscle insertions and the ora serrata is clinically important, as a malpositioned bridle suture could pass through the insertion of the superior rectus muscle and perforate the retina.[6]

### Retractors

The retractors of the upper eyelid are the levator muscle, the levator aponeurosis, and the sympathetically innervated superior tarsal muscle (Müller's muscle).[5] In the lower eyelid, the retractors are the capsulopalpebral fascia and the inferior tarsal muscle (Müller's muscle).[5]

### Levator Muscle

The levator palpebrae superioris muscle originates in the apex of the orbit from the periorbita of the lesser wing of the sphenoid, just above the annulus of Zinn.[5] The body of the levator muscle overlies the superior rectus as it travels anteriorly toward the lid. The levator muscle and its tendon in adults is 50 to 60 mm long. The muscle portion, which is approximately 40 mm long, is innervated by the superior division of the oculomotor nerve and elevates the upper eyelid. The levator palpebra is often called the *seventh extraocular muscle*. The superior transverse ligament (Whitnall's ligament) is a condensation of the sheath of the levator muscle located in the approximate area of the transition from levator muscle to levator aponeurosis.[5] Whitnall's ligament functions primarily as a suspensory support for the upper eyelid and the superior orbital tissues.[5] Its analog in the lower eyelid is Lockwood's ligament.[5] As the levator aponeurosis continues forward, it inserts into the anterior surface of the tarsus and by medial and lateral horns into the canthal tendons.[5, 6] The lateral horn of the levator aponeurosis is strong, and it divides the lacrimal gland into orbital and palpebral lobes, attaching firmly to the orbital tubercle.[5] As mentioned, the superior tarsal muscle (Müller's muscle) also inserts on the superior tarsal border, and this muscle provides approximately 2 mm of lift for the upper eyelid. If this muscle is paralyzed, as in Horner's syndrome, a mild proptosis will result.[5]

## Lower Eyelid Retractors

The capsulopalpebral fascia is the lower eyelid analog to the levator palpebra muscle and aponeurosis.[5] It is a layer of dense connective tissue that originates at the capsulopalpebral head from the terminal muscle fibers and tendon of the inferior rectus muscle.[5] The capsulopalpebral head divides into two portions as it encircles and fuses with the sheath of the inferior oblique muscle. Anterior to the inferior oblique muscle, the two portions of the capsulopalpebral head join to form Lockwood's suspensory ligament, where it becomes known as the *capsulopalpebral fascia*.[5] The capsulopalpebral fascia fuses with the orbital septum. This fused fascial layer proceeds upward to insert on the inferior tarsus.[5]

## Movements of Eyelid and Eyeball

The levator palpebra superioris is the main, striated voluntary muscle that elevates the upper eyelid. It is opposed by the orbicularis oculi.[1, 6] When the smaller inferior stratum of nonstriated Müller's muscle is denervated, it is responsible for the ptosis in Horner's syndrome. Blinking results in distribution of the lacrimal secretions. The height at which the upper lid is maintained is in part related to the brightness of the light entering the eye. In very bright conditions, the lid is lower, thereby limiting glare.

Within its fascial sheath, the eyeball is rotated by the extraocular muscles, which displace the gaze upward (elevation), downward (depression), medially (adduction), and laterally (abduction). Rotation about an anteroposterior axis (torsion) may also occur.[11, 12, 14, 15] The actions of the medial and lateral recti are adduction and abduction, respectively. They are antagonists, and by reciprocal adjustment of their lengths, the visual axis can be swept through a horizontal arc. The superior rectus muscle's primary action is elevation. This muscle also has a secondary, less powerful action of medial rotation (adduction).[1, 12] Its primary antagonist is the inferior rectus, which depresses and adducts the eyeball. The superior oblique muscle acts on the eyeball from the trochlea. Because the attachment of the inferior oblique is for practical purposes vertically inferior to this, both muscles approach the eyeball at the same angle, being attached in approximately similar positions in the superior and inferior posterolateral quadrants of the eyeball.[1] From these attachments, it is easy to understand that the inferior oblique elevates the gaze and the superior oblique depresses it. Both oblique muscles produce abduction.[1, 12] Like the superior and inferior recti, the two oblique muscles have opposed forces with respect to the other (antagonist). However, acting together, they can assist the lateral rectus in abduction of the visual axis.[1]

## Blood Supply to the Extraocular Muscles

The blood supply for the extraocular muscles is derived from the inferior and superior muscular branches of the ophthalmic artery, the lacrimal artery, and the infraorbital artery. Except for the lateral rectus muscle, each rectus muscle receives two anterior ciliary arteries that communicate with the major arteriole circle of the ciliary body. The lateral rectus is supplied by a single vessel derived from the lacrimal artery.

## OPTIC NERVE

The optic nerve is not a nerve but actually a nerve fiber tract of the central nervous system formed by over 1 million axons that originate in the ganglion cell layer of the retina.[6, 16] The nerve has an organization similar to that of the white matter of the brain. Its fibers are surrounded by glial rather than Schwann cell sheaths.[6, 16] The optic nerve (Fig. 9-6), along with the ophthalmic artery, traverses the optic canal and passes forward and laterally within the cone of rectus muscles to enter the eyeball just medial to its posterior pole. The optic nerve is about 3.5 to 5.5 cm long and about 3 to 4 mm in diameter.[3, 6] It is divided into four portions: intraocular (1 mm), intraorbital (3 cm), intracanalicular (5 to 6 mm), and intracranial (1 cm).[3] The intraocular portion can be divided into three parts: (1) prelaminar, (2) laminar, and (3) retrolaminar. The surface of the prelaminar portion is visible ophthalmoscopically. It is a $1.5 \times 1.75$ mm oval with a disc-shaped depression (the physiologic cup) located slightly temporal to its geometric center.[5, 6] The optic nerve head (optic disc) is composed of nonmyelinated axons from the retinal ganglion cells, blood vessels, and astrocytes that form a thin basal lamina on its inner surface. Myelinated nerve fibers in the retina result from oligodendrocytes that have migrated beyond the lamina cribrosa and have formed a lamellar envelope around ganglion cell axons.[5, 6] As ganglion cell axons enter the optic nerve head, they become segregated into bundles or fascicles by neuroglial cells. These astrocytes enclose groups of nerve fibers throughout the ocular and orbital portions of the optic nerve.[5] The bundles continue to be separated by connective tissue all the way to the chiasm. This connective tissue is derived from the pia mater and is known as the *septal tissue*.[5, 6] The retinal layers terminate as they approach the edge of the optic disc. The laminar portion of the optic disc is composed of astrocytes, elastic fibers, collagenous connective tissue from the scleral lamina, and small blood vessels. The lamina cribrosa functions as a scaffold for the optic nerve axons. The retrolaminar portion extends from the lamina cribrosa to the apex of the orbit. From the lamina cribrosa centrally, the retinal ganglion cells become myelinated as the cross-sectional diameter of the nerve increases to approximately 3 mm. After passing through the optic canal, the optic nerves lie above the ophthalmic arteries, and above and medial to the internal carotid artery. The anterior cerebral arteries cross over the optic nerves and are joined by the anterior communicating artery. The optic nerves then pass posteriorly to join in the optic chiasm.

## Meningeal Sheaths (Dura, Arachnoid, Pia)

The dura, the outer layer, is composed of collagenous connective tissue. The arachnoid is made up of fine collagenous fibers arranged in a loose meshwork lined by endothelial cells. The innermost layer, the pia, is made up of fine collagenous and elastic fibers and is highly vascularized. Elements from both the arachnoid and the pia are continuous with the optic nerve septa. The pial septa, which originate in the region of the posterior lamina cribrosa, enclose all neurofascicles. The septa continue throughout the orbital and intracanalicular portion of the nerve and end in the intracranial portion. They are composed of collagen, elastic tissue, fibroblasts, nerves, and small arterioles and venules. They provide mechanical support for the nerve bundles and nutrition to the axons and glial cells. Meningothelial cells cover the pia mater. The arachnoid mater is continuous with the subarachnoid space. It ends at the level of the lamina cribrosa. It is composed of collagenous tissue, small amounts of elastic tissue, and meningothelial cells. The dura mater encases the optic nerve and comprises the outer layer of the meningeal sheaths. It is 0.3 to 0.5 mm thick and consists of dense bundles of collagen and elastic tissue fused anteriorly with the outer layers of the sclera. The meninges of the optic nerve are supplied by sensory fibers, which accounts for the pain experienced by patients with inflammatory optic nerve diseases.

## Blood Supply of the Optic Nerve

The prelaminar and lamina cribrosa regions are supplied by branches of the posterior ciliary arteries, while the surface of the optic disc is supplied by retinal arterioles that are branches of the central retinal artery or from branches of small cilioretinal arteries.[5, 6, 16] The intraorbital part of the optic nerve is supplied by intraneural branches of the central retinal artery and multiple recurrent pial branches arising from both the peripapillary choroid and the central retinal and ophthalmic arteries.[5] The intracanalicular portion of the optic nerve is supplied almost exclusively by the ophthalmic artery. The intracranial portion of the optic nerve is supplied primarily by branches of both the internal carotid artery and the ophthalmic artery. The actual distance from the back of the globe to the orbital apex is 20 mm. Thus, from the optic foramen, the optic nerve takes a tortuous, S-shaped course to the back of the globe. This longer length of the optic nerve allows movement of the eye without tension on the nerve. As mentioned, the intraorbital portion of the optic nerve increases to 3 mm in diameter due to myelination of the nerve fibers and surrounding meningeal sheaths. The orbital portion of the optic nerve lies within the muscle cone. Before passing into the optic canal, the nerve is surrounded by the annulus of Zinn, formed by the origins of the rectus muscles. The superior and medial rectus muscles partially originate from the sheath of the optic nerve. This may explain why patients with retrobulbar

neuritis complain of pain when moving their eyes.[5] As previously mentioned, the optic nerve is covered by three layers: the pia mater, the arachnoid, and the dura, which sheathe the nerve and extend from the optic canal forward to the globe. The pia mater is highly vascular and is attached tightly to the optic nerve.[16, 17] The subarachnoid space is filled with CSF in continuity with the intracranial subarachnoid space. The subdural space surrounding the optic nerve, however, has no direct connection to the intracranial subdural space.[16, 17] The optic nerve is fixed to the apex of the orbit by fusion of the pia mater, the arachnoid membrane, and the dura mater to the periosteum at the optic canal.[17] At the optic canal, the dural sheath of the nerve fuses to the periosteum so that the nerve is completely immobilized.[5] The ophthalmic artery is encased by dura in the optic canal, where it lies inferolateral to the nerve. At the orbital end of the canal, it loses the dural coat and crosses medially in the intraconal space.[17]

## PERIPHERAL NERVES

Several nerves reach the orbit from the middle cranial fossa and the pterygopalatine fossae. The optic nerve traverses the optic canal. Other nerves gain access to the orbit through the orbital fissures.

## SENSORY INNERVATION

The major sensory innervation of the orbit is via the ophthalmic ($V_1$) and maxillary ($V_2$) divisions of the trigeminal nerve. The trigeminal nerve is the largest cranial nerve and possesses both sensory and motor divisions. The sensory portion ($V_1$ and $V_2$) subserves the greater part of the scalp, forehead, face, eyelids, eyes, lacrimal gland, extraocular muscles, ears, and dura. The motor portion innervates the muscles of mastication and the tensor tympani through the branches of the mandibular nerve. The trigeminal nuclear complex extends from the midbrain to the upper cervical segments, often as caudal as $C_4$.[5, 6] The cell bodies of the ophthalmic nerve are in the semilunar (Gasserian) ganglion. From the ganglion, the nerve courses along the lateral wall of the cavernous sinus, below the oculomotor and trochlear nerves, and enters the orbit through the superior orbital fissure. The ophthalmic nerve, before entering the orbit, divides into lacrimal, frontal, and nasociliary nerves, each of which enters the orbit through the superior orbital fissure.[3, 6] The frontal (largest branch) and lacrimal (smallest branch) branches of the ophthalmic nerve enter the orbit outside of the annulus of Zinn and run forward between the periorbita and the levator complex to supply the forehead and lacrimal gland. The nasociliary branch is intraconal, crosses medially over the optic nerve, continues forward along the medial wall of the orbit below the superior rectus and superior oblique muscles, and terminates as the ethmoidal (anterior and posterior) and infratrochlear nerves.[6] Its branches include one to the ciliary ganglion and two long ciliary nerves.[3, 6] The long ciliary nerves carry sympathetic vasoconstrictor fibers to supply vessels within the eyeball.[6]

# MOTOR INNERVATION

## Oculomotor Nerve (III)

The nucleus of the oculomotor nerve is in the midbrain tegmentum. The nerve appears in the interpeduncular fossa, courses above the other nerves in the most cephalic, lateral wall of the cavernous sinus, and enters the orbit through the superior orbital fissure. It has superior and inferior divisions, which are often formed before entering the orbit.[6] The nerve enters the muscle cone within the annulus of Zinn as a superior division (supplying the levator and superior rectus) and an inferior division (supplying the medial and inferior recti and the inferior oblique).

## Trochlear Nerve (IV)

The nucleus of the trochlear nerve is in the midbrain tegmentum. Its fibers leave the central nervous system through the anterior medullary velum dorsally, cross to the opposite side, and pass rostrally and caudally to run in the lateral wall of the cavernous sinus between the oculomotor (III) and ophthalmic ($V_1$) nerves. The trochlear nerve then crosses the oculomotor nerve and passes through the superior orbital fissure above the other nerves to supply the superior oblique muscle.[5, 6]

## Abducens Nerve (VI)

The nucleus of the abducens nerve is in the tegmentum of the pons. Its fibers leave the central nervous system in the ventral groove between the medulla and pons, and pass through the cavernous sinus between the internal carotid artery and the ophthalmic nerve ($V_1$). The abducens nerve then enters the orbit through the superior orbital fissure and passes forward on the inner surface of the lateral rectus, which it supplies.[5, 6]

# OTHER NERVES

The seventh cranial nerve is the motor supply for the orbicularis oculi and its sensory division; the nervus intermedius gives the parasympathetic supply to the lacrimal gland. The facial nerve enters the parotid gland and then divides into upper temporal facial and lower cervical facial branches. It innervates the orbicularis via the upper division, which forms the temporofrontal and zygomatic branches.[3]

# AUTONOMIC NERVES

The ciliary ganglion lies 1.5 to 2 cm behind the eyeball, lateral to the optic nerve and medial to the lateral rectus muscle. The ciliary ganglion measures about 1 to 2 mm in diameter. It receives sensory fibers from the nasociliary nerve, parasympathetic fibers from the oculomotor nerve, and sympathetic fibers from the internal carotid plexus in the cavernous sinus (via the superior orbital fissure).[3, 6] Only the parasympathetic fibers synapse in the ganglion. The sensory root subserves the cornea, iris, and ciliary body through short ciliary nerves that pass from the anterior part of the ciliary ganglion into the eyeball.[6] The parasympathetic fibers supply the ciliary muscle and iris sphincter (constricts pupil). The preganglionic fibers of the parasympathetics to the sphincter muscle arise in the Edinger-Westphal nucleus of the midbrain, travel with the oculomotor nerve, and run in its inferior division to end by synapsing in the ciliary ganglion. The postganglionic fibers arise from cells of the ciliary ganglion and leave the ganglion by short ciliary nerves that pierce the sclera and run to the iris. The sympathetic fibers supply ocular vessels, the iris dilator (by means of the ciliary nerves), the lacrimal gland, and the sympathetic muscles (Müller's muscles) of the upper and lower eyelids. The sympathetic fibers to the dilator pupillae muscle pass through the ciliary ganglion without synapse and run with the short ciliary nerves. The preganglionic fibers of the sympathetics to the dilator pupillae arise in the intermediolateral gray column of the upper thoracic cord, enter the sympathetic trunk, and ascend in the cervical sympathetic trunk to end by synapses in the superior cervical ganglion.[5] The postganglionic fibers arise in cells of the superior cervical ganglion and ascend through the carotid and cavernous nervous plexuses. Some fibers join the ophthalmic nerve to continue in its nasociliary branch and are carried to the eye with the long ciliary branches of this nerve. Other fibers from the cavernous plexus enter the sympathetic "root" of the ciliary ganglion, pass through this ganglion without synapse, and run with the short ciliary nerves.[5] Still other intraorbital sympathetic fibers travel with the oculomotor nerve to the smooth muscle component of the levator palpebrae superioris and inferior recti (Müller's muscles).[6]

The preganglionic parasympathetic fibers of the lacrimal gland arise from cells in the superior salivatory nucleus and run in the nervus intermedius with the facial nerve. They then leave the facial nerve, at the geniculate ganglion, as the greater superficial petrosal nerve, which becomes part of the nerve of the pterygoid (vidian) canal, to enter and synapse in the pterygopalatine ganglion. The postganglionic fibers arise from the cells of the pterygopalatine ganglion, pass through the pterygopalatine nerves to the maxillary nerve, and then pass through the zygomatic branch of this nerve.[5] These fibers then enter the zygomaticotemporal branch of the zygomatic nerve in the orbit and communicate with the lacrimal branch of the ophthalmic nerve to reach the lacrimal gland. The preganglionic sympathetic fibers of the lacrimal gland arise in the intermediolateral gray column of the upper thoracic cord, enter the sympathetic trunk, ascend in the cervical sympathetic trunk, and end by synapses in the superior cervical ganglion.[5] The postganglionic sympathetic fibers arise in cells of the superior cervical ganglion, pass through the carotid plexus, and continue rostrally in the deep petrosal nerve, to join the superficial greater petrosal nerve to become the pterygoid (vidian) nerve. Then the fibers pass through the pterygopalatine ganglion, without synapse, and are distributed in a manner similar to that of the postganglionic parasympathetic fibers to reach the lacrimal gland.[5]

## VASCULAR ANATOMY

The major arterial supply to the orbit is from branches of the ophthalmic artery. This artery usually arises from the distal end of the cavernous sinus segment of the internal carotid artery. Rarely, it may arise from the middle meningeal artery and enter the orbit through the superior orbital fissure.[3] In the optic canal, it courses below and lateral to the optic nerve within the dural sheath, and at the orbital apex it penetrates laterally through the dura. In 82.6% of subjects it crosses to the medial orbit over the optic nerve, and in the remaining 17.4% of subjects the artery courses under the nerve.[3] The branches of the ophthalmic artery, with some variations in origin, are the lacrimal, supraorbital, anterior and posterior ethmoidal, nasofrontal, and dorsonasal arteries. The branches for the eyeball include the central artery of the retina and the ciliary arteries. The central artery of the retina is the first branch of the ophthalmic artery.[6] It crosses the optic nerve, pierces it, and runs in its center to spread over the retina.[5] The ciliary arteries are arranged in three groups: short posterior ciliary, long posterior ciliary, and anterior ciliary arteries.[5] The posterior ciliary arteries supply the globe via 15 to 20 short (to the choroid and ciliary processes and the optic nerve head) and 2 long (to the ciliary muscle, iris, and the anterior choroid) branches.[3] The long posterior ciliary arteries enter the sclera on either side of the optic nerve and run between the choroid and sclera to the ciliary body, where their branches form the anterior major arterial circle. The anterior ciliary arteries arise from the muscular branches that run with the tendons of the recti muscles and form the vascular zone under the conjunctiva. These arteries then pierce the sclera to join the major arterial circle.[5] The lacrimal artery branches into the recurrent meningeal, zygomatic, glandular, and lateral palpebral arteries (which form the arcades of the lid). The ophthalmic artery frequently has anastomotic branches to the external carotid system, by means of the middle meningeal and lacrimal arteries, which pass through the superior orbital fissure, and by means of the anterior deep temporal, superficial temporal, and lacrimal arteries.[3]

## VENOUS DRAINAGE OF THE ORBIT AND EYEBALL

The venous blood from the eyeball and adjacent structures drains into the valveless inferior and superior ophthalmic veins. The superior ophthalmic vein drains into the cavernous sinus via the superior orbital fissure. The inferior ophthalmic vein passes through the inferior orbital fissure, anastomosing with the pterygoid venous plexus.[1, 3, 6] Both the superior and inferior ophthalmic veins communicate with the veins of the face.[1, 6] The superior ophthalmic vein is the larger of these two veins and arises behind the medial part of the upper eyelid by the union of a branch from the supraorbital vein and a branch from the facial vein (angular, supraorbital). The branch from the supraorbital vein enters the orbit through the supraorbital notch, while the branch from the facial vein pierces the orbital septum. The superior ophthalmic vein receives tributaries that correspond to most of the branches of the ophthalmic artery.

It communicates with the central vein of the retina, and near the apex of the orbit it commonly receives the inferior ophthalmic vein. The superior ophthalmic vein also receives the two vorticose veins from the upper part of the eyeball (the vorticose veins correspond to the posterior ciliary veins). It has three sections, the first extending posterolaterally to the medial border of the superior rectus. The second section enters the muscle cone and passes superolaterally to the optic nerve and beneath the superior rectus muscle. The third section extends posteromedially along the lateral border of the superior rectus and extends to the superior orbital fissure.[3] The more variable inferior ophthalmic vein arises from a venous plexus on the anterior part of the floor of the orbital cavity. It communicates with the facial vein over the inferior orbital margin and with the pterygoid venous plexus through the inferior orbital fissure. It passes posteriorly in the orbital fat on the inferior rectus muscle and receives muscular branches and the two inferior vorticose veins from the lower part of the eyeball. The inferior ophthalmic vein often forms inferolaterally as a plexus and passes posteriorly adjacent to the inferior rectus muscle. It anastomoses with the superior ophthalmic vein and has a similar branch that connects with the pterygoid plexus through the inferior orbital fissure.[3] It may pass through the lower part of the superior orbital fissure and empty directly into the cavernous sinus.

## LACRIMAL APPARATUS

The lacrimal gland lies in the superolateral angle of the orbit, in a shallow fossa (lacrimal fossa) behind the upper eyelid, and is deeply indented by the lateral border of the tendon of the levator palpebra superioris (Fig. 9-8).[1, 3, 17] The gland weighs 78 g and measures $20 \times 12 \times 5$ mm.[3] It is divided into palpebral and orbital (larger) lobes by the lateral border of the levator aponeurosis.[3] The orbital lobe is superior to the palpebral lobe. Small ducts (10 to 12) open from the deep surface of the gland into the conjunctival sac, and resection of the palpebral lobe functionally destroys the gland.[3] This is important to remember when attempting to biopsy the lacrimal gland. The borders of the gland are related anteriorly to the orbital septum, posteriorly to the periorbital fat, and medially to the superior rectus, globe, and lateral rectus (Fig. 9-8). The inferior surface rests on the lateral rectus.[3] The lacrimal gland is a serous gland. The gland has a nodular surface with a fine connective tissue pseudocapsule.[3] The gland is supported by Whitnall's ligament and by septal attachments to the superior periorbita. The lacrimal artery penetrates it posteriorly, and the vein from it drains into the superior ophthalmic vein. Its lymphatic drainage is by means of the lid and conjunctiva to the preauricular nodes.[3] The lacrimal nerve, and sometimes branches of the zygomatic nerve, carry the sensory afferents. The parasympathetic efferents are by the nervus intermedius, facial, greater superficial petrosal, vidian, sphenopalatine ganglion, infraorbital, and lacrimal nerves.[1, 3] The sympathetic efferents are from the internal carotid plexus through the sphenopalatine (pterygopalatine) ganglion. In addition to the main lacrimal gland, there are accessory glands (of Krause and Wolfring) in the lids and conjunctiva.

There are 20 to 40 glands of Krause in the upper fornix and 6 to 8 in the lower fornix. The glands of Wolfring are fewer, consisting of three at the upper border of the superior tarsus and one at the lower border of the inferior tarsus.[3] Tears produced by the gland pass medially toward the lacrimal puncta across the surface of the cornea, assisted by blinking of the eyelids. Evaporation of the fluid is retarded by the oily secretion of the tarsal glands. Tears are drained into the lacrimal sac through the lacrimal canaliculi of the upper and lower lids. The canaliculi originate at the puncta and have a 2 mm vertical portion and an 8 mm horizontal portion, which join into a common canaliculus. The superior canaliculus first is directed upward, then medially and downward. The inferior canaliculus first descends and then is directed medially. The common canaliculus enters the lateral wall of the lacrimal sac by means of the valve of Rösenmuller, which prevents reflux.[3] The lacrimal sac lies in the lacrimal groove, which is formed by the lacrimal bone and the frontal process of the maxillary bone.[1] The lacrimal canaliculi are lined by squamous epithelium, whereas the sac and nasolacrimal duct are lined by columnar epithelium, goblet cells, and ciliated cells. The lacrimal sac is 13 to 15 mm in vertical length. The tears drain through the nasolacrimal duct just beneath the inferior turbinate through a fold in the duct (called the *valve of Hasner*) in the lateral wall of the nasal cavity (also see Chapter 10).[3]

## TECHNIQUE FOR ORBITAL CT AND MR IMAGING

### General Considerations

CT and MR imaging are the two modalities commonly used for imaging the orbit. Each has advantages and disadvantages. In general, CT is the modality of choice for bony detail and for detecting calcifications and foreign bodies, but irradiation to the orbital structures is a disadvantage. The radiation dose to the lens, although less than that of a complex motion tomography orbital series, averages about 5 cGy per imaging plane. MR imaging, on the other hand, has no known biologic side effects and is superior to CT when evaluating soft-tissue detail in the globe. MR imaging is generally considered equivalent to or slightly better than CT when evaluating the orbital soft tissues. However, MR imaging should not be used for the evaluation of the orbit whenever a ferromagnetic foreign body is suspected to be present.

### Computed Tomography

A routine CT examination of the orbits includes contiguous axial and coronal sectioning with a 3 mm slice thickness. When there is a suspicion of a smaller lesion, thinner sections (two 1 mm sections) should be obtained. Such thin sections are essential for optimal demonstration of the optic nerve's anatomy and pathology. Thin slices have the advantage of less volume averaging and thus provide finer spatial resolution. The radiologist should always tailor the examination according to the clinical information and the preliminary diagnosis. For foreign bodies, it is important

to obtain 1.0 to 1.5 mm axial sections to increase the sensitivity for detection of smaller objects. Provided there is no patient motion, it is often unnecessary to obtain additional direct coronal sections for the localization of foreign bodies because the use of computer reformatting is helpful in producing images in other planes, especially if a multidetector scanner is utilized. For foreign bodies or lesions at the 6 or 12 o'clock position in a coronal view, it may be advisable to obtain direct coronal sections. However, the use of multidetector CT may obviate the need for such multiplanar acquisitions. For lesions of the globe, thin sectioning (1.0 to 1.5 mm) is exceedingly important, because one can easily miss an ocular lesion on routine 5 mm sections.[17] For bony lesions or orbital fractures, in addition to the routine study, retrospective high-resolution extended bone scale images should be obtained (4000 ms window width, 700 to 800 window level).[17]

For orbital CT scanning, the need for intravenous (IV) contrast medium administration should be determined by the clinical information and is best left to the discretion of the radiologist. Contrast material uniformly increases the density of most intraorbital soft-tissue structures.[18] Although it is not always easy to discriminate between orbital lesions based on their patterns of enhancement, contrast material is often necessary to evaluate their vascular characteristics and, more importantly, to evaluate any intracranial extension of an orbital lesion. Not uncommonly, an apical orbital mass may be an extension of an intracranial lesion such as a meningioma, which can be readily missed on a noncontrast CT study. In general, a contrast medium is not used when evaluating for foreign bodies, uncomplicated orbital fractures, uncomplicated thyroid ophthalmopathy, morphologic changes in or variations of the extraocular muscles, dermoid cysts (noninfected and unruptured), and bony lesions such as osteoma, osteoid osteoma, fibrous dysplasia, and Paget's disease. Contrast-enhanced CT is usually necessary in patients with osteogenic or chondrogenic sarcomas or metastatic bone disease.

The axial sections normally are obtained roughly parallel to the infraorbital-meatal line.[17, 18] This can be easily determined by obtaining a lateral digital scout view (scanogram). The inferior section should include the upper portion of the maxillary sinuses, and the upper section should include the sella and the entire frontal sinuses. For all orbital and ocular tumors, additional postcontrast 10 mm axial sections of the remainder of the head are usually obtained. Although brain metastasis from orbital and ocular tumors is uncommon, the additional sections may provide information about unsuspected lesions (meningioma, aneurysm, and arteriovenous malformation).[17] The coronal sections are obtained roughly perpendicular to the infraorbital-meatal line. However, in many instances, the angle of the coronal sections is made more oblique (semicoronal) when the patient has many dental fillings or other metallic prostheses. Patient positioning for imaging in the coronal plane can be in either the prone or supine position, and as for the axial sections, the coronal plane study can be determined easily by obtaining a lateral digital scout view of the orbit. The coronal examination of the orbits should be tailored according to the clinical information and the findings on the axial sections. In patients suffering from visual loss and when evaluating the intracranial extension of an apical lesion, the coronal sections should be extended posteriorly to include the optic chiasm. For lesions involving the anterior ethmoid air cells and nasal cavity, and for lesions arising from the nasolacrimal sac and duct, coronal sections should be extended anteriorly to include the nasal bones.

Almost all CT scanners are capable of performing computer reformation of compiled data from axial sections into coronal, sagittal, or oblique planes. Although the quality of the images may be inferior to those obtained with direct scanning, in many instances additional information can be obtained, particularly if high-quality, thin (1.5 to 3 mm) direct axial or coronal sections are available. It should be noted, however, that the quality of such images on the newer multidetector CT scanners is excellent. If a multidetector scanner is not available, direct sagittal plane scans of the craniofacial structures can be achieved by laying the patient on a separate support and using a special head holder that is fitted to the standard tabletop.[19, 20]

## MR Imaging Techniques

Almost all of the MR images presented in this section were obtained with a 1.5 Tesla Signa unit (General Electric, Milwaukee). Using a head coil, single echo spin-echo (SE) pulse sequences were obtained with a repetition time (TR) of 400 to 800 ms and an echo time (TE) of 20 to 25 ms (TR/TE, 400 to 800/20 to 25 ms). Multiecho SE pulse sequences were obtained with a TR of 1500 to 2800 ms and a TE of 20 to 100 ms. Although each examination should be specifically tailored to the patient's problem, the routine MR imaging examination of the orbit should include short TR, short TE sagittal images, 4 to 5 mm in thickness with 1 to 1.5 mm intersection spacing, using the routine head coil. These studies were most often performed with one excitation, a $256 \times 192$ or $256 \times 256$ matrix size, and a 20 to 24 cm field of view. Following the sagittal T1-weighted scans, an axial multiecho SE sequence (TR/TE 2000 to 2800/20, 80 ms) was obtained to include the entire orbital structures. For this multiecho SE pulse sequence, a section thickness of 4 to 5 mm with a 1.5 to 2.5 mm intersection gap was used, with a matrix size of $256 \times 192$ and a 20 cm field of view. An additional single echo or multiecho SE sequence in the coronal plane was obtained according to the findings on the sagittal and axial sections. Because T1-weighted images provide more spatial resolution than T2-weighted images, if more anatomic detail is essential, coronal T1-weighted images are preferred. On the other hand, T2-weighted images provide more contrast resolution than T1-weighted images, and if there is a need for more pathologic detail, coronal multiple SE pulse sequences are obtained (TR/TE, 2000/20, 80 ms). For optic nerve lesions, additional parasagittal images are obtained by using a head coil. For some of the orbital lesions, additional images were obtained using a surface coil. Images with a surface coil provide better spatial resolution than images obtained with a head coil. However, because of signal dropout, an apical lesion or intracranial extension of an orbital lesion cannot be fully evaluated. Paramagnetic contrast material, a gadolinium complex of diethylenetriamine pentaacetic acid (Gd-DTPA), should be used for suspected orbital abscesses,

meningiomas, schwannomas, neurofibromas, hemangiopericytomas, fibrous histiocytomas, lacrimal gland tumors, metastases, lymphomas, pseudotumors, other specific or nonspecific orbital masses, and optic nerve lesions including optic neuritis. Contrast-enhanced, T1-weighted studies were obtained with an axial SE 600 to 800/20 (TR/TE) sequence with four excitations, a 16 to 20 cm field of view, and a $256 \times 128$ matrix size. Section thickness was 3 mm with a 0.5 mm intersection gap. A precontrast T1-weighted axial SE sequence was always obtained. This pulse sequence was identical to the postcontrast T1-weighted sequence, except that two rather than four excitations were used.

### Inversion Recovery and Application of Fat-Suppression Technique

Short tau inversion recovery (STIR) images result in very high lesion conspicuity by suppressing the signal from fat and by adding T1-weighted and T2-weighted information together. Because most pathology has a long T1 and T2 relaxation time, pathology appears with a high signal intensity on STIR. Further, the lower fat signal intensity makes any pathology stand out. The optimal TI (time of inversion) for fat suppression may vary from one individual to another, depending on coil loading and fat composition. The optimal TI for fat suppression at 1.5 Tesla is in the 145 to 170 ms range. Usually the STIR image is obtained with a TR of 2000, a TI of 150 to 160, and a TE of 20 ms.

### T1-Weighted Fat-Suppression Technique

Fat-suppressed T1-weighted images may be obtained using various techniques.[21, 22] In this chapter, fat-suppressed T1-weighted images were obtained using a presaturation technique. Before imaging, the spectral fat peak was determined in each patient. Subsequently, an RF pulse was applied, centered at the resonant frequency of fat. The RF pulse was followed by a spoil gradient. This fat-suppression technique (chemsat) is a standard feature on the Signa system and can be easily applied in the same time required for a standard T1-weighted sequence. After the postcontrast fat-suppressed images were obtained, a standard T1-weighted sequence in either the axial or coronal plane, with the same parameters used for the fat-suppressed T1-weighted images, was immediately obtained. This was done because the fat-suppression pulse sequences are more sensitive to magnetic susceptibility artifacts.[21–23] In addition, the enhancement of the extraocular muscles, and in particular the lacrimal glands, is exaggerated on the fat-suppressed images. There is thus the possibility of misinterpreting a lesion if it is adjacent to the lacrimal gland, the extraocular muscles, or the walls of the sinuses (air–bone–soft-tissue interface).[17]

## Normal CT and MR Imaging Anatomy

The bony landmarks can be visualized best on CT with the aid of the bone extended scale and bone window technique (Fig. 9-9). The optic canal can be seen on both axial and coronal scans. The lateral and medial bony orbital margins, the superior and inferior orbital fissures, the lacrimal fossa, lacrimal sac, nasolacrimal canal, infraorbital canal, and paranasal sinuses are also equally well seen on

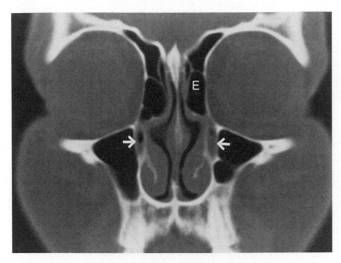

**FIGURE 9-9** Nasolacrimal canals. Coronal CT scan shows nasolacrimal canals (*arrows*). Note the anterior ethmoid cells (*E*).

axial or coronal scans (Fig. 9-9). Coronal scans are best for assessing the floor and roof of the orbits. The lamina papyracea is a paper thin plate of bone that forms most of the medial orbital wall, separating it from the adjacent ethmoid air cells. This plate often appears to be dehiscent on CT, and therefore care should be taken not to make an erroneous diagnosis of bone destruction or fracture.

### Extraocular Muscles

The extraocular muscles are well visualized on CT, and they are uniformly enhanced on postcontrast CT scans (Figs. 9-10 to 9-13). These muscles are also seen well on MR imaging (Figs. 9-14 to 9-26). The extraocular muscles generally have a course parallel to that of the adjacent orbital wall. Consequently, only the horizontal recti (lateral and medial) may be seen in their entirety in the axial plane (Figs. 9-12 and 9-16). Likewise, the vertical recti (inferior and superior) may be seen best in the parasagittal (oblique) plane (Figs. 9-6, 9-7, and 9-27). The tapering of these muscles in

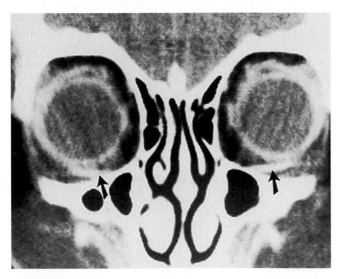

**FIGURE 9-10** Inferior oblique muscles. Coronal CT scan shows inferior oblique muscles (*arrows*).

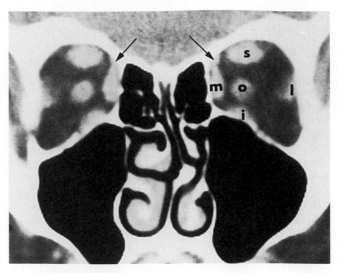

**FIGURE 9-11** Extraocular muscles. Coronal CT scan shows inferior rectus muscle (*i*); lateral rectus muscle (*l*); medial rectus muscle (*m*); and superior rectus muscle (*s*). Note the superior oblique muscles (*arrows*) and optic nerve (*o*).

their tendinous portions and their origins at the annulus of Zinn are seen well in the parasagittal (vertical recti) and axial (horizontal recti) planes (Figs. 9-6 and 9-16). The superior and inferior recti are only partially visualized in any one axial plane (Figs. 9-14, 9-15, 9-20, and 9-21). On coronal scans, all of the recti muscles are seen in an oblique cross section (Figs. 9-22 and 9-24) related to their slanted orientation to the coronal plane as the walls of the orbit slant toward the orbital apex. For accurate determination of the cross-sectional size of these muscles, reformatted images or direct oblique MR imaging would have to be done separately for each muscle. This is obviously not practical, nor is it necessary unless there is a critical situation requiring the precise size of a particular muscle.[15] The levator palpebrae superioris is closely approximated to the superior rectus muscle, and it is identified as a separate muscle only on anterior coronal images (Fig. 9-22), where it diverges from the superior rectus. These two muscles can be visualized as separate muscles on sagittal and parasagittal (oblique) MR imaging (Fig. 9-27). The muscle portion of the superior oblique muscle can be visualized best on coronal scans, and its tendinous portion is seen best on axial scans (Figs. 9-11, 9-13, and 9-23). The reflected portion of the superior oblique muscle and its tendon are seen best on axial scans (Figs. 9-13 and 9-20). The trochlea is seen well on axial scans, and it is occasionally calcified. The inferior oblique muscle is seen best on coronal, sagittal, and parasagittal scans (Fig. 9-10). On axial scans the muscle belly is poorly seen, but its insertion is well visualized.

### Orbital Compartments

In descriptive terms, the orbit has been divided into the extraperiosteal, subperiosteal, extraconal, conal, and intraconal spaces (Boxes 9-1 to 9-3). The intraconal space is separated from the other spaces by the rectus muscles and their intermuscular septa, which are denser in the anterior orbit and are seen best on coronal scans (Figs. 9-22 and 9-23). Because certain lesions have a predilection to present

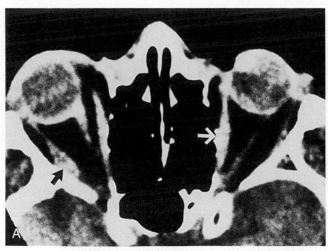

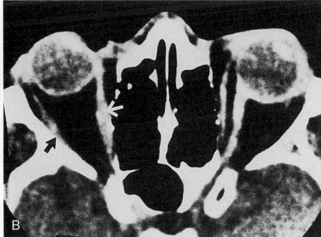

**FIGURE 9-12** Demonstration of Sherrington's law of reciprocal innervation. **A,** Axial CT scan obtained during right lateral gaze. Note that the right lateral rectus muscle (*black arrow*) and the left medial rectus muscle (*white arrow*) contract, and the right medial and left lateral rectus muscles relax (lengthen). **B,** Axial CT scan obtained during left lateral gaze. Right medial rectus muscle (*white arrow*) and left lateral rectus muscle are contracted, and right lateral rectus muscle (*black arrow*) and left medial rectus muscle are relaxed (lengthened). (From Mafee MF et al. CT in the evaluation of Brown's superior oblique tendon sheath syndrome. Radiology 1985;154:691–695.)

in a specific orbital space, the concept of the orbital spaces has some practical value. It is useful for radiologic differential diagnosis and for surgical planning, and these lesions are discussed later in this chapter. The distinction of intraocular and extraocular locations within the orbit is also useful when evaluating metastatic and dystrophic orbital calcifications (Boxes 9-4 and 9-5).

### Lacrimal Gland

With the exception of a portion of the superior ophthalmic vein, the lacrimal glands are the only prominent structures readily identified in the superolateral extraconal space.[18] Each lacrimal gland is about the size and shape of an almond. It is adjacent to the tendons of the superior and lateral rectus muscles and is separated from the globe by the lateral rectus muscle (Figs. 9-10, 9-13, and 9-19). The more anterior palpebral lobe is separated from the deeper orbital lobe by the lateral horn of the levator muscle aponeurosis.[24]

### Vascular and Neural Structures

Although the vascular structures in the orbit frequently can be seen on noncontrast CT, they are highlighted with

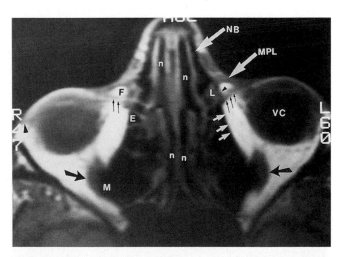

**FIGURE 9-14** Normal MR imaging anatomy. T1-weighted MR image shows the nasal bone (*NB*); nasal cavities (*n*); medial palpebral ligament (*MPL*); lacrimal portion of the orbicularis oculi and orbital septum (*small black arrows*); lacrimal sac (*L*); lacrimal fascia (*small arrowhead*); periorbita (periosteum) (*three white arrows*); inferior rectus muscle (*large black arrows*); maxillary sinus (*M*); ethmoid air cells (*E*); nasal bone (*NB*); vitreous chamber of the eye (*VC*); fat pad (*F*) adjacent to the lacrimal sac; and the lateral palpebral ligament (*large black arrowhead*). The lacrimal sac is about 12 cm long, is situated in the lacrimal fossa, and is enclosed by the lacrimal fascia (*small black arrowhead*), which is attached behind to the posterior lacrimal crest of the lacrimal bone and in front to the anterior lacrimal crest of the maxilla. The fascia is formed from the periorbita (*three white arrows*).

**FIGURE 9-13** Normal superior oblique muscles. Axial CT scan demonstrates the superior oblique tendon (*crossed arrows*); trochlea (*arrowhead*); reflected portion of the superior oblique muscle's tendon (*white arrows*); medial rectus (*hollow arrow*); and lacrimal glands (*curved arrow*). (From Mafee MF et al. CT in the evaluation of Brown's superior oblique tendon sheath syndrome. Radiology 1985;154:691–695.)

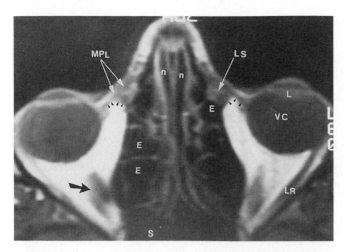

**FIGURE 9-15** Normal MR imaging anatomy. T1-weighted MR image obtained 3 mm superior to the view in Figure 9-14 shows the medial palpebral ligament (*MPL*); lacrimal sac (*LS*); medial check ligament (*arrowheads*); nasal cavities (*n*); ethmoid air cells (*E*); sphenoid sinus (*S*); inferior rectus muscle (*black arrow*); and lateral rectus muscle (*LR*).

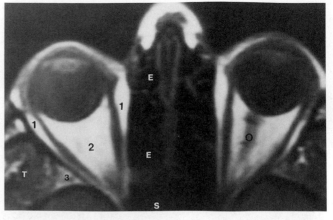

**FIGURE 9-17** Normal MR imaging anatomy. T1-weighted MR image obtained 3 mm superior to the view in Figure 9-16 shows the optic nerve (*0*); extraconal fat (*1*); intraconal fat (*2*); bone marrow of the greater wing of the sphenoid (*3*); temporalis muscle (*T*); ethmoid (*E*); and sphenoid (*S*) sinuses.

contrast. On MR imaging the larger vessels usually have low signal intensity (signal void). The ophthalmic artery can be seen in the apex of the orbit on the inferior aspect of the optic nerve and then as it swings laterally before looping around and over the optic nerve to its superior medial aspect (Fig. 9-24). Several of its branches, including the anterior and posterior ethmoidal and posterior ciliary branches, usually can be identified.[3, 25, 26]

The superior ophthalmic vein originates in the extraconal space, in the anteromedial aspect of the orbit. It then courses near the trochlea to pass through the muscle cone beneath the superior rectus muscle and above the optic nerve. It then exits the intraconal space through the superior orbital fissure

(Figs. 9-19 and 9-20). This vein is routinely identified in axial, coronal, sagittal, and parasagittal images. The inferior ophthalmic and connecting veins are seen inconsistently.[3] The intraconal and extraconal components of the small nerves of the orbit, particularly the frontal, supraorbital, and inferior divisions of the third nerve, as well as the infraorbital nerve, may be identified on CT. These nerves are identified better on MR imaging. The position of these nerves may be variable.[3] The frontal nerve can be seen between the levator palpebrae superioris muscle and the orbital roof (Figs. 9-22 and 9-23). Most of these small nerves can be seen on coronal scans of the orbital apex (Fig. 9-22 ).[26]

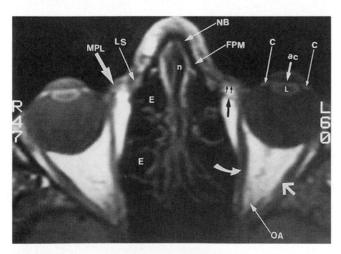

**FIGURE 9-16** Normal MR imaging anatomy. T1-weighted MR image obtained 3 mm superior to view in the view in Figure 9-15 shows the nasal bone (*NB*); frontal process of the maxilla (*FPM*); ciliary body (*C*); anterior chamber (*ac*); lens (*L*); lacrimal sac (*LS*); medial palpebral ligament (*MPL*); ethmoid sinuses (*E*); medial rectus muscle (*curved arrow*); and lateral rectus muscle (*straight arrow*). Notice the expansion of the fascial sleeve of the medial rectus muscle as it forms the medial check ligament (*black arrow*). The medial check ligament is attached to the lacrimal bone. The orbital septum (*small black arrows*) is seen anterior to the medial check ligament.

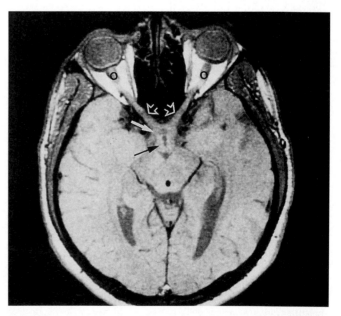

**FIGURE 9-18** Normal MR imaging anatomy. PW MR image shows the intraorbital segment of the optic nerves (*o*); intracanalicular segment of the optic nerves (*hollow arrows*); chiasm (*white arrow*); and hypothalamus (*black arrow*).

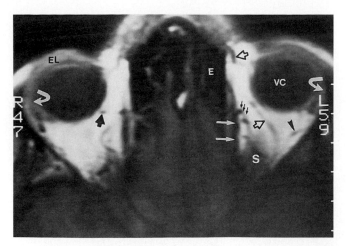

**FIGURE 9-19**   Normal MR imaging anatomy. T1-weighted MR image obtained 6 mm superior to the view in Figure 9-17 shows the superior rectus muscle (*S*); lacrimal vein (*arrowhead*); lacrimal glands (*curved arrows*); superior ophthalmic vein (*hollow arrows*); medial ophthalmic vein (*three small arrows*); superior oblique muscle (*white arrows*); presumed vorticose vein (*solid black arrow*); eyelid (*EL*); and vitreous chamber (*VC*).

## Optic Nerve

The optic nerve arises from the ganglionic layer of the retina and consists of coarse myelinated fibers, like the white matter of the central nervous system.[1, 6, 16] The orbital segment of the optic nerve is 3 to 4 mm in diameter and 20 to 30 mm long (Fig. 9-18). It has a serpiginous course (with minimal inferior and lateral bowing in its midportion) in the orbit, which allows unrestricted movement of the globe. From its insertion on the posterior globe, it courses posteriorly, medially, and superiorly to exit the orbit at the optic canal. The optic nerve is covered by layers of pia, subarachnoid membrane, and dura mater. All these layers fuse as they approach the globe, becoming continuous with the sclera. The intracranial subarachnoid space extends around the optic nerve, ending at the sclera. The subdural space is a potential space and is not considered to be continuous with the intracranial subdural space. At the superior aspect of the intracanalicular portion of the optic nerve, the three layers of covering are fused to each other and to the optic nerve. The dural layer is fixed to the periosteum of the optic canal, protecting it from back-and-forth motion.[17] The intracranial segment of the optic nerve is located medially and then above the internal carotid artery in the suprasellar region (Fig. 9-18). The optic nerves join in the suprasellar cistern to form the optic chiasm (Fig. 9-18). The subarachnoid space around the optic nerve sheath has a low density on CT and can be imaged during the course of iodinated contrast cisternography. The meningeal layers of the optic nerve show enhancement on postcontrast CT. On coronal scans, immediately posterior to the globe, a small central density within the nerve represents the central retinal artery and vein.[3] The optic nerve and sheath measure 3 to 5 mm in the axial plane and 4 to 6 mm in the coronal plane.[17] The intracanalicular and prechiasmatic portions of the optic nerve are particularly well demonstrated by MR imaging (Fig. 9-18). Generally, on T1-weighted, proton density, and T2-weighted images, the optic nerve has signal intensities similar to those of normal white matter.[27] A ring of T1-weighted hypointensity and T2-weighted hyperintensity, representing CSF within the nerve sheath, is frequently seen on coronal sections. This should not be confused with well-defined areas of hypointensity bordering the nerve, which are caused by chemical shift artifact.

## Globe

The three ocular coats (sclera, choroid, and retina) form a well-defined line on CT that enhances with IV contrast. The lens is normally hyperdense on CT, and the vitreous appears hypodense and shows no contrast enhancement. On MR imaging the ocular coats appear as a hypointense ring, and the vitreous has characteristics very similar to those of CSF. The lens is isointense to vitreous (low signal intensity) on T1-weighted images and has very low signal intensity on T2-weighted images. These signal intensities reflect the high

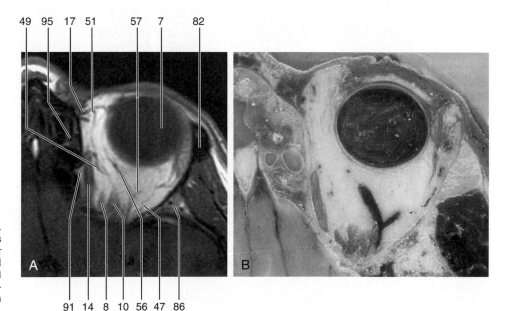

**FIGURE 9-20**   Normal MRI anatomy. T1-weighted MRI obtained 3 mm shows superior muscle complex (*S*); superior ophthalmic vein (*hollow arrows*); lacrimal artery (*LA*); lacrimal vein (*LV*); lacrimal gland (*curved arrow*); and reflected portion of superior oblique muscle tendon (*black arrows*).

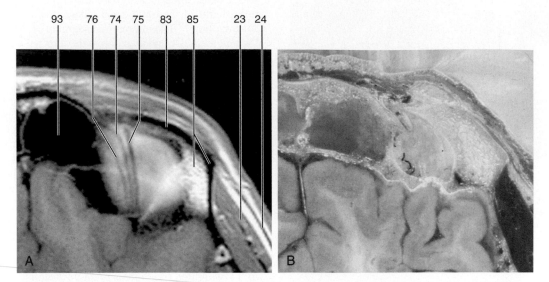

**FIGURE 9-21** Normal MRI anatomy. T1-weighted MRI obtained 3 mm superior to view in Figure 9-20 shows superior rectus–levator palpebrae complex (*SMC*); superior ophthalmic vein (*SOV*); presumed frontal nerves (*hollow arrows*); presumed lacrimal nerve (*arrowheads*); lacrimal glands (*curved arrows*); sclera (*S*); trochlea (*white solid arrow*); presumed supratrochlear nerve (*two small black arrows*); frontal bone (*FB*); frontal sinus (*FS*); orbital septum (*curved black arrow*); and orbicularis oculi (*four black arrows*).

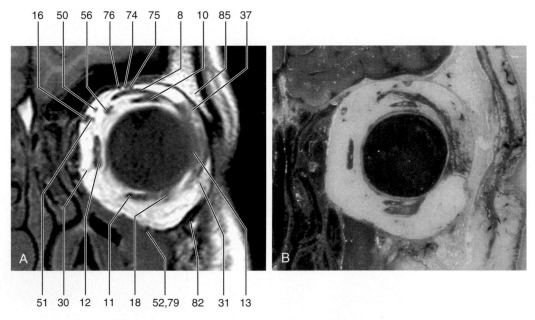

**FIGURE 9-22** Normal MRI anatomy. Coronal T1-weighted MRI shows medial rectus muscle (*1*); superior oblique muscle tendon (*2*); superior ophthalmic/supratrochlear vein (*3*); levator palpebrae superioris (*4*); tendon of superior rectus (*single short arrow*); tendon of superior oblique muscle (*5*); inferior oblique muscle (*6*); tendon of inferior rectus muscle (*7*); tendon lateral rectus muscle (*8*); palpebral portion of lacrimal gland (*9*); supraorbital nerve (*white arrowhead*); and intermuscular septum (*black arrows*).

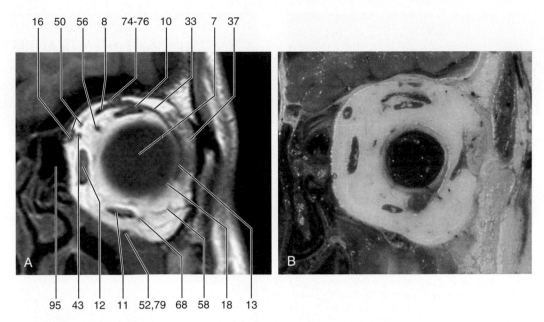

**FIGURE 9-23**   Normal MRI anatomy. Coronal T1-weighted MRI shows inferior rectus muscle (*1*); medial rectus muscle (*2*); superior oblique muscle (*3*); superior rectus muscle (*4*); levator palpebrae superioris (*5*); partially volumed lacrimal gland (*6*); lateral rectus (*7*); presumed branch of oculomotor nerve (*8*); collateral vein (*small arrowheads*); medial ophthalmic vein (*solid black arrow*); frontal nerve/supraorbital nerve (*hollow arrow*); supraorbital/ophthalmic artery (*single arrowhead*); vitreous (*V*); and maxillary antrum (*M*).

protein and liquid crystal composition of the lens. The imaging of the globe is discussed in detail in Chapter 8.

## BONY INTERORBITAL DISTANCE

The distance between the orbits and their individual dimensions are important in the diagnosis of craniofacial anomalies. The orbits are often involved in craniofacial malformations, which include orbital clefts, orbital hypo-

telorism, and hypertelorism, and measurement of the bony interorbital distance (BID) is useful in establishing the severity of hypertelorism. This distance between orbits is commonly measured at the interdacryon level, the dacryon being the point of junction of the nasal bone, lacrimal bone, and maxilla.[19] Before CT, most observers relied on standard radiographs for measuring the BID, and normal values for adults and the younger age groups are available.[28-32] The BID was first defined by Cameron, in a small number of dried skulls, as the maximum distance between the medial

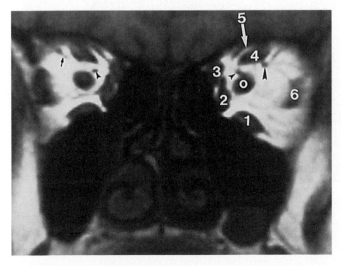

**FIGURE 9-24**   Normal MR imaging anatomy. T1-weighted MR coronal image shows the inferior rectus muscle (*1*); medial rectus muscle (*2*); superior oblique muscle (*3*); superior rectus muscle (*4*); levator palpebrae superioris (*5*); lateral rectus muscle (*6*); optic nerve (*o*); superior ophthalmic vein (*large arrowhead*); ophthalmic artery (*small arrowhead*); and lacrimal nerve (*black arrow*).

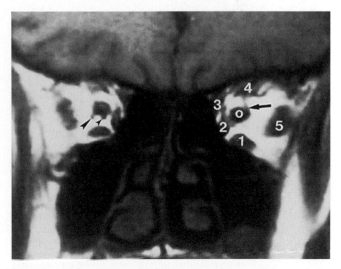

**FIGURE 9-25**   Normal MR imaging anatomy. T1-weighted MR coronal image shows the inferior rectus muscle (*1*); medial rectus muscle (*2*); superior oblique muscle (*3*); superior rectus muscle (*4*); lateral rectus muscle (*5*); optic nerve (*o*); long posterior ciliary arteries (*arrowheads*); and presumed ciliary ganglion (*arrow*).

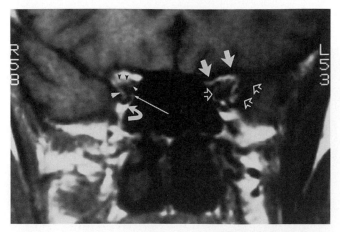

**FIGURE 9-26** Normal MR imaging anatomy. T1-weighted MR coronal image shows the lesser (*double solid arrows*) and greater (*double hollow arrows*) wings of the sphenoid bone, medial rectus muscle (*single hollow arrow*); inferior rectus muscle (*long arrow*); lateral rectus muscle (*large white arrowhead*); superior muscle complex (*black arrowheads*); optic nerve (*short white arrowhead*); and fat in the apex of the orbit, along with the inferior orbital fissure (*curved arrow*). The common tendon of Zinn is seen as areas of hypointensity between the rectus muscles. The relative position of the nerves, veins, and ophthalmic artery entering orbital cavity through superior orbital fissure cannot be precisely resolved with current MR imaging technology.

## BOX 9-1
## INTRACONAL (CENTRAL ORBITAL) LESIONS

| More Common | Less Common |
|---|---|
| Cavernous hemangioma | Capillary hemangioma |
| Optic nerve meningioma | Peripheral nerve tumors |
| Optic nerve glioma |   Neurofibroma |
| Optic nerve granulomatous disease (sarcoid) |   Schwannoma |
| Optic neuritis (multiple sclerosis) | Leukemia |
| Lymphoma | Hematocele |
| Pseudotumor | Optic nerve sheath cyst |
| Lymphangioma | Colobomatous cyst |
| Venous angioma | Hemangioblastoma (optic nerve) |
| Varix | Chemodectoma (ciliary ganglion) |
| Arteriovenous malformation | Necrobiotic xanthogranuloma |
| Carotid cavernous fistula | Lipoma |
| Hemangiopericytoma | Amyloidosis |
| Rhabdomyosarcoma | |
| Metastasis | |
| Orbital cellulitis and abscess | |

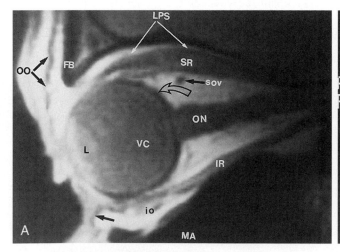

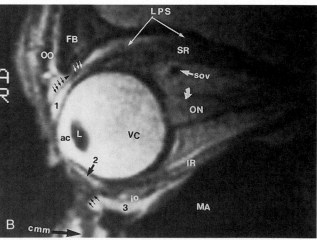

**FIGURE 9-27**   **A,** Normal MR imaging anatomy. Sagittal PW MR image shows fibers of the orbicularis oculi (*OO*); frontal bone (*FB*); levator palpebrae superioris (*LPS*); superior rectus muscle (*SR*); superior ophthalmic vein (*SOV*); sclera and Tenon capsule (*curved arrow*); optic nerve (*ON*); inferior rectus muscle (*IR*); maxillary antrum (*MA*); inferior oblique muscle (*io*); vitreous chamber (*VC*); lens (*L*); and orbital septum (*straight arrow*). **B,** Sagittal T2-weighted MR image shows fibers of the orbicularis oculi (*OO*); frontal bone (*FB*); levator palpebrae superioris (*LPS*); superior rectus muscle (*SR*); superior ophthalmic vein (*SOV*); optic nerve (*ON*); CSF along the optic nerve (*curved arrow*): inferior rectus muscle (*IR*); maxillary antrum (*MA*); inferior oblique muscle (*io*); extraconal fat (*3*); orbital septum (*three small arrows*); complex muscle of mouth (*cmm*); inferior (*2*) and superior (*1*) fornices; anterior chamber (*ac*); lens (*L*); and vitreous chamber (*VC*). Note the tendon of insertion of the levator palpebrae superioris (*small white arrows*). This tendon is an aponeurosis that descends posterior to the orbital septum. The orbital septum is depicted in this section as an ill-defined image (*arrowhead*). The tendinous fibers of the superior palpebrae muscle pierce the orbital septum and become attached to the anterior surface of the superior tarsal plate (*four black arrows*).

## BOX 9-2
## COMMON CAUSES OF ENLARGED EXTRAOCULAR MUSCLES AND SUBPERIOSTEAL LESIONS

**Enlarged Extraocular Muscle**

Graves' myositis
Inflammatory myositis, including cysticercosis
Granulomatous myositis (less common)—sarcoidosis
Pseudotumor (myositic type)
Lymphoma
Vascular lesions (hemangioma, arteriovenous malformation)
Aromegaly
Pseudorheumatoid nodule
Metastasis (breast, lung)

**Orbital Subperiosteal Lesions**

Subperiosteal cellulitis
Subperiosteal abscess
Infiltration of neoplastic lesions of paranasal sinuses

Infiltration of meningiomas (en plaque meningiomas)
Lymphomas
Leukemia
Plasmacytomas

Lacrimal gland tumors
Dermoid and epidermoid
Hematoma and hematic cyst
Cholesterol granuloma
Fibrous histiocytoma

Primary osseous or cartilaginous tumors
Metastasis (neuroblastoma)

## BOX 9-3
## EXTRACONAL PERIPHERAL ORBITAL LESIONS

**More Common**

Capillary hemangiomas
Cholesterol granulomas
Dermoids and epidermoids
Lacrimal gland lesions
 Inflammation
 Lymphoma
 Pseudotumor
 Sarcoidosis
Epithelial tumors
Lymphangiomas
Peripheral nerve tumors
Plasmacytomas
Rhabdomyosarcomas
Sarcoidosis

**Less Common**

Amyloidosis
Fibrous histiocytoma
Hemangiosarcoma
Hemangiopericytoma
Hematic cyst
Lipoma
Orbital encephalocele
Wegener's granulomatosis

## BOX 9-4
## DIFFERENTIAL DIAGNOSIS OF METASTATIC ORBITAL CALCIFICATION

Congenital
 Fanconi's syndrome (proximal renal tubular dysfunction)
 Milk-alkali syndrome
 Renal tubular acidosis
Endocrine
 Hyperparathyroidism, primary or secondary
 Hypoparathyroidism
 Pseudohypoparathyroidism
Idiopathic—sarcoidosis
Infectious
 Cytomegalovirus
 Leprosy
 Osteomyelitis
 Syphilis
 Toxoplasmosis
 Tuberculosis
Toxic
 Excessive ingestion of calcium phosphate or alkali
 Vitamin D intoxication
Traumatic—immobilization
Neoplastic
 Bronchogenic carcinoma
 Metastatic involvement of bone
 Multiple myeloma
 Parathyroid adenoma
 Parathyroid carcinoma

Modified from Froula PD et al. The differential diagnosis of orbital calcifications, as detected on computed tomographic scans. Mayo Clin Proc 1993;68:256-257.

walls of the bony orbits measured at the juncture of the crista lacrimalis posterior with the frontolacrimal suture.[31] Currarino and Silverman, in their studies of arhinencephaly and trigonocephaly, measured the BID between the medial walls at what was described to be the junction between each medial angular process of the frontal bone with the maxillary and lacrimal bones.[28]

To provide a statistically more reliable standard, Gerald and Silverman repeated the original work of Currarino and Silverman, using the same technical factors, and studied 100 patients at each year of age from birth to 12 years.[28, 29] Hansman, using radiographs of the skull and paranasal sinuses in a large group of healthy subjects, presented measurements of the BID and the thickness of the skull.[32] According to him, from infancy to adulthood, the BID for girls is consistently narrower than for boys. Starting at 1 year 6 months, there is a gradual increase in the size of the BID for both sexes. At about 13 years of age, girls' growth begins to level off. Since boys' growth continues to increase to the age of about 21 years, the measurements in girls fall more markedly below those of boys as growth is completed. The average adult measurement in women is 25 mm and in men is 28 mm.[32]

CT of the orbit provides, along with other information, an opportunity to evaluate the distance between the orbits and, if necessary, any other linear and angular measurements. On

CT, the lacrimal bones and orbital plates of the ethmoid (lamina papyracea) are seen as a thin line of bone, and the BID can be measured at any desired point.[19] From the CT studies of 400 adults (200 men aged 18 to 82, average age 52; 200 women aged 17 to 88, average age 54), the BID was measured between the medial walls of the orbits, along with certain other linear and angular measurements; these data are given in Table 9-1. These data were collected from patients with normal orbits who were studied because of a suspected diagnosis of brain infarction, hearing loss, or brain tumor. None of these patients had any underlying craniofacial anomaly or congenital malformation. The patients were Caucasian, except for a few who were Asian. In this study, data were collected only from nonrotated axial sections in the plane of the optic nerve (Fig. 9-28). On similar CT sections through the orbits, there are two configurations of the medial orbital walls. The first is a parallel separation of the medial orbital walls, and the second is a fusiform or lateral spread of the ethmoidal air cells, with the widest separation of the orbital walls occurring posterior to the posterior pole of the globe.[19] The distance between the medial walls of the bony orbits at various points, and other linear and angular measurements, are illustrated in Figure 9-28A,B. Several reference points have been used. The anterior pole ($A$) is applied to the central point of the anterior curvature of the eyeball, and the posterior pole ($P$) is the central point of its posterior curvature. A line joining the two poles forms the optic axis ($AP$), and the primary axes of the two globes are nearly parallel. The cranial opening of the optic canal is well demonstrated in Figure 9-28A. The optic canal lies between the root of the lesser sphenoid wing and the body of the sphenoid bone (Fig. 9-28A and 9-29). The anterior root is broad and flat and is continuous with the planum sphenoidale (Figs. 9-26 and 9-28A). The posterior root is shorter and thicker (optic strut), and is connected to the body of the sphenoid opposite the posterior border of the sulcus chiasmatis.[19]

As seen in Table 9-1, the normal BID, measured at the posterior border of the frontal processes of the maxilla on nonrotated CT scans in the plane of the optic nerve, ranges from 2.29 to 3.21 cm (average, 2.67 cm) in men and 2.29 to 3.20 cm (average, 2.56 cm) in women. The widest interorbital distance lies behind the posterior poles of the globes. This ranges from 3.16 to 4.10 cm (average, 3.37 cm) in men and 2.93 to 3.67 cm (average, 3.20 cm) in women. A line joining the lateral orbital margins in the axial plane (line DD in Table 9-1 (Figs. 9-26 and 9-28B) normally intersects the globe near its midportion, with at least one third of the globe posterior to this line.

## PATHOLOGY

### Hypertelorism, Hypotelorism, Exophthalmos, and Exorbitism

The terminology used to describe abnormalities of the orbit is complicated and may be confusing[33] to those unfamiliar with it. It will therefore be briefly reviewed. *Hypertelorism* is literally translated from Greek as "increased distance" (*hyper* meaning "over" and *tele* meaning

**Table 9-1**
**CT ORBITAL MEASUREMENTS IN 400 ADULTS**

| Line, Description | Measurement (cm) | | | | | |
|---|---|---|---|---|---|---|
| | Minimum | | Maximum | | Mean | |
| | Male | Female | Male | Female | Male | Female |
| AA, Approximates interpupillary distance | 6.26 | 6.21 | 7.51 | 7.50 | 6.78 | 6.63 |
| BB, BID measured at posterior border of frontal processes of maxillae | 2.29 | 2.29 | 3.21 | 3.20 | 2.67 | 2.56 |
| CC, BID measured posteriorly or at level of orbital equator (useful orbits) | 2.63 | 2.56 | 3.50 | 3.30 | 2.80 | 2.83 |
| DD, Distance between anterior margin of frontal processes of zygomatic bones at level of plane of optic nerves | 9.18 | 9.29 | 10.13 | 11.00 | 9.73 | 9.97 |
| EE, Distance between optic nerves where they enter eyeballs | 5.16 | 4.78 | 6.40 | 6.00 | 5.43 | 5.27 |
| FF, BID measured at level of posterior poles of eyeballs | 2.87 | 2.56 | 3.70 | 3.51 | 3.10 | 2.97 |
| GG, BID measured at its widest part (usually posterior to FF line) | 3.16 | 2.93 | 4.10 | 3.67 | 3.37 | 3.20 |
| HH, BID measured at its most posterior part (apex of bony orbit) | 2.16 | 2.43 | 3.37 | 3.23 | 2.73 | 2.80 |
| II, Distance between superior orbital fissures at apex of bony orbit | 2.90 | 2.70 | 3.83 | 3.63 | 3.10 | 3.00 |
| JJ, Distance between central portion of cranial opening of optic canals | 2.20 | 2.01 | 2.73 | 2.70 | 2.30 | 2.20 |
| KK, Distance between tips of anterior clinoid processes | 2.31 | 2.43 | 3.21 | 3.16 | 2.80 | 2.83 |
| EI, Length of intraorbital part of optic nerve: | | | | | | |
|     Right | 2.70 | 2.40 | 3.80 | 3.23 | 3.10 | 2.90 |
|     Left | 2.60 | 2.40 | 3.80 | 3.21 | 3.20 | 2.80 |
| AP, Anteroposterior diameter of eyeball: | | | | | | |
|     Right | 2.50 | 2.39 | 2.90 | 2.70 | 2.80 | 2.50 |
|     Left | 2.40 | 2.40 | 2.80 | 2.80 | 2.70 | 2.63 |
| TT, Transverse diameter of eyeball: | | | | | | |
|     Right | 2.50 | 2.40 | 2.80 | 2.90 | 2.70 | 2.71 |
|     Left | 2.50 | 2.50 | 2.90 | 2.90 | 2.80 | 2.83 |
| Angle between optic nerve axes (in degrees) | 35° | 36.5° | 50° | 51.5° | 41° | 42.3° |

Note: *BID* = bony interorbital distance.

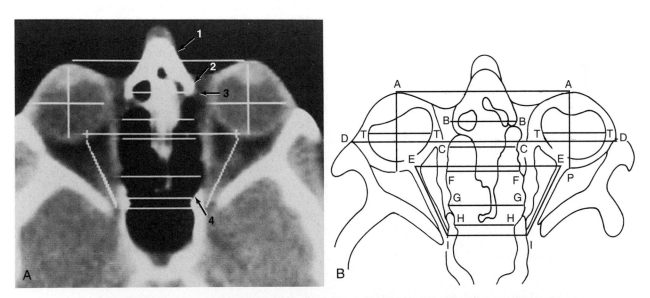

**FIGURE 9-28**   **A,** Axial CT scan of the orbits at the level of the plane of the optic nerves shows the outline of the globes, lenses, and vitreous bodies; level of the medial check ligament (*3*); medial and lateral rectus muscles; optic nerves; and retroorbital fat compartments. Note the nasal bone (*1*) and frontal process of the maxilla (*2*) on either side. The lamina papyracea is seen as a very thin density hardly distinguishable from the medial aspect of the medial rectus muscle. Posterior to that is the most posterior part of the medial wall of the bony orbit (*4*), which is related to the anterior part of the sphenoid sinus. **B,** Diagram shows different points selected for various measurements presented in Table 9-1. (From Mafee MF et al. CT in the evaluation of the orbit and the bony interorbital distance. AJNR 1986;7:265.)

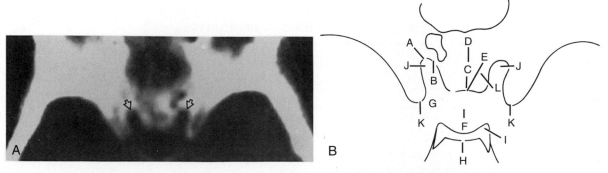

**FIGURE 9-29** **A,** Axial CT scan of the head at the level of the planum sphenoidale and anterior roots of the lesser wings of the sphenoid bone shows the cranial openings (*arrows*) of the optic canals. **B,** Diagram shows structures in **A.** *A,* Cranial opening of the optic canal; *B,* anterior root of the lesser wing of the sphenoid; *C,* posterior border of the chiasmatic groove; *D,* planum sphenoidale; *E,* tuberculum sellae; *F,* pituitary fossa; *G,* middle clinoid; *H,* dorsum sellae; *I,* posterior clinoid; *J,* midportion of the cranial opening of the optic canal; *K,* anterior clinoid; *L,* anterior border of the chiasmatic groove. (From Mafee MF et al. CT in the evaluation of the orbit and the bony interorbital distance. AJNR 1986;7:265.)

"distant"). Orbital hypertelorism describes the anatomic situation in which the medial walls of the orbits are farther apart than normal.[33-35]

Patients with orbital hypertelorism almost always have eyes that are spaced more widely apart than normal. Telecanthus is a condition that may clinically mimic orbital hypertelorism. In telecanthus the distance between the apices of the medial canthal ligaments is increased, and the eyes are spaced more widely apart than normal. However, the BID is not increased; these patients do not have orbital hypertelorism. They do have medial canthal hypertelorism. Telecanthus may be congenital or acquired; when acquired, it is often a consequence of trauma.[33]

Orbital *hypotelorism* refers to a decrease in the BID. Patients with this condition may appear clinically to have either narrowly spaced or normally spaced eyes; surprisingly, they may even appear to have widely spaced eyes. For example, patients with Down's syndrome and trisomy 13 syndrome were classically described as having hypertelorism on the basis of clinical evaluation. However, in fact, these patients have orbital hypotelorism.[33, 35]

*Exophthalmos* describes abnormal prominence of the globe, and proptosis emphasizes abnormal protrusion of the globe. *Exophthalmos* and *proptosis*, however, commonly are used as synonyms. *Exorbitism*, on the other hand, refers to a decrease in the volume of the orbit. The orbital contents are greater in volume than the orbital capacity and generally protrude anteriorly (proptosis), causing the globe to be unusually prominent (exophthalmos).

## Congenital and Developmental Abnormalities

There are many hereditary and sporadic abnormalities that involve the orbits, globe, adjacent orbital tissues, and other craniofacial and skeletal structures. The embryology of the eyes and orbits is presented in Chapter 8 and earlier in this chapter. The embryology of the midface is presented in Chapter 1. The study of these congenital and developmental conditions is complicated by the variety of names used for the same syndrome and by the overlapping criteria used to establish the diagnosis of a syndrome.[36] To list all of the congenital malformations or syndromes is beyond the scope of this chapter. Many excellent books have detailed descriptions of these disorders.[34-39] The eyes are often involved in craniofacial malformations, including orbital clefts and orbital hypotelorism and hypertelorism. CT and MR imaging have proven to be very useful in the preoperative evaluation of such patients, and imaging may show an encephalocele or a porencephalic cyst as an additional feature of the malformation.[19] The surgical treatment of hypertelorism involves translocation of the globes toward the midline by lateral wall osteotomy at a point posterior to the equator of the eye.[19]

## Anatomic and Developmental Considerations

Congenital abnormalities of the orbit and eyes result from faulty development of the embryo and fetus, and the eighth week of gestation is the last week of true embryonic development.[36, 40-46] By the third week of gestation, the optic pits appear, one on either side of the forebrain. Disturbance of the prosencephalic organizing center (prechordal mesoblast) can cause cyclopia, synophthalmia, or arhinencephaly. Anophthalmia occurs as a result of failure of the neuroectoderm of the optic pit to develop from the anterior portion of the neural plate. A variety of ocular and systemic abnormalities may be seen with an optic nerve coloboma. These conditions have been described in Chapter 8. Craniosynostosis is due to abnormal development of the blastemic stage of the skull bone, including the basicranium. Mandibulofacial dysostosis and otocephaly probably are due to inhibition of mesodermal differentiation of the facial structures derived from the first branchial (visceral) arch. These conditions are discussed in Chapter 1.[36]

Under normal conditions, the eye directs orbital growth.

During the first year of life, the eye practically doubles in volume and attains more than 50% of its adult volume.[47] By the end of the third year, 75% of the adult volume is achieved (similar to neural growth).[47] The shape of the orbital cranial junction is also influenced by the development of the brain and skull.[47] When the brain is underdeveloped but the eye is normal, the orbital plate of the frontal bone is usually elevated into the anterior fossa of the skull.[19] In microcephaly the orbits are usually circular and the roofs are highly arched.[48] When the eye is underdeveloped but the brain is normal, the orbital plate of the frontal bone appears hypoplastic and the vertical or cranial part is usually normal (Fig. 9-30). Enucleation of the globe in infancy and early childhood, if untreated with a prosthesis, leads to arrested development of the orbit, resulting in a small orbit.[36]

In coronal suture synostosis, the orbit on the side of the fusion is elongated superiorly and laterally, imparting a harlequin appearance (Fig. 9-31). Correction of the cranial deformity can lead to spontaneous correction of the orbital deformity in some instances.[49, 50] In mandibulofacial dysostosis, the orbits may be defective inferolaterally because of malar bone hypoplasia. In cases of severe malar hypoplasia, the lateral wall of the orbit is formed by the greater wing of

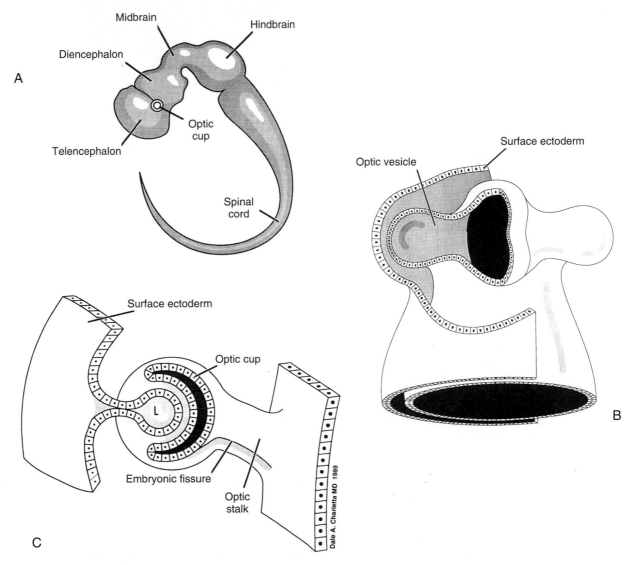

**FIGURE 9-30**   **A,** A 5-mm developing human embryo (4 weeks of gestation). By 3 weeks of gestation two indentations appear, one on either side of the neural groove. These are optic pits, which deepen to form the optic vesicles, one on either side of the forebrain. The optic vesicles give rise to an optic stalk and optic cup on either side. **B,** Development of the posterior ocular structures. In the 4 mm embryo, lateral diverticula on either side of the forebrain have given rise to two optic vesicles. The distal portions of the optic vesicles expand, and the proximal portions become the tubular optic stalks. **C,** At the 5 mm stage, the external surface of each optic vesicle invaginates to form the optic cup. The inner wall of the optic cup (formerly the outer wall of the optic vesicle) gives rise to the retina, and the outer wall of the cup becomes the retinal pigment epithelium. The optic vesicle is covered by a layer of surface ectoderm, which forms the lens (*L*). Note the embryonic fissure, through which mesenchyme extends into the optic stalk and cup. Failure of the embryonic fissure to close causes typical ocular colobomas. (From Mafee MF et al. CT of optic nerve colobomas, morning glory anomaly, and colobomatous cyst. Radiol Clin North Am 1987;25:693.)

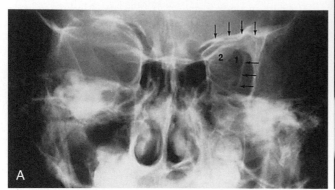
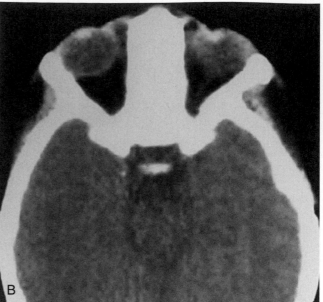

**FIGURE 9-31**   **A,** Microphthalmia. Posteroanterior view of the skull. The lesser wing of the sphenoid (*2*) and the left maxillary sinus are hypoplastic; superior orbital fissures are asymmetric (*1*). Note the difference between the oblique lines (*horizontal arrows*), which represent cortices of the temporal surface of the greater wings of the sphenoid bone. Notice the hypoplasia of the roof of the left orbit (*vertical arrows*). **B,** Microphthalmia. Four-year-old boy born without a nose and with left microphthalmos and apparent hypertelorism. The left globe is smaller than the right. Increased soft tissue between the medial wall or orbit and the globe anteriorly has the clinical appearance of hypertelorism. In fact, the interorbital bony distance is normal. (From Mafee MF et al. CT in the evaluation of the orbit and the bony interorbital distance. AJNR 1986;7:265.)

the sphenoid and the zygomatic process of the frontal bone (also see Chapter 1).

## Bony Abnormalities

Minor degrees of facial and orbital asymmetry are the most common causes of pseudoproptosis.[4] For the most part, these patients have minor degrees of asymmetry involving all of the hemifacial structures.[3] However, in a few instances, the asymmetry may be related to maxillary hypoplasia resulting in a relatively retroplaced orbit on the affected side. In many cases, familial asymmetry may be evident when the siblings or parents are examined. These minor developmental abnormalities of the orbit are considered anatomic variations. Anomalies of ossification may result in accessory sutures and supernumerary ossicles in the orbital walls.[36] On rare occasions, congenital absence of bone in the frontal, maxillary, and orbital regions may result in deformity of the bony orbit. Asymmetric enlargement of one bony orbit may be due to eccentrically located lesions such as neurofibroma, hemangioma, lymphangioma, dermoid, and other slow-growing processes. A small orbit is seen in anophthalmia, microphthalmia, and postenucleation of the globe in infancy, if not followed by prompt prosthetic treatment.

## Bony Orbit in Craniofacial Dysostosis

Craniofacial dysostosis and developmental anomalies may result in profound orbital abnormalities. Orbital malformations in craniofacial dysostosis result chiefly from coronal synostosis. Premature closure of one or more cranial sutures, termed *craniosynostosis* or *craniostenosis*, is the common denominator of many patients with craniofacial anomaly.[51–58]

## Primary Congenital Isolated Craniosynostosis

Any cranial suture may undergo premature closure, but several patterns are recognizable more commonly than others.[50] The incidence of congenital suture synostosis reported by Harwood-Nash,[51] derived from a composite of his experience and from two large series reported by Anderson and Geiger[52] and Shillito and Matson,[53] is as follows: sagittal, 56%; single coronal, 11%; bilateral coronal, 11%; metopic suture, 7%; lambdoid, 1%; and three or more sutures, 14%. Depending on the suture that is prematurely closed, the skull and orbit, including the interorbital distance, have a characteristic shape. These can be grouped as follows: (1) metopic; trigonocephaly (triangular head); hypotelorism is a constant feature of the trigonocephaly;[48] (2) sagittal, scaphocephaly (dolichocephaly), in which the anteroposterior diameter of the bony orbit is usually increased and the vertical and transverse diameters of the bony orbit are usually decreased; (3) unilateral coronal or lambdoid; plagiocephaly; in this condition, if the coronal suture is involved, there is characteristic deformity of the bony orbit, which will be discussed later; (4) bilateral coronal or lambdoid, resulting in brachycephaly; (5) coronal and sagittal; oxycephaly or acrocephaly (turricephaly); and (6) coronal, lambdoid, and sagittal;

cloverleaf skull (kleeblattschädel). Primary craniosynostosis may be associated with congenital syndromes. These conditions include the following: Crouzon's disease (craniofacial dysostosis), Apert's disease (acrocephalosyndactyly, type I), Saethre-Chotzen syndrome (acrocephalosyndactyly, type II), Carpenter's syndrome (acrocephalopolysyndactyly), chondrodystrophia calcificans congenita (Conradi's syndrome, or punctate epiphyseal dysplasia), Brachmann-de Lange syndrome, Laurence-Moon-Biedl-Bardet syndrome, Treacher Collins syndrome (mandibulofacial dysostosis), and craniotelencephalic dysplasia.[39, 48, 50]

## Orbit in Plagiocephaly

Plagiocephaly is due to unilateral closure of one of the paired sutures of the skull, frequently the coronal or lambdoid but rarely the temporosquamous sutures. Each produces a characteristic deformity of the skull. In practice, most of the time, plagiocephaly is seen in patients with hemicoronal premature synostosis, in which there is an ipsilateral elevation of the lesser wing of the sphenoid associated with upward extension of the superior lateral portion of the orbit, imparting a harlequin appearance to the orbit (Fig. 9-32A).[50] The flattening of the ipsilateral frontal bone is also characteristic of premature coronal synostosis (Fig. 9-32B). The volume of the anterior cranial fossa on the side of fusion is decreased. The greater wing of the sphenoid is expanded, displaced forward and downward, and forms a relatively large middle cranial fossa (Fig. 9-32B,C). This occurs in addition to upward elevation of the roof of the orbit, which produces a shallow orbit. The ethmoidal plate (roof of the ethmoidal sinus) also is elevated on the side of fusion (Fig. 9-32A). The nasal septum, crista galli, and ethmoidal complex are tilted to the side of fusion (Fig. 9-32A).

Premature fusion of both coronal sutures may occur with or without any other associated abnormality. This may result in marked shortening of the anterior cranial fossa and orbital depth, and the brain impressions become more prominent on the inner table of the frontal bone (Fig. 9-33). Both a harlequin appearance of the orbit and the bony changes of the unilateral coronal synostosis are duplicated in this bilateral form of premature fusion (Fig. 9-33). Lombardi noted a connection between sagittal or lambdoid synostosis, or both, in half of the reported cases of coronal suture synostosis.[55]

## Orbit in Crouzon's and Apert's Diseases

Crouzon's disease, also known as *craniofacial dysostosis*, is an autosomal dominant disorder with considerable variability in expression.[50] Apert's disease, also known as *acrocephalosyndactyly type I*, is transmitted as an autosomal dominant disorder. The cranial and facial characteristics of Crouzon's disease are somewhat similar to those of Apert's syndrome, including brachycephaly, hypertelorism, bilateral exophthalmos, parrot-beaked nose, maxillary hypoplasia, relative prognathism, and a drooping lower lip that produces a half-open mouth. Bilateral exophthalmos is essentially a consequence of exorbitism, which in turn is a consequence

of several factors that combine to produce a decrease in orbital volume. On the basis of the skull shape alone, Crouzon's and Apert's diseases cannot be distinguished.[50]

In any large series of patients with Crouzon's disease, there is no regular pattern of calvarial deformity. Oxycephaly, brachycephaly, scaphocephaly, and trigonocephaly may be present. In fact, there is too much heterogeneity to allow for a simplistic description. Generally, in Crouzon's disease, brachycephaly, or oxycephaly, is most often observed. Apert's disease is characterized by irregular craniostenosis with an acrobrachycephalic skull and syndactyly of the hands and feet. Associated skeletal abnormalities such as ankylosis of the elbow, hip, and shoulder, as well as malformations of the cardiovascular, gastrointestinal, and genitourinary systems, may be present.

The orbital malformation in Crouzon's and Apert's diseases is due mainly to premature coronal synostosis. A striking harlequin appearance of the orbits is seen that results from elevation of the roof and lateral walls of the orbits (Fig. 9-34). The supraorbital rim is recessed, and the infraorbital rim is hypoplastic. The orbital depth is markedly reduced as the result of verticalization of the roof (upward tilt of the lesser wing and orbital plate of the frontal bone). Displacement of the greater wing of the sphenoid into a more coronal orientation, which is referred to as *frontalization* of the greater wing of the sphenoid, and ballooning of the ethmoid are other factors contributing to exotropia. Hypoplasia of the maxilla and the intermaxillary component contributes in part to the exophthalmos and relative prognathism (Figs. 9-34 and 9-35). Hypoplasia of the maxilla causes recession of the infraorbital rim and foreshortening of the orbital floor.[50] The optic canal in Crouzon's and Apert's diseases is usually narrow. This may lead to optic atrophy.[3] The distance between the intracranial openings of the optic canals is usually normal, and this finding forms the basis for surgical procedures designed to correct orbital hypertelorism by moving the bony orbits closer together without damaging the optic or oculomotor nerves.[50] Of particular importance to the surgeon contemplating surgical correction of orbital hypertelorism are the orientation and degree of foreshortening of the lateral wall of the orbit. The type of lateral wall osteotomy performed (sagittal split or total mobilization) often depends on these anatomic factors.[33, 34] Patients with craniosynostosis syndromes may have marked extraocular muscle anomalies ranging from an apparent absence of ocular muscles to abnormally inserted muscles or very small extraocular muscles (Figs. 9-34 to 9-36).

## Saethre-Chotzen Syndrome (Acrocephalosyndactyly Type II)

Saethre-Chotzen syndrome was described by Saethre in 1931 and in 1932 by Chotzen.[50, 55-57] The first family with this disease to be reported in the United States was described in 1970 by Bartsocas et al.[58] Saethre-Chotzen syndrome is characterized by synostotic malformation of multiple sutures, facial asymmetry, mild midface hypoplasia, ptosis of the eyelids, an antimongoloid slant of the palpebral fissures, a beaked nose, a low-set frontal hairline, variable brachycephaly, and variable cutaneous syndactyly, particularly of the second and third fingers. Other associated abnormalities

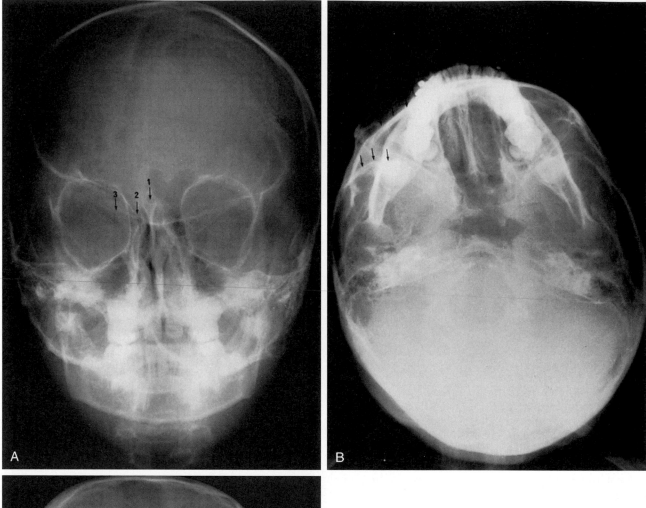

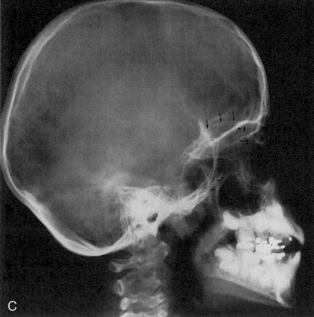

**FIGURE 9-32** Plagiocephaly. **A,** Cauldoid view. Premature fusion of the right coronal suture. Note the elevation of the right roof of the orbit, giving a harlequin appearance to the right eye. The right lesser wing of the sphenoid (*3*) and the right ethmoidal plate (fovea ethmoidal [roof]) (*2*) are elevated. The right lateral margin of the orbit is flattened, particularly in the superior portion. Digital markings are somewhat increased on the right side. Note the shift of the crista galli (*1*), ethmoid complex, and nasal septum to the right. The volume of the right anterior cranial fossa is decreased, usually a characteristic of premature coronal synostosis. **B,** Submentovertical view of the same patient as in **A.** Note flattening of the right frontal bone (*upper arrows*), expansion of the right greater wing of the sphenoid (*lower arrows*), and tilting of the ethmoid complex to the involved side. Note the anterior displacement of the right petrous bone and right temporomandibular joint and flattening of the right side of the occipital bone. **C,** Lateral view of same patient as in **A** and **B.** Note the anterior displacement of the right greater wing of the sphenoid (*lower arrows*), elevation of the orbital surface of the right anterior cranial fossa (*upper arrows*) and the bony ridge along the right (*1*) and left (*2*) medial borders of orbital roof. (From Mafee MF et al. Radiology of the craniofacial anomalies. Radiol Clin North Am 1982;14:939–988.)

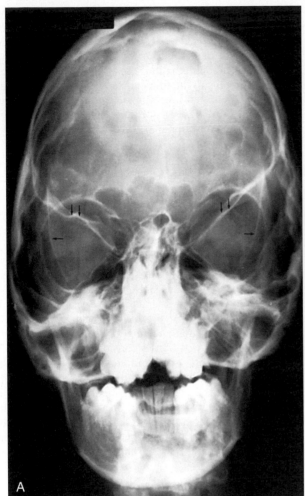

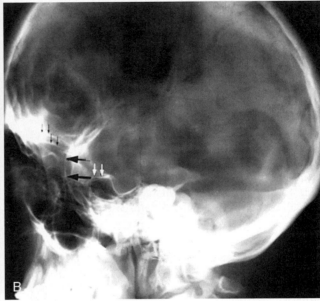

**FIGURE 9-33** Craniosynostosis caused by bilateral premature fusion of coronal sutures. **A,** Posteroanterior view of skull shows hyperteloric orbits and markedly increased digital markings. Note elevation of the lesser wings of the sphenoid (*vertical arrows*) and harlequin appearance of both orbits. Note the stretched and laterally placed oblique lines (*horizontal arrows*) and flattening of the lateral wall of the orbits with a recessed lateral orbital rim. **B,** Lateral skull view of the same patient as in **A** shows absence of sutural lines, increased digital markings, downward and forward displacement of the greater wings of the sphenoid bone (*large black arrows*), elevation of the roof of the orbits (*small black arrows*), and low position of the planum sphenoidale (*white arrows*).

include a high-arched palate, cleft palate, and deformity of the external ear. The orbital abnormalities in these patients are similar to those in Crouzon's and Apert's diseases.

## Neurofibromatosis

The classic description of neurofibromatosis was published by Friedrich Daniel von Recklinghausen in 1882. Clinical criteria for diagnosing neurofibromatosis include (1) six or more café-au-lait spots, each greater than 1.5 cm in diameter; (2) axillary or other intertriginous freckles; (3) cutaneous neurofibromas; and (4) one or more unequivocally affected parents or siblings.[59] The disease itself is characterized by abnormalities of both ectodermal and mesodermal origin. It is transmitted as an autosomal dominant disorder of variable penetrance.[33] The incidence of neurofibromatosis is approximately 1 in 3000 live births.[60] About 50% of these patients have a positive family history of the disease, and the other 50% are the result of a spontaneous mutation; the mutation rate is about 10:4.[61] The incidence of central nervous system tumors, including acoustic neuromas, gliomas, meningiomas, and ependymomas, is six times that of the general population.[62] Often multiple central nervous system tumors are present. Al-

though 25% to 35% of neurofibromas occur in the head and neck region, orbital abnormalities are relatively uncommon.[60] Orbital abnormalities are often associated with exophthalmos, which may be pulsatile and generally can be classified into one of four categories: (1) orbital neoplasms; (2) plexiform neurofibromatosis; (3) orbital osseous dysplasia (Fig. 9-37); and (4) congenital glaucoma.[60] The most common orbital neoplasm seen in association with neurofibromatosis is optic glioma (Fig. 9-37A). Meningioma is not unusual. Both optic gliomas and meningiomas may occur bilaterally. Bilateral optic gliomas are almost pathognomonic of neurofibromatosis (Fig. 9-38), whereas bilateral meningiomas are only suggestive of neurofibromatosis. Orbital schwannoma, neurofibroma, and neurofibrosarcoma also can be seen in these patients.

## Orbital (Mesodermal) Defects

Osseous dysplasia of the cranial bones, in particular the bony orbit, may be part of the abnormality associated with von Recklinghausen's disease. The orbital defect is a consequence of partial or complete absence of the greater or lesser wing of the sphenoid bone, or both. The body of the sphenoid bone may also be involved, producing an abnormal and dysplastic sella turcica (Fig. 9-37).[33, 60] These osseous abnormalities allow the adjacent temporal lobe of the brain and its overlying, often thickened dural membrane to herniate anteriorly into the posterior aspect of the orbit, causing anterior displacement of the globe (Fig. 9-37). The normal CSF pulsations are transmitted to the globe, resulting in pulsatile exophthalmos. Associated findings include hypoplasia of the ipsilateral frontal and maxillary sinuses and hypoplasia of the adjacent ethmoid air cells.[33, 60]

## Mandibulofacial Dysostosis

### Orbital Defects

The malformation known as *mandibulofacial dysostosis* (MFD) was first reported in 1889 by an ophthalmologist, G.A. Berry.[63] Treacher Collins, whose name is attached to the disease of MFD, described the disease and noted the characteristic malar hypoplasia and the associated flattening of the cheeks.[64] In 1923, Pires de Lima and Monteior stated that MFD probably is due to a developmental defect affecting the branchial arches (the hallmark of MFD is its varied expressivity).[65] Franceschetti and Klein, who coined the name *mandibulofacial dysostosis*, classified the syndrome into five separate categories: complete, incomplete, abortive, unilateral, and atypical.[66] Gorlin et al. stated that there is no unilateral form of the syndrome

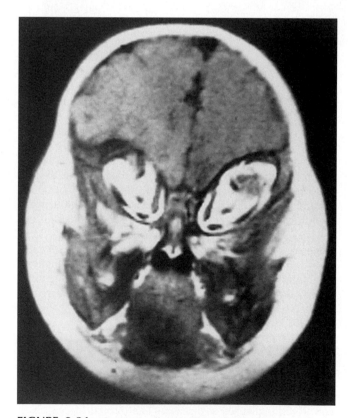

**FIGURE 9-34** Crouzon's disease. Coronal MR image shows the striking harlequin appearance of the orbits caused by elevation of the roofs and lateral walls or orbits. Note the deformity of the extraocular muscles and hypoplasia of the midface. One or more extraocular muscles may be absent in Crouzon's or Apert's disease.

and that such cases are better classified as hemifacial microsomia.[37] Poswillo, in his experimental study of a teratogenically induced phenocopy of MFD in an animal model, showed that the disorder results from disorganization of the preoptic neural crest at about the time of migration of cells to the first and second branchial arches.[67] There are now several recognized malformations in which abnormalities of the eye and associated abnormalities of structures derived from the first and second branchial arches are found.

### Bony Orbital Defects

In MFD the maxilla and malar bones are usually poorly developed, with small antra and shallow or incomplete orbital floors (Fig. 9-39A).[50] The malar bones are hypoplastic, and the zygomatic arches are usually incomplete. The development of the zygomatic process of the maxilla varies among the cases described, and it may not be developed. The radiographic orbital characteristics of MFD are the downward-sloping floors of the orbits in line medially with a beak-like bony nasal contour. The lateral and lower rim of the orbit is often defective (Fig. 9-39A). CT shows the deficiency of the lateral orbital floor as an orbital cleft that varies considerably in degree. The greater wings of the sphenoid may be hypoplastic, and therefore the lateral orbital wall may be defective (Fig. 9-39A). Herring et al. reported a patient with MFD who had hypoplasia of the greater wing of the sphenoid and in whom the temporal squamous bone extended anteriorly, beyond its usual boundaries, to replace the very hypoplastic greater wing of the sphenoid.[68] The squamous bone articulated directly with the frontal bone, at the anterior end of the temporal fossa, and formed a section of the lateral orbital wall. In MFD the infraorbital foramen may be absent, the fossa of the lacrimal sac may be larger than normal, and the nasolacrimal canal is usually short.[68] The lacrimal bones are normal.

## Bony Orbit in Craniofacial Microsomia

Craniofacial microsomia is known by many names, including *first and second branchial syndrome, otomandibular dysostosis,* and *oculoauriculovertebral dysplasia.*[37, 50, 69] In general, among the congenital oculoauriculocephalic syndromes, the term *first and second branchial arch syndrome* designates a characteristic congenital malformation that is usually unilateral but occasionally is bilateral. The term *hemifacial microsomia* was advocated by Gorlin et al. to refer to patients with unilateral microtia, microsomia, and failure of formation of the mandibular ramus and condyle.[37] Hemifacial microsomia includes as a variant of this complex such malformations as Goldenhar's syndrome and oculoauriculovertebral dysplasia, previously described as separate entities.[37] About 10% of the patients have bilateral involvement, but the disorder is nearly always more severe on one side.[37] The associated eye findings that are considered variable features of this syndrome include epibulbar dermoids or lipodermoids, microphthalmia, coloboma of the choroid and iris, and deformity of the bony orbit similar to MFD as a result of hypoplasia of the maxilla and malar bone.

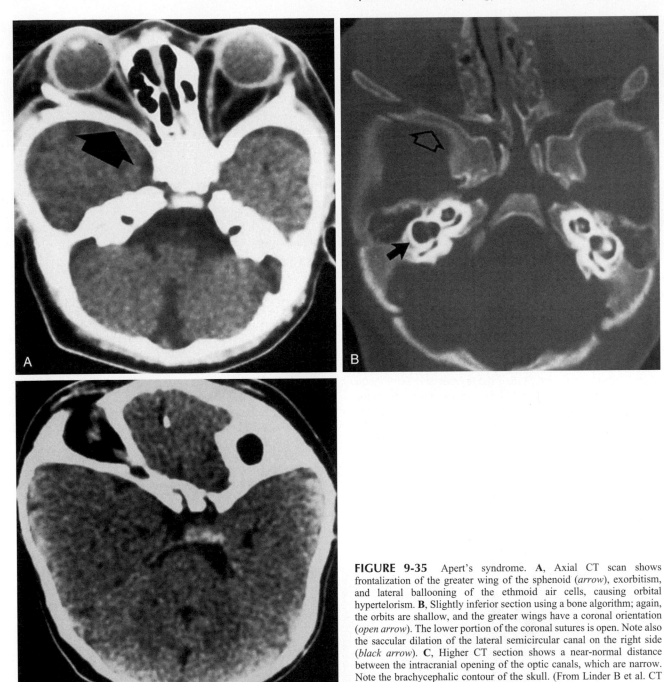

**FIGURE 9-35**  Apert's syndrome. **A**, Axial CT scan shows frontalization of the greater wing of the sphenoid (*arrow*), exorbitism, and lateral ballooning of the ethmoid air cells, causing orbital hypertelorism. **B**, Slightly inferior section using a bone algorithm; again, the orbits are shallow, and the greater wings have a coronal orientation (*open arrow*). The lower portion of the coronal sutures is open. Note also the saccular dilation of the lateral semicircular canal on the right side (*black arrow*). **C**, Higher CT section shows a near-normal distance between the intracranial opening of the optic canals, which are narrow. Note the brachycephalic contour of the skull. (From Linder B et al. CT and MRI of orbital abnormalities in neurofibromatoses and selected craniofacial anomalies. Radiol Clin North Am 1987;25:787–802.)

## Developmental Orbital Cysts

The most frequent developmental cysts involving the orbit and periorbital structures are the dermoid and epidermoid cysts, choristomas, and teratomas.[3, 8, 17, 70, 72] The relative frequency of these cysts compared to other orbital lesions is shown in Table 9-2. The age distribution of the common orbital diseases is shown in Table 9-3. Choristoma is a focus of tissue histologically normal for an organ or part of an organ at a site other than the site at which it is located.[5, 6, 73] A dermoid or epidermoid cyst is a choristoma that may be found in several locations in the orbit. Lipodermoids are solid tumors that are usually located beneath the conjunctiva over the lateral surface of the globe.[5, 6] A conjunctival lipodermoid is a true choristoma, since (adipose) fatty tissue usually is not found in this region. Conjunctival choristomas are relatively common congenital lesions that possess little growth potential. They contain both dermal and epidermal elements that are not normally found in the conjunctiva.[74] Three types of conjunctival choristomas are found—the solid limbal dermoid, the more diffuse dermolipoma, and the complex choristoma. Solid limbal dermoids typically occur unilaterally, at the inferotemporal limbus. Dermolipomas (lipoder-

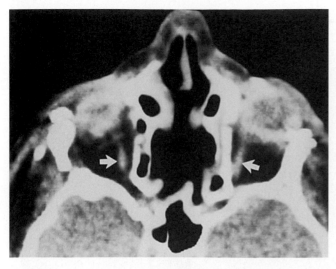

**FIGURE 9-36**  Crouzon's syndrome. CT scan shows the small inferior rectus muscles (*arrows*). Note the hypertelorism and postsurgical changes of the lateral orbital walls.

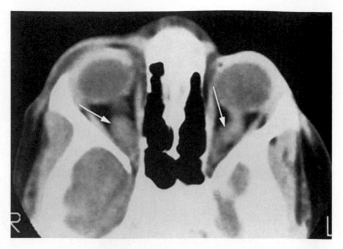

**FIGURE 9-38**  Axial CT scan. Neurofibromatosis with bilateral optic nerve gliomas (*arrows*).

moids) are less dense than solid dermoids and contain more adipose tissue. Typically they are found on the superior temporal bulbar conjunctiva near the levator and extraocular muscles[5, 6] (Fig. 9-40). These masses can extend from the limbus anteriorly to the posterior aspect of the globe and orbit between the superior and lateral rectus.[74] Care must be taken during surgical removal to avoid rupture of the cyst, with deposition of cells at the operative sites, and in particular not to damage the palpebral portion of the lacrimal gland, extraocular muscles, or levator palpebrae superioris.[73, 74] Bilateral limbal dermoids or dermolipomas are found in children who have Goldenhar's syndrome. Complex choristomas consist of variable combinations of ectopic

tissues such as ectopic lacrimal gland, respiratory, eyelid gland, or brain tissues. Epibulbar osseous choristomas are solitary nodules that resemble dermoids. They are composed of mature, compact bone along with other typical choristomatous elements such as pilosebaceous units and hair follicles.[74] Dermoid and epidermoid cysts are choristomas that are among the most common orbital tumors of childhood. Both may be found in several locations in the orbit, most frequently superior and temporal. The tumor is congenital but may not be noted at birth. Many become evident only in the second and third decades.[6] Both result from the inclusion of ectodermal elements during closure of the neural tube. The dermal elements that are pinched off along the suture lines, diploe, or within the meninges or scalp in the course of embryonic development give rise to

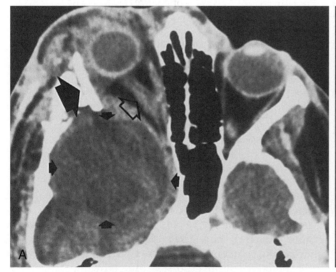

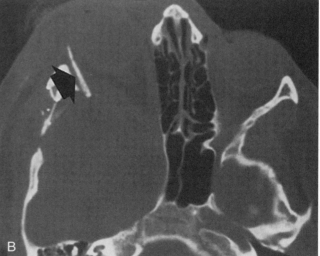

**FIGURE 9-37**  Neurofibromatosis. The patient had previous surgery for correction of an orbital deformity. **A**, Axial CT scan. Note the bone graft along the lateral margin of the right orbit (*large black arrow*). Note the normal left and dysplastic right greater wing of the sphenoid bone, with anterior herniation of the porencephalic cyst of the temporal lobe (*small arrows*) covered by dura. The right optic nerve is enlarged (*open arrow*), and the right globe is proptotic. Enlargement of the optic nerve is thought to be caused by optic nerve glioma. **B**, Osseous abnormalities are better seen on this bone detail image. (From Linder B et al. CT and MRI of orbital abnormalities in neurofibromatosis and selected craniofacial anomalies. Radiol Clin North Am 1987;25:787.)

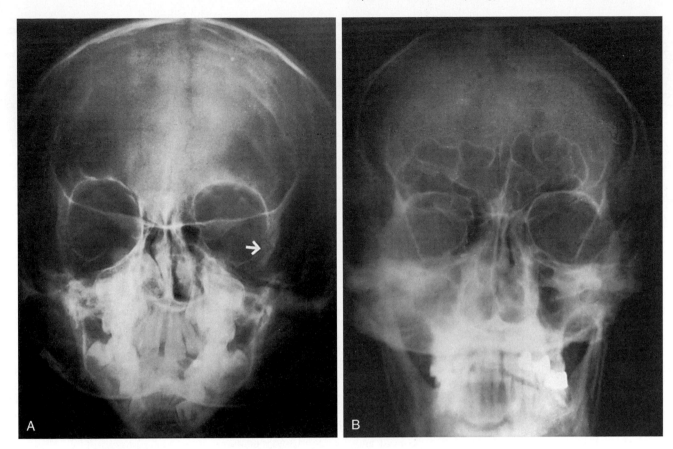

**FIGURE 9-39**   **A**, Mandibulofacial dysostosis. Posteroanterior (PA) view of the skull shows a hypoplastic mandible, hypoplastic malar bones, hypoplastic maxillary antra, and hypoplastic lateral wall of the orbits (*arrow*). Oblique (innominate) lines are not visible because of hypoplasia of the greater wing of the sphenoid. **B**, Normal PA view of the skull for comparison.

these cysts.[6, 71] Both have a fibrous capsule with varying degrees of thickness. The epidermoid has a lining of keratinizing, stratified squamous epithelium. The dermoid contains one or more dermal adnexal structures such as sebaceous glands and hair follicles. Some dermoid cysts

**Table 9-2**
**FREQUENCY OF ORBITAL LESIONS BY MAJOR DIAGNOSTIC GROUP**

| Diagnostic Group | Frequency (%) |
| --- | --- |
| Thyroid orbitopathy | 47 |
| Cystic lesions | 8 |
| Inflammatory lesions | 8 |
| Vascular lesions | 5 |
| Lacrimal gland lesions | 4 |
| Lymphoproliferative lesions | 4 |
| Secondary tumors | 4 |
| Myxomatous and adipose lesions | 3 |
| Mesenchymal lesions | 2 |
| Metastatic tumors | 2 |
| Optic nerve tumors | 1 |
| Fibrous and connective tissue lesions | 1 |
| Osseous and fibroosseous lesions | 1 |
| Histiocytic lesions | <1 |
| Other and unclassified | 17 |

From Dutton J. Orbital diseases. In: Yanoff M, Duker JS, eds. Ophthalmology. St. Louis: CV Mosby, 1999;14.1–14.7.

may also contain lobules of fat. These dermoid cysts should be considered well-differentiated teratomas, because they contain tissue derived from more than a single embryonic germ layer. Teratomas are choristomatous tumors that contain tissues representing two or more germ layers. Endodermal derivatives such as gut or respiratory epithelium, ectodermal tissues such as skin and its appendages, and neural and mesodermal tissues such as connective tissues, smooth muscles, cartilage, bone, and vessels may be present. These developmental cysts represent 24% of all orbital and lid masses, 6% to 8% of deep orbital masses, and 80% of cystic orbital lesions.[75] These cysts may contain fluid or solid components.[73, 76] Teratomas are evident at birth as grossly visible cystic orbital masses.[8, 71] Teratomas are tumors composed of cells originating from more than one embryonic germ layer and situated in a site that is not the normal location for the cells.[73] Orbital teratomas may arise from pluripotential stem cells delivered to the orbit hematogenously or from stem cells displaced during their migration.[73] The tumors can be both solid and cystic. However, they are usually cystic and can cause dramatic exophthalmos at birth. Although teratomas in other sites such as testes are commonly malignant, teratomas within the orbit are rarely malignant.[73] Orbital teratomas tend to affect girls, are unilateral, grow rapidly, and are not associated with other anomalies. Although exenteration is sometimes performed

**Table 9-3**
**AGE DISTRIBUTION OF COMMON ORBITAL DISEASES**

| Diagnostic Group | Frequency (%) | | |
| --- | --- | --- | --- |
| | Childhood and Adolescence (0–20 Years) | Middle Age (21–60 Years) | Later Adult Life (61+ Years) |
| Thyroid orbitopathy | 10 | 59 | 40 |
| Infectious process | 7 | 3 | 3 |
| Inflammatory lesions | 6 | 5 | 9 |
| Cystic lesions | 12 | 3 | 4 |
| Vascular neoplastic lesions | 15 | 2 | 1 |
| Other vascular lesions | 7 | 2 | 3 |
| Trauma | 7 | 4 | 2 |
| Secondary orbital malignancies | 1 | 2 | 9 |
| Metastatic malignancies | 1 | 1 | 8 |
| Mesenchymal lesions | 9 | 1 | 1 |
| Lymphangiomas | 6 | 1 | 0 |
| Lymphoproliferative diseases | 1 | 3 | 12 |
| Optic nerve lesions | 5 | 1 | 1 |
| Other neurogenic lesions | 5 | 3 | 2 |
| Lacrimal gland fossa | 1 | 1 | 1 |
| Other | 7 | 8 | 4 |

From Dutton J. Orbital diseases. In: Yanoff M, Duker JS, eds. Ophthalmology. St. Louis: CV Mosby, 1999;14.1–14.7.

because of the fear of malignancy, cystic teratomas can sometimes be removed with preservation of the eye.[6] Intraocular teratomas are distinctly rare and may appear similar to the teratoid medulloepithelioma, a usually benign tumor of the ciliary body and rarely of the optic disc and nerve, which is seen in young children. The dermoid and epidermoid cysts favor the upper portion of the orbit for their growth (Figs. 9-41 and 9-42). They grow slowly; however, at times these cysts can grow rapidly, particularly in adults.[72] They are most frequently located at the superior temporal quadrant of the orbit, where they are fixed to the periosteum near the frontozygomatic suture line (Figs. 9-41 and 9-42A,B).[70–72] Occasionally, they can be found at the frontoethmoidal or frontonasal sutures and can simulate an encephalocele (Fig. 9-42C).[6] These cysts may be entirely confined to the orbital adnexal tissues. Most of them appear clinically during childhood and present as subcutaneous nodules near the orbital rim. In adults the cysts most commonly arise behind the orbital rim, often near the lacrimal gland, and may be difficult to distinguish from lacrimal gland tumors.[71, 72] The cysts may contain cystic or solid components.

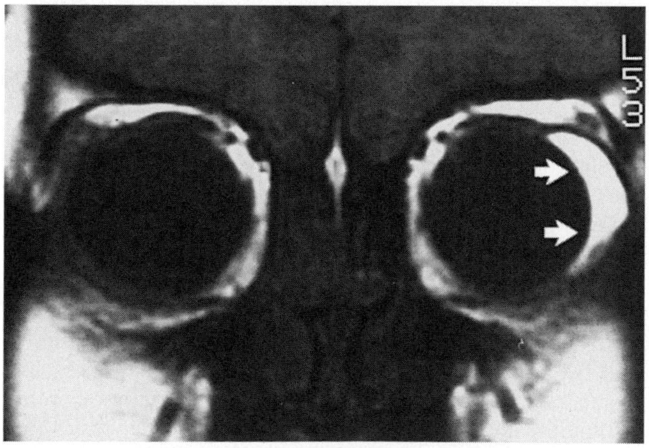

## Diagnostic Imaging

The imaging modality of choice depends on the entity being considered. When a prominent feature of the suspected lesion is bone remodeling, bone destruction, bone or calcium deposition, or intralesional fat, CT scanning is indicated (Fig. 9-41). MR imaging may provide information about the characteristics of fluid and tissues within the cystic lesion. Both epidermoid and dermoid cysts appear on CT as unenhanced, well-circumscribed, smoothly margin-ated, low-density masses (Figs. 9-41, 9-42). If a dermoid cyst contains fatty tissues (well-differentiated teratomas), it has fat density on CT (Fig. 9-42A). Similarly, calcifications may be seen within these dermoid cysts. Calcification is not a feature of epidermoids. Although rare, we have seen calcification in intracranial epidermoid but not in orbital epidermoid cysts. Fat-fluid levels may be present in dermoid cysts. A ruptured dermoid/epidermoid cyst shows surrounding inflammatory changes. Some dermoid cysts may appear moderately to markedly hyperdense on CT scans. On MR imaging, dermoid and epidermoid cysts have low signal intensity on T1-weighted MR images and high signal intensity on T2-weighted, flair as well as diffusion-weighted MR images (Fig. 9-41B). A dermoid cyst that contains significant fatty tissue demonstrates the MR characteristics of fat (Fig. 9-42B). Both dermoid and epidermoid cysts may demonstrate marginal enhancement of their wall on postcontrast CT and MR images. The CT and MR imaging features of these lesions are shown in Table 9-4.

**FIGURE 9-40**   Coronal T1-weighted MR image shows a hyperintense mass (*arrows*) compatible with a dermolipoma. (From Kaufman LM et al. Diagnostic imaging of cystic lesions in the child's orbit. Radiol Clin North Am 1998;36:1149–1163.)

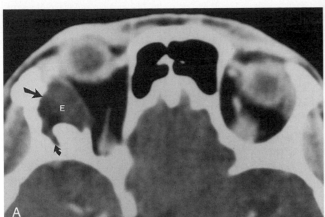

**FIGURE 9-41** Epidermoid cyst. **A**, Postcontrast axial CT scan shows a nonenhanced low-density mass (*E*) compatible with an epidermoid cyst. Notice the scalloping of the lateral orbital wall (*arrows*). **B**, T2-weighted MR scan. The epidermoid cyst (*E*) appears as a homogeneous hyperintense mass.

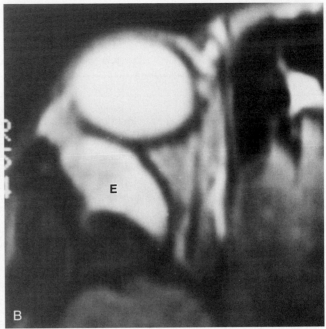

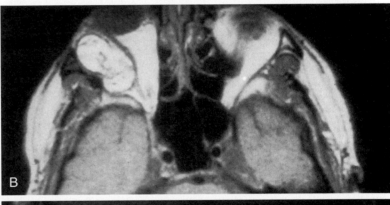

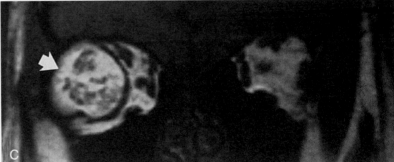

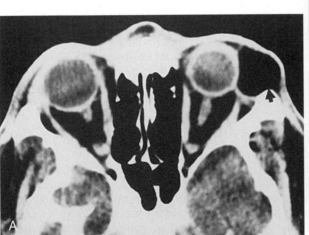

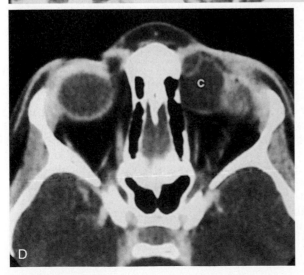

**FIGURE 9-42** **A**, Dermoid. Axial CT scan shows a fat-containing lesion (*arrow*) compatible with an orbital dermoid. **B**, Another patient. Dermoid. PW axial MR image and T2-weighted coronal MR image (**C**) show a giant dermoid (*arrow*). The lesion is inhomogeneous and contains hyperintense areas caused by fat. The lesion is nearly isointense to fat on the T2-weighted MR image. **D**, Axial-enhanced CT scan shows a well-circumscribed, rounded, low-density dermoid cyst (*C*) in the nasal aspect of the anterior orbit. (From Kaufman LM et al. Diagnostic imaging of cystic lesions in the child's orbit. Radiol Clin North Am 1998;36:1149–1163.)

**Table 9-4**
**CT AND MR IMAGING FEATURES OF ORBITAL CYSTS**

| Diagnostic Group | CT Characteristics | MR Imaging Characteristics |
|---|---|---|
| Epidermoid cyst | Nonenhancing mass with or without bone erosion<br>Scalloping with sclerosis of the adjacent bone may be present<br>No calcification<br>Minimal enhancement of the capsule may be present | Hypointense on T1-weighted and hyperintense on T2-weighted images<br>Minimal enhancement of capsule may be present<br>Associated orbital inflammatory changes, when cyst is ruptured |
| Dermoid cyst | Nonenhancing mass with or without bone erosion<br>Scalloping with sclerosis of the adjacent bone may be present<br>Calcification, if present, is a characteristic feature<br>Hypodensity (fat), if present, is characteristic (adipose tissue)<br>Fat-fluid level may be present and is characteristic<br>Minimal enhancement of the capsule may be present | Hypointense on T1-weighted and hyperintense on T2-weighted images<br>Those containing fat demonstrate signal characteristics of fatty tissue<br>Minimal enhancement of capsule may be present<br>Associated orbital inflammatory changes, when cyst is ruptured |
| Conjunctival choristoma (dermolipoma) | Density of adipose tissue | Intensity of adipose tissue |
| Cholesterol granuloma (chronic hematic cyst) | Nonenhancing mass with or without bone erosion<br>Lytic lesion with ragged bone destruction<br>Often isodense to brain<br>No sclerotic margin | High signal on T1-weighted and T2-weighted images<br>Often homogeneous in signal characteristics<br>Heterogeneous signal, particularly on T2-weighted images |
| Enterogenous cysts | Isodense or hyperdense, depending on the mucous content of the cyst | Hypointense or hyperintense on T1-weighted images, depending on the mucous content of the cyst, and hyperintense on T2-weighted images |
| Other orbital epithelial and appendage cysts, including implantation cysts | Nonenhancing low-density mass | Nonenhancing, hypointense on T1-weighted and hyperintense on T2-weighted images |
| Congenital cystic eye | Nonenhancing low-density mass | Hypointense on T1-weighted and hyperintense on T2-weighted images<br>Nonenhancing mass |
| Dacryocele | Nonenhancing (unless infected) low-density mass | Hypointense on T1-weighted and hyperintense on T2-weighted images; nonenhancing mass, unless infected |
| Parasitic cysts (hydatid, cysticercosis) | Cystic lesions within or near an EOM<br>Some degree of enhancement around the cyst wall<br>Scolex can be identified<br>Diffuse myositis may be present<br>Cystic lesion within or near lacrimal gland or other part of the orbit | Cystic lesions within or near an EOM<br>Hypointense on T1-weighted and hyperintense on T2-weighted images<br>Some degree of enhancement around the cyst wall<br>Scolex can be identified<br>Diffuse myositis may be present |

## Other Less Common Congenital Anomalies and Acquired Cysts of the Orbit and Optic System

The orbit develops from mesodermal tissues, and the globe and optic pathway develop from ectodermal tissues. Developmental defects of the eyeball result in a small orbit. The majority of orbital changes are found in association with deformities of the skull (Fig. 9-30) and skeleton.[36] Cyclopia, synophthalmia, clinical anophthalmia, and microphthalmia (Figs. 9-30 and 9-31) are developmental anomalies of the globe that are seen in the fetal central system anomalies associated with problems in forebrain differentiation (holoprosencephaly). MR imaging is particularly noteworthy in the detection of these anomalies. In general, a variety of cysts and cyst-like lesions involve the orbit. The list includes developmental anomalies as well as acquired lesions arising in the orbit or in adjacent structures.[73] A *cyst* is defined as a closed sac with a membranous or cellular lining and a luminal space containing air, fluid, semifluid, or solid materials. Cysts typically result from developmental anomalies, obstruction of ducts, or parasitic infections or trauma, as listed in Table 9-5.

## Congenital Cystic Eye

Congenital cystic eye is a rare congenital anomaly resulting from failure of the optic vesicle to invaginate during the fourth week of embryogenesis.[73] It presents at birth as a complex cyst occupying the orbit, without any vestige of a globe (Fig. 9-43). The cyst wall is lined by cells derived from undifferentiated retina and retinal pigment epithelium. Some remnant of an optic nerve–like structure and extraocular muscles may be present.[73] CT and MR imaging generally show an enlarged orbit containing a rounded or ovoid, septated cyst (Fig. 9-43). The superior orbital fissure may be enlarged (widened) ipsilaterally. On MR imaging, the signal intensity of the cyst may not be equal to that of the normal vitreous, because the cyst is generally filled with serum. A rudimentary connection to a thinned optic nerve may be seen. A nodular focus may be seen adjacent to the cyst wall, representing primitive ectopic lens tissue.[73] In the colobomatous orbital cyst, unlike the congenital cystic eye, the globe and optic nerve are seen on CT and MR imaging. The globe is, however, microphthalmic (Fig. 9-44). Orbital colobomatous cysts are described in Chapter 8.

# Other Orbital Cysts

## Optic Nerve Sheath Meningocele

Optic neural sheath meningocele (optic nerve sheath cyst, arachnoid cyst, perioptic hygroma, and dural ectasia, among others) is a saccular dilatation of the meninges surrounding the orbital portion of the optic nerve.[77] These meningoceles may occur primarily or secondarily in association with other orbital processes, such as meningioma, optic nerve pilocytic astrocytoma, and hemangioma. Clinically, these meningoceles may present with changes in visual acuity, visual field, and optic nerve appearance. The CT and MR imaging appearance of optic nerve meningocele or ectasia is that of a prominent focal or segmental enlargement of the dural arachnoid sheath around the optic nerve (Fig. 9-45). The optic nerve dural ectasia may be associated with an empty sella and enlarged subarachnoid cisterns, such as gasserian cisterns (Fig. 9-46).

Cephaloceles include meningocele, encephalocele, meningoencephalocele, and porencephalic cyst.[73] A cephalocele is a cyst-like herniation of brain or meningeal tissues into adjacent structures. The lesions are commonly congenital but can also be due to acquired defects in the bony orbit. The herniated tissue may be limited to meninges (meningocele); brain parenchyma (encephalocele); brain and meninges (meningoencephalocele); or expanding porencephalic cysts. Brain tissue may herniate into the orbit via natural orbital foramina, such as the superior orbital fissure; through dehiscences of the cranial sutures; or through bony orbital defects, such as those seen in patients with neurofibromatosis type 1. When a cleft associated with a midline craniofacial dysraphism affects the nose, there is an increased incidence of frontonasal and intraorbital encephaloceles,

anophthalmos, or microphthalmos. Hypertelorism and a broad nasal root are also found in nearly all affected individuals.[73] MR imaging remains the study of choice to illustrate cephaloceles.

## Enterogenous Cysts

Enterogenous cysts are rare congenital choristomatous cysts of the central nervous system. They contain a single layer of mucin-secreting epithelial cells that resemble gastrointestinal epithelium. The lower cervical and cervicothoracic regions are the more common sites of the lesion. An orbital location is extremely rare.[78] Occasionally these cysts may be seen in the anterior cranial fossa and extending into the orbit. CT shows a well-circumscribed, homogeneous, rather hyperdense, lobular, nonenhancing mass. Extension through the superior orbital fissure may be present. Bony erosion due to compressive bone atrophy or bony remodeling including the greater wing of the sphenoid bone and ethmoid roof may be present. On MR imaging, the lesion usually appears hyperintense on T1-weighted images due to the mucous secretions elaborated by the epithelial lining cells. The T2-weighted MR images may show variable signal intensity, depending on the protein content of the fluid within the cyst. Enhancement of the mucosal rim may be seen on enhanced CT and MR images.[78]

## Dentigerous Cysts

Dentigerous cysts, fluid-filled and lined by keratinizing (keratogenic cysts) or nonkeratinizing, stratified squamous epithelium, arise from the jaw. Infrequently, the cyst can enlarge into the maxillary sinus and erode into the orbit. These cysts appear as a nonenhancing low-density mass on CT scans. On MR imaging they appear with a low to intermediate signal on T1-weighted MR images and hyperintense on T2-weighted MR images. The signal characteristics on T1-weighted MR images depend on the cyst's protein content.

## Cystic Vascular Lesions: Lymphangioma, Varix, Chocolate Cyst

Lymphangioma and varix will be described later in this chapter. Lymphangiomas contain numerous variably sized cystic spaces. Acute hemorrhage into these cystic spaces, whether spontaneous or after minor trauma, results in chocolate cysts. A varix is a venous anomaly and may include a single smooth-contoured, dilated vein. Intralesional hemorrhage in an orbital varix may result in the formation of a chocolate cyst.[73]

## Epithelial and Appendage Cysts

Various acquired cysts involving the eyelids or superficial orbit may derive from the skin of the eyelids, the skin appendages (glands and cilia), or the conjunctiva.[73] Common in children is the chalazion, a cystic expansion at the meibomian sebaceous gland due to a blockage of its excretory duct. Other cysts include apocrine hidrocystoma (sudoriferous cyst), originating from a blocked excretory duct of Moll's apocrine sweat gland; eccrine hidrocystoma, derived from the lid eccrine sweat gland; sebaceous cyst (pilar cyst, retention cyst of the pilosebaceous structure); milia (cystic expansion of the pilosebaceous structure due to obstruction of the orifice); epidermal inclusion cyst (cutane-

---

**Table 9-5**
**ORBITAL CYST**

I. Developmental
   Choristoma (epidermal, dermoid, dermolipoma)
   Teratoma
   Colobomatous cyst
   Congenital cystic eye
   Optic nerve sheath meningocele
   Congenital dacryocele (mucocele)

II. Cysts of Adjacent Structures
   Cephalocele (meningocele, encephalocele, meningoencephalocele, porencephalic cyst)
   Enterogenous cyst
   Dentigerous cyst

III. Acquired Orbital Cyst
   Mucocele
   Mucopyocele
   Dacryocele
   Cystic vascular lesions (lymphangioma, orbital varix)
   Chocolate cyst (hemorrhagic cyst)
   Epithelial and appendage cysts
   Epithelial implantation cysts
   Lacrimal gland cyst
   Lacrimal sac cyst (dacryocele), mucocele
   Hematic cyst (subperiosteal)
   Cholesterol granulomatous cyst
   Aneurysmal bone cyst
   Cystic myositis
   Orbital abscess
   Parasitic cyst (hydatid cyst, cysticercoses)

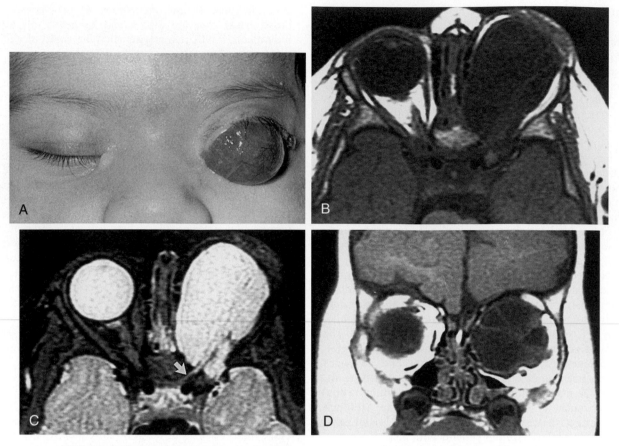

**FIGURE 9-43**    Congenital cystic eye. **A**, Four-month-old girl with a congenital cystic eye associated with Goltz's syndrome. **B**, Axial T1-weighted MR image through the orbit shows a large orbital cyst, an enlarged orbit, and no discernible normal bulbar structures on the left. **C**, Axial T2-weighted MR image shows a rudimentary optic nerve (*arrow*) leading into the lesion. Signal intensity is homogeneously high. **D**, Coronal contrast-enhanced, T1-weighted MR image shows thin, enhancing strands and a more focal amorphous tissue mass in the posterior aspect of the lesion (probably dysmorphic retinal tissue). (From Kaufman LM et al. Diagnostic imaging of cystic lesions in the child's orbit. Radiol Clin North Am 1998;36:1149–1163.)

ous or subcutaneous cyst lined by stratified squamous epithelium with a keratin-filled lumen); pilomatrixoma (calcifying epithelioma of Malherbe, a solid or cystic mass derived from hair matrix cells); and conjunctival inclusion cyst (a thin-walled, fluid-filled cyst lined by stratified, nonkeratinizing, cuboidal epithelium containing mucus-secreting goblet cells). Because most epithelial and appendage cysts remain small (less than 1 cm) and limited to the eyelid and the superficial orbit, medical imaging studies are rarely ordered by the ophthalmologist.

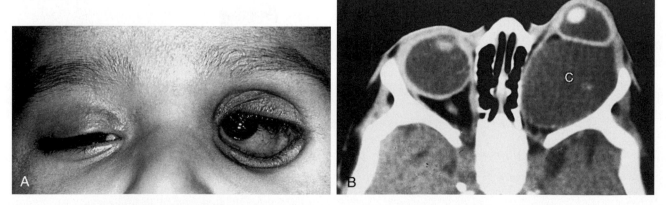

**FIGURE 9-44**    **A**, Six-month-old girl with proptosis of a microphthalmic eye with colobomatous cyst. **B**, CT image shows a large, low-density retrobulbar cyst (*C*) and a microphthalmic eye. The connection between the cyst and the globe is not evident in this image. (From Kaufman LM et al. Diagnostic imaging of cystic lesions in the child's orbit. Radiol Clin North Am 1998;36:1149–1163.)

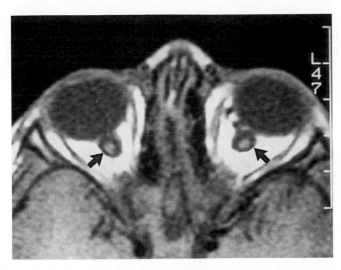

**FIGURE 9-45**   Ectasia of the optic nerve sheath (meningocele). Axial T1-weighted MR image shows the prominence of the subarachnoid space around the nerves (*arrows*). (From Kaufman LM et al. Diagnostic imaging of cystic lesions in the child's orbit. Radiol Clin North Am 1998;36:1149–1163.)

### Epithelial Implantation Cysts

Epithelial implantation cysts are derived from cells of the cutaneous epithelium, conjunctival epithelium, or respiratory epithelium that are traumatically displaced under the skin of the eyelid or into the orbit. The CT and MR imaging appearance of these cysts is nonspecific and similar to that of any simple cyst (Fig. 9-47). A nonenhanced cystic orbital mass following orbital surgery or enucleation should raise the question of the presence of an epithelial implantation cyst.

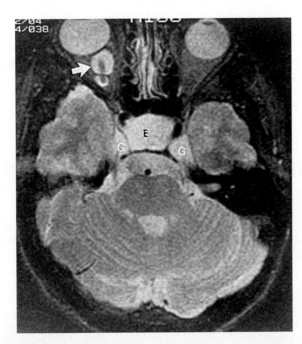

**FIGURE 9-46**   Ectasia of the optic nerve sheath. T2-weighted MR image shows marked expansion of the subarachnoid space around the right optic nerve (*arrow*). Note the empty sella (*E*) and dilated Gasserian cisterns (*G*). (From Kaufman LM et al. Diagnostic imaging of cystic lesions in the child's orbit. Radiol Clin North Am 1998;36:1149–1163.)

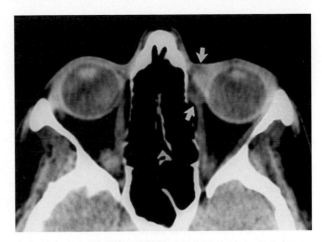

**FIGURE 9-47**   Axial CT scan shows a well-defined mass (*arrows*) compatible with an epithelial implantation cyst. (From Kaufman LM et al. Diagnostic imaging of cystic lesions in the child's orbit. Radiol Clin North Am 1998;36:1149–1163.)

### Lacrimal Gland Cysts

Cysts of the lacrimal glands can be due to blockage of the gland's excretory ducts.[73] The cyst is then located in either the orbital or the palpebral lobe of the main lacrimal gland, or in the conjunctival fornices due to blockage of the accessory lacrimal glands of Krause and Wolfring.[73] The CT and MR imaging appearance of lacrimal gland cysts is similar to that of any simple cyst (Figs. 9-48 and 9-49).

### Dacryoceles

A dacryocele (lacrimal sac mucocele) is a cystic expansion of the nasolacrimal sac or a diverticulum of the sac. The expansion is caused by a proximal or distal block of the nasolacrimal duct. Dacryoceles are considered a congenital anomaly of the lacrimal drainage system and are usually apparent in the first few days of life. On CT and MR imaging, dacryoceles appear as well-circumscribed, rounded lesions centered in the nasolacrimal sac region. On CT scans, the density of the lesion is homogeneous when noninfected. On MR imaging, a dacryocele appears hy-

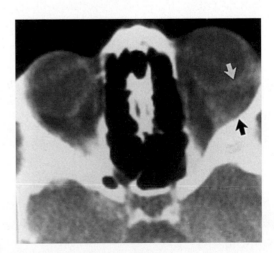

**FIGURE 9-48**   CT scan shows a low-density image (*arrows*) compatible with a lacrimal gland cyst. (From Kaufman LM et al. Diagnostic imaging of cystic lesions in the child's orbit. Radiol Clin North Am 1998;36:1149–1163.)

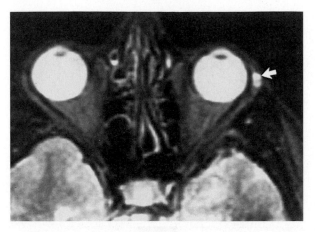

**FIGURE 9-49**    Axial T2-weighted MR image shows a lacrimal gland cyst (*arrow*). (From Kaufman LM et al. Diagnostic imaging of cystic lesions in the child's orbit. Radiol Clin North Am 1998;36:1149–1163.)

pointense on T1-weighted and hyperintense on T2-weighted images. If it is infected, there may be a rim of contrast enhancement (Fig. 9-50).

### Hematic Cysts and Cholesterol Granuloma

Most orbital hematomas, like other localized collections of blood, resolve within days. The hematic cyst (organizing hematoma, hematocele), is a cyst-like mass that develops slowly as an acute orbital hemorrhage, is incompletely absorbed, and undergoes organization.[73] There may be a fibrous cyst wall with a lumen composed of degraded blood products, cholesterol, hemosiderin, hematoidin crystals, erythrocytes, histiocytes, giant cells, and granuloma tissue. The hematic cyst may occur anywhere in the orbit or in the orbital bones (cholesterol granuloma).[73, 79] The subperiosteal compartment of the orbit, a potential space, is an important entity due to its unique anatomy, location, and susceptibility to various pathologic processes, such as

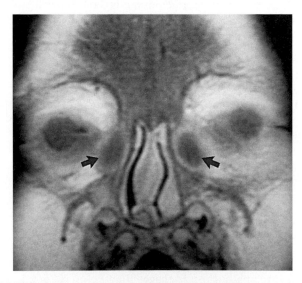

**FIGURE 9-50**    Enhanced coronal T1-weighted MR image shows bilateral dacryoceles (*arrows*). (From Kaufman LM et al. Diagnostic imaging of cystic lesions in the child's orbit. Radiol Clin North Am 1998;36:1149–1163.)

hemorrhage, infection, infiltration of lymphoproliferative disorders, infiltration of en plaque meningiomas, and metastasis.[17, 79] The etiology of subperiosteal hematomas is either traumatic or spontaneous. Traumatic hemorrhage is most common, but the time interval between the traumatic episode and the clinical manifestation may vary from immediate to months or years.[17, 79] Spontaneous hemorrhage can occur as a complication of leukemia, thrombocytopenia, blood dyscrasia, hemophilia, anticoagulant use, and other hemorrhagic systemic diseases, including sickle cell anemia.[79] Subperiosteal hematomas can be of several varieties. Acute subperiosteal hematoma is a rare complication of trauma, presenting as painful unilateral proptosis.[79] It may also develop so insidiously as to defy explanation, especially when there is no definite history of injury. Usually it is the result of bleeding from the subperiosteal blood vessels.[79] It may also develop as an extension of a subgaleal hematoma. At times it is continuous with an epidural hematoma after head trauma. In cases of trauma, blood tends to collect in the subperiosteal location superiorly, as the frontal bone is the largest continuous concave surface of the orbit and has a loose periosteal attachment.[79]

#### Diagnostic Imaging

CT is a very accurate diagnostic method to evaluate subperiosteal hematomas. Coronal sections, either direct or reformatted, are essential for accurate diagnoses. The CT appearance of acute and subacute subperiosteal hematomas is that of a sharply defined extraconal, homogeneous, high-density, nonenhancing mass with a broad base abutting the bone and displacing the peripheral orbital fat toward the center of the orbit (Figs. 9-51 to 9-53). The mass, like other subperiosteal lesions, is fusiform or biconvex, is confined by the sutures (frontozygomatic or frontoethmoidal), and is best seen in coronal or sagittal images. Prompt aspiration of the hematoma can lead to early decompression and prevent serious late sequelae. A chronic subperiosteal hematoma appears on CT as a heterogeneous, relatively hypodense, sharply defined extraconal mass with a broad base (Fig. 9-54). Long-standing chronic hematic cysts, the so-called cholesterol granulomas, appear as cystic lesions, associated with compression bone atrophy as well as expansion and erosions of adjacent bone (Fig. 9-55). On a CT scan, chronic hematic cysts may not be differentiated from epidermoid-dermoid cysts (Fig. 9-10). However, they can be easily differentiated by MR imaging (Fig. 9-56).

#### MR Imaging Findings in Various Stages of Orbital Hematoma

The diagnosis of hematoma is greatly aided by MR imaging, which can characterize all stages of blood degradation. The iron atoms of hemoglobin have a different magnetic effect, depending on the physical and oxidative state of the hemoglobin itself.[80] Fresh (hyperacute) oxygenated blood (hemorrhage no more than a few hours old) has approximately the same MR imaging characteristics as water, being hypointense on T1-weighted and hyperintense on T2-weighted images, using a high field (1.5 Tesla) MR unit. Acute hemorrhages (1 to 7 days old), because of the paramagnetic effect of deoxyhemoglobin, have a low signal on T1-weighted and in particular on T2-weighted images

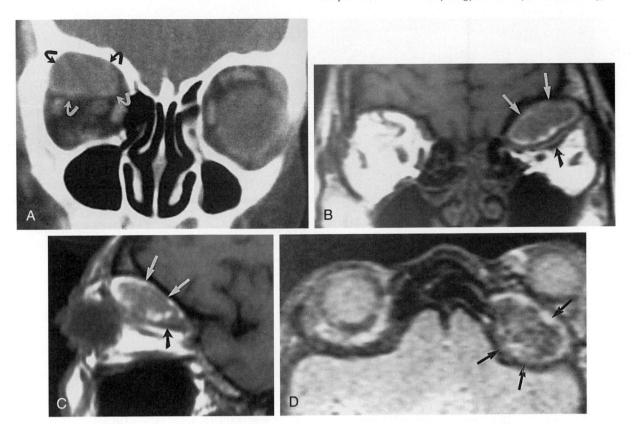

**FIGURE 9-51** Acute subperiosteal hematoma. **A,** Coronal CT scan through the orbit showing a hyperdense acute subperiosteal hematoma (*arrows*) along the roof of the orbit and displacing the orbital contents inferiorly. **B,** Coronal T1-weighted (500/20, TR/TE) MR image in another patient showing the intermediate signal intensity of an acute subperiosteal hematoma (*white arrows*). Note the displaced periosteum (*black arrow*). **C,** Sagittal T1-weighted (600/20, TR/TE) MR image of the same patient in **B** showing the acute subperiosteal orbital hematoma (*white arrows*). Note the displaced periosteum (*black arrow*). **D,** Axial T2-weighted (200/80, TR/TE) MR image of the same patient in **B** through the orbit. Note the low signal intensity of the acute hematoma (*arrows*) on the T2-weighted image. (From Dobben GD et al. Orbital subperiosteal hematoma, cholesterol granuloma, and infection. Evaluation with MR imaging and CT. Radiol Clin North Am 1998;36:1185–1200.)

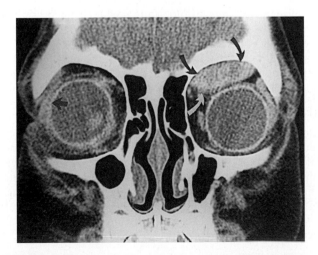

**FIGURE 9-52** Acute subperiosteal hematoma. Coronal CT scan through the orbit of an 8-year-old boy showing an acute subperiosteal hematoma (*curved arrows*). Note its hyperdense nature and fusiform shape. Note the normal lacrimal gland (*arrow*) on the opposite side. (From Dobben GD et al. Orbital subperiosteal hematoma, cholesterol granuloma, and infection. Evaluation with MR imaging and CT. Radiol Clin North Am 1998;36:1185–1200.)

(Fig. 9-51). With progressive oxidation of deoxyhemoglobin to methemoglobin, hemorrhages older than 7 days become hyperintense on T1-weighted images (Fig. 9-56). The signal on T2-weighted MR images remains low if the methemoglobin is still intracellular (i.e., if oxidation occurred before erythrocyte lysis), therefore having limited motion. The signal is high if the methemoglobin has become extracellular (Fig. 9-56). Hemosiderin, which causes a low signal on both T1-weighted and T2-weighted sequences, is encountered in scars or organized hematoma.[80] The MR imaging of hematoma is presented in Table 9-6.

### Orbital Cholesterol Granuloma

Cholesterol granulomas are bone-pushing and bone-destroying lesions characterized by granulomatous infiltration surrounding cholesterol crystals. The cholesterol granuloma may be etiologically related to the loss of aeration of normally pneumatized bone, such as the petromastoid bone. Negative pressure develops, leading to tissue edema and hemorrhage. Rupture of red blood cell membranes results in precipitation of cholesterol and membrane phospholipids. This crystallized cholesterol, in turn, acts as a foreign body and elicits a giant cell

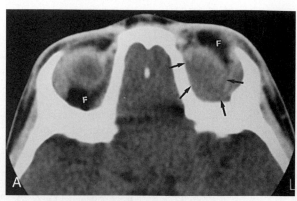

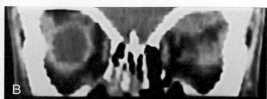

**FIGURE 9-53**    Subacute subperiosteal hematoma (less than 7 days). **A,** Axial CT scan of the orbit in a 2-year-old child. Note the subacute subperiosteal hematoma (*arrows*) and displacement of the peripheral orbital fat (F). **B,** Coronal reformatted images of the same patient showing the subacute hematoma. (From Dobben GD et al. Orbital subperiosteal hematoma, cholesterol granuloma, and infection. Evaluation with MR imaging and CT. Radiol Clin North Am 1998;36:1185–1200.)

granulomatous reaction. Histologically, there are no epithelial elements in the cholesterol granuloma. Histologically, the tissues consist of foci of reactive xanthogranulomatous infiltrates, cholesterol crystals, giant cells, and hemosiderin surrounded by a fibrous capsule (Fig. 9-55B). The initiating factors must be different in the lesions arising in nonpneumatized bone from those in the orbital region. In the orbit, cholesterol granulomas are secondary lesions that are formed due to a posttraumatic, postsurgical, or postinflammatory event. Various terms have been used to describe cholesterol granuloma including *lipid granuloma, cholesteatoma, xanthomatosis, histiocytic granuloma,* and *chronic hematic cyst.* Cholesteatomas are considered epidermoid cysts and should not be confused with cholesterol granulomas.

**Diagnostic Imaging.** On CT, cholesterol granulomas are seen as lytic lesions, usually with ragged bone destruction,

that invariably extend extraperiosteally into the orbit, causing proptosis (Fig. 9-55A). Extension into the anterior and middle cranial fossae occurs less frequently.[79] On CT scans, the density of a cholesterol granuloma is approximately isodense with the brain, with the attenuation values ranging from 25 to 45 HU (mean, 34 HU). Unlike epidermoid cyst, no sclerotic margin is seen between the mass and normal diploic bone. The lesion demonstrates no enhancement on postcontrast CT scans. The differential diagnosis on the basis of CT scanning is limited to epidermoid and dermoid cysts or aneurysmal bone cyst. Aneurysmal bone cysts occur almost exclusively in children.[79] MR imaging can be of most value in the diagnosis of cholesterol granuloma. These lesions give rise to high signal on T1-weighted and T2-weighted sequences, characteristic of chronic hemorrhage (Fig. 9-57).[79]

### Aneurysmal Bone Cysts

The term *aneurysmal bone cyst* (ABC) is a misnomer, because the lesion is histologically neither an aneurysm nor a cyst. Infrequently, ABC of the facial bones may involve the orbit in children.[73] ABC has been described as a benign lesion of bone characterized by a blood-filled cyst-like expansion within the bone. The expansion may be complex and multilobular, with septae of bony trabeculae, fibrous tissues, and stromal giant cells. The lesions remodel adjacent bone, but the surrounding periosteum remains intact. ABC is not an entity by itself but is always secondary to an underlying bony or fibroosseous condition, such as nonossifying fibroma, ossifying fibroma, fibrous dysplasia, juvenile pseudomonatous active (aggressive) ossifying fibroma (Fig. 9-58), chondroblastoma, chondromyxoid fibroma, osteoblastoma, giant cell tumor (osteoclastoma), fibrosarcoma, osteochondrosarcoma, hemangioendothelioma, or hemangioma.[73]

### Cystic Myositis

Infrequently, nonspecific orbital myositis may result in cyst-like changes in an extraocular muscle.[73] These cysts may respond to treatment with oral corticosteroids, suggest-

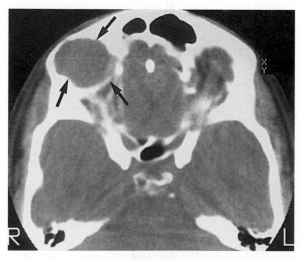

**FIGURE 9-54**    Chronic subperiosteal hematoma (cholesterol granuloma). Axial CT scan shows an expansile mass (*arrows*) compatible with a chronic hematic cyst. (From Dobben GD et al. Orbital subperiosteal hematoma, cholesterol granuloma, and infection. Evaluation with MR imaging and CT. Radiol Clin North Am 1998;36:1185–1200.)

ing that the cysts do not have a parasitic origin and probably represent edema in the muscles.[73]

### Orbital Abscesses (Inflammatory Orbital Cysts)

Orbital abscesses are cyst-like pus pockets that develop subperiosteally, or in the orbit or lids, in association with orbital or preseptal cellulitis most often associated with sinonasal infections (Fig. 9-59). The CT and MR imaging of orbital abscesses will be described in a following section.

### Parasitic Cysts
#### Hydatid Cysts

The occurrence of parasitic orbital cysts is limited to endemic regions with poor sanitation. The hydatid cyst is related to infection by the larval form of a parasitic tapeworm, *Echinococcus granulosus*. The adult worm lives in the intestines of carnivores (usually dogs but not humans). The infected carnivore passes the worm's ova in its feces. Grazing animals, acting as intermediate hosts, ingest the

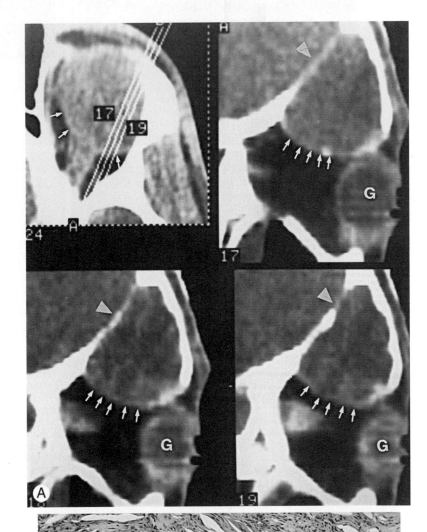

**FIGURE 9-55**   Chronic hematic cyst (cholesterol granuloma). **A**, Axial CT scan with oblique sagittal reformatting showing a cholesterol granuloma (*arrows*) of the left orbit. Note the displacement of the globe (*G*) inferiorly. The lesion, which is almost isodense with brain, has caused ragged bony destruction (*arrowheads*). On the axial image, the lesion may be mistaken for a lacrimal gland mass. **B**, Histopathologic examination of a cholesterol granuloma showing abundant cholesterol cells (*arrows*), foreign-body giant cells (*arrowheads*), and inflammatory cells (hematoxylin-eosin, original magnification ×40). (From Dobben GD et al. Orbital subperiosteal hematoma, cholesterol granuloma, and infection. Evaluation with MR imaging and CT. Radiol Clin North Am 1998;36:1185–1200.)

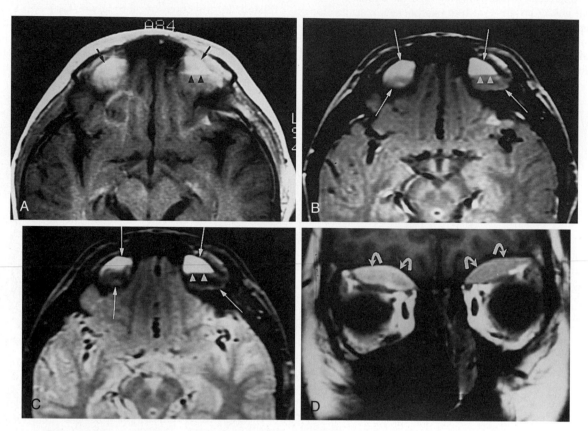

**FIGURE 9-56** Subacute subperiosteal hematoma. **A,** Axial contrast-enhanced T1-weighted (350/16, TR/TE) MR image shows a subacute subperiosteal hematoma (*arrows*) in an 8-year-old child. Note the high to mixed signal intensity pattern on the T1-weighted sequence. Note the fluid-fluid level (*arrowheads*). **B,** Axial proton-density (2300/30, TR/TE) MR image of the same patient showing a fluid-fluid level (*arrowheads*) within the hematoma (*arrows*). **C,** Axial T2-weighted (2300/80, TR/TE) MR image showing a mixed signal intensity pattern with hypointensity images related to the intracellular methemoglobin portion of the subacute hematoma (*arrows*). Note the fluid-fluid level (*arrowheads*). **D,** Coronal T1-weighted (600/12, TR/TE) MR image reveals an excellent demonstration of the subacute subperiosteal hematoma (*arrows*). Note the high to intermediate signal intensity of the hematoma. (From Dobben GD et al. Orbital subperiosteal hematoma, cholesterol granuloma, and infection. Evaluation with MR imaging and CT. Radiol Clin North Am 1998;36:1185–1200.)

### Table 9-6
### MR IMAGING STAGING OF ORBITAL HEMATOMA

| Stage | Hyperacute | Acute | Subacute | Subacute-Chronic | Chronic |
|---|---|---|---|---|---|
| Time | Few hours | 1–3 days | 3–7 days | 7 days–weeks | Months–years |
| Type | Fresh blood | Early clot | Before cell lysis | After cell lysis | Organized/scars |
| Content | Oxyhemoglobin | Deoxyhemoglobin | Intracellular methemoglobin | Extracellular methemoglobin | Hemosiderin |
| T1-weighted MR image | Low-high | Low-iso | High | High | Low |
| T2-weighted MR image | High | Low | Low | High | Low |

From Flanders AE, Espinosa GA, Markiewicz DA, et al. Orbital lymphoma. Radiol Clin North Am 1987;25:601-612.

ova, which develop into larval forms in the hosts' muscles. Humans are infected by eating the undercooked meat of an infected grazing animal. Traveling via the bloodstream, the hydatid can lodge in the orbit, resulting in a well-defined cystic mass with or without a fluid-fluid level containing the parasite. Clinically, patients present with slowly progressive, painless orbital signs.[73, 81]

### Cysticercosis

Cysticercosis is a disease due to infestation by *Cysticercus cellulosae*, the larval form of the parasitic tapeworm *Taenia solium*. Clinically, patients present with either a visible subconjunctival cyst or orbital signs due to an extraocular muscle cyst that is unresponsive to treatment with oral corticosteroids.

### Diagnostic Imaging

The CT and MR imaging characteristics of most parasitic cysts are nonspecific. There may be some degree of enhancement around the cyst wall.[73, 81] Nearly all patients

with orbital cysticercosis examined by CT show a cystic lesion near or within an extraocular muscle. An intraocular mass or cyst may be present.[82] A scolex can be identified within the cystic lesions in nearly one half of patients by CT or MR imaging and is diagnostic (Fig. 9-60). CT or MR imaging evidence of a cystic lesion without a scolex or diffuse myositis in the presence of a positive enzyme-linked immunosorbent assay for anticysticercal antibodies is also diagnostic. Concurrent neurocysticercosis and orbital cysticercosis appear uncommonly (Fig. 9-60). Neurocysticercosis is generally associated with more morbidity than orbital cysticercosis.[73]

## INFLAMMATORY DISEASES

Orbital infections account for about 60% of primary orbital disease processes.[3] The infection may be acute, subacute, or chronic. The majority of acute inflammatory disorders are of paranasal sinus origin. However, the

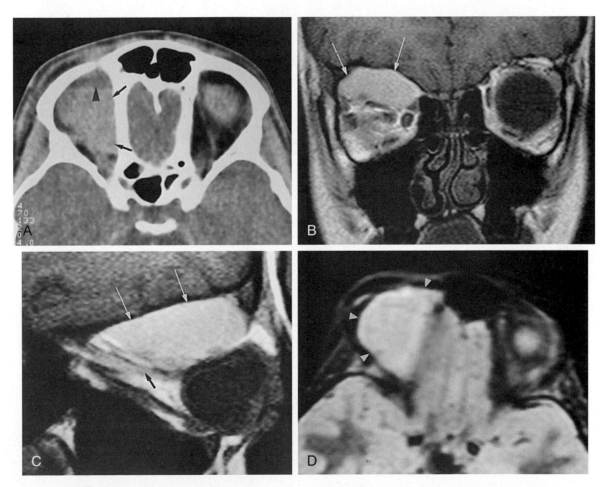

**FIGURE 9-57**   Chronic subperiosteal hematoma (about 12 days). **A**, Axial CT scan of the orbit showing a chronic subperiosteal hematoma (cholesterol granuloma) (*arrows*) seen as an isodense lesion with a fluid-fluid level (*arrowhead*). **B**, Coronal T1-weighted (500/20, TR/TE) MR image showing the cholesterol granuloma (*arrows*) in the same patient in **A** as a high-signal lesion, indicating its chronic nature. **C**, Sagittal T1-weighted (500/20, TR/TE) MR image illustrates the high signal pattern of the subperiosteal hematoma (*white arrows*), resulting in downward displacement of the optic nerve (*black arrow*). **D**, Axial proton density (2000/40, TR/TE) MR image shows this chronic hematoma (cholesterol granuloma) as a hyperintense lesion (*arrowheads*). (From Dobben GD et al. Orbital subperiosteal hematoma, cholesterol granuloma, and infection. Evaluation with MR imaging and CT. Radiol Clin North Am 1998;36:1185–1200.)

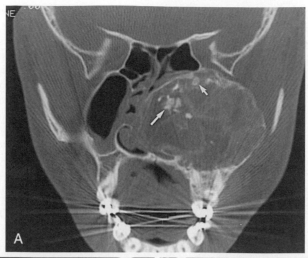

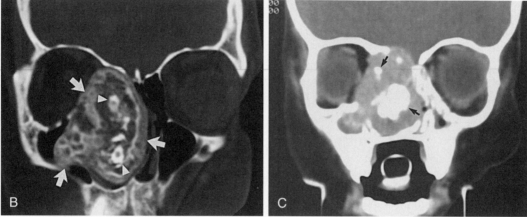

**FIGURE 9-58** Aggressive psammomatoid ossifying fibroma. **A,** Coronal CT scan shows a large, expansile mass of mixed intensity. Note the psammomatoid bodies (*arrows*). **B,** Coronal CT scan in another patient shows an ossifying fibroma (*arrows*). The lesion is less aggressive than the lesion shown in **A.** Note the CT appearance of the psammomatoid bodies (*arrowheads*). **C,** Coronal CT scan in a 18-month-old child shows a soft-tissue mass, with involvement of the medial wall of the orbit as well as the roof of the ethmoid bone. Note the intralesional islands of calcification (*arrows*). Pathologic diagnosis was felt to be most consistent with an aggressive fibro-osseous lesion (fibrous dysplasia versus ossifying fibroma). (From Mafee MF et al. Fibro-osseous, osseous, and cartilaginous lesions of the orbit and paraorbital region. Radiol Clin North Am 1998;36:1241.)

infection may develop from infectious processes of the face or pharynx, trauma, or foreign bodies, or it may be secondary to septicemia. Nearly two thirds of orbital infections are estimated to occur secondary to sinusitis, and about one fourth of the infections are due to orbital foreign bodies. The bacteria most commonly involved are *Staphylococcus*, *Streptococcus*, *Pneumococcus*, *Pseudomonas*, Neisseriaceae, *Haemophilus*, and mycobacteria.[83, 84] Herpes simplex and herpes zoster are the major viral infections of the orbit. In immune-suppressed or immunocompromised patients and poorly controlled diabetic patients, opportunistic infections such as fungal and parasitic pathogens may be responsible for severe sinonasal-orbital infections. Acute inflammation is characterized by rapid onset associated with soft-tissue swelling and infiltration, loss of the normal soft tissue planes, local soft-tissue destruction, and abscess formation. The location of the process is clinically important because a preseptal infection (Fig. 9-61) rarely affects orbital functions. On the other hand, a retroseptal (postseptal) infection (Fig. 9-61) may have a profound and sudden

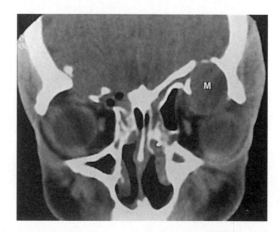

**FIGURE 9-59** Extension of a supraorbital ethimoid mucocele into the orbit. Coronal CT scan shows an orbital cystic mass (*M*) related to extension of a mucocele. Note the postoperative changes of the contralateral orbital roof. (From Kaufman LM et al. Diagnostic imaging of cystic lesions in the child's orbit. Radiol Clin North Am 1998;36:1149–1163.)

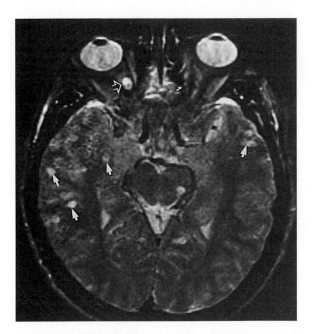

**FIGURE 9-60**   Cysticercosis. Axial T2-weighted MR image shows multiple intracranial abscesses (*arrows*) and an orbital abscess (*hollow arrow*). The orbital cyst shows a fluid-fluid level. Scolices are seen within the abscesses as tiny hypointense areas. (From Kaufman LM et al. Diagnostic imaging of cystic lesions in the child's orbit. Radiol Clin North Am 1998;36:1149–1163.)

effect on optic nerve and orbital motility function. Pathologically, in acute bacterial inflammation, polymorphonuclear leukocytes are usually the dominant cells, which, along with their pharmacologic intermediates, lead to necrosis and rapid involvement and destruction of tissue planes.

## Orbital Cellulitis and Sinusitis

Sinusitis is the most common cause of orbital cellulitis. Even though antibiotics have reduced the incidence of complicated sinusitis with orbital involvement, it still occurs and may be the first sign of sinus infection in children.[71, 83, 84] In the preantibiotic era, morbidity and mortal-

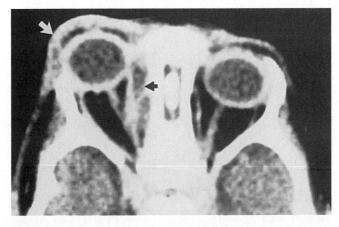

**FIGURE 9-61**   Preseptal and retroseptal orbital inflammation. Axial CT scan shows periorbital soft-tissue infiltration and edema (*white arrow*) and retroseptal subperiosteal inflammation and edema (*black arrow*).

ity from orbital cellulitis were significant, with 17% of cases resulting in death and 20% resulting in blindness. Orbital cellulitis is probably the most common cause of proptosis in children.[6] Pathophysiologically, infection originating within the sinuses can spread readily to the orbit via the thin and often dehiscent bony orbital walls and their many foramina or by means of the interconnecting valveless venous system of the face, sinuses, and orbit.[3] The classification of orbital cellulitis includes five categories or stages of orbital involvement: (1) inflammatory edema; (2) subperiosteal phlegmon and abscess; (3) orbital cellulitis; (4) orbital abscess; and (5) ophthalmic vein and cavernous sinus thrombosis.[3, 71, 84] Limiting a particular inflammatory lesion to one of these categories is often difficult because they tend to overlap.[71, 84]

## Bacterial Orbital Cellulitis Classification

Based upon the anatomy and the presumed pathogenesis of orbital cellulitis of Chandler et al.,[85] classification of the orbital complications of sinus infections is recognized as most useful in clinical situations. The Chandler et al.[85] classification was devised prior to the advent of newer orbital imaging techniques, and modifications that make use of information obtained from these imaging techniques are indicated. We therefore recommend the classification scheme of periorbital infections,[86] outlined in Table 9-7.

## Bacterial Preseptal Cellulitis and Preseptal Edema

Preseptal cellulitis defines infections limited to the skin and subcutaneous tissues of the eyelid anterior to the orbital septum.[86] Clinically, the patient has erythema and swelling

**Table 9-7**
**STAGING OF ORBITAL CELLULITIS**

| State | Clinical Findings |
| --- | --- |
| Inflammatory edema | Eyelid swelling and erythema |
| Preseptal cellulitis | Eyelid swelling and erythema associated with inflammatory soft-tissue thickening of the orbit anterior to the orbital septum |
| | Chemosis may be present |
| Postseptal cellulitis | Edema of the orbital contents; proptosis, chemosis, and decreased extraocular movement |
| | Visual loss (unusual) |
| Subperiosteal abscess | A collection of inflammatory infiltrates and pus between the periorbita and involved sinuses |
| | Globe proptotic and displaced by abscess |
| | Visual loss with progression of the disease |
| Orbital abscess | Marked proptosis, ophthalmoplegia, and visual loss associated with abscess formation within the orbital fat or muscles |
| Cavernous sinus thrombosis | Proptosis and ophthalmoplegia with development of similar signs on the contralateral side associated with cranial nerve palsies (nerves III, IV, V, VI) and visual loss |

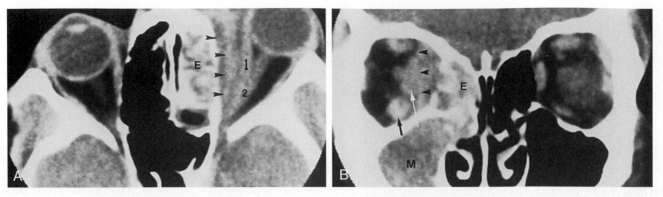

**FIGURE 9-62** Orbital subperiosteal phlegmon. **A**, Axial CT scan shows proptosis of the left eye with mucoperiosteal thickening of the left ethmoid sinus (*E*), with soft-tissue induration in the medial subperiosteal space (*arrowheads*). Note the lateral displacement of the inflamed left medial rectus muscle (*1*). Optic nerve (*2*). **B**, Coronal CT scan, same patient as in **A**, shows clouding of the right ethmoid (*E*) and maxillary (*M*) sinuses, with subperiosteal soft-tissue induration (*arrowheads*) and swelling of the right medial rectus muscle (*white arrow*) and right inferior rectus muscle (*black arrow*). (From Mafee MF et al. CT assessment of periorbital pathology. In: Gozalez CA, Beeker MH, Flanagan JC, eds. Diagnostic Imaging in Ophthalmology. New York: Springer-Verlag, 1985;281–302.)

of the eyelids. There is no proptosis, chemosis, or limitation of ocular motility.[86] At a slightly more advanced stage, chemosis occurs. It is unusual for a preseptal infection to traverse the orbital septum and result in postseptal cellulitis.[86] Preseptal edema is the first stage of infection secondary to sinusitis. It is often clinically misdiagnosed as orbital or periorbital cellulitis. The infection in this early stage actually is still confined to the sinus; however, there is swelling of the eyelids with mild orbital edema reflecting congestion of the venous outflow of the eyelid. Usually the upper medial eyelid is affected, and if untreated, preseptal cellulitis will develop. CT or MR imaging demonstrates the eyelid edema and the inflammatory paranasal sinus disease.[8, 84]

## Postseptal Orbital Cellulitis

Postseptal orbital cellulitis is an infectious process that occurs within the orbit proper, behind the orbital septum, and within the bony walls of the orbit.[86] Inflammatory edema characterizes the earliest stage of postseptal orbital infection. There is diffuse edema of the orbital contents with inflammatory cells and fluid, but no abscess formation.[86] The swelling of orbital tissues occurs when an increase in sinus venous pressure is transmitted to the orbital vasculature, resulting in transudation and leakage through the vessel walls.[86] Clinically, the patient has eyelid edema, mild proptosis, and chemosis. In severe cases, there may be generalized limitation of motility; however, visual acuity is not impaired.[86] Although contrast-enhanced diagnostic imaging of an isolated preseptal cellulitis usually is not clinically indicated, it can be useful in cases in which the clinical differentiation of preseptal and postseptal cellulitis is impossible or when the diagnosis is unclear.[86] It is important to recognize that based solely on CT and MR imaging, the differentiation between a cellulitis and allergic eyelid edema is impossible, particularly if the paranasal sinuses appear to be clear. The history is always essential in these cases. The CT and MR imaging findings include

soft-tissue thickening of the eyelids. Usually the process is diffuse, and a localized eyelid abscess cavity is not seen. In postseptal orbital cellulitis, orbital imaging is indicated and a contrast-enhanced study is necessary to differentiate inflammatory edema, cellulitis, orbital phlegmon, and orbital abscess (Figs. 9-62 to 9-67).

## Subperiosteal Phlegmon and Abscess

As the reaction of the orbital periosteum begins and gradually advances, the edema of the eyelids and conjunctivae becomes more generalized and the eye begins to protrude. Inflammatory tissue and edema collect beneath the periosteum to form a subperiosteal phlegmon (Fig. 9-62), which, subsequently, may develop into a subperiosteal abscess (Fig. 9-63). As the disease progresses, the inflammatory process infiltrates the periorbital and retroocular fat, giving rise to a true orbital cellulitis (Figs. 9-64, 9-66, and 9-67). The subperiosteal abscess and orbital cellulitis frequently coexist.[71, 84] At this stage, extraocular motility becomes progressively

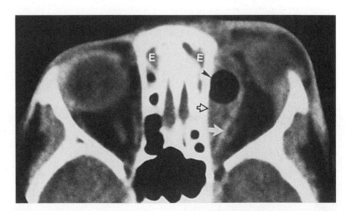

**FIGURE 9-63** Orbital subperiosteal abscess. CT scan shows proptosis of the left eye with mucosal thickening of the ethmoid air cells (*E*), with subperiosteal abscess (*hollow arrow*). Note the air bubble (*arrowhead*) within the abscess and the swollen left medial rectus muscle (*arrow*).

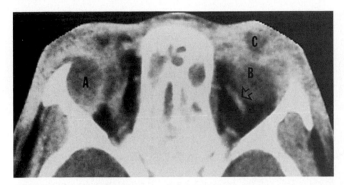

**FIGURE 9-64**   Orbital cellulitis and abscesses. CT scan shows right periorbital cellulitis and three abscesses. (*A*), Right retroseptal abscess. (*B*), Left retrobulbar abscess. (*C*), Left eyelid abscess. Note slightly engorged left superior ophthalmic vein (*hollow arrow*).

impaired. With severe involvement, visual disturbances can result from optic neuritis or ischemia (Fig. 9-62A). Progression of intraorbital cellulitis or spread from the subperiosteal space leads to intraconal or extraconal loculation and abscess formation (Fig. 9-64).[3, 71, 84] Progression of disease may lead to ophthalmic vein thrombosis (Fig. 9-68), cavernous sinus thrombosis, and associated mycotic aneurysm of the internal carotid artery (Fig. 9-69), all dire complications of orbital and sinonasal infections.

## Cavernous Sinus Thrombosis

Cavernous sinus thrombosis (CST) arises from an infection in an area having venous drainage to the cavernous sinus.[83] Thus, the source infection is usually in the sinonasal cavities, in the orbits, and from infections involving the middle third of the face.[86] CST may develop from a septic thrombophlebitis arising in the ophthalmic vein (Fig. 9-68). Proptosis and ophthalmoplegia are common. Offending organisms may be aerobic or anaerobic, with *Staphylococcus aureus* and anaerobic streptococci being the most common organisms. Clinically, patients with CST are extremely ill, demonstrating signs of meningitis and multiple cranial nerve palsies bilaterally.[86] These patients usually have a headache, fever and chills, and an elevated white blood cell count with positive blood cultures.[83] The ophthalmologic findings include edema of the lids, exophthalmos, chemosis, paralysis of the eye muscles, engorgement of the retinal veins, and low-grade papilledema.[83] On contrast-enhanced CT scans, the normal cavernous sinus is seen as an enhancing parasellar structure with a sharply defined lateral border that is either straight or concave toward the adjacent middle cranial fossa. The internal carotid artery cannot normally be separated from the opacified venous sinuses within the cavernous sinus. When thrombosis is present, the cavernous sinus often has a low-attenuation, nonenhancing appearance. The lateral border may bow laterally toward the middle cranial fossa, and the contrast-enhanced internal carotid artery may be seen as a contrast-enhanced tubular structure within the cavernous sinus (Figs. 9-69B,C). Often the superior ophthalmic vein is markedly enlarged and possibly thrombosed. False-negative CT scans are common until late in the course of the disease.[86] Thrombosis of the superior ophthalmic vein (SOV) is seen on MR imaging as an enlarged vein that appears less hypointense than the vein on the normal opposite side. On T1-weighted and T2-weighted MR images, the thrombosed SOV may be seen as a hyperintense area within the lumen of the vein.[87–89] CST results in

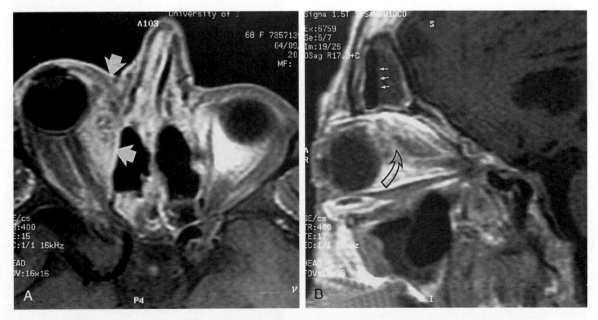

**FIGURE 9-65**   Orbital cellulitis. **A**, Enhanced, fat-suppressed, axial T1-weighted MR image showing diffuse enhancement of pre- and postseptal orbital tissue (*arrows*). **B**, Enhanced, fat-suppressed, sagittal T1-weighted MR image shows an air-fluid level in the frontal sinus (*arrows*) and diffuse orbital enhancement (*curved arrow*). There is no orbital abscess formation. (From Eustis HS et al. MR imaging and CT of orbital infections and complications in acute rhinosinusitis. Radiol Clin North Am 1998;36:1165–1183.)

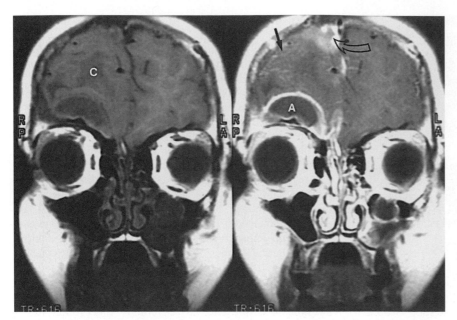

**FIGURE 9-66** Epidural abscess, cerebritis, and meningitis in a child with acute sinusitis. Pre- and postcontrast-enhanced coronal MR image showing epidural abscess (*A*), edema adjacent to focal cerebritis (*C*), and leptomeningeal enhancement (*straight arrow*) related to meningitis. Note the enhancement of focal cerebritis (*curved arrow*). (From Eustis HS et al. MR imaging and CT of orbital infections and complications in acute rhinosinusitis. Radiol Clin North Am 1998;36: 1165–1183.)

engorgement of the cavernous sinus and ophthalmic veins and usually engorgement of the extraocular muscles.[86] MR imaging and MR venography are more sensitive than CT for revealing CST.[88] On MR imaging there is deformity of the cavernous portion of the internal carotid artery. The signal from the abnormal cavernous sinus is heterogeneous, and there is an obvious hyperintense signal intensity representing the thrombosed vascular sinus that often is seen on all pulse sequences. Mycotic (septic) aneurysm of the internal carotid artery is a serious complication of orbital infection. This can be suspected on CT or MR imaging and confirmed by MR angiography or standard angiography (Fig. 9-69).

## Mycotic Infections

Orbital cellulitis secondary to infection with mycotic organisms occurs less frequently than bacterial infections, and usually these patients have a history of uncontrolled diabetes mellitus or are immunocompromised. Immunocompromised patients are particularly susceptible to infection by fungi such as *Candida* species, *Histoplasma capsulatum*, *Coccidioides immitis*, *Mucor*, and *Aspergillus* species.[86] *Mucor* and *Aspergillus* are by far the most

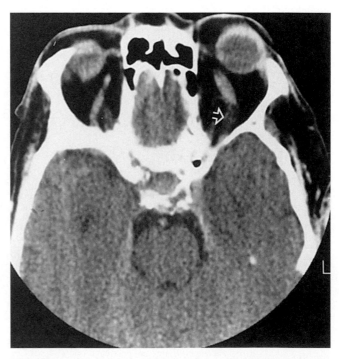

**FIGURE 9-68** Thrombosis of the superior ophthalmic vein. Axial CT scan shows an engorged left superior ophthalmic vein with a filling defect (*arrow*), which was caused by a sphenoid sinus infection (moniliasis).

**FIGURE 9-67** Sphenoid sinus abscess and subperiosteal abscess. Enhanced coronal T1-weighted MR image in a 12-year-old girl showing a sphenoid abscess (*A*) and a subperiosteal abscess (*arrows*). The patient lost her vision completely on the right. (From Eustis HS et al. MR imaging and CT of orbital infections and complications in acute rhinosinusitis. Radiol Clin North Am 1998;36:1165–1183.)

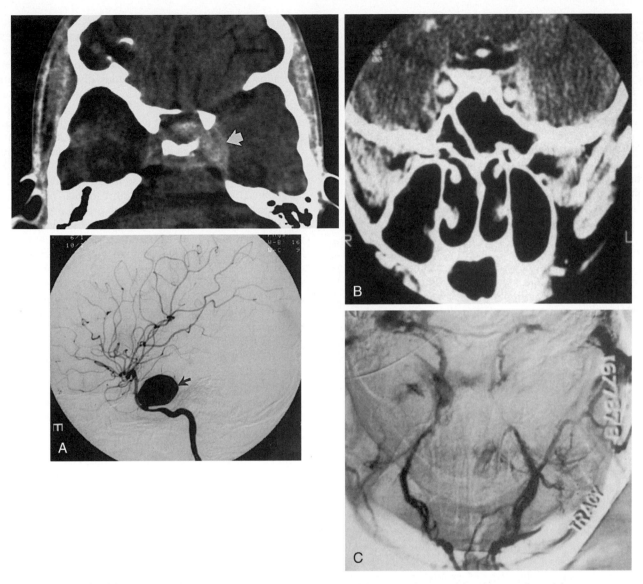

**FIGURE 9-69**   **A,** Mycotic (septic) aneurysm. **1,** Enhanced axial CT scan shows an enhancing mass (*arrow*) in the left cavernous sinus related to a mycotic artery. **2,** Lateral angiogram shows a large aneurysm (*arrow*) of the cavernous portion of the internal carotid artery. (From Eustis HS et al. MR imaging and CT of orbital infections and complications in acute rhinosinusitis. Radiol Clin North Am 1998;36:1165–1183.) **B,** Bilateral cavernous sinus thrombosis. Coronal CT section through the cavernous sinus following bolus injection reveals opacification of the internal carotid arteries bilaterally. The cavernous sinus reveals decreased attenuation in keeping with cavernous sinus thrombosis. Note enhancement of the dura bordering the left cavernous sinus. **C,** Right cavernous sinus thrombosis. Orbital venogram in the axial projection shows obstruction of the cavernous sinus on the right, secondary to thrombosis. Note the filling of the normal left cavernous sinus. (**B** and **C** from Weber AL, Mikulis DK. Inflammatory disorders of the paraorbital sinus and their complications. Radiol Clin North Am 1987;25:615–630.)

common fungal organisms incriminated. The fungi responsible for mucormycosis are ubiquitous and normally saprophytic in humans; they rarely produce severe disease, except in those with predisposing conditions.[71, 83, 90] There are four major types of mucormycosis: rhinocerebral, pulmonary, gastrointestinal, and disseminated, the most common of which is the rhinocerebral form.[90] The infection usually begins in the nose and spreads to the paranasal sinuses; then it extends into the orbit and cavernous sinuses.[71, 90] Orbital involvement results in orbital signs such as ophthalmoplegia, proptosis, ptosis, loss of vision, and orbital cellulitis.[71] The inflammatory process soon extends along the infra-

orbital fissure into the infratemporal fossa (Fig. 9-70) and may extend into the cavernous sinuses.

Black necrosis of a turbinate is a diagnostic clinical sign, but it may not be present until late in the course of the disease.[71, 90] The pathologic hallmark of mucormycosis is invasion of the walls of small vessels. For this reason, when the cavernous sinus is invaded, particularly in patients with mucormycosis and aspergillosis, rapid brain infarction may develop.[91]

*Aspergillus* is a ubiquitous fungus found primarily in agricultural dust. It may produce rhinocerebral disease and orbital involvement similar to that of mucormycosis, although hematogenous spread from the lungs to the brain is more common.[90] This fungus also has a well-known propensity for invading blood vessels, including the internal carotid artery.[71] One important but not pathognomonic MR imaging finding of mycotic infections is the hypointensity of mycetoma on T2-weighted MR images (Fig. 9-71). This is thought to be due to paramagnetic materials produced by the fungi and the semisolid, cheesy nature of the mycetoma.

In general, and in the appropriate clinical setting, a multicentric or unicentric sinusitis with or without bone destruction, and orbital tissues with or without vascular thrombosis, should strongly raise the possibility of sino-orbital mycosis.[86] Although the combination of orbital and sinus involvement is not pathognomonic of rhinocerebral mucormycosis or aspergillosis, awareness of these diagnoses, particularly when any predisposing factors are present, helps establish an early diagnosis. Rapid diagnosis is important because early aggressive treatment is necessary to minimize morbidity and mortality from these usually fatal diseases. The main contribution of CT and MR imaging is their clear demonstration of the relationship between sinonasal, orbital, and intracranial disease (Fig. 9-71). One should realize that the CT and MR imaging findings of invasive aspergillosis are indistinguishable from those of mucormycosis and that advanced sino-orbital mucormyosis and invasive aspergillosis mimic aggressive tumors on CT and MR imaging.

## Acute, Subacute, and Chronic Idiopathic Orbital Inflammatory Disorders (Pseudotumors)

Idiopathic inflammatory syndromes usually are referred to as *orbital pseudotumors*, a clinically and histologically confusing category of lesions.[3] In general, orbital pseudotumors represent a nongranulomatous inflammatory process in the orbit or eye with no known local or systemic causes.[92–94] This is a diagnosis of exclusion based on the history, the clinical course of the disease, the response to steroid therapy, laboratory tests, and biopsy in a limited number of cases.[92] There is a group of diverse disease entities that can mimic pseudotumors such as lymphoma, sarcoidosis, and other granulomatous diseases. By definition, the diagnosis excludes orbital inflammatory disease caused by entities such as Wegener's granulomatosis, retained foreign bodies, sclerosing hemangioma, trauma, and sinusitis. Among orbital disorders, after Graves' disease, pseudotumor is the next most common ophthalmologic disease. Pseudotumors account for 4.7% to 6.3% of orbital disorders, and the disease usually affects adults but may also affect children.[92] Pediatric orbital pseudotumor encompasses almost 6% to 16% of orbital pseudotumors. There is a higher incidence of bilateral orbital involvement, with approximately one third of the pseudotumors being bilateral.[92] Such pseudotumors are rarely associated with systemic disease. Children with orbital pseudotumor may also exhibit papillitis or iritis.[5, 6] Bilateral orbital pseudotumors in adults suggest the possibility of systemic vasculitis or a systemic lymphoproliferative disorder.[5, 6] Patients with pseudotumor typically present with the acute onset of orbital pain, restricted eye movement, diplopia, proptosis, and impaired vision from perioptic nerve involvement. Conjunctival vascular congestion and edema, as well as lid erythema and swelling, are common.[5, 6] Pseudotumors are often multicentric. In addition to the variety of classification systems and diagnostic criteria that have been offered over the years, the disease can include a wide range of clinical presentations and many of the symptoms are nonspecific. Pain is an important feature of pseudotumors; however, not all patients with pseudotumors present with pain.[5, 6] Some may have minimal proptosis or may even present with a totally scarred lesion (sclerosing pseudotumor) within a single muscle or in the retrobulbar fat pad.[5, 6]

### Histopathology

The condition was first described in 1905 by Birch-Hirschfield[95] and has remained somewhat of an enigma in

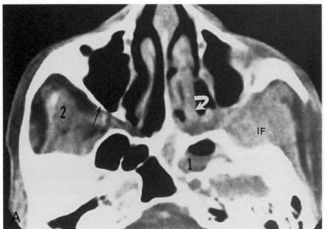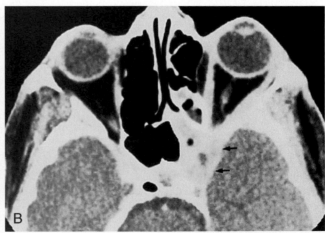

**FIGURE 9-70**    Mucormycosis. **A**, Axial CT scan shows soft-tissue induration in the left nasal cavity (*curved arrow*) and left infratemporal fossa (*IF*). Note the air-fluid level in the left sphenoid sinus (*1*). Fascial planes in the left infratemporal fossa (*IF*) region, compared with the right side (*2*), are obliterated. Note the rarefaction of the posterior wall of the left maxillary sinus compared with the normal right side (*black arrow*). **B**, Axial CT scan, same patient as in **A**, shows involvement of the left cavernous sinus (*arrows*) with enlargement (engorgement) of the left lateral and medial rectus muscles.

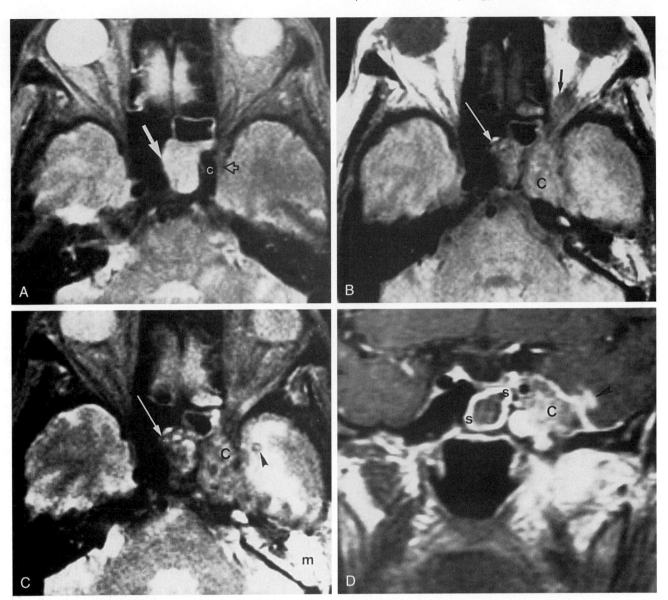

**FIGURE 9-71**    Aspergillosis. **A**, Axial T2-weighted MR image shows soft-tissue induration in the left sphenoid sinus (*white arrow*). Note the internal carotid (*C*) and early soft-tissue infiltration of the left cavernous sinus (*hollow arrow*). **B**, Axial PW MR image follow-up scan. **C**, Axial T2-weighted MR image follow-up scan. Scans show progression of the pathologic process, with marked infiltration of the left cavernous sinus (*C*) and formation of the left temporal lobe abscess (*arrowhead*) with marked peripheral edema. Note apical infiltration into the left orbit (*black arrow* in **B**) and inflammatory mycotic tissue in the left sphenoid sinus (*white arrow*). The mycotic process appears rather hypointense on the T2-weighted MR image, a not uncommon finding with fungal infections. Note the nonvisualization of the left internal carotid artery (compare with **A**); this results from invasion of the mycotic process, a finding confirmed by angiography and surgery. The mycotic process (*m*) has extended over the left petrous apex. **D**, Postcontrast (Gd-DTPA) coronal MR image shows enhancement of mucosal thickening of the left sphenoid sinus (*S*) and infiltrative process of the left cavernous sinus (*C*) and the temporal lobe abscess (*arrowhead*).

the ophthalmology, radiology, and pathology literatures.[94] The histopathology can vary from polymorphous inflammatory cells and fibrosis with a matrix of granulation tissue, eosinophils, plasma cells, histiocytes, lymphoid follicles with germinal centers and lymphocytes to a predominantly lymphocytic form (lymphoid hyperplasia) embedded in a loose fibrous stroma. It is the chronic lymphocytic variety that is related to lymphoma.[94] Many cases have been reported of lymphocytic pseudotumor that over a period of time are found to harbor a malignant lymphoma without any

evidence of systemic lymphoma. The presence of germinal follicles and increased vascularity is indicative of a reactive lesion, often associated with a favorable prognosis and responsiveness to steroids. An association has been noted between diffusely distributed lymphoblasts, unresponsiveness to steroids, and a probable neoplastic lymphoid lesion.[94] However, not all steroid-resistant pseudotumors are destined to become lymphomatous. The peculiar behavior of pseudotumors has led some authors to speculate that some forms of pseudotumor are the result of an autoimmune process.[94, 96] Pseudotumors are often multicentric, presenting with myositis, dacryoadenitis, sclerotenonitis (Tenon fasciitis), and inflammation of the dural sheath of the optic nerve and surrounding connective tissue.[5, 6] Pseudotumors may be classified as (1) acute and subacute idiopathic anterior orbital inflammation; (2) acute and subacute idiopathic diffuse orbital inflammation; (3) acute and subacute idiopathic myositic orbital inflammation; (4) acute and subacute idiopathic apical orbital inflammation; (5) idiopathic dacryoadenitis; and (6) perineuritis. Tolosa-Hunt syndrome (painful ophthalmoplegia) is a variant of pseudotumor in which the inflammatory process is restricted to the vicinity of the superior orbital fissure, the optic canal, or the cavernous sinus.[5, 6]

### Anterior Orbital Inflammation

In the anterior orbital pseudotumor group, the main focus of inflammation involves the anterior orbit and adjacent globe.[3] The major features at presentation are pain, proptosis, lid swelling, and decreased vision. Other findings may be ocular and include uveitis, sclerotenonitis (Tenon's capsule), papillitis, and exudative retinal detachment. Extraocular muscle (EOM) motility is usually unaffected. CT and MR imaging show thickening of the uveal-scleral rim with obscuration of the optic nerve junction, which enhances with contrast infusion on CT (Fig. 9-72).[94] These findings are due to leakage of proteinaceous edema fluid into the interstitium of the uvea and Tenon's capsule secondary to the inflammatory reaction.[94] Fluid in Tenon's capsule has been well documented with ultrasound (the T sign). Patients with posterior scleritis can develop retinal detachment and fundal masses, which simulate intraocular tumors.[94] The differential clinical diagnosis of anterior orbital pseudotumor includes orbital cellulitis, ruptured dermoid cyst, or hemorrhage within a vascular lesion (hemangioma, lymphangioma), collagen vascular disease, rhabdomyosarcoma, and leukemic infiltration.

### Diffuse Orbital Pseudotumor

Diffuse orbital pseudotumor is similar in many respects to acute and subacute anterior inflammation, with more

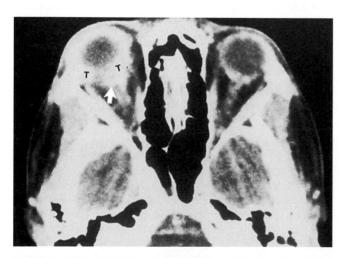

**FIGURE 9-72**   Pseudotumor: periscleritis/perineuritis. Postcontrast axial CT scan shows diffuse thickening of the scleral coat with inflammatory infiltration into Tenon's space (*T*) and perineuritis (*arrow*).

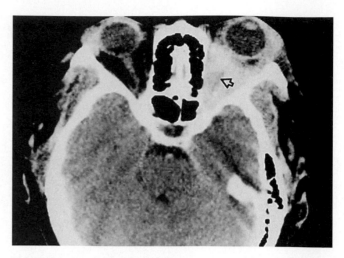

**FIGURE 9-73**   Pseudotumor. Axial CT scan shows diffuse infiltration of the entire retrobulbar space. The optic nerve appears as a lucent band (*arrow*) embedded within the lesion. (From Curtin HD. Pseudotumor. Radiol Clin North Am 1987;25:583.)

severe signs and symptoms.[3] The diffuse, tumefactive, or infiltrative type of pseudotumor may fill the entire retrobulbar space and mold itself around the globe while respecting its natural shape. Even the largest mass usually does not invade or distort the shape of the globe or erode bone (Figs. 9-73 and 9-74). This type of disease can be very difficult to differentiate from lymphoma. These large, bulky masses can be intraconal, extraconal, or involve both spaces. This disease must be differentiated from true tumors of the orbit such as cavernous hemangioma, hemangiopericytoma, optic nerve sheath meningioma, optic nerve glioma, orbital schwannoma, and metastasis.[94] True tumors usually do not respect the boundaries of the globe, indenting or deforming its surface. Also, bone erosion and extraorbital extension are more typical of true tumors than of pseudotumors.

### Orbital Myositis

Idiopathic orbital myositis is a condition in which one or more of the EOMs are primarily infiltrated by an inflammatory process (Figs. 9-75 to 9-79). The myositis can be acute, subacute, or recurrent, and the patient usually presents with painful extraocular movements, diplopia, proptosis, swelling of the lid, conjunctival chemosis, and inflammation over the involved EOM.[3, 94] This disorder may be bilateral. The most frequently affected muscles are the superior complex and the medial rectus (Fig. 9-75). The major differential diagnosis is Graves' disease. However, dysthyroid myopathy is usually painless in onset, asymmetric, slowly progressive, and associated with a systemic diathesis.[3] Trokel and Hilal state that the typical CT finding in orbital myositis is enlargement of the EOMs, which extends anteriorly to involve the tendon insertion (Figs. 9-75 and 9-76).[97] Other helpful indicators of inflammatory orbital myositis include a ragged, fluffy border of the involved muscle, with infiltration and obliteration of the fat in the peripheral surgical space between the periosteum of the orbital wall and the muscle cone. Also observed is an inward bowing of the medial contour of the muscle belly, forming a shoulder as it passes behind the globe (Fig. 9-75). All these findings can be attributed to local tendinitis, fasciitis, and

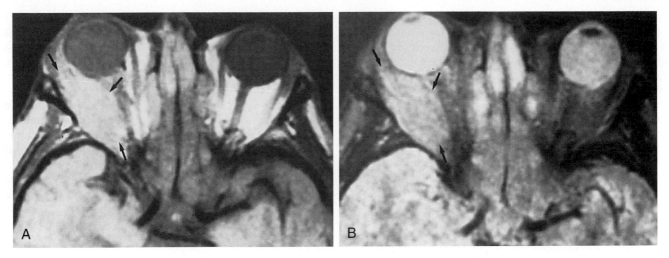

**FIGURE 9-74**   Pseudotumor. **A**, Axial PW MR image. **B**, Axial T2-weighted MR image. Scans show infiltrative process (*arrows*) compatible with pseudotumor. The lesion is isointense to brain on PW and T2-weighted MR scans. (From Curtin HD. Pseudotumor. Radiol Clin North Am 1987;25:583.)

myositis of the involved muscle. In contrast, the fusiform appearance of an enlarged muscle in thyroid myopathy is produced by a myositis without involvement of the muscle tendon insertion. The muscle borders are sharply defined, the fat in the peripheral surgical space is preserved, and there is no medial muscle bowing. Less common causes of EOM enlargement include arteriovenous fistula (e.g., carotid-cavernous fistula), granulomatous disease, and neoplasm (primary or metastatic).[94]

### Perineuritis and Periscleritis

Idiopathic perineuritis (inflammation of the sheath of the optic nerve) can simulate optic neuritis by presenting with orbital pain, pain with extraocular motility, decreased visual acuity, and disc edema. In contrast to optic neuritis, pain is exacerbated with retrodisplacement of the globe, and there is mild proptosis.[94] CT and MR imaging show a ragged, edematous enlargement of the optic nerve sheath complex (Fig. 9-79A). If periscleritis is present, the inflammation involves the tissues immediately contiguous to the sclera (Fig. 9-79B).

### Lacrimal Adenitis

Acute idiopathic lacrimal adenitis (pseudotumor) presents with tenderness in the upper outer quadrant of the orbit in the region of the lacrimal gland.[24, 94] Viral dacryoadenitis may present in a similar manner, although it is commonly associated with an etiology such as mumps, mononucleosis, or herpes zoster virus infection. Adenopathy and lymphocytosis can be present in these latter cases. The differential diagnosis of nonspecific lacrimal adenitis includes viral and bacterial dacryoadenitis, rupture of a dermoid cyst in the lacrimal gland region, specific lacrimal gland inflammations such as sarcoidosis and Sjogren's disease, lymphoproliferative disorders, cysts, and neoplasia in this region. Because of the wide variety and incidence of pathology that can involve the lacrimal gland, biopsy of this accessible site is necessary to obtain a definitive diagnosis (Fig. 9-80).[3]

### Apical Orbital Inflammation

Pseudotumor may present with infiltration of the orbital apex, and these patients present with a typical orbital apex syndrome consisting of pain, minimal proptosis, and painful ophthalmoplegia. The CT and MR imaging findings include an irregular infiltrative process of the orbital apex with extension along the posterior portion of the EOMs or the optic nerve. Sarcoidosis (Fig. 9-81) and other granulomatous processes including Wegener's granulomatosis may be responsible for similar clinical and imaging presentations.

### Painful External Ophthalmoplegia (Tolosa-Hunt Syndrome)

In 1954, Tolosa described a patient with unilateral recurrent painful ophthalmoplegia involving cranial nerves III, IV, VI, and V1.[98] Carotid arteriography in this case

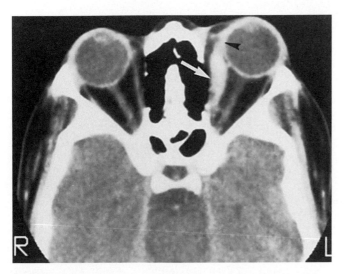

**FIGURE 9-75**   Myositic pseudotumor. Postcontrast Axial CT scan shows marked thickening and enhancement of the left medial rectus muscle (*arrow*). Note extension of the process into its tendinous insertion on the globe (*arrowhead*). (From Flanders AE et al. CT characteristics of orbital pseudotumor and other orbital inflammatory processes. J Comput Assist Tomogr 1989;13:40–47.)

showed segmental narrowing in the carotid siphon. The patient died after surgical exploration, and a postmortem study showed adventitial thickening in the cavernous carotid artery surrounded by a cuff of nonspecific granulation tissue that also involved the adjoining cranial nerve trunks. In 1961, Hunt et al. reported six patients, with similar clinical symptoms and signs.[99] After reviewing Tolosa's slides, these authors proposed a low-grade, nonspecific inflammation of the cavernous sinus and its walls as the cause of the syndrome. They also emphasized that angiography was essential to rule out an aneurysm or neoplasm.[99] In 1966, Smith and Taxdal applied the term *Tolosa-Hunt syndrome* to this entity.[100] They described five additional cases and stressed the diagnostic usefulness of the dramatically rapid therapeutic response to corticosteroids. In 1973, Sondheimer and Knapp reported three patients with Tolosa-Hunt

syndrome on whom orbital venography was performed.[101] These investigators observed that the superior ophthalmic vein on the affected side was occluded in the posterior portion of the muscle cone in each case and that there was partial or complete obliteration of the ipsilateral cavernous sinus.

Painful external ophthalmoplegia, or Tolosa-Hunt syndrome, is now considered an idiopathic inflammatory process and a regional variant of idiopathic orbital pseudotumors that, because of its anatomic location (superior orbital fissure, cavernous sinus, or both), produces typical clinical manifestations.[98, 102] The disease manifests as recurrent attacks of a steady, dull, retroorbital pain, palsies of the third, fourth, or sixth cranial nerve and the first or second divisions or both of the trigeminal nerve, and venous engorgement. It is usually unilateral, but bilateral cases do

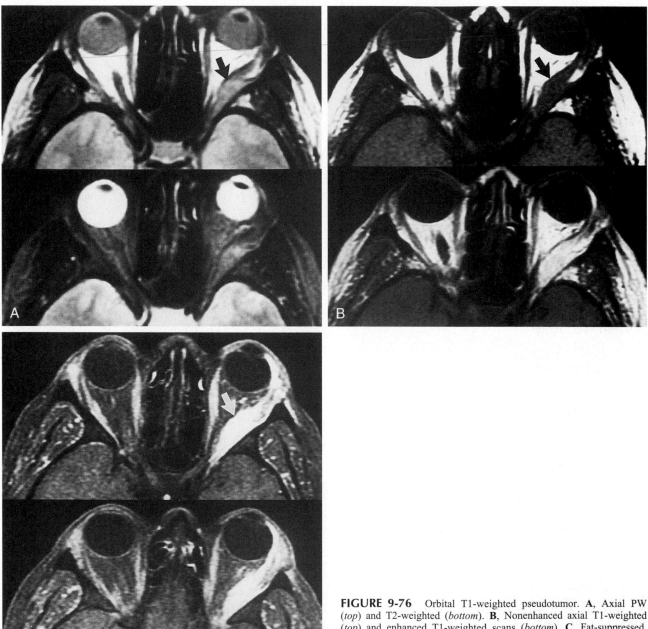

**FIGURE 9-76** Orbital T1-weighted pseudotumor. **A,** Axial PW (*top*) and T2-weighted (*bottom*). **B,** Nonenhanced axial T1-weighted (*top*) and enhanced T1-weighted scans (*bottom*). **C,** Fat-suppressed, enhanced, axial T1-weighted MR scans show an infiltrative process involving the left lateral rectus and adjacent extraorbital fat (*arrows*).

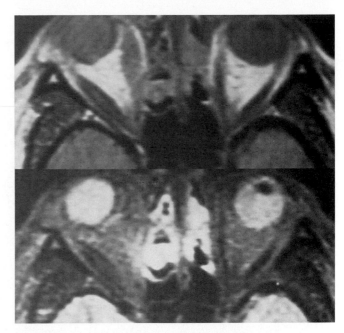

**FIGURE 9-77** Pseudotumor (myositic type), axial PW (*top*) and T2-weighted (*bottom*) MR scans in another patient show enlargement of the right lateral and medial rectus muscles.

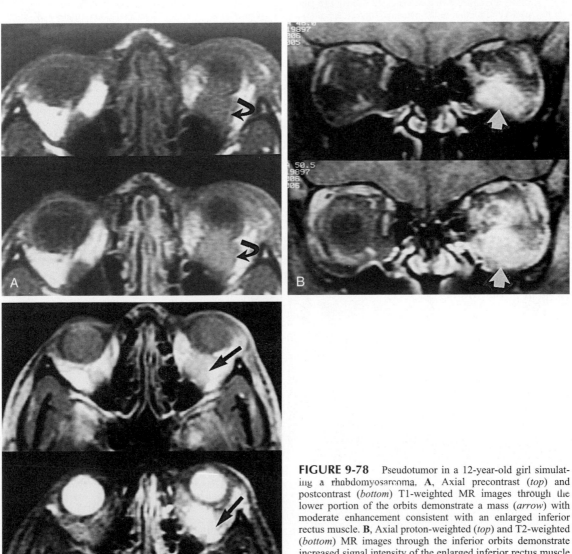

**FIGURE 9-78** Pseudotumor in a 12-year-old girl simulating a rhabdomyosarcoma. **A**, Axial precontrast (*top*) and postcontrast (*bottom*) T1-weighted MR images through the lower portion of the orbits demonstrate a mass (*arrow*) with moderate enhancement consistent with an enlarged inferior rectus muscle. **B**, Axial proton-weighted (*top*) and T2-weighted (*bottom*) MR images through the inferior orbits demonstrate increased signal intensity of the enlarged inferior rectus muscle (*arrows*). **C**, Coronal postcontrast, fat-suppressed, T1-weighted MR images through the orbits reveal diffuse enhancement of the enlarged inferior rectus muscle (*arrows*).

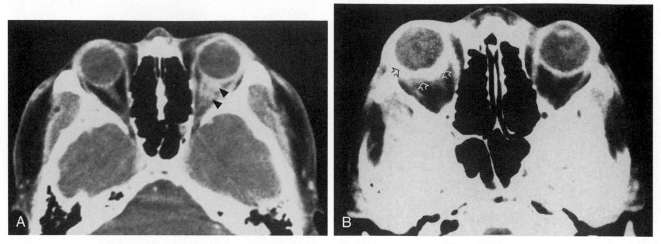

**FIGURE 9-79** **A**, Pseudotumor (perineuritis type). Axial CT scan shows the intraconal region of infiltration (*arrowheads*) surrounding the left optic nerve. Slight thickening of the posterior sclera indicates posterior scleritis and fluid (exudate) in Tenon's space. **B**, Pseudotumor (scleritis and episcleritis type). Postcontrast axial CT scan shows a prominent ring of increased density and enhancement (*arrows*) due to reactive inflammatory effusion as well as infiltration in the potential Tenon's space (fasciitis). (**B** from Mafee MF et al. Lacrimal gland tumors and simulating lesions. Radiol Clin North Am 1999;37:219–239.)

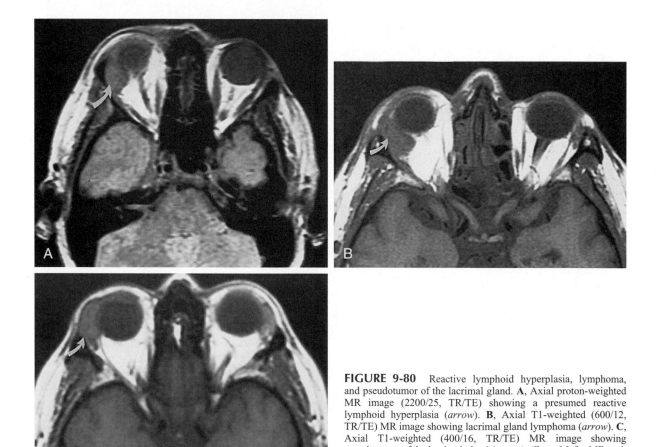

**FIGURE 9-80** Reactive lymphoid hyperplasia, lymphoma, and pseudotumor of the lacrimal gland. **A**, Axial proton-weighted MR image (2200/25, TR/TE) showing a presumed reactive lymphoid hyperplasia (*arrow*). **B**, Axial T1-weighted (600/12, TR/TE) MR image showing lacrimal gland lymphoma (*arrow*). **C**, Axial T1-weighted (400/16, TR/TE) MR image showing pseudotumor of the lacrimal gland (*arrow*). (From Mafee MF et al. Lacrimal gland tumors and simulating lesions. Radiol Clin North Am 1999;37:219–239.)

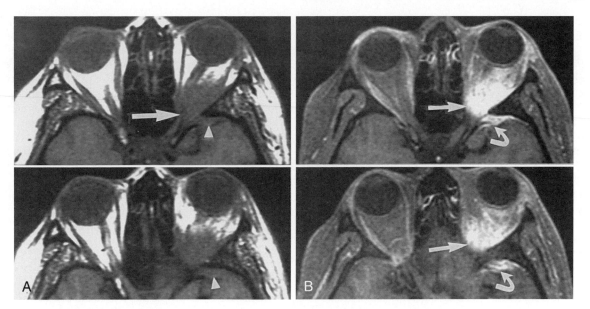

**FIGURE 9-81**  Orbital sarcoidosis presenting as superior orbital fissure syndrome. **A,** Unenhanced axial T1-weighted (400/25, TR/TE) MR images. Note the infiltrative process involving the orbital apex on the left side (*large arrow*). Note extension through the superior orbital fissure into the left temporal epidural space (*arrowheads*). **B,** Enhanced axial fat-suppressed, T1-weighted MR images show marked enhancement of this sarcoid granulomatous infiltration (*straight arrows*). Note the abnormal enhancement in the left temporal fossa (*curved arrows*). (From Mafee MF et al. Sarcoidosis of the eye, orbit, and central nervous system. Role of MRI. Radiol Clin North Am 1999;37:73–87.)

occur.[92] Immediate relief of symptoms following high doses of steroid therapy differentiate pseudotumor of the orbital apex and cavernous sinus from other lesions causing a superior orbital fissure syndrome.

Pathologically there is an infiltration of lymphocytes and plasma cells along with thickening of the dura matter, and it is important to exclude the possibility of a neoplastic (Fig. 9-82A), inflammatory (particularly mycotic) (Figs. 9-70 and 9-71), or vasogenic lesion. Carotid angiography and MR imaging are most useful in excluding an aneurysm as a cause of the clinical signs and symptoms.[103] Certain cavernous sinus, orbital apex, and parasellar lesions such as lymphoma, including Burkitt's lymphoma, leukemic infiltration, granulomatous diseases, pituitary adenomas, meningiomas, craniopharyngiomas, neurogenic tumors, dermoid cysts, orbital/sinonasal and nasopharyngeal carcinomas, invasive mycotic infections, aneurysm, and metastatic lesions (melanoma, lung, breast, kidney, thyroid, and prostate cancers) may produce similar symptoms.[103]

## Thyroid Orbitopathy (Graves' Dysthyroid Ophthalmopathy)

Thyroid orbitopathy, or Graves' dysthyroid ophthalmopathy, is the most common cause of unilateral and bilateral exophthalmos in the adult population.[6, 103] The disease usually has its onset between the ages of 20 and 45 years.[6] The mean age of presentation for Graves' thyroid disease is 41 years, and the orbital disease occurs, on average, 2 to 5 years afterward.[104] Even though the disease is more common in women, its severity tends to be greater in men and in patients more than 50 years of age.[104] Graves' disease is a multisystem disease of unknown cause

characterized by one or more of the three pathognomonic clinical entities: (1) hyperthyroidism associated with diffuse hyperplasia of the thyroid gland; (2) infiltrative ophthalmopathy; and (3) infiltrative dermopathy.[6] Thyroid orbitopathy (Graves' disease) includes any of the orbital and eyelid manifestations of this disorder. Among these clinical features are upper and lower eyelid retraction, exophthalmos, limitation of eye movements, eyelid edema, and epibulbar vascular congestion.[6] Although the majority of patients with thyroid orbitopathy have hyperthyroidism, the orbital manifestations of the disease may occur in individuals who are hypothyroid or euthyroid.[6] Occasionally, Graves' ophthalmopathy occurs in patients with Hashimoto's thyroiditis.[103]

### Pathology
#### Immunopathology

Thyroid orbitopathy is presumed to be an autoimmune disease.[6, 103] It is postulated that the immune complexes (thyroglobulin and antithyroglobulin) reach the orbit via the superior cervical lymph channels that drain both the thyroid and the orbit.[6] These complexes bind to extraocular muscles and stimulate acute inflammation characterized by an influx of lymphocytes, plasma cells, mast cells, and fibroblast proliferation, glycosaminoglycan overproduction, and orbital congestions.[6, 103, 104] Circulating autoantibodies against a human eye muscle-soluble antigen have been detected in a significant percentage of patients with thyroid orbitopathy, and both humoral and cell-mediated immune mechanisms have been implicated.[6, 103] Immunohistochemical analysis and histologic findings have shown orbital infiltration with mononuclear cells sensitized to retro-orbital antigens.[103] Cytokines released by the infiltrating monocytes may stimulate immunomodulatory protein expression, glycosaminoglycan production, and proliferative activity from orbital fibroblasts.

### Histopathology

Generally, as in other forms of inflammatory myositis, the histopathology in Graves' ophthalmopathy consists early on of inflammatory cell infiltration, mucopolysaccharide deposition, and increased water content.[103] The EOMs are infiltrated by lymphocytes and contain an increased amount of hyaluronic acid, which binds to water and accounts for some of the orbital congestion.[6] In the chronic stage of the disease, the EOMs undergo degeneration of the muscle fibers and replacement fibrosis.[6, 103] Restrictive myopathy is caused by this fibrosis.

### Diagnosis

The diagnosis of thyroid orbitopathy is based primarily on the patients' symptoms and clinical findings. Laboratory testing, including imaging studies, often is valuable in confirming the diagnosis.[6] The active phase of inflammation

and progression tends to stabilize spontaneously 8 to 36 months after onset.[103] Exophthalmos, lid retraction, lid lag, prominence of the episcleral vessels, and lid edema are important clinical findings. In some patients, the disease is characterized by the gradual onset of primarily verical gaze diplopia.[11] In patients with Graves' ophthalmopathy, the forced duction test result is almost always abnormal, and limitation is the most common disturbance of ocular motility.[11, 14] The exophthalmos is the result of enlargement of the EOMs and/or increased orbital fat volume.[103] The exophthalmos is almost always bilateral and usually relatively symmetric, although occasionally it may be quite asymmetric.[103] The inferior rectus muscle is involved most commonly, followed by the medial rectus and the superior rectus.[103]

### Diagnostic Imaging

CT and MR imaging in the acute congestive phase may show only markedly swollen retrobulbar orbital contents causing bilateral proptosis. The muscle bellies need not be

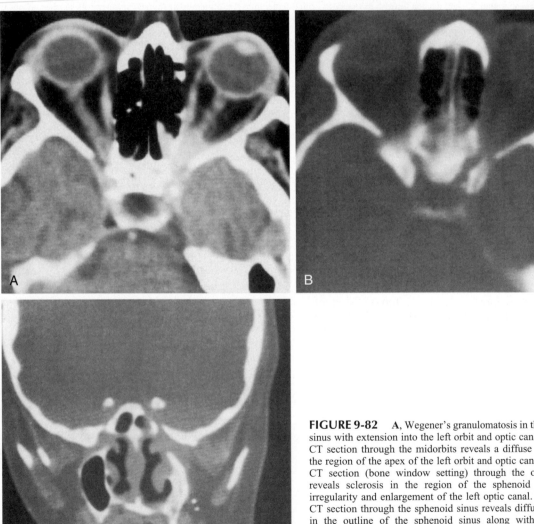

**FIGURE 9-82** **A**, Wegener's granulomatosis in the sphenoid sinus with extension into the left orbit and optic canal. **A**, Axial CT section through the midorbits reveals a diffuse infiltrate in the region of the apex of the left orbit and optic canal. **B**, Axial CT section (bone window setting) through the optic canals reveals sclerosis in the region of the sphenoid sinus with irregularity and enlargement of the left optic canal. **C**, Coronal CT section through the sphenoid sinus reveals diffuse sclerosis in the outline of the sphenoid sinus along with soft-tissue thickening in the sphenoid sinus, especially on the left. Note destruction in the left lateral wall of the sphenoid sinus. (From Weber AL, Mikulis DK. Inflammatory disorders of the paraorbital sinus and their complications. Radiol Clin North Am 1987;25:615–630.) **B**, Neurosarcoidosis.

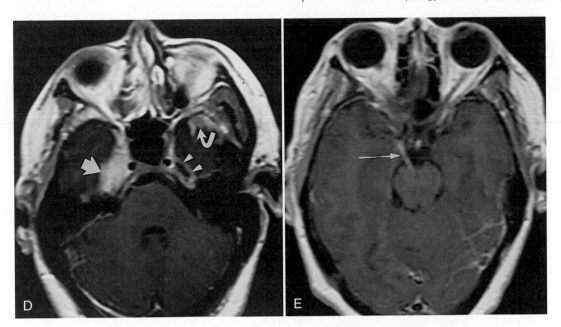

**FIGURE 9-82**   *Continued.* **D**, Enhanced axial T1-weighted (4501/11, TR/TE) MR image shows sarcoid granuloma involving the right Gasserian cistern (*large arrow*) and adjacent cavernous sinus, normal left Gasserian cistern (*arrowheads*), and abnormal enhancement in the left temporal fossa (*curved arrow*). **E**, Enhanced axial T1-weighted (450/11, TR/TE) MR image shows enhancement of the cisternal segment of the right third cranial nerve (*arrow*). The lateral gaze of the right eye is caused by the right oculomotor nerve palsy. (From Mafee MF et al. Sarcoidosis of the eye, orbit, and central nervous system. Role of MRI. Radiol Clin North Am 1999;37:73–87.)

enlarged. However, in this early stage of the disease, there also may be enlargement of the EOMs, and the coronal view is especially valuable in evaluating the degree of muscle enlargement and any optic nerve compression at the orbital apex. The increased orbital fatty reticulum results in anterior displacement of the orbital septum and at times prolapse of lacrimal glands. Strangulation of the optic nerve is seen best on axial CT scans.[3, 11]

About 90% of patients with thyroid orbitopathy have bilateral CT or MR imaging abnormalities (Figs. 9-83 and 9-84), even if the clinical involvement is unilateral.[3] Typically, enlargement involves the muscle belly, sparing the anterior tendinous insertion. However, there are rare patients who show thickening of the tendinous portion of the muscle.[3] Another helpful finding in thyroid myopathy is the presence of low-density areas within the muscle bellies. These are probably the result of focal accumulation of lymphocytes and mucopolysaccharide deposition.[3] Other CT and MR imaging findings in thyroid orbitopathy are increased orbital fat, enlargement (engorgement) of the lacrimal glands, edema (fullness) of the eyelids, proptosis, anterior displacement of the orbital septum, and stretching of the optic nerve with or without associated "tenting" of the posterior globe. On T2-weighted MR images, areas of high signal intensity may be present within the involved muscle. These areas presumably represent inflammation, and it is in these patients that a good clinical response to a trial of steroid therapy occurs. Later, a more chronic noncongestive phase follows, in which a restrictive type of limited eye movement often develops, secondary to fibrosis of the EOMs and to subsequent loss of elasticity.[11] At this stage, CT and MR imaging may show fatty replacement of the EOMs (Fig. 9-84B) or a string-like appearance of the

EOMs (Fig. 9-84C). Although the muscles may be moderately to markedly attenuated, the orbital fatty reticulum volume remains increased, as may be evidenced by exophthalmos, anterior displacement of the orbital septum, and prolapse of the lacrimal glands. The differential diagnosis of Graves' dysthyroid orbitopathy on a clinical basis includes tumors that may be primary or metastatic, orbital inflammation including pseudotumor, and carotid cavernous or dural shunt fistulas. All of these conditions can usually be distinguished from Graves' orbitopathy on CT or MR images. However, at times, orbital myositis secondary to an inflammatory sinusitis, trichinosis, or a myositis due to

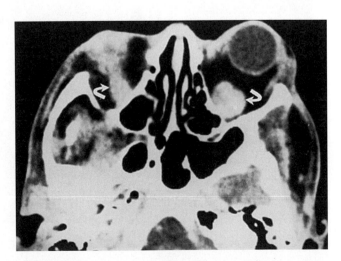

**FIGURE 9-83**   Thyroid myopathy. Axial CT scan shows enlargement of the inferior rectus muscles (*arrows*).

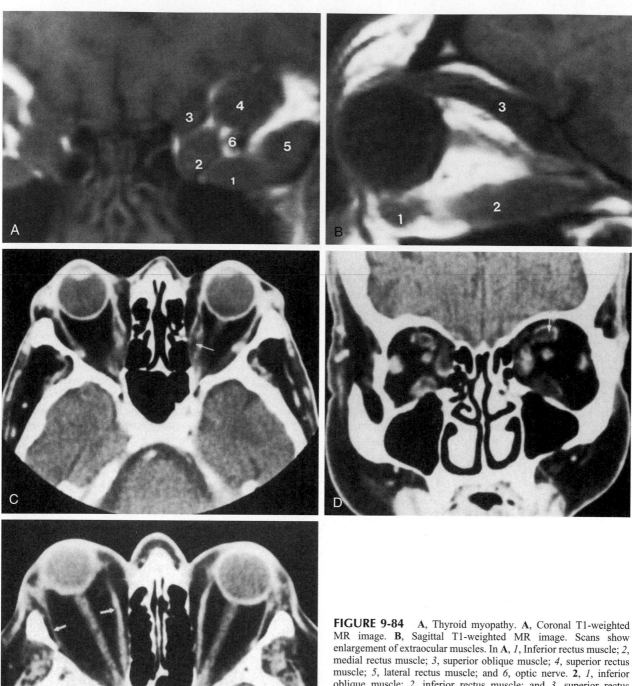

**FIGURE 9-84** **A,** Thyroid myopathy. **A,** Coronal T1-weighted MR image. **B,** Sagittal T1-weighted MR image. Scans show enlargement of extraocular muscles. In **A,** *1,* Inferior rectus muscle; *2,* medial rectus muscle; *3,* superior oblique muscle; *4,* superior rectus muscle; *5,* lateral rectus muscle; and *6,* optic nerve. **2,** *1,* inferior oblique muscle; *2,* inferior rectus muscle; and *3,* superior rectus muscle. **C,** Graves' dysthyroid orbitopathy. Lucency seen within the extraocular muscle seen on axial (**C**) and coronal (**D**) views. The muscles are again enlarged, with sparing of the tendinous insertions. **E,** Graves' dysthyroid orbitopathy. Axial slice shows an absolute increase in the amount of orbital fat with pronounced proptosis. There is stretching of the extraocular muscles, which appear to be smaller than usual (*small arrows*). There is also stretching of the optic nerve. (**B** and **C** from Curtin HD. Pseudotumor. Radiol Clin North Am 1987;25:583.)

systemic diseases such as Crohn's disease or Wegener's granulomatosis, pseudotumor, lymphoma, and even metastases to extraocular muscles may be difficult to differentiate on imaging studies.

## Sarcoidosis

Sarcoidosis is a granulomatous systemic disease that occurs worldwide, affecting persons of all races, both sexes, and all ages. It has a particular proclivity for adults under the age of 40 and for certain ethnic and racial groups. Estimates of the prevalence of sarcoidosis range from fewer than 1 to 40 cases per 100,000 population, with an age-adjusted annual incidence rate in the United States of 10.9 per 100,000 for whites and 35.5 per 100,000 for African Americans.[105] Higher annual incidence rates have been reported in other studies among African Americans, Irish, and Scandinavians. Sarcoidosis affects African Americans more acutely and more severely than it does people of other races. The cause of sarcoidosis remains obscure. The diagnosis of sarcoidosis is generally based on a biopsy finding of noncaseating granulomas with no other explanation.[3, 105]

The presenting features of sarcoidosis are protean, ranging from asymptomatic with abnormal findings on chest radiography in many patients to progressive multiorgan failure. Ophthalmic lesions develop in approximately 25% of patients, and virtually any part of the globe or orbit may be involved. There may be uveitis, chorioretinitis, and keratoconjunctivitis, and conjunctival inflammatory nodules may be seen.[3] The most common form of orbital involvement in sarcoidosis is chronic dacryoadenitis. This may be unilateral and may easily mimic a lacrimal gland tumor (Fig. 9-85A). Involvement of the lacrimal glands may also be very extensive (Fig. 9-85B), and when it occurs bilaterally in the lacrimal and salivary glands, it causes a Mikulicz-like

syndrome of dry eyes and xerostomia.[17, 105] Sarcoid may also involve the optic nerve, and when this occurs, it may clinically resemble a primary neoplasm of the optic nerve (Fig. 9-86).[106, 107]

The classic symptoms of anterior uveitis have a rapid onset, with blurred vision, photophobia, and excessive lacrimation. These symptoms usually clear spontaneously within a year. Sarcoidosis may affect virtually any part of the nervous system. Among the 5% of patients so affected, involvement of the facial nerve is the most common and bilateral facial nerve palsy should be considered highly suspicious for sarcoidosis or Lyme disease. Any cranial nerve can be affected. The most common cranial nerves to be affected are the optic nerve, facial nerve, trigeminal nerve, acoustic nerve, oculomotor nerve, and abducens nerve in decreasing order of involvement. The illness can be self-limited or chronic, with episodic recrudescence and remissions.

It is not clear why some patients recover spontaneously, whereas others worsen. Visual system abnormalities are the most common extrathoracic manifestations of sarcoidosis. In addition to the globe, the conjunctiva, EOMs, retrobulbar space, lacrimal gland, optic nerve, chiasm, and optic radiations (meningovascular infiltration) may be affected.[105] These patients may present with confusing clinical and radiologic findings, especially if ophthalmic and neurologic involvement precedes systemic symptoms. Several investigators have characterized the MR imaging findings in neurosarcoidosis and in orbital and optic pathway sarcoidosis.

### Pathologic and Immunologic Features

Sarcoidosis is a disorder mediated by excess helper T-lymphocyte activity at sites of disease activity. The noncaseating granulomas consist of mononuclear inflammatory cells, histiocytes, lymphocytes, plasma cells, and multinucleated giant cells.[105] Some of the granulomas may

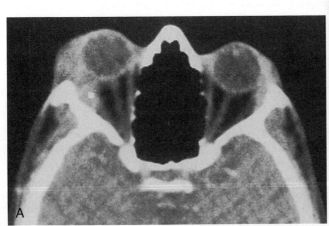
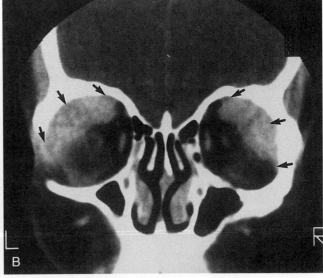

**FIGURE 9-85**   **A,** Sarcoidosis chronic dacryoadenitis. Axial CT scan shows enlargement of the right lacrimal gland. Note the mild enlargement of the left lacrimal gland. **B,** Sarcoidosis. Coronal-enhanced CT scan shows moderate enhancement of markedly enlarged lacrimal glands (*arrows*).

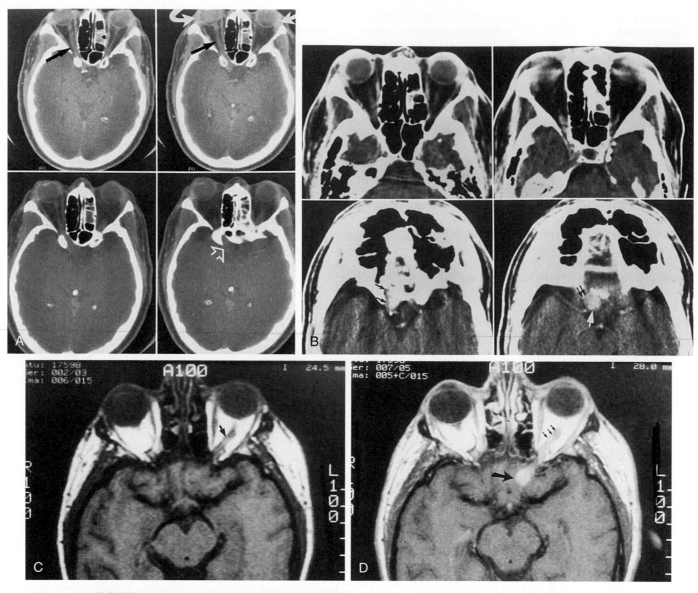

**FIGURE 9-86**   Sarcoidosis with optic nerve involvement. **A,** Serial axial CT scans show enlargement of the right optic nerve (*arrows*), including its intracranial segment. Note the soft-tissue mass in the right side of the chiasmatic cisterns (*hollow arrow*) and slight bilateral enlargement of the lacrimal glands (*curved arrows*). **B,** Serial axial CT scans obtained for soft-tissue detail, same patient as in **A,** show enhancing granulomas (*arrows*). **C,** Sarcoidosis-granuloma of the optic nerve. Axial T1-weighted MR scan shows no obvious lesion. There is a suggestion of slight thickening of the left optic nerve (*arrow*). **D,** Sarcoidosis-granuloma of the optic nerve. Enhanced axial T1-weighted MR scan shows increased enhancement of the left optic nerve (*arrows*) and a large granuloma involving the intracranial segment of the left optic nerve (*single arrow*).

have necrotic centers. Once mononuclear inflammatory cells accumulate in the target organ, macrophages aggregate and differentiate into epithelioid and multinucleated giant cells. Significant CD4 (helper-inducer) T cells are interspersed among these inflammatory cells. In time, CD4 and CD8 lymphocytes, and to a lesser extent B lymphocytes, form a rim around the granuloma. Except in the earliest stages of the granuloma, a dense band of fibroblasts, mast cells, collagen fibers, and proteoglycans begins to encase the cluster of cells in the granuloma. Fibrosis is an unfortunate outcome for many patients with sarcoidosis. Macrophages have a critical role in inducing fibroblasts to proliferate and to produce fibronectin and collagen in the lung. Most cells

also contribute to the chronic fibrotic response in the granulomas.

### Clinical Features

The clinical presentation of sarcoidosis may range from widespread disease to involvement of only one organ system at a time. Many asymptomatic cases are discovered during screening chest radiography, and these patients may or may not progress to clinically symptomatic disease. The majority of patients, however, present with systemic symptoms. In the United States, more than 50% of patients present with chronic respiratory symptoms and few constitutional symptoms. Lofgren's syndrome is referred to as the *constellation of erythema nodosum, bilateral hilar adenopathy,* and *polyarthralgias.* Uveitis and parotiditis are referred to as *uveoparotid fever* or *Heerfordt's syndrome.* Lupus pernio is referred to as *nasal sarcoidosis.*[105]

There are no definitive diagnostic blood, skin, or radiologic imaging tests specific for the disorder. Although an elevated angiotensin converting enzyme (ACE) level helps to establish a diagnosis of sarcoidosis, measurement of serum ACE activity and gallium-67 scanning add little diagnostic value because of their lack of specificity.[105] Oksanen reviewed 50 cases of neurosarcoidosis and found that the ACE in the CSF was elevated in 18 of the 31 patients in whom it was measured.[105] The Kveim-Siltbach skin test is not widely available and is not approved for general use by the Food and Drug Administration. Respiratory tract involvement occurs at some time in the course of nearly all cases of sarcoidosis. Pulmonary involvement in sarcoidosis is typically bilateral, with four radiographic patterns: (1) bilateral lymphadenopathy without parenchymal abnormalities; (2) bilateral hilar lymphadenopathy with diffuse parenchymal changes; (3) diffuse parenchymal changes without hilar lymphadenopathy; and (4) diffuse parenchy-mal changes without hilar lymphadenopathy with upper lobe retraction. Hilar adenopathy is frequently accompanied by right paratracheal lymphadenopathy. Atypical radiographic presentations include unilateral lung or lobar infiltrates, unilateral lymphadenopathy, and predominant upper lobe involvement.[105]

Intrathoracic and peripheral lymphadenopathy are common, with radiographic evidence of hilar node enlargement in up to 90% of patients. Peripheral lymphadenopathies are typically nontender. Approximately 25% of patients have one or more skin manifestations. Dermatologists frequently detect sarcoidosis during a biopsy of atypical skin lesions. Lupus pernio produces indurated violaceous lesions principally on the cheeks, nose, lips, and ears.[105]

As mentioned, the ophthalmic lesions include uveitis (Fig. 9-87), infiltration of the lids, optic nerve (Fig. 9-88), orbit and EOMs (Fig. 9-81), granulomatous infiltration of lacrimal glands (Figs. 9-89 and 9-90), retinal vasculitis, uveitis, uveoretinitis, and vitritis. Dykhuizen and associates[108] reported a case of sarcoidosis that presented with recurrent headaches, transient right hemiparesis, and left-sided ophthalmoplegia. An excised left retrobulbar lesion demon-

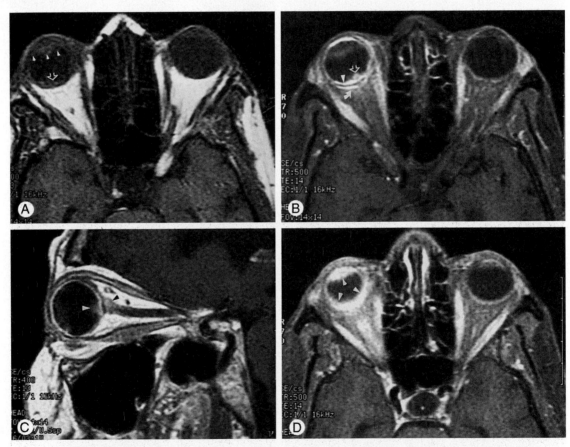

**FIGURE 9-87**    Ocular sarcoidosis panuveitis. **A,** Unenhanced, axial, T1-weighted (500/13, TR/TE) MR image shows nodular thickening of the posterior aspect of the right globe (*arrow*) and thickening of the anterior segment (*arrowheads*) of the right globe. **B,** Enhanced, axial, fat-suppressed T1-weighted (500/13, TR/TE) MR image shows nodular enhancement of the posterior aspect of the right globe (*arrowhead* and *open arrow*), related to granulomatous involvement of the choroid. Note enhancement of the anterior segment of the right globe. Notice abnormal enhancement of the Tenon's capsule (*curved arrow*). **C,** Enhanced, sagittal T1-weighted (400/13, TR/TE) MR image shows granuloma at the optic disc (*white arrowhead*) as well as involvement of the optic nerve (*black arrowhead*). **D,** Enhanced, axial, fat-suppressed T1-weighted (500/14, TR/TE) MR image shows enhancement of markedly thickened uveal tract (*arrowheads*). (From Mafee MF et al. Sarcoidosis of the eye, orbit, and central nervous system. Role of MRI. Radiol Clin North Am 1999;37:73–87.)

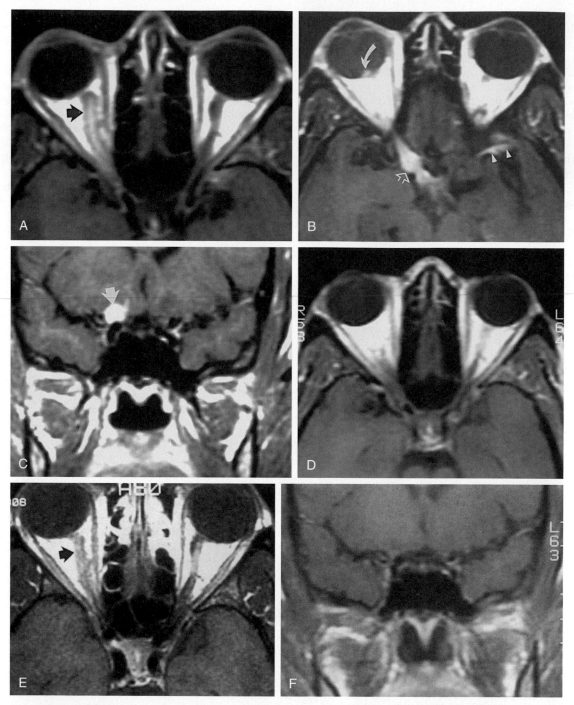

**FIGURE 9-88**    Optic nerve sarcoidosis. **A,** Enhanced, axial, T1-weighted (600/20, TR/TE) MR image shows increased enhancement of the right optic nerve (*arrow*). **B,** Enhanced, axial, T1-weighted (600/20, TR/TE) MR scan, taken 3 mm superior to **A.** Note nodular enhanced lesion (granuloma) involving right globe (*curved arrow*), enhancement of thickened intracranial segment of right optic nerve (*open arrow*), and abnormal enhancement along the anterior left sylvian fissure (*arrowheads*). **C,** Enhanced, coronal T1-weighted (650/20, TR/TE) MR image shows enlargement as well as marked enhancement of intracranial segment of the right optic nerve (*arrow*). **D,** Enhanced, axial, T1-weighted (600/20, TR/TE) MR image after corticosteroid treatment. Note absence of abnormal enhancement of the right globe as well as left anterior sylvian fissure (compare with **B**). **E,** Enhanced, axial, T1-weighted (612/25, TR/TE) MR image after corticosteriod treatment. Note decreased right optic nerve enhancement (*arrow*). **F,** Enhanced, coronal, T1-weighted (867/20, TR/TE) MR image. Note absence of enhancement of intracranial segment of right optic nerve, which was seen in **C.** (From Mafee MF et al. Sarcoidosis of the eye, orbit, and central nervous system. Role of MRI. Radiol Clin North Am 1999;37:73–87.)

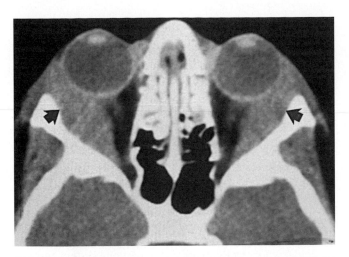

**FIGURE 9-89**   Presumed sarcoidosis of the lacrimal gland. Axial CT scan in this 7-year-old African American child shows marked enlargement of the lacrimal glands (*arrows*). (From Mafee MF et al. Sarcoidosis of the eye, orbit, and central nervous system. Role of MRI. Radiol Clin North Am 1999;37:73–87.)

strated sarcoid granulomatosis. Twelve years later, the patient developed a mass in the right lung. The excised lung mass was similar histologically to the previously removed left orbital mass. Idiopathic orbital inflammation displays a granulomatous inflammatory pattern that may mimic sarcoidosis. Raskin and associates[109] reported 12 patients with a diagnosis of sarcoidosis or another noninfectious granulomatous process involving the orbit. Five of these patients were diagnosed with sarcoidosis on histologic examination. In these patients, evaluation failed to reveal evidence of systemic involvement. The authors suggested that the clinicians should be aware of the existence of granulomatous idiopathic orbital inflammation not associated with systemic sarcoidosis as a distinct clinicopathologic entity. Monfort-Gouraud and associates[110] reported an inflammatory pseudotumor of the orbit and suspected sarcoidosis in a 13-year-old boy who had uveitis and symptoms of unilateral orbital inflammation. Mombaerts and associates[111] reported seven patients with unilateral idiopathic granulomatous orbital inflammation. Histopathologic analysis showed a spectrum of granulomatous inflammation admixed with nongranulomatous inflammation and fibrosis. They concluded that based on their study and review of the literature,

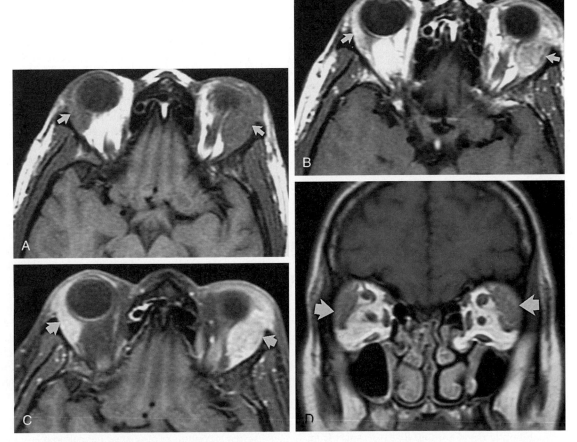

**FIGURE 9-90**   Sarcoidosis of lacrimal gland. Unenhanced, axial, T1-weighted (500/17, TR/TE) (**A**), enhanced, axial, T1-weighted (500/17, TR/TE) (**B**), enhanced, axial, fat-suppressed T1-weighted (500/17, TR/TE) (**C**), and enhanced, coronal, T1-weighted (600/18, TR/TE) (**D**) MR images show enlargement as well as increased enhancement of both lacrimal glands (*arrows*), more so on the left side. (From Mafee MF et al. Sarcoidosis of the eye, orbit, and central nervous system. Role of MRI. Radiol Clin North Am 1999;37:73–87.)

it appears that idiopathic granulomatous orbital inflammation is more closely related to orbital pseudotumor than to orbital sarcoidosis.

Carmody et al.[112] reported the MR imaging scans of 15 patients, 3 with presumed and 12 with proven orbital or optic pathway sarcoidosis. Eight patients had MR imaging evidence of optic nerve involvement by sarcoid granuloma. Perineural enhancement was seen in four cases and optic atrophy in one. Nine patients had optic chiasmal involvement. One patient had increased T2-weighted signal intensity in the optic radiations. Three patients had orbital masses that had MR imaging signal characteristics similar to those of idiopathic pseudotumor. Five patients had periventricular white matter abnormalities closely resembling multiple sclerosis.

Recently, Ing et al.[113] reported a 22-year-old white woman with optic nerve sarcoidosis without evidence of systemic or ocular disease. The authors found 17 cases similar to hers, with the diagnosis proved by optic nerve biopsy, reported in the English-language literature. In all of them, extensive prospective investigations revealed no systemic sarcoidosis. Most of these cases were initially mistaken for optic nerve sheath meningioma.

Neurosarcoidosis may produce anosmia and is frequently associated with ocular findings. In many cases of neurosarcoidosis, a diagnosis of meningioma is suspected preoperatively. Hypothalamic involvement in sarcoidosis is not uncommon and may mimic hypothalamic glioma. Lymphoma and Castleman's disease may involve the central nervous system including leptomeninges mimicking neurosarcoidosis and meningioma. Lymphoma may have primary intraorbital, intraocular, and intracranial involvement. Involvement of the optic nerve and other cranial nerves by angiocentric T-cell lymphoma, also known as *lymphomatoid granulomatosis*, has been reported.[105] Castleman's disease, a benign lymphoproliferative disorder related to lymphoma, is characterized by hyperplastic lymphoid follicles with capillary proliferation. This disorder was initially observed by Castleman in the mediastinum, but later reports described involvement elsewhere, including orbital and intracranial involvement.

Neurologic involvement with sarcoidosis takes two forms. In acute sarcoidosis, there tends to be involvement of a peripheral nerve, especially a cranial nerve and in particular the facial nerve. The optic nerve (which is not a peripheral nerve) is involved next most frequently. As mentioned, sarcoid uveitis in combination with a facial nerve palsy and fever is known as *Heerfordt's syndrome* or *uveoparotid fever*. The second form of nervous system sarcoidosis occurs in the chronic form of the disease with central nervous system involvement. Involvement of the optic nerve is more common in this form.[105] The involvement may be at the chiasm or in the intracanalicular or intraorbital segments of the optic nerve. Optic neuritis, granulomatous protrusions from the optic nerve head into the vitreous, and optic atrophy are manifestations of central nervous system and optic nerve sarcoid disease. Apart from the involvement of the lacrimal gland, involvement of the orbital tissues by true systemic sarcoidosis is rare.

Orbital pseudotumor may have a granulomatous pattern, which can easily be mistaken for sarcoidosis. Sarcoidosis-like lesions can be found in patients with syphilis, lymphogranuloma venereum, leprosy, tularemia, torulosis, histoplasmosis, blastomycosis, and coccidioidomycosis. The early lesions of sarcoidosis are much more likely to respond to corticosteroid therapy than are the late, fibrotic, hyalinized lesions. Lesions that demand systemic corticosteroid therapy are uveitis, optic neuritis, diffuse pulmonary and central nervous system lesions, persistent facial palsy, persistent hypercalcemia, and cutaneous lesions.

### Optic Nerve Sarcoidosis

Certain inflammatory conditions, such as syphilis, tuberculosis, or sarcoidosis, may be responsible for a chronic and progressive loss of vision. Chronic optic neuropathy, however, is more frequently due to a compressive lesion, such as meningioma (intracanalicular, intraorbital, or tuberculum sellae), pituitary tumor, or paraclinoid aneurysm. Sarcoidosis frequently involves the nervous system and can present as an abrupt or chronic visual loss, with or without disc changes. In one series of 11 cases of sarcoidosis of the optic nerve in patients ranging in age from 16 to 48 years, only two patients were previously known to have the disorder.[114] Four patients showed disc granulomas, four had optic nerve granulomas, and five had posterior uveitis and retinitis. In this series, chest radiographs were characteristically abnormal in 8 of the 11 patients.[114] Only one third had elevated serum levels of ACE. CT scans in these 11 patients infrequently showed enlarged nerves or other findings. Although sarcoidosis is classically believed to commonly not involve the optic nerves, increasing numbers of cases of presumed optic nerve sarcoidosis have been seen on MR images and CT scans, some of them with histologic confirmation. Although neuroimaging does not distinguish optic nerve sheath meningioma from sarcoid of the optic nerve, in the absence of uveitis and systemic sarcoid disease certain imaging features should raise the possibility of optic nerve sarcoidosis, prompting a trial of corticosteroid therapy before proceeding to biopsy. Imaging features that may favor a diagnosis of sarcoidosis of the optic nerve include (1) enhancement of the optic nerve associated with prominent enlargement of the intracranial segment of this nerve; (2) enlargement of the intracranial segment of the optic nerve associated with contrast enhancement; and (3) abnormal enhancement of the optic nerve associated with abnormal dural and leptomeningeal enhancement. Bilateral optic nerve enlargement along with abnormal enhancement has not been seen. This finding should favor optic nerve sheath meningioma, demyelinating disease, optic glioma, lymphoma, leukemic infiltration, or pseudotumor. Optic nerve sarcoidosis in persons under age 16 years is extremely rare.[105] Enlargement and enhancement of the optic nerve in children is seen with optic nerve glioma, extension of retinoblastoma along the optic nerve, leukemic infiltration, and in very rare cases of optic nerve sheath meningioma and optic nerve medulloepithelioma.[105]

### Diagnostic Imaging in Optic Nerve Sarcoidosis

When an ophthalmologist or neurologist suspects that an optic nerve is involved by sarcoidosis or that there is sarcoid of the central nervous system, a chest radiograph can be very useful. Active pulmonary sarcoidosis characteristically shows bilateral hilar adenopathy, with or without parenchymal disease. The nodes characteristically stand out from the right heart border, and there is associated right paratracheal nodal involvement. Chest abnormalities are found in about 80% of patients with ocular sarcoidosis (uveitis). Gallium scintigraphy is more sensitive than chest radiography for showing pulmonary involvement in patients with sarcoidosis.[105] It lacks specificity, however, because other pulmonary diseases also show similar uptake. Lacrimal gland uptake of gallium-67 also occurs in more than 80% of patients with active sarcoidosis. This uptake is also nonspecific.[105]

In patients with ocular, orbital, and optic nerve sarcoidosis as well as neurosarcoidosis, MR imaging remains the imaging study of choice. Gadolinium-enhanced T1-weighted pulse sequences are the most informative part of the MR imaging study (Fig. 9-88), and enhanced fat-suppressed, T1-weighted MR images are essential for the diagnosis of optic nerve sarcoidosis or simulating lesions.[105]

## Sjogren's Syndrome

Sjogren's syndrome is an autoimmune disorder characterized by keratoconjunctivitis sicca and xerostomia. Patients may have an associated autoimmune disease such as rheumatoid arthritis, systemic lupus erythematosus, polymyositis, scleroderma, or vasculitis. The lacrimal and salivary glands are initially infiltrated by periductal lymphocytes, and eventually atrophy of the acini with hyalinization and fibrosis occurs. The early disappearance of lysozymes from the tears in Sjogren's syndrome may help distinguish it from sarcoidosis, a disease in which the lysosomes in the tears are actually increased.

## Vasculitides (Angiitides)

The vasculitides are an immunologically complex-mediated group of diseases that include a variety of inflammatory angiodestructive processes. Clinically, the vasculitides may show features of acute, subacute, and chronic inflammatory and vaso-obstructive signs and symptoms.[3] This group of diseases includes a wide variety of disorders that are usually classified on the basis of the symptoms they produce and the organs affected, as well as their histopathologic features.[3] The major ophthalmic or orbital diseases include polyarteritis nodosa, Wegener's granulomatosis, T-cell or B-cell lymphoma (previously called *idiopathic midline destructive disease, malignant midline reticulosis,* or *polymorphic reticulosis*), giant cell arteritis (temporal arteritis), hypersensitivity (leukocytoclastic) angiitis, and connective tissue disease, including systemic lupus erythematosus, rheumatoid arthritis, scleroderma, and polymyositis.

### Wegener's Granulomatosis
Wegener's granulomatosis is a multisystem disease characterized by a triad of necrotizing granulomas in the upper and lower respiratory tracts, necrotizing vasculitis (focal necrotizing angiitis of small arteries and veins) of the lung, upper respiratory tract, and other sites, and glomerulonephritis.[3, 107] If left untreated, the disease is often fatal. The introduction of combined corticosteroid cyclophosphamide

treatment has proven very successful.[3] The main chronic inflammatory or granulomatous processes that involve the sinus and the orbit include Wegener's granulomatosis and sarcoidosis.[102] Wegener's granulomatosis often mimics inflammatory, infectious, or malignant diseases and clinically involves the respiratory tract and kidneys.[102] However, ocular involvement is also common, occurring in 18% to 50% of the cases.[102] The disease may cause scleritis, episcleritis, uveitis, retinal vasculitis, and, rarely, conjunctival involvement. The condition is characterized by pain, proptosis, motility disturbance, chemosis, papilledema, and erythematous edema of the eyelids.[3, 107] Characteristically, ocular and orbital involvement is bilateral and either nonresponsive or transiently responsive to corticosteroids, often providing a clue to the diagnosis.[3] Involvement of the ocular adnexa includes lacrimal gland enlargement, nasolacrimal obstruction, and eyelid fistula formation.[3] The disease most commonly spreads from the paranasal sinuses to the orbit and produces pain, ophthalmoplegia, and loss of vision.[102] Although Wegener's granulomatosis characteristically occurs in the fifth decade of life, it has been documented in children.[102]

Orbital involvement with Wegener's granulomatosis should be differentiated from idiopathic pseudotumors, lymphoreticular proliferative disorders, and metastatic carcinoma.[107] The CT and MR imaging appearance of Wegener's granulomatosis is similar to that of pseudotumor and lymphoma (Figs. 9-91 and 9-92), and nasal and paranasal sinus involvement is present in the majority of cases (Fig. 9-82A). These diseases are definitively differentiated by biopsy, and a high titer of serum antineutrophil cytoplasmic antibodies is highly indicative of Wegener's granulomatosis. Treatment of the disease with glucocorticoids and cyclophosphamide results in complete remission in 75% of patients and partial remission in another 15%.[109]

### B-Cell and T-Cell Lymphoma[109]
B-cell or T-cell lymphoma was formerly referred to as *idiopathic midline destructive disease, lethal midline granuloma, malignant midline reticulosis,* and *polymorphic reticulosis.* This disease is a clinical entity characterized by extensive destructive lesions of the nose, paranasal sinuses, and pharynx, often with associated involvement of the orbit and central facial bones. It has some similarity to Wegener's granulomatosis, but pulmonary disease is rare and renal involvement is absent.[107] This disease, which is not necessarily midline,[102, 115] is characterized by progressive unrelenting ulceration and necrosis, with destruction of the nasal septum. Most of these tumors are classified as T-cell lymphomas and are associated with Epstein-Barr virus infection.[102, 115] If the biopsy result indicates granulomatous vasculitis, the preferred treatment is cyclophosphamide and corticosteroids, as used for Wegener's granulomatosis. If the biopsy shows a lymphomatous process, radiotherapy is considered the treatment of choice.[107]

### Periarteritis Nodosa (Polyarteritis Nodosa)
This condition is a vasculitis of the medium-sized and small arteries, adjacent veins, and occasionally arterioles and venules. The disease is segmental and leads to nodular aneurysms. The major ophthalmologic manifestations are retinal and choroidal infarcts that lead to exudative retinal

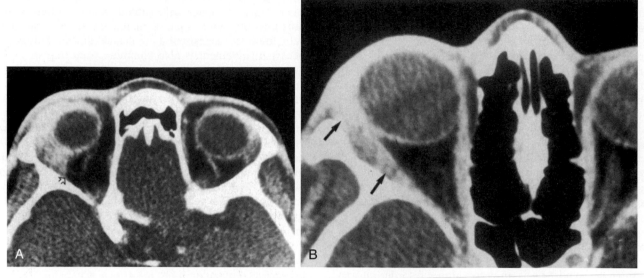

**FIGURE 9-91**  **A**, Wegener's granulomatosis with involvement of the lacrimal gland. Axial postcontrast CT scan shows diffuse enlargement of the right lacrimal gland. The lesion involves both palpebral and orbital lobes. Notice the rather straight configuration of the posterior aspect of the lesion (*hollow arrow*). In epithelial tumors of the lacrimal gland, the posterior border of the tumor has a rounded configuration. In Wegener's granulomatosis, enlargement of the lacrimal gland may be symmetric and extensive. Notice the slight enlargement of the involved left lacrimal gland in this patient. (From Mafee MF et al. Lacrimal gland and fossa lesions: role of computed tomography. Radiol Clin North Am 1987;25:767–779.) **B**, Wegener's granuloma. Axial CT scan showing an infiltrative process involving the right lacrimal gland and extending along the extraorbital space (*arrows*). (From Mafee MF et al. Orbital space-occupying lesions: role of CT and MRI: an analysis of 145 cases. Radiol Clin North Am 1987;25:529–559.)

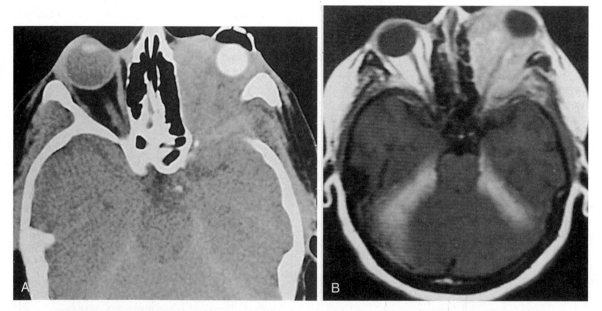

**FIGURE 9-92**  Progressive Wegener's granulomatosis of the left orbit. **A**, Axial CT scan demonstrates a diffuse homogeneous infiltrate obliterating the left orbit following exenteration of the left orbital contents. Note the anteriorly displaced prosthesis and a surgical defect in the lateral wall of the left orbit from previous surgery. **B**, Axial postcontrast T1-weighted MR image through the midorbits demonstrates marked enhancement of the inflammatory granulomatous process, which completely obliterates the left orbit, with stretching and anterior displacement of the globe. Note the diffuse enhancement of the tentorium cerebelli. (From Weber AL et al. Pseudotumor of the orbit: clinical, pathologic, and radiologic evaluation. Radiol Clin North Am 1999;37:151–168.)

detachment. Proptosis may occur secondary to severe inflammation of the orbital arteries, often leading to necrosis of the orbital connective tissues.[3, 107]

### Hypersensitivity (Leukocytoclastic) Angiitis

This condition resembles periarteritis nodosa microscopically, but it affects smaller vessels. Pathologically, the arterioles, venules, and capillaries are usually but not necessarily necrotic, or they may simply have perivascular infiltration, with neutrophils undergoing karyolysis (leukocytoclasis). The spectrum of clinical disease varies from widespread multisystem involvement to primary dermatologic lesions.[3]

### Lupus Erythematosus

Any of the connective tissue disorders may be associated with systemic vasculitis. The most common ones include systemic lupus erythematosus, rheumatoid arthritis, and dermatomyositis. Systemic lupus erythematosus is an autoimmune disease that affects many organs. It has a female/male ratio of 9:1 and occurs primarily in the second and third decades of life.[3] Histologically, the vasculitides in the connective tissue diseases resemble hypersensitivity angiitis.[3]

Evidence of antinuclear antibodies is universally present in this disorder. Of these patients, 20% have ocular involvement, primarily affecting the retinal vessels.[3] Orbital involvement is rare and is believed to be secondary to severe orbital vasculitis.[107] The CT and MR imaging appearance of orbital lupoid disease may resemble that of the pseudotumors and lymphoreticular proliferative disorders.

## Amyloidosis

Amyloidosis is caused by deposition of an amorphous hyaline material (amyloid) in various tissues such as muscle, skin, nerve, submucosa, adrenal gland, and the orbit. Involvement of the orbit and ocular adnexa may occur as part of primary hereditary systemic amyloidosis, as part of secondary amyloidosis, or as a localized isolated process.[17, 83, 116] The clinical features of orbital and adnexal amyloidosis include blepharoptosis, caused by infiltration of the levator muscle of the upper eyelid, and oculomotor palsies resulting from involvement of multiple extraocular muscles. When the lacrimal gland is involved, the disease resembles a lacrimal gland tumor. On CT, amyloid deposits (homogeneous eosinophilic protein) simulate pseudotumors, vascular malformation, and other mass lesions, and the deposits can occasionally calcify (Figs. 9-93 and 9-94A).[83] On MR imaging, the amyloid deposits have signal intensities similar to those of skeletal muscle on all imaging sequences (Fig. 9-94B). Localized amyloid infiltrations may affect the paranasal sinuses, and bone destruction has been reported.[83]

## MISCELLANEOUS GRANULOMATOUS AND HISTIOCYTIC LESIONS

A number of pathologic entities are recognized that, except for fibrous histiocytoma, rarely involve the orbit.

These include histiocytosis X (Langerhans' histiocytosis), Erdheim-Chester disease, juvenile xanthogranuloma, pseudorheumatoid nodules, necrobiotic xanthogranuloma, and fibrous histiocytoma.[3] All of these lesions bear a common feature based on local or systemic infiltration by histiocytes.[3] Fibrous histiocytoma is the most common tumor in this category.[5]

## Langerhans' Cell Histiocytosis

A granulomatous disease that occurs in children more often than sarcoidosis or Wegener's granulomatosis is Langerhans' cell histiocytosis; the disease has a predilection for children between 1 and 4 years of age.[102] The term *histiocytosis X* was coined to describe a group of histiocytic conditions, with the letter X indicating their unknown nature.[116] It is now known that these histiocytic conditions result from the proliferation and infiltration of abnormal histiocytes within various tissues. These cells are morphologically and immunologically similar to Langerhans' cells, leading to the name *Langerhans' cell histiocytosis* (*Hand-Schuller-Christian disease*, *Letterer-Siwe disease*, and *eosinophilic granuloma*).[117] Hand-Schuller-Christian disease typically involves the triad of diabetes insipidus, proptosis, and destructive bone lesions, often involving the sphenoid bone. Letterer-Siwe disease is seen in children under 2 years of age and is characterized by an acute disseminated form of Langerhans' cell histiocytosis associated with hepatosplenomegaly, adenopathy, fever, thrombocytopenia, anemia, and cutaneous lesions. The diagnostic feature is the presence of abnormal aggregates of Langerhans' cells. These cells, unlike other histiocytes, are characterized by immunochemical positivity for S-100 protein and CD1a and by the ultrastructural presence of membranous cytoplasmic structures, 200 to 400 mm in width and shaped like tennis rackets, that are known as *Birbeck granules*.[102]

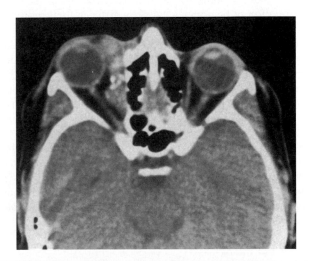

**FIGURE 9-93**   Amyloidosis of the right orbit with calcification. Axial CT section without infusion of contrast material reveals a mass in the extraconal space of the right orbit with a slight bulge into the intraconal space. Note the speckled calcifications within the amyloid deposit. The adjacent ethmoid sinus is normal. (From Weber AL, Mikulis DK. Inflammatory disorders of the paraorbital sinus and their complications. Radiol Clin North Am 1987;25:615–630.)

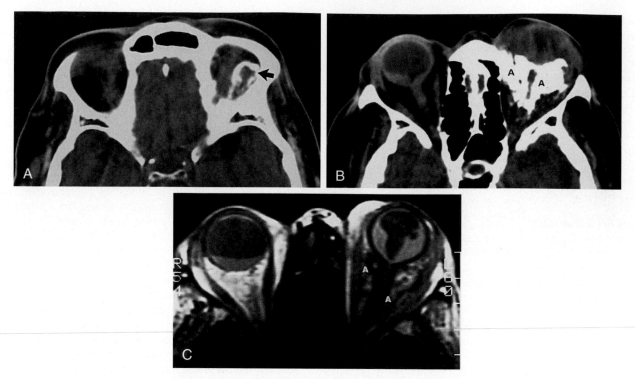

**FIGURE 9-94**    Amyloidosis of the lacrimal gland and orbit. **A,** Axial CT scan shows marked calcification of the left lacrimal gland (*arrow*). **B,** Axial CT scan shows a prominent cast-like calcification in the retrobulbar space caused by amyloidosis (*A*). Note the retinal detachment of the right eye. **C,** Axial T1-weighted (600/25, TR/TE) MR image shows hypointensity of the amyloid deposit (**A**). Note the bilateral exudative retinal detachment. The amyloid deposit appeared markedly hypointense on T2-weighted MR images (not shown). (From Mafee MF et al. Lacrimal gland tumors and simulating lesions. Radiol Clin North Am 1999;37:219–239.)

It is generally agreed that histiocytic disorders can be divided into two general categories: (1) X histiocytic (Langerhans' cell), Langerhans' cell histiocytosis (LCH), and (2) non–X histiocytic (monocyte-macrophage type) proliferation, including juvenile xanthogranuloma (JXG).[118] All of these disorders are characterized by a localized proliferation of histiocytes, but they differ in their morphology, histochemical and immunohistochemical staining patterns, and electron microscopic features.[119] Furthermore, they differ in their clinical presentation and radiologic appearance. Recently, the Histiocyte Society has redefined the classification of the histiocytoses of childhood. Class I includes LCH; class II includes all the histiocytoses of the mononuclear phagocytes other than Langerhans' cells, such as juvenile JXG; and class III includes the malignant histiocytic disorders. Orbital histiocytic disorders are classified as LCH (histiocytosis X); sinus histiocytosis with massive lymphadenopathy (Rosai-Dorfman syndrome); JXG; Erdheim-Chester disease; necrobiotic xanthogranuloma (NXG); pseudorheumatoid nodule; and sarcoidosis.[118]

### Historical Background

In 1953, Lichtenstein[116] introduced the term *histiocytosis X* for a group of diseases that include eosinophilic granuloma, Hand-Schuller-Christian disease, and Letterer-Siwe disease. He believed that the pathologic common denominator of all three conditions was a distinctive and specific inflammatory histiocytosis. The letter X was used to

underscore the unknown nature of the disease. Using the Birbeck granule as a marker, Nezelof and Barbey[117] in 1985 reported that the lesions of histiocytosis X were the result of inappropriate proliferation and infiltration of various tissues with abnormal histiocytic cells that are morphologically and immunologically similar to Langerhans' cells of the Langerhans' cell system. Consequently, the name of the disease was changed to *Langerhans' cell histiocytosis*.[118–120] This is a disease of unknown etiology. Some investigators suggested that LCH may be a disorder of immune regulation; however, recently, some investigators have provided strong evidence that all forms of LCH are a clonal proliferative disease.[119, 121]

### Clinical Features

The disease has a predilection for children 1 to 4 years old.[102, 119] Lesions in children are most commonly located in bone or bone marrow. Although LCH is a rare disease, in patients with the disease orbital involvement is not uncommon, and with few exceptions it is usually seen in the chronic form of the disease, especially eosinophilic granuloma. The overall incidence of orbital involvement in a series of 76 children with LCH was 23%.[118] The most common signs and symptoms of orbital LCH were unilateral or bilateral proptosis, edema, erythema of the eyelid, and periorbital pain. Other signs and symptoms were ptosis, optic nerve atrophy, and papilledema. The frontal bone was most commonly involved by LCH, and the lesions were usually seen in the superior or superolateral wall of the orbit

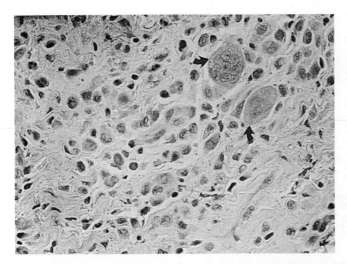

**FIGURE 9-95**   Langerhans' cell histiocytosis of the orbit. In addition to the mononuclear histiocytes, there are two multinucleated giant cells at the upper-right corner (*arrows*). "Coffee bean" nuclei are seen within the giant cells (hematoxylin-eosin, original magnification ×390). (From Hidayat AA et al. Langerhans' cell histiocytosis and juvenile granuloma of the orbit. Radiol Clin North Am 1998;36:1229–1240.)

in a rather anterior location. On rare occasions, the tumor may be noted in the orbital apex and superior orbital fissure without bone involvement. Classic cases of Hand-Schuller-Christian disease (the chronic disseminated form of LCH) with bilateral proptosis, diabetes insipidus, and bony defects of the skull are very rare.[118]

### Ocular Manifestations

Intraocular involvement by LCH is rare and usually occurs as part of an acute disseminated form of the disease (i.e., Letterer-Siwe disease). In these cases, the uveal tract, particularly the choroid, is affected.[118]

### Histopathologic Features

Grossly, the lesions are usually described as consisting of soft, friable, hemorrhagic, tan-yellow tissue. Histologically, the tumors are composed of sheets of large histiocytes with interspersed eosinophils, lymphocytes, and a few multinucleated giant cells (Fig. 9-95).

### Immunohistochemistry

LCH cells are usually positive for the following immunologic markers: S-100 protein, peanut lectin, and CD1a (OKT-6).

### Diagnostic Imaging

CT and MR imaging provide the most diagnostic assistance. Most lytic bony defects seen on standard plain films have been described as being irregular, serrated, and beveled, with or without a narrow zone of sclerosis. Orbital involvement may vary, but the most common orbital manifestation is a solitary lesion. In the typical case of orbital involvement, CT and MR imaging show an osteolytic lesion, commonly in the superior or superotemporal orbital region (Figs. 9-96 and 9-97). There is a fairly well-defined or diffuse soft-tissue mass encroaching on the lacrimal gland, the lateral rectus, or even the

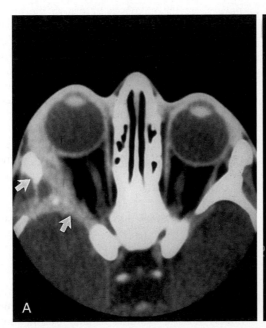
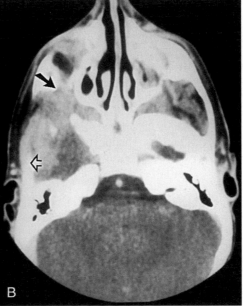

**FIGURE 9-96**   **A**, Langerhans' cell histiocytosis. Four-year-old boy with a history of gradual proptosis, diabetes insipidus, and skin lesions consistent with Hand-Schüller-Christian disease. Postcontrast axial CT scan shows replacement of the greater wing of the sphenoid bone (*arrows*) by soft tissue, which demonstrates marked enhancement. **B**, Langerhans' cell histiocytosis. Postcontrast axial CT scan in the same patient as in **A** showing a destructive lesion involving the squama of the right temporal bone (*hollow arrow*) as well as the posterior wall of the right maxillary sinus (*solid arrow*). Notice the marked soft-tissue infiltration into the right temporal fossa (*hollow arrow*). (From Hidayat AA et al. Langerhans' cell histiocytosis and juvenile granuloma of the orbit. Radiol Clin North Am 1998;36:1229–1240.)

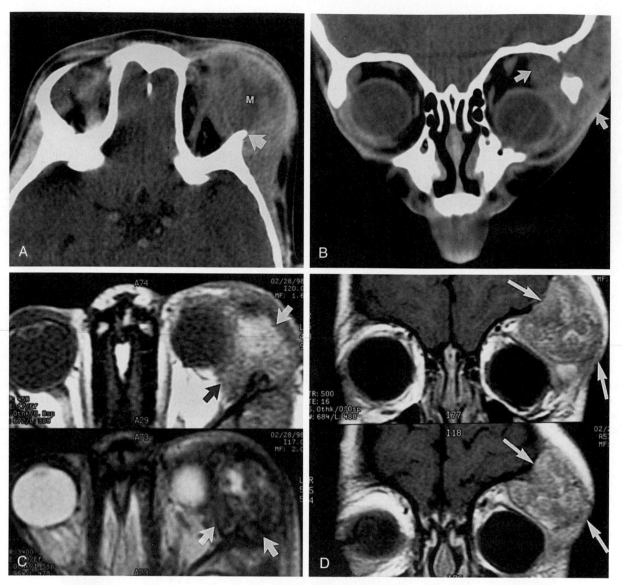

**FIGURE 9-97** Langerhans' cell histiocytosis. **A**, Enhanced axial CT scan shows a prominent soft-tissue mass (*M*) with destruction of the orbital wall (*arrow*). **B**, Enhanced coronal CT scan shows a destructive mass involving the superolateral orbit (*arrows*). **C**, Axial proton-weighted (*top*) and T2-weighted (*bottom*) MR images show the mass (*arrows*). The mass appears hypointense on T2-weighted MR images caused by recent traumatic hemorrhage confirmed at surgery. **D**, Gadolinium contrast-enhanced, coronal T1-weighted MR images show marked enhancement of the lesion (*arrows*). (From Hidayat AA et al. Langerhans' cell histiocytosis and juvenile granuloma of the orbit. Radiol Clin North Am 1998;36:1229–1240.)

globe. There may be extension of the soft tissue into the epidural space, as well as into the temporal fossa. There may be marked infiltration of temporalis muscles (Fig. 9-96). At times, multiple lesions may be present, resulting in multiple bony defects, particularly in the superolateral orbital roof region. Similar osseous lesions may be seen in the sphenoid, ethmoid, temporal, occipital, and parietal bones, as well as in the facial bones. Rarely, the lesion may be totally extraosseous. On postcontrast CT and MR imaging, lesions demonstrate moderate to marked enhancement (Fig. 9-97). The differential diagnosis of LCH from an imaging viewpoint includes rhabdomyosarcoma, juvenile fibrosarcoma, aggressive fibromatosis, lacrimal gland tumors, lymphoma, pseudotumor, leukemic infiltration, granulocytic sarcoma or chloroma, sinus histiocytosis, metastatic neuroblas-

toma, metastatic Wilms' tumor, and metastatic Ewing's sarcoma.

## Juvenile Xanthogranuloma

Juvenile xanthogranuloma (JXG) (nevoxanthoendothelioma)[121] is a benign, usually self-healing disorder of infants, children, and occasionally adults. The disease is of unknown etiology and pathogenesis and represents a proliferation of non-Langerhans' (monocyte-macrophage) types of cells. The term *juvenile xanthogranuloma* was first introduced in 1936, but recognition of the entity did not occur until 1954.[118] Recently, the Histiocyte Society has redefined the classification of the histiocytoses of childhood and included JXG in class II.[118]

### Clinical Features

Characteristically, the disease affects children, particularly infants, and is sometimes noted at birth. Adults are affected less frequently. The most common site is the skin, where spontaneous resolution is frequent.

Orbital involvement with JXG is rare, with only 15 patients having been described in the English literature, mostly as case reports, except for the series of 5 infantile cases in Zimmermans's[121] report and 5 adult cases reported by Jakobiec and coworkers.[122] Eight of these patients were infants, mostly less than 9 months old. In four of these infants, the orbital lesion was present since birth. In 7 of the 15 orbital cases, the patients were adults ranging from 22 to 60 years of age (average, 45 years).

Inside the eye, the most common sites of involvement are the iris and the ciliary body.[118] The retina, choroid, and optic nerve are rarely involved. In the eye, the presenting clinical signs, as described by Zimmerman,[121] are (1) asymptomatic localized or diffuse tumor of the iris; (2) congenital or acquired heterochromia of the iris; (3) unilateral glaucoma; (4) spontaneous hyphema; and (5) a red eye with signs of uveitis.[118, 121]

Central nervous system involvement by JXG has been reported with associated seizures, ataxia, subdural effusions, increased intracranial pressure, developmental delay, diabetes insipidus, and other neurologic deficits.[118] T1-weighted MR imaging of the brain showed solid, gadolinium-enhancing masses without evidence of cerebral edema or displacement.

### Histopathologic Features

Histologically, the lesions are composed of foamy histiocytes, epithelioid monocytes, lymphocytes, plasma cells, eosinophils, Touton giant cells, and spindle cells (Fig. 9-98).[118] Touton giant cells are multinucleated cells with the nuclei grouped in a wreath-like arrangement around a small central island of nonfoamy cytoplasm (Fig. 9-98). In contrast, the peripheral cytoplasm is foamy. The numbers of the different histiocytic cells are variable and form four distinctive patterns with varying degrees of overlap: (1) xanthomatous, (2) xanthogranulomatous, (3) fibrohistiocytic, and (4) combined patterns. It should be noted that the number of foamy or lipidized cells can be few, and Touton giant cells can be rare or absent in some cases, thus making the histologic diagnosis extremely difficult, as noted in one of the reported cases of orbital JXG.[121] In that case, there were many eosinophils and the lesion closely resembled those of LCH. Histologically, the differential diagnosis of orbital JXG includes Erdheim-Chester disease, particularly in adult patients. In both conditions there are Touton giant cells and foamy histiocytes. The only subtle difference between these disorders is the increased amount of fibrosis with collagenization and cholesterol clefts in Erdheim-Chester disease. In such cases, the clinical and paraclinical data, such as metaphyseal radiopacities, pulmonary infiltration and fibrosis, cardiac decompensation, chronic lipogranulomatous pyelonephritis, retroperitoneal xanthogranuloma, and hyperlipidemia in Erdheim-Chester disease, are extremely important for establishing the correct diagnosis.[123, 124] Inflammatory pseudotumor does not show xanthoma or Touton giant cells histologically. The differential diagnosis also includes LCH. In both lesions eosinophils are present, but the histiocytes are different morphologically

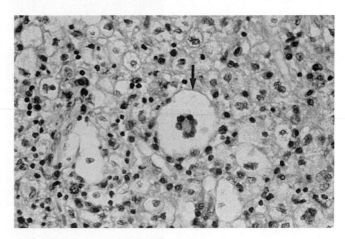

**FIGURE 9-98**   JXG of the orbit. Centrally, there is a characteristic multinucleated Touton giant cell (*arrow*), with the nuclei grouped in a wreath-like arrangement around a central small island of nonfoamy cytoplasm. The peripheral cytoplasm of the giant cell is pale and foamy. Other cells include xanthoma cells (lipidized histiocytes), with pale, foamy cytoplasm. A few lymphocytes are also present (hematoxylin-eosin, original magnification ×390). (From Hidayat AA et al. Langerhans' cell histiocytosis and juvenile granuloma of the orbit. Radiol Clin North Am 1998;36:1229–1240.)

and immunohistochemically. Touton giant cells are present only in JXG. The foamy histiocytes and Touton giant cells are negative for S-100 protein; however, a few S-100-positive dendritic cells were reported in the peripheral areas of JXG lesions.

### Diagnostic Imaging

Radiologically, the most common ocular finding is involvement of the anterior portion of the eye (Fig. 9-99). It is important to know that the bony wall of the orbit may be involved.[119] These changes included simple erosions of the superior orbital rim in one patient, radiolucency in the malar eminence in another patient, and marked destruction of the roof and lateral wall of the orbit and of the greater wing of the sphenoid in a third patient.[119] Those cases with bone involvement may not be distinguished from LCH radiologically. There has also been a case in which the clinical and radiologic findings were typical of LCH (Hand-Schuller-Christian disease) in a 3-year-old girl who had bilateral proptosis and diabetes insipidus. However, the histopathology was more consistent with JXG (Fig. 9-100). Furthermore, the histiocytes were negative for the immunologic marker S-100 protein, and no Birbeck granules were found when electron microscopy was performed. The CT characteristics of orbital involvement of JXG in an adult are shown in Figure 9-101. It is important to realize that the inflammatory process, including the granulomatous disease involving the orbit, may simulate LCH. A case of orbital involvement by tuberculosis simulating LCH or JXG is shown in Figure 9-102.

## Erdheim-Chester Disease

Erdheim-Chester disease is a peculiar form of systemic xanthogranulomatosis that occurs in adults.[123, 124] Most patients do not have orbital involvement. The first two cases

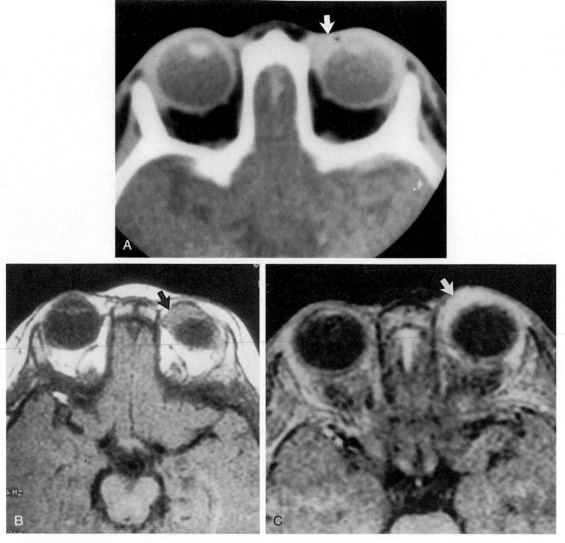

**FIGURE 9-99**    JXG of the orbit. **A,** Enhanced axial CT scan shows an enhancing infiltrative process involving the medial orbital region (*arrow*). **B,** Axial T1-weighted MR image shows the lesion (*arrow*) to be isointense to brain. **C,** Gadolinium-enhanced, fat-suppressed axial MR image shows marked enhancement of the orbital lesion (*arrows*). The lesion was adherent to the sclera. (From Hidayat AA et al. Langerhans' cell histiocytosis and juvenile granuloma of the orbit. Radiol Clin North Am 1998;36:1229–1240.)

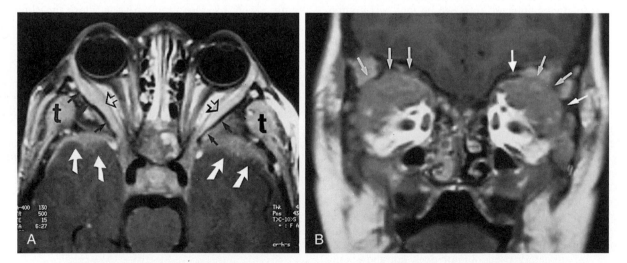

**FIGURE 9-100**    JXG. **A,** Enhanced axial T1-weighted MR image shows an enhanced soft-tissue infiltrative process involving the lateral orbital walls (*open arrows*), epidural space (*white arrows*), and temporal fossa (*t*). **B,** Enhanced coronal T1-weighted MR image shows marked soft-tissue infiltration of both orbits (*arrows*), as well as involvement of the frontal bone on both sides. (From Hidayat AA et al. Langerhans' cell histiocytosis and juvenile granuloma of the orbit. Radiol Clin North Am 1998;36:1229–1240.)

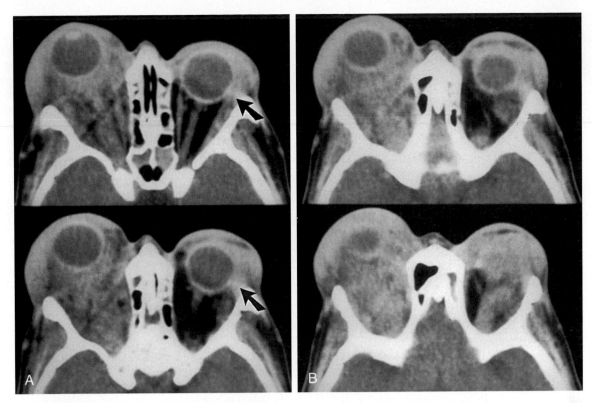

**FIGURE 9-101**   JXG of the orbit in an adult. **A,** Axial enhanced CT scans show proptosis and a diffuse infiltrative process involving the right orbit. There is abnormal soft-tissue thickening (*arrows*) of the left orbit as well. **B,** Enhanced axial CT scans show a marked infiltrative process involving the right orbit and, to a lesser extent, the left orbit. The differential CT diagnosis is bilateral pseudotumor, lymphoma, Wegener's granulomatosis, and necrobiotic xanthogranuloma. (From Hidayat AA et al. Langerhans' cell histiocytosis and juvenile granuloma of the orbit. Radiol Clin North Am 1998;36:1229–1240.)

were reported by Shields et al.[124] This disease is characterized by the infiltration of many organs including the lung, kidney, heart, bones, orbit, and retroperitoneal tissues. Orbital involvement tends to be bilateral. These patients present with progressive bilateral exophthalmos, which may lead to ophthalmoplegia, and visual loss secondary to compressive optic neuropathy.[92] CT and MR imaging may show extensive soft-tissue infiltration of the orbital fatty reticulum (Fig. 9-103).[107, 125] There may be no enhancement following the administration of Gd-DTPA contrast material.

## Pseudorheumatoid Nodules

Pseudorheumatoid nodules usually occur as focal masses in the dermis of children. This disease may involve the

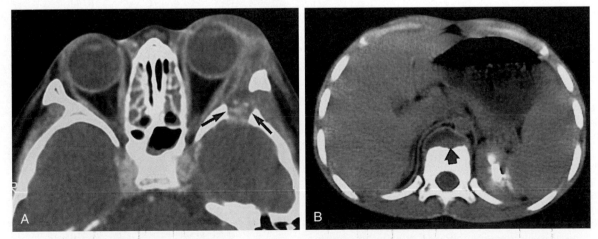

**FIGURE 9-102**   Tuberculosis. **A,** Enhanced axial CT scan shows a destructive lesion involving the left orbit (*arrows*). **B,** Axial CT scan through the abdomen shows a prevertebral tuberculous abscess (*arrows*). (From Hidayat AA et al. Langerhans' cell histiocytosis and juvenile granuloma of the orbit. Radiol Clin North Am 1998;36:1229–1240.)

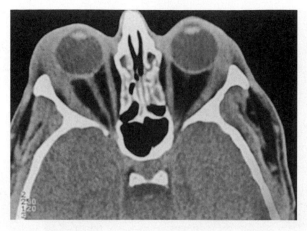

**FIGURE 9-103**   Erdheim-Chester disease of both orbits. Axial CT scan through the midorbits reveals a diffuse infiltrate around the right globe laterally with extension into the lateral rectus muscles. A similar infiltrate is noted along the lateral part of the left globe and adjacent rectus muscle. (From Weber AL et al. Pseudotumor of the orbit: clinical, pathologic, and radiologic evaluation. Radiol Clin North Am 1999;37:151–168.)

anterior orbit and periorbital region. The subcutaneous nodules consist of zonular granulomas surrounding necrobiotic collagen. These are thought to be more common in sites of previous trauma and are easily managed by simple excision[3] (Fig. 9-104).

## Necrobiotic Xanthogranuloma

Necrobiotic xanthogranuloma is a histocytic disease characterized by multiple indurated xanthomatous subcutaneous nodules in patients with paraproteinemia and proliferative disorders such as multiple myeloma and leukemia.[3, 107, 126] Pathologically, a zonular granulomatous inflammatory infiltrate, with Touton giant cells and xanthoma cells, surrounds an area of necrobiosis. Ophthalmic manifestations are common and include xanthogranulomas involving the eyelid, orbit, conjunctiva, and orbital fatty reticulum.

## TUMORS

### Orbital Lymphoma

Orbital lymphomas are solid tumors of the immune system composed primarily of (monoclonal) B cells. The extranodal presentation of non-Hodgkin's lymphoma is common, with an incidence ranging from 21% to 64%. Roughly 10% of the cases of non-Hodgkin's lymphoma present in the head and neck region, and lymphoid tumors account for 10% to 15% of orbital masses.[89]

Lymphoid neoplasms of the orbit span a large continuum of various classifications ranging from the malignant lymphomas, to the benign pseudolymphomas or pseudotumors, to the reactive and atypical lymphoid hyperplasias.[91] There are no absolute imaging, clinical, or even laboratory tests that distinguish all types of benign orbital lymphoid lesions from orbital lymphomas or lesions that can simulate

them.[91-93] A pleomorphic cellular infiltrate is correlated with more benign biologic activity, and the more uniform the cellular appearance, the greater the likelihood that a malignancy is present.[91] Of all patients with orbital lymphoma, 75% have or will have systemic lymphoma.[91] There is extensive overlap histologically from one type to another, and some forms of the benign process can transform over time into a more aggressive variety of lymphoma. True lymphoid tissue in the orbit is found in the subconjunctival and lacrimal glands, and these two areas account for most of the lymphoreticuloses developing in the orbit.[91, 94] The most common cytologic forms of malignant lymphoma involving the orbit are histiocytic and lymphocytic, with various degrees of differentiation. Both benign and malignant lymphoid tumors of the orbit occur predominantly in adults and are extremely rare in children.[6] The two main types of lymphoid tumor that ophthalmologists deal with are reactive lymphoid hyperplasia, a localized benign disease of unknown cause, and malignant lymphoma, which may either arise in and be limited to the orbit, may arise in the sinonasal cavities and extend into the orbit, or may be one focus of a systemic lymphoma.[6] Clinically, both malignant lymphoma and reactive lymphoid hyperplasia can produce a painless progressive proptosis accompanied by extraocular motility disturbance, visual disturbance, and lacrimal gland enlargement.[6] Any orbital tissue or combination of tissues may be involved in either disease process.[6] All patients with benign and malignant lymphoid lesions of the orbit should be subjected to systemic evaluation to rule out a systemic lymphoproliferative disorder. Intracranial involvement is extremely uncommon in patients with lymphoma at the time of presentation, but such involvement occasionally occurs in some patients with persistent disease.[102] A few patients with Hodgkin's disease, Burkitt's lymphoma, and other non-Hodgkin's lymphomas have presented with the Tolosa-Hunt syndrome.[102] Outside the original lymphoid tissue of Waldeyer's ring, there is a mixed population of lymphocytes

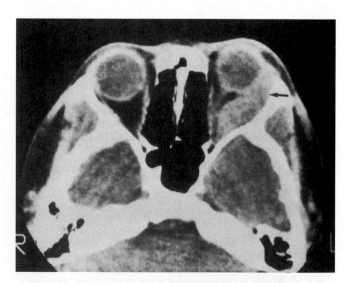

**FIGURE 9-104**   Pseudotumor. Axial CT scan showing an extraconal infiltrative lesion (*arrow*) displacing the lateral rectus muscle medially. Histologic study showed a pseudorheumatoid nodule. (From Mafee MF et al. Orbital space-occupying lesions: role of CT and MRI: an analysis of 145 cases. Radiol Clin North Am 1987;25:529–559.)

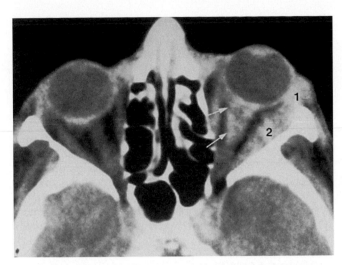

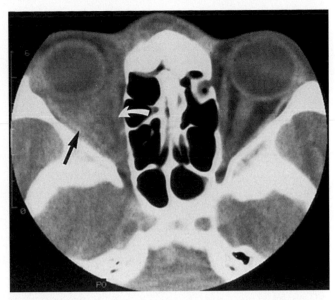

**FIGURE 9-105**   Lymphoma. Postcontrast axial CT scan shows an infiltrative process involving the left lacrimal gland (*1*), lateral orbital compartment (*2*), and perioptic nerve region (*arrows*).

**FIGURE 9-106**   Lymphomatoid granulomatosis. Contrast-enhanced axial CT scan shows diffuse infiltration of the intraconal space of the right orbit (*arrows*) with putty-like molding of the process around the posterior globe. CT features of this T-cell lymphoma precursor are virtually identical to those of true lymphoma, pseudotumor, lupoid infiltration, and metastatic carcinoma associated with marked proliferation of dense connective tissue surrounding malignant cells, such as in scirrhous carcinoma (breast, stomach).

that reside in the subepithelial area of the nasal cavity. A smaller population of lymphocytes is scattered among the submucosal glands and within the deep vascular stroma; extranodal B-cell non-Hodgkin's lymphoma derives from these cells.[115] In most cases, multiple sinuses are affected. Involvement of one or more paranasal sinuses is more typical of B-cell lymphoma, whereas involvement of the nasal cavity is more typical of T-cell lymphoma.[102] Less commonly, the lymphomas (generally those of a T-cell phenotype) invade adjacent sites such as the orbit, and patients present with diplopia, blurred vision, and paralysis of the cranial nerves.[102]

### Diagnostic Imaging

Ultrasound, CT, and MR imaging can be used to evaluate orbital lymphomas. CT and MR imaging have made it possible to make a strong presumptive diagnosis of orbital lymphoma, especially when the CT and MR imaging

features are examined in conjunction with the clinical signs and symptoms.[131] The CT and MR imaging findings are usually nonspecific, and based solely on imaging, it may be impossible to differentiate the lymphomas from orbital pseudotumors (Figs. 9-105 to 9-107), lacrimal gland tumors (Fig. 9-107), optic nerve tumors, Graves' orbitopathy, primary orbital tumors, or orbital cellulitis.[127–131] Orbital lymphomas are homogeneous masses of relatively high density and sharp margins, which are more often seen in the anterior portion of the orbit, the retrobulbar area (Fig. 9-108), or in the superior orbital compartment. CT and MR

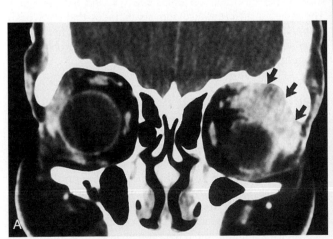

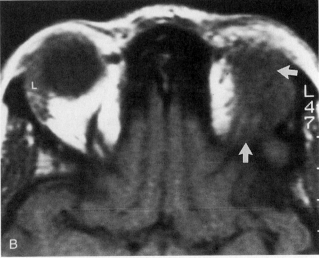

**FIGURE 9-107**   Orbital pseudotumor. **A,** Enhanced coronal CT scan. **B,** Axial T1-weighted axial MR scan showing an irregular mass involving the left lacrimal gland and adjacent orbital tissues (*arrows*).

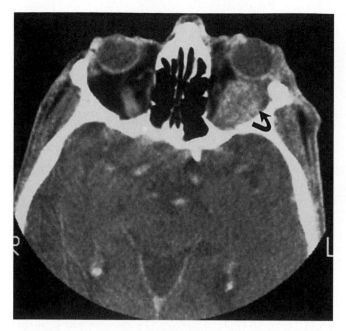

**FIGURE 9-108** Lymphoma. Postcontrast axial CT scan shows a soft-tissue mass (*arrow*) in the left retrobulbar region.

imaging may reveal a putty-like molding of the tumor to preexisting structures without eroding the bone or enlarging the orbit.[127, 128] Mild to moderate enhancement is usually present (Figs. 9-106 to 9-108).[127, 131]

All orbital lymphoid tumors tend to mold themselves around the orbital structures without producing bony erosion (Figs. 9-108 and 9-109). Specifically, a bulky lesion in the region of the lacrimal fossa that does not produce bony erosion is most likely to be either inflammatory or lymphoid in character (Figs. 9-109 and 9-110).[17, 131] However, the aggressive malignant lymphomas can produce frank destruction of bone.[131] Lacrimal gland lymphoma displaces the globe medially and forward and appears as a moderately enhancing mass that diffusely involves the gland (Figs. 9-110 and 9-111).[127] Deformity of the globe's shape is rare.

MR imaging has proven to be as sensitive as CT for the diagnosis of orbital lymphoma and pseudotumors. Both pseudotumors and lymphoma may have intermediate or low signal intensity on T1-weighted and proton density images and appear isointense to fat on T2-weighted images (Figs. 9-111 and 9-112).[127]

## Lymphoplasmacytic Tumor (Plasma Cell Tumor)

Tumors composed purely of plasma cells (plasmacytomas) and those composed of B lymphocytes and plasma cells (lymphoplasmacytoid tumors) are closely related to the various lymphomas.[3, 107] The plasma cell is actually a B lymphocyte that has become modified to produce large quantities of immunoglobulin.[107] These so-called plasmacytoid lymphomas may secrete IgM paraprotein in sufficient quantities to cause a monoclonal peak in the serum; this is

classically seen in Waldenstrom's macroglobulinemia.[3] One of the important tumors composed of plasma cells is multiple myeloma (Fig. 9-113). There are also solitary forms of extramedullary plasmacytomas, which are not associated with systemic multiple myeloma.[107] These plasma cell tumors, particularly as they affect the orbit and ocular structures, display the same spectrum of clinical involvement seen in the lymphoproliferative disorders (Fig. 9-113).[3] Both isolated plasmacytoma and Waldenstrom's macroglobulinemia can produce a mass that can be visualized by both CT and MR imaging. The mass may be lobulated, densely enhancing, and well defined, and can be present with or without bone erosion (Fig. 9-114).[3] In systemic myelomatosis, a permeative or moth-eaten pattern of bone destruction or gross destruction may be present.[71]

## ORBITAL LEUKEMIA

Leukemia is one of the most common childhood cancers. It is estimated that of the approximately 7100 cases of childhood cancer in the United States each year, 35% are leukemia.[107, 126] Leukemic disorders in children fall mainly into the lymphoid and myeloid groups. About 75% of the cases are acute lymphoblastic leukemia, 20% are acute myelogenous leukemia (AML), and 5% are chronic myelogenous leukemia.[107] Chronic lymphocytic leukemia is a disease of adulthood and almost never affects children.[107] The eye and adnexa are not infrequently involved (Fig. 9-115). Orbital involvement with leukemia is the result of direct infiltration of the orbital bone or soft tissue by leukemic cells (Fig. 9-116). In patients with AML, such infiltration most often occurs in the form of a granulocytic sarcoma (Fig. 9-117). A granulocytic sarcoma is commonly called a *chloroma* because the myeloperoxidase within the tumor imparts a green hue to it, as seen on gross examination.[107] This may be the first manifestation of AML in many patients. The lesion typically involves the orbital subperiosteal space, usually affecting the lateral wall of the orbit, with extensions to the temporal fossa. Medial orbital wall disease also occurs with involvement of ethmoid air cells, the cribriform plate, and the anterior cranial fossa. There may be dural or leptomeningeal infiltration, demonstrating enhancement on enhanced CT and MR imaging. The imaging differential diagnosis includes rhabdomyosarcoma, LCH, subperiosteal abscess, subperiosteal hematoma, lymphoma, pseudotumor, and metastasis (neuroblastoma, Ewing's sarcoma, and Wilms' tumor).

## ORBITAL VASCULAR CONDITIONS

Vascular lesions of the orbit represent an important group of orbital pathologies, particularly in infants and children. They also are the most controversial group of lesions because of confusion regarding their nature, and a debate continues as to the classification of the various vascular malformations that may involve the orbit.[132] In general, orbital vascular lesions include capillary hemangioma, cavernous hemangioma (cavernoma, a venous malformation), varices (venous malformation), lymphangioma, lymph-

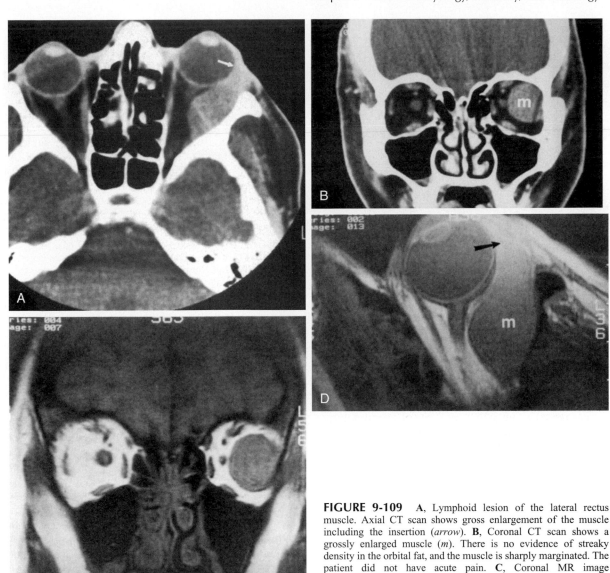

**FIGURE 9-109** **A,** Lymphoid lesion of the lateral rectus muscle. Axial CT scan shows gross enlargement of the muscle including the insertion (*arrow*). **B,** Coronal CT scan shows a grossly enlarged muscle (*m*). There is no evidence of streaky density in the orbital fat, and the muscle is sharply marginated. The patient did not have acute pain. **C,** Coronal MR image demonstrating the enlarged muscle with its sharp margin and the normal orbital fat. **D,** Surface coil MR image showing the enlarged muscle (*M*) and the enlarged insertion (*arrow*). (From Curtin HD. Pseudotumor. Radiol Clin North Am 1987;25:583.)

angiovenous (venolymphatic) malformation, arteriovenous malformation, "sclerosing hemangioma," hemangiopericytoma, and hemangioendotheliomas (angiosarcomas).

## Capillary Hemangioma (Benign Hemangioendothelioma)

Capillary hemangiomas are tumors that occur primarily in infants during the first year of life. The tumor often increases in size for 6 to 10 months and then gradually involutes.[8, 17, 132, 133] It occurs most commonly in the superior nasal quadrant. Microscopically, the tumor is composed of endothelial and capillary vessel proliferations with benign endothelial cells surrounding small, capillary-sized vascular spaces.[8, 17, 132] Capillary hemangiomas in and

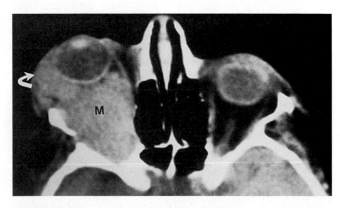

**FIGURE 9-110** Lymphoma. Postcontrast axial CT scan shows a large mass (*M*) involving the right lacrimal gland (*arrow*) and retrobulbar region.

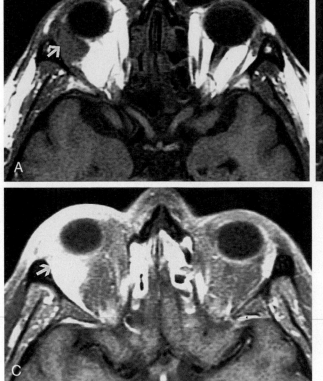

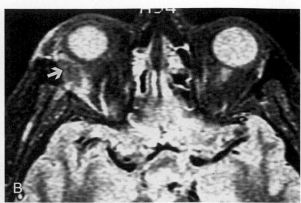

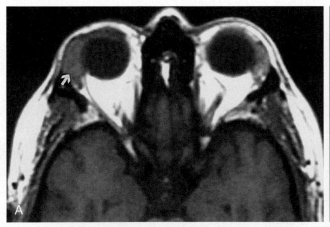

**FIGURE 9-111** Axial T1-weighted MR (**A**), axial T2-weighted MR (**B**), and postcontrast axial, fat-suppressed, T1-weighted MR scans (**C**). There is a large mass (*arrow*) in the region of the right lacrimal gland, which in the T2-weighted MR image becomes bright at the periphery but remains dark in its central portion. The mass undergoes prominent enhancement. The appearance of the lesion may mimic that of a pseudotumor. Note also the enhancement of the right eyelid. Note that the apparently prominent enhancement of the neoplasm is partly caused by the technique of fat suppression. This technique, besides causing increased dynamic range of the gray scale, results in increased signal of the normal lacrimal gland as well as the extraocular muscles. (From Valvassori GE et al. Imaging of orbital lymphoproliferative disorders. Radiol Clin North Am 1999;37:135–150.)

around the orbit may have an arterial supply from either the external carotid or internal carotid arteries, and these tumors are capable of bleeding profusely.[8, 132, 133] These hemangiomas may extend intracranially through the superior orbital fissure (Fig. 9-118), optic canal, and orbital roof. On CT these lesions are seen as fairly well-marginated (Fig. 9-118) to poorly marginated, irregular, enhancing lesions. Most are extraconal, although some of them may be seen in the intraconal space (Fig. 9-119). On dynamic CT, capillary hemangiomas characteristically show intense homogeneous enhancement (Fig. 9-120). On MR imaging, capillary hemangiomas appear as hypointense or slightly hyperintense to brain on T1-weighted images and hyperintense to brain on proton density and T2-weighted images. They show intense enhancement following the intravenous injection of Gd-DTPA contrast material. On MR angiography (MRA) the vascularity of these lesions may not be appreciated. Therefore, at present, one should not rely only on MRA for the diagnosis of these capillary hemangiomas.

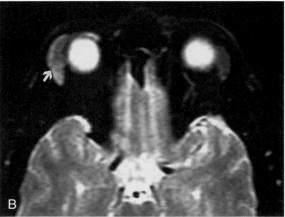

**FIGURE 9-112** Pseudotumor. Axial T1-weighted MR (**A**) and axial T2-weighted MR (**B**) images. The right lacrimal gland is enlarged (*arrows*). The peripheral portion of the gland becomes brighter in the T2-weighted MR images, mimicking a lymphoma. (From Valvassori GE et al. Imaging of orbital lymphoproliferative disorders. Radiol Clin North Am 1999;37:135–150.)

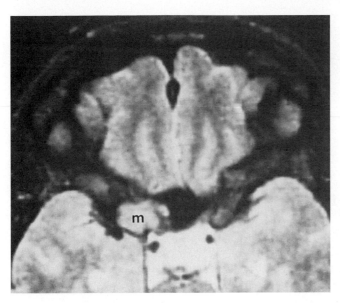

**FIGURE 9-113**    Multiple myeloma. Axial T2-weighted MR scan shows a mass (*m*) involving the right lesser wing and optic canal.

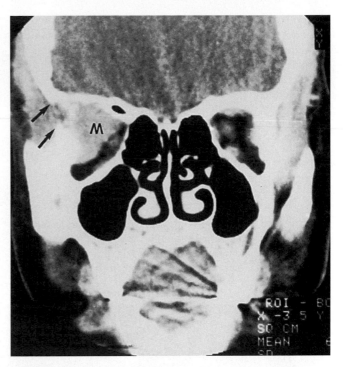

**FIGURE 9-114**    Orbital myeloma. Postcontrast coronal CT scan shows bone destruction of the superolateral aspect of the right orbit (*arrows*), with a large orbital mass (*M*). This patient initially showed symptoms of proptosis. Biopsy of this mass revealed features compatible with lymphoplasmacytic tumor.

## Cavernous Hemangioma

Cavernous hemangioma of the orbit, the most common orbital vascular tumor in adults, has distinctive clinical and histopathologic features.[7, 17, 132] It tends to occur in the second to fourth decades of life. These tumors show a slowly progressive enlargement distinct from that of capillary hemangiomas, which gradually diminish in size. In contrast to capillary hemangiomas, a prominent arterial supply is usually absent.[8] Cavernous hemangiomas possess a distinct fibrous pseudocapsule and therefore, on CT and MR imaging, appear as well-defined masses (Figs. 9-121 and 9-122). This observation, in addition to the fact that they are usually independent of the general circulation, enables excision of the entire lesion without fragmentation.[8] These hemangiomas may be located anywhere in the orbit but frequently (83%) occur within the retrobulbar muscle cone (Figs. 9-121 to 9-123). On CT, cavernous hemangiomas appear as well-defined, smoothly marginated, homogeneous, rounded, ovoid, or lobulated soft-tissue masses of increased density and variable contrast enhancement (Fig. 9-121). Unless they are ruptured or surgically violated, cavernous hemangiomas always respect the contour of the globe (Fig. 9-124). The MR imaging characteristics of hemangiomas are shown in Figure 9-122. Histologically, cavernous hemangiomas are composed of large, dilated vascular channels (sinusoid-like spaces) lined by thin, attenuated endothelial cells.[8, 17, 132] At times, intraconal cavernous hemangiomas may be difficult to differentiate

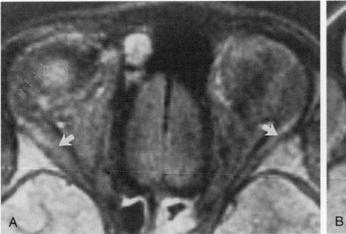

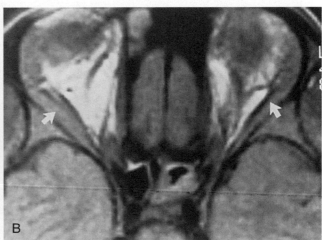

**FIGURE 9-115**    **A**, Axial PW scan. **B**, Axial T2-weighted MR imaging scan. Leukemic infiltration. Scans show bilateral subperiosteal leukemic infiltration (*arrows*).

from other intraconal lesions such as meningiomas, hemangiopericytomas, and schwannomas.[8, 17, 132] Uncommonly, an intramuscular hemangioma may occur (Fig. 9-125). Orbital bone modeling is not uncommon in cavernous hemangiomas, and at times, calcification may be seen in these lesions. *Sclerosing hemangioma* is another less well defined term used to describe hemangiomas that show prominent sclerosis. These lesions often show foci of calcification (Fig. 9-126).

## Lymphangioma

Although the origin of lymphangioma may remain controversial, the lesion is an unencapsulated mass consisting mostly of bloodless vascular and lymph channels.[73] Connective tissue between the channels may contain foci of lymphoid cells that proliferate in viral infections, resulting in the clinical finding of worsening proptosis when the child has an upper respiratory tract infection.[73] Orbital lymphangiomas occur in children and young adults. In contrast to the rapid, self-limited growth of infantile capillary hemangiomas, lymphangiomas gradually and progressively enlarge during the first two decades of life.[8, 132] Cavernous lymphangiomas are composed of delicate endothelium-lined, lymph-filled sinuses (filled with clear fluid or chocolate-colored, unclotted fluid) that invade the surrounding connective tissue stroma.[8, 73, 132] The interstitial tissue often shows lymphoid follicles and lymphocytic infiltration.[8] Spontaneous (or after minor trauma) hemorrhage within the lesion is common, resulting in a chocolate cyst.[8, 17] Lymphangiomas may have distinct borders but are typically diffuse and not well encapsulated (Figs. 9-127 and 9-128), with portions of the lesion infiltrating normal tissues of the lid and orbit.[8, 17] They are usually multilobular (Fig. 9-128), and because complete surgical excision is seldom

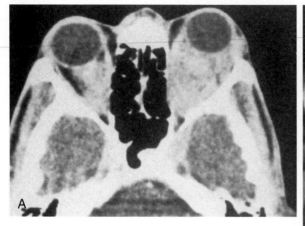

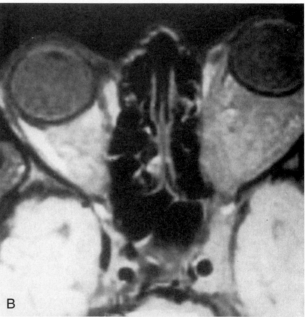

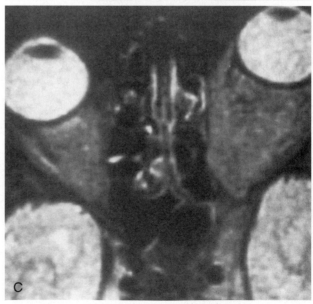

**FIGURE 9-116**  Leukemia. Axial CT scan (**A**) showing a bilateral intraconal infiltrative process. Axial MR (2000/20) scan (**B**) showing hypointensity of the lesion in relation to the fat. MR (2000/80) T2-weighted scan (**C**) showing hyperintensity of the lesion in relation to the fat. The lesion is hypointense to brain in both early and late echoes (**C**). (From Mafee MF et al. Orbital space-occupying lesions: role of CT and MRI: an analysis of 145 cases. Radiol Clin North Am 1987;25:529.)

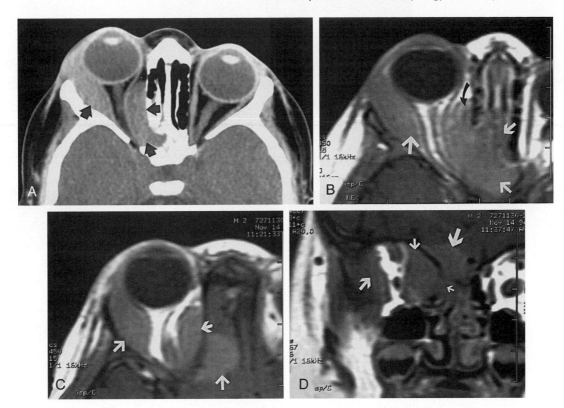

**FIGURE 9-117**   Granulocytic sarcoma (leukemia). Axial CT (**A**), postcontrast axial T1-weighted (**B** and **C**), and postcontrast coronal T1-weighted (**D**) MR scans demonstrate an extraconal infiltration involving both the medial and lateral aspects of the orbit (*arrows*). The lesion erodes into the ethmoid air cells and erodes the cribriform plate, with extension into the anterior cranial fossa. (From Valvassori GE et al. Imaging of orbital lymphoproliferative disorders. Radiol Clin North Am 1999;37:135–150.)

accomplished, recurrence is common.[8, 132] They are more common in the extraconal space.[8]

On CT these lymphangiomas appear as poorly circumscribed, often heterogeneous masses of increased density in

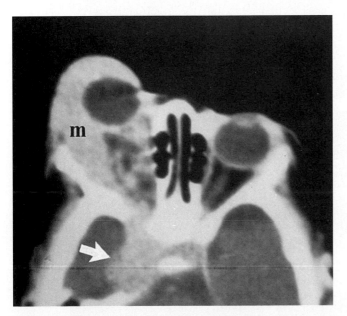

**FIGURE 9-118**   Capillary hemangioma. Postcontrast axial CT scan shows an enhancing mass (*m*) with involvement of the eyelid and extension into the right cavernous sinus (*arrow*).

the extraconal or intraconal space (Fig. 9-127). Bony remodeling may be present, calcification is rare, and minimal to marked contrast enhancement may be present (Fig. 9-127). On MR imaging, lymphangiomas are relatively hypointense or hyperintense to brain on T1-weighted images and usually very hyperintense on T2-weighted images (Figs. 9-128 and 9-129). Fluid-fluid levels related to hemorrhages of various ages are characteristic of lymphangioma. Their MR imaging characteristics should help differentiate them from pseudotumors and hemangiomas (Fig. 9-129).[8]

## Orbital Varix

Primary orbital varices are congenital venous malformations characterized by proliferation of venous elements and massive dilation of one or more orbital veins, presumably associated with congenital weakness in the venous wall.[8, 17, 73, 134] A varix may include a single smooth-contoured, dilated vein, a single vessel with segmental dilatation, or a tangled mass of venous channels.[73] Varices within the orbit may appear to have both cystic (chocolate) and solid components.[73] Orbital varices are the most common cause of spontaneous orbital hemorrhage.[135] Clinically, proptosis or globe displacement increases during a Valsalva maneuver, reflecting the varix's connection to the venous system.[73] The CT appearance of orbital varix may be normal in axial sections (Fig. 9-130A), but because of increased venous pressure, it is quite abnormal in coronal

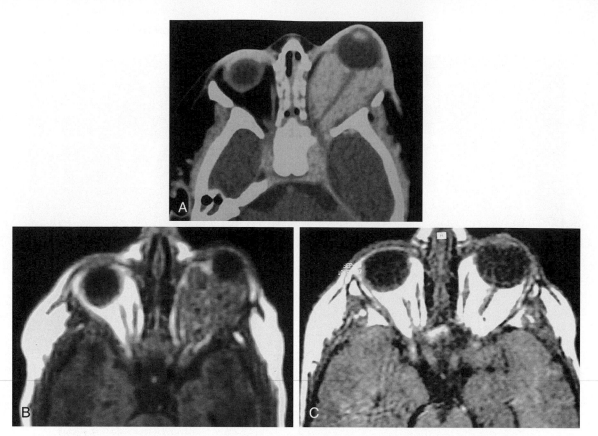

**FIGURE 9-119** A baby boy with a left orbital capillary hemangioma that presented shortly after birth. **A,** Axial contrast-enhanced CT scan shows a mass filling and expanding the left orbit. The hemangioma appears to extend through the superior orbital fissure into the left cavernous sinus. The mass encircles and stretches the optic nerve sheath complex. Biopsy was performed but was inconclusive, and there was some discussion about further surgery. MR findings convinced the clinicians that this was a capillary hemangioma and the patient was treated with steroids instead. **B,** Axial T1-weighted MR image reveals a large, heterogeneous, finely lobulated mass expanding the left bony orbit. The focal regions of hypointensity are consistent with flow voids attributable to vessels. **C,** Axial T1-weighted MR scan shows that the capillary hemangioma involuted completely 2 years after the initial presentation. (From Bilanuik LT. Orbital vascular lesions: role of imaging. Radiol Clin North Am 1999;37:169–183.)

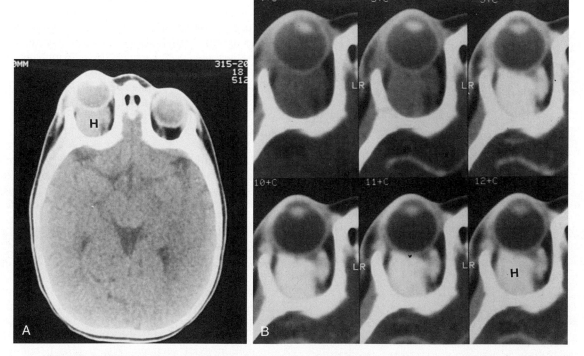

**FIGURE 9-120** Capillary hemangioma. **A,** Enhanced axial CT scan showing a large retrobulbar mass compatible with a capillary hemangioma (*H*). **B,** Dynamic axial CT scanning reveals rapid wash-in of contrast in hemangioma (*H*). (From Mafee MF et al. Rhabdomyosarcoma of the orbit: evaluation with MR imaging and CT. Radiol Clin North Am 1998;36:1215–1227.)

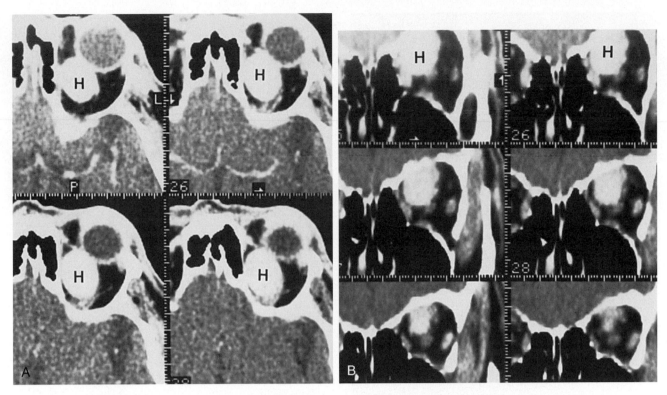

**FIGURE 9-121**   Cavernous hemangioma. **A,** Serial axial CT scan. **B,** Reformatted coronal CT scans. **A** and **B** show a well-defined intraconal markedly enhancing hemangioma (*H*).

sections, particularly those obtained in the prone position (Figs. 9-130B and 9-131). Because the varix may be completely collapsed or barely visible when the patient is lying quietly supine, any time an orbital varix is suspected, it is recommended that additional CT sections be obtained during a Valsalva maneuver. In a patient suspected of having an orbital varix, MR imaging also should be performed with the patient in the prone position. Some varices may have such a small communication with the systemic venous system that they are undistensible. Because they have

stagnant blood flow, they manifest themselves by thrombosis and hemorrhage.[132] Venous anomalies of the orbit including varices may be associated with contiguous or noncontiguous intracranial venous anomalies.[132] Orbital varices may also be secondary to intracranial vascular malformations, particularly arteriovenous shunts.[172] MR imaging of orbital varices usually shows a varix to be hyperintense on T1-weighted, proton density, and T2-weighted images (Fig. 9-132). At times, an orbital varix may have the same MR imaging characteristics as a cavernous

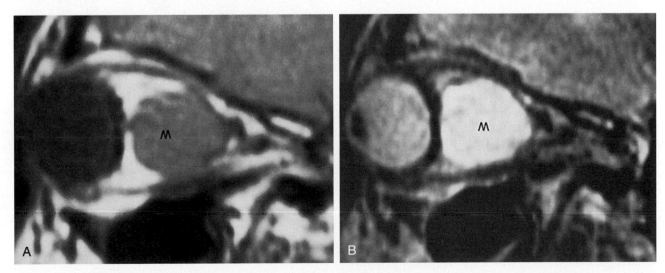

**FIGURE 9-122**   Cavernous hemangioma. **A,** Satittal PW MR scan. **B,** Sagittal T2-weighted MR scan. Scans show an intraconal mass (*M*), which was presumed to be a cavernous hemangioma.

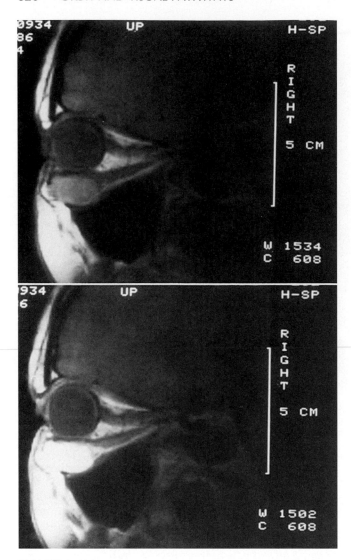

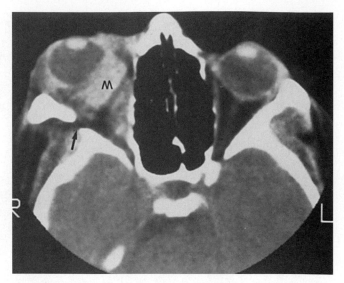

**FIGURE 9-124** Cavernous hemangioma. Postcontrast axial CT scan shows an inhomogeneous enhancing mass (*M*) indenting the nasal aspect of the right globe. Note surgical defect (*arrow*).

**FIGURE 9-123** Orbital hemangioma. Sagittal MR images obtained without (*top*) and with (*bottom*) intravenous Gd-DTPA show a hemangioma in the anterior floor of the orbit. (Courtesy of Dr. August F. Markl.)

hemangioma or other orbital masses, being hypointense on T1-weighted, hyperintense on T2-weighted, and enhanced on postcontrast T1-weighted MR images. An orbital varix may also be seen as several round or tubular structures with associated calcifications (phleboliths) (Fig. 9-133).[8]

## Carotid Cavernous Fistulas and Arteriovenous Malformations

Carotid cavernous fistulas produce proptosis, chemosis, venous engorgement, pulsating exophthalmos, and an auscultable bruit. Ischemic ocular necrosis resulting from a carotid-cavernous fistula has also been reported.[17, 136] A carotid cavernous fistula may result from trauma or surgery, or it may occur spontaneously. Spontaneous carotid-cavernous fistulas have been reported in patients with osteogenesis imperfecta, Ehlers-Danlos syndrome, and pseudoxanthoma elasticum. In these cases, the fistula probably

resulted from weakness of the vessel walls related to the connective tissue disease.[136] CT and MR imaging demonstrate proptosis, with engorgement of the superior ophthalmic vein and frequent enlargement of the ipsilateral extraocular muscles (Fig. 9-134). There may be CT or MR imaging evidence of venous thrombosis in the lumen of the superior ophthalmic vein or cavernous sinus. Arteriovenous shunts within the orbit itself are rare.[132] At times, anomalous intracranial venous malformations, as well as dural vascular malformations and fistulas, may mimic the imaging appearance of carotid cavernous fistulas (Fig. 9-135).[136] Angiographic demonstration of the exact location of the carotid-cavernous fistula is essential to plan definitive therapy.

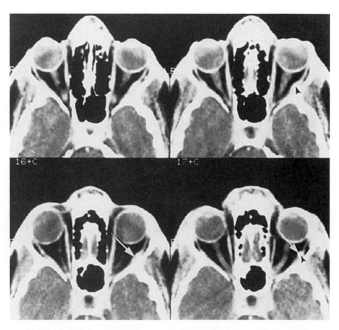

**FIGURE 9-125** Hemangioma. Serial axial contrast-enhanced CT scans show an intramuscular hemangioma (*arrows*).

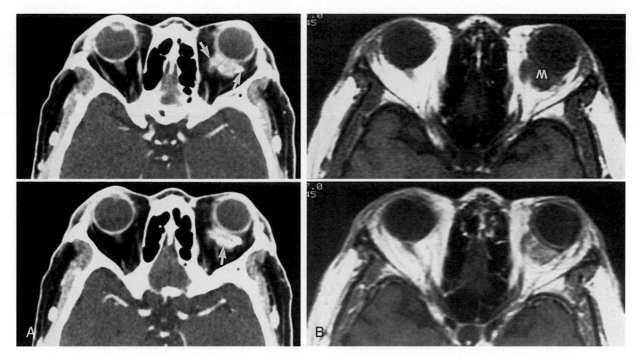

**FIGURE 9-126**    Sclerosing hemangioma. **A,** Axial-enhanced CT scans show an enhancing intraconal mass. Note several areas of calcifications. At histologic examination, there were foci of amyloidosis present in addition to calcifications. **B,** Axial T1-weighted (*top*) and enhanced T1-weighted (*bottom*) MR images show an intraconal mass (*M*) with moderate enhancement. (From Valvassori GE et al. Imaging of orbital lymphoproliferative disorders. Radiol Clin North Am 1999;37:135–150.)

## Hemangiopericytoma

Hemangiopericytomas are rare, slow-growing vascular neoplasms that arise from unique cells called *pericytes of Zimmermann*, which normally envelop capillaries and postcapillary venules of practically all types of tissues.[8, 137–139] Histologically, these tumors are composed of scattered, capillary-like spaces surrounded by proliferating pericytes.[8] Hemangiopericytomas may be divided into lobules by fibrovascular septa.[8, 137] About 50% of the cases are malignant, and distant metastases, although uncommon, occur via the vascular and lymphatic routes.[8, 140] Most such metastases go to the lungs.[8, 137, 139] If not excised completely, these lesions tend to recur, and wide surgical excision is the treatment of choice.

On CT, the margins of an orbital hemangiopericytoma, in contrast to those of a cavernous hemangioma, may be slightly less distinct owing to its tendency to invade the adjacent tissues (Fig. 9-136).[8, 17] Erosion of the underlying bone may be present (Fig. 9-137), and marked contrast enhancement favors a diagnosis of hemangiopericytoma. MR imaging may not differentiate these tumors from cavernous hemangiomas, neurogenic tumors, meningiomas, and other lesions (Fig. 9-138), but angiography may

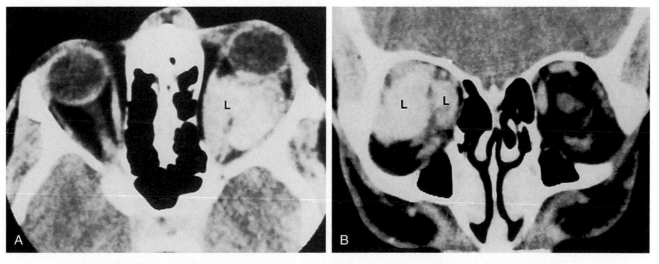

**FIGURE 9-127**    Lymphangioma. **A,** Contrast-enhanced axial CT scan. **B,** Coronal CT scan. **A** and **B** show a large lobulated lymphangioma (*L*).

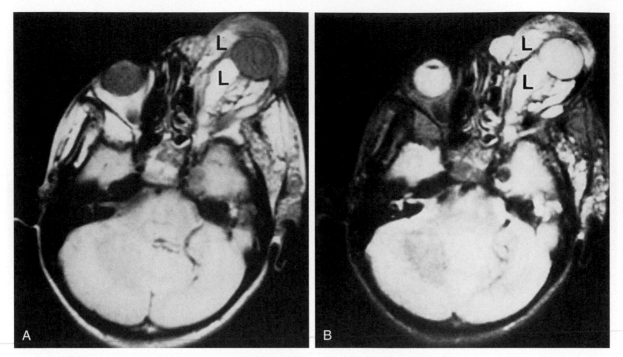

**FIGURE 9-128**   Lymphangioma. **A**, Axial PW MR scan. **B**, Axial T2-weighted MR scan. **A** and **B** show a large lymphangioma (*L*).

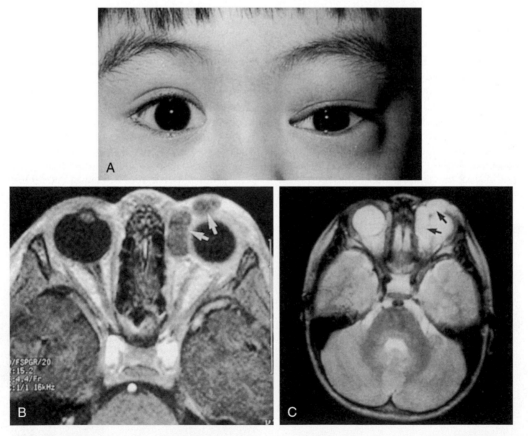

**FIGURE 9-129**   **A**, Clinical photograph of an 8-year-old boy who presented with acute upper-lid fullness on the left and inferior displacement of the globe caused by hemorrhage within a lymphangioma. **B**, Axial-enhanced T1-weighted MR image shows a lobular mass (*arrows*) in the anteromedial left orbit. The signal intensity of the lesion is hyperintense to vitreous and isointense to brain. There is no contrast enhancement. **C**, Axial T2-weighted MR image shows that the lesion (*arrows*) is homogeneously hyperintense to brain and isointense to vitreous. (From Kaufman LM et al. Diagnostic imaging of cystic lesions in the child's orbit. Radiol Clin North Am 1998;36:1149–1163.)

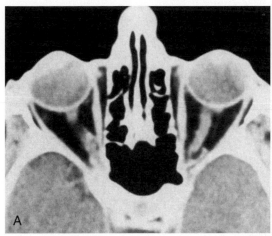
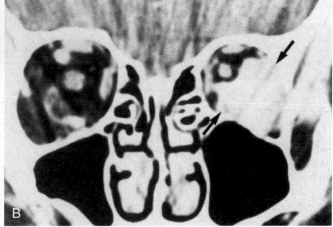

**FIGURE 9-130**   **A,** Orbital varix. Axial CT scan shows no obvious lesion. **B,** Coronal CT scan shows a large mass (*arrows*). (From Mafee MF et al. Orbital space-occupying lesions: role of CT and MRI: an analysis of 145 cases. Radiol Clin North Am 1987;25:529.)

differentiate the tumors from cavernous hemangiomas, meningiomas, and schwannomas.[8] Hemangiopericytomas usually have an early florid blush (Fig. 9-136C), and cavernous hemangiomas show a late minor pooling of contrast or often appear as avascular masses.[8, 134, 141]

Meningiomas may show multiple tumor vessels and a late blush, and schwannomas may show no tumor blush.[8, 17, 140, 141] Hemangiopericytomas may be difficult to differentiate from other rare vasculogenic tumors such as angioleiomyomas, malignant hemangioendotheliomas (angiosarcomas), and fibrous histiocytomas.[8] Follow-up CT or MR imaging is extremely important to diagnose tumor recurrences (Fig. 9-137B).

## NEURAL LESIONS

### Orbital Schwannoma

The orbit is host to many peripheral nerves. Approximately 4% of all orbital neoplasms are peripheral nerve tumors and consist primarily of neurofibromas and neu-

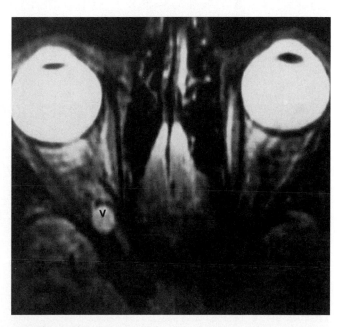

**FIGURE 9-132**   Orbital varix. Axial T2-weighted MR scan shows a round, hyperintense mass compatible with surgically proved orbital varix (*V*).

**FIGURE 9-131**   Orbital varix. Coronal contrast-enhanced CT scan shows several round, enhancing masses compatible with orbital varix (*V*).

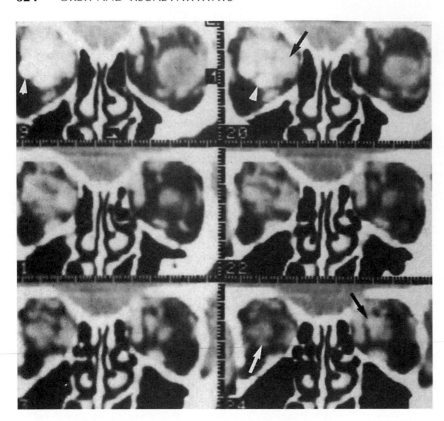

**FIGURE 9-133** Orbital varix. Serial reformatted coronal sections showing multiple dilated veins in both eyes (*arrows*). Notice the calcifications (*arrowheads*). (From Mafee MF et al. Orbital space-occupying lesions: role of CT and MRI: an analysis of 145 cases. Radiol Clin North Am 1987;25:529.)

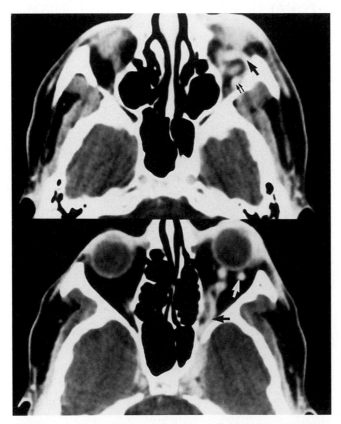

**FIGURE 9-134** Carotid cavernous fistula. Enhanced axial CT scan shows enlarged intraorbital veins (*arrows*) and an enlarged left cavernous sinus.

rilemmomas or schwannomas.[142] Of these, 2% of the lesions are plexiform neurofibromatosis, 1% are isolated neurofibromas, and 1% are schwannomas.[142] Malignant peripheral nerve tumors (malignant schwannoma, neurofibrosarcoma) are extremely rare in the orbit.[142]

## Neurofibroma

Neurofibromas may occur in one of four patterns: (1) plexiform, (2) diffuse, (3) localized or circumscribed, and (4) postamputation neuromas.[142] When most of the fascicles in a segment of peripheral nerve are involved, cylindrical enlargement of the entire nerve segment is observed. This clinical and gross pathologic configuration is referred to as *plexiform neurofibroma*.[7, 17, 142] Plexiform neurofibromas present in infancy or childhood and most commonly involve the eyelids. The tumor consists of cords and nodules giving rise to a "bag of worms" on palpation, and a plexiform neurofibroma involving the eyelid is considered to be virtually pathognomonic for neurofibromatosis (Von Recklinghausen's disease).[142] Diffuse neurofibromas have an appearance similar to that of plexiform neurofibromatosis, with infiltration of the orbital fat and EOMs, but these lesions are less likely to be associated with Von Recklinghausen's disease.[142] Circumscribed or localized neurofibromas often present as slow-growing tumors that exert a mass effect, with displacement of the globe. The tumor may occur along any sensory nerve but is more common in the superior quadrants. When arising from the lacrimal nerve, it may have the clinical appearance of a lacrimal gland tumor.

Histologically, plexiform neurofibromas are unencapsulated and have an organoid appearance, with proliferating units surrounded by perineurium enclosing axons, Schwann cells, and endoneurial fibroblasts. There is a marked increase in vascularity, which leads to profuse bleeding at the time of surgery.

This increased vascularity is responsible for marked contrast enhancement on CT and MR imaging. The CT and MR imaging appearance of plexiform neurofibromatosis in infants and children may be identical to that of a capillary hemangioma. Solitary neurofibromas often demonstrate a pseudocapsule, but a true perineurium is not seen. They are composed of wavy bundles of peripheral nerve sheath cells with comma-shaped nuclei and hyaluronic acid and collagen

in the stroma.[142] The CT and MR imaging characteristics of neurofibroma are shown in Figures 9-138 to 9-140.

Schwannomas are benign, slow-growing nerve sheath tumors that account for 1% of all orbital tumors.[7,106, 107, 142] They may arise anywhere within the orbit, although they are most common in the intraconal space.[7] Their malignant counterpart, the malignant schwannoma (malignant neurolemma, neurogenic sarcoma, and fibrosarcoma of the nerve sheath), is exceedingly rare in the orbit.[7, 142] In general, neurofibromas and schwannomas are two benign tumors originating from Schwann cells that occur in the orbit as isolated lesions or in association with neurofibromatosis. The optic nerve has no Schwann cells; therefore, orbital schwannomas must arise from peripheral nerve fibers of

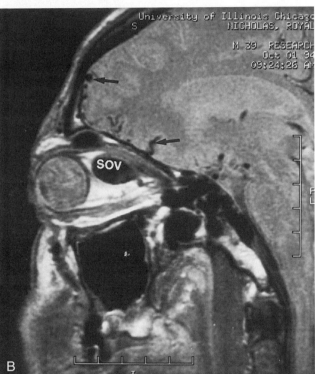

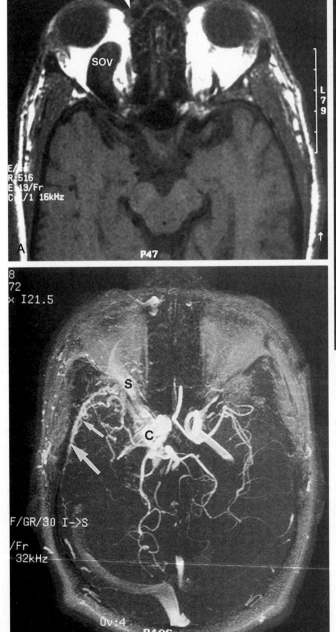

**FIGURE 9-135** Intracranial vascular malformation mimicking carotid cavernous fistula. **A,** Axial T1-weighted MR image shows an enlarged superior ophthalmic vein (*SOV*) and engorged veins over the nose (*arrows*). **B,** Sagittal PW MR image shows an engorged superior ophthalmic vein (*SOV*) and engorged intracranial vessels (*arrows*). **C,** Three-dimensional time of flight MR angiogram shows abnormal tortuous dural vessels (*arrows*), large superior ophthalmic vein (*S*), and enlargement of the right cavernous sinus (*C*).

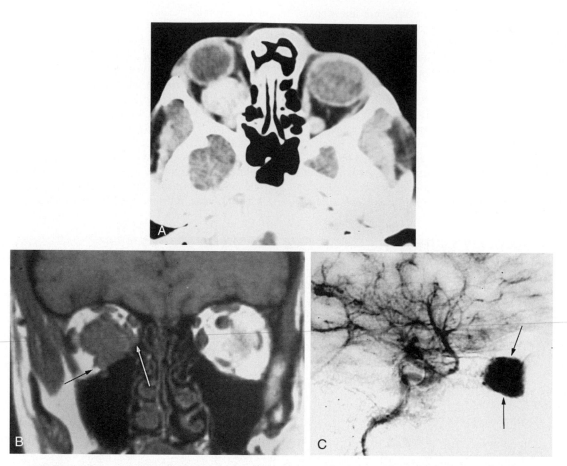

**FIGURE 9-136** Hemangiopericytoma in a woman. **A,** Axial contrast-enhanced CT scan shows a large, enhancing mass in the right orbit that scallops the medial wall of the orbit and appears to have an irregular interface with the posterior right globe. **B,** Coronal T1-weighted MR image shows that the mass is irregular in outline, invades the inferior rectus muscle (*black arrow*), and extends around the left medial rectus muscle to infiltrate the extraconic fat (*white arrow*). **C,** Sagittal subtraction image of a conventional angiogram reveals marked enhancement of the hemangiopericytoma (*arrows*). This is an important differentiating point from a cavernous hemangioma, which usually shows no contrast pickup or a minimal amount in the venous phase. (Courtesy of Mahmood Mafee, MD, University of Illinois at Chicago, Chicago, Illinois. From Bilaniuk LT. Orbital Vascular Lesions: Role of Imaging. Radiol Clin North Am 1999 Jan;37(1):181.)

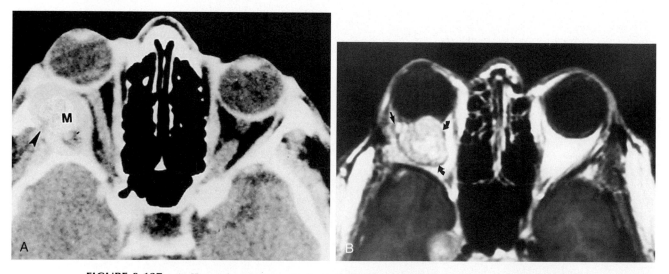

**FIGURE 9-137** **A,** Hemangiopericytoma. Contrast-enhanced axial CT scan shows an enhancing mass (*M*) compatible with hemangiopericytoma. Note the erosion of the lateral orbital wall (*arrowhead*). **B,** Recurrent hemangiopericytoma. Enhanced axial T1-weighted MR scan shows a heterogeneously enhancing mass (*arrows*) compatible with recurrent hemangiopericytoma. (Courtesy of Dr. Michael Rothman.)

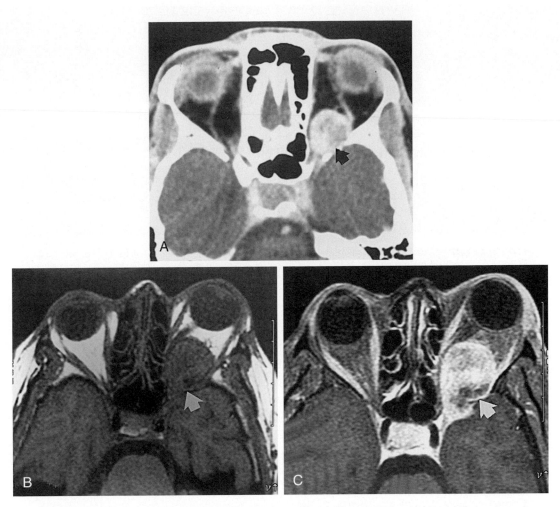

**FIGURE 9-138**   **A**, Postcontrast axial CT scan demonstrating a well-enhanced intraconal neurofibroma (*arrow*) of the posterior orbit. **B**, Axial T1-weighted MR scan of a posterior neurofibroma (*arrow*) as in **A**. Tumor is isointense to brain and hypointense to orbital fat. **C**, Axial fat-suppressed T1-weighted MR image of the tumor seen in **A** and **B** demonstrating the marked contrast enhancement of a posterior neurofibroma (*arrow*). (Courtesy of Mahmood Mafee, MD, University of Illinois at Chicago, Chicago, Illinois. From Carroll GS, Barrett GH, Fleming JC, et al. Peripheral Nerve Tumors of the Orbit. Radiol Clin North Am 1999 Jan;37(1):200.)

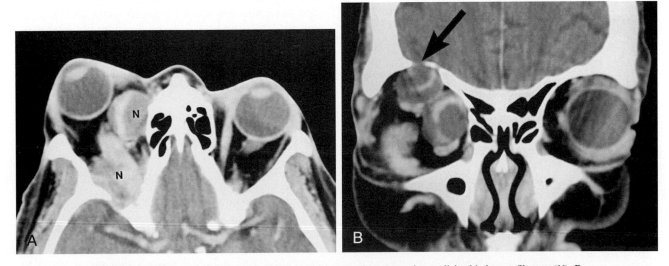

**FIGURE 9-139**   **A**, Axial postcontrast CT scan demonstrating an anterior medial orbital neurofibroma (*N*). **B**, Coronal CT scan of the tumor in **A** showing its multinodular configuration not readily seen in a single axial view. Note the compression atrophy of the orbital roof (*arrow*). (From Carroll GS, Barrett GH, Fleming JC, et al. Peripheral Nerve Tumors of the Orbit. Radiol Clin North Am 1999 Jan;37(1):198.)

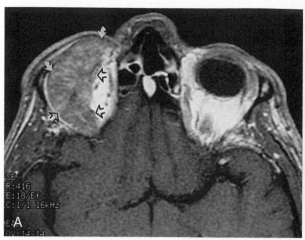

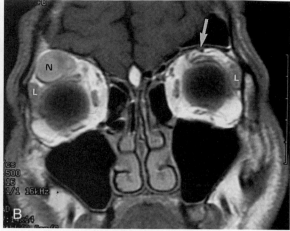

**FIGURE 9-140**   Neurofibroma of the frontal nerve. **A**, Axial-enhanced T1-weighted (416/18, TR/TE) MR image shows a large orbital mass (*arrows*), which shows moderate enhancement. **B**, Coronal-enhanced T1-weighted (500/16, TR/TE) MR image shows moderate enhancement of a neurofibroma (*N*). Note the normal lacrimal glands (*L*) and normal left frontal nerve (*arrow*). (From Mafee MF et al. Lacrimal gland tumors and simulating lesions. Radiol Clin North Am 1999;37:219–239.)

nerves III, IV, V, VI, VII, and the autonomic nerves. Schwannomas and neurofibromas are differentiated primarily on the basis of histopathology. Schwannomas are well encapsulated by the perineurium of the nerve of origin and, in contrast to neurofibromas, display clear evidence of Schwann cell origin.[142] Histologically, they are surrounded by a thin fibrous capsule that is formed by compression of perineural tissue. The tumor is composed of compactly arranged spindle-shaped cells that interlace in cords and whorls frequently oriented with their long axis parallel to one another. This cellular pattern is referred to as *Antoni type A*.[7, 107, 142] Commonly, the Antoni type B part of the tumor has a less cellular pattern characterized by haphazardly distributed cells in a collagenous matrix.[7, 17, 107, 142] On CT and MR imaging, orbital schwannomas appear as sharply marginated, oval or fusiform, intraconal or extraconal masses that demonstrate moderate to marked enhance-

ment (Figs. 9-141 and 9-142). The optic nerve is always displaced and may be engulfed by the tumor (Fig. 9-141). The differential diagnosis includes cavernous hemangioma, meningioma, fibrous histiocytoma, neurofibroma, fibrocystoma, hemangiopericytoma, and metastasis.

## TUMORAL AND NONTUMORAL ENLARGEMENT OF THE OPTIC NERVE SHEATH

Optic nerve sheath meningiomas and gliomas are the most common tumors involving the optic nerves, resulting in localized or diffuse enlargement of the optic nerve sheath complex (see Chapter 11). Primary or secondary involvement of the optic nerve in cases of lymphoma (Fig. 9-85), sarcoid (Fig. 9-86), leukemia, tuberculosis, toxoplasmosis, and syphilis has been reported.[16, 17, 27, 83] Optic nerve sarcoid manifesting as an enhanced tumor on CT and MR imaging scans can be easily mistaken for optic nerve sheath meningioma (Figs. 9-86, 9-88). Other rare causes of enlargement of the optic nerve include intradural cavernoma of the optic nerve and hemangioblastoma of the optic nerve, characteristically seen in patients with von Hippel-Lindau disease (Fig. 9-143).

## OPTIC NEURITIS

This condition is an acute inflammatory process involving the optic nerve that may present as optic nerve enlargement.[16] Multiple sclerosis is the most common cause of optic neuritis and visual loss is typically unilateral, although it may be bilateral.[143] Optic neuropathies following chicken pox, rubella, rubeola, mumps, herpes zoster, mononucleosis, and viral encephalitis are referred to as *parainfections*, as opposed to those caused by direct tissue infiltration by microorganisms.[143] Visual loss is typically bilateral, occurring 10 to 14 days after the primary illness.

**FIGURE 9-141**   Orbital schwannoma. Contrast-enhanced axial CT scan shows a large enhancing mass (*M*).

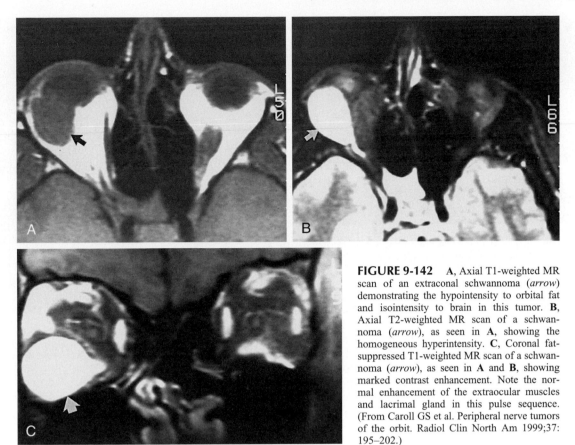

**FIGURE 9-142**   **A**, Axial T1-weighted MR scan of an extraconal schwannoma (*arrow*) demonstrating the hypointensity to orbital fat and isointensity to brain in this tumor. **B**, Axial T2-weighted MR scan of a schwannoma (*arrow*), as seen in **A**, showing the homogeneous hyperintensity. **C**, Coronal fat-suppressed T1-weighted MR scan of a schwannoma (*arrow*), as seen in **A** and **B**, showing marked contrast enhancement. Note the normal enhancement of the extraocular muscles and lacrimal gland in this pulse sequence. (From Caroll GS et al. Peripheral nerve tumors of the orbit. Radiol Clin North Am 1999;37: 195–202.)

This delay suggests a cascade of autoimmune mechanisms. Optic neuritis in patients with systemic lupus erythematosus or other autoimmune states is referred to as *autoimmune optic neuritis*.[143] Infective causes of optic neuritis include syphilis (neuroretinitis, papillitis, and perineuritis); toxoplasmosis; toxocariasis (papillitis); and, uncommonly, borreliosis (Lyme disease) and other granulomatous diseases.[143] Radiation optic neuropathy is another cause of optic neuritis. Optic neuritis in children differs from that in adults, including a greater incidence of disc swelling and a tendency toward bilateral simultaneous involvement.[143] Optic neuritis is often an early manifestation of multiple

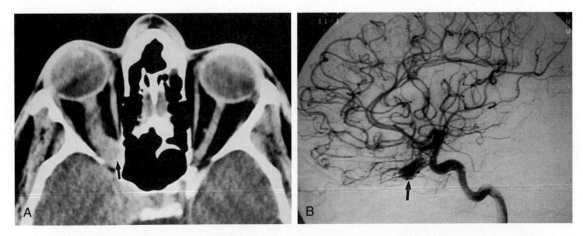

**FIGURE 9-143**   Optic nerve hemangioblastoma. Enhanced axial CT scan (**A**) and lateral angiogram (**B**) showing an optic nerve hemangioblastoma (*arrows*). (From Mafee MF et al. Optic nerve sheath meningiomas: role of MR imaging. Radiol Clin North Am 1999;37:37–58.)

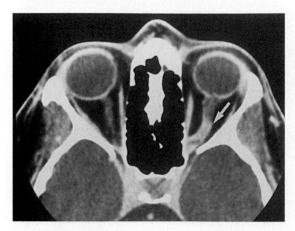

**FIGURE 9-144** Optic neuritis. Enhanced axial CT scan shows enhancement of the left optic nerve (*arrow*). This may not be differentiated from sarcoidosis or meningioma.

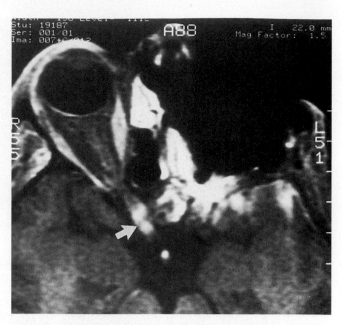

**FIGURE 9-146** Postradiation optic neuritis. Enhanced, fat-suppressed, axial T1-weighted MR image shows enhancement of the intracanalicular segment of right optic nerve (*arrow*). Notice the postorbital exenteration on the left side.

sclerosis, and on CT there may be some enlargement of the optic nerve, usually with some degree of contrast enhancement (Fig. 9-144). On MR imaging the optic nerve may appear thickened and hyperintense on T2-weighted images (Fig. 9-145), and the MR visualization of multiple sclerosis plaques may be accentuated by inversion recovery (STIR) technique.[16, 83] Postcontrast fat-suppressed, T1-weighted MR images may be the best technique to demonstrate optic neuritis, and localized or diffuse areas of enhancement are typically seen within the nerve (Figs. 9-146 and 9-147). In general in patients with optic neuritis, contrast enhancement on CT and MR imaging is often subtle or present in a short segment of the optic nerve, particularly in the intracanalicular portion of the nerve (Fig. 9-146).

# PNEUMOSINUS DILATANS

Pneumosinus dilatans is a rare condition in which dilated paranasal sinuses lined by normal mucosa are present. In these hyperpneumatized paranasal sinuses, excessive pneumatization can lead to thinning and gross dehiscence of the bony wall. When there is actual bone dehiscence, the lesion is usually referred to as a *pneumocele* (see Chapter 5). The frontal sinus is most commonly affected, but the sphenoid sinus is the most important for visual loss because of its intimate relation with the optic canal.[144] Sphenoidal or sphenoethmoidal pneumosinus dilatans may be associated with visual symptoms.[144] Pneumosinus dilatans has been associated with meningioma and fibroosseous lesions, and pneumosinus dilatans without an associate pathologic process rarely causes visual loss (Fig. 9-148). The mechanism leading to optic neuropathy is uncertain, although with

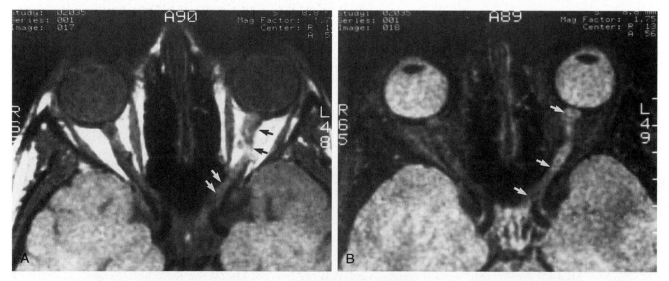

**FIGURE 9-145** Optic neuritis. Axial PW (**A**) and T2-weighted (**B**) MR images show enlargement of the left entire optic nerve (*arrows*) in this 14-year-old girl with left optic neuritis.

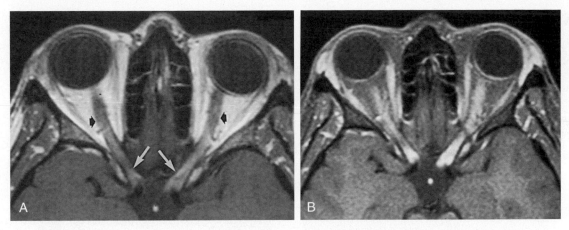

**FIGURE 9-147**   Optic neuritis. (**A**) Enhanced axial T1-weighted (600/18, TR/TE) and (**B**) enhanced axial fat-suppression T1-weighted (500/15, TR/TE) MR scans showing marked enhancement of intraorbital (*black arrows*) and intracanalicular segments (*white arrows*) of optic nerves. Biopsy revealed a demyelinating process. (From Mafee MF et al. Optic nerve sheath meningiomas: role of MR imaging. Radiol Clin North Am 1999;37:37–58.)

direct communication between the sinus and the optic canal present, one could postulate a direct compressive effect by mucosa or air leading to ischemic nerve damage.[144] It has been suggested that sudden elevation of the intrasinus pressure, as with sneezing or with altitude change (in airplanes), may cause direct damage to an exposed optic nerve.[144]

## FIBROUS TISSUE TUMORS OF THE ORBIT

Fibrous tumors of the orbit are a group of lesions that present a confusing clinical, histologic, and imaging spectrum of disease. These include fibroma, fibrous histiocytoma, fibrocystoma, aggressive fibromatosis, nodular fasciitis, and fibrosarcoma. Fibrohistiocytic tumors are more common than fibroblastic (fibroma, fibromatosis) tumors.[145]

## Fibrous Histiocytoma

Fibrous histiocytoma is a mesenchymal tumor that involves the fascia, muscle, and soft tissues of the body.[3, 145–148] It is considered by some authors to be the most common mesenchymal tumor of the orbit.[146] The neoplasm is made up of fibroblasts, myofibroblasts, undifferentiated mesenchymal cells, and fibrous-appearing histiocytic cells that tend to form a characteristic cartwheel or storiform pattern.[3, 145–148] Fibrous histiocytoma probably arises from a fibroblast precursor, and it bears no relationship to the systemic reticuloendothelioses or malignant histiocytoses. The tumor may be either benign or malignant.[146, 147] Malignant fibrous histiocytomas produce bone erosion. Benign lesions cause a mass effect with compressive bone atrophy (remodeling).[7] Fibrous histiocytomas are seen on CT and MR imaging as well-circumscribed masses that may be intraconal or extraconal and demonstrate

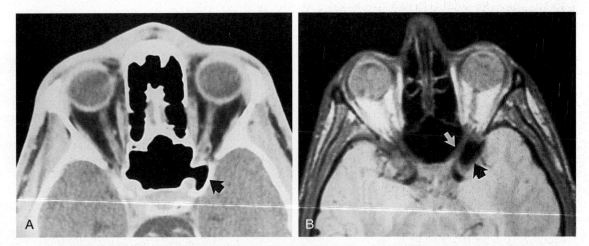

**FIGURE 9-148**   **A**, Sphenoid pneumosinus dilatans. Axial CT scan shows extension of sphenoid sinus pneumatization into the left lesser wing of sphenoid (*arrow*). **B**, Proton-weighted (2400/20, TR/TE) axial MR scan shows normal optic nerve (*white arrow*) and pneumatized lesser wing of sphenoid (*black arrow*). (From Mafee MF et al. Optic nerve sheath meningiomas: role of MR imaging. Radiol Clin North Am 1999;37:37–58.)

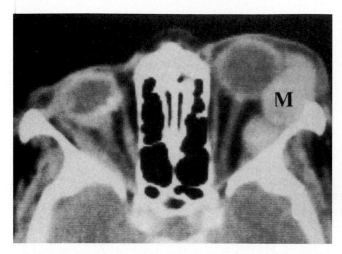

**FIGURE 9-149**   Fibrous histiocytoma. Axial postcontrast CT scan showing a bilobed enhancing mass (*M*) involving the peripheral orbital space. Notice the deformity of the right globe with calcifications representing pthisis bulbi. (From Mafee MF et al. Orbital space-occupying lesions: role of CT and MRI: an analysis of 145 cases. Radiol Clin North Am 1987;25:529–559.)

moderate to marked contrast enhancement (Figs. 9-149 and 9-150).[145] Some of the tumors may be bilobed. Some of the densely cellular fibrous histiocytomas may appear moderately to markedly hypointense on T2-weighted images, and these lesions may not be differentiated on imaging from some of the neurofibromas and other fibrous lesions (Fig. 9-151). The differential diagnosis should include cavernous hemangioma, hemangiopericytoma, schwannoma, meningioma, neurofibroma, fibrocystoma, vasculogenic leiomyoma, lymphoma, and metastasis. Malignant fibrous histiocytomas may be seen following irradiation of the orbit for retinoblastoma.[17]

## Fibroma and Fibrosarcoma

Fibroma is the least common fibrous tumor of the orbit and is found mostly in young adults.[145] It is usually encapsulated and grows slowly over several years. It arises from the fascia of the EOMs or Tenon's capsule in the orbit. Fibrosarcoma is also rare in the orbit. Congenital, infantile, juvenile, and adult forms of fibrosarcoma are recognized.[145] Aggressive fibromatosis is a benign but locally invasive fibroblastic lesion lying clinically and pathologically in the spectrum between fibrosis and low-grade fibrosarcoma. Infantile deep (desmoid type), infantile myofibromatosis (congenital generalized fibromatosis), and adult (deep or musculoaponeurotic) forms are recognized (Fig. 9-152).

The lesion may be (1) solitary in about 73%; (2) multicentric, involving subcutaneous tissues, skeletal muscle, and the ends of long bones; or (3) generalized, with cutaneous, musculoskeletal, and visceral involvement.[145] Orbital involvement may rarely be bilateral.[145] Fibromatosis tends to be locally infiltrative and grows rapidly, which may cause it to be considered as a low-grade fibrosarcoma. Histologically, it is composed of well-differentiated, uniform fibroblasts, appearing similar to smooth muscle, but electron microscopy reveals that the lesion contains fibro-

blasts and myofibroblasts. Treatment is wide surgical excision. Fibromatosis recurs locally in 25% to 65% of cases and can be fatal. CT and MR imaging may show a lesion with either benign-appearing or invasive characteristics (Fig. 9-152).

## Nodular Fasciitis

Nodular fasciitis is a common fibrous tumor found elsewhere in the limbs and trunk of adults, but head and neck involvement is seen more commonly in infants and children.[145] Orbital involvement may develop in the lid, conjunctiva, Tenon's capsule, or the deep orbit.[145] Microscopically, plump fibroblasts have a stellate appearance. Normal mitosis is present. The pathologic differential diagnosis should include fibromatosis, fibrosarcoma, leiomyoma, neurofibroma, schwannoma, myxofibrosarcoma, and myxoid liposarcoma.[145] Nodular fasciitis is best treated with complete excision and has a recurrence rate of 1% to 2%.[145] CT and MR imaging findings are nonspecific and similar to those of aggressive fibromatosis (Fig. 9-153).

## RHABDOMYOSARCOMA OF THE ORBIT

Although rhabdomyosarcoma (RMS) is a rare tumor, it is still the most common primary orbital malignancy in children and the most common soft-tissue malignancy of childhood. Soft-tissue sarcomas account for 6% of all childhood cancers, and RMS accounts for approximately 50% of all pediatric soft-tissue sarcomas and 15% of all pediatric solid tumors.[149–153] Approximately 250 new pediatric patients are diagnosed with RMS each year in the United States. The head and neck area accounts for 35% of all RMS, the genitourinary system for 23%, and the extremities for 17%. The remainder are found in the trunk, retroperitoneum, chest, perineum, and gastrointestinal tract.[149–153] RMS occurs primarily in patients from ages 2 to 5; however, the tumor may occur at any age from birth to adulthood. In most cases, the average age at diagnosis is 7 to 8 years. RMS can be further divided into bimodal age peaks, depending on the histology. The embryonal and alveolar subtypes present in children, and the pleomorphic type presents more commonly in adults. The tumor may even be present at birth.[149] Orbital RMS is invariably unilateral, and although the tumor may involve any part of the orbit and adnexa, it tends to involve the superior portion of the orbit. The most characteristic presenting features of orbital RMS are a fairly rapid onset and progression, with proptosis and displacement of the globe.

RMS originates from embryonic tissue, either from immature prospective muscle fibers or pluripotential embryonic mesenchymal tissue, with a potential for aberrant differentiation into muscle fibers. Cytogenic analysis has found that many of these patients have a translocation between chromosomes 2 and 13 and abnormalities of chromosome 11.[149–153] This tumor does not originate from preformed extraocular striated muscles. The differential diagnosis also includes leukemic and metastatic deposits (neuroblastoma), lymphoma, LCH, aggressive fibromatosis, plexiform neurofibromatosis, ruptured dermoid cyst, subperiosteal hematoma after trauma, and a chocolate cyst related to hemorrhage in a lymphangioma. RMSs are pleomorphic tumors, and the cells may be anaplastic. On the basis of their histopathologic characteristics, RMSs are classified into one of three histologic types: (1) embryonal, (2) differentiated, and (3) alveolar. Differentiated RMS is the least frequent type and is rarely misdiagnosed because cells with eosinophilic cytoplasmic fibrils that are usually

cross-striated are used to identify the tumor. Embryonal RMS, the most common histologic subtype, is believed to arise from the primitive muscle cell, because it is found in 7- to 10-week-old fetuses. The histologic differentiation between embryonal and alveolar RMS may be difficult. It has been estimated that up to 50% of proved cases of RMS are misdiagnosed on initial biopsy.[149]

RMS of the sinonasal tract and orbit often presents as a

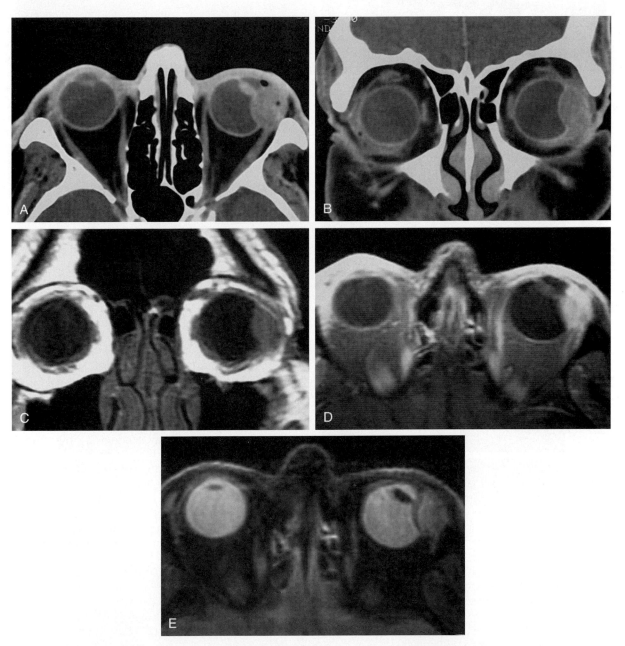

**FIGURE 9-150**   Malignant fibrous histiocytoma. Axial (**A**) and coronal (**B**) contrast-enhanced CT. The contrast-enhanced CT studies on this 58-year-old man demonstrate a well-defined, moderately enhancing mass at the left lateral globe margin, which indents the globe without visibly invading the dense sclera. A small amount of gas is present in the mass after needle biopsy. **C,** Coronal T1-weighted image (TR/TE = 600/12) reveals that the mass is intermediate in signal intensity. **D,** Axial, fat-saturation, T1-weighted image (600/12) shows moderate gadolinium enhancement. **E,** Axial, conventional, STIR (TR/TE/T1 = 2000/43/170) image shows that the mass is hyperintense to temporalis muscle, slightly hypointense to the vitreous, and separated from the globe contents by the hypointense band of sclera. At surgery, it arose from the ciliary body near the tendinous insertion of the lateral rectus muscle. (From Dalley RW. Fibrous histiocytoma and fibrous tissue tumors of the orbit. Radiol Clin North Am 1999;37:185–194.)

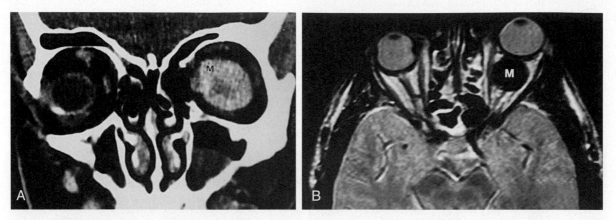

**FIGURE 9-151**    Fibrocytoma. **A**, Coronal contrast-enhanced CT scan shows moderately enhancing intraconal mass (*M*). **B**, Axial T2-weighted MR image shows markedly hypointense mass (*M*). This is related to marked dense collagen content. (From Dalley RW. Fibrous histocytoma and fibrous tissue tumors of the orbit. Radiol Clin North Am 1999;37:185–194.)

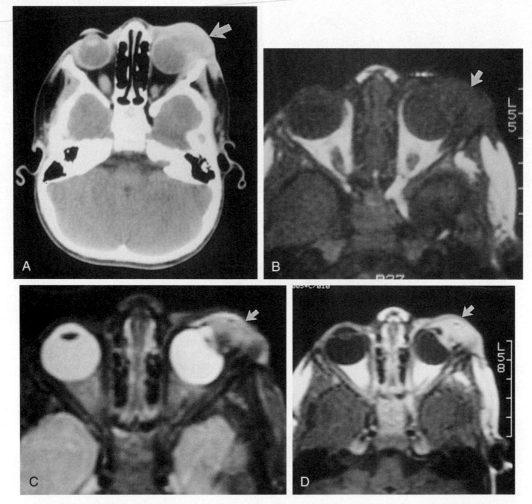

**FIGURE 9-152**    Aggressive fibromatosis. **A**, Enhanced axial CT scan shows a mass (*arrow*) with moderate enhancement. **B**, Axial T1-weighted MR image. The mass (*arrow*) is isointense to brain tissue. **C**, Axial T2-weighted MR image. The mass (*arrow*) appears hyperintense to muscles. **D**, Enhanced fat-suppression axial T1-weighted MR image. The mass (*arrow*) shows marked enhancement. Note invasion of the globe. (From Mafee MF et al. Rhabdomyosarcoma of the orbit: evaluation with MR imaging and CT. Radiol Clin North Am 1998;36:1215–1227.)

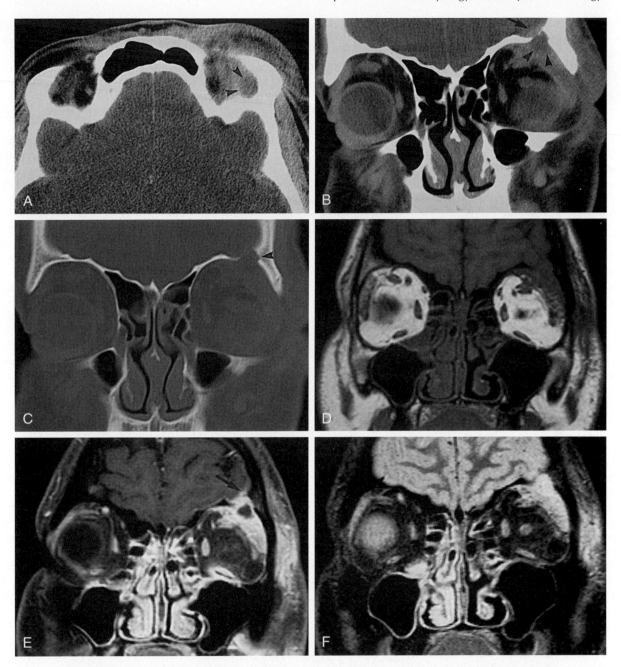

**FIGURE 9-153**   Nodular fasciitis. A 36-year-old man presented with an apparent inflammatory left orbital mass, which was unresponsive to 3 weeks of antibiotics. Axial (**A**) and coronal (**B**) contrast-enhanced CT. Soft-tissue windows show an ill-defined, enhancing, extraconal or subperiosteal soft-tissue mass in the left superior-lateral orbit, with a low-attenuation central area (*arrowheads*). Note the subtle enhancement along the anterior cranial fossa (*arrow*). **C,** Coronal CT bone windows demonstrate focal erosion in the frontal bone adjacent to this low-attenuation region (*arrowhead*). **D,** Coronal T1-weighted image (600/15) reveals an intermediate intensity extending lateral to the orbital rim in addition to eroding the frontal bone. **E,** Coronal, fat-saturation, postgadolinium, T1-weighted image (650/15). After gadolinium, most of the mass enhances, with a central, nonenhancing focus adjacent to the bone erosion. Note the intracranial dural reaction (*arrow*). **F,** Coronal, fast-STIR (2000/12/160) image. The mass is isointense to gray matter, with a focal area of hyperintensity corresponding to the cystic-appearing region on the postgadolinium image. The preoperative diagnosis was ruptured dermoid cyst or an aggressive lacrimal region abscess with osteomyelitis. (From Dalley RW. Fibrous histiocytoma and fibrous tissue tumors of the orbit. Radiol Clin North Am 1999;37:185–194.)

relatively innocuous problem (e.g., recurrent sinusitis, proptosis, or a small nasoorbital mass). Secondary sinonasal tumors may arise from adjacent orbital spread of orbital or pharyngeal RMS. RMSs are aggressive bone-destroying and bone-pushing lesions. Although RMS of the orbit is most

often seen in children and in adults under 20 years of age, at times it affects older patients.

RMS, nonrhabdomyosarcomatous soft-tissue sarcoma, and Ewing's sarcoma occur frequently in the head and neck of children. The nonrhabdomyosarcomatous sarcomas include fibrosarcoma, angiosarcoma, malignant fibrous histiocytoma, malignant schwannoma and neurofibroma, leiomyosarcoma, hemangiopericytoma, synovial sarcoma, and other less common sarcomas. Rao et al.[154] reported 110 cases of nonrhabdomyosarcomatous soft-tissue sarcomas. Head and neck sites accounted for only 15% of these tumors. The head and neck sites can be divided into three broad groups: (1) cranial parameningeal, (2) orbital, and (3) nonorbital-nonparameningeal.[149] Parameningeal RMS refers to those tumors arising in the nasopharynx, paranasal sinuses, nose, middle ear, temporal fossa, and pterygopalatine fossa. Nonorbital-nonparameningeal head lesions include superficial and deeply placed tumors, including tumors of the scalp and face, as well as deep tumors arising in the buccal mucosa, parapharyngeal space, larynx, salivary gland, and neck.[149]

Proptosis is an uncommon finding in children, but the vast majority of space-occupying lesions in the orbit causing proptosis in children are benign. These include inflammatory lesions (infection, abscess, and idiopathic orbital inflammation); developmental cysts (teratoma, dermoid, epidermoid); subperiosteal hematoma; benign and malignant mesenchymal tumors (osteogenic, chondrogenic, histiocytomatous, fibromatous [aggressive fibromatosis], lipomatous, myxomatous, rhabdomyomatous); tumors of vascular origin (hemangioma and lymphangioma); metastases; and neurogenic tumors (neurofibroma, plexiform neurofibromatosis, optic nerve glioma). Although malignant lesions are rare, clinically they can mimic more common benign processes, creating difficulty in diagnosis. Other orbital malignancies include lymphoma (including Burkitt's lymphoma), leukemia, extension of retinoblastoma, metastatic neuroblastoma, and secondary involvement by Ewing's sarcoma. Radiologic imaging is an essential aid to the clinician in differentiating the diagnostic possibilities.

Orbital RMS generally presents painlessly with rapidly progressive unilateral exophthalmos or, less commonly, as a superficial swelling with a palpable mass and proptosis. Patients may even present with a confusing or misleading history, such as recent trauma. Orbital RMS usually affects young children or adolescents up to age 16 years, with an average age of 7 years, but has been reported in older children and adults. Most tumors are retrobulbar, resulting in proptosis, but they can arise extraconally, especially superiorly or supranasally. They have also been reported to arise intraocularly from the ciliary body.[149] Tumors arising in the paranasal sinuses, nasal cavity, pterygopalatine fossa, nasopharynx, and parapharyngeal space may secondarily invade the orbit, and RMS arising elsewhere can metastasize to the orbit.[149]

Of the head and neck sites, orbital RMS has a better outlook, presumably because of the paucity of lymphatics and tumor confinement by the bony orbit. Parameningeal involvement is associated with the poorest outcome, presumably because of abundant lymphatics and the lack of confinement to prevent extension into the surrounding tissues.

## Diagnostic Imaging

CT and MR imaging play an important role in the preoperative evaluation and staging of these tumors.

Imaging should include CT and MR imaging of the primary and metastatic sites (i.e., lung, liver, brain, and so forth). CT and MR imaging are also important in evaluating recurrent and residual disease, and a baseline CT or MR imaging study is essential following completion of treatment. Without a baseline CT or MR scan, the follow-up studies may not be specific for tumor recurrence. Because of the dramatic improvement in survival of patients treated promptly with appropriate chemotherapy and radiation therapy, these tumors must be diagnosed as soon as possible.

On CT images, the RMSs are isodense in relation to normal muscles and appear as homogeneous, well-defined soft-tissue masses without bone destruction (Fig. 9-154). Larger tumors appear as less well defined soft-tissue masses with bone destruction or invasion of surrounding structures (Fig. 9-155). Tumors that have focal hemorrhage appear heterogeneous on CT scans. All tumors demonstrate moderate to marked contrast enhancement.[149]

On T1-weighted MR images, the RMSs are isointense or slightly hypointense compared with brain. On T2-weighted MR images, they appear to have increased signal intensity compared with brain (Fig. 9-156). Tumors that have chronic or subacute areas of hemorrhage demonstrate focal areas of increased signal on T1-weighted and T2-weighted images.[152] RMS demonstrates enhancement on contrast-enhanced CT and MR images (Fig. 9-157).[149] With the fat-suppression technique, T1-weighted images demonstrate marked expansion of the gray scale, with apparently increased signal intensity of the normal EOMs and lacrimal glands. Therefore, these normal structures should not be mistaken for tumor. The tumors appear more hyperintense on postcontrast fat-suppressed, T1-weighted images than on postcontrast non-fat-suppressed T1-weighted images.

When the diagnosis is suspected, cross-sectional imaging primarily with CT or MR imaging is performed to confirm the presence of an infiltrative mass and evaluate the extent of involvement of adjacent structures, including the brain. Although both may be equivalent in detecting an abnormal mass and determining its origin, MR imaging better delineates the full extent of involvement due to its superior soft-tissue contrast (Fig. 9-158).

Concomitant reactive sinus disease can be differentiated on MR imaging by differences in signal intensity on SE and postcontrast images. Superimposed fungal infection, during or following radiation therapy and chemotherapy, may pose

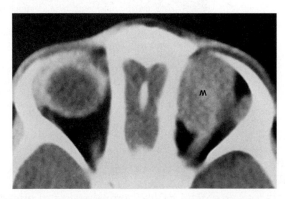

**FIGURE 9-154** Rhabdomyosarcoma (5-year-old boy). Enhanced axial CT scan shows an orbital mass (*M*) with moderate contrast enhancement. (From Mafee MF et al. Rhabdomyosarcoma of the orbit: evaluation with MR imaging and CT. Radiol Clin North Am 1998;36:1215–1227.)

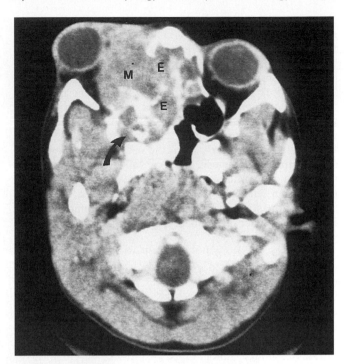

**FIGURE 9-155** Rhabdomyosarcoma. Axial enhanced CT scan shows a large mass (*M*) in the right orbit extending into the right ethmoid air cells (*E*) and right infratemporal fossa (*arrow*).

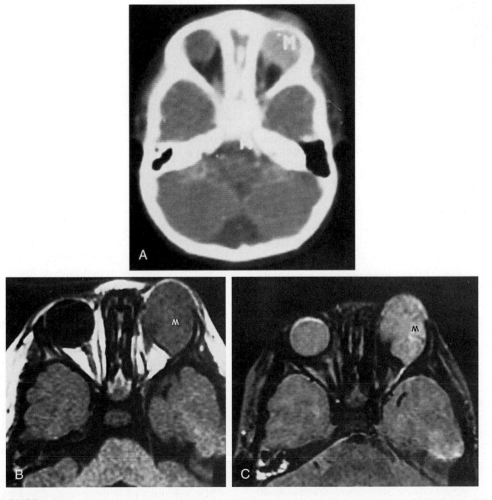

**FIGURE 9-156** Rhabdomyosarcoma (2-year-old boy). **A**, Enhanced axial CT scan shows an orbital mass (*M*) that demonstrates moderate contrast enhancement. **B**, Axial T1-weighted MR image shows the mass (*M*), which is slightly hypointense to the brain. **C**, Axial T2-weighted MR image. The mass (*M*) appears hyperintense relative to the brain. (From Mafee MF et al. Rhabdomyosarcoma of the orbit: evaluation with MR imaging and CT. Radiol Clin North Am 1998;36:1215–1227.)

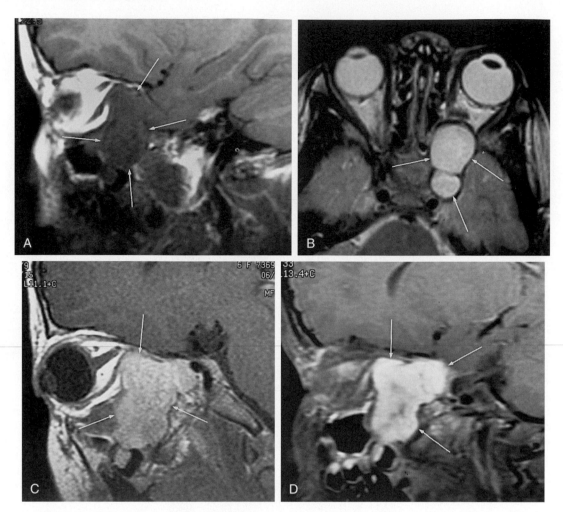

**FIGURE 9-157** Rhabdomyosarcoma (6-year-old girl). **A**, Sagittal T1-weighted MR image shows a large mass (*arrows*) in the pterygopalatine fossa and infratemporal fossa. **B**, Axial T2-weighted MR image shows extension of tumor into the left orbital apex. Lesion appears hyperintense to brain. **C**, Enhanced sagittal T1-weighted MR image shows marked enhancement of tumor (*arrows*). Note extension into the orbital apex with elevation of the inferior rectus. Note also extension into the anterior aspect of the cavernous sinus. **D**, Enhanced fat-suppression sagittal T1-weighted MR image. Note apparent marked enhancement of tumor (*arrows*). (From Mafee MF et al. Rhabdomyosarcoma of the orbit: evaluation with MR imaging and CT. Radiol Clin North Am 1998;36:1215–1227.)

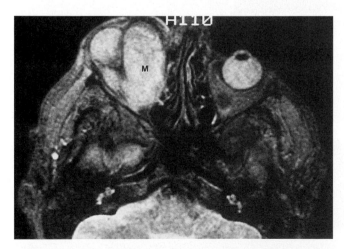

**FIGURE 9-158** Rhabdomyosarcoma. Axial T2-weighted MR image shows a large orbital mass (*M*) in this 60-year-old man compatible with rhabdomyosarcoma.

a problem for the radiologist in distinguishing residual tumor from invasive fungal infection. The resultant bone destruction or remodeling about the orbit and cranium is common with advanced disease and is best evaluated with CT. It is still possible, however, to detect bony invasion by the distortion of the bone marrow signal on MR imaging, especially after the administration of contrast.

Many common and less common orbital and head and neck neoplasms, however, such as hemangiomas, lymphangiomas, lymphoma, leukemic infiltration, plexiform neurofibromatosis, aggressive fibromatosis, pseudorheumatoid nodule, and pseudotumor, can appear similar to RMS, with similar CT and MR imaging characteristics. Thus, the findings are nonspecific in many cases, necessitating a tissue diagnosis. Subperiosteal hematoma in children may simulate RMS. MR imaging in these cases may be extremely valuable to make the correct diagnosis. Orbital pseudotumors in children can simulate orbital RMS (Fig. 9-159), as can aggressive fibromatosis RMS (Fig. 9-152). Capillary hem-

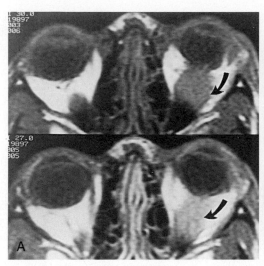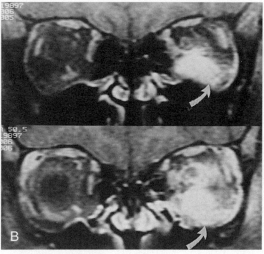

**FIGURE 9-159**   Pseudotumor. **A,** Nonenhanced (*top*) and enhanced (*bottom*) axial T1-weighted MR images showing thickening and enhancement of the left inferior rectus (*arrows*). **B,** Enhanced fat-suppression coronal T1-weighted MR images showing marked enhancement of this pseudotumor (*arrows*). This MR appearance can easily simulate rhabdomyosarcoma. (From Mafee MF et al. Rhabdomyosarcoma of the orbit: evaluation with MR imaging and CT. Radiol Clin North Am 1998;36:1215–1227.)

angiomas and other vasculogenic lesions (Fig. 9-160), including vascular malformations, may also simulate RMS, and dynamic CT may be very helpful in the diagnosis of capillary hemangiomas. At times, RMS may present with a clinical picture and imaging features of an orbital subperiosteal abscess.[155] In adults, lymphoma and primary and secondary orbital tumors should be included in the differential diagnosis (Fig. 9-161).

Imaging also allows planning of biopsy and surgery. Although superficial disease is easily accessible to the clinician, deeply seated masses present technical difficulties. Radiologic guidance (i.e., CT) may be used to direct aspiration biopsy safely, with minimal risk and morbidity. Further workup for staging should be performed including chest radiographs, a blood count, liver function tests,

skeletal survey, bone marrow biopsy, etc. Surgery is performed to remove the maximum amount of tumor tissue that is safely feasible while minimizing the resulting deformity. Thus, staging depends on resection of the primary mass, the amount of residual tumor, and the presence of distant metastases, which usually involve the lung, bone marrow, lymph nodes, and brain. Due to the absence of lymphatics about the orbit, regional lymph nodes tend not to be involved, at least until advanced spread has occurred.

Once the diagnosis is confirmed by pathologic analysis, prompt treatment is initiated to maximize the patient's chances of survival. Currently, treatment includes biopsy or excision and radiation therapy with adjuvant chemotherapy. Smaller focal lesions may be entirely removed safely, whereas larger masses or metastatic lesions usually have

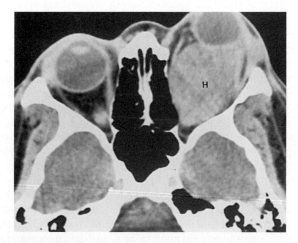

**FIGURE 9-160**   Sclerosing hemangioma (16-year-old girl). Enhanced axial CT scan shows a large, moderately enhancing intraconal mass compatible with hemangioma (*H*). (From Mafee MF et al. Rhabdomyosarcoma of the orbit: evaluation with MR imaging and CT. Radiol Clin North Am 1998;36:1215–1227.)

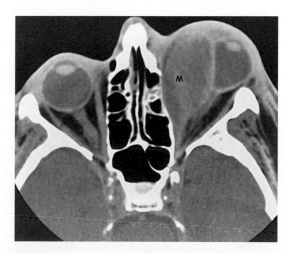

**FIGURE 9-161**   Malignant melanoma. Enhanced axial CT scan shows a large mass (*M*). This was diagnosed as primary orbital malignant melanoma, because no other primary could be identified. (From Mafee MF et al. Rhabdomyosarcoma of the orbit: evaluation with MR imaging and CT. Radiol Clin North Am 1998;36:1215–1227.)

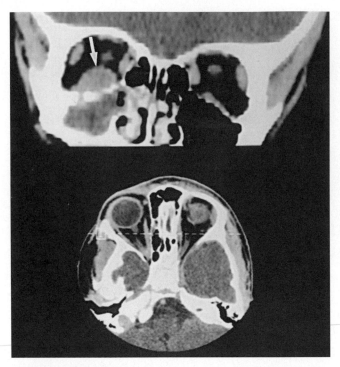

**FIGURE 9-162** Axial CT scans with coronal reconstruction show recurrence of rhabdomyosarcoma in a 5-year-old girl. (From Mafee MF et al. Rhabdomyosarcoma of the orbit: evaluation with MR imaging and CT. Radiol Clin North Am 1998;36:1215–1227.)

residual disease after extirpation. Regardless, radiation therapy helps control the local residual tumor, which may be microscopic and/or due to incomplete excision. The addition of combination chemotherapy has been shown to improve survival. Complete resection of a local tumor or minimal residual tumor after removal of regional disease allows 90% or greater survival after 5 years. With significant residual tumor, the prognosis drops to 35%. The major side effects of therapy are vision problems due to cataracts, retinopathy, and corneal scarring from keratoconjunctivitis. Other late side effects include bony orbital deformity and enophthalmos, secondary malignancy (leukemia), and leukoencephalopathy. Improvements in treatment regimens and decreases in radiation doses have decreased secondary complications.

After treatment is instituted, cross-sectional imaging can be used to objectively monitor tumor regression or residual and recurrent disease (Figs. 9-162 and 9-163). In fact, an increased risk of relapse is associated with posttreatment residual tissue, and residual tissue can be shown with CT or MR imaging prior to any clinical relapse. A relapse, in turn, denotes a poor prognosis; thus, early detection is essential. Clinical abnormalities and symptoms usually occur with recurrence, initiating further imaging to confirm the suspicion. Recurrent disease usually occurs locally in the surgical bed or regionally in the adjacent central nervous system. It is difficult to differentiate fibrosis and scarring from active tumor with CT and MR imaging, particularly if no baseline study is available. On the other hand, healing of bone destruction may signify a response to therapy and can be easily evaluated by CT. Furthermore, MR imaging of the brain may be helpful to monitor for, or follow up on,

associated parenchymal leukoencephalopathic changes resulting from chemotherapy and radiation therapy, which may be subtle in the early stages. CT is less sensitive in this latter situation.

## MESENCHYMAL CHONDROSARCOMA OF THE ORBIT

Extraskeletal malignant cartilaginous tumors are subdivided into two major categories: mesenchymal and myxoid chondrosarcoma. Mesenchymal chondrosarcomas commonly occur within the bones. Extraskeletal locations include the head and neck, the cranial and spinal dura mater, and, less frequently, the leg, especially the thigh.[156] Orbital mesenchymal chondrosarcoma (OMC) remains an extremely rare entity occurring more frequently in young women.[156–159] The most common presenting symptom of OMC is proptosis, with orbital pain, diplopia, and headache. Histologically, OMC is relatively distinct, containing islands of chondroid tissue. The cartilaginous areas have the appearance of mature cartilage. Most of them contain amorphic calcification and foci of ossification of the cartilaginous matrix.[156, 158] Other areas of undifferentiated mesenchymal tissue are seen, with a predominance of spindle-shaped cells. Mitoses are not frequent. In addition, areas of dilated vascular channels in the stroma can be seen that histologically resemble hemangiopericytoma.[156–159]

CT imaging characteristics include a relatively well-defined soft-tissue mass with areas of mottled, coarse calcification (Fig. 9-164A), and moderate, delayed contrast enhancement is noted. MR imaging characteristics include a signal intensity lower than or equal to that of brain on T1-weighted images and isointense to brain on T2-weighted images, with moderate enhancement after gadolinium contrast administration (Fig. 9-164B-F). The calcified component of the tumor shows low signal on both T1-weighted and T2-weighted MR images (Fig. 9-164B,F). On enhanced T1-weighted MR images, however, mild enhancement is seen even within the calcified components (Fig. 9-164D,E).[156]

The differential diagnosis for an intraorbital calcified mass includes meningioma, sclerosing hemangioma, hemangiopericytoma, vascular malformation, varix, and orbital amyloidosis.[8, 156] Calcification in cavernous hemangioma, fibrous histiocytoma, fibrocystoma, schwannoma, neurofibroma, and optic glioma is extremely rare. Hemangiopericytomas may occasionally demonstrate dystrophic calcification, which is usually seen after recurrence of the lesion.[156] Fibrous histiocytomas are the most common adult mesenchymal tumors of the orbit, presenting as well-circumscribed intraconal or extraconal masses with moderate to marked enhancement. The more cellular fibrous histiocytomas may have moderately or markedly low signal intensity on T2-weighted MR images.[156] This MR appearance may mimic that of OMC; however, unlike OMC, fibrous histiocytomas do not show calcification on CT scans. Orbital amyloidosis demonstrates a soft-tissue mass with coarse, streaky, amorphous calcification diffusely scattered throughout the lesion (Figs. 9-93 and 9-94). In addition, certain areas that appear to be calcific density actually represent amyloid (Figs. 9-93 and 9-94).[156]

## LACRIMAL GLAND AND FOSSA LESIONS

The lacrimal gland is about the size and shape of an almond and is located in the superolateral extraconal orbital fat in the lacrimal fossa, adjacent to the tendons of the superior and lateral rectus muscles. The more anterior palpebral lobe is separated from the deeper orbital lobe by the lateral horn of the levator muscle aponeurosis.[24, 120] The lacrimal gland is a modified salivary gland, and it can be involved by a wide spectrum of orbital pathology. Meticulous clinical and preoperative imaging of these patients is imperative so that an inappropriate incisional biopsy is avoided. This situation is especially true when a benign mixed tumor of the lacrimal gland is suspected. This tumor requires en bloc excision through a lateral orbitotomy to ensure complete extirpation and prevent late recurrences.[24] If an incisional biopsy of a benign mixed tumor is performed, there is an increased likelihood of operative tumor spillage and thus late recurrences.[24, 160, 161] The excellent prognosis of benign mixed tumor, provided that it is completely removed at the first surgery, is now widely accepted.

Lesions of the lacrimal gland and fossa present special problems in diagnosis and management. Because of the importance of preoperative diagnosis, all clinical ancillary findings should be integrated into the assessment of individual cases. In general, epithelial tumors represent about 50% of the masses involving the lacrimal gland. The remaining 50% of lacrimal gland masses are either lymphoid or inflammatory in nature.[24, 160] Metastasis to the parenchyma of the lacrimal gland is rare.[24] Dermoid cysts are not true lacrimal gland tumors; rather, they arise from epithelial rests located in the orbit, particularly in the superolateral quadrant. Epithelial cysts, on the other hand, are intrinsic lesions that result from dilation of the lacrimal ducts.[24, 160]

Inflammatory diseases of the lacrimal gland can be divided into two categories, acute and chronic.[24] Acute dacryoadenitis (bacterial or viral) is more commonly seen in children and in younger people.[24, 156, 162, 163] It may be related to trauma and clinically is associated with local

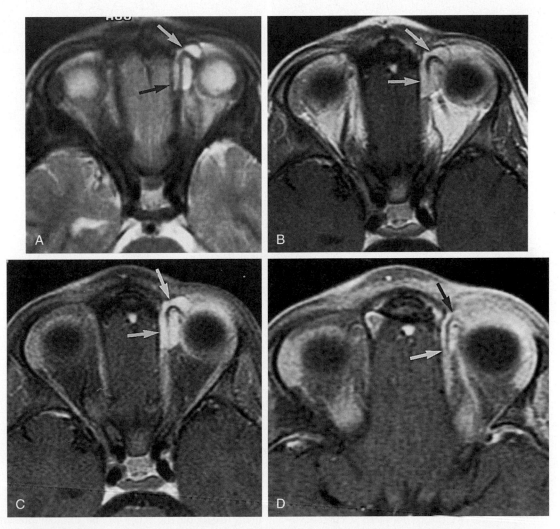

**FIGURE 9-163**   Rhabdomyosarcoma (4-year-old boy). **A,** Axial T2-weighted MR image shows a predominantly hyperintense mass (*arrows*). **B,** Enhanced axial T1-weighted MR image. Note enhancement of tumor (*arrows*). Enhanced, fat-suppressed T1-weighted image. Note enhancement of tumor (*arrows*). Enhanced fat-suppression axial T1-weighted MR images (**C** and **D**), taken 6 months after completion of chemotherapy and radiation therapy. Note decreased size of mass (*arrows*). (From Mafee MF et al. Rhabdomyosarcoma of the orbit: evaluation with MR imaging and CT. Radiol Clin North Am 1998;36:1215–1227.)

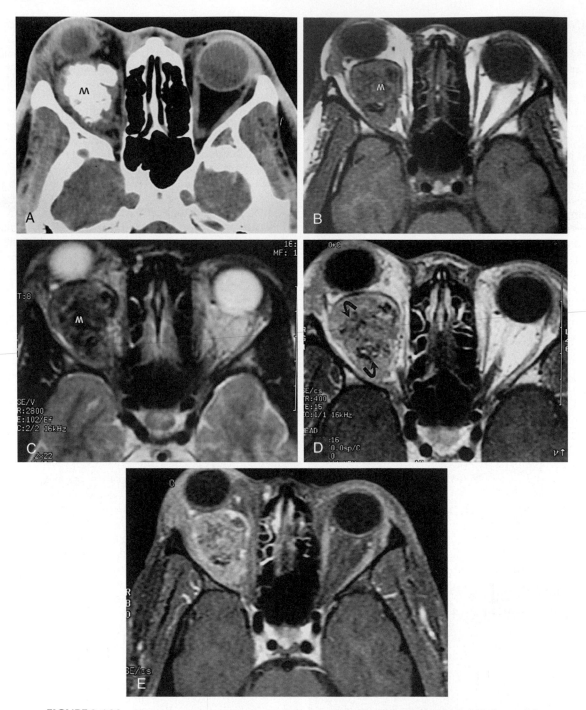

**FIGURE 9-164** Mesenchymal chondrosarcoma. **A,** Enhanced axial CT scan shows a heavily calcified mass (*M*) in the right retrobulbar space. **B,** Axial nonenhanced T1-weighted MR image shows that the mass (*M*) is isointense to brain. Note areas of hypointensity related to more dense calcification. **C,** Axial, fast spin-echo, T2-weighted MR image shows that the mass (*M*) is heterogeneous but markedly hypointense, related to intratumoral foci of calcifications. **D,** Axial-enhanced T1-weighted MR image shows that the mass is rather hypervascular, as evidenced by marked contrast enhancement. The calcified component of the mass shows less enhancement (*arrows*). **E,** Axial fat-suppressed, enhanced T1-weighted MR image shows marked tumor enhancement. (From Koeller KK. Mesenchymal chondrosarcoma and simulating lesions of the orbit. Radiol Clin North Am 1999;37:203–217.)

tenderness, erythema, lid swelling, conjunctival chemosis, discharge or suppuration, enlarged preauricular and cervical nodes, and systemic findings.[24, 156] Acute dacryoadenitis is usually unilateral and tends to respond very rapidly to therapy.[24, 156] It may be part of the spectrum of idiopathic inflammatory orbital pseudotumor, and this diagnosis is made often on the basis of the clinical presentation, CT findings, and the prompt and favorable response to the administration of systemic corticosteroids.[24, 156, 163, 164]

Chronic dacryoadenitis may follow acute infection or may be caused by sarcoidosis (Fig. 9-165), thyroid ophthalmopathy, Mikulicz's syndrome, Sjogren's syn-

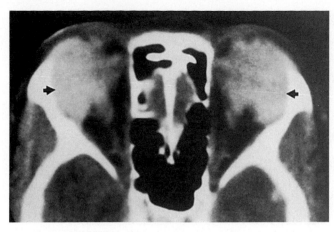

**FIGURE 9-165** Sarcoidosis. Axial CT scan shows bilateral diffuse enlargement of entire lacrimal glands (*arrows*).

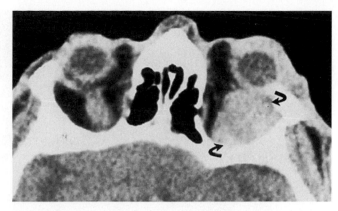

**FIGURE 9-167** Lymphoma. Axial postcontrast CT scan shows a large mass in the superior temporal quadrant extending posteriorly to the orbital apex (*arrows*); the lacrimal gland is totally involved. Note the postsurgical changes in the lateral wall of the left orbit.

drome, "sclerosing pseudotumors" (Fig. 9-166), and Wegener's granulomatosis. In sarcoid there is usually bilateral disease, with either symmetric or asymmetric lacrimal gland enlargement (Fig. 9-165). Mikulicz's syndrome is a nonspecific swelling of the lacrimal gland and salivary glands associated with conditions such as leukemia, lymphoma, pseudotumor, tuberculosis, syphilis, and sarcoidosis. In Sjogren's syndrome, there is enlargement of and lymphocytic infiltration of the lacrimal glands. Half of these patients have a connective tissue disease such as rheumatoid arthritis, systemic lupus erythematosus, scleroderma, or polymyositis. Inflammatory pseudotumor in the region of the lacrimal gland accounts for about 15% of all orbital pseudotumors (Fig. 9-107).[156, 164] Although this disease is rare in the very young, the age variation is quite wide. The most common symptoms include proptosis, swollen lids,

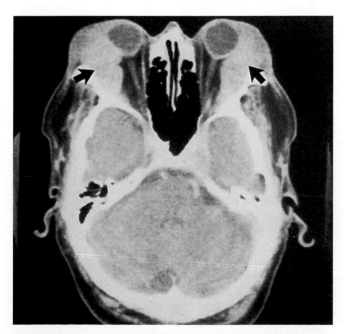

**FIGURE 9-166** Lacrimal gland pseudotumor. An 80-year-old patient with swelling of both eyes. Axial postcontrast CT scan shows bilateral lobular enlargement of the lacrimal glands (*arrows*).

pain, and diplopia, and in the majority of patients the duration of symptoms is less than 6 months. Wegener's granulomatosis is characterized by necrotizing granulomas of the respiratory tract, renal failure, and a disseminated focal necrotizing angiitis of small arteries and veins.[24, 82, 165] Ocular involvement in Wegener's granulomatosis is common, affecting 40% of patients with generalized disease.[24, 82] Involvement of the lacrimal gland is not uncommon (Fig. 9-91). Histologic examination of involved lacrimal glands shows infiltration with histiocytes, plasma cells, lymphocytes, polymorphs, and eosinophils, with giant cell formation.[24, 164] Massive enlargement of lacrimal glands may be present and has been demonstrated on CT.[24, 164] Lymphomatous lesions of the lacrimal gland include a broad spectrum ranging from reactive lymphoid hyperplasia to malignant lymphomas of various types (Fig. 9-167). It can be very difficult to differentiate pathologically between benign lymphocytic infiltration and lymphoma other than to note in a general way that lymphomas tend to occur in older patients. Shield et al., in a review of 645 space-occupying orbital lesions that underwent biopsy, found 71 cases of lymphocytic and plasmacytic lesions.[165, 166] Of these, 12 were located in the lacrimal gland.

Benign mixed lacrimal gland tumors tend to occur in patients in the third to sixth decades of life. The tumors present with slowly progressive, painless upper lid swelling, proptosis, or both, without inflammatory symptoms or signs (Fig. 9-168). Malignant tumors also occur but may not be diagnosed as such on imaging unless there is adjacent bone destruction.

## Diagnostic Imaging

Inflammatory lesions of the lacrimal gland cause diffuse enlargement of the gland. Contrast enhancement may be marked, and there may be associated acute lateral rectus muscle myositis. There may be associated scleritis with fluid in Tenon's space and a ring of uveoscleral enhancement. In chronic dacryoadenitis, the gland also shows diffuse oblong enlargement (Figs. 9-165 and 9-166). The glands may be massively enlarged in cases of sarcoidosis (Figs. 9-165), or in other conditions such as Mikulicz's syndrome, pseudotu-

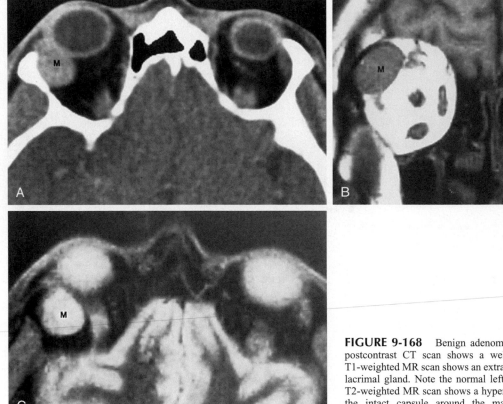

**FIGURE 9-168**  Benign adenoma of the lacrimal gland. **A,** Axial postcontrast CT scan shows a well-defined mass (*M*). **B,** Coronal T1-weighted MR scan shows an extraconal mass (*M*) involving the right lacrimal gland. Note the normal left lacrimal gland (*arrow*). **C,** Axial T2-weighted MR scan shows a hyperintense lacrimal mass (*M*). Notice the intact capsule around the mass, which is delineated by the hypointensity of the surrounding orbital fat and lateral orbital bone.

mor (Fig. 9-166), and Wegener's granulomatosis.[24, 82, 164] However, in these patients, scleral enhancement is not an associated feature, as it is in patients with acute inflammation.

Benign and malignant lymphoid tumors situated in the lacrimal gland also display diffuse enlargement with oblong contouring of the gland (Fig. 9-107).[24, 164] However, these lesions are usually bulky (Fig. 9-110), frequently have anterior and posterior extension, and mold and drape themselves on the globe. In general, inflammatory processes and lymphomas tend to involve all aspects of the lacrimal

gland, often including its palpebral lobe (Figs. 9-107 and 9-110). By comparison, neoplastic lesions rarely originate in the palpebral lobe of the gland, and therefore there is often only posterior extension of the mass rather than anterior growth beyond the orbital rim (Figs. 9-168 to 9-170).

Because the lacrimal gland is histologically similar to a salivary gland, the diseases that affect these glands are similar and epithelial tumors represent 50% of the masses involving the lacrimal gland.[24, 160, 164] Half of these tumors are pleomorphic (benign mixed) adenomas, and the other half are malignant lesions. Of the malignant tumors,

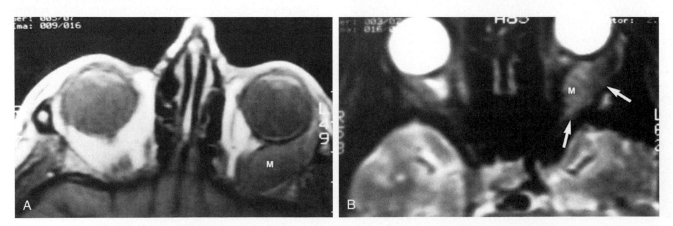

**FIGURE 9-169**  Adenocarcinoma of the lacrimal gland. **(A)** Axial T1-weighted MR scan and **(B)** Axial T2-weighted MR scan show a large mass (*M*). The lateral orbital wall is irregular (*arrows*). CT scans showed erosion of bone.

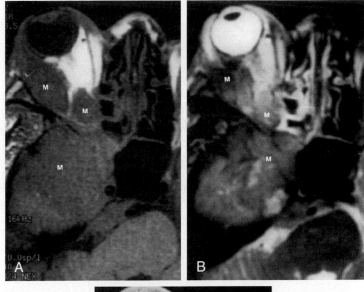

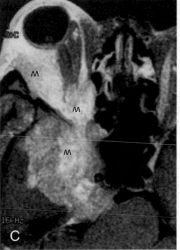

**FIGURE 9-170**   Adenoid cystic carcinoma of lacrimal gland. A 42-year-old man with decreased vision and painless proptosis of the right eye. A presumptive diagnosis of cavernous meningioma was made based on MR study (not shown). **A**, One year later, the patient returned for a follow-up study. Clinically, the right eye was grossly proptotic. Unenhanced axial T1-weighted MR image shows infiltrating soft-tissue mass (*M*) extending into right middle cranial fossa with involvement of adjacent cavernous sinus. **B**, Axial T2-weighted MR image shows that the mass (*M*) is isointense to brain. **C**, Axial-enhanced T1-weighted MR image shows diffuse enhancement of the mass (*M*). (From Mafee MF et al. Lacrimal gland tumors and simulating lesions. Radiol Clin North Am 1999;37:219–239.)

adenocystic carcinoma is the most common, followed by pleomorphic (malignant mixed tumor, carcinoma ex-pleomorphic adenoma), mucoepidermoid carcinoma, adenocarcinoma (Fig. 9-167), squamous cell carcinoma, and undifferentiated (anaplastic) carcinoma. A significant number of these tumors arise within pleomorphic adenomas as carcinoma ex-pleomorphic adenomas.[24, 158] Benign mixed tumors may undergo spontaneous malignant degeneration and are increasingly likely to undergo such malignant degeneration the longer they exist.[158, 161, 165] In such a malignant mixed tumor, the malignant cell clone develops from the preexisting benign mixed tumor, and the malignancy is often a poorly differentiated adenocarcinoma or an adenoid cystic carcinoma.[24, 164] In general, patients with these carcinomas have a poor prognosis.[24, 157]

In 1979 Stewart et al. described a scheme for the clinical diagnosis and management of lacrimal fossa pathology that classified these lesions using distinguishing clinical features and plain film radiographs.[157] Jakobiec et al.[161] performed a study evaluating the clinical and CT findings in 39 patients with four different kinds of lacrimal gland swelling. Sixteen of these patients had a parenchymal benign or malignant tumor. This study added a new diagnostic criterion, the

"contour analysis" of the shape of the mass, as a factor to be combined with the clinical history. Stewart et al. reviewed 31 cases of benign and malignant lacrimal gland masses.[157] Fourteen patients had benign mixed lacrimal gland tumors, and 13 had pressure changes characterized by enlargement of the lacrimal fossa without destruction of bone. Sclerosis of bone was present in one patient. Malignant neoplasms accounted for 17 of the 31 tumors. Twelve patients had pressure changes, two had no bone changes, and three showed destructive changes. Three patients with pressure changes and malignant tumors had calcification in the lacrimal gland fossa. Two patients had sclerosis of bone adjacent to the lacrimal fossa.

In the series of Jakobiec et al.,[161] benign tumors had smooth, encapsulated outlines, whereas the malignant tumors displayed microserrations indicative of infiltration. In their series, inflammatory conditions demonstrated diffuse, compressed, and molded enlargement of the lacrimal gland in an oblong fashion, and there were no associated bone defects. This study concluded that well-encapsulated, rounded masses of long duration were likely to be benign mixed tumors. The epithelial neoplasms probably began unicentrally within the lacrimal gland and

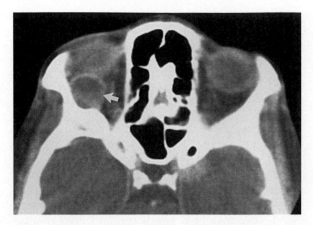

**FIGURE 9-171**    Lacrimal gland cyst. Axial CT scan shows a lacrimal gland cyst (*arrow*). This epithelial cyst developed in the orbital component of the lacrimal gland. (From Mafee MF et al. Lacrimal gland tumors and simulating lesions. Radiol Clin North Am 1999;37:219–239.)

grew in a centrifugal fashion in all directions, sometimes indenting the globe, distorting its muscle cone, and creating fossa or bone destruction in the orbital walls.[161] By contrast, inflammatory and lymphoid lesions of the lacrimal gland were seen as diffuse expansions of the lacrimal gland, and the lesions molded themselves to preexisting orbital structures without eroding bone or enlarging the orbit.[161, 164] The study found that the stroma of the epithelial tumors was often hyalinized or even cartilaginous and that this tissue was less likely than inflammatory or lymphoid tissue to mold, in a putty-like fashion, to the isthmus between the globe and the orbital bone.[161, 164]

Bony changes in the lacrimal gland fossa may be produced by either benign or malignant epithelial tumors.[24] However, bone changes also can be produced by a lacrimal gland cyst (Fig. 9-171) and by other orbital lesions such as schwannoma, neurofibroma, fibrous histiocytoma, and lesions originating within the subperiosteal space or bone such as a benign orbital cyst, hematic cyst (Fig. 9-172), cholesterol granuloma, LCH (in particular eosinophilic granuloma), dermoid cyst, epidermoid cyst, or metastatic carcinoma.[161] Lymphoid and inflammatory processes rarely produce bone changes.[24]

## MISCELLANEOUS LACRIMAL GLAND LESIONS

### Amyloid Tumor of the Lacrimal Gland

Infiltration of the lacrimal gland with amyloid is a very uncommon disorder.[164] Amyloidosis of the lacrimal gland and orbit usually is associated with the primary localized variant of the disorder, although it can be seen as a secondary form of the disease due to degeneration and amyloid depositions.[164] Isolated lacrimal gland involvement is rare and may mimic inflammatory, infiltrative, and even neoplastic diseases of the lacrimal gland. The CT and MR imaging findings of lacrimal gland amyloidosis consist of an enlarged lacrimal gland with or without calcification. Amorphous calcification of the lacrimal gland should raise the possibility of

lacrimal amyloidosis (Fig. 9-94A), and calcifications may also be multiple, resembling phleboliths.[164]

### Kimura's Disease

Kimura's disease is a chronic self-limited inflammatory condition of unknown etiology and a rare cause of a tumor-like mass in the head and neck.[164] Kimura et al.[167] reported this entity in 1948. Kimura's disease was long regarded as synonymous with angiolymphoid hyperplasia with eosinophilia; however, it is now clear that they are separate entities despite having some similar histologic features (also see Chapter 36).[164] Patients typically present with painless tumor-like nodules in the head and neck region, often associated with regional lymphadenopathy. Peripheral blood eosinophilia and an elevated serum level of IgE are almost always present.[164] Histologically, Kimura's disease is characterized by a mixed lymphoeosinophilic infiltration, reactive lymphoid follicles, ill-defined fibrosis, and capillary proliferation. Major salivary glands as well as the lacrimal gland may be involved in Kimura's disease.[164] The CT appearance of Kimura's disease is shown in Figure 9-173. The differential diagnosis of Kimura's disease of the lacrimal gland includes dacryoadenitis, sarcoidosis, pseudotumor, lymphoma, and lacrimal gland and fossa tumors.[164]

## SECONDARY ORBITAL TUMORS

Malignant tumors of the sinonasal cavities may invade the orbit directly. Tumors of the skin of the face, such as basal cell and squamous cell carcinomas and malignant melanoma, can invade the orbit. The inferior orbital fissure is a pathway for tumors arising from or extending into the pterygopalatine or infratemporal fossae. Adenoid cystic tumors of the oral cavity and sinonasal cavities, as well as squamous cell carcinoma and lymphoma of the sinonasal-oral cavities, can extend along the perineural-perivascular pathways into the pterygopalatine fossa and then into the

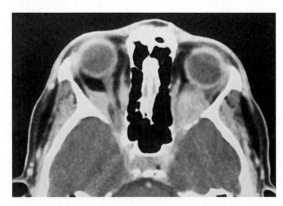

**FIGURE 9-172**    Bilateral orbital metastases from a carcinoma of the breast. Axial postcontrast CT scan through the midorbits demonstrates a homogeneous mass in the retrobulbar space of the left orbit with no bony involvement. Note partial obliteration of the extraocular muscles and the optic nerve. There is asymmetric enlargement of the mid- to posterior portion of the right lateral rectus muscle. (Courtesy of Mahmood Mafee, MD, University of Illinois at Chicago, Chicago, Illinois. From Carroll GS, Barrett GH, Fleming JC, et al. Peripheral Nerve Tumors of the Orbit. Radiol Clin North Am 1999 Jan;37(1):166.)

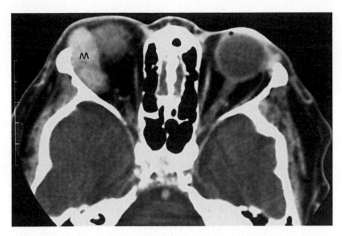

**FIGURE 9-173**   Kimura disease. Axial-enhanced CT scan shows moderate enhancement of a right lacrimal gland mass (*M*). This may not be differentiated from lymphoma, pseudotumor, sarcoid, Wegener's granuloma and even epithelial tumor of lacrimal gland. (From Mafee MF et al. Lacrimal gland tumors and simulating lesions. Radiol Clin North Am 1999;37:219–239.)

orbit. Intracranial lesions such as meningioma may extend through the posterolateral wall of the orbit, the optic canal, the sphenoid fissures, the ethmoidal foramina, or less resistant bony walls such as the lamina papyracea and orbital roof. Metastases to the orbit are most commonly the result of breast carcinoma in women (Fig. 9-172) and carcinoma of the lung, kidney, or prostate in men (Fig. 9-174). In children, metastases are from primary neuroblastoma, Ewing's sarcoma, and Wilms' tumor. Metastases can simulate primary tumors, myositis, or diffuse orbital pseudotumor (notably breast carcinoma), and a multiplicity of lesions can be helpful in suggesting the diagnosis of metastatic disease. Metastatic lesions may occur in any of the orbital compartments.[168] At times, a metastatic deposit may be single and well defined, simulating benign orbital tumors. This appearance has been seen in patients with known or unknown primary malignant melanoma and carcinoid tumor. In patients who have undergone enucleation for malignant uveal melanoma, retinoblastoma, and ocular medulloepithelioma, any tumor mass within the surgical bed should be considered a metastatic recurrence.

## ADDITIONAL PATHOLOGIES OF THE EXTRAOCULAR MUSCLES

### Ocular Motility Disorders

Ocular muscle disturbances (strabismus) are relatively common, occurring at a rate of approximately 2% to 4%.[15] While the onset is usually in infancy or early childhood, acquired forms may occur at any age. If the object being viewed does not fall on the macula of both eyes, strabismus exists and the position of the nonaligned eye determines the description of the type of deviation (esotropia = inward deviation, exotropia = outward deviation; vertical imbalance described as hyper- or hypotropia).[15]

Strabismus is frequently divided into two types based on the diagnostic and therapeutic implications. In comitant

types of strabismus, movement is not limited in any field of gaze, nor is there evidence of a paretic muscle. The etiology is thought to be abnormalities in higher brain centers. By contrast, noncomitant strabismus is characterized by limited ocular movement due to lesions involving the brainstem, cerebral centers, or cranial nerves; to muscle damage; or to any process causing restricted movement of the EOMs and resulting in asymmetric movements. These two possible etiologies of noncomitant strabismus, neurologic and restrictive, can often be distinguished by a forced duction test that shows no impediment to passive movement of the eye with forceps when there is neurologic damage compared to limitation on attempted movement of the globe in restrictive disease of the EOM. For example, in a diabetic lateral rectus palsy, the eye may be passively moved freely, whereas in thyroid myopathy, when an attempt is made to rotate the eye with a forceps, the examiner experiences restriction to movement in one or more fields of gaze.[15]

The use of CT and MR imaging has improved our understanding of many congenital and acquired conditions causing strabismus. This results in more appropriate therapeutic intervention and gives insight into the pathophysiology of these conditions.[15]

When evaluating the relative size of EOMs, particularly the horizontal muscles (the medial rectus and lateral rectus), it is important to know where the patient is fixing his or her gaze at the time of scanning. The Sherrington law of reciprocal innervation states that when the agonist muscle contracts, an inhibitory impulse is sent to the antagonist muscle, which then relaxes and lengthens. These actions are essential for normal full range of ocular movement. Therefore, when the patient is looking at the right field of gaze, there is an increase in the size of the contracting right lateral and left medial rectus muscles and a decrease in the relaxed left lateral and right medial rectus muscles. If this is not appreciated when analyzing the CT scan, an inappropriate diagnosis of an enlarged muscle can be made (Fig. 9-12). In most clinical situations, it is preferable to have the patient fix his or her gaze in the straight-ahead position, and it is

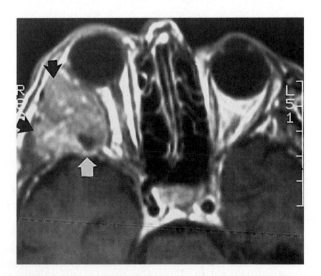

**FIGURE 9-174**   Orbital metastasis from a malignant histiocytoma. Axial-enhanced T1-weighted MR image shows a metastatic deposit involving the lateral wall of the right orbit (*arrows*).

useful to place some fixation target at a center point in the scanner unit.

## Acquired Ocular Motility Disturbances Associated with Orbital Pathology

Many patients with classic hyperthyroidism show no ocular muscle involvement; conversely, patients manifesting severe eye muscle restriction often have normal thyroid function but are considered to have a form of euthyroid myopathy. Progressive limitation of movement may occur many years after active thyroid disease, or it may be the presenting symptom of thyroid dysfunction. Orbital myositis is a nonspecific orbital inflammation involving one or more EOMs, with characteristic clinical and CT findings, and it is often very responsive to systemic corticosteroids. Patients with orbital myositis or other conditions may present with an onset of limitation of ductions (monocular movement in test fields of gaze) in one or both eyes, with variable signs of inflammation and proptosis.[15] These conditions include carotid-cavernous fistula, infectious cellulitis, lymphomas, retrobulbar masses such as cavernous hemangioma, and occasional metastatic disease. In patients with carotid-cavernous sinus fistula resulting from an abnormal communication between the carotid arterial system and the cavernous sinus, orbital venous congestion occurs, with subsequent swelling of the EOMs and mechanical interference with movement. There may also be an associated neurologic palsy, especially of the sixth cranial nerve. CT and MR imaging may demonstrate enlarged EOMs in these patients with generalized ophthalmopathy that will revert to normal after closure of the fistula. Other lesions of the cavernous sinus such as aneurysm may also be responsible for limitation of ductions.[15]

### Brown's Superior Oblique Tendon Sheath Syndrome

In 1973, Brown described a clinical syndrome (superior oblique tendon sheath or Brown's syndrome) characterized by an impaired ability to raise the eye in adduction. Typically, the patient may have straight eyes or a hypotropia (one eye lower in the primary position). Brown further classified this condition into true and simulated syndromes.[169] True (congenital) Brown's syndrome includes only those patients with a congenitally short or taut superior oblique tendon sheath complex. Patients with simulated (acquired) Brown's syndrome acquire the clinical features of the syndrome secondary to a variety of etiologies. Most authors, including Brown, have postulated that acquired Brown's syndrome is primarily a disease of the tendon sheath–trochlear complex of the superior oblique muscle secondary to an inflammatory process of the adjacent tissues.

Normal ocular movement of the superior oblique muscle requires a loose sheath and free movement of the tendon in the sheath. When the eye is adducted, the primary action of the inferior oblique muscle is elevation. When the eye is elevated in the adducted position, the superior oblique muscle normally relaxes, causing its tendon to lengthen and slide freely through the trochlea. If the superior oblique muscle cannot relax or its tendon cannot lengthen, the eye cannot be elevated while adducted. This limitation of elevation in adduction simulates an inferior oblique palsy, although the pathologic process is postulated to be located primarily in the superior oblique complex. This restriction in the physiologic passage of the tendon through the trochlea may be permanent or occur on an intermittent basis in the acquired form.

In acquired Brown's syndrome, the symptoms and findings often are intermittent. Affected patients usually complain of intermittent double vision (diplopia) on upward gaze and sometimes a "clicking" sensation in the area of the trochlea when attempting to look up (Fig. 9-175).

The CT appearance may show abnormalities in the area of the trochlea in acquired Brown's syndrome (Figs. 9-175 and 9-176). One patient who had a history of head trauma showed significant thickening of the reflected portion of the superior oblique tendon in the involved eye (Fig. 9-175), which was confirmed at the time of surgery.[169] The association of acquired Brown's syndrome and rheumatoid arthritis has been well documented in the literature and may spontaneously disappear (Fig. 9-177).

The CT scan enables an evaluation of three features of the superior oblique muscle: (1) the angle that the reflected tendon makes with the medial wall of the orbit; (2) the thickness of the tendon; and (3) the density of the tendon compared with that of surrounding tissues.[170] Under normal circumstances, these characteristics are nearly equal in both eyes. The CT scan makes this comparison of both eyes possible in a manner that no other procedure allows. The angle of the reflected tendon may be altered by surgery. CT scanning may also be used to compare the angle of the reflected tendon with the clinical function of the superior oblique muscles and to determine damage to the trochlear region. However, in congenital Brown's syndrome, relatively little abnormality of the superior oblique tendon has thus far been demonstrated by CT scan.

### Double Elevator Palsy

Double elevator palsy is a weakness of both elevators of the same eye (weakness of superior rectus and inferior oblique muscles is almost always congenital and is characterized by limited elevation through the entire upper field). There have been very few descriptions of CT findings in these patients, but two interesting cases showed a small superior rectus muscle, although the inferior oblique muscle could not be definitely identified (Fig. 9-178). Interestingly, one patient also had a large inferior rectus muscle. It is not known whether the size change is primary or secondary in nature. Congenital double elevator palsy must be differentiated from acquired conditions that cause a restriction in upward gaze, such as a blowout fracture of the orbital floor, a downwardly displaced superior orbital wall fracture with impingement on the globe, atypical Brown's syndrome, or endocrine myopathy with involvement of the interior rectus. This differentiation can be aided by forced duction testing and the radiographic findings. Patients with symptomatic double elevator palsy may require muscle-transposing surgery in the affected eye.

### Other Causes

Myositis of the EOMs with proptosis and signs of orbital inflammation have also been reported with systemic lupus erythematosus; proptosis has been noted with dermatomyo-

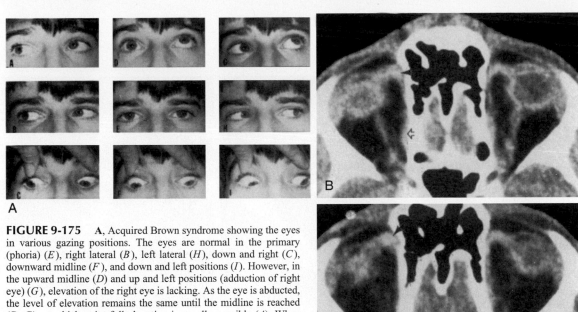

**FIGURE 9-175** **A,** Acquired Brown syndrome showing the eyes in various gazing positions. The eyes are normal in the primary (phoria) (*E*), right lateral (*B*), left lateral (*H*), down and right (*C*), downward midline (*F*), and down and left positions (*I*). However, in the upward midline (*D*) and up and left positions (adduction of right eye) (*G*), elevation of the right eye is lacking. As the eye is abducted, the level of elevation remains the same until the midline is reached (*D, G*), at which point full elevation is usually possible (*A*). When the eye is adducted nasally (*G*) from the primary position (*E*), the primary action of the inferior oblique muscle is elevation; thus, lack of elevation of the right eye during adduction (*G*), as in this patient, simulates paralysis of the right inferior oblique tendon, which is the hallmark of Brown syndrome. This actually represents "pseudoparalysis" because the cause is not dysfunction of the right inferior oblique muscle but rather inadequate relaxation of its antagonist, the right superior oblique muscle. **B,** Axial CT scan demonstrates thickening of the reflected portion of the right superior oblique tendon (*arrowhead*). The belly of the superior oblique muscle can be seen on each side (*hollow arrow*). **C,** Scan taken 1.5 mm higher demonstrates marked thickening of the reflected tendon (*arrow*). (From Mafee MF, Folk ER, Langer BG, et al.: Computed tomography in the evaluation of Brown syndrome of the superior oblique tendon sheath. Radiology 1985;154:691–695.)

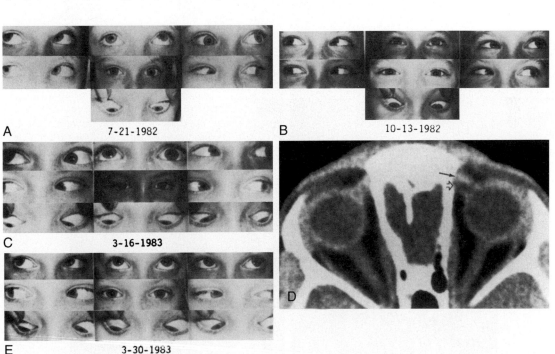

**FIGURE 9-176** **A,** Congenital Brown syndrome showing the eyes in various gazing positions. Note the markedly limited elevation of the right eye in the upward midline position (*top middle*), which is even more pronounced on adduction of the right eye (*top right*). **B,** Eleven months after tenotomy of the right superior oblique muscle, elevation is markedly improved on both adduction and abduction. **C,** Acquired Brown syndrome developed on the opposite side following trauma. Note the limited elevation of the left eye in the straight-up position (*top middle*) and during adduction (*top right*). **D,** Axial CT scan demonstrates slight thickening of the reflected portion of the left superior oblique tendon (*arrow*). The open arrow points to area of edema. **E,** After 2 weeks of steroid therapy, elevation is markedly improved on both adduction and abduction. (From Mafee MF, Folk ER, Langer BG, et al.: Computed tomography in the evaluation of Brown syndrome of the superior oblique tendon sheath. Radiology 1985;154:691–695.)

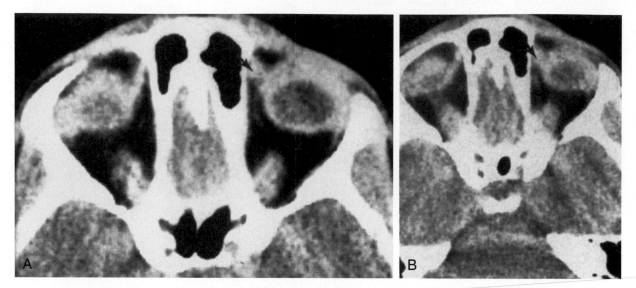

**FIGURE 9-177**   **A**, Axial CT scan demonstrates thickening of the reflected portion of the left superior oblique tendon (*arrow*). **B**, Scan taken 1.5 mm higher confirms the marked tendon thickening (*arrow*). (From Mafee MF, Folk ER, Langer BG, et al.: Computed tomography in the evaluation of Brown syndrome of the superior oblique tendon sheath. Radiology 1985;154:691–695.)

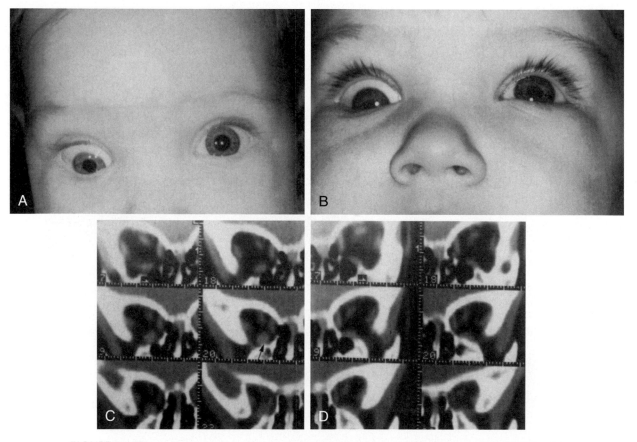

**FIGURE 9-178**   **A**, Double elevator palsy. Right hypotropia in the primary position in a patient with congenital double elevator palsy of the right eye. (Courtesy of D. Mittelman, MD.) **B**, Note limitation of elevation of the right eye. (Courtesy of D. Mittelman, MD.) **C**, Double elevator palsy. Serial reformatted coronal images showing enlarged right inferior rectus muscle. The superior rectus muscle is quite thin and hardly recognized as a distinct image. **D**, Serial reformatted coronal images of the normal left eye of the same patient in **C** for comparison.

sitis. Other rare causes of EOM enlargement include Crohn's colitis, sarcoidosis, cysticercosis, and carcinoma metastatic to an ocular muscle. CT studies have shown large EOMs in many cases of acromegaly. The increased size appeared to be related to the disease duration but not to growth hormone levels. These muscle findings have been observed even in treated cases.

Tychsen and coworkers described a group of patients with tenderness over the trochlea and discomfort on movement of the eye. CT scans demonstrated a soft-tissue density in the area of the trochlea that was believed to represent a localized subtype of idiopathic orbital inflammation.[171]

## Traumatic Injury of Ocular Muscles

### Blowout Fracture

The classic blowout fracture involves the floor of the orbit, usually sparing the orbital rim (see Chapter 7). Frequently, orbital tissues are trapped in the fracture site and ocular motility disturbances have been ascribed to entrapment of one or both inferior EOMs, but clinical and surgical experience has not supported the entrapment etiology of restricted ocular movement in many cases. Early positive forced duction tests do not necessarily prove entrapment, and these disturbances may be the result of hematoma or inflammation. Soft-tissue damage may play a significant role in causing the typical findings of a blowout fracture.

## Congenital Anomalies of the Extraocular Muscles

### Congenital Syndromes

Ocular motility disturbances frequently occur in craniosynostosis syndromes, and the observed patterns of abnormal movement are characteristically predictable. This is particularly true for the craniosynostosis syndromes of Apert and Crouzon. The type of abnormal movement noted in these two groups may be affected by mechanical factors induced by abnormal anatomy but also may show abnormalities in the size of muscles and the location of insertion.

Apert's and Crouzon's syndromes usually show strabismus in the primary position in addition to the presence of a V pattern, with an exotropia in the up position and straight eyes or esotropia in the down position, thus producing a V configuration. Most patients also have an associated overaction of the inferior oblique muscles and show limitation of movement in the field of action of the superior rectus and superior oblique muscles. This pattern (V) of ocular muscle imbalance is not unique to patients with certain craniofacial anomalies; it is present in many patients without bony abnormalities. What is unparalleled is the frequency of craniosynostosis patients who manifest this abnormality.

Another somewhat unexpected and well-documented finding in vertical ocular muscle imbalance in craniosynostosis patients is abnormal insertion or structure of the muscle. A number of case reports have noted the apparent absence of vertically acting muscles at the time of surgery. Diamond and coworkers reported EOM anomalies (primarily of the inferior and superior rectus muscles) in 42% of their patients with craniofacial dysostosis. Orbital high-resolution CT scanning with thin cuts (1 to 1.5 mm) demonstrates changes in the location and/or the size of EOMs. Axial, coronal, and sagittal projections are useful in obtaining an accurate estimate of the degree of abnormality. Patients with gross limitation of movement are most likely to demonstrate CT scan abnormalities. This type of evaluation is indicated to plan appropriate surgical procedures if ocular motility surgery is contemplated or to plan alternatives if the ocular muscles cannot be located.

## Noncomitant Strabismus Without Associated Malformations

A few studies have utilized CT analysis of the EOMs in normal subjects, with attention to variation in size and location. This method of analysis has also been used to evaluate the position or slippage of the muscles as the eyes move to different gaze positions.

In some types of routine comitant strabismus, the degree of horizontal deviation is noted to change when the patient looks up and down. If there is a significant difference in the amount of esotropia (or exotropia) in upgaze and downgaze, the patient is described as having an A or V syndrome. Since a V pattern has been observed in most patients with craniosynostosis deviation, it has been postulated that this may be caused or enhanced by an abnormal vertical insertion of the horizontal recti. Following this reasoning, some strabismus patients who manifested a V or A pattern of horizontal strabismus, but did not have any evidence of craniofacial anomalies, were evaluated by CT. One group of investigators noted some change in the position of the horizontal recti in these patients. Further data are necessary to understand these relationships.

Diagnostic imaging studies such as CT and MR imaging are invaluable tools to demonstrate orbital and EOM anatomy in cases of strabismus following trauma or surgery, or loss of rectus muscle function following strabismus surgery, retinal detachment surgery, or ocular trauma. Traumatic disruption of the orbital tissues can simulate a lost muscle by many different mechanisms: severed nerves, neuropraxia, muscle crush, muscle entrapment in an orbital wall fracture, muscle slippage, muscle fibrosis and contracture, edema, hemorrhage, and adhesions. When an EOM is surrounded by tissue edema, hemorrhage, granulation tissue, or scar tissue, there may not be sufficient contrast to differentiate muscle from adjacent tissue by CT and MR imaging. When diagnostic imaging fails to reveal the muscle in question, however, exploratory surgery should still be considered before the diagnosis of lost muscle is accepted.

## REFERENCES

1. Warwick R, Williams PL. Gray's Anatomy, 35th British ed. Philadelphia: WB Saunders, 1973;145–147.
2. Snell RS, Lemp MA (eds). Clinical Anatomy of the Eye. Boston: Blackwell Scientific, 1989;1–15.
3. Rootman J, ed. Diseases of the Orbit. Philadelphia: JB Lippincott, 1988.

4. Reeh MJ, Wobij JL, Wirtschafter JD. Ophthalmic Anatomy: A Manual with Some Clinical Applications. San Francisco: American Academy of Ophthalmology, 1981;11–54.

5. Smith MF. Orbit, eyelids, and lacrimal system. Basic and Clinical Science Course. San Francisco: American Academy of Ophthalmology, 1987–1988.

6. Wilson FM. Fundamentals and principles of ophthalmology. Basic and Clinical Science Course. San Francisco: American Academy of Ophthalmology, 1991–1992.

7. Daniels DL, Yu S, Pech P, et al. Computed tomography and magnetic resonance imaging of the orbital apex. Radiol Clin North Am 1987;25:803–817.

8. Mafee MF, Putterman A, Valvassori GE, et al. Orbital space-occupying lesions: role of CT and MRI, an analysis of 145 cases. Radiol Clin North Am 1987;25:529–559.

9. Canalis RF, Burstein FD. Osteogenesis in vascularized periosteum. Arch Otolaryngol 1985;3:511–518.

10. Duhamel HL. Sur le development et la crue des os des animax. Mem Acad R Sci 1742;55:354–370.

11. Mafee MF, Miller MT. Computed tomography scanning in the evaluation of ocular motility disorders. In: Gonzalez CF, Becker MH, Flanagan JC, eds. Diagnostic Imaging in Ophthalmology. New York: Springer-Verlag, 1985;39–54.

12. Dale RT, ed. Fundamentals of Ocular Motility and Strabismus. New York: Grune & Stratton, 1982.

13. Helveston EM, Merriam WW, Ellis FD, et al. The trochlea: a study of the anatomy and pathology. Ophthalmology 1982;89:124–133.

14. Fink WH. The anatomy of the extrinsic muscles of the eye. In: Allen JH, ed. Strabismus Ophthalmic Symposium. St. Louis: CV Mosby, 1950;17–62.

15. Miller TM, Mafee MF. Computed tomography scanning in the evaluation of ocular motility disorders. Radiol Clin North Am 1987;25:733–752.

16. Snell RS, Lemp MA, eds. Clinical Anatomy of the Eye. Boston: Blackwell Scientific, 1989.

17. Mafee MF. Imaging of the orbit. In: Valvassori GE, Mafee MF, Carter B, eds. Imaging of the Head and Neck. Stuttgart: Georg Thieme, 1995;248–327.

18. Zonneveld FW, Koorneef L, Hillen B, et al. Direct Multiplanar, High Resolution, Thin-Section CT of the Orbit. Eindhoven: Philips Medical Systems, 1986.

19. Mafee MF, Pruzansky S, Corrales MM, et al. CT in the evaluation of the orbit and the bony interorbital distance. AJNR 1986;7:265–269.

20. Mafee MF, Kumar A, Tahmoressi CN, et al. Direct sagittal CT in the evaluation of temporal bone disease. AJNR 1988;9:371–378.

21. Barakow JA, Dillon WP, Chew WM. Orbit, skull base and pharynx: contrast-enhanced fat suppression MR imaging. Radiology 1991;179:191–198.

22. Tien RD, Hesselink JR, Szumowski J. MR fat suppression combined with Gd-DTPA enhancement in optic neuritis and perineuritis. J Comput Assist Tomogr 1991;15:223–227.

23. Tien RD, Chu PK, Hesselink JR, et al. Intra- and paraorbital lesions: value of fat-suppression MR imaging with paramagnetic contrast enhancement. AJNR 1992;12:245–253.

24. Mafee MF, Haik BG. Lacrimal gland and fossa lesions: role of computed tomography. Radiol Clin North Am 1987;25:767–779.

25. Langer BG, Mafee MF, Pollack S, et al. MRI of the normal orbit and optic pathway. Radiol Clin North Am 1987;25:429–446.

26. Zonneveld FW, Koornneef L, Hiller B, et al. Normal direct multiplanar CT anatomy of the orbit with correlative anatomic cryosections. Radiol Clin North Am 1987;25:381–407.

27. Ettl A, Salomonowitz E, Koornneef L, Zonneveld FW. High resolution MR imaging anatomy of the orbit. Correlation with comparative cryosectional anatomy. Radiol Clin North Am 1998;36:1021–1045.

28. Currario G, Silverman FN. Orbital hypotelorism, arhinencephaly, and trigoncephaly. Radiology 1960;74:206–216.

29. Gerald BE, Silverman FN. Normal and abnormal interorbital distances with special reference to mongolism. AJR 1956;95:154–161.

30. Morin J, Hiu J, Anderson J, et al. A study of growth in the interorbital region. Am J Ophthalmol 1936;56:895–901.

31. Cameron J. Interorbital width: new cranial dimension, its significance in modern and fossil man and in lower mammals. Am J Phys Anthropol 1931;15:509–515.

32. Hansman CF. Growth of interorbital distance and skull thickness as observed in roentgenographic measurements. Radiology 1966;86:87–96.

33. Linder B, Campos M, Schafer M. CT and MRI of orbital abnormalities in neurofibromatosis and selected craniofacial anomalies. Radiol Clin North Am 1987;25:787–802.

34. Converse JM, McCarthy JG. Orbital hypertelorism. Scand J Plast Reconstr Surg 1985;15:265–276.

35. DeMyer WM. Neurologic evaluation associated forebrain maldevelopment and orbital hypotelorism. In: Symposium on Diagnosis and Treatment of Craniofacial Anomalies, Vol. 20. St. Louis: CV Mosby, 1979;153–163.

36. Becker MH, McCarthy JG. Congenital abnormalities. In: Gonzalez CF, Becker MH, Flanagan JC, eds. Diagnostic Imaging in Ophthalmology. New York: Springer-Verlag, 1985;115–187.

37. Gorlin RJ, Pindberg JJ, Cohen MM Jr. Syndromes of the Head and Neck, 2nd ed. New York: McGraw-Hill, 1976.

38. Smith DW. Recognizable Patterns of Human Malformation. Philadelphia: WB Saunders, 1970.

39. Taybi H. Radiology of Syndromes and Metabolic Disorders, 2nd ed. St. Louis: CV Mosby, 1983.

40. Mafee MF, Jampol LM, Langer BG, et al. Computed tomography of optic nerve colobomas: morning glory anomaly, and colobomatous cyst. Radiol Clin North Am 1987;25:693–699.

41. Mann I. Developmental Abnormalities of the Eye, 2nd ed. Philadelphia: JB Lippincott, 1957;74–78.

42. Mann I. The Development of the Human Eye. New York: Grune & Stratton, 1969.

43. Brown G, Tasman W, eds. Congenital Anomalies of the Optic Disc. New York: Grune & Stratton, 1983;97–191.

44. Arey LB. Developmental Anatomy, 6th ed. Philadelphia: WB Saunders, 1970.

45. Duke-Elder S, Wybar KC. System of Ophthalmology: The Anatomy of the Visual System, Vol. 2. St. Louis: CV Mosby, 1961.

46. Hamilton WJ, Boyd JD, Mossman HW, eds. Human Embryology: Development of Form and Function, 3rd ed. Baltimore: Williams & Wilkins, 1962.

47. Tessier P. The definitive plastic surgical treatment of the severe facial deformities of craniofacial dysostosis: Crouzon's and Apert's diseases. Plast Reconstr Surg 1971;48:419–442.

48. Campbell JA. Craniofacial anomalies. In: Newton TH, Potts DG, eds. Radiology of the Skull and Brain, Vol. 1, Book 2. St. Louis: CV Mosby, 1971;571–633.

49. Pruzansky S. Time: the fourth dimension in syndrome analysis applied to craniofacial malformations. Birth Defects 1977;13:3–28.

50. Mafee MF, Valvassori GE. Radiology of the craniofacial anomalies. Otolaryngol Clin North Am 1981;14:939–988.

51. Harwood-Nash DC. Coronal sysostosis. In: Rogers LF, ed. Disorders of the Head and Neck Syllabus. Second Series. Chicago: American College of Radiology. 1977.

52. Anderson FM, Geiger L. Craniosynostosis: a survey of 204 cases. J Neurosurg 1965;22:229–240.

53. Shillito J Jr, Matson DD. Craniosynostosis: a review of 519 surgical patients. Pediatrics 1968;41:829–853.

54. Crouzon O. Dysostose cranio-faciale hereditaire. Bull Mem Soc Med Hop (Paris) 1912;33:545–555.

55. Lombardi G. Radiology in Neuro-Ophthalmology. Baltimore: Williams & Wilkins, 1967.

56. Saethre H. Ein beitrag zum turnschadel problem (pathogenese, erblickeit und symptomatologie). Deutsch Z Nervenh 1931;119:533–555.

57. Chotzen F. Eine eigenartige familiare entwicklungsstorung (akrocephalo-syndaktylie), dysostosis craniofacialis und hypertelorisms). Mschr Kinder 1932;55:97–122.

58. Bartsocas CS, Weber AL, Crawford JD. Acrocephalosyndactyly type 3: Chotzen's syndrome. J Pediatr 1970;77:267–272.

59. Lewis A, Gerson P, Axelson K, et al. Von Recklinghausen neurofibromatosis II. Incidence of optic glioma. Ophthalmology 1984;91:929–935.

60. Zimmerman RA, Bilaniuk LT, Mezger RA, et al. Computed tomography of orbitofacial neurofibromatosis. Radiology 1983;146:113–116.

61. Kobrin JL, Block FC, Wiengiest TA. Ocular and orbital manifestations of neurofibromatosis. Surv Ophthalmol 1979;24:45–51.

62. Jacoby CG, Go RT, Beren RA. Cranial CT of neurofibromatosis. AJR 1980;135:553–557.
63. Berry GA. Note on a congenital defect (? coloboma) of the lower lid. R Lond Ophthalmol Hosp Rep 1889;12:225.
64. Treacher Collins E. Case with symmetrical congenital notches in the outer part of each lower lid and defective development of the malar bones. Trans Ophthalmol Soc 1900;20:190–191.
65. Pires de Lima JA, Monteior HB. Aparello branquiale suas pertur-bacoes evolutivas. Arch Anat Anthrop (Lisboa) 1923;8:185.
66. Francheschetti A, Klein D. The mandibulo-facial dysostosis, a new hereditary syndrome. Acta Ophthalmol 1949;27:141–224.
67. Poswillo D. The pathogenesis of the Treacher-Collins syndrome (mandibulofacial dysostosis). Br J Oral Surg 1975;13:1–26.
68. Herring SW, Rowlatt UF, Pruzansky S. Anatomical abnormalities in mandibulofacial dysostosis. Am J Med Genet 1979;3:225–259.
69. Pruzansky S, Miller M, Krammer JF. Ocular defects in craniofacial syndromes. In: Goldberg MF, ed. Genetic and Metabolic Eye Disease. Boston: Little, Brown, 1974;487, 498.
70. Henderson JW. Orbital Tumors. Philadelphia: WB Saunders, 1973;116–123.
71. Mafee MF, Dobben GD, Valvassori GE. Computed tomography assessment of paraorbital pathology. In: Gonzalez CA, Becker MH, Flanagan JC, eds. Diagnostic Imaging in Ophthalmology. New York: Springer-Verlag, 1985;281–302.
72. Grove AS. Giant dermoid cysts of the orbit. Ophthalmology 1979;86:1513–1520.
73. Kaufman LM, Villablanca JP, Mafee MR. Diagnostic imaging of cystic lesions in the child's orbit. Radiol Clin North Am 1998;36:1149–1163.
74. Rubenstein J. Disorders of the conjunctiva and limbus. In: Yanoff M, Duker JS, eds. Ophthalmology. St. Louis: CV Mosby, 1999;1.1–1.21.
75. Dutton J. Orbital diseases. In: Yanoff M, Duker JS, eds. Ophthalmology. St. Louis: CV Mosby, 1999;14.1–14.7.
76. Chang DF, Dallow RL, Walton DS. Congenital orbital teratoma: report of a case with visual preservation. J Pediatr Ophthalmol Strabismus 1980;17:88.
77. Garrity JA, Trautmann JC, Bartley GB, et al. Optic nerve sheath meningoceles: clinical and radiographic features in 13 cases with a review of the literature. Ophthalmology 1990;97:1519.
78. Laventer DB, Merriman JC, Defendini R, et al. Enterogenous cysts of the orbital apex and superior orbital fissure. Ophthalmology 1994;101:1614.
79. Dobben GD, Philip B, Mafee MF, et al. Orbital subperiosteal hematoma, cholesterol granuloma, and infection. Evaluation with MR imaging and CT. Radiol Clin North Am 1998;36:1185–1200.
80. Polito E, Leccisotti A. Diagnosis and treatment of orbital hemorrhagic lesions. Ann Ophthalmol 1994;26:85–93.
81. Gomez-Morales A, Croxatto JO, Croxatto L, et al. Hydatid cysts of the orbit: a review of 35 cases. Ophthalmology 1988;95:1027.
82. Mafee MF, Atlas SW, Galetta SL. In: Atlas SW, ed. Magnetic Resonance Imaging of the Brain and Spine, 3rd ed. Philadelphia: Lippincott Williams & Wilkins, 2002;1433–1524.
83. Weber AL, Mikulis DK. Inflammatory disorders of the paraorbital sinuses and their complications. Radiol Clin North Am 1987;25:615–630.
84. Hawkins DD, Clark RW. Orbital involvement in acute sinusitis. Clin Pediatr 1977;16(5):464–471.
85. Chandler JR, Langenbrunner DJ, Stevens ER. The pathogenesis of orbital complications in acute sinusitis. Laryngoscope 1970;80:1414.
86. Eustis HS, Mafee MF, Walton C, Mondonca J. MR imaging and CT of orbital infections and complication in acute rhinosinusitis. Radiol Clin North Am 1998;36:1165–1183.
87. Dolan RW, Choudhury K. Diagnosis and treatment of intracranial complications of paranasal sinus infection. J Oral Maxillofac Surg 1995;53:1080.
88. Igarishi H, Igarishi S, Fujio N, et al. Magnetic resonance imaging in the early diagnosis of cavernous sinus thrombosis. Ophthalmologica 1995;209:292.
89. Saah D, Schwartz A. Diagnosis of cavernous sinus thrombosis by magnetic resonance imaging using flow parameters. Ann Otol Rhinol Laryngol 1994;103:487.
90. Centeno RS, Bentson RJ, Mancuso AA. CT scanning in rhinocerebral mucormycosis and aspergillosis. Radiology 1981;140:383–389.
91. Courey WR, New PFJ, Price DL. Angiographic manifestations of craniofacial phycomycosis: report of three cases. Radiology 1972;103:329–334.
92. Weber AL, Vitale Romo L, Sabates NR. Pseudotumor of the orbit. Clinical, pathologic, and radiologic evaluation. Radiol Clin North Am 1999;37:151–168.
93. Blodi FC, Gass JDM. Inflammatory pseudotumor of the orbit. Br J Ophthalmol 1968;52:79–93.
94. Flanders AE, Mafee MF, Rao VM, et al. CT characteristics of orbital pseudotumors and other orbital inflammatory processes. J Comput Assist Tomogr 1989;13(1):40–47.
95. Birch-Hirschfield A. Zur diagnostik and pathologie der orbital-tumoren. Deutsche Ophth Ges 1905;32:127–135.
96. Motto-Lippa L, Jakobiec FA, Smith M. Idiopathic inflammatory orbital pseudotumor in childhood. II. Results of diagnostic tests and biopsies. Ophthalmology 1981;88:565–574.
97. Trokel SL, Hilal SK. Recognition and differential diagnosis of enlarged extraocular muscles in computed tomography. Am J Ophthalmol 1979;87:503–512.
98. Tolosa E. Periarthritic lesions of the carotid siphon with the clinical features of a carotid infraclinoid aneurysm. J Neurol Neurosurg Psychiatry 1954;17:300–302.
99. Hunt WE, Meagher JN, LeFever HE, et al. Painful ophthalmoplegia. Neurology 1961;11(Suppl):56–62.
100. Smith JL, Taxdal DSR. Painful ophthalmoplegia: the Tolosa-Hunt syndrome. Am J Ophthalmol 1966;61:1466–1472.
101. Sondheimer FK, Knapp J. Angiographic findings in the Tolosa-Hunt syndrome: painful ophthalmoplegia. Radiology 1973;106:105–112.
102. Hurwitz CA, Faquin WC. Case record 5-2002. N Engl J Med 2002;346(7):513–520.
103. Rubin RM, Sadun AA. Ocular myopathies. In Yanoff M, Duker JS, eds. Ophthalmology. St. Louis: CV Mosby, 1999;11.18.1–11.18.8.
104. Kendler DL, Lippa J, Rootman J. The initial clinical characteristics of Graves' orbitopathy vary with age and sex. Arch Ophthalmol 1993;111:197–201.
105. Mafee MF, Dorodi S, Pai E. Sarcoidosis of the eye, orbit, and central nervous system: role of MR imaging. Radiol Clin North Am 1999;37:73–87.
106. Mafee MF. Case 25: optic nerve sheath meningioma. In: Head and Neck Disorders (fourth series) test and syllabus. Reston, VA: American College of Radiology, 1992;552–595.
107. Shields JA, ed. Diagnosis and Management of Orbital Tumors. Philadelphia: WB Saunders, 1989.
108. Dykhuizen RS, Smith C, Kennedy MM, et al. Necrotizing sarcoid granulomatosis with extrapulmonary involvement. Eur Respir J 1997;10:245–247.
109. Raskin EM, McCormick SA, Maher EA, et al. Granulomatous idiopathic orbital inflammation. Ophthalmol Plast Reconstr Surg 1995;11:131–135.
110. Monfort-Gouraud M, Chokre R, Dubiez M, et al. Inflammatory pseudotumor of the orbit and suspected sarcoidosis. Arch Pediatr 1996;3:697–700.
111. Mombaerts I, Schlingemann RO, Goldschmeding R, Koornep L. Idiopathic granulomatous orbital inflammation. Ophthalmology 1996;103:2135–2141.
112. Carmody RF, Mafee MF, Goodwin JA, et al. Orbital and optic pathway sarcoidosis: MR findings. AJNR 1994;15:775–783.
113. Ing EB, Garrity JA, Gross SA, Ebersold MJ. Sarcoid masquerading as optic nerve sheath meningioma. Mayo Clinic Proc 1997;72:38–43.
114. Beardsley TL, Brown SV, Sydner CF, et al. Eleven cases of sarcoidosis of the optic nerve. Am J Ophthalmol 1984;97:67–77.
115. Vidal RW, Devaney K, Ferlito A, et al. Sinonasal malignant lymphomas: a distinct clinicopathological category. Ann Otol Rhinol Laryngol 1999, 108:411–419.
116. Lichtenstein L. Histiocytosis X: integration of eosinophilic granuloma of bone, "Letterer-Siwe disease" and "Hand Schuller-Christian disease" as related manifestations of a single nosologic entity. Arch Pathol 1953,56:84–102.
117. Nezelof C, Barbey S. Histiocytosis: nosology and pathobiology. Pediatr Pathol 1985;3:1–41.
118. Hidayat AA, Mafee MF, Laver NV, Noujaim S. Langerhans' cell histiocytosis and juvenile xanthogranuloma of the orbit. Clinicopathologic, CT, and MR imaging features. Radiol Clin North Am 1998;36:1229–1240.

119. Stanley SS. Taking the X out of histiocytosis X. Radiology 1997;204: 322–324.

120. Nezelof C, Basset F. Langerhans' cell histiocytosis research: past, present, and future. Hematol Oncol Clin North Am 1998;12: 385–406.

121. Zimmerman LE. Ocular lesions of juvenile xanthogranuloma. Neoxanthoendothelioma. Trans Am Acad Ophthalmol Otolaryngol 1965;69:412–442.

122. Jakobiac FA, Mills MD, Hidayat AA, et al. Periocular xanthogranulomas associated with severe adult-onset asthma. Trans Am Opthalmol Soc 1993;91:99–129.

123. Alper MG, Zimmerman LE, LaPiana FG. Orbital manifestations of Erdheim-Chester disease. Trans Am Ophthalmol Soc 1983;8:64–68.

124. Shields AK, Karcioglu ZA, Shields C, et al. Orbital and eyelid involvement with Erdheim-Chester disease: a report of two cases. Arch Ophthalmol 1991;109:850–854.

125. Tien RD, Brasch RC, Jackson DE, et al. Cerebral Erdheim-Chester disease: persistent enhancement with Gd-DTPA on MR images. Radiology 1989;172:791–792.

126. Mafee MF. Eye and orbit. In: Som PM, Curtin HD, eds. Head and Neck Imaging. St. Louis: Mosby-Yearbook, 1996;1009–1128.

127. Flanders AE, Espinosa GA, Markiewicz DA, et al. Orbital lymphoma. Radiol Clin North Am 1987;25:601–612.

128. Peyster RG, Hoover ED. Computerized Tomography in Orbital Disease and Neuro-Ophthalmology. Chicago: CV Mosby, 1984;21–56.

129. Fitzpatrick PJ, Macko S. Lymphoreticular tumors of the orbit. Int J Radiat Oncol Biol Phys 1984;10:333–340.

130. Yeo JH, Jakobiec FA, Abbott GF, et al. Combined clinical and computed tomographic diagnosis of orbital lymphoid tumors. Am J Ophthalmol 1982;94:235–245.

131. Valvassori GE, Sabnis SS, Mafee RF, et al. Imaging of orbital lymphoproliferative disorders. Radiol Clin North Am 1999;37:135–150.

132. Bilaniuk LT. Orbital vascular lesions: role of imaging. Radiol Clin North Am 1999;37:169–183.

133. Mafee MF, Miller MT, Tan WS, et al. Dynamic computed tomography and its application to ophthalmology. Radiol Clin North Am 1987;25:715–731.

134. Ruchman MC, Stefanyszn MA, Flanagan JC, et al. Orbital tumors. In: Gonzalez CA, Becjer MH, Flanagan JC, eds. Diagnostic Imaging in Ophthalmology. New York: Springer-Verlag, 1985;201–238.

135. Krohel GB, Wright JE. Orbital hemorrhage. Am J Ophthalmol 1979;88:254–258.

136. Tan WS, Wilbur AC, Mafee MF. The role of the neuroradiologist in vascular disorders involving the orbit. Radiol Clin North Am 1987;25:849–861.

137. Panda A, Dayal Y, Singhal V, et al. Hemangiopericytoma. Br J Ophthalmol 1984;68:124–127.

138. Stout AP. Tumors featuring pericytes, glomus tumor and hemangiopericytoma. Lab Invest 1956;5:217–223.

139. Stout AP, Murray MR. Hemangiopericytoma. Ann Surg 1972;116: 26–32.

140. Bockwinkel KD, Diddams JA. Hemangiopericytoma: report of care and comprehensive review of literature. Cancer 1970;25:896–901.

141. Rootman J, Goldberg C, Robertson W. Primary orbital schwannomas. Br J Ophthalmol 1982;66:194–204.

142. Carroll GS, Haik BG, Fleming JC, et al. Peripheral nerve tumors of the orbit. Radiol Clin North Am 1999;37:195–202.

143. Mafee MF, Goodwin J, Dorodi S. Optic nerve sheath meningiomas: role of MR imaging. Radiol Clin North Am 1999;37:37–58.

144. Skolnick CA, Mafee MF, Goodwin JA. Pneumosinus dilatans of the sphenoid sinus presenting with visual loss. J Neuro-Ophthalmol 2000;20(4):259–263.

145. Dalley R. Fibrous histiocytoma and fibrous tissue tumors of the orbit. Radiol Clin North Am 1999;37:185–194.

146. Font RL, Hidayat AA. Fibrous histiocytoma of the orbit: a clinicopathologic study of 150 cases. Hum Pathol 1982;13:199.

147. Ros PR, Kursunoglu S, Batle JF, et al. Malignant fibrous histiocytoma of the orbit. J Clin Neuroophthalmol 1985;5:116.

148. Jacomb-Hood J, Moseley IF. Orbital fibrous histiocytoma: computed tomography in 10 cases and a review of radiological findings. Clin Radiol 1991;43:117–120.

149. Mafee MF, Pai E, Philip B. Rhabdomyosarcoma of the orbit. Evaluation with MR imaging and CT. Radiol Clin North Am 1998;36:1215–1227.

150. Vade A, Armstrong D. Orbital rhabdomyosarcoma in childhood. Radiol Clin North Am 1987;25:701–714.

151. Mafee MF. Case 10: myositic orbital pseudotumor. In: Head and Neck Disorders (fourth series) tested syllabus. Reston, VA: American College of Radiology, 1992;213–259.

152. Mafee MF. The orbit proper. In: Som PM, Bergeron RT, eds. Head and Neck Imaging. St. Louis: Mosby-Yearbook, 1991;747–813.

153. Mafee MF. Orbital and intraocular lesions. In: Edelman RR, Hesselink JR, Zlatkin MC, eds. Clinical Magnetic Resonance Imaging. Philadelphia: WB Saunders, 1995;985–1020.

154. Rao BN, Santana VM, Fleming ID, et al. Management and prognosis of head and neck sarcomas. Am J Surg 1989;158:373–377.

155. Seedat RY, Hamilton PD, deJager LP, et al. Orbital rhabdomyosarcoma presenting as an apparent orbital subperiosteal abscess. Int J Pediatr Otorhinolaryngol 2000;52:177–181.

156. Shinaver CN, Mafee MF, Choi KH. MRI of mesenchymal chondrosarcoma of the orbit: case report and review of the literature. Neuroradiology 1997;39:296–301.

157. Stewart WB, Krohel GB, Wright JE. Lacrimal gland and fossa lesions: an approach to diagnosis and management. Ophthalmology 1979;86:886–895.

158. Wright JE. Factors affecting the survival of patients with lacrimal gland tumors. Can J Ophthalmol 1982;17:3–9.

159. Koeller KK. Mesenchymal chondrosarcoma and simulating lesions of the orbit. Radiol Clin North Am 1999;37:203–217.

160. Zimmerman LE, Sanders LE, Ackerman IV. Epithelial tumors of the lacrimal gland: prognostic and therapeutic significance of histologic types. Int Ophthalmol Clin 1962;2:337–367.

161. Jakobiec FA, Yeo JH, Trokel SL, et al. Combined clinical and computed tomographic diagnosis for primary lacrimal fossa lesions. Am J Ophthalmol 1982;94:785–807.

162. Hesselink J, Davis K, Dallow R, et al. Computed tomography of masses in the lacrimal gland region. Radiology 1979;131:143–147.

163. Jones BR. Clinical features and etiology of dacryoadenitis. Trans Ophthalmol Soc UK 1955;75:435–452.

164. Mafee MF, Edward DP, Koeller KK, Dorodi S. Lacrimal gland tumors and simulating lesions. Clinicopathologic and MR imaging features. Radiol Clin North Am 1999;37:219–239.

165. Hoffman GS, Kerr GS, Leavitt RY, et al. Wegener granulomatosis: an analysis of 158 patients. Ann Intern Med 1992;116:488–498.

166. Shield SJA, Bakewell B, Augsburger JJ, et al. Classification and incidence of space-occupying lesions of the orbit: a survey of 645 biopsies. Arch Ophthalmol 1984;102:1606–1611.

167. Kimura T, Yoshimura S, Ishikawa E. Eosinophilic granuloma with proliferation of lymphoid tissue. Trans Soc Pathol Jpn 1948;37:179.

168. Char DH, Unsöld R. Computed tomography: ocular and orbital pathology. In: Newton TH, Bilaniuk LT, eds. Radiology of the Eye and Orbit. New York: Raven Press, 1990;9.1–9.64.

169. Brown HW. True and simulated superior oblique tendon sheath syndromes. Doc Ophthalmol 1973;34:123, 134.

170. Mafee MF, Folk ER, Langer BG, et al. CT in the evaluation of Brown syndrome of the superior oblique tendon sheath. Radiology 1985;154:691–695.

171. Tychsen L, Tse DT, Ossoining K, Anderson RL. Trochleitis with superior oblique myositics. Ophthalmology 1984;91:1075–1079.

# 10

# Lacrimal Apparatus

## Edward E. Kassel and Charles J. Schatz

## INTRODUCTION

Abnormalities of the nasolacrimal drainage system (NLDS) bring many patients to the eye clinic. The majority of these patients present with epiphora (tearing), with a smaller number presenting with swelling, discomfort, or a mass in the inferomedial orbit, the area of the lacrimal sac. Multiple diverse etiologies, intrinsic or extrinsic to the NLDS, may be responsible. To assess for causative factors, the clinician augments the clinical examination with specific clinical tests and/or an imaging referral to document the anatomy and functional capabilities, degrees and levels of patency of the NLDS itself, or to visualize the tissues extrinsic and adjacent to the NLDS.

This chapter will outline the various imaging tests available for such patients. Discussions of dacryocystogra-

655

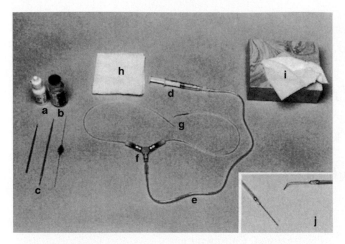

**FIGURE 10-1**   Equipment used in DCG: *a*, topical ophthalmic anaesthetic; *b*, low-osmolar, water-soluble contrast material; *c*, lacrimal dilators; *d*, 3 to 5 ml syringe; *e*, low-pressure tubing; *f*, Y-connector; *g*, lacrimal cannula; *h*, gauze pad; *i*, paper tissues; *j* (*inset*), magnified view of a commercially available lacrimal cannula. The cannula tip may be bent if clinically desired.

phy, dacryoscintigraphy, computed tomography, magnetic resonance imaging, and CT and MR imaging with topically or cannula introduced contrast media or solutions will outline the indications for and relative benefits of these various tests in specific patient populations. Radiographic anatomy, the more common pathologic processes, and their correlative imaging will be discussed in reference to the patient presenting with epiphora or a mass lesion of the inferomedial orbit. Applicable surgical procedures and the more recent experience with alternative dacryocystoplasty or stenting procedures provide a perspective on the current treatment options available to the patient.

## CONTRAST DACRYOCYSTOGRAPHY

The radiographic evaluation of the NLDS by contrast dacryocystography (DCG) was first described by Ewing, and remains the definitive and usually the primary study in the evaluation of patients with tearing (epiphora) (Figs.

10-1[4] to 10-10).[1] Epiphora is a common cause of referral to the general ophthalmologist, and the treatment often requires surgery. DCG is capable of determining the patency of the canaliculi, lacrimal sac, and nasolacrimal duct. When disease is present, the site and degree of obstruction or stenosis or the presence of fistulae, diverticula, and concretions are well evaluated by DCG (Fig. 10-10).

## Equipment

The equipment commonly used is illustrated in Figure 10-1. A dacryocystogram needle can be made by grinding off the sharp point of a 27-gauge lymphangiogram needle; the tip should be rounded and polished so that no metallic burrs remain. An alternative to this needle is a tapered catheter, as described by Iba and Hanafee,[2] made from no. 18 Teflon tubing, or commercially available Rabinov sialography catheters with a fine metallic cannula of 0.016 inch (27 gauge) diameter (Cook, Inc, Bloomington, Indiana). A punctal or lacrimal dilator (sharp or blunt Nettleship dilator) is also utilized, and for simultaneous injection and visualization of bilateral studies, a Y-connector may be helpful.

## Contrast Materials

A variety of opaque contrast media have been used. Ewing used bismuth subnitrate in liquid petrolatum. Since then, ethiodized oil (ethiodol), iodized oil (lipiodol), and iophendylate (Pantopaque) have also been used.[1, 3–5] Such oil-based contrast media, (e.g., ultrafluid lipiodol) were felt to better fill the NLDS than water-soluble agents, were less irritating, and were undiluted by tears, offering better opacification. Such contrast entered the NLDS at negligible pressure, minimizing the chances of extravasation. However, oil-based agents have disadvantages in the NLDS. First, if extravasated, oily contrast can remain in the soft tissues for many years, inciting a granulomatous inflammatory response.[6] Second, oily opaque material is not completely miscible with tears and can fail to fill or coat the entire NLDS, limiting diagnostic capabilities. Third, oily

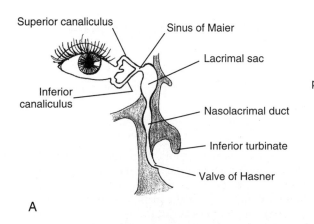

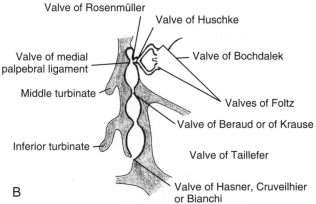

**FIGURE 10-2**   **A**, Anatomy of the NLDS. Right eye, frontal view. **B**, Drawing of the valves of the NLDS. Left eye, frontal view. (Modified from Warwick R. Eugene Woolf's Anatomy of the Eye and Orbit, 7th ed. Philadelphia: WB Saunders, 1976;232.)

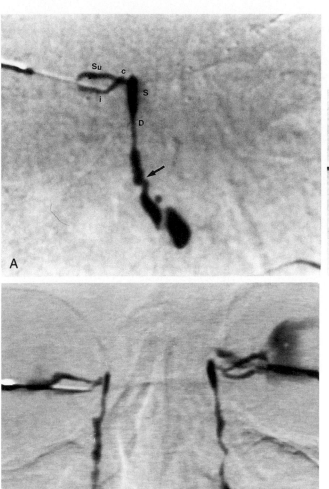

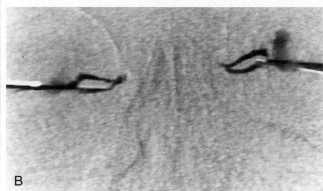

**FIGURE 10-3**   Radiographic anatomy: DCG. **A**, Normal right digital subtraction DCG, frontal view, cannula in inferior canaliculus. Superior (*Su*), inferior (*i*), and common (*c*) canaliculi visualized. Lacrimal sac (*S*) and nasolacrimal duct (*D*) visualized with contrast material entering nasal cavity through the valve of Hasner (*arrow*). **B** and **C**, Another patient. Early image (**B**) and later image (**C**) of DCG. Bilateral DCG utilizing the digital subtraction (DS-DCG) technique allows rapid imaging demonstrating the upper drainage system before possible reflux into the conjunctival sac obscures canalicular information. The later phase (**C**) shows the lacrimal sac and nasolacrimal duct with drainage into the nasal cavity.

*Illustration continued on following page*

contrast is more viscous than tears and often requires heating (especially with iodized oil) to reduce its viscosity before being injected.[7] If not heated, oily material requires a greater injection pressure than aqueous contrast material. Physiologic aqueous solution in the form of methylglucamine diatrizoate 40% (methylglucamine iodipamide 20%, Sinografin) was proposed by Sargent and Ebersole[6] as an excellent dacryocystographic contrast agent that was nonirritating, water soluble, miscible with tears, and similar in viscosity and pH to tears. Nonionic or lower osmolar aqueous solutions provide variable levels of iodine concentration and decreased viscosity, and are preferred for use when combining dacryocystography with digital subtraction techniques (see the section on Digital Subtraction (Macro) Dacryocystography). Munk et al.[8] noted some patient discomfort (a burning sensation) with sinografin and the nonionic solutions of 300 mg iodine per milliliter. Lipiodol offered the highest level of comfort and was the only

"tasteless" solution. All the aqueous solutions have a disagreeable or mildly unpleasant taste but are safe to swallow.

## Radiographic Techniques

Since the original description of Ewing,[1] many radiographic techniques for DCG have been described. The following are the more commonly used techniques:

- Macrodacryocystography, which uses a magnification (two and a half diameters optimum) technique after van der Plaat's description of radiographic magnification procedures.[9, 10]
- Kinetic DCG, which uses a cinematography format for evaluating the anatomy and function of the nasolacrimal apparatus.[11, 12]

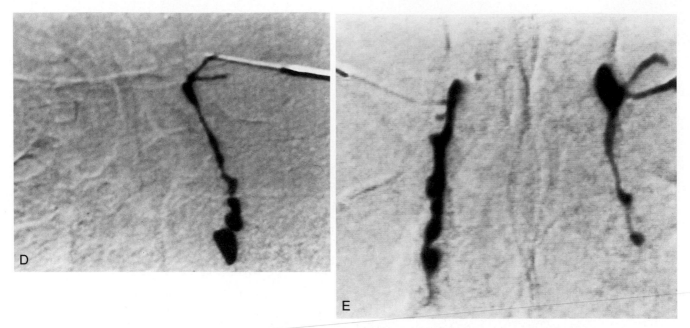

**FIGURE 10-3**    *Continued.* **D**, Anatomic variant with the left common canaliculus draining into the fundus of the lacrimal sac. **E**, Left common canaliculus empties into the lacrimal sac more inferiorly than usual. The left lacrimal sac is mildly dilated, with slight delay of drainage into the nasolacrimal duct.

- Distention DCG, which involves plain radiographs that are obtained during injection of the contrast material to better fill (distend) the NLDS.[2]
- Intubation macrodacryocystography, which combines distention DCG and macrodacryocystography.[13]
- Subtraction DCG, which combines intubation macrodacryocystography with a standard photographic subtraction technique.[14, 15]
- Tomographic DCG, which uses complex motion tomography to offer finer detail of the nasolacrimal apparatus. Thin-section images can be obtained in the frontal and lateral planes with improved detail compared to the above techniques[16] (Figs. 10-4 to 10-6).
- Digital subtraction DCG, which combines the techniques of dacryocystography with digital subtraction fluoroscopic capabilities.[17, 18] With the availability of higher-resolution digital capabilities, this technique has become the routine dacryocystographic study and is described separately in this chapter.

## Injection Techniques

The study is performed with the patient supine on the examination table, and initial preliminary films are obtained to ensure patient positioning and image quality. The procedure is not uncomfortable, and in many patients no topical anesthetic is necessary. However, to make the patient more relaxed and to decrease blinking and lacrimation, one may instill into the conjunctival sac a very short-acting topical ophthalmic anesthetic (e.g., 0.5% proparacaine [Ophthaine]). Oxybuprocaine 0.4% is a very short-acting topical anesthetic that does not require shielding of the eye following the procedure, thus making it especially advantageous for bilateral studies. Approximately 2 ml of the radiopaque contrast material is drawn into a small syringe, which is then connected to the lacrimal cannula and tubing, and the system is cleared of any air bubbles. The inferior punctum is then dilated with a lacrimal dilator, with the lower lid slightly everted and with minimal lateral traction to help stabilize the punctum. To avoid damage (false passage) to the canaliculus, the dilator, and subsequently the cannula, are positioned initially perpendicular to the lid margin and then rotated 90° horizontally to be directed medially along the horizontal component of the canaliculus (with the lower lid stretched laterally). The lacrimal sac and medial canthus are then palpated to detect any mass lesion, fullness, or tenderness and to express any fluid present in the sac through the punctum or into the nose. Ideal procedure includes pre-DCG irrigation and careful expression of the lacrimal sac to flush out accumulation of thickened mucus within the duct system. Failure to irrigate the nasolacrimal duct system (NLDS) or express the lacrimal sac contents may lead to interpretive difficulties, including improper estimation of the size of the lacrimal sac or misdiagnosis of obstructions proximal to a stenosing lesion due to the retained secretions.[19] Residual fluid in the sac causes oil-based contrast media to form globules, giving a false impression of a polycystic sac or diverticula.[9] The lacrimal cannula is then placed into the inferior punctum just far enough to remain stable during the study, and the tubing is taped to the patient's face. Care should be taken to avoid a common error, which is placement of the cannula too far into the inferior canaliculus. Frontal projection images approximating the Water's projection (40° occipitomental projection) are used to bring the nasolacrimal duct parallel to the imaging plane in an attempt to eliminate any distortion of the nasolacrimal duct. In this projection, the inferior orbital rim is approximately at the level of the junction of the middle and upper third of the nasolacrimal duct.[9] A coned occipitomental view is also obtained, centered midline at the inferior orbital margin. The injection is then made, and films

are immediately obtained. If distention DCG, intubation DCG, or digital subtraction DCG is used, the films are obtained during the injection. Initial or subsequent cannulation of the superior punctum may be appropriate when there is difficulty with cannulation of the inferior punctum or when further assessment is required following the initial injection of the inferior punctum. A delayed upright film should be taken, especially if obstruction is suspected, to assess possible delayed drainage into or through the inferior drainage system.

The decision to perform specific unilateral or routine bilateral DCG varies with the individual or institutional philosophy. Routine bilateral DCG may be justified by the

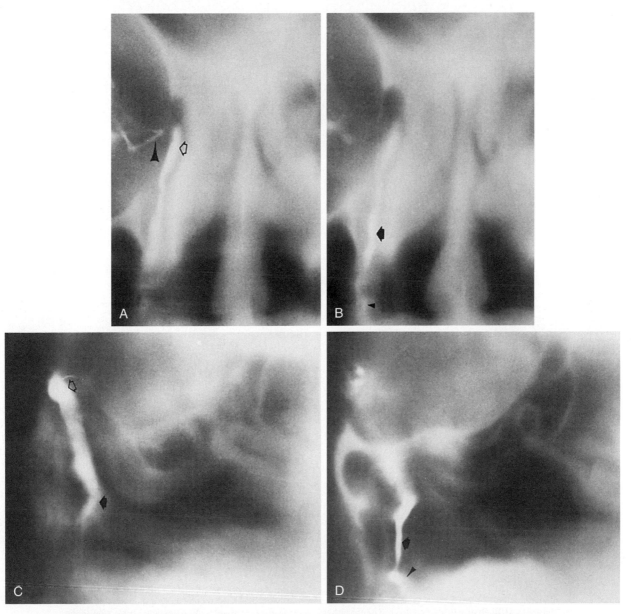

**FIGURE 10-4**   Tomographic DCG, which provides superb anatomic detail. **A**, Frontal plane tomography. Anterior section shows the canaliculi (*arrowhead*) and lacrimal sac (*open arrow*). **B**, More posterior tomographic section shows the nasolacrimal duct (*arrow*) and contrast material in the nasal cavity (*arrowhead*). **C** and **D**, Lateral tomograms show the lacrimal sac (*open arrow*), nasolacrimal duct (*closed arrow*), and contrast material in the nose (*arrowhead*). (See also Fig. 10-6.)

relative ease of the procedure; the lack of additional radiation, since the contralateral orbit is frequently included in the field of study; and the frequent finding of abnormalities in the clinically "asymptomatic" side.[20] Bilateral simultaneous injection, using a Y-connector, allows comparative flow characteristics through the NLDS. Other centers restrict the cannulation and visualization to those NLDSs that are symptomatic, eliminating any potential for iatrogenic insult to the noninvolved tear duct system.

## DIGITAL SUBTRACTION (MACRO) DACRYOCYSTOGRAPHY

In contrast to intubation macrodacryocystography using a serial film changer, digital subtraction dacryocystography (DS-DCG) allows, under fluoroscopic control, proper positioning and subsequent real-time imaging during the introduction of contrast medium. Images are usually taken every 1 to 2 seconds and can be terminated as soon as

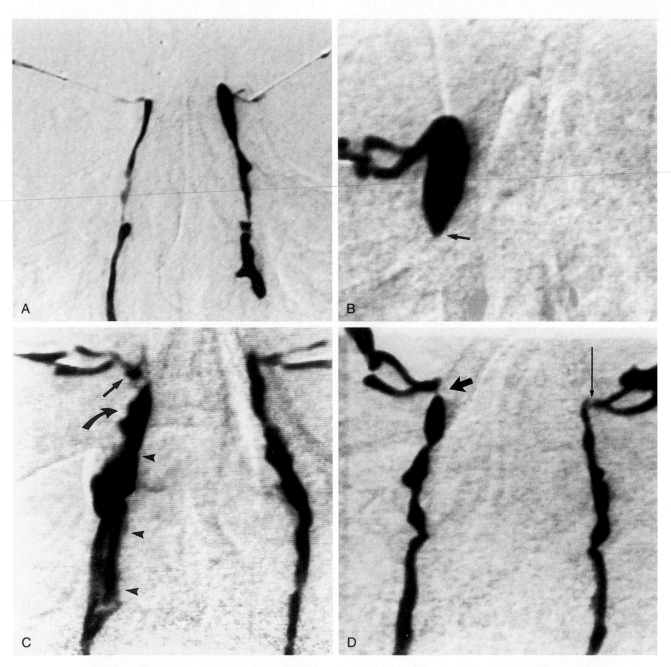

**FIGURE 10-5**   Stenosis-obstruction: DCG of the NLDS. Multiple patients. **A,** DCG with normal drainage bilaterally. Early distention of the left lacrimal sac compared with the more tubular configuration of the right lacrimal sac. Lack of reflux of contrast material into the right superior canaliculus. **B,** Complete obstruction of the distal lacrimal sac (*arrow*) at the junction with the nasolacrimal duct (*NLD*). Dilation (mucocele) of the lacrimal sac is present. **C,** Markedly irregular right lacrimal sac, contracted superiorly (*straight arrow*) and dilated inferiorly (*curved arrow*). The right NLD is also irregular and dilated (*arrowheads*). The left side is normal. Right chronic dacryocystitis is present. **D,** Stenosis at the junction of the right common canaliculus and lacrimal sac with contracture (*short arrow*) of the superior aspect of the lacrimal sac. Focal stenosis (*thin arrow*) is seen in the medial aspect of the left common canaliculus.

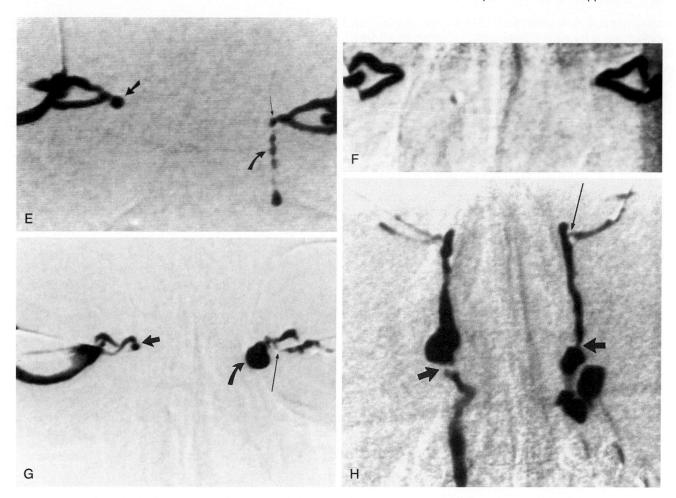

**FIGURE 10-5**   *Continued.* **E**, Bilateral DCG with an obstructed, cicatrized right lacrimal sac (*oblique arrow*). The left lacrimal sac is also scarred down (*thin arrow*), with irregularity and focal stenoses of the nasolacrimal duct (*curved arrow*). **F**, Bilateral obstruction of the lateral aspect of the common canaliculus with dilatation of the superior and inferior canaliculi bilaterally. **G**, Bilateral obstruction on DCG. Right cicatrized lacrimal sac (*straight arrow*). Left lacrimal sac mucocele (*curved arrow*). Stenosis also is present in the left inferior canaliculus (*thin arrow*). **H**, Stenosis at the valve of Hasner (*short arrows*), with distention of the distal right nasolacrimal duct. Mild stenosis in the left common canaliculus (*thin arrow*) with no reflux to the superior canaliculus.

*Illustration continued on following page*

patency or obstruction is defined. Fewer images (4 to 6) are usually acquired than for conventional DCG (6 to 10 images).[17] Digital adjustment of the data provides the most desired image quality on the "hard copy" film. The subtraction image is also digital, avoiding the time-consuming process of conventional photographic subtraction. The radiation dose to the lens is less in DS-DCG than in conventional DCG. Lead eye protection can reduce lens dosage, with further reduction achieved by noting early ductal patency using the real-time imaging capability of DS-DCG.[18, 21] The use of a carefully collimated high-kilovoltage primary beam; lead eye shields, which do not compromise the diagnostic quality of the study (placed lateral and anterior to the NLDS); and 30° oblique lateral projections for simultaneous bilateral DCG are simple measures that decrease by 97% the lens dosage required with conventional techniques. With these techniques, the radiation dosage for bilateral DCG can be limited to less than 1 mGy (1 mGy = 100 mrad) to the lens.[21] For conventional DCG, the patient lies supine, and the x-ray source is anterior to the patient. With DS-DCG the patient is

also supine. However, the x-ray source is posterior to the patient, so that the cranium acts as a "radiation shield" to the lens. Galloway et al.[17] found the actual lens radiation dose/exposure to be 13 times greater for conventional DCG than for DS-DCG (270 vs. 20 mrad), with the total lens radiation dose per study (six exposures each) being 1644 versus 126 mrad. King and Haigh's[18] study had a mean radiation dose/DS-DCG run of 0.68 mSv compared with 1.53 mSv (1 mSv = 100 mrem) for conventional two-film DCG, with the latter patients studied in the uncommon occipitomental position, and therefore having a lower reading than for the mentooccipital position usual for conventional DCG. Repeat studies needed as a result of suboptimal radiographic exposure factors were also obviated. Similarly, the ability to visualize the early flow of contrast medium through the canaliculi and upper drainage system obviates the need to repeat studies in which reflux into the conjunctival sac obscures information of canalicular patency.

In the early phase of injection, reflux can be minimized by an initial slow injection rate. Subsequently, the rate can be increased to achieve greater sac distention or to overcome resistance caused by partial obstruction.[17] The ability of DS-DCG to clearly demonstrate the upper drainage system, especially the common canaliculus, further reduces the relative radiation exposure of conventional DCG by obviating the need for tomographic DCG. DS-DCG has also dramatically decreased the need for lateral radiographic images. In the majority of studies, a single dynamic injection is required. In those departments where lacrimal imaging is infrequently performed, the advantages of DS-DCG become more apparent in both radiation reduction and study quality.[18]

With the newer digital units, spatial resolution is superb, approaching that of conventional radiography, while the contrast resolution of digital imaging is markedly superior to that of conventional imaging. The immediate viewing (or reviewing) of DS-DCG images significantly reduces the proportionate length of the study, allowing more efficient use of time for the radiologist and the patient. The increased contrast sensitivity of digital imaging allows for greater flexibility of choice of contrast agents, with water-soluble agents being preferred because of their lower viscosity, greater miscibility with tears, and easier flow through the NLDS. These agents usually require smaller volumes and have lower iodine content than the agents used for conventional DCG. For appropriate DS-DCG images, the patient must be fully cooperative, and be able to lie still and follow instructions, although manipulation of the computed data can offset minor degrees of movement. The use of topical anesthetic and the choice of catheters and their placement within the canaliculus are similar to those of conventional DCG.

Inclusion of a late (delayed) image, after the patient has been in the upright position for 5 minutes, increases the sensitivity of DCG or DS-DCG, with the specific intention to assess for failure of gravitational drainage of contrast medium from the nasolacrimal duct system (NLDS). This delay also allows DCG and DS-DCG, more anatomically orientated imaging procedures, to offer a physiologic component to the procedure, augmenting the value of DCG and DS-DCG in the evaluation of patients with functional nasolacrimal duct obstruction (FNLDO).[22] (In the section on Dacryoscintography, see also Incomplete Obstruction and Functional Nasolacrimal Duct Obstruction.) FNLDO is diagnosed if there is poor emptying, with residual contrast material present in the lacrimal sac or nasolacrimal duct on the delayed image. In the normal patient, contrast medium almost immediately disappears from the NLDS with the patient placed in the upright position. Issues with viscosity and surface tension may affect contrast drainage. Oil-based contrast may be more easily detected as small droplets within the duct system.[22] Water-soluble contrast, although safer, may be partially absorbed by the epithelium of the NLDS during the delayed period. Although Zinreich et al.[23] have attempted contrast DCG by simply placing the radiographic contrast agent into the conjunctival sac, the display of anatomic structures is less detailed than with DCG using cannulation despite the sensitivity of digital subtraction imaging. The hope that such a topically applied contrast

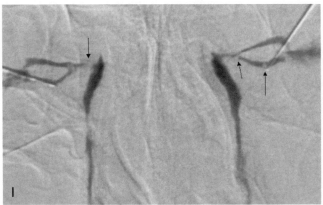

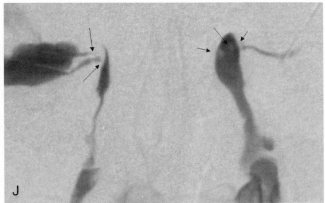

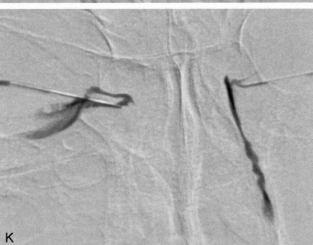

**FIGURE 10-5** *Continued.* **I,** Stenosis (mild) in the right common canaliculus. Small dacryoliths in the left inferior canaliculus and at the junction of the left inferior and common canaliculi, with no obstruction to drainage bilaterally. **J,** Bilateral tearing. Stenosis of the medial aspect of the right superior canaliculus and common canaliculus. Two subtle stones are seen in the superior left lacrimal sac and a small stone appears at the junction of the left common and superior canaliculi, blocking contrast reflux into the superior canaliculus. **K,** Right tearing. Complete obstruction at the right common canaliculus. At surgery, lymphoma of the lacrimal sac infiltrating into the common canaliculus was found.

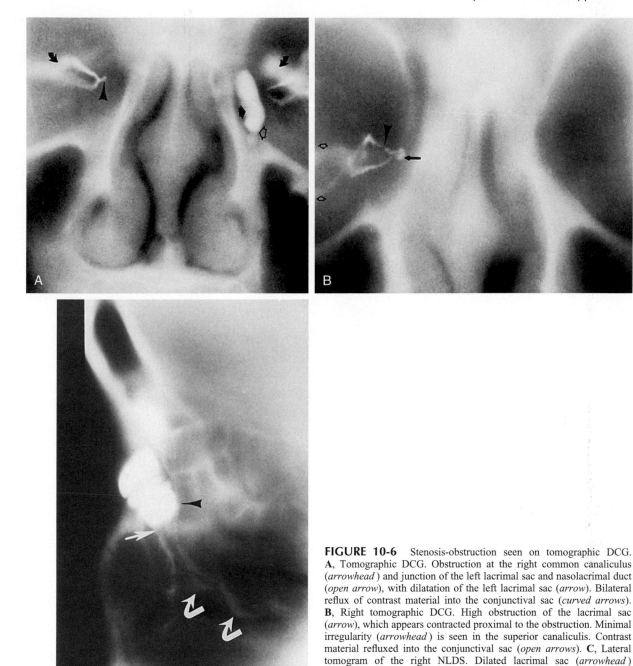

**FIGURE 10-6**  Stenosis-obstruction seen on tomographic DCG. **A,** Tomographic DCG. Obstruction at the right common canaliculus (*arrowhead*) and junction of the left lacrimal sac and nasolacrimal duct (*open arrow*), with dilatation of the left lacrimal sac (*arrow*). Bilateral reflux of contrast material into the conjunctival sac (*curved arrows*). **B,** Right tomographic DCG. High obstruction of the lacrimal sac (*arrow*), which appears contracted proximal to the obstruction. Minimal irregularity (*arrowhead*) is seen in the superior canaliculis. Contrast material refluxed into the conjunctival sac (*open arrows*). **C,** Lateral tomogram of the right NLDS. Dilated lacrimal sac (*arrowhead*) proximal to partial obstruction at the junction of the lacrimal sac and the nasolacrimal duct (*arrow*). Contrast material is seen in the nose (*curved arrows*).

DCG may allow the physiologic advantage of dacryoscintigraphy to be combined with the anatomic detail of cannulated DCG has yet to be fulfilled. The main acceptance of this technique is in its application to CT-dacryocystography or MR-dacryocystography techniques.

## CLINICAL TESTS

Before referral for DCG, most patients are seen by an ophthalmologist, who performs a number of tests to assess epiphora.

## Probing

Multiple calibers of fine flexible probes (Bowman probes 0000 to 0) may be used to "palpate" the nasolacrimal drainage lumen. Such probes can be passed to a "hard stop" representing the medial wall of the lacrimal sac. Slight withdrawal and downward angulation of the probe may allow entry into the nasolacrimal duct. A feeling of "give" or loss of resistance may be felt as the probe passes through the valve of Hasner. The upper drainage system is considered patent if a No. 0 probe passes through to the medial wall of the lacrimal sac.[24]

*Text continued on page 669*

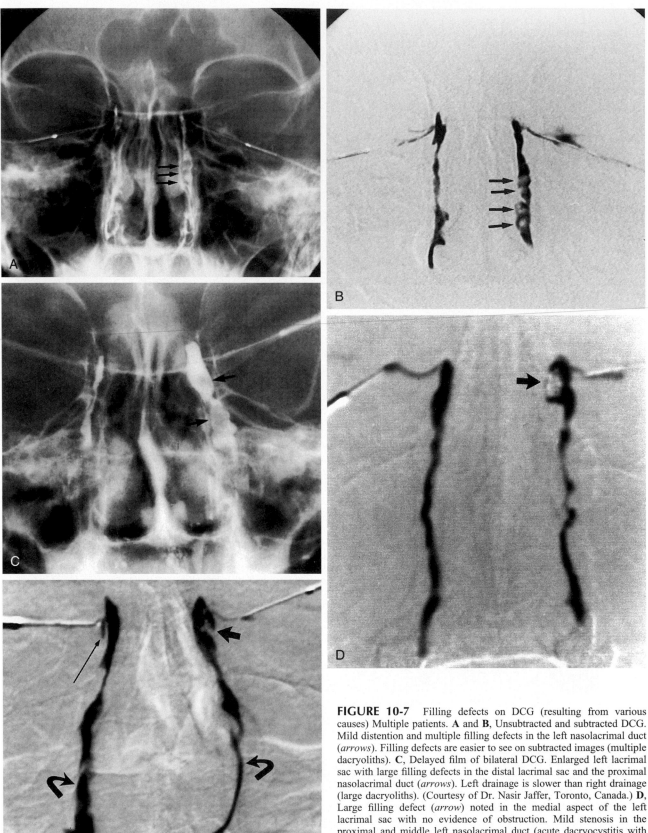

**FIGURE 10-7** Filling defects on DCG (resulting from various causes) Multiple patients. **A** and **B**, Unsubtracted and subtracted DCG. Mild distention and multiple filling defects in the left nasolacrimal duct (*arrows*). Filling defects are easier to see on subtracted images (multiple dacryoliths). **C**, Delayed film of bilateral DCG. Enlarged left lacrimal sac with large filling defects in the distal lacrimal sac and the proximal nasolacrimal duct (*arrows*). Left drainage is slower than right drainage (large dacryoliths). (Courtesy of Dr. Nasir Jaffer, Toronto, Canada.) **D**, Large filling defect (*arrow*) noted in the medial aspect of the left lacrimal sac with no evidence of obstruction. Mild stenosis in the proximal and middle left nasolacrimal duct (acute dacryocystitis with dacryolith). **E**, Ill-defined, irregularly shaped filling defect (*short arrow*) in the lateral aspect of the left lacrimal sac caused by hypertrophied mucosa. Note the extreme variability of the contrast medium pathway within the nasal cavity (*curved arrows*). The right cannula is placed too medially. A small diverticulum (*thin arrow*) extends inferiorly from the right common canaliculus.

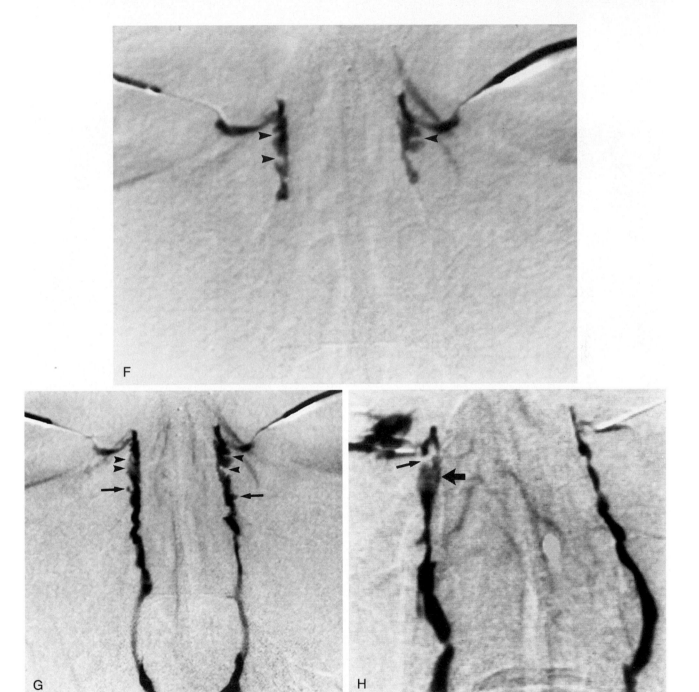

**FIGURE 10-7**   *Continued.* **F** and **G**, Early and late films of bilateral DCG. Lateral filling defects (*arrowheads*) and small diverticuli (*arrows*) are noted in the lacrimal sac and nasolacrimal duct bilaterally. Hypertrophic mucosal changes. **H**, Immediate drainage of the nasolacrimal system bilaterally. Filling defect in the right lacrimal sac (*thin arrow*) and decreased density in the inferior aspect of the right lacrimal sac (*short arrow*) caused by hematoma in the right lacrimal sac wall (pedestrian struck by a car).

*Illustration continued on following page*

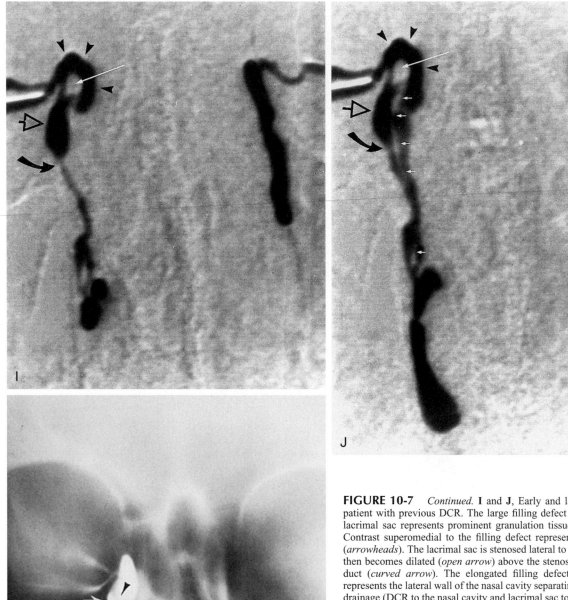

**FIGURE 10-7** *Continued.* **I** and **J**, Early and late DCG images in a patient with previous DCR. The large filling defect in the abnormal right lacrimal sac represents prominent granulation tissue (*long white arrow*). Contrast superomedial to the filling defect represents the DCR pathway (*arrowheads*). The lacrimal sac is stenosed lateral to granulation tissue and then becomes dilated (*open arrow*) above the stenosis of the nasolacrimal duct (*curved arrow*). The elongated filling defect (*tiny white arrows*) represents the lateral wall of the nasal cavity separating the two channels of drainage (DCR to the nasal cavity and lacrimal sac to the nasolacrimal duct to the nasal cavity). **K** and **L**, AP and lateral tomographic DCG in a patient with a 10-year history of epiphora. Filling defect (*arrowhead*) in the dilated lacrimal sac (*arrow*) represents concretion of *Actinomyces israelii* (found at surgery). Lateral view shows contrast material in the inferior meatus (*open arrow*).

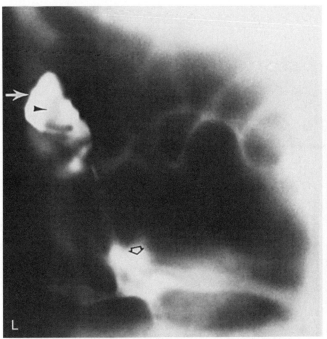

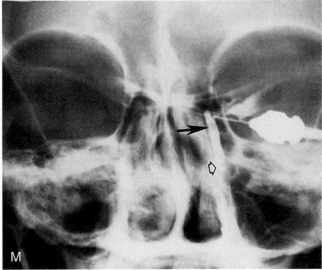

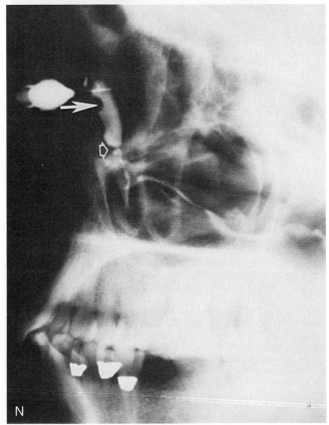

**FIGURE 10-7**   *Continued.* **M** and **N,** Left DCG, frontal view, and cross-table lateral projection. Air bubbles are present as a filling defect in the dilated lacrimal sac (*arrow*). On the cross-table lateral film, air bubbles rise in the lacrimal sac to differentiate it from concretions. Partial obstruction at the junction of the lacrimal sac and nasolacrimal duct (*open arrow*). (See also Figs. 10-17 to 10-19).

*Illustration continued on following page*

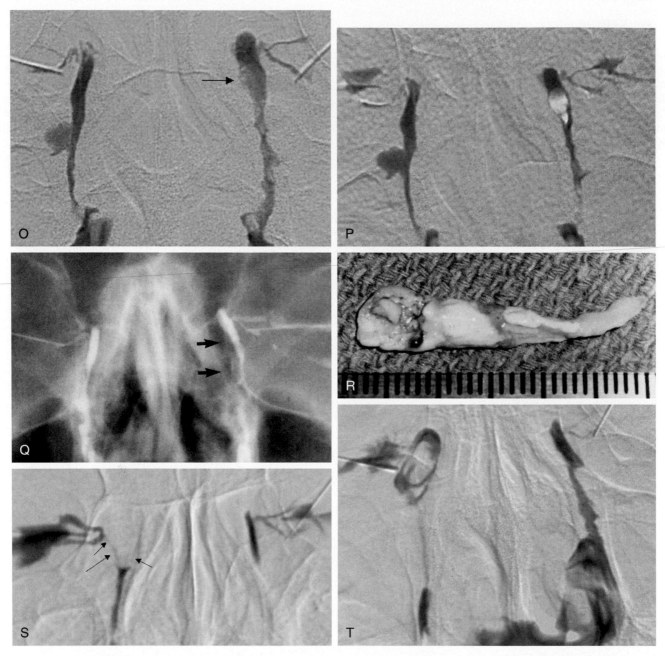

**FIGURE 10-7**   *Continued.* **O** and **P**, Tearing. Previous patency on irrigation. Recent intermittent patency. **O**, Subtle filling defect (*arrow*) is seen in the distended left lacrimal sac. **P**, Fourteen months later, a large dacryolith was more easily seen in the lacrimal sac. Incidental diverticulum at the junction of the right lacrimal sac and nasolacrimal duct. **Q** and **R**, Calculus in the left NLDS. The patient presented with tearing and patency on syringing. **Q**, DCG shows no evidence of obstruction. Contrast medium column is deflected laterally (*arrows*) from the expected position of the lacrimal sac. **R**, At surgery (DCR), a large stone was seen filling the entire sac and superior aspect of the nasolacrimal duct. **S**, Right tearing. Large filling defect distending the right lacrimal sac (*arrows*), with minimal contrast seen only peripherally. Common canaliculus not identified. Pathology: lymphoma lacrimal sac. (See also Fig. 10-5K). **T**, Large filling defect (dacryolith) in the right lacrimal sac, with limited contrast into the nasolacrimal duct. (**Q** and **R** From Hurwitz JJ, Kassel EE. Dacryocystography. In: Hurwitz JJ, ed. The Lacrimal System. Philadelphia: Lippincott-Raven, 1996;71.)

## Irrigation

Standard lacrimal cannulation and irrigation are performed using saline solution. The patient is usually inclined forward, in a sitting position, to allow the irrigating solution to be readily assessed exiting from the nostrils. False-negative or false-positive tests may partly result from the variable ability (subjective) of the patient to detect the presence of saline entering the nasopharynx. A small amount of fluoroscein may be added to the saline to assist in the detection of patency of the drainage system. Syringing of the lacrimal system correlates poorly with DCG[25] and shows an 18% discordance with dacryoscintigraphy (DSG)[26] in detecting obstruction.

## Dye Tests

### Jones 1 Test

The fluoroscein 2% dye test (the primary dye test) detects functional obstruction, that is, defines the inability of the drainage apparatus to pump tears from the eye to the nose.[27] Two drops of dye placed into the conjunctival cul de sac should reach the nasal cavity within 1 to 3 minutes (positive test). It should be noted that in the Jones tests, a normal result is referred to as a positive test, unlike in most imaging examinations. The dye may be retrieved on a nasal applicator or confirmed by nose blowing or by nasal irrigation with saline.

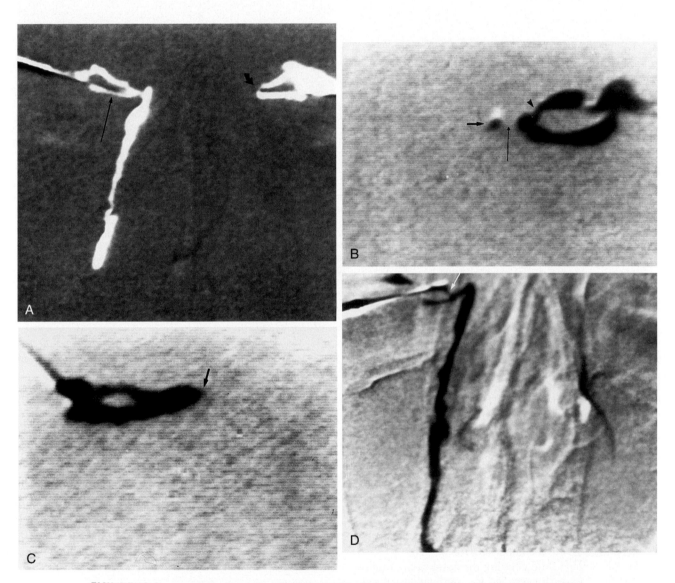

**FIGURE 10-8**   Canalicular obstruction. **A,** Bilateral DCG with complete obstruction of the lateral (proximal) left common canaliculus (*short arrow*). Mild stenosis of the distal right inferior canaliculus (*thin arrow*). **B,** Left superior canalicular injection shows severe stenosis of the medial left common canaliculus (*thin arrow*) with minimal contrast reaching the lacrimal sac (*short arrow*), which may be fibrosed. Mild stenosis of the medial aspect of the left superior canaliculus (*arrowhead*). **C,** Right DCG shows complete obstruction at the medial (distal) aspect of the common canaliculus (*arrow*). **D,** Superior canalicular injection. Focal tight stenosis (*arrow*) of the medial aspect of the superior canaliculus. No reflux into superior canaliculus had been seen from an inferior canalicular injection.

*Illustration continued on following page*

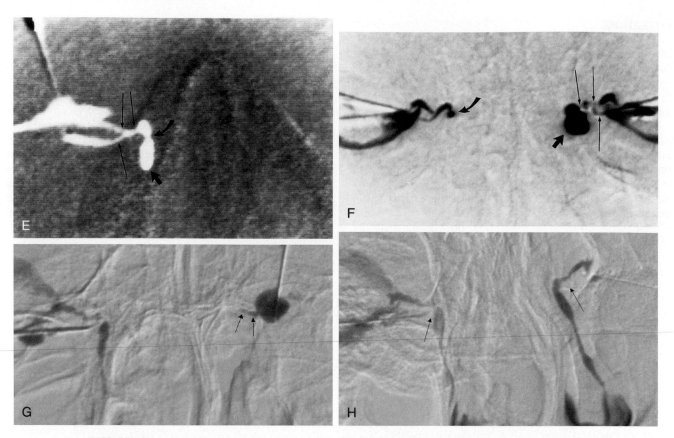

**FIGURE 10-8** *Continued.* **E,** Superior canalicular injection. Mild stenosis (*thin arrows*) of the medial common canaliculus and the medial aspect of the right superior and inferior canaliculi. Obstruction of the distal right lacrimal sac (*short arrow*). Narrowed segment (*curved arrow*) of the lacrimal sac is due to fibrosis. **F,** Distended lobulated left lacrimal sac (mucocele) with outlet obstruction (*short arrow*). Severe stenosis (*thin arrows*) of the left common canaliculus (with focal dilatation) and inferior and superior canaliculi medially. Cicatrized right lacrimal sac (*curved arrow*). **G** and **H,** Bilateral tearing. **G,** Irregular dilated right superior canaliculus and stenosis at the junction of the common canaliculus and lacrimal sac, with contrast refluxing into the conjunctival sac. Obstruction at the medial aspect of the left inferior canaliculus (*arrows*), with contrast refluxing into the conjunctival sac. **H,** Repeat injection. The right cannula was moved closer to the punctum to better visualize the stenosis in the medial aspect of the right inferior canaliculus (*arrow*). Left injection through the superior punctum shows no obstruction to drainage. No reflux into the obstructed inferior canaliculus (*arrow*).

### Jones 2 Test

If the Jones 1 test is negative (no dye reaches the nasal cavity), the Jones 2 test is performed by irrigating the NLDS with a saline solution (1 ml) after the conjunctival application of fluoroscein dye has been irrigated out of the conjunctival sac.[27]

1. Lack of fluid entering the nose is evidence of complete obstruction in the drainage system (negative test).
2. The presence of clear saline in the nasal cavity implies that the fluoroscein did not reach the lacrimal sac. The test is negative (abnormal). The canaliculi may be open, but they are not functioning, and the abnormality is localized to the upper NLDS.
3. Deeply stained fluid entering the nasal cavity implies that the fluoroscein reached the lacrimal sac physiologically but did not drain any further. The test is positive (the lacrimal pump and canaliculi are functioning, so that the lacrimal sac fills). There is incomplete obstruction of the nasolacrimal duct.

If both the Jones 1 and 2 tests fail to detect fluoroscein in the nasal cavity (negative tests), the lacrimal system is irrigated with fluoroscein to confirm total obstruction.[28]

## Schirmer's Test

Schirmer's test is a measure of the eye's ability to produce tears in response to an external stimulus and can be estimated by the amount, in millimeters, of filter paper wetting by lacrimal fluid in 5 minutes. A dry eye may intermittently produce a large amount of tears, simulating epiphora. The test can differentiate hyposecretion and pseudoepiphora from normal secretions.[27]

## Valsalva DCR Bubble Test

The Valsalva DCR bubble test offers confirmation of patency of a dacryocystorhinostomy site. A drop of saline is placed at the inner canthus, and the patient is asked to perform the Valsalva maneuver. The formation of a bubble in the region of the punctum indicates a positive test.[29] Again as in the Jones test, the normal test is referred to as positive.

## INDICATIONS FOR DACRYOCYSTOGRAPHY

DCG is indicated to investigate patients with epiphora after the clinical examination suggests a mechanical obstruction. Campbell[9] outlined the three fundamental principles in interpretation of DCG: (1) to describe the level of the obstruction, (2) to state whether the obstruction is complete or incomplete, and (3) to determine the cause of the obstruction. The suspected obstruction may be associated with various clinical conditions, including congenital obstructions, supernumerary canaliculi, lacrimal fistula or diverticula, concretions (dacryoliths), neoplastic or inflammatory processes, or posttreatment changes. When there is clinically assessed chronic obstruction, surgical or interventional treatment is indicated and DCG should offer maximum information to allow the appropriate procedure.

## SURGICAL PROCEDURES FOR EPIPHORA

The most common surgical procedure for epiphora is a dacryocystorhinostomy (DCR), in which the medial wall of the lacrimal sac is opened into the nasal cavity, with specific attention being devoted to appropriate removal of adjacent bone (osteotomy) and suturing of the lacrimal sac and nasal mucosal flaps.[30] DCR is the procedure of choice to treat epiphora secondary to obstruction or severe stenosis of the distal lacrimal sac and the nasolacrimal duct. Stenoses or occlusion within the upper drainage system, proximal to the lacrimal sac, may require placement of fine stents (silastic or rubber) within the canaliculi to complement the DCR. Alternatively canaliculo-DCR may be performed, with resection of a canalicular stenotic segment and anastomosis to the lacrimal sac and incorporation into the DCR.[31] These stents are placed on a temporary basis. Construction of a conjunctival tract with insertion of permanent glass tubes (Pyrex) to bypass an occluded canaliculus (conjunctival DCR) has long-term implications for care and maintainance.[32] A limited canthocystostomy (lacrimal sac opened into the conjunctival fornix) procedure may be performed when the lacrimal sac and lower NLDS are intact and

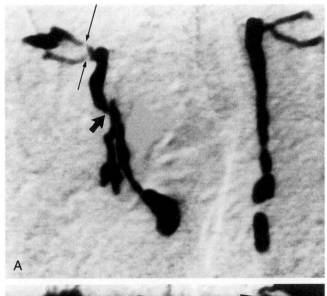

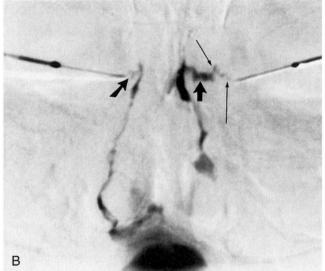

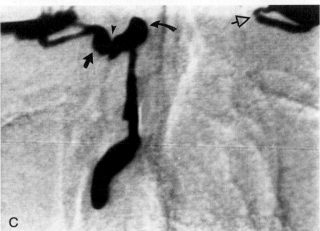

**FIGURE 10-9**   Post-DCR studies on different patients. **A,** Previous right DCR. Contrast material extends from the distal right lacrimal sac (*short arrow*) into the nasal cavity. Strictures in the medial aspect of the superior and inferior canaliculi (*thin arrows*). Normal left side. **B,** Previous left DCR with left inferior (*vertical thin arrow*) and common (*oblique thin arrow*) canaliculi markedly stenotic and irregular. No reflux to the superior canaliculus. Medial contrast collection toward the nasal midline (*short arrow*) is consistent with scarring. On the right, a small filling defect (*oblique arrow*) within the inferior canaliculus is seen. **C,** Previous bilateral DCR. Distended right lacrimal sac (*short arrow*) with large lobulation (*curved arrow*) medial to the DCR site (*arrowhead*) before emptying into the nasal cavity. Medial lobulation suggests synechia to the midline nasal septum. Complete obstruction at the proximal left common canaliculus (*open arrow*). (See also Figs. 10-7I,J, 10-20, 10-28A,B.)

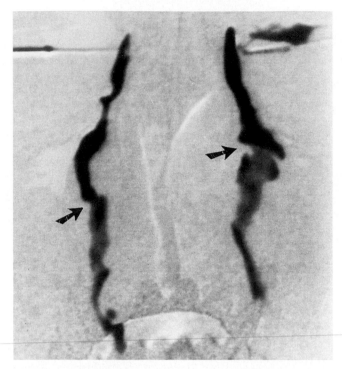

**FIGURE 10-10**   Shortened left nasolacrimal duct. Contrast material enters the left nasal cavity (*arrow*) more superiorly than usual (compare with the right side). There was previous resection of a left maxillary sinus neoplasm.

patent.[9] A canthoplasty (lateral) with resection and tightening of the preseptal and pretarsal orbicularis muscle may correct abnormal positions of the lid and allow tears to enter the punctum.

The increasing trend of minimally invasive surgical techniques, combined with the advancing technology of endoscopic visualization, has also been applied to the lacrimal patient. Endoscopic dacryocystoplasty (endonasal DCR), utilizing an endonasal endoscope to make an anastomosis (using traditional bone-removing instruments or a laser) between the lacrimal sac and the nasal cavity, circumvents the external approach (Toti's operation). With no external scar, the endoscopic approach offers better cosmesis. There is preservation of lacrimal pump function of the orbicularis oculi muscle, the presaccal fibers, the medial canthal tendon and their osseous supporting structures by approaching the lacrimal sac from the nasal cavity.[33–35] Compared to external DCR, endonasal DCR is less traumatic and offers minimal morbidity, less intraoperative bleeding, a shorter operative time, and a low complication rate.[36] Endoscopic DCR is a more difficult procedure to learn, is more technically challenging, and has the disadvantage of a smaller anastomotic opening and a higher recurrence rate of epiphora. Bone removal by drilling or by laser may cause overheating and increase the risk of postoperative fibrosis and closure of the lacrimal window.[35] As for external DCR, scarring of the ostium and errors in ostium location are the major reasons for surgical failure.[37] Epithelial anastomosis and continuous fluid flow are necessary for maintaining a patent surgical rhinostoma. For this purpose, a silicone stent is placed and is usually kept in place for at least 2 months.[36] Conversely, Kong et al.[38] suggest removal of the silicone tubes before 8 weeks to prevent granuloma formation and closure of the osteotomy site. Premature tube dislodgement may be associated with surgical failure.

Microendoscopy of the NLDS, endocanalicular and translacrimal DCR,[39] and fiberoptic laser probing are less frequently used surgical procedures for the treatment of lacrimal sac and nasolacrimal duct obstruction. Translacrimal and endocanalicular laser DCR techniques offer the advantage of less surgical dissection. The laser energy is directed away from the eye, avoiding the risks of laser injury to the globe that may occur with laser-assisted endonasal DCR.[39, 40] Thermal injury of the lacrimal sac may increase postoperative scarring and reduce patency.[41] (See also the section on Endoscopy of the Lacrimal Drainage System later in this chapter.)

## THE NORMAL DACRYOCYSTOGRAM

### Anatomy

The lacrimal system consists of the inferior canaliculus, superior canaliculus, common canaliculus, lacrimal sac, and nasolacrimal duct (Figs. 10-2 to 10-4). Tears from the conjunctival sac enter the punctum of both the inferior and superior canaliculi approximately 6 mm lateral to the medial canthus, briefly travel through a 2 mm vertical segment, and then turn abruptly medially to continue in the longer (7 to 10 mm) horizontal canalicular segment. There is a slight dilation, the ampulla, at the junction of the vertical and horizontal components of each canaliculus.[42] The superior and inferior canaliculi merge to form the common canaliculus (common ampulla) and enter a small diverticulum of the lateral wall of the lacrimal sac, the sinus of Maier. Occasionally the canaliculi enter the sinus of Maier separately. The upper canaliculus is slightly shorter and straighter than the lower, and the canalicular diameter is 0.5 mm, with a punctal diameter of 0.3 mm. The thin, elastic walls of the canaliculi allow the canaliculi to be dilated three times their normal diameter or to be straightened by lateral tension on the eyelid, an anatomic feature of significance for probing or instrumentation.[42] The punctal region is relatively avascular and therefore paler than adjacent tissues. This contrast is accentuated by lateral tension on the lid margin, helping to locate a stenosed punctum. The normal close contact between the puncta and the conjunctival tear fluid is essential (and should be noted for normal function) since the canaliculi fill by capillary extraction.

The common canaliculus is 1 to 5 mm in length and terminates medially through flaps of mucosa created by the acute angle with which the sinus of Maier enters the lacrimal sac. The superior flap is called the valve of Rosenmüller, and the inferior flap is called the valve of Huschke. The canaliculus enters the lateral aspect of the nasolacrimal sac just above the junction of its upper and middle thirds (i.e., 3 mm from the dome of the sac).[27]

In 1911, Schaeffer[43] described three different ways in which the canaliculi communicate with the lacrimal sac: (1) they can drain through a common canaliculus; (2) they can empty separately into a diverticulum of the lacrimal sac (sinus of Maier); or (3) in rare cases, they can empty separately into the lacrimal sac, with no common canaliculus or diverticulum present. Variations in the configuration

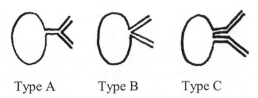

Type A          Type B          Type C

**FIGURE 10-11**   Forms of canalicular connection to the lacrimal sac. **Type A**: Upper and lower canaliculi join the common canaliculus. **Type B**: Upper and lower canaliculi join at the lacrimal sac wall to form a common opening. **Type C**: Upper and lower canaliculi enter the lacrimal sac separately. (Adapted from Yazici B, Yacizi Z. Frequency of the common canaliculus. A radiological study. Arch Ophthalmol 2000;118:1381–1385.)

of the common canaliculus have been noted. Approximately 90% of individuals have the typical configuration, that is, a common canaliculus clearly defined between the merged inferior and superior canaliculi laterally and the entry point into the lateral wall of the lacrimal sac medially.

For the 10% of the population for whom a common canaliculus is not present, there has been no clear description of how the canaliculi terminate. Jones and Wobig[27] reported that in 10% of individuals, the canaliculi actually open separately into a ''sinus of Maier,'' which in turn opens into the tear sac, implying only one common internal opening, also celled the inner punctum, into the tear sac. The term *sinus of Maier* is somewhat confusing since it has been used to describe three different anatomic entities: (1) the common canaliculus itself; (2) the terminal dilation of a common canaliculus; and (3) the lacrimal sac diverticulum into which the canaliculi open separately.[27, 42, 44] Yacizi and Yacizi[44] propose a functional term, *common opening*, to describe the configuration in which the common canaliculus is absent and the canaliculi unite at the sac wall and drain by one ostium. In a smaller number of patients, the upper and lower canaliculi drain separately and distinctly into the lacrimal sac.

In a recent study of 341 digital subtraction macrodacryocystograms on patients with obstructive epiphora, Yacizi and Yacizi[44] noted that 94.1% had the typical common canaliculus configuration (type A). In this study, 3.8% had an absent common canaliculus, with the lower and upper canaliculi united at a common opening in the lacrimal sac wall and draining into the lacrimal sac through this opening (type B). In only 2% of the studies did the upper and lower canaliculi drain separately into the lacrimal sac (type C) (Fig. 10-11).

In type B, the upper and lower canaliculi joined at a narrow angle at the lacrimal sac wall for a common opening. This pattern was unlikely to be confused with type C since the type C canaliculi maintained nearly parallel courses as they approached and maintained separate openings into the lacrimal sac. The authors[44] emphasize analysis of the early images of canalicular filling before a distended lacrimal sac may obscure a short common canaliculus and resemble a type B or type C pattern. There is no evidence that the presence or type of canalicular drainage affects the clinical course of nasolacrimal duct obstruction. Nasolacrimal duct obstruction, with resultant lacrimal sac distention, causes kinking of the common canaliculus (and probably of the superior and inferior canaliculi in type B and C configurations) due to compression by the lacrimal sac and may better explain further sac enlargement. Anatomic configurations

have surgical implications for planned probings or silicone intubations at the time of DCR or for repairs of traumatized (lacerated) canaliculi to prevent the creation of false canalicular passages.

Review of the functional anatomy of the lacrimal outflow system at the junction of the common canaliculus and lacrimal sac may also be warranted. Mucosal folds at the superior and inferior borders of the common canaliculus–lacrimal sac junction have been described and respectively named the valve of Rosenmüller and the valve of Huschke. These valves have been seen or described inconsistently and occasionally have been omitted in the literature. Only the Hasner valve at the distal nasolacrimal duct has been shown to be a functional barrier to retrograde flow or reflux of fluid. However, the belief that the Rosenmüller valve prevents tear reflux from the lacrimal sac to the common canaliculus has persisted as the only explanation for the lack of reflux of lacrimal sac contents. The theory holds that the valve may become tighter with edema, inflammation, and distortion related to dacryocystitis, explaining the difficulty of cannulating the lacrimal sac in cases of dacryocystitis, dacryocystocele, or acute dacryocystic retention.[45]

Tucker et al.[46] have hypothesized that the Rosenmüller valve alone may be insufficient to explain the functional valve mechanism and offer an alternative finding and theory from their study of casts of lacrimal outflow systems. A consistent canaliculi configuration of an initial posterior vector at the level of the eyelids, followed by an anterior vector after passing posterior to the medial canthal tendon, with continuation in this anterior direction to enter the lacrimal sac at an acute angle suggests functional significance. The authors have postulated that the angle of entry of the common canaliculus into the lacrimal sac may explain the lack of reflux in pathologic conditions associated with an enlarged sac. As the lacrimal sac increases in size, its expansion is limited medially and posteriorly by the bony lacrimal sac fossa. Thus there is more expansion laterally and anteriorly. The lateral expansion may cause kinking of the canaliculus, which functionally blocks the canaliculus–sac junction (Fig. 10-12). External pressure applied to the sac may accentuate the functional valve. In patients with

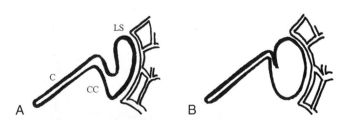

**FIGURE 10-12**   Pattern of angulation within the canalicular system at the canaliculus–lacrimal sac junction: hypothesis for one-way valve phenomenon. **A** and **B**, Looking at the right eye from above (i.e., anterior aspect is at the bottom of the image); the medial aspect (ethmoid sinuses) is at the right side of the image. **A**, Normal lacrimal anatomy. Canaliculi (*c*) bend posteriorly to pass behind the medial canthal tendon, and the common canaliculus (*cc*) bends anteriorly directly behind the medial canthal tendon to enter the lacrimal sac (mean angle of 58° to the lateral wall of the sac). **B**, Kinking and collapse of the common canaliculus at its junction with the lacrimal sac may occur with sac enlargement, leading to a one-way valve effect, preventing reflux of sac contents in certain cases of dacryocystitis, lacrimal sac mucoceles, and acute dacryocystic retention. (Adapted from Tucker NA, Tucker SM, Linberg JV. The anatomy of the common canaliculus. Arch Ophthalmol 1996;114:1231–1234.)

dilated lacrimal sacs not exhibiting a functional valve, the angulation of the common canaliculus, as it enters the sac, may not be acute enough to have a valve effect.[46]

Malik et al.[47] reported radiographic measurements of the lacrimal sac and nasolacrimal duct (Table 10-1). Any distention of the sac greater than 4 mm on the frontal radiograph is considered pathologic. The lacrimal sac ends in a slight taper inferiorly caused by a mucosal fold, the valve of Krause, just above the inferior rim of the orbit. The nasolacrimal duct, which extends 15 to 20 mm in length, begins at this level and may have a small portion of its course within the orbit before entering the bony canal (intraosseous component). This intraorbital segment is approximately 1 cm in length. Within the nasolacrimal duct there is a midsection mucosal constriction, the valve of Taillefer, just superior to the inferior turbinate bone, and a distal constriction, the valve of Hasner. The duct empties through the valve of Hasner into the inferior meatus of the nose, beneath the inferior turbinate. This inferior, or meatal, component usually opens into the nasal cavity 5 mm below the vault of the inferior meatus (anterior aspect) but may extend more inferiorly down the lateral wall of the inferior meatus before entering the nasal cavity. Such inferiorly located valves tend to have a more slit-like opening rather than the fold of mucosa forming Hasner's valve seen in the more superiorly located valves.

In the normal DCG, the canaliculi, lacrimal sac, and nasolacrimal duct are not dilated. On the frontal images, the lacrimal sac and nasolacrimal duct have a linear configuration. The fascia of the orbicularis oculi, which splits to enclose the lacrimal duct and sac, is thick and taut and indents the lumen at the junction of the lacrimal sac and nasolacrimal duct 0.7 cm above the bony canal opening.[9] On the lateral film, the nasolacrimal duct is seen to change direction slightly, inclining posteriorly. This marks the site of the valve of Krause. This combination of indentation and mild kinking caused by the change in nasolacrimal duct system (NLDS) direction may explain why the junction of the lacrimal sac and duct is the most frequent site of obstruction. A second change in direction, more acute, and also posteriorly inclined, is noted at the valve of Taillefer. On a lateral film, the course of the lacrimal sac and nasolacrimal duct should extend along a line from the medial canthus to the first maxillary molar.[42] The lacrimal sac may normally be three times as wide on the lateral image as on the frontal image.[9] Contrast material is identified entering the nasal cavity. In a patent system, the contrast

medium will immediately drain from the nose into the pharynx and onto the base of the tongue, with the patient tasting the solution within a few moments. Normally 0.5 to 1.0 ml of contrast medium is injected per side. There should be free flow of contrast through the NLDS into the nasal cavity (inferior meatus). A mild increase in injection pressure may overcome an area of "relative" obstruction that may represent secretions or a partial stenosis, which would otherwise have been incorrectly interpreted as obstruction, with implications for treatment decisions. Three anatomic narrowings normally occur and may be noted: at the junction of the common canaliculus and lacrimal sac (valve of Rosenmüller or "inner punctum"; at the junction of the distal lacrimal sac and nasolacrimal duct (valve of Krause); and at the distal valve of Hasner. These physiologic narrowings must not be mistaken for strictures or obstructions that are also more commonly located at these same sites.

Various mechanisms have been proposed to explain the drainage of tears. These anatomic and physiologic mechanisms, or their dysfunction, are poorly assessed by imaging modalities. Recent interest in the specialized vascular plexus, including cavernous tissue, which closely surrounds the lacrimal sac and nasolacrimal duct and connects caudally with the cavernous body of the nasal inferior turbinate, offers a further theory of tear outflow.[48, 49] Congestion within the vascular plexus affects the tear outflow system, allowing either obstruction or rapid transit of tear fluid. Paulsen et al.[50] propose that the previously described NLDS valves (Rosenmüller, Aubaret, Beraud, Krause, and Taillefer) may be based on different states of swelling of the cavernous body network and should be considered speculative (which may partly explain their inconsistent descriptions in the literature). (In the section Dacryoscintigraphy, see Normal Examination for further discussion of tear outflow.)

## PATHOLOGY OF THE NASOLACRIMAL DRAINAGE SYSTEM

The lacrimal gland situated laterally and superiorly to the globe secretes tears. Under normal circumstances, the tears either evaporate from the surface of the globe or drain into the nasolacrimal passages and pass into the inferior meatus of the nose. Tearing may have several causes.[9] Excessive lacrimation may result in inadequate evaporation or drainage caused by a greater than normal volume of tears. In this situation, the DCG will appear normal. Much more commonly, excessive tearing represents obstructive epiphora, which results from complete or incomplete obstruction or from a functionally inefficient lacrimal system that cannot adequately handle the normal flow of tears. When there is an obstruction or stenosis, the DCG is abnormal. In a symptomatic patient, if contrast medium does not reflux into the superior canaliculus of an otherwise normal NLDS, a repeat study with cannulation of the superior canaliculus should be performed (Fig. 10-8D). There may be an inadequate or altered relationship of the puncta to the ocular surface or an abnormally small punctum inhibiting the transmission of tears into the lacrimal drainage system. In

**Table 10-1**
**NORMAL LACRIMAL DIMENSIONS**

| Area | Dimension (mm) | Mean (mm) | Range (mm) |
|---|---|---|---|
| Lacrimal sac | Vertical diameter | 11.10 | 6–14 |
| | Lateral diameter | 2.43 | 1–4 |
| | Anteroposterior diameter | 4.00 | 1–6 |
| Nasolacrimal duct | Vertical diameter | 20.97 | 13–26 |
| | Lateral diameter | 2.30 | 1–4 |
| | Anteroposterior diameter | 2.84 | 1–4 |

From Malik SRK, Gupta AK, Chaterjee S, et al. Dacryocystography of normal and pathological lacrimal passages. Br J Ophthalmol 1969;53:174–179.

such circumstances, the DCG will be normal. It must be emphasized that the introduction of a cannula into the puncta does not allow radiographic or physiologic assessment of the puncta. Observations regarding laxity of the lower lid, scarring or stenosis of the puncta, or other abnormalities of the lid may be better assessed clinically and should be commented on during the performance of the DCG. Such relationships may require functional assessment, such as with DSG. Permeable (patent) passageways, normal on DCG, may be functionally inefficient and better assessed with DSG. Finally, nasal obstruction may cause epiphora, occluding the valve of Hasner or the adjacent nasolacrimal canal. The venous plexus surrounding the NLDS is in direct communication with the venous plexus of the nasal mucosa. Edema within the nasal mucosa leads to venous plexus engorgement and secondary compression of the nasolacrimal duct.

Obstruction of the nasolacrimal duct system (NLDS) in the great majority of patients is due to idiopathic inflammation and scarring, which causes a spectrum of clinical symptoms ranging from partial occlusion to total obstruction.[51] Clear epiphora, secondary to nasolacrimal duct obstruction, represents a milder presentation. Mucoid epiphora results if bacterial overgrowth occurs in the stagnant fluid of the lacrimal sac. Clinical deterioration will include further signs of dacryocystitis (inflammation of the lacrimal sac) such as a medial canthal mass with increasing tenderness, mucopurulent discharge, secondary conjunctivitis, periorbital cellulitis, and a walled-off abscess in the lacrimal sac. The radiologist investigating the NLDS should be aware of this clinical spectrum and should understand that subtle cases of dacryocystitis require careful physical examination, including lacrimal irrigation.[51]

Dacryocystitis occurs because of obstruction of the flow of tears from the lacrimal sac. The obstructive etiology may be congenital or acquired, including inflammatory, infectious, infiltrative, traumatic, or neoplastic causes. All such processes must be considered as possible underlying factors in the presentation of dacryocystitis. In patients with nasolacrimal duct obstruction, the inflammation and fibrosis may be secondary to coexisting infectious colonization within the lumen of the lacrimal sac. Culture results of conjunctival and nasal specimens have not been predictive of lacrimal sac flora.[52] Assessment of the bacterial flora at the inferior lacrimal sac–nasolacrimal junction, using direct biopsy methods during 132 DCR procedures, to explore the possibility of primary bacteriologic etiology of the inflammatory response, gave positive culture results in 41.7% of the obstructed nasolacrimal duct systems undergoing DCR.[53] Of the isolates cultured, 78.5% were gram-positive bacteria (of this group 76.5% were *Staphylococcus* sp.) and 21.5% were gram-negative bacteria. Nine specimens yielded more than one organism. These organisms were found in patients with and without a history of infection, dacrycystitis, or the presence of a mucocele. Of the isolates, 69.2% were from patients with no history of dacryocystitis or mucocele, suggesting that the infection may have been the primary cause of the nasolacrimal duct obstruction. Conversely, the lack of positive cultures in a significant proportion of the above patients suggests etiologies other than bacterial invasion as the primary cause of obstruction, and organisms isolated may represent resident flora and not be causative.[54] DeAngelis et al.[53] have

noted a greatly diminished prevalence of *Streptococcus pneumoniae* over the past 10 years. Others have noted a higher proportion of gram-negative bacteria associated with chronic dacryocystitis.[55]

One should try to distinguish between acute and chronic bacterial dacryocystitis. Acute dacryocystitis manifests as a painful swelling of the lacrimal sac, with surrounding erythema and edema. Pus may be expressible by pressure over a tender lacrimal sac. The bacteria reside in the wall of the sac, and treatment should be via the systemic route.[56] Complications include orbital cellulitis (usually limited to preseptal tissues), corneal involvement, lacrimal sac mucocele, and, rarely, orbital abscesses. The most common organisms implicated are *Staphylococcus aureus* in acquired cases and *S. pneumoniae* in congenital cases, although, due to the large number of potential causative organisms (gram positive or gram negative, aerobic or anaerobic), cultures and smears of expressed punctal secretions are desirable.

Chronic dacryocystitis is characterized by swelling of the lacrimal sac, which may or may not be painful, and with minimal if any surrounding inflammation. The bacteria reside in the lumen of the sac, necessitating treatment by local irrigation as well as by the systemic route.[56] A history of previous attacks of acute dacryocystitis may be present. Patients with chronic dacryocystitis and incomplete obstruction of the nasolacrimal duct may have superimposed bouts of acute dacryocystitis if duct patency is altered by swelling or debris in the duct system. For proper eradication of infection and resolution of dacryocystitis, the lacrimal obstruction must be eliminated to ensure adequate drainage of the nasolacrimal system. Chronic or recurrent dacryocystitis may require DCR. An obstructed lacrimal sac or lacrimal sac distention alone must be differentiated from dacryocystitis and its associated inflammatory changes.

Acute dacryocystitis is commonly associated with preseptal cellulitis. Infection of the lacrimal sac will preferentially localize in the preseptal space since the orbital septum inserts at the posterior lacrimal crest and acts as a significant anatomic barrier to prevent infections extending from the lacrimal sac posteriorly into the orbit. Orbital cellulitis rarely and orbital abscess very rarely result from acute dacryocystitis.[57, 58] The onset of a lacrimal sac abscess must be treated aggressively to prevent possible extension to adjacent tissues as an extraconal or intraconal orbital abscess.[57–60]

In a review of 148 patients with orbital abscesses, acute dacryocystitis was not the source of infection for a single patient.[61] Acute drainage of a lacrimal sac abscess is indicated, especially if it may be the source of orbital infection. In hyperacute dacryocystitis, treatment, although controversial, favors external drainage rather than intranasal (DCR) drainage. A DCR performed following resolution of the acute inflammation reduces the otherwise high risk of late failure due to extensive scarring.[58]

An intraconal abscess in a 1-month-old infant with congenital nasolacrimal duct obstruction (congenital dacryocystitis) suggests that anatomic barriers to infection may be less well defined in neonates than in adults.[62]

Subacute to chronic dacryocystitis may represent later stages of acute dacryocystitis that do not respond sufficiently to antibiotics or that may develop owing to persistent obstruction of the lacrimal system distal to the lacrimal sac.

A chronic lacrimal sac abscess (with the lacrimal sac swollen and filled with pus) or low-grade chronic dacryocystitis with intermittent exacerbations may result. Failure of antibiotic treatment of a lacrimal abscess due to chronic or subacute dacryocystitis is associated with obstruction of the lacrimal drainage system distal to the lacrimal sac, preventing drainage of pus from the lacrimal sac. Janssen et al.[60] have presented a subgroup of such patients who may be offered an alternative to DCR such as temporary stent placement within the nasolacrimal duct, along with systemic and topical broad-spectrum antibiotic coverage. This allows drainage of pus from the sac and relief of the infection, with no incidence of exacerbations or extension of the active inflammatory process. Long-term patency of the lacrimal duct system was not ensured by dacryocystoplasty. Surgical DCR was considered if reobstruction of the lacrimal duct system occurred.

Swelling (with or without fluctuance), erythema, and tenderness in the medial canthal area, extending inferior to the medial canthal tendon, simulating acute dacryocystitis or lacrimal sac abscess, may result from anterior ethmoiditis.[63, 64] Such cases of pseudodacryocystitis may be distinguished by the lack of a purulent discharge in the tear reflux, lack of a previous history of epiphora, or failure to note tearing between episodes of inflammation. Probing, irrigation, or DCG will confirm patent lacrimal systems. Inflammatory disease within the anterior ethmoid air cells may be noted on CT or MR imaging, with bone dehiscence of the lacrimal sac fossa better identified on CT. Such inner canthal fistulae associated with ethmoiditis are rare and tend to develop above the level of the medial palpebral ligament,[65] in contrast to acute dacryocystitis or lacrimal sac abscess, which extend inferior to the medial canthal tendon. An ethmoidectomy procedure rather than DCR is the treatment of choice for patients with primary sinonasal disease.

## Obstruction

Obstruction may be due to various causes, including congenital stenosis, inflammatory diseases, calculi, trauma including foreign bodies, and tumors. Filling defects may be associated with an inflammatory process (see the section on Chronic Canaliculitis). DCG can assess both complete and incomplete obstructions (Figs. 10-5 to 10-8). The most common site of obstruction is the neck of the lacrimal sac, at its junction with the nasolacrimal duct, and it is usually due to inflammation (chronic dacryocystitis) and scarring of the nasolacrimal duct. Marked dilatation of the sac is usually clinically noted inferior to the level of the medial canthal tendon. Dilatation of the canaliculi is often associated with a dilated sac. Obstructions of the sac may be associated with a membrane at the medial end of the common canaliculus. Such a membrane must be identified and removed for a dacryocystorhinostomy (DCR) to be successful.[66] With pure sac obstructions, DCR should be successful in 100% of the cases, without the need for temporary intubation. Of the failed DCRs, 12% to 40% were due to common canaliculus problems.[66, 67] Thus high-quality images, especially of the canaliculi, are necessary to predict which patients will do poorly with simple DCR. The size of the lacrimal sac

mucosal flap needed for the DCR may also be predicted from the DCG.

DCG may also define a cicatrized lacrimal sac, seen in chronic dacryocystitis. A cicatrized sac is more difficult to operate on, and is associated with poorer results than normal or enlarged lacrimal sacs when treated by endoscopic intranasal DCR in either primary treatment or revision patient populations. In these patients, the DCG can suggest that an external DCR should be the treatment procedure of choice.[37]

The next most frequent site of obstruction is the common canaliculus.[9, 16, 47] Common canalicular obstructions are most frequently related to chronic dacryocystitis or a ball valve effect of dacryoliths.[68] Accurate localization of canalicular obstruction has treatment implications (Fig. 10-8). Two thirds of common canalicular obstructions occur at the medial end, at the junction with the lacrimal sac, where a thin membrane, as a complication of inflammation within the sac, is present.[69] The common canaliculus appears as a well-defined structure on DCG. Treatment includes excision of the membrane and a DCR with temporary intubation (3 months) of the canaliculus. One third of common canalicular obstructions occur at its lateral end, as a result of mucosal obstruction where the superior and inferior canaliculi join. The entire common canaliculus is dissected out before mobilizing the lacrimal sac or periosteum. The scarred (stenosed) segment of canaliculus is excised, and the canaliculi are reanastomosed into the lateral wall of the lacrimal sac as a canaliculo-DCR. Occlusions or stenosis of the inferior or superior canaliculus may be due to traumatic laceration, canaliculitis, canalicular papillomas, and chronic pilocarpine or phospholine iodide use, and can be treated with DCR and temporary or permanent canalicular tubes or canaliculo-DCR reconstructive surgery.[68] Preoperative DCG diagnosis, with the exact location and length of occlusions/stenoses, therefore aids surgical planning and treatment decisions.

Less frequently, obstructions occur within the superior aspect of the lacrimal sac. Noncongenital obstructions of the distal nasolacrimal duct tend to be incomplete and are more frequently associated with adjacent sinus disease, inflammatory or neoplastic, than with intrinsic pathology of the nasolacrimal duct.[9] Neoplasms of the nasolacrimal duct (or sac) are rare, usually arise from pseudostratified columnar epithelium, and cause duct obstruction (Fig. 10-13A-C). On DCG, irregular duct obstruction, although nonspecific, should suggest or include this diagnostic possibility.[70]

Radiographically, the lacrimal sac above the obstruction will usually be dilated and have an ovoid or rounded configuration rather than a normal linear shape. The dilated sac or "mucocele of the lacrimal sac" is palpable below the medial canthus.[9] Occasionally the lacrimal sac will be constricted above the obstruction because of a cicatricial inflammatory response or fibrosis.[71]

Reflux of contrast medium into the conjunctival sac through the uncannulated punctum will occur when obstruction is present. This occurs early during the injection of a small volume of contrast medium. When the obstruction is incomplete, the DCG usually demonstrates dilation of the lacrimal sac above the incomplete obstruction. Contrast material must be visualized entering the nasal cavity to confirm the incomplete nature of the obstruction. Dilated

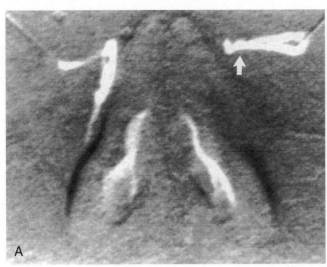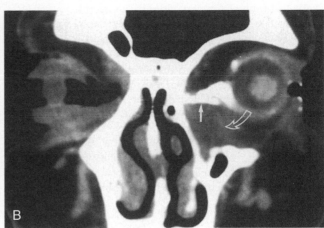

**FIGURE 10-13**   CT-DCG of mass lesions: inner canthus. CT-DCG allows better assessment of the extent of adjacent tissue involvement than DCG alone and better assessment of NLDS involvement than CT alone. **A** to **C**, Patient presents with left inner canthus prominence and epiphora. **A**, DCG shows superior displacement of the left canaliculi (*arrow*) with no visualization of the left lacrimal sac or nasolacrimal duct. **B**, Coronal CT-DCG shows displacement of the proximal NLDS (*solid arrow*) by a soft-tissue mass in the inner canthus (*open arrow*).

*Illustration continued on following page*

lacrimal sacs, distorted by fibrosis, must be differentiated from distended cystic diverticula or true cysts of the lacrimal sac (Fig. 10-14). Traumatic dislocation of the lacrimal sac must also be considered.

Obstructions in the lower part of the nasolacrimal duct occur less frequently. The diameter of the bony canal is one of the contributing factors for occurrence of strictures at this site. Women are affected much more frequently than men (up to 80%), probably related to their narrower bony canal.

## Fistulae

Congenital lacrimal sac fistulae are relatively uncommon, estimated to occur in 1 per 2000 births.[72] Fistulae may also be postinflammatory (chronic dacryocystitis), posttraumatic, or postsurgical.[42, 72, 73] The fistula most commonly originates from the lacrimal sac (lacrimal sac-cutaneous fistula) but may arise from the canaliculi or nasolacrimal duct. Most of the fistulae are unilateral and located inferonasal to the medial canthus. Patients may be asymptomatic and overlooked for some time after birth or may demonstrate tearing from the fistula. the eye, or both.[74] Fistulae are usually associated with long-standing obstruction of the nasolacrimal drainage system (Fig. 10-15). A previous DCR may have been performed without recognition of the fistula's presence. The majority of patients present with epiphora, which may be delayed in onset; occasionally an inflammatory lesion of the lower lid may be the presenting sign.

Congenital lacrimal fistulae probably result from failure of involution of the lacrimal anlage, the thickened surface ectoderm of the nasooptic fissure, which becomes buried in the mesenchyme between the nasal and maxillary processes to form the nasolacrimal drainage system. Instead, this anlage proliferates, canalizes, and forms a fistula, whose cutaneous opening is just medial and inferior to the medial canthus.[27] The fistulous tract may also be incomplete and end blindly in the subcutaneous tissues near the lacrimal sac.[75] Welham and Bergin[76] have proposed that a congenital fistula may be caused by aberrant budding of the canaliculi, with the fistula representing a supernumerary or aberrant canaliculus. Absence of a superior or inferior canaliculus or absence of a punctum has been noted to be associated with lacrimal fistulae.[76, 77] The epithelial lining of the fistula is identical to that of a normal canaliculi.[75] A hereditary or familial pattern of presentation of lacrimal fistulae has also been noted.[27]

If the fistula is not clearly demonstrated by the DCG, placement of a lacrimal probe into the external opening, in conjunction with the DCG, may help show its origin from the nasolacrimal drainage system. Recommended treatment includes DCR, common canalicular dissection, fistula excision, and temporary canalicular intubation to bypass the distal obstruction and prevent common canalicular obstruction and recurrence of the fistula.[76] Others recommend excision alone or with nasolacrimal intubation, without DCR if there is no evidence of nasolacrimal obstruction.[74] Patients with very minor or no symptoms may simply be kept under observation.

## Diverticula

Diverticula represent outpouchings of a lacrimal drainage pathway and are usually the result of a long-standing obstruction (Fig. 10-7F,G). They are most commonly asymptomatic, small, and clinically undetected. Occasionally they may be associated with episodic or permanent symptoms of nasolacrimal duct obstruction (chronic tearing discharge) and may present as a mass lesion without associated nasolacrimal duct obstruction.[78] Less often, they may present as an acute infection, either diverticulitis or dacryocystitis secondary to duct obstruction. Congenital lacrimal sac diverticula most frequently result from the spontaneous rupture (outpouching) of the lacrimal sac wall in acute dacryocystitis associated with congenital nasolacrimal duct obstruction.[79]

Acquired lacrimal sac diverticula most commonly result from a weakening of the lacrimal sac wall after inflammation or trauma, including probing or irrigation, or after incision and drainage procedures for dacryocystitis.[78]

Diverticula of the lacrimal sac may be associated with dacryoliths, which may intermittently obstruct the opening of the lacrimal sac and increase the pressure of fluid within the sac, with resultant weakening of the lacrimal sac wall and diverticular formation in an asymptomatic patient.

Epiphora, associated with these diverticula, may result from mechanical pressure on the lacrimal drainage system rather than a primary intraluminal blockage of a duct or sac. Slow evolution of a lacrimal sac diverticulum is typical.[80] The most common location is at the junction between the lacrimal sac and the nasolacrimal duct. The communication between the diverticulum and the lacrimal sac may be clearly open or may be valvular and limited, limiting diverticular drainage. The relative rarity of reports of lacrimal diverticula in the literature more likely reflects their

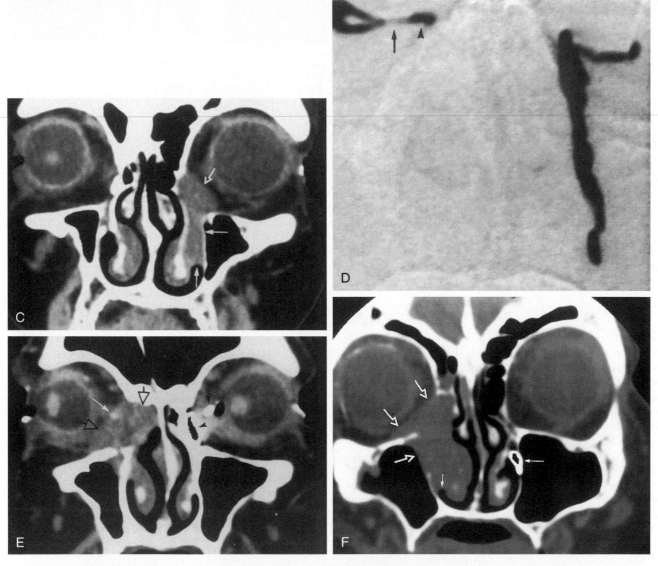

**FIGURE 10-13** *Continued.* **C,** More posterior coronal image shows the soft-tissue mass (*open arrow*) extending into and widening the left nasolacrimal canal (*horizontal arrow*), reaching the inferior meatus (*vertical arrow*). CT-DCG offered significant information beyond that available by DCG alone. Pathology: transitional cell carcinoma in the left lacrimal sac. **D** to **F,** Right inner canthus mass with epiphora. **D,** DCG. Superior displacement of the right proximal NLDS (*arrow*). Only the most superior aspect of the lacrimal sac is visualized (*arrowhead*). **E,** Coronal CT-DCG. Large soft-tissue mass (*open arrows*) in the right medial canthus and adjacent ethmoid sinus, with destruction of the medial orbit wall. The lacrimal sac containing contrast medium is displaced laterally and superiorly (*thin arrow*). Normal left NLDS (*arrowheads*). **F,** Bone windows of a slightly more posterior coronal CT scan shows extension of the mass (*open arrows*) along the path of the nasolacrimal canal to the inferior meatus (*vertical arrow*) with adjacent bone destruction. Contrast material in the left inferior meatus (*horizontal arrow*). Pathology: squamous cell carcinoma.

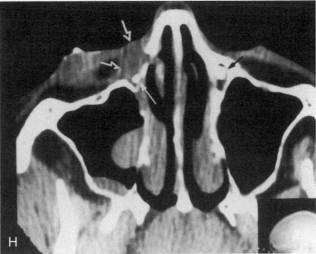

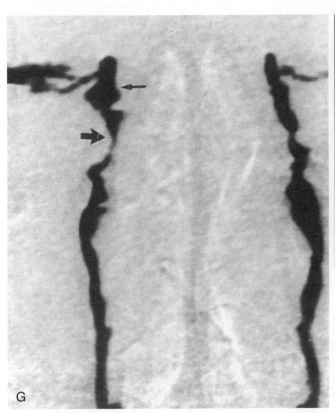

**FIGURE 10-13**  *Continued.* **G** and **H**, Mild prominence of the right inner canthus. **G**, DCG. Mass indenting the proximal right nasolacrimal duct (*larger arrow*) from the lateral aspect with mild distention of the lacrimal sac (*thin arrow*). **H**, Axial CT-DCG shows a soft-tissue mass in the right inner canthus (*open arrows*) displacing the lacrimal sac (*thin arrow*) posteromedially within the nasolacrimal fossa. Normal left NLDS (*black arrow*). Pathology: lymphocytic lymphoma in the wall of the lacrimal sac and duct. (Note also the nasopharyngeal lymphomatous mass.) (Courtesy of Dr. Nasir Jaffer, Toronto, Canada.)

frequently asymptomatic nature and difficulty in demonstrating them routinely by DCG. In many cases, only the obstruction or impression on the lacrimal sac due to the mechanical pressure of the diverticulum is noted. Only DCG or ultrasonography may reveal the narrow communication, while CT/MR imaging may better display the size, extent, and cyst-like characteristics of the diverticula, and their relationship to the nasolacrimal drainage system, for those lesions unable to be directly visualized by DCG.[78, 80]

Diverticula of the canaliculi, lacrimal sac, or nasolacrimal duct are usually the result of a long-standing obstruction (Fig. 10-7F,G), and the diverticula will remain until adequate drainage of the obstructed or partially obstructed nasolacrimal system is restored. It is not possible to diagnose diverticula preoperatively without a DCG. Clinically, distended cystic diverticula may resemble a dilated lacrimal sac or a true cyst of the lacrimal sac, which does not communicate with the NLDS.

## Lacrimal Sac Cysts

Cysts arising from the lacrimal sac epithelium are rare. Although these cysts may be congenital, inflammatory, or traumatic in origin, most think they arise from diverticula of the lacrimal sac, with the cyst forming when the communication to the lacrimal sac closes off.[81] The cyst may communicate directly with the sac or may be anatomically separate. Lacrimal sac cysts usually present as a nonreducible, well-defined, slow-growing, painless mass in the inner canthus, below the level the medial canthal tendon.[82] Epiphora, which may be secondary to pressure on the sac, is a common symptom, and/or the cyst may be associated with a patent nasolacrimal drainage system.[81] Pressure over the mass will not alter the size of a lacrimal sac cyst but may reduce the size of a diverticulum. The pathologic description of a cystic cavity lined by columnar to cuboidal epithelium may not help differentiate a lacrimal sac cyst from a diverticulum or mucocele of lacrimal sac etiology. Treatment consists of total excision of the cyst. If there is any communication with the lacrimal sac, lacrimal sac wall repair and simultaneous DCR is indicated.

## Lacrimal Calculi

Lacrimal sac dacryoliths may be present in 10% to 30% of patients presenting with chronic dacryocystitis.[83–85] In addition to tearing, patients with lacrimal sac calculi may present with a history of mucopurulent discharge, lacrimal sac distention, tenderness in the medial canthal region, and recurrent dacryocystitis. The frequency of partial nasolacrimal duct obstruction with dacryocystitis has been reported in as many as 65% to 70% of patients.[83, 84, 86, 87] Primary and secondary dye tests indicate partial obstruction of the nasolacrimal duct (Figs. 10-7, 10-16C,D, 10-17D,E, and 10-18A-C).[85]

Wilkins and Pressly[86] stressed the intermittent but chronic nature of tearing unresponsive to treatment in patients with lacrimal calculi. There may be a history of repeated, painful lacrimal probings, occasionally with transient relief caused by either repositioning or fragmentation of the stone. The extreme inconsistency of nasolacrimal irrigation in patients with lacrimal calculi is most impressive, and by itself may suggest the diagnosis. Such variability of results may occur within a short period (minutes), with one irrigation showing reflux and suggesting obstruction and a second irrigation showing normal flow into the nasal cavity. Friable or fragmented calculi within the

sac are subject to the currents produced by an irrigation, and cranial movement of the calculus will allow free flow, while caudal movement of the lacrimal sac calculus creates a ball-valve effect and complete nasolacrimal occlusion.[86] Weber et al.[88] have noted that dacryoliths do not change in size or shape, representing permanent filling defects in the DCG. Dacryoliths should be differentiated from retained thick secretions or air bubbles. Air bubbles injected into the nasolacrimal system represent an artifact that can simulate a concretion, although bubbles tend to be rounder and more sharply defined. A cross-table lateral view will demonstrate the air bubble floating in the lacrimal sac, while concretions tend to settle in the more dependent inferior posterior aspect of the sac and do not change location with altered positions of the head as quickly as air bubbles (Figs. 10-7M,N and

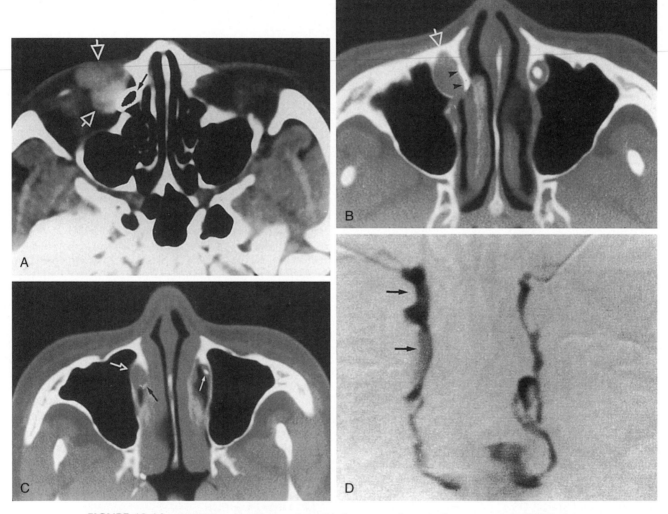

**FIGURE 10-14**  CT-DCG to identify the relationship between an inner canthus mass and the NLDS. **A** to **D**, Patient with a 2-year history of swelling of the right inner canthus. No epiphora. **A** to **C**, Axial CT-DCG scan from the superior to the inferior location. **A**, Large lobulated mass seen in the right inner canthus (*open arrow*) displacing the lacrimal sac (filled with contrast and seen as black because of density misregistration) (*solid arrow*) posteriorly within the nasolacrimal fossa. **B**, Enlarged right nasolacrimal canal (*open arrow*) with a contrast-filled nasolacrimal duct is compressed medially (*arrowheads*), resembling the bony wall of the canal. Normal left NLDS. **C**, At the level of the inferior meatus, normal termination of the left NLDS (*thin arrow*). Soft tissue on the right (*arrow*) displaces the contrast-filled nasolacrimal duct (*black arrow*) posteromedially. **D**, DCG. Prior to CT, only lateral indentation (*upper arrow*) of the dilated lacrimal sac was discussed, with less attention to the medial displacement of the nasolacrimal duct (*lower arrow*). Pathology: benign lacrimal sac cyst (from the wall of the lacrimal sac).

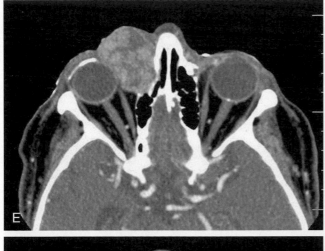

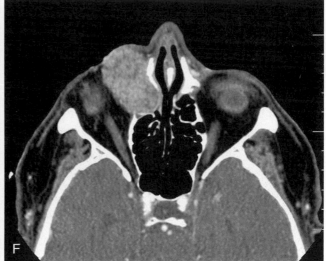

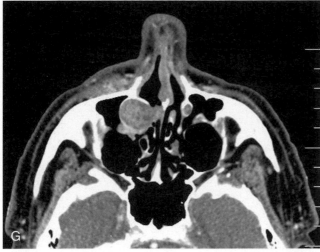

**FIGURE 10-14** *Continued.* **E** to **L**, Second patient: right inner canthus swelling for 2 years. **E**, to **G**, Axial enhanced images, plus topical contrast, show a large, solid, well-defined mass in the right inner canthus displacing the globe laterally and extending into the nasolacrimal canal.

*Illustration continued on following page*

10-19A). Lacrimal sac calculi are often unsuspected at the time of surgery even though they are a common cause of epiphora. Preoperatively, such a diagnosis should be more strongly suspected in the younger patient (under age 50 years) with no obvious cause of epiphora.[86] In Jones'[84] and Wilkins and Pressly's series,[86] 65% and 53% of patients, respectively, under age 50 with epiphora of unknown etiology had calculi detected during DCR. Several reports have noted dacryoliths to be more common in younger and female patients. Reports indicate that 58% to 80% of patients with dacryoliths are under 50 years of age.[83, 84, 86, 87] Between 68% and 95% of patients with dacryoliths are female.[83, 84, 86, 87]

Most reports indicate that the frequency of lacrimal sac stones between 6% and 18% in patients undergoing dacryocystorhinostomy (DCR) for nasolacrimal duct obstruction. Yazici et al.'s[89] of 163 DCR cases noted a difference in the frequency of lacrimal sac dacryoliths in patients subcategorized as to etiology of obstruction. They report that 9.2% of the cases with primary acquired (idiopathic) nasolacrimal duct obstruction (PANDO) had dacryoliths. However, no dacryoliths were noted in a smaller group (38 cases) with a known cause of obstruction (congenital, traumatic, sinonasal surgery), a finding also noted in other series.[83, 84, 86] In analyzing the symptoms of patients with PANDO and dacryoliths compared to those

without dacryoliths, Yazici et al.[89] noted the increased likelihood of acute medial canthal swelling (lacrimal sac distention or acute dacryocystic retention) without infection in patients with dacryoliths. They emphasized the distinction between lacrimal sac distention (no erythema or extreme tenderness, with a mucoid but not a purulent discharge) and dacryocystitis. Forty-two percent of the 12 patients with dacryoliths had simple acute lacrimal sac distention versus 5% of the 103 patients without dacryoliths. The previously reported greater frequency of acute dacryocystitis with dacryoliths may not have considered the distinction between lacrimal sac distention (retention) and acute dacryocystitis.

In these patients[89] with PANDO requiring DCR, the presence of lacrimal sac distention and male gender were more frequently associated with dacryoliths. There was no statistical significance related to age. Partial nasolacrimal duct obstruction and a history of cigarette smoking were relative risk factors for stone formation. Other studies[83, 84, 86] have noted a higher incidence of calculi in younger patients (under age 50) and in females.

The calculi may be fragmented, especially if the lacrimal drainage system has been probed. At surgery (DCR) the lacrimal sac must be carefully assessed and the puncta irrigated to ensure that all fragments are removed. Although the etiology of lacrimal calculi is obscure, predisposing factors such as stasis and infection are frequently associated with calculus formation. An obstruction allowing partial drainage may facilitate the accumulation of debris. The etiology of dacryoliths, however, is more complex, with dacryolith formation noted in patients with no narrowing or compromise of the drainage system. The dacryolith is typically friable, often molding itself to the sac and duct. This friability helps explain the spontaneous passage of

large dacryoliths through obstructed or anatomically narrowed ducts.[90, 91] The calculus consists of lamellae of cellular breakdown products and mucoproteins with or without calcium or ammonium salts.[89] Eyelashes, and occasionally particles of makeup, may be found in dacryoliths and may have acted as a nidus for dacryolith formation.[92–94] Herzig and Hurwitz,[95] in a series of 246

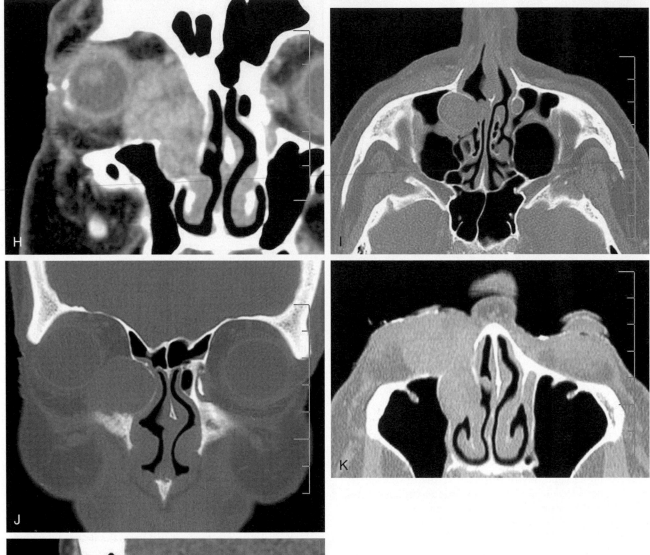

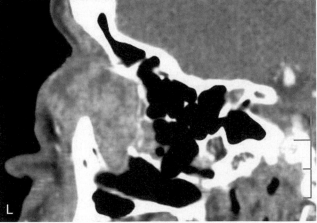

**FIGURE 10-14** *Continued.* **H,** Coronal reformation shows the mass extending into the widened nasolacrimal canal. **I** to **K,** Bone algorithm images. Axial (**I**), coronal (**J**), and coronal oblique reformations (**K**) show remodeling and displacement of the adjacent bony wall of the orbit and the widened nasolacrimal canal. **L,** Sagittal reconstruction through the left nasolacrimal canal shows a mass extending to reach the inferior meatus. Topical contrast present in the left NLDS on several images but not entering the right NLDS. Pathology: squamous papilloma. (See also Figs. 10-13, 10-17A, 10-18, 10-20B.)

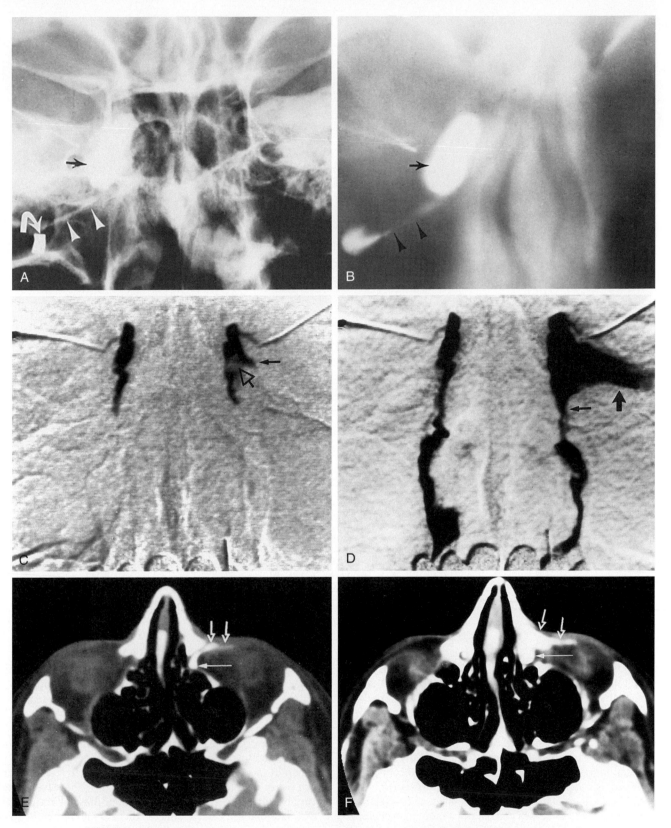

**FIGURE 10-15** Fistulas and sinus tracts in preseptal tissues. **A** and **B**, Patient with epiphora and dacryocutaneous fistula draining below the inferior orbital rim. **A**, DCG, frontal view. **B**, Tomographic image. Dilated lacrimal sac (*arrow*). Fistula (*arrowheads*) seen extending from the distal lacrimal sac to the metallic marker on the skin surface at the cutaneous end of the fistula (*curved arrow*). **C** to **F**, Patient with a 2-year history of intermittent swelling of the left inferior eyelid causing closure of the eye and epiphora. Sinus tract into the lower lid in a patient with Crohn's disease. **C**, Early DCG image shows a suspicious ill-defined filling defect (*open arrow*) of the inferior left lacrimal sac, just above the origin of the nasolacrimal duct. Abnormal projection of contrast material in the lateral wall of the left lacrimal sac (*thin arrow*). **D**, Later DCG image. A large amount of contrast material extends inferolaterally toward the lower lid (*vertical arrow*). Contrast also enters the nasolacrimal duct (*horizontal arrow*) to empty into the nasal cavity. **E**, Axial CT-DCG shows contrast material extending from the lacrimal sac (*thin arrow*) to enter the soft tissues of the lower lid (*open arrow*). **F**, More inferior axial image shows the abnormal location of contrast material in the left inner canthus and lower lid (*open arrows*) and an enlarged collection of contrast material in or surrounding the left lacrimal sac (*thin arrow*).

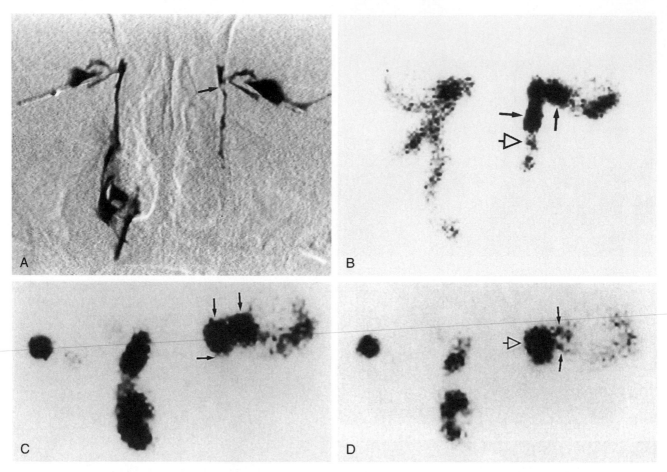

**FIGURE 10-16** Comparison of DCG and DSG. **A** and **B**, Patient with left epiphora. **A**, DCG of the normal right side. Small filling defect of the distal left lacrimal sac (*arrow*) with delayed drainage into the nasolacrimal duct. **B**, DSG at 20 minutes. Normal drainage on the right side with decreased isotope activity within the NLDS. Persistent increased activity within the left lacrimal sac and canaliculi (*solid arrows*) with minimal activity entering the nasolacrimal duct (*open arrow*). **C** and **D**, Patient with left epiphora and a bloody discharge from the left tear duct. **C**, DSG at 15 minutes. Inferior portion of the left lacrimal sac is not seen (*horizontal arrow*). Increased activity in the proximal lacrimal sac and canaliculi (*vertical arrows*). Normal right drainage. **D**, Postrub DSG. Decreased activity in the right NLDS. Persistent increased activity in the left lacrimal sac (*open arrow*), superior canaliculus, and inferior canaliculus (*solid arrows*) caused by obstruction to outflow in the left lacrimal sac. Dacryolith in the left lacrimal sac. (See Fig. 10-18A-C for DCG and CT of the same patient.)

patients treated surgically, of whom 14 had calculi, were unable to demonstrate any systemic electrolyte abnormality predisposing to stone formation. They noted no abnormality of tear or serum calcium, phosphorus and uric acid concentrations, tear to serum calcium ratios or calcium-phosphate products. Accumulation (supersaturation) of electrolytes in an obstructed tear sac eventually leads to precipitation of a stone. Such precipitation can occur when obstruction is sudden (as in trauma or nasal surgery) or when obstruction is long-standing and associated with infection. The great majority of stones consist of calcium phosphate.[95]

The presence of a dacryolith, with persistent clinical features not responding to conservative treatment and requiring a DCR, may make endoscopic DCR more difficult or necessitate a larger opening for lacrimal sac exploration. An external approach may be necessary.[96]

Fungi have been noted in canalicular concretions but less frequently in lacrimal sac concretions. Anaerobic infection (*Actinomyces israelii*) is more common in canalicular stones (Fig. 10-7K,L), whereas *Candida*, an aerobic fungus, has

been noted in lacrimal sac concretions.[97, 98] The relatively large size of fungi probably acts as the nidus, which, in a setting of chronic stasis, promotes or initiates calculus formation. The stasis, in a significant number of patients, is midlevel in the sac and probably results from the nature of the split fascia of the orbicularis muscle at this level, causing chronic dacryocystitis. The occurrence of lacrimal calculi is generally more frequent in female patients, but in at least one series male predominance was noted.[89] There have been variable results in identifying bacteria or fungi in association with lacrimal sac calculi. Jones[84] did not find any infectious agents in his results, while Berlin et al.[83] found bacteria or fungi rather commonly in lacrimal sac stones. They used routine hematoxylin-eosin stains as well as special fungal stains and recommended cultures for aerobes, anaerobes, and fungi. They noted DCG filling defects within the lacrimal sac in 4 of 11 patients found to have dacryoliths of the lacrimal sac at DCR.

Cast-like fungus obstruction of the nasolacrimal duct is uncommon.[98] When fungi occlude the lacrimal drainage

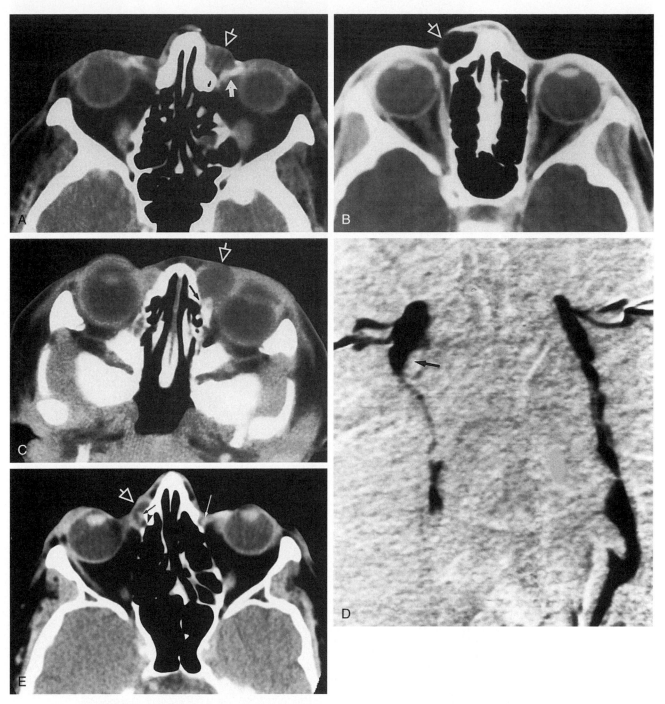

**FIGURE 10-17**   Cystic lesions of the inner canthus, CT-DCG. **A**, Mass in the left inner canthus (*open arrow*) is well defined and lies anterior to the left inferior canaliculus, which is filled with contrast medium (*closed arrow*). **B**, Well-defined right inner canthus mass (*arrow*) overlying the nasal bones. Tissue characteristics (-100 HU). Dermoid tumor. **C**, Neonate with a prominent left inner canthus. Hypodense mass (*open arrow*) contiguous with the nasolacrimal fossa (*solid arrow*). Dacryocystocele. **D** and **E**, DCG and enhanced axial CT in a patient with right epiphora and a questioned inner canthus mass. **D**, Mass indenting the medial aspect of the lacrimal sac inferiorly (*arrow*) with resultant dilation of the right lacrimal sac and a slight delay in drainage. **E**, Hypodense mass with a well-defined capsule (*open arrow*) extends into the nasolacrimal fossa (*arrowhead*) and represents a dilated lacrimal sac. Hyperdensity (*thin black arrow*) represents dacryolith in the medial wall of the sac, explaining the filling defect on DCG. Normal left lacrimal sac (*white thin arrow*). Pathology: chronic dacryocystitis with dacryolith. (See also Fig. 10-33, dacryocystocele.)

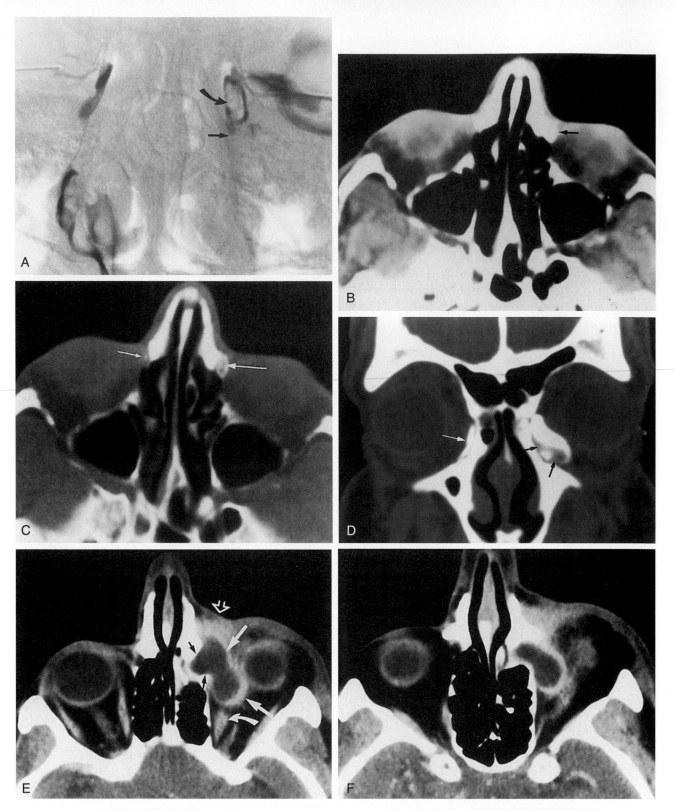

**FIGURE 10-18** CT-DCG of intraluminal lesions. Multiple patients. **A,** Patient with a bloody discharge from the left tear duct. DCG shows a large filling defect (*curved arrow*) of the left lacrimal sac with a thin rim of contrast material peripherally. The nasolacrimal duct does not fill (*straight arrow*). **B,** CT-DCG. Soft-tissue window. See the prominent hyperdensity in the region of the left nasolacrimal fossa (*arrow*) compared with the right. **C,** Wider window of **B** shows a filling defect (*long arrow*) centrally in the enlarged left lacrimal sac within the nasolacrimal fossa. Contrast is faintly seen in the right lacrimal sac (*short arrow*). Pathology: dacryolith associated with gram-positive cocci. See Figure 10-16C,D for DSG on the same patient. **D,** Different patient with left inner canthus swelling. Coronal image shows a filling defect (*black arrows*) in the inferomedial aspect of the dilated left lacrimal sac. Normal right lacrimal sac (*white arrow*). Pathology: acute and chronic dacryocystitis with marked mucoid and cellular debris in a very distended lacrimal sac. **E** and **F,** Different patient. Cellulitis and chronic dacryocystitis with a lacrimal sac mucocele. **E,** Well-defined lobulated hypodensity of a lacrimal sac mucocele (*long arrows*) intimately associated with and enlarging the left nasolacrimal fossa (*short arrows*). The left globe is displaced laterally by the mass, which also abuts the optic nerve (not shown on this image). Preseptal soft-tissue swelling is present (*open arrow*). The medial rectus muscle is enlarged (*curved arrow*), representing a component of postseptal inflammatory involvement. **F,** More inferiorly located axial image emphasizes the relationship of the mucocele with the enlarged nasolacrimal fossa. Mucocele should not be mistaken for abscess cavity.

system, it is usually by formation of a stone or cast. *Aspergillus fumigatus* is an extremely rare cause of canalicular or lacrimal sac obstruction. *Aspergillus* produces hyphae, forming a ball or plug that obstructs the lacrimal system by mechanical obstruction without invading the surrounding tissues. Many cases have concomitant keratoconjunctivitis.[99] A lacrimal sac *Aspergillus* plug, presenting with initial intermittent obstruction and progressing to total obstruction, with discharge from the lacrimal punctum and extreme discomfort, may show no involvement of adjacent tissues (CT, operative and pathologic assessment), with CT only displaying an enlarged lacrimal sac. The discomfort is presumed to be caused by the stretched lacrimal sac capsule.[99] In patients with mechanical obstruction (i.e., plug) as an etiologic consideration, the planned DCR may be initiated with lacrimal sac exploration prior to osteotomy of the lacrimal fossa. The DCR may be abandonned if unnecessary.[99]

Calculi related to the canaliculi are discussed in the next section.

Since stasis secondary to an anatomic obstruction is likely to be the precipitating factor,[95] massaging, probing, or irrigation techniques to flush out the dacryoliths are restricted to incomplete obstructions and are limited in success due to the persistent stenosis of the nasolacrimal duct system (NLDS) or the increased size of the prestenotic dacryolith. Surgical removal of the dacryolith, in conjunction with an external DCR, is the standard treatment. The presence of calculi in the NLDS represents a limitation for endonasal DCR treatment. There have been attempts at nonsurgical management of dacryolithiasis using stent placement to correct an obstruction at the lacrimal sac–nasolacrimal junction. After fragmentation of the stones during stent implantation, the fragments passed through the stent with saline irrigation.[100]

In cases of dacryolithiasis associated with incomplete

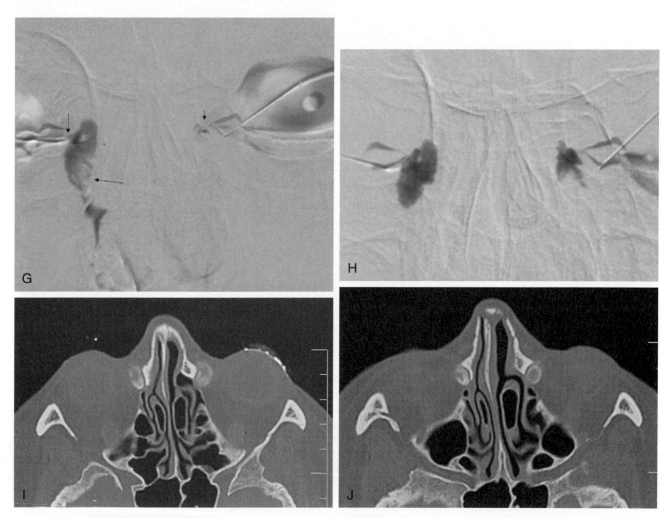

**FIGURE 10-18**   *Continued.* **G** to **N**, Lupus patient with bilateral tearing and intermittent facial swelling. **G**, DCG shows minimal filling of a stenosed left common canaliculus (*short arrow*). Contrast refluxes into the conjunctival sac. The right lacrimal sac is distended with secretions and debris (*horizontal arrow*) in the inferior medial aspect of the sac. Stenosis of the right superior canaliculus (*vertical arrow*). **H**, Repeat DCG study. Left lacrimal sac was distended and irregular, with a filling defect in the inferior aspect. Distended irregular right lacrimal sac. Contrast was not entering the nasolacrimal duct bilaterally. **I** and **J**, CT-DCG. Axial images show filling defects within the right and left lacrimal sacs.

*Illustration continued on following page*

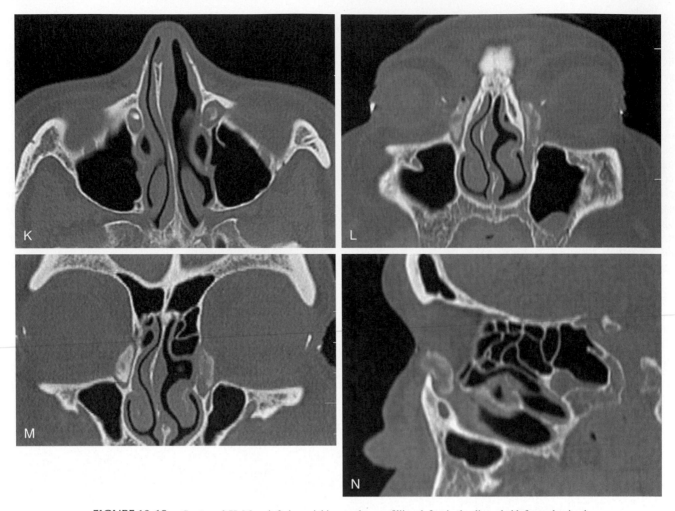

**FIGURE 10-18** *Continued.* **K**, More inferior axial image shows a filling defect in the distended left nasolacrimal duct. **L** to **N**, Coronal (**L** and **M**) and left sagittal (**N**) reformations show intraluminal filling defects that lack sharp margins or definition. Pathology: chronic dacryocystitis with extensive mucoid and cellular debris.

(eight patients) or complete (two patients) obstructions, Wilhelm et al.[101] have performed balloon dilatation of the NLDS, principally to widen the stenosed obstructing segment, so that the dacryoliths may pass more easily into the nasal cavity during forced irrigation with saline. If stone passage was not achieved because of persistent stenosis or large dacryolith size, further balloon dilatation (eight patients) was used to crush the calculi. Incomplete washout of calculi by forced irrigation was supplemented by retrograde passage of a 6.3F sheath across the stenosis. With the tip inferior to the dacryolith, repeat forced irrigation is performed, with active aspiration of the fragments through the sheath. In two patients, additional fragmentation of the dacryolith with a gooseneck Amplatz snare, passed retrograde through the sheath, was followed by successful irrigation combined with aspiration. Attempts at stone removal may be unsuccessful when bending of the sheath occurs or if fragments are too large to pass through the sheath.[101] For those patients with preintervention complete obstruction, stent implantation was initially necessary to restore drainage function. Stone removal itself, by such nonsurgical techniques, should not be considered without concomitant treatment of the stenosis or obstruction.[100, 101]

(See the section on Dacryocystoplasty and Stent Placement for a more detailed procedural discussion.)

## Chronic Canaliculitis

Chronic infective canaliculitis, although relatively uncommon, is significant because of its specific radiologic and clinical features (Fig. 10-8). In 1854, von Graefe[102] was the first to attribute this condition to an infectious source. Although chronic canaliculitis was called *streptothrix,* since the anaerobic bacterium *A. israelii* was the most frequent causative agent. Numerous other anaerobic agents have been identified, including *Nocardia* and *Fusobacterium* species, *Arachnia propionica,* and *Bacteroides,* as well as aerobic fungi, including *Candida, Aspergillus,* and *Blastomyces,*[83, 103] emphasizing the need for both anaerobic and aerobic cultures. Secondary bacterial infections should be treated independently.

Chronic canaliculitis, as with most lacrimal drainage afflictions, affects women more often than men and the lower canaliculus more than the upper.[103] Involvement of more than one canaliculus rarely occurs,[104] and the disease

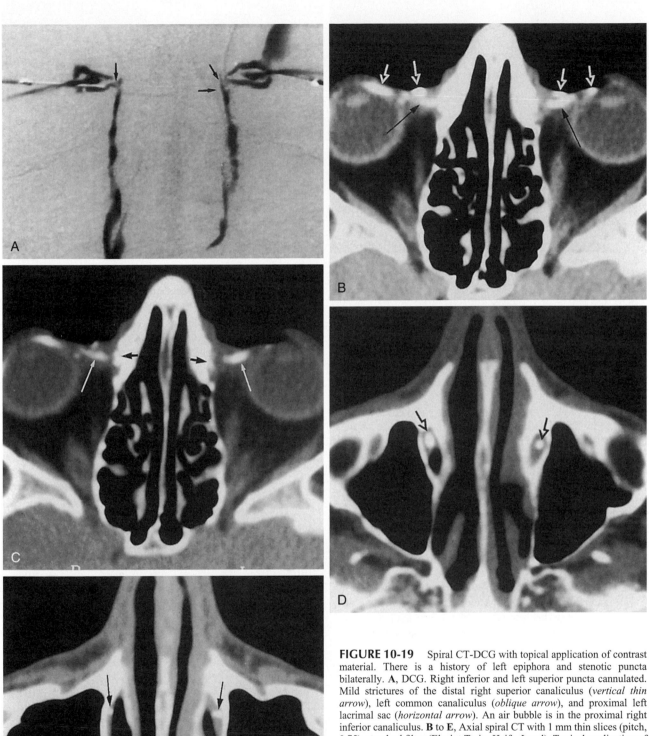

**FIGURE 10-19**   Spiral CT-DCG with topical application of contrast material. There is a history of left epiphora and stenotic puncta bilaterally. **A**, DCG. Right inferior and left superior puncta cannulated. Mild strictures of the distal right superior canaliculus (*vertical thin arrow*), left common canaliculus (*oblique arrow*), and proximal left lacrimal sac (*horizontal arrow*). An air bubble is in the proximal right inferior canaliculus. **B** to **E**, Axial spiral CT with 1 mm thin slices (pitch, 0.75), standard filter (Elscint Twin; Haifa, Israel). Topical application of Isovue 200 (200 mg I/ml [Squibb Diagnostics, Princeton, New Jersey]). Two drops per eye are instilled every minute for 4 minutes. **B**, Contrast material seen in the canaliculi bilaterally (*thin arrows*) directed toward the lacrimal sac. Contrast material in the conjunctival sac (*white open arrows*). **C**, Wider window at the level of the lacrimal sac. Normal medial position of the lacrimal sac (*short arrows*) within the nasolacrimal fossa (*thin arrows*, inferior canaliculi). **D**, Nasolacrimal duct (*arrows*) is clearly identified within the nasolacrimal canal bilaterally. **E**, Right and left nasolacrimal ducts (*arrows*) seen submucosally at the level of the inferior meatus.

*Illustration continued on following page*

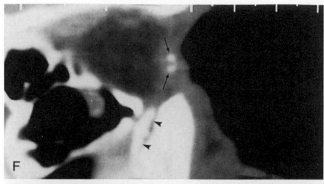
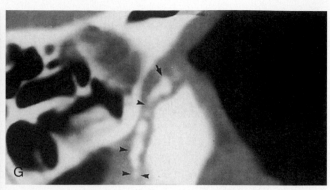
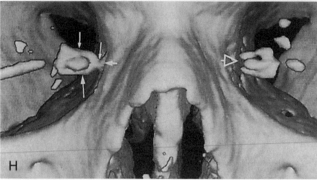

**FIGURE 10-19** *Continued.* **F** to **H**, Image reformation from volume data acquisition during axial imaging. **F**, Sagittal reformation of the left inner canthus lateral to the lacrimal sac. Superior and inferior canaliculi seen in cross section (*arrows*) just proximal to the common canaliculus (*arrowheads,* nasolacrimal canal). **G**, Sagittal reformation through the left nasolacrimal canal. Contrast material extends from the lacrimal sac superiorly (*arrow*) through the nasolacrimal duct (*arrowheads*) toward the nasal cavity. **H**, Three-dimensional reformation (anterior view). Right superior, inferior, and common canaliculi filled with contrast material, clearly defined (*thin arrows*), entering the lacrimal sac (*short arrow*). Left superior and inferior canaliculi also are shown. Failure to show the left common canaliculus (*open arrow*) may correlate with the stenosis seen on DCG.

is almost always unilateral.[83, 103] Clinically, the affected lid is swollen from the lacrimal punctum to the medial canthus, with a chronic mucopurulent discharge or particulate matter expressed (with difficulty) from a pointing dilated punctum. Erythema and induration over the canaliculus may be noted. Demonstration of concretions within the canaliculus virtually establishes the diagnosis, although concretions can also form around small foreign bodies or hair (eyelash) in the canaliculi.[94, 103] Organisms such as *Actinomyces* or, less frequency, *S. aureus*, form filamentous aggregates (sulfur granules), which distend the canaliculus and impede the drainage of tears. However, the canaliculus is often patent to syringing, obscuring the correct diagnosis.[85] Adequate treatment requires complete removal of concretions, material that has accumulated within the canaliculus. Expression and curettage may be adequate, but often incision and debridement of the affected canaliculus is necessary. Antibiotics used without surgical correction are unsuccessful. Such patients therefore usually present with an extensive list of previously prescribed medications. Chronic unilateral conjunctivitis should always suggest the possibility of canaliculitis.

DCG shows dilation and irregularity of the affected canaliculi, with an appearance of sacculation, beading, or diverticula. Such dilation is nonspecific and may be noted proximal to any obstructive or stenosing lesion. Dilation without stenosis or the presence of irregular filling defects (due to concretions) within the canaliculi is more specific for a chronic infectious etiology such as actinomycosis. Filling defects in the absence of concretions or sulfur granules may represent actinomycotic filaments. The degree of dilation is related to the presence of filling defects and is unrelated to the infective organism.[103] Classically, the distal nasolacrimal system fills and is normal, with no evidence of inflammatory change despite the severity of the proximal

canalicular duct involvement. The extent of involvement is characteristically limited to the proximal canaliculi such that the common canaliculus and lacrimal sac are usually normal (e.g., the common canaliculus was normal in 15 of 18 patients in one series).[103]

Concretions (dacryoliths) are more frequent in the lacrimal sac. Such concretions are less consistently associated with chronic infection than are concretions in the canaliculi.[83, 86] Chronic viral canaliculitis (e.g., ocular vaccinia, herpes zoster, or simplex ophthalmicus, viral conjunctivitis) tends to cause scarring, with stenosis or occlusion of the puncta and/or canaliculi, and therefore differs from the classic description of chronic infective canaliculitis.[105] Obstruction of the medial half of both canaliculi is often herpetic or trachomatous in origin.[106] In contrast to conjunctival infections caused by microbes, certain viral infections extend deeper into the stratified squamous epithelium of the canaliculi to involve the elastic layer, with resultant scarring and stenosis.[105]

## Posttreatment Considerations

### Postsurgical Considerations

Radiopaque tubes between the nasal cavity and medial canthus may be used in conjunction with DCR (canaliculo-DCR) to maintain patency within the canaliculi (Figs. 10-7I-J, 10-9, 10-20). Surgical clips may occasionally be present in the region of the medial canthus, and their relationship to the nasolacrimal drainage system may be important in cases of postsurgical obstruction. The relationship of the nasolacrimal sac to the DCR osteotomy site is assessed by CT. DCR is a relatively successful surgical procedure in 85% to 90% of cases, with an average failure rate of approximately 10%.[30, 107–110] DCR failure may be due to delayed obstruction at the surgical anastomosis by granulation tissue, fibrosis, or osteogenic activity or by secondary stenosis of the canaliculi. The failed DCR patient will have recurrence of epiphora and frequently recurrent dacryocystitis. DCG shows DCR failure to be related to problems distal to the common canaliculus in 60% of cases.[66] A residual inferior portion of the sac, with its bony covering (incomplete osteotomy), may produce inadequate drainage requiring a direct surgical approach on the anastomosis. This is in contrast to a canaliculo-DCR, which is required in 12% to 40% of failed DCRs where the obstruction is in the common canaliculus.[66, 67] It may not be possible on DCG to differentiate an obstruction of the common canaliculus from a closed osteotomy site in patients with a previous DCR.[107] Scarring of the ostium (rhinostomy site) and errors in ostium location are the major causes of surgical failure.[111, 112] Adhesions to the nasal septum (synechia) from the rhinotomy site may case obstruction and DCR failure. These adhesions are detectable on CT.[111] On DCG, lacrimal sac diverticula, directed medially toward the midline, may suggest adhesions between the ostium and the nasal septum.[111]

The relatively increasing percentage of patients with postsurgical canalicular problems may reflect increasing attention to the lacrimal flap/osteotomy site and/or reflect the iatrogenic effects of dilations and probings of the canaliculi preoperatively or during surgery.

Hurwitz et al.[113] studied the effects of surgery and/or radiation treatment for paranasal sinus tumors on the NLDS of 19 patients. Of those patients treated surgically, the majority (75%) did not develop obstruction even though the NLDS was anatomically altered, with the nasolacrimal duct frequently being shortened and the lacrimal sac displaced (Fig. 10-10). During maxillary sinus surgery, the lacrimal bone and nasolacrimal canal are frequently removed, and these patients tended to have obstruction in the lower part of the NLDS and were amenable to treatment by DCR. Stenosis or irregularity of the lacrimal sac or one of the canaliculi may develop secondary to scar tissue formation but does not tend to cause obstruction.

### Postirradiation Considerations

Patients treated with postoperative radiotherapy tended to have more profound abnormalities of the lacrimal system than those treated by surgery alone, with the delicate structure of the canaliculi most susceptible to irradiation injury and subsequent obstruction.[105, 106, 113] Such patients may need to be treated by prolonged intubation of the canaliculi (silicone tubing) or (canaliculodacryocystorhinostomy), with a success rate of only 60% to 70% versus 80% to 95% for uncomplicated lower NLDS obstruction.[114] Doucet and Hurwitz[114] postulated whether or not prophylactic placement of intubation tubes (silicone or glass stents) at the time of surgery would be beneficial for patients undergoing postoperative radiation therapy to prevent the canalicular stenosis or obstruction.

### Postchemotherapy Considerations

The onset of epiphora, due to the development of punctal and canalicular fibrosis, soon after the weekly administration of docetaxel, an effective first- or second-line antineoplastic agent for the treatment of breast or prostate cancer,

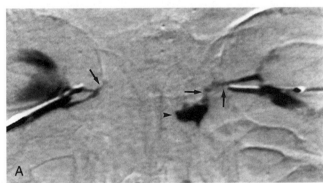
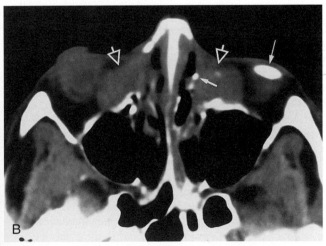
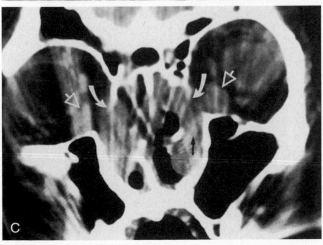

**FIGURE 10-20** Bilateral inner canthal masses: previous bilateral DCG recurrent right epiphora. **A,** DCG. Right superior canalicular injection shows severe stenosis of the common canaliculus (*oblique arrow*), reflux into the inferior canaliculus, and no filling of the lacrimal sac. Left inferior canaliculus shows stenosis medially (*vertical arrow*) and a fibrosed lacrimal sac (*horizontal arrow*), with contrast entering the nasal cavity through the previous DCR (*arrowhead*) at the inferior aspect of the lacrimal sac. **B,** Axial CT-DCG shows bilateral inner canthus soft-tissue masses (*open arrow*). Contrast material is seen in the left NLDS (*solid arrow*) and conjunctival sac (*thin arrow*). **C,** Coronal CT-DCG (artifact from dental restorations). Inner canthus masses (*open arrows*) appear to be contiguous with soft-tissue densities of the nasal cavity through previous DCR osteotomy sites (*curved arrows*) and the left nasolacrimal canal (*black arrow*).

*Illustration continued on following page*

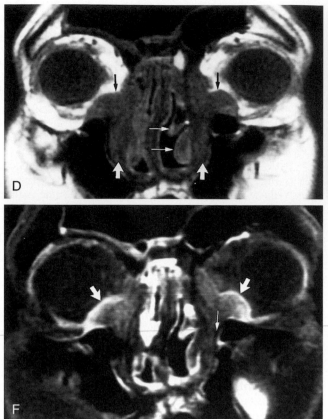

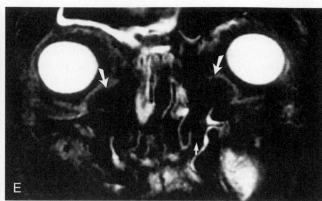

**FIGURE 10-20** *Continued.* **D**, Coronal T1-weighted image shows bilateral masses of the inferomedial orbit (*black arrows*) extending inferolaterally to the middle and inferior turbinate bones (*horizontal arrows*) along the course of the nasolacrimal canal (*vertical white arrows*). **E**, Coronal T2-weighted images shows hypointense inner canthus masses bilaterally (*diagonal arrows*). Left nasolacrimal canal appears widened (*small vertical arrow*). **F**, Postgadolinium coronal T1-weighted anterior image with fat suppression shows inner canthal masses to be well defined, but enhancement is more peripheral (*oblique arrows*). Left inner canthal mass extends into the nasolacrimal duct (*thin arrow*). Pathology: exuberant chronic granulation tissue and nodular fibrosis. (See also Fig. 10-7I,J.)

has recently been described in three patients.[115] The pattern of fibrosis involved all four puncta and canaliculi. Discontinuation of the agent led to resolution of symptoms in only one of the three patients (who may have had less advanced fibrosis). The mechanism of canalicular stenosis may be secondary to secretion of the chemotherapeutic agent in the tear film, with fibrosis resulting from the direct contact (local) of the agent in the canaliculi. Alternatively, the mucous membrane lining the puncta and canaliculi may undergo fibrosis secondary to systemic effects of the drug, similar to the widespread edema and fibrosis noted elsewhere within the body.

Canalicular stenosis had previously been described in association with other chemotherapeutic agents, such as 5-fluorouracil.[116, 117] Screening for epiphora and canalicular stenosis has been advocated for this patient population, with early treatment consideration of silicone intubation or punctoplasty, while the patient is receiving the chemotherapeutic agent, to prevent complete closure of the canaliculi and the need for conjunctivo-DCR and Jones tube placement.

## DACRYOSCINTIGRAPHY

In 1972, Rossomondo et al.[118] introduced a radionuclide technique to assess the lacrimal passages (Figs. 10-16, 10-21, and 10-22). This technique offers a more physiologic, less expensive, more sensitive, and more comfortable modality for assessing epiphora.[119–122] The ease of performance and the noninvasive nature of the procedure tend to

encourage routine bilateral studies. DSG can also provide a quantitative dynamic analysis of tear drainage physiology. DCG, although the most commonly used imaging technique for evaluating the anatomy and pathology of the lacrimal drainage system, does not provide physiologic information.[113, 123] Because the pressure required to inject the DCG contrast material overcomes any functional occlusion of the NLDS, a normal DCG in a patient with epiphora offers no information related to functional stenosis or obstruction.

## Technique

The patient is placed in a modified sitting position so that the head rests on a modified slit-lamp support that includes a chin rest, forehead support, and straps to immobilize the head for the study. Just before the instillation of radionuclide, manual pressure over the inner canthus empties the lacrimal sacs. With the head tilted back, a drop (approximately a 10 µl aliquot) of the solution technetium 99m pertechnetate or 99m-Tc-sulfur colloid is placed in the lateral conjunctival sac using an automatic micropipette. Instillation of larger volumes will simply overfill the conjunctival sac, resulting in spillage onto the face.[124] The patient's head is then placed within the supporting frame, and a micropinhole (1 mm) collimator is placed just anterior (e.g., 8 to 9 cm) to the nasion and between the two orbits in the upper central field of the gamma camera. Dynamic acquisition of scintigraphic images starts immediately after instillation of the radiopharmaceutical. Patients are instructed to blink every 5 seconds during data acquisition. A computer is set up for a two-phase dynamic acquisition with the following protocol: phase 1 (stimulated phase, 0 to 2 minutes), 5 second scans for 24 frames; phase 2 (initial drainage phase, 2 to 12 minutes), 10 to 15 second scans for 40 frames. A variation of this technique has the patient remain still but blink normally, with the dynamic acquisition of tracer distribution imaged every 10 seconds for the first 160 seconds.[22] Static views are then taken routinely at 5, 10, 15, and 20 minutes.

An alternative technique includes an 8 μl drop of 99m-technetium-tin colloid, containing no more than 4 MBq and capturing 48 consecutive 15 second images, using a 2 mm pinhole collimator placed 2 cm from the eye, centered on the medial canthus.[26] Using this technique, each eye is imaged separately. The 2 mm aperture offers a preferred balance between resolution and increased sensitivity (sampling of radiation emitted). Other authors favor a 3 mm aperture or vary the distances (e.g., 1 cm subject to collimator, 5 cm nasion to collimator, or 8 cm subject distance).[125–127]

The passage of radioactivity is followed on a video display unit. An area of interest (e.g., interpalpebral fissure and canaliculi) can be outlined on a rapid-sequence video display terminal and quantitative data analysis achieved by the computer interfaced to the gamma camera (Fig. 10-22).

Radiopharmaceutical activity enters the canaliculi rapidly and then progresses along the NLDS, with activity increasing in the lacrimal sac and decreasing in the canaliculi. Data analysis and time activity curves for the radiopharmaceutical to leave an area of interest (various constructed points along the NLDS) can be obtained. The $T_{1/2}$ (the time required for one half of the radioactive dose to disappear) for a specific site can be estimated by finding the slope of the curve plotting the natural logarithm of counts per second from the region of interest against time.[128] The examination is terminated when the radiopharmaceutical reaches the nasal cavity. Residual radioactivity is flushed out by a saline eye bath at the end of the study (Fig. 10-16D). The radiation dose to the lens (4 to 21 mrad) is minimal, 1% of that from a DCG[129] or less than 2% of the radiation from an anterioposterior skull film (i.e., 4 vs. 200 to 370 mrad).[118, 130] The usual aliquot administered contains between 50 and 100 μCi of 99m-Tc.[118] The radiation dose will be increased if the lacrimal drainage system is blocked. If lacrimal fluid turnover is minimal and disappearance occurs only by physical decay, the maximum absorbed dose to the nearpoint of the lens will be 400 mrad.[129]

## Normal Examination

Both lid margins are visualized, and the canaliculi are seen after approximately 10 seconds. The radiopharmaceu-

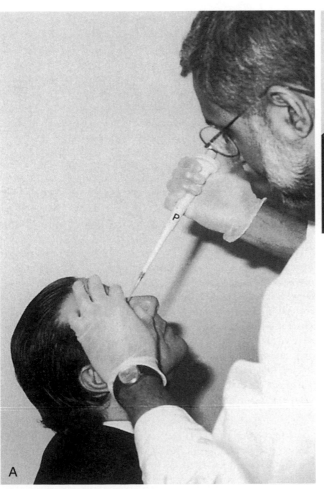

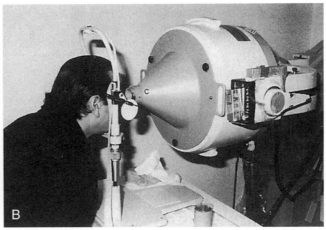

**FIGURE 10-21**   DSG. Technique and equipment. **A,** With the head tilted back, an automatic micropipette (*P*) is used to place a specific volume (10 μl aliquot) of radioisotope into the lateral conjunctival sac. **B,** Patient is positioned with the chin on the slit lamp support, with the micropinhole collimater (*c*) 8 cm anterior to the nasion.

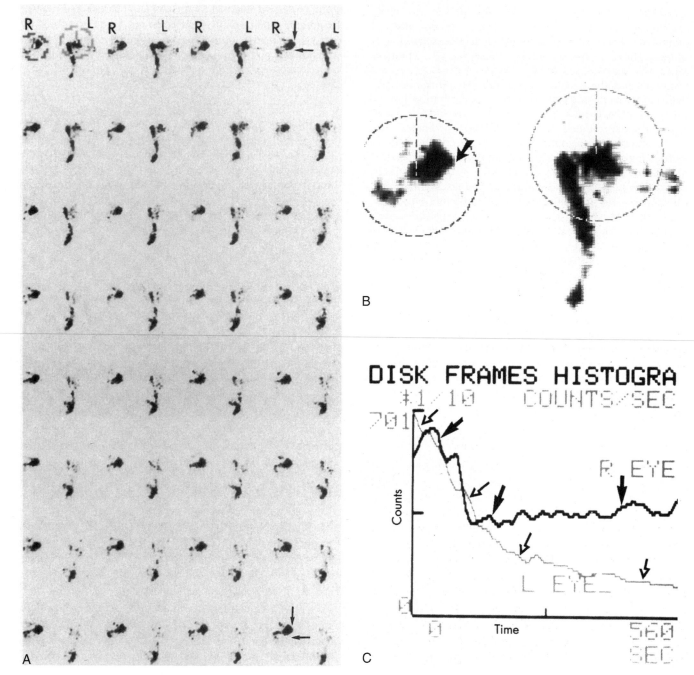

**FIGURE 10-22** Bilateral DSG demonstrating isotope time activity patterns (normal and abnormal). **A,** Representative collection of images (each gathered at 10 second intervals) shows progression of activity (from superior to inferior) on the left (normal drainage). Obstruction at the right lacrimal sac (*vertical arrow*) with persistent proximal activity and no distal activity (*horizontal arrow*). **B,** Magnified image. The area of interest is outlined (*circles*) for the time–activity curve. Obstruction of the right lacrimal sac (*arrow*). **C,** Histogram of counts (activity) versus time. Normal slope indicates proper drainage from the left eye (*open arrows*). Right eye time–activity curve (*solid arrows*) shows failure of the normal slope, indicating a lack of drainage. ($T_{1/2}$ is beyond the limits of the scan time.)

tical can be seen progressively in the lacrimal sac and nasolacrimal duct, terminating in the nasal cavity. The valve of Hasner is usually seen as a reduction of scintillations at the lower end of the tracer column. A significant proportion of normal volunteers showed delayed passage of the radiopharmaceutical between the lacrimal sac and the nasal cavity, such that dacryoscintigraphy (DSG) is deemed

unreliable for assessing the nasolacrimal duct, that is, the drainage system inferior to the lacrimal sac.[20, 125, 127] The flow of tears (radiopharmaceutical) from the conjunctival cul-de-sac to the lacrimal sac occurs in approximately 12 seconds, yet the radiopharmaceutical may not reach the nasal cavity for 10 to 20 minutes.[125] The elimination of tears is affected by the blink-driven ''lacrimal pump,'' which depends on the muscular blinking action of the eyelids, that is, the superficial and deep insertions of the preseptal and pretarsal orbicularis oculi of the lower and upper eyelids.[131] This component of the orbicularis envelops the lacrimal system, thus transmitting pressure through the tear outflow tract. With the eyelids closed, the ampulla and canaliculi are shifted medially, shortened, and compressed, and the tear fluid is driven into the lacrimal sac, which has a negative pressure. When the eyelids are open, pressure in the ampulla decreases and the pressure in the lacrimal sac increases, expelling fluid out through the nasolacrimal duct.[132]

The lacrimal pump can exert a suction effect at the punctum on the lacrimal secretions during blinking (Fig. 10-23)[124, 133, 134] Transit times of radioisotope to the lacrimal sac may be greatly prolonged in patients who do not blink but rather keep their eyelids closed. Occasional exceptions occur in patients with orbicularis contractions during lid closure. The elderly, with open lacrimal passages but inefficient tear fluid transportation, may also show delayed transit.[135] The greatest decay of tracer from the conjunctival sac occurs within the first few blinks.[136, 137] The relative drainage to the inferior and superior canaliculi remains controversial. Several studies concluded that activity was greater in the inferior than the superior canaliculus.[26, 128, 138] White et al.[126] showed that the superior and inferior canaliculi are of equal importance in lacrimal drainage and that no statistical difference exists between the amounts of tears that drain into either canaliculus. Similarly, Daubert et al.[139] showed no significant difference in tear flow between the upper and lower canaliculi in normal, patent, asymptomatic systems. If one canaliculus was blocked in an anatomically healthy NLDS, a compensatory increase in tear flow might occur in the other canaliculus such that no significant difference (statistical analysis $p < 0.05$) in time activity would be noted for $T_{1/2}$ of the interpalpebral fissure radioactivity (overall tear flow).[139] A single (upper or lower) canaliculus is sufficient for basal tear drainage but will not be sufficient to drain reflex tear secretion in 50% of cases.[140] The lacrimal drainage system is a closed system with a negative pressure, and occlusion of one canaliculus increases the suction effect and the subsequent increased tear flow through the patent canaliculus.[139]

The drainage of tears involves a number of different mechanisms including capillary action,[131, 133, 134] aided by contraction of the lacrimal part of the orbicularis oculi with blinking,[131, 141, 142] and craniocaudad distention of the sac with passive wringing of the sac because of its medial attachment and helically arranged fibrillar structure.[49] A vascular plexus, comparable to a cavernous body and embedded in the wall of the lacrimal sac and nasolacrimal duct, contains specialized blood vessels including regulatory arteries, a dense network of capillaries, capacitance veins, and cushion veins, which can reduce or interrupt venous blood outflow to allow large amounts of blood to accumulate inside the capacitance veins.[50] This cavernous body, which connects to that of the inferior turbinate of the nasal cavity, may facilitate closure and opening of the lumen of the nasolacrimal duct system (NLDS) by swelling and shrinkage of the cavernous body, with consecutive regulation of the tear outflow. When the net outflow of blood from the

cavernous body is less than its inflow, there is mucosal expansion, functionally decreasing tear outflow. This represents a protective mechanism against foreign bodies or toxic stimuli that enter the conjunctival sac. In addition to increased lacrimal gland tear production, the decreased tear outflow, by the cavernous body response allows the increased tear pool to flush out the conjunctival sac while protecting the NLDS. The pathophysiology of functional lacrimal drainage insufficiency (epiphora despite a patent

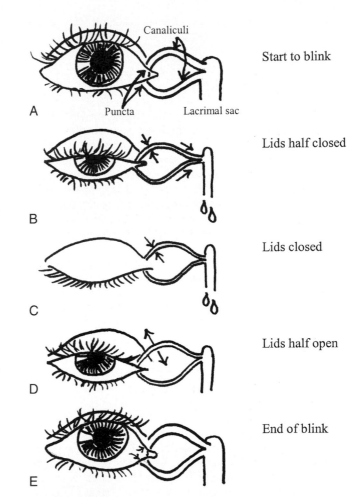

**FIGURE 10-23** Lacrimal pump theory of Doane. **A,** Start of blink. The canaliculi and sac contain tear fluid from the previous blink. **B,** Lids half closed. As the upper lid descends, papillae containing punctal openings elevate from the medial lid margin, forcefully meeting the opposing lid margin, occluding the puncta, and preventing fluid regurgitation. Further lid closure squeezes the canaliculi and sac (through the action of the orbicularis oculi), forcing the contained tear fluid into the nasolacrimal duct. **C,** Lids closed. Maximum compression of the canaliculi and sac, with all fluid expressed into the nasal cavity. **D,** Lids half open. Puncta still occluded by opposing medial lid margins. Release of pressure by the orbicularis oculi with cessation of compression action. Elastic walls of the passages try to expand to their normal shape, with a resultant partial vacuum and negative pressure and with a suction effect forming within the canaliculi and sac. **E,** End of blink. As lid separation progresses, suction force holding the punctal region together is released and the punctal papillae "pop" apart, with negative intraluminal pressure drawing tear lake fluid into the canaliculi and sac. (Redrawn adaptation from Doane MG. Blinking and the mechanics of the lacrimal drainage system. Ophthalmology 1981;88:844–851 and adaptation of the above by Dale DL. Embryology, anatomy, and physiology of the lacrimal drainage system. In: Stephensen CM, ed. Ophthalmic, Plastic, Reconstructive, and Orbital Surgery. Boston: Butterworth-Heineman, 1997;19–30.)

NLDS during syringing) may be explained by the presence of the cavernous body.[50] Malfunctions within the vascular bed may lead to disturbances in the tear outflow cycle, ocular congestion, or total occlusion of the NLDS and may be caused more acutely by allergic conjunctivitis, rhinitis, or hay fever, or more chronically, as with stenoses after dacryocystitis or dacryolithiasis.[50] Persistent epiphora after dacryocystorhinostomy (DCR) may be due to destruction of the surrounding cavernous body. The cavernous body may also play a role in the absorption of tear fluid by the NLDS epithelial lining mucosa and alternative draining by the surrounding venous plexus before reaching the nasal cavity.[48]

## Complete Obstruction

Total obstruction, if present, is identified on DSG (Fig. 10-16). Even though the lacrimal sac may be filled with lacrimal secretions, debris, or even concretions, there is physiologic reflux of the secretions into the conjunctival sac.[143, 144] Therefore, fresh secretions or radiopharmaceutical from the DSG will enter the lacrimal sac. The study is sensitive to the site of obstruction so that the appropriateness of surgery, such as DCR, or placement of drainage tubes can be determined. The smaller pinhole aperture helps improve resolution that may still be suboptimal in differentiating canalicular from proximal lacrimal sac pathology. However, DCG will provide anatomic information to complement DSG when necessary. If a DSG shows obstruction proximal to the lacrimal sac, the common canaliculus or the inferior and superior canaliculi or puncta may be obstructed.

## Incomplete Obstruction: Functional Nasolacrimal Duct Obstruction

Patients with epiphora who have a normal DCG or a normal clinical lacrimal irrigation test usually have physiologic obstruction to the drainage of tears. FNDLO has been interpreted to mean symptomatic epiphora, with a lacrimal system patent to syringing and no detectable cause of epiphora external to the lacrimal drainage system (no cause for increased lacrimation and no lid abnormality present).[22] The main level of functional blockage (lacrimal drainage delay) in the lacrimal system was easier to detect objectively with DSG than with DCG. When discrepancies in the identified level of functional block occurred (41% of combined DSG-DCG studies of FNLDO patients), Wearne et al.[22] noted that the DSG detected an obstruction at a more proximal level in 16 of 20 patients. DSG/DCG discrepancies were most likely due to the pressure injection of DCG contrast dilating lesser degrees of more proximal stenosis. Positive scintigrams were subdivided into those demonstrating prelacrimal sac delay (13%), delay at the lacrimal sac–nasolacrimal duct junction (35%), or delay within the nasolacrimal duct (42%). Prelacrimal sac delay was defined as holdup at the inner canthus or failure of the tracer to reach the lacrimal sac by the end of the dynamic phase (160 seconds). Delay at the lacrimal sac–nasolacrimal duct junction (35%) was defined as preductal delay with early

filling of the lacrimal sac but no sign of sac emptying on the static image at 5 minutes. Delay within the nasolacrimal duct (42%) was defined as intraductal delay with tracer noted in the upper part of the nasolacrimal duct at 5 minutes but no further drainage over the next 15 minutes. Of note, 72% of patients in the above series had clinically bilateral FNLDO.[22] The transit time through the distal part of the nasolacrimal duct and into the nasal cavity, known to show marked variability in normal individuals, was not calculated in their study. It is interesting to speculate whether the marked variability in transit time of normal individuals and patients with FNLDO may be related to functionality of the surrounding vascular plexus (cavernous body) or to variability of resorption of the tear fluid by the NLDS mucosa, as outlined by Paulsen et al.[50] (In the section Dacryoscintigraphy, see Normal Examination for further discussion.) Simultaneous bilateral DSG studies can compare and evaluate the delay in transit of the radiopharmaceutical on the involved side. Frequently, however, the clinically normal side will also reveal abnormal flow. Amanat et al.[20] noted in their patients with a clinically unilateral abnormality that 42% had an abnormal flow pattern by DSG on the contralateral side. Thus the contralateral side was clinically silent relative to the increased symptoms on the primary symptomatic side.

## Sensitivity of Dacryoscintigraphy

DSG is more sensitive for detecting obstruction than macro-DCG.[127] Normal DSG was always associated with duct patency on DCG, allowing a protocol specifying that DSG should be the first investigation; if it is normal, DCG is unnecessary. In Rose and Clayton's series,[127] 26% of the NLDS showing obstruction on DSG had a normal DCG. In a series[22] limited to patients with a clinical diagnosis of FNLDO, both DSG and DCG were very sensitive in detecting abnormalities (95% and 93%, respectively), with DCG including the performance of a delayed upright 5 minute film and DSG results including quantitative analysis.[121] Hanna et al.,[26] in comparing syringing to DSG in patients with epiphora, found that 65% of apparently patent systems on syringing demonstrated abnormalities on DSG. Abnormalities included 40% with decreased entry into the NLDS or canalicular obstruction on DSG. In those patients with abnormal syringing, the most common site of obstruction on DSG was at the lacrimal sac outflow. In these patients, canalicular obstruction was seen with almost the same frequency as in those with patent syringing (35% vs. 33%).[26] Both DCG and syringing require cannulation. Either lid puncta and proximal canalicular functional or anatomic abnormalities may be missed on the basis of the cannulation or the pressure of the injection or irrigation.

In syringing, false negatives or false positives may result partly from the subjective nature of the patient's ability to interpret or be aware of saline entering the nasopharynx. In the Hanna et al. series, 18% of those who had a positive syringing test had a negative DSG.[26]

Weber et al.[88] found the greatest application for DSG to include children; puncta unable to be cannulated after surgery; posttrauma; and functional obstructions, especially if the DCG was normal.

## COMPUTED TOMOGRAPHY

DCG cannot display information beyond that of the drainage lumen proper. Although displacement of the NLDS may be shown by DCG, the peripheral extent of mucosal or periductal disease cannot be defined. In these cases, CT may be indicated either initially or as a complementary study. The understanding that epiphora (or dacryostenosis) results from a multitude of etiologies should suggest a more selective imaging approach for each patient. When appropriate imaging studies are performed, diagnostic accuracy in dacryostenosis may be significantly improved, ensuring that diagnosis is not delayed and that the appropriate operation is done or that surgery can be avoided if contraindicated.[63, 145] Classifications of acquired lacrimal drainage obstruction further emphasize the need to understand the etiology of dacryostenosis.[145–148] Appropriate decisions are based on whether or not signs or symptoms result from processes arising outside the NLDS or whether abnormalities outside the NLDS are present that could adversely affect the outcome of the proposed lacrimal surgery. If such factors cannot be determined through clinical means, imaging tests should be performed that will limit surprises at the time of surgery.[149] Specific patients with epiphora and all patients presenting with an inferomedial orbital mass lesion are candidates for CT. The broader base of anatomic and pathophysiologic relationships to adjacent tissues offered by CT becomes helpful in making treatment decisions. As noted by others,[145, 150] dacryostenosis may be much more closely related to local nasal or sinus problems than has been previously emphasized. Similarly, the etiology of FNDLO and its relation to sinonasal disease has been largely unappreciated. High-resolution, thin-section CT imaging (1.0 to 2.5 mm slice thickness) may be an appropriate and useful modality for assessing the NLDS, its immediate bony confines, the lacrimal fossa, the adjacent orbit, the facial skeleton, paranasal sinuses (especially the agger nasi and ethmoid bulla air cells), and the nasal cavity. The increasing capabilities of volume acquisition thin-slice CT, with multiplanar and 3D reconstruction availability and shorter time acquisition, offer excellent imaging resolution and patient compliance. Anatomic depiction of the nasolacrimal sac and duct is well seen in the axial plane. Coronal assessment may be helpful, especially to display the junction of the lacrimal sac and duct and the relationship of the medial orbital floor or nasal cavity structures to the NLDS. Intravenous enhancement is routinely used (except in the trauma patient), since one is frequently assessing the possibility or the extent of an inflammatory or neoplastic lesion. The radiation dose absorbed by the lens during spiral CT for assessment of the NLDS has been measured at 1.8 to 2.6 mSv[151] compared to 0.68 mSv for DS-DCG.[18]

## Radiographic Anatomy

Plain or intravenous enhanced CT (Fig. 10-24) does not identify the superior and inferior canaliculi or the common canaliculus. The canaliculi may be visualized by placement of topical contrast medium into the conjunctival sac (see the section on Combined CT-Dacryocystography).

The normal lacrimal sac and duct may be either tear-filled (soft-tissue density) or air-filled (Fig. 10-25). The lacrimal sac will normally not exceed a 2 mm diameter unless distended with air.[152] The sac itself is a membranous structure, noted within the bony lacrimal fossa.

The frontal process of the maxillary bone and the lacrimal bone form the lacrimal sac fossa. The fossa is a clearly demarcated depression bound anteriorly by the anterior lacrimal crest, contiguous with the inferior orbital rim, and posteriorly by the posterior lacrimal crest, a linear elevation along the anterior aspect of the lacrimal bone. The frontal process of the maxillary bone and the lacrimal bone contribute varying proportions to the formation of the lacrimal sac fossa. The anteroposterior position of the vertical suture between these components is variable. The lacrimal bone separates the upper half of the lacrimal fossa from anterior ethmoid air cells and the inferior part from the middle meatus of the nasal cavity. Closely surrounding the lacrimal sac is a rich venous plexus separating the sac from the adjacent lacrimal fascia, an anterior extension of the orbital periosteum, which splits at the posterior lacrimal crest to invest the lacrimal sac.

Enhancement of the venous plexus or the closely associated superficial and deep heads of the orbicularis oculi may help identify the lacrimal sac within the soft-tissue density of the medial canthal structures if the lacrimal sac is not air-filled. Horner's muscle represents the lacrimal component of the superficial and deep heads of the orbicularis oculi muscle attaching to the anterior and posterior lacrimal crests, respectively. These fibers act as a muscle envelope, surrounding the lacrimal fascia and sac. They are not distinguishable on CT from the anteriorly placed medial palpebral ligament, the subjacent lacrimal fascia, or the posteriorly positioned orbital septum.[42, 153]

The medial canthal ligament attaches to the anterior lacrimal crest and forms an anterior margin to the lacrimal sac. The medial orbital septum attaches just posterior to the posterior lacrimal crest. The lacrimal fossa and sac are therefore preseptal structures. Below the level of the medial palpebral ligament, the lacrimal sac is not enveloped by the orbicularis oculi muscle and therefore is potentially weaker at this site, offering less resistance to intraorbital spread of infection[153] or possibly to perforation by antegrade manipulation of instruments within the nasolacrimal drainage.[154]

In DCR, the opening in the bony wall between the lacrimal sac and the nasal cavity is initiated with perforation of the thin lacrimal bone at the inferior portion of the lacrimal sac fossa. In external DCR, a large bony opening measuring 1.5 cm is produced through the nasal wall of the lacrimal fossa, including the anterior lacrimal crest (thicker frontal process of the maxillary bone).[30] In endonasal DCR, the bony opening, at the same site, tends to be smaller and does not include the anterior lacrimal crest.[33] Because of the increasing popularity and frequency of use of endonasal DCR, using various laser and endoscopic techniques (and to a lesser extent endocanalicular laser DCR techniques), attention to the anatomic structures that need to be penetrated by the procedures has grown. Lacrimal bone thickness and variations in sinonasal configuration that may limit access or the feasibility of specific surgical approaches (endonasal or endocanalicular) have clinical treatment implications.[155, 156] The ability of various lasers to penetrate

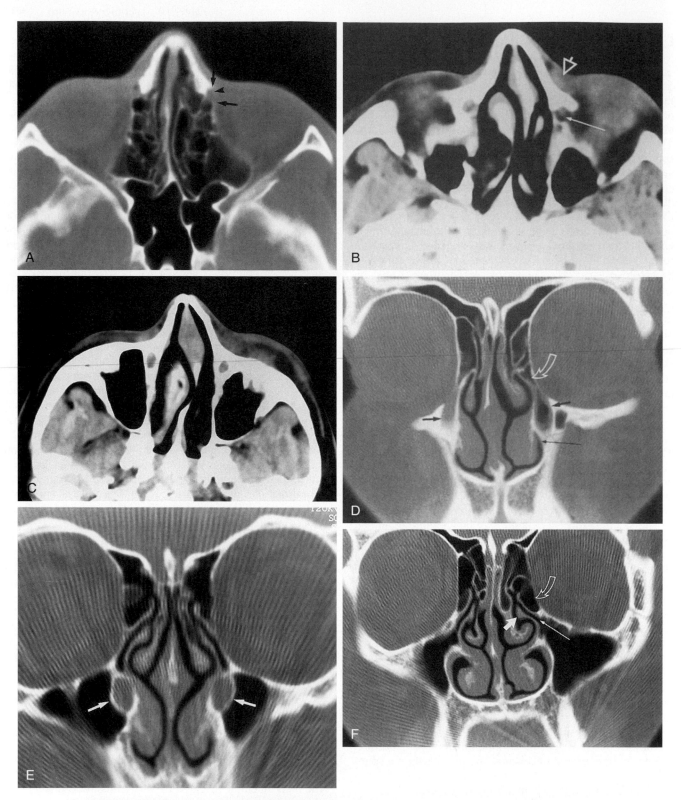

**FIGURE 10-24**  Normal CT anatomy. **A** to **C**, Axial. **A**, High-resolution axial CT scan shows the nasolacrimal fossa (*arrowhead*) and anterior and posterior lacrimal crests (*arrows*). **B** and **C**, Study done to assess preseptal lymphoma of the left orbit, noted as a soft-tissue density (*open arrow* in **B**) on both images. **B**, Fat-density tissue plane surrounding the lacrimal sac and proximal nasolacrimal duct (*thin arrow on the left*), which frequently is not identified (as in the nasolacrimal canal on the right) because of surrounding venous plexus, decreased fat content within the confined space, and artifact from adjacent bone. **C**, One slice, more inferiorly, is unable to define the nasolacrimal duct within the nasolacrimal canal. Compare this with the MR image of the nasolacrimal duct (Fig. 10-26). **D** to **F**, Coronal. **D**, Nasolacrimal canal (*short arrows*) is seen bilaterally lateral to the middle meatus and is directed inferiorly toward the inferior meatus (*thin arrow*). Note the normal cortical margin to the canal. Ethmoid bullae (*open arrow*) lie just medial to the superior aspect of the nasolacrimal canal. **E**, Nasolacrimal canals are oriented postinferiorly from superior to inferior. Depending on the angulation of coronal imaging, the canal may be obliquely transected (*arrows*). **F**, Just posterior to the nasolacrimal canal, a coronal image shows the osteomeatal unit. Ethmoid bulla (*open arrow*), infundibulum (*thin arrow*), and uncinate process (*short arrow*) are seen.

bone is less than that of the traditional mechanical instruments, especially when the fiberoptic laser is used through the endocanalicular route.[155]

Hartikainen et al.[155] noted the mean thickness of the lacrimal bone at the lacrimal fossa to be 106 μm, with 67% of patients having a mean thickness of less than 100 μm. Only 4% of patients had a mean thickness greater than 300 μm. A slightly decreased thickness of bone with increasing age was not significant. The lacrimal bone, although variable, tends to be thin, about 0.1 mm on average, and so can be easily penetrated with most surgical instruments. The osteotomy is then enlarged to include the thicker bone (frontal process of the maxilla) to the appropriate size required by the DCR technique.[155] Of 48 lacrimal patients with fossa dissections, only 1 displayed a significant anatomic variant, with no real lacrimal fossa bilaterally. The lacrimal sac was bounded, nasally and inferiorly, entirely by the frontal process of the maxillary bone, and the vertical suture was situated temporal to the tiny posterior lacrimal crest. Such a variation makes endoscopic or endocanalicular DCR techniques difficult or impossible.[155]

Yung and Logan,[156] in a smaller cadaveric series, reported an average thickness of 57 μm in nine dissections, excluding one abnormally thick lacrimal bone (296 μm). In all cases, the part of the lacrimal passage covered by the thin lacrimal bone corresponded to the upper part of the nasolacrimal duct and the lower part of the lacrimal sac. The thin lacrimal bone covered the posteromedial part of the upper nasolacrimal duct, with the thicker frontal process of the maxilla still covering the main part of the nasolacrimal duct. The authors note that the lacrimal bone is always situated immediately anterior to the mid-third of the uncinate process, an anatomic landmark in endonasal DCR procedures. An extremely large anterior ethmoidal air cell, the agar nasi, can be juxtaposed completely between the nasal cavity and the entire lacrimal fossa, leading to considerable confusion during DCR.[157]

A light source positioned within the lacrimal sac will transmit through the tiny lacrimal bone but not the thicker maxillary bone. Such transillumination can assist placement of the DCR osteotomy during endonasal DCR. Therefore, any surgical process (e.g., laser beam) directed at the area of maximum illumination (from the light source) tends to only remove the bone at the posteromedial portion of the inferior lacrimal sac–superior nasolacrimal duct rather than its entire width, with a resultant small lacrimal window.[156]

The lacrimal sac tapers inferiorly and is continuous with the nasolacrimal duct. The fascia investing the lacrimal sac also continues inferiorly to invest the nasolacrimal duct and become continuous with the periosteum surrounding the inferior meatus. The entire lacrimal drainage system remains continuous with the preseptal space even though the nasolacrimal duct is directed posteriorly and inferiorly.

The valve-like folds of mucosa (valves of Krause) separating the lacrimal sac from the nasolacrimal duct are not recognized on CT. An encircling bony canal along the medial aspect of the maxilla identifies the intraosseous component of the duct. The duct itself is usually collapsed and occupies only a small portion of the cross-sectional diameter of the bony canal. The most inferior portion of the nasolacrimal duct, approximately 5 mm in length, represents the membranous (or meatal) portion of the canal, passing beneath the nasal mucosa before emptying into the inferior meatus through a slit-like or funnel-shaped opening, the valve of Hasner.

The nasolacrimal canal represents the bony canal, which encloses and protects the nasolacrimal duct, connecting the inferior aspect of the lacrimal sac fossa to the inferior meatus of the nose. The maxilla contributes the greatest component, with the formation of a longitudinal groove, the lacrimal sulcus. The gap between the lips of this groove is completed by the articulation of two other component bones, the descending process of the lacrimal bone from above and the lacrimal process of the inferior nasal concha from below.[158] The form, dimension, and direction of the bony lacrimal

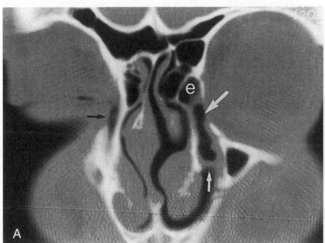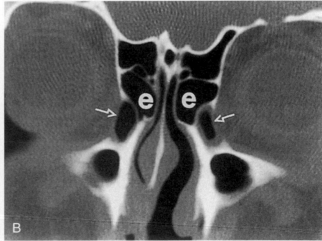

**FIGURE 10-25**  Air within the NLDS as a normal variant. **A,** Distended left nasolacrimal duct (*oblique arrow*) with air extending to the valve of Hasner (*vertical arrow*). Air also in the right lacrimal sac (*horizontal arrow*). Ethmoid agger nasi (*e*) immediately medial to the superior aspect of the lacrimal sac. **B,** Bilateral air-filled lacrimal sacs (*arrows*). Note the intimate relationship of the anterior ethmoid air cells (agger nasi) (*e*) and its importance in DCR planning. (See also Fig. 10-30C,D.)

**Table 10-2**
**CAUSES OF SECONDARY ACQUIRED NASOLACRIMAL DUCT OBSTRUCTION**

| Primary Neoplasms | Inflammation |
|---|---|
| Papilloma | Granulomatous pseudotumor |
| Squamous cell carcinoma | Sarcoidosis |
| Hemangiopericytoma | Wegener's granulomatosis |
| Fibrous histiocytoma | |
| Oncocytic adenocarcinoma | |
| Melanoma | |
| Fibroma | |
| **Secondary Involvement by Neoplasm** | **Infections** |
| Lymphoma | Trachoma |
| Leukemia | Leprosy |
| Lethal midline lymphoma | Tuberculosis |
| Basal cell carcinoma | Rhinosporidiosis |
| Neurofibroma | |
| Maxillary sinus tumors | |

From Linberg JV, McCormick SA. Primary acquired nasolacrimal duct obstruction: a clinicopathologic report and biopsy technique. Ophthalmology 1986;93:1055–1063.

passages show considerable variation, mainly due to the extent to which the individual bones participate in their formation, with the lacrimal bone being the most variable.[158]

The bony nasolacrimal canal has been reported to be a structure highly variable in size, with differences associated with age, sex, and race. There has been recent interest in CT imaging of the bony nasolacrimal canal to assess normal CT values and to establish values that may be causative or a component of factors leading to nasolacrimal duct obstruction. Assessment of an epiphora patient population with PANDO may indicate minimal bone canal diameter acceptable for balloon dacryocystoplasty (DCP) versus DCR.[159–161] PANDO is an idiopathic process, whereas secondary obstructions are attributed to a recognized causative factor.[146, 161] See Table 10-2. The prevalence of PANDO in women has generated interest in possible etiologies. Proposed mechanisms include heightened levels of inflammation in women, leading to tissue swelling and obstruction; hormonal imbalances causing transient changes in the mucous membranes; and anatomic differences between men and women.[146, 150, 161] A narrower bone environment, combined with inflamed mucosal tissues, would place the raw mucosal surfaces in close proximity, enhancing the chance that the mucosal walls will stick together, forming an obstruction secondary to scar tissue.[160] Generalized deepithelialization of mucous membranes occurs during the menstrual cycle, with smaller nasolacrimal passages being more easily obstructed with epithelial debris. Osteoporotic changes may also be a factor in the female predilection for PANDO. Chronic allergy or maxillary sinusitis may percolate through the porotic bony wall of the sinus and nasolacrimal duct, causing inflammatory changes in the canal and duct, leading to blockage.[162]

Groessl et al.[160] noted that women have significantly smaller anteroposterior dimensions in the inferior nasolacrimal fossa and the midnasolacrimal canal. Janssen et al.,[159] using 2 mm axial CT images photographed on bone windows to measure the minimal transverse diameter of the bony nasolacrimal canal, studied a control group of 50 men and 50 women, as well as a patient group with epiphora and PANDO treated by balloon DCP. The longer anteroposterior diameter of the canal (ranging in size from an average normal of 2.84 mm[47] to an upper limit of 8 mm[158]) was felt to be less useful due to the oblique posteroinferior orientation (15° to 25°) of the nasolacrimal canal relative to the axial image.[159] The smallest diameter of the bony canal appears to be the most relevant measure for ascertaining the origin of an obstruction of the lacrimal drainage system.[159] This smallest diameter is generally found midway along the canal.[160] The mean minimum transverse diameters of the bony canal in the control groups were 3.7 mm and 3.35 mm for men and women, respectively.[159] These measurements are considerably smaller than previously measured transverse diameters of 4 to 6 mm[158, 163] but correlate with the 3 mm diameter[157] or 2.3 mm[47] measurements of other studies, with variations reflecting the different measuring techniques or modalities used. The mean minimal diameter in the epiphora patient group was 3.0 mm, considerably smaller than that of the control groups, suggesting a relationship between a narrower bony canal and obstruction of the NLDS. The broad range of diameters found in the control group (1.5 to 6.3 mm) showed complete overlap with the range found in the symptomatic group (2.0 to 4.2 mm), suggesting that a relatively small minimal diameter of the bony canal is not the sole etiologic factor in PANDO.[159] Further research is needed to ascertain whether a minimum threshold value of the diameter of the bony canal can be determined, below which balloon DCP as a treatment for lacrimal obstruction is contraindicated, making surgical DCR the preferred treatment.[159]

While the majority of patients with clinically suspected PANDO will have histopathologic findings of inflammation and fibrosis, there is a low incidence of significant other pathology of the lacrimal sac, such as neoplasm. These cases can only be identified by biopsy of the lacrimal sac during DCR.[150, 161, 164] Malignant tumors, especially epitheliomas and lymphomas, may first appear as simple dacryocystitis for prolonged periods.[165] Defining the true incidence of unsuspected lacrimal sac neoplasms presenting clinically as PANDO has specific implications in determining whether routine biopsy during DCR is warranted. This would also determine if there is a significant risk of missing an underlying lacrimal sac tumor in patients not undergoing surgical intervention but having procedures such as DCP, or in those undergoing laser DCR, where direct visualization and biopsy of the lacrimal sac are not possible.[164]

When an asymptomatic, exceptionally enlarged nasolacrimal canal is observed, concern for the presence of a relatively uncommon lacrimal sac tumor is raised, since these tumors may grow down into and expand the nasolacrimal canal. Associated CT signs of lacrimal sac tumors should be sought, including a soft-tissue mass of the lacrimal sac, bone erosion, and extension of the mass into adjacent tissues.

There may be variable amounts of air or soft tissue within the confines of the nasolacrimal canal, with air occasionally extending from the inferior meatus to the lacrimal sac. In a large population of patients scanned for other reasons, soft-tissue opacification restricted to the nasolacrimal canal is routinely noted and is considered a normal variant. In 200 nasolacrimal ducts studied by coronal CT, 72% were opaque.[166] Of those ducts associated with normal paranasal sinuses, 79% had an opacified nasolacrimal duct. However, in the lacrimal patient, soft-tissue opacity of the nasolacrimal duct may have more significance and reflect pathologic characteristics of the nasolacrimal duct itself, such as PANDO, or adjacent inflammatory or neoplastic processes extending to the nasolacrimal canal from the lacrimal sac, orbital origins, or sinonasal origins.[145] One should assess the tissues adjacent to the nasolacrimal canal and examine for prominence or abnormal thickness of the lacrimal sac wall. While the lacrimal patient may display soft-tissue opacification of the nasolacrimal canal more frequently on the side of epiphora,[145] the exact significance if this finding is unclear. With such opacification as the only CT finding, the need for further imaging investigations, such as DCG or CT-DCG, must be based on clinical correlation. Obstruction of the nasolacrimal duct with dilatation of the lacrimal sac (lacrimal sac mucocele, dacryocele, dacryocystocele) may cause pressure erosion and enlargement of the nasolacrimal canal, depending on the degree of lacrimal sac enlargement and the level of distal obstruction within the canal. The pressure within the obstructed NLDS results from obstruction at both the proximal and distal aspects and tends to be most profound in congenital dacryocystocele (nasolacrimal mucocele). In congenital dacryocystocele the distal obstruction tends to be at the valve of Hasner, with the classic triad of cystic dilatation of the lacrimal sac, a dilated nasolacrimal duct/canal, and an intranasal cystic mass from the inferior imperforate membrane ballooning into the nasal cavity. In two patients presenting with an intermittent obstruction, Rheeman and Meyer[167] hypothesized that the intraluminal pressure, great enough to cause pressure erosion and dilation of the bone canal, may also reach a level high enough to overcome the obstruction intermittently. Significant nasolacrimal canal enlargement may occur as an incidental normal variant, without evidence of erosion, displacement, or mass lesions. Such findings in asymptomatic patients usually warrant no further investigation. A DCR may help exclude any small neoplastic lesion of the lacrimal sac and nasolacrimal duct. A follow-up CT scan to show lack of change may be justified. Biopsy of the lacrimal sac or duct is not warranted in the absence of any clinical or radiologic evidence of tumor.[167]

Coronal CT (direct or reformatted) may better display the longitudinal course of the nasolacrimal canal but will not directly assess the membranous nasolacrimal duct (compare this to MR imaging of the nasolacrimal canal [Fig. 10-26] or CT-DCG [Figs. 10-19 to 10-27]).

## CT Pathology

Dacryocystitis (inflammation and dilation of the lacrimal sac) is usually diagnosable clinically unless associated preseptal or periorbital cellulitis limits an adequate clinical assessment. Enhanced imaging studies are most useful and help differentiate preseptal inflammatory lesions from more specific acute and/or chronic dacryocystitis. CT demonstrates an enlarged lacrimal sac centered around the lacrimal fossa (Figs. 10-17 and 10-28 to 10-30). Axial CT (and/or MR imaging) also distinguishes the postseptal inflammatory lesions (periorbital or orbital abscess), which require urgent surgical intervention, from acute dacryocystitis, a preseptal

inflammatory process that is treated nonsurgically (Fig. 10-29). Extrinsic compression or infiltration by an adjacent inflammatory, neoplastic, or traumatic process of the nasolacrimal duct or sac may result in obstruction, enlargement, or dilation of the lacrimal sac and must be considered in the differential diagnosis of medial canthal mass lesions. Mass lesions in the region of the medial canthus and lacrimal sac may represent lacrimal sac diverticula. While these lesions are most commonly small and asymptomatic, they may present as cystic mass lesions, with or without mechanical obstruction of the NLDS. DCG or ultrasound infrequently demonstrates the communication between the lacrimal sac lumen and the diverticulum, such that only indirect signs of compression, displacement, or obstruction are visualized on the DCG. The most common location of these diverticula is at the junction of the lacrimal sac and the nasolacrimal duct. Those larger clinically apparent cystic diverticula tend to appear tense and fluctuant, affixed to the deep tissues but not to the skin.[78] They are almost always located lateral to the lacrimal sac, frequently coursing along the inferior orbital rim deep to the medial aspect of the lower eyelid.[78] With gentle pressure, some may be decompressed through the punctum or into the nose if the communication between the diverticulum and the lacrimal system is patent. Air may be trapped in a diverticulum, enabling a pneumatocele to develop.

Pneumatocele should always be considered in this location, especially with a well-circumscribed roundish or cystic-appearing mass that may contain air or have an air-fluid level. There are usually no associated inflammatory changes and no evidence of lacrimal drainage system obstruction. In contrast to chronic dacryocystitis, which demonstrates a thick-walled lacrimal sac, diverticula tend to be surrounded by an extremely thin fibrous or epithelial/fibrous layer that may not be apparent on CT.[80] These masses do not enhance and suggest a cystic lesion rather than a neoplastic process. Lacrimal sac mucoceles and true lacrimal sac cysts may be difficult to differentiate by imaging. The tendency of lacrimal sac diverticula to extend more laterally at the inferior sac–duct junction, with thinner capsule, may help differentiate these lesions from the lacrimal sac mucocele that tends to expand more superiorly and to have a thicker, enhancing wall and an obstructed nasolacrimal system clinically. Topical administration of contrast medium (DCG-CT) may help define the lacrimal system's patency, as well as the possibility of contrast extending into the diverticulum. However, the communication between the lacrimal system and the diverticulum may be progressively sealed by chronic inflammation, forming an independent cyst (lined by lacrimal epithelium) containing increased caseous or proteinaceous content, and with inflammatory changes thickening its capsule, obscuring its more cystic nature and resembling a more solid mass. MR imaging may better demonstrate the cystic nature of the lesion in such a circumstance.

Lacrimal sac diverticula may be treated by ligation and excision. Those lesions (congenital or postinflammatory) located at the inferior lacrimal sac or nasolacrimal duct and causing obstruction are better treated by DCR.

Lesions arising within the orbit, paranasal sinuses, or nasal cavity may mimic lesions of the nasolacrimal drainage apparatus and present clinically with the same symptomatol-

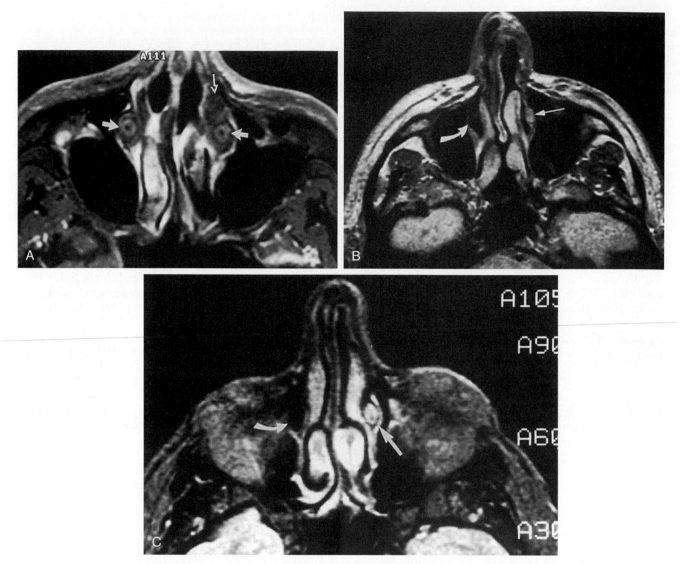

**FIGURE 10-26**   Nasolacrimal canal assessed by MR imaging. **A**, Patient with chronic inflammatory disease of the NLDS. Axial T1-weighted postgadolinium image shows mucosal enhancement of the nasolacrimal duct epithelium (*white arrows*). Nasal polypoid tissue is anterior to the nasolacrimal duct (*open arrow*). **B** and **C**, Another patient. **B**, Axial proton density image at the level of the inferior meatus shows the left nasolacrimal duct (*thin arrow*) just proximal to the valve of Hasner. Air in the right nasolacrimal canal is seen as signal void (*curved arrow*). **C**, Axial T2-weighted image scan shows the left nasolacrimal duct (*straight arrow*) within the canal. Air in the right nasolacrimal canal is seen as signal void (*curved arrow*). (See also Fig. 10-25.)

ogy as mass lesions of the inner canthus or inferomedial orbit (Fig. 10-30).[145, 152, 153]

A wide variety of neoplasms (benign and malignant) of the adjacent nasal cavity, maxillary, ethmoid, or even frontal sinuses may manifest as medial canthal masses. (See Table 10-3.) Squamous cell carcinoma and, less commonly, adenocarcinoma represent a majority of the malignant lesions. Inverted papilloma may arise within the lacrimal sac, although more commonly such tumors arise within the adjacent nasal cavity and paranasal sinuses and directly invade the lacrimal sac or spread from the nasal cavity up the nasolacrimal duct to reach the lacrimal sac and inner canthus.

Mucoceles arising in the anterior ethmoid air cells have an intimate relationship with the lacrimal fossa. CT may show opacified expanded anterior ethmoid air cells with

thinning and remodeling of bone. Any bone destruction caused by pressure erosion, if present, will be more extensive than that seen with lacrimal sac dilations and will be eccentric relative to the nasolacrimal fossa. In these cases, the lamina papyracea bows toward the orbit.

Dermoids are well-defined lesions of the orbit that result from sequestration of ectodermal elements trapped along lines of embryonic fusion. Such masses tend to localize adjacent to suture lines. Although they are located most frequently adjacent to the frontozygomatic suture, a medial (nasal) extraconal location is also common. The presence of fat density, a fat-fluid level, or rim calcification may help suggest this diagnosis and differentiate a dermoid from a dilated lacrimal sac. Medial orbital or nasal dermoids also tend to be more superomedial. Unlike dacryocystitis or mucoceles of the nasolacrimal sac, such lesions do not

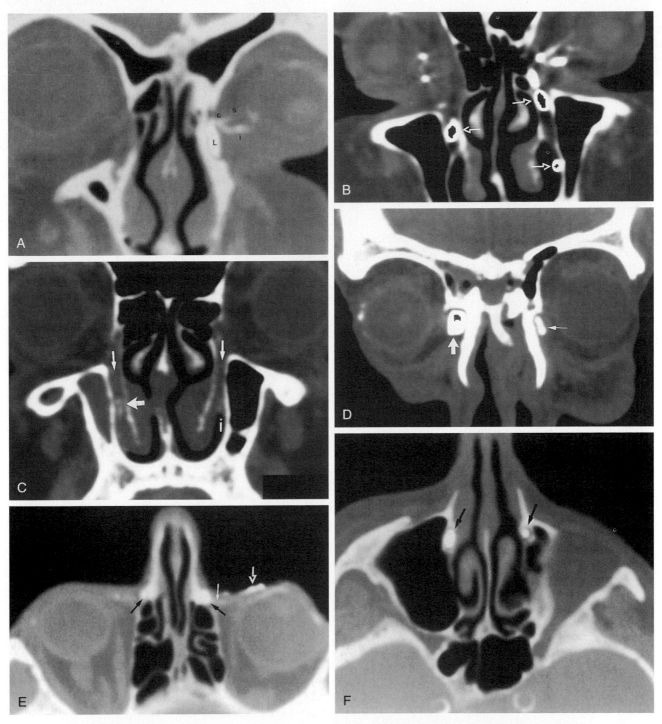

**FIGURE 10-27**   CT-DCG of normal anatomy. **A** to **D**, Coronal images of different patients. **E** and **F**, Axial images of the same patient. **A**, Coronal CT shows contrast in the left superior (*s*) and inferior (*i*) canaliculi, sinus of Maier (common canaliculus) (*c*), and lacrimal sac (*L*). **B**, Contrast material is seen in the proximal left nasolacrimal canal, left inferior meatus, and right distal nasolacrimal canal (*arrows*). Density artifact misregistration causes contrast material to appear black. The upper drainage system is not labeled. **C**, Coronal slice through the nasolacrimal canals bilaterally (*vertical arrows*) shows a small amount of contrast in the distal right nasolacrimal canal (*horizontal arrow*). *i*, Inferior meatus. **D**, Dilatation of the right lacrimal sac (*vertical arrow*) compared with the normal left sac (*horizontal arrow*). **E**, Left common canaliculus (*vertical arrow*) filled with contrast material. Slight prominence of the left lacrimal sac compared with the right (*black arrows*). *Open arrow*, Conjunctival sac. **F**, More inferior slice through the nasolacrimal canal shows contrast material within the nasolacrimal duct bilaterally (*arrows*). Normal variation with asymmetry in the diameter of the ducts. (See also Fig. 10-19.)

extend into the nasolacrimal duct. Coronal CT may be diagnostic by displaying continuity between the lacrimal sac and the nasolacrimal duct. Encephaloceles or meningoceles may present in the inner canthus as well-defined masses. Their extension superiorly within the nasoorbital tissues should suggest this diagnosis, and a defect in the skull base should be carefully sought. Hemangioma, lymphangioma, and neurofibroma are frequent benign tumors of the orbit. They may be associated with a mass effect and pressure erosion, but they do not cause bone invasion. Occasionally, an isolated varix of the angular vein may manifest as a medial canthal mass or may simulate a lacrimal sac mass.

The patient usually presents with intermittent swelling. Tearing may be present if there is compression of the lacrimal drainage system. Regression of the mass with gentle pressure, or an alteration in the size of the mass with Valsalva maneuvers, or with alteration in head position, should suggest this diagnosis.[168, 169]

Malignant lesions arising within the orbit that may present as inner canthal masses include lymphoma, rhabdomyosarcoma, and metastases. Preseptal malignancies, including basal cell and squamous cell carcinomas of the skin and non-Hodgkin's lymphoma, commonly invade the medial canthal tissues. Rarely, plasmacytomas

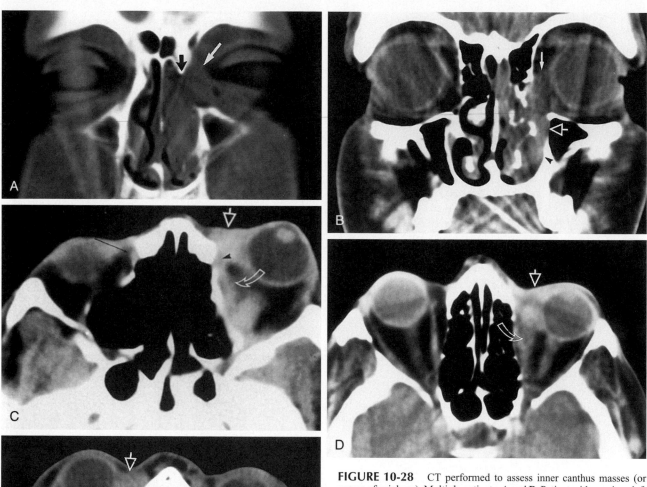

**FIGURE 10-28** CT performed to assess inner canthus masses (or causes of epiphora). Multiple patients. **A** and **B**, Patient with previous left DCR and DCR revision has persistent left epiphora. **A**, Coronal CT scan shows an adequate osteotomy defect (*black arrow*) from previous left DCR. Soft-tissue swelling within the inner canthus and nasal cavity (*white arrow*). **B**, Slightly more posterior coronal image shows soft-tissue density of the inferomedial orbit (*solid arrow*) extending into the left nasolacrimal canal (*open arrow*) to the inferior meatus (*arrowhead*). Biopsy of the left nasolacrimal sac revealed inverted papilloma. **C**, Second patient. Mass in the left inner canthus (*open arrow*) is poorly defined and extends to involve the retrobulbar tissues medially (*curved arrow*). Loss of the fat tissue plane surrounding the lacrimal sac (*arrowhead*) compared with the normal contralateral side (*thin arrow*). Biopsy showed sarcoid. **D**, Third patient. Mass of the left inner canthus (*open arrow*) infiltrates the preseptal tissues, displaces the globe laterally, and extends posteriorly to involve the medial rectus muscle (*curved arrow*). Biopsy revealed basal cell carcinoma. **E**, Fourth patient. Mass of the right inner canthus (*arrow*) obscures insertion of the medial rectus into the globe. Biopsy found orbital pseudotumor. (See also Fig. 10-20.)

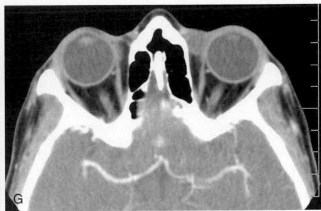

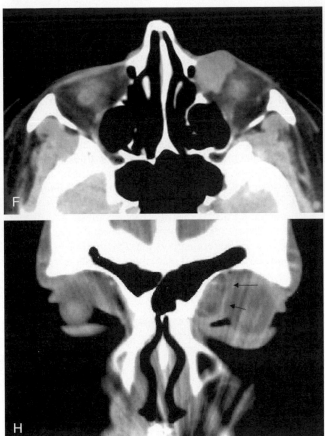

**FIGURE 10-28** *Continued.* **F,** Fifth patient. Mass in the left inner canthus abuts the lacrimal sac, which is not compressed. Deeper borders of the mass are well defined. Mass extends to preseptal tissues, with suspected skin fixation. Pathology: melanoma. **G** and **H,** Sixth patient. Palpable mass just superior to the medial canthal tendon. Axial and coronal CT scans show a hypodense mass with a faint capsule (*arrows*) remaining superior to the lacrimal sac fossa. Pathology: dermoid tumor (compare with Fig. 10-25G).

and malignant fibrous histiocytomas may present at this location.

Orbital pseudotumor, especially if the medial rectus is primarily involved, can extend from the tendinous insertion to the adjacent lacrimal fossa. Radiographically, pseudotumor may be difficult to differentiate from malignant involvement, especially lymphoma. Sarcoidosis and other granulomatous inflammatory processes occasionally will be localized in the inferomedial orbit or within the nasolacrimal drainage apparatus (Fig. 10-20).

### Lacrimal Sac Tumors

Tumors of the lacrimal sac are rare.[165, 170] These include a wide variety of epithelial and nonepithelial tumors (see Table 10-4). Epithelial neoplasms are subdivided histopathologically according to the Ryan and Font classification.[171] Benign epithelial tumors include papillomas (squamous, transitional, mixed) and are subdivided into exophytic or inverted growth patterns: oncocytomas, and benign mixed tumors. Malignant epithelial tumors (carcinomas) include squamous and transitional carcinomas, adenocarcinoma, oncocytic adenocarcinoma, and mucoepidermoid and adenoid cystic carcinomas, as well as poorly differentiated carcinoma and papilloma with carcinoma. Malignancies have been subdivided into those arising de novo or arising within or from a benign papilloma[170] (Fig. 10-13A-C).

There is a 55% malignancy rate for all tumors arising within the lacrimal sac.[170] Most tumors arise from the pseudostratified columnar epithelial lining of the sac. Epithelial tumors therefore predominate, representing 75%

of all reported cases, with nonepithelial tumors accounting for the remaining 25%.[172] Poorly differentiated squamous cell (epidermoid) carcinomas, followed by transitional cell and mucoepidermoid carcinomas, are the most common malignancies. Benign epithelial masses, mainly papillomas, occur less than one third as frequently as the malignant epithelial tumors.

Nonepithelial tumors include those of mesenchymal origin (fibrous histiocytoma, hemangiopericytoma, lipoma); lymphoid lesions; reactive hyperplasia or malignant melanoma; granulocytic sarcoma (prior to peripheral blood or bone marrow involvement); and neural tumor. Fibrous histiocytoma and lymphoma are the most common nonepithelial tumors of the lacrimal sac. Fibrous histiocytoma displays varying patterns, fibroblastic to histiocytic predominance, and varying degrees of aggressiveness.

Lacrimal sac tumors present insidiously, with nonspecific symptoms of dacryostenosis or dacryocystitis. The tumors may be undiagnosed for months or years.[173] Treatment for a presumed infection may transiently improve swelling of the lacrimal sac and give a false impression of a clinical response, obscuring the underlying neoplastic disease.

The most common presenting signs and symptoms associated with lacrimal sac neoplasms include epiphora (53% of patients) with a mean duration of 3 years; dacryocystitis (38%, often chronic and irrigates freely); a mass or mucocele of the lacrimal sac (36%)[170]; and extension above the medial canthal tendon.[164] In 43% of patients in the Stefanyszyn et al. series,[170] the tumor was inadvertently found at the time of DCR for presumed dacryostenosis. Bleeding from the puncta, either spontaneously or on applied pressure to the lacrimal sac, or bleeding from the nose was noted in 8% of patients, as an early sign in one patient with melanoma and as a late sign in all other neoplasms. The average duration of symptoms in this series preoperatively was 3 years. In a small percentage of cases, metastatic lymph nodes may be the initial manifestation of a malignant lacrimal sac tumor.[174]

The usual sequence of events with a lacrimal sac tumor begins with epiphora, followed by recurrent bouts of dacryocystitis, development of a nonreducible mass in the area of the lacrimal sac, with eventual extension outside the sac, and, later, in certain cases, epistasis, ulceration over the sac, regional nodal involvement (preauricular, submandibular, cervical) in approximately 28% and metastases.[170, 174, 175] Eyelid and orbital extension, with proptosis and decreased ocular motility, may then be noted in a high percentage of patients with malignant epithelial neo-

plasm.[174, 175] Signs to complement a high index of suspicion, necessary for an early diagnosis, include a painless, nonreducible, firm mass in the lacrimal sac region, especially if the mass extends superior to the medial canthal tendon,[164, 176] compared to the slightly lower position of the lacrimal sac mucocele associated with chronic dacryocystitis. There is a tendency for melanoma of the lacrimal sac to bleed (punctal or epistaxis) and disperse pigment.[176]

DCG tends to display findings earlier with a distended lacrimal sac and a filling defect, as well as mottled density (intraluminal growth), in conjunction with delayed drainage of the contrast material, when CT may still be negative. In early stages of tumor growth, the lacrimal drainage system will be patent.[176] DCG may be a more effective study for differentiating dacryocystitis from neoplasia and differentiating extrinsic from intrinsic lacrimal sac pathologic processes. CT better displays the extraluminal component of the soft-tissue lacrimal sac mass and its extension into

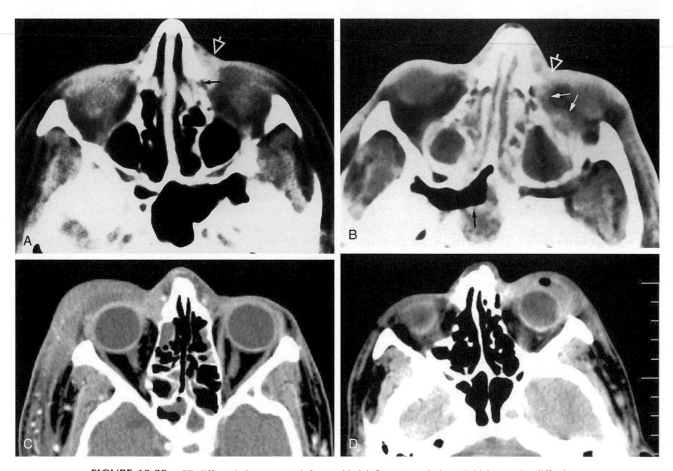

**FIGURE 10-29** CT differentiating preseptal from orbital inflammatory lesions (which may be difficult on clinical examination). Multiple patients. **A,** Soft-tissue mass in the left inner canthus (*open arrow*) with faint peripheral enhancement contiguous with the left nasolacrimal fossa (partially obscured by beam-hardening artifact) (*thin arrow*). Mass is localized to the preseptal tissues. Pathology: chronic dacryocystitis with mucocele formation. **B,** Soft-tissue prominence (*open arrow*) of the left inner canthus, clinically noted on axial CT to involve the medial orbital soft tissues and inferior rectus muscle (*thin white arrows*). Pansinus opacification with fluid level in the right sphenoid sinus (*black arrow*). Sinusitis with left orbital cellulitis. **C,** Second patient. Preseptal orbital cellulitis secondary to dacryocystitis. Note the sharp posterior border of the inflammatory process due to orbital septum attachment to the posterior lacrimal crest. **D** and **E,** Third patient. Axial (**D**) and coronal (**E**) CT scans show a preseptal left orbital abscess containing air and pus. Soft-tissue edema extends medially to abut the normal air-containing lacrimal sac.

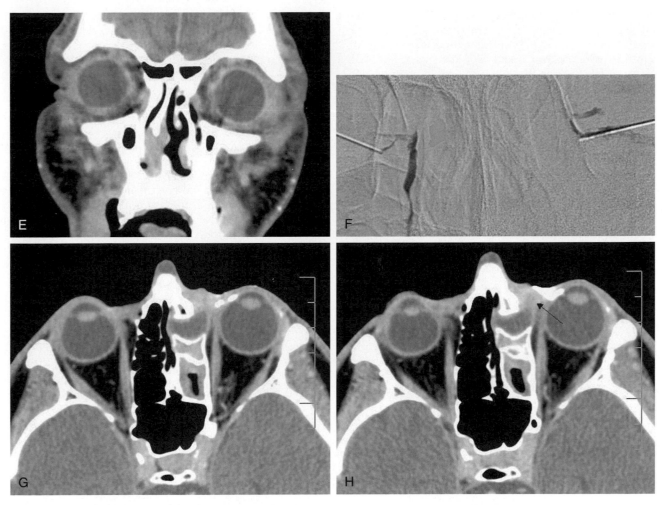

**FIGURE 10-29**    *Continued.* **F** to **J**, Fourth patient. Anterior ethmoid mucocele. **F**, DCG shows blocks at the common canaliculus, with dilatation of the superior and inferior canaliculi suggesting chronic canalicular inflammatory changes. **G** and **H**, Axial-enhanced CT scan shows a cystic mass centered within the anterior ethmoid air cell and projecting into the lacrimal sac fossa. Soft-tissue swelling of the left inner canthus and enlarged lacrimal sac (*arrow*).

*Illustration continued on following page*

surrounding tissues, bone erosion, or infiltration of the lacrimal sac fossa, nasolacrimal canal, or adjacent orbit and paranasal sinuses. CT-DCG will offer further information about the lacrimal sac lumen, allowing better assessment of the thickness or irregularity of the lacrimal sac wall (intramural growth) and the nasolacrimal duct than CT alone. MR imaging, with its superior soft-tissue resolution, may better display neoplastic extension of the lacrimal sac tumor into the nasolacrimal canal or into the adjacent soft tissues of the orbit.[177] Because of the desire for both bone and soft-tissue detail, CT usually is the primary modality for assessment, with MR imaging playing an adjunctive role in selective cases.

While benign lesions may allow a local resection, epithelial malignancies tend to grow along the epithelium of the lacrimal drainage system. Cure, therefore is dependent on a wide surgical excision of the lacrimal sac mass and the entire lacrimal drainage system (canaliculi, sac, and nasolacrimal duct), combined with a lateral rhinostomy and radiation ther-

apy. CT remains the preferred posttreatment modality for follow-up of these patients. Persistent epiphora is frequently seen in the postradiation nonsurgical patient (e.g., with lymphoma). Postirradiation nasolacrimal duct stenosis is a frequent complication[178] that may be prevented by the insertion of nasolacrimal stents.[177] Epithelial carcinomas of the lacrimal sac have a recurrence rate of 50%.[171] The overall mortality of those treated with a combination of wide surgical excision and radiation is 37.5%.[174, 179]

CT findings of sac enlargement (dacryocystitis as a complication) should be distinguishable from the findings of solid tumor. Intraductal tumor and its relationship to the nasolacrimal bony canal or nasolacrimal fossa is best seen on CT, which also allows extracanalicular tumor spread to be assessed.[70] Bone destruction of the lacrimal fossa is common with intraductal malignant neoplasms.[152] DCG alone or in combination with CT may help better define small tumors arising from the lacrimal sac fundus or show the lumen irregularity caused by the tumor.[180]

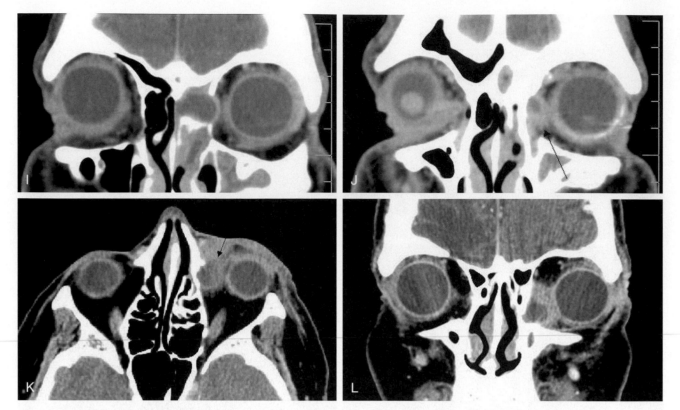

**FIGURE 10-29** *Continued.* **I** and **J**, Coronal CT scans shows lateral displacement of the lamina papyracea and lacrimal fossa bed, as well as inflammatory changes of the lacrimal sac and surrounding tissues (*arrow*), with loss of normal tissue planes. Pathology: dacryocystitis secondary to anterior ethmoid inflammatory disease—mucocele. **K** and **L**, Fifth patient. Axial and coronal CT scans show a distended lacrimal sac with thickened walls, extensive preseptal swelling, and loss of adjacent tissue planes (*arrow*). Incidental right frontal lobe encephalomalacia. Pathology: lacrimal sac abscess.

Granulomatous pseudotumors, sarcoidosis, or other less common inflammatory or infiltrative diseases may involve the lacrimal sac and should be considered in the differential diagnosis.[181]

### Facial Trauma

Traumatic lacerations of the canaliculi are poorly visualized by CT, and if clinical assessment is indefinite, DCG is the definitive study (Fig. 10-31). Similarly, CT may be insufficient to differentiate NLDS obstruction caused by acute edema or ecchymosis of adjacent tissues.[173] Persistent tearing (after subsidence of soft-tissue swelling) or recurrent dacryocystitis suggests a probable obstruction of the nasolacrimal duct system (NLDS) and the need for further assessment.

Fractures of the lacrimal fossa and nasolacrimal canal may lead to an acute and/or delayed obstruction of the nasolacrimal system. Such fractures or bone displacements are best assessed by CT, which may also help prevent a closed manipulation of a sharp, displaced fracture fragment that could further harm the lacrimal sac or duct. Demonstration of such bone fragments suggests that exploration and open reduction is a more prudent treatment.

Approximately 85% of obstructions associated with trauma occurred at the junction of the lacrimal sac and nasolacrimal duct. CT may suggest the level of obstruction by noting the location of fracture fragments. However, DCG remains a more exact and definitive method for locating the point of obstruction.

There is a relative infrequency of epiphora associated with severe facial trauma.[182] Campbell[9] noted only a 12% incidence in 100 cases of central midfacial fractures and postulated several reasons. In both the cranofacial (LeFort III)- and pyramidal (LeFort II)-type fractures, the lacrimal fossa and nasolacrimal canal tend to escape the fracture lines centered more superiorly at the nasofrontal suture and extending lateral to the nasolacrimal fossa and canal. The anterior and posterior lacrimal crests deflect the pyramidal fractures superior and then posterior to the lacrimal fossa into the orbital plate of the ethmoid. The transverse (LeFort I)-type fracture usually involves the lateral wall of the nasal cavity immediately above the floor of the nasal fossa, thereby sparing the nasolacrimal canal. Fistulae of the nasolacrimal duct into the maxillary antra may result from LeFort I type fractures.

Several series documenting orbital findings relative to facial fractures have noted symptomatic lacrimal obstruction in 0.2% of nasal fractures, 3.4% of LeFort II or III fractures, and 17% to 21% of nasoorbital-ethmoidal fractures.[182–187] Unger[188] noted that fractures involving the bony nasolacrimal fossa and canal were associated with simple unilateral facial fractures as well as the more complex midface fractures. Three patterns of fractures were noted: avulsion of the lacrimal sac fossa, comminuted fractures of the lacrimal

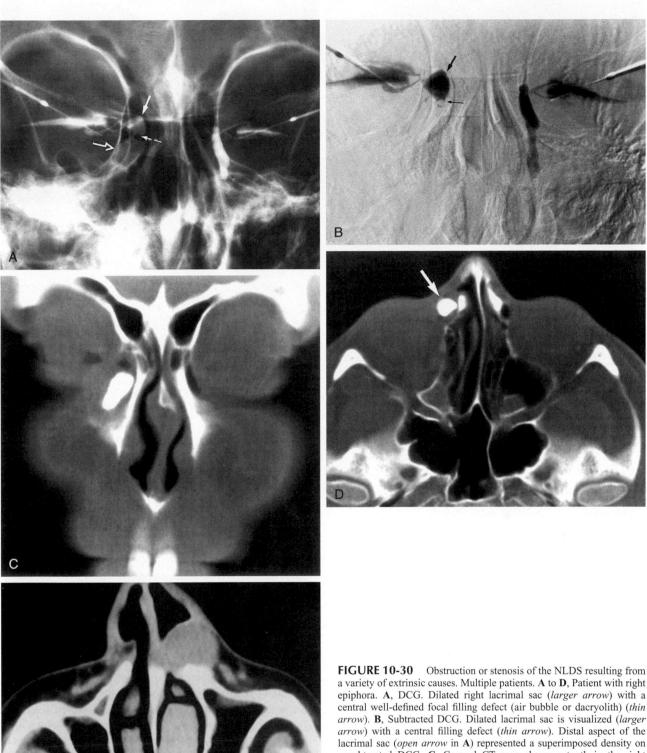

**FIGURE 10-30** Obstruction or stenosis of the NLDS resulting from a variety of extrinsic causes. Multiple patients. **A** to **D**, Patient with right epiphora. **A**, DCG. Dilated right lacrimal sac (*larger arrow*) with a central well-defined focal filling defect (air bubble or dacryolith) (*thin arrow*). **B**, Subtracted DCG. Dilated lacrimal sac is visualized (*larger arrow*) with a central filling defect (*thin arrow*). Distal aspect of the lacrimal sac (*open arrow* in **A**) represented a superimposed density on unsubtracted DCG. **C**, Coronal CT scan shows a tooth in the right nasolacrimal fossa causing compression of the lacrimal sac. **D**, Axial image (for nonbelievers) shows the tooth (*arrow*) causing pressure erosion with broadening of the nasolacrimal fossa. Pathology: ''eye tooth.'' **E** and **F**, Second patient with soft-tissue mass in the left nasolabial angle and epiphora. **E**, Well-defined soft-tissue mass (nasolabial cyst) causing mild pressure erosion in the left maxilla (the cyst does not explain the epiphora).

*Illustration continued on following page*

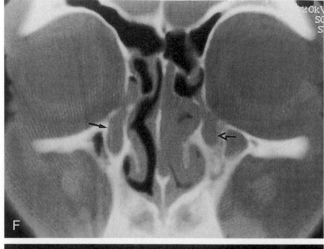

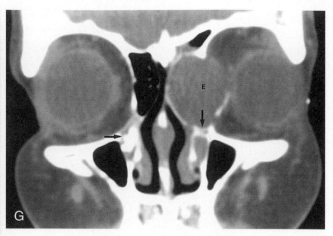

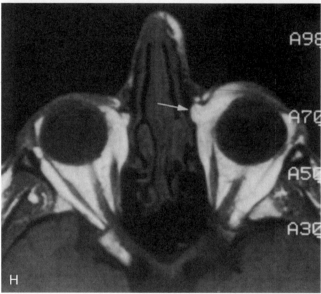

**FIGURE 10-30**   *Continued.* **F,** Coronal CT scan shows demineralization with loss of cortical bone of the left nasolacrimal canal (*open arrow*) compared with the normal right side (*solid arrow*). Pathology: posttraumatic inclusion cyst and suspected osteitis in the anterior maxilla. **G,** Soft-tissue mass centered about and expanding the left side of the ethmoid sinus (*E*). Medial wall of the orbit is displaced laterally, in contrast to a mass arising within the orbit. Bony partition (*vertical arrow*) is present between the mass and the nasolacrimal canal, in contrast to the mass arising in the nasolacrimal fossa. Contrast medium in the right nasolacrimal canal (*horizontal arrow*). Pathology: ethmoid mucocele. **H,** Intermittent left epiphora. Axial T1-weighted image shows increased fat content in the left inner canthus (compared with the right), with fat tissue herniating into and filling the left nasolacrimal fossa (*arrow*). (Courtesy of Dr. George Wortzman, Toronto, Canada.)

sac fossa or nasolacrimal canal, and linear fractures of the nasolacrimal canal. Fractures involving the nasolacrimal fossa most commonly were avulsions of an intact nasolacrimal fossa, with comminution of the nasolacrimal fossa being less frequent. Linear fractures of the fossa are rare. The anterior (frontal process of the maxilla) and posterior (lacrimal bone) lacrimal crests fortify the nasolacrimal fossa such that it maintains its integrity when displaced from the more fragile components of the adjacent orbital and nasal structures.[188] This CT finding correlates with the clinical observations that direct lacerations of the lacrimal sac are rare and that obstruction at the junction of the lacrimal sac and nasolacrimal duct is common.[189]

Although the superior aspect of the nasolacrimal canal is also formed by the lacrimal bone and maxilla, most of the canal continues within the medial (nasal) wall of the maxilla, which progressively thins toward the nasolacrimal canal opening just inferior to the inferior turbinate. The majority of fractures involving the nasolacrimal canal are comminuted, with the comminution being more common and more extensive where the bone is thinner at the more inferior aspect of the canal. Linear fractures of the nasolacrimal

canal are relatively uncommon. Complication of drainage (epiphora) was seen in only 5 of 25 patients.[188]

Previous facial fracture repairs may add complexities to the performance of lacrimal surgery.[189] Bone grafts used in reconstruction may alter anatomic landmarks.[183, 190] Metallic plates, wires, and silastic or mesh sheets used for fracture repair may impede the lacrimal surgery or be causative factors in the lacrimal drainage symptoms and may require removal during the surgical repair or DCG.[183, 190] CT remains the primary modality of investigation for assessing facial fractures, malalignments, residual deformities, previous instrumentation, and their relationship to the NLDS. CT can also be used to show the bony anatomy in patients after surgery such as DCR (Fig. 10-32).

## COMBINED CT-DACRYOCYSTOGRAPHY

DCG is the best modality to demonstrate obstruction of the NLDS itself, and CT is valuable in imaging the surrounding bone and soft-tissue structures of the face, sinuses, and orbit. Conventional CT alone cannot provide

**Table 10-3**
**MASS LESIONS OF THE INNER CANTHUS**

**I. Nasolacrimal Drainage System**
  A. Inflammatory/obstructive:
    1. lacrimal sac mucocele
    2. dacryocystitis
    3. lacrimal sac abscess
    4. cyst of the lacrimal sac
    5. granulomatous pseudotumor including sarcoid/Wegener's
  B. Benign tumors*
    1. Epithclial: inverting papilloma, benign mixed tumor
    2. Mesenchymal: fibroma, histiocytoma, hemangioma, neurogenic
  C. Malignant tumors*
    1. epithelial carcinomas
    2. lymphoma
    3. melanoma
    4. hemangiopericytoma
    5. granulocytic sarcoma

**II. Orbit**
  A. Preseptal
    1. Inflammatory: cellulitis, abscess
    2. Benign tumor: inclusion cysts, sebaceous cysts, dermoid
    3. Malignant skin or eyelid neoplasms: basal cell carcinoma, squamous cell carcinoma, meibomian gland carcinoma, sebaceous cell carcinoma, lymphoma, schwannoma
  B. Postseptal
    1. Inflammatory, including lymphatic: cellulitis, abscess, medial periorbital abscess, nasolabial pseudotumor, myositis
    2. Benign: dermoid, hemangioma
    3. Malignant: lymphoma, rhabdomyosarcoma, extramedullary plasmacytoma

**III. Sinonasal**
  A. Inflammatory: sinusitis, orbital cellulitis, periorbital abscess, orbital abscess, mucocele, ethmoid, frontal chronic granulation tissue
  B. Benign: polyposis, papilloma, oncocytoma
  C. Malignant: carcinoma (squamous cell, adenoca, minor salivary gland, etc.), lymphoma, melanoma, esthesioneuroblastoma

**IV. Local—From Above (Skull Base, Dura, Brain)**
  A. Meningioma
  B. Meningocele
  C. Encephalocele

**V. Local Bone—Cartilage**
  A. Fibro-osseous osteoma
  B. Osteosarcoma
  C. Chondrosarcoma
  D. Myeloma/plasmacytoma

**VI. Geographic—Local Soft Tissues**
  A. Neurogenic: neurofibroma
  B. Vascular: varix malformations, hemangioma, developmental or fissural cysts

**VII. Trauma**
  A. Hematoma: edema
  B. Displaced bone fragments
  C. Instrumentation of implants

**VIII. Systemic**
  A. Metastases
  B. Lymphoma, myeloma
  C. Histiocytosis

*See Table 10-4 for tumors of the lacrimal sac.

adequate information to suggest a focus of obstruction in the epiphora patient. Combining these two modalities shows the relationship between the NLDS and the surrounding soft tissue or bony structures to better advantage. This combined study (CT-DCG) is indicated in the assessment of more complex lacrimal problems such as medial canthal tumors, midface trauma, or previous lacrimal or adjacent sinonasal surgery (Figs. 10-13 to 10-15, 10-18, 10-19, and 10-27). The combined study can more confidently show masses to be intrinsic (e.g., dacryolith) or extrinsic to the duct system, and the full extent of an extrinsic mass can be more properly

defined during CT-DCG. Either axial or coronal imaging may be preferred. Frequently these views are complementary. The continuing advances of spiral (volumetric) imaging with thinner overlapping slices allow improved image data accumulation in the axial plane. Reconstruction capabilities allow selective sagittal or coronal oblique images exactly along the axis of the NLDS. Reformatted studies reduce the total radiation exposure for such studies compared to direct imaging in multiple planes.

CT-DCG may better demonstrate the exact relationship of the lacrimal sac to the paranasal sinuses and advise the

**Table 10-4**
**TUMORS OF THE LACRIMAL SAC (HISTOPATHOLOGIC CLASSIFICATION)**

**I. Epithelial Tumors**
  A. Benign
    1. Papilloma: squamous, transitional
    2. Oncocytoma
    3. Benign mixed tumors
  B. Malignant epithelial tumors
    1. Papilloma with carcinoma
    2. Carcinoma: squamous, transitional adenocarcinoma, oncocytic adenocarcinoma, mucoepidermoid, poorly differentiated, adenoid cystic

**II. Nonepithelial Tumors**
  A. Mesenchymal
    1. Fibrous histiocytoma
    2. Hemangiopericytoma
    3. Hemangioma
    4. Lipoma
  B. Lymphoma
    1. Reactive
    2. Malignant
  C. Melanoma
  D. Granulocytic sarcoma
  E. Neurogenic
    1. Neurofibroma
    2. Neurilemmoma

Adapted from Stefanyszym MA, Hidayat AA, Pe'er JJ, Flanagan JC. Lacrimal sac tumors. Ophthal Plast Reconstr Surg 1994;10:169–184.

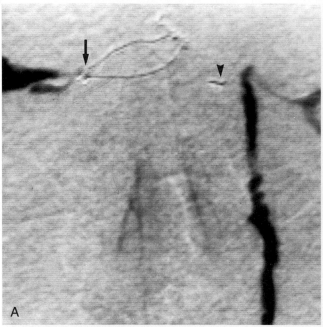

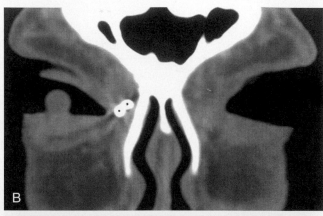

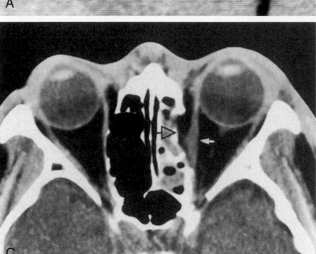

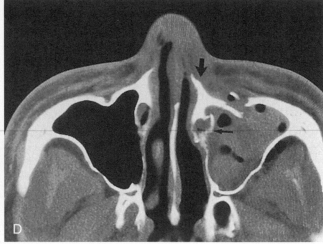

**FIGURE 10-31**   Trauma of the NLDS. **A** and **B**, Old medial orbital fracture and persistent right epiphora. **A**, DCG. Wire ligature occludes the right common canaliculus (*arrow*). Fine ligature is noted medial to the left nasolacrimal sac (*arrowhead*). **B**, Coronal CT scan shows the wire ligature to be too lateral within the right inner canthus. **C** and **D**, Acute face trauma with left epiphora. **C**, Medial blowout fracture (*open black arrow*) with a contused medial rectus muscle (*white arrow*). **D**, Fracture involves the nasolacrimal canal, with buckling of the medial and lateral walls (*horizontal arrow*), resulting from posterior displacement of an anteromedial maxillary fragment (*vertical arrow*). (**C** and **D** Courtesy of Dr. Lyne Noël de Tilly, Toronto, Canada.)

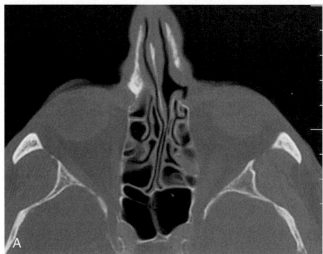

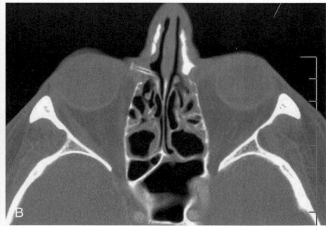

**FIGURE 10-32**   **A**, Typical bone defect from previous left external DCR. Open communication between the nasal cavity and lacrimal sac outlined by the presence of air. **B**, Canaliculo-DCR for reconstruction of the canaliculi, with postsurgery bone changes and the presence of a Jones tube (see "Surgical Procedures for Epiphora" in text).

surgeon whether the ethmoid sinus will be encountered in the course of the dacryocystorhinostomy (DCR). The most anterior ethmoid cells, the agger nasi cells, extend into bone adjacent to the lacrimal sac in 94% to 98.5% of patients, overlying the superior half of the lacrimal sac fossa.[191] Inappropriate osteotomy placement or inadvertent anastomosis of the lacrimal sac to an ethmoid air cell, rather than to the nasal mucosa, can lead to DCR failure.[191–193]

The location of the bony opening in patients who have undergone previous unsuccessful DCR is frequently invisible on DCG, but this surgically important information may be attained by CT-DCG.[194] Welham and Wulc's study[112] of 208 DCR failures, problems with the bony ostium were present in over half of the cases and represented the most common cause of DCR failure. Glatt et al.[194] emphasized the use of CT-DCG to show the relationship between the bony ostium of the failed DCR and the lacrimal sac, filled with radiographic contrast medium. Improper placement of the ostium, including too anterior, too inferior, or too small (improper size), was noted in their study. A proper osteotomy for external DCR should be relatively large, measuring at least 15 mm in diameter, all bone between the lacrimal sac and nasal mucosa should be removed, and no bone should be left within 5 mm of the common canaliculus.[24, 107, 112] A smaller bony ostium (5 to 7 mm in diameter) may be successful and appropriate for a transnasal laser DCR.[195] Bone regrowth at the osteotomy site after DCR is unusual, but may occur in children and can be a cause of DCR failure at the osteotomy site.[112] CT-DCG may show bone regrowth between the lacrimal sac and nasal cavity. Linberg et al.[196] showed that the average diameter of the intranasal ostium postoperatively shrinks to 2% of the original operative diameter, mainly because of soft-tissue scarring. CT or CT-DCG with proper use of bone and soft-tissue windows facilitates reoperation after DCR failure by determining what modifications are required in the bony ostium.[194] Such studies can also show whether anterior ethmoid air cell resection is required to allow proper mobilization of lacrimal and nasal mucosal flaps and appropriate internal anastomosis and drainage into the nasal cavity. Similarly, anatomic variants of the nasal cavity, anterior middle turbinate, inferior turbinate, or nasal septum may be noted. CT-DCG best shows the relationship of surgical clips, sutures, and fixation plates to the nasolacrimal sac or the osteotomy site. On routine intravenous enhanced CT or during surgery, it may be very difficult to identify the lacrimal sac on DCR failure patients because of exuberant granulation tissue or scarring and attenuation of anatomic landmarks. Such soft-tissue proliferation at the internal anastomosis may represent inadequate mucosal end-to-end suturing between the lacrimal sac and the nasal cavity.[112] CT-DCG facilitates the treatment of these more difficult patients by identifying the lacrimal sac's shape, location, and relationship to surrounding structures, especially the ostium and/or surgical clips. The more recent transnasal endoscopic approach to DCR failures requires knowledge that the bony ostium is of adequate size and location before considering this approach.

CT-DCG was more sensitive than MR-DCG in differentiating high-grade stenosis from total obstruction of the NLDS.[151] In the presence of postoperative scarring, MR-DCG was less helpful in assessing the site and size of a bone defect after rhinostomy. CT-DCG is preferred for such patients, better differentiating soft tissue from bone obstructions. Epiphora is a common complication following medial maxillectomy for lateral nasal wall neoplasms. Outlining the NLDS with contrast, in conjunction with CT, may better assess patients with poor lacrimal drainage and may differentiate possible causes including residual tumor, inflammatory changes, fibrosis, and postsurgical or postradiation effects on the sinus, the nasal cavity, or the NLDS itself.

In patient with a lacrimal outflow symptoms after trauma, CT-DCR offers all the advantages of routine CT with the additional benefits of more exact localization of the lacrimal drainage system. CT-DCR can assess the possible complexities of the lacrimal surgery (usually DCR) resulting from distorted anatomy secondary to trauma or previous reconstructions including grafting. Adjacent anatomic variations (anterior ethmoid air cells, proximity of the anterior middle turbinate process, or deviated nasal septum) are visualized, as are the locations of previous placed miniplates, wire, or silastic sheets that may need to be removed because of interference with lacrimal flow.[51]

Ashenhurst et al.[197] performed CT-DCG immediately following standard intubation macro-DCG. They left the DCG lacrimal cannula in place, with contrast medium reinjected just before CT scanning (Fig. 10-27). Images were obtained in the coronal and/or axial plane, depending on clinical and DCG information. Glatt et al.[194] similarly used an oil-based radiopaque contrast medium injected via an inferior canalicular catheter insertion and recommended CT-DCG immediately following the injection of contrast. In the assessment of failed DCRs, they found coronal images to be more helpful. Imaging should be obtained in both bone and soft-tissue modes for proper assessment of the soft tissues and adjacent bony landmarks. CT-DCG can be performed using water-soluble contrast medium eye drops placed into the conjunctival cul-de-sac.[23, 197–200] Although such topical application of contrast material may be less predictable in demonstrating the NLDS than cannulation CT-DCG, several advantages may be realized. Topical CT-DCG allows a more physiologic evaluation of the NLDS and increases patient comfort, tolerance, and acceptance of the study. The ease of the procedure obviates the need for skilled personnel to perform the lacrimal cannulation and eliminates any risk of procedural iatrogenic injury from the cannulation or injection of contrast medium. The increased sensitivity of CT for detection of subtle attenuation changes of contrast medium within the NLDS has allowed the option of decreased volumes and concentrations of such agents. The topically applied contrast used is low-osmolar, non-ionic, and water soluble, with a concentration of 200 mg I/ml. One to two drops per minute, per eye, is given for 2 to 3 minutes before actual scanning starts. The patient is kept in a supine position for axial imaging or turned prone just before direct coronal imaging.

In a study[199] comparing instillation of topically applied contrast agents into the tear lake, iopamidol (Isovue 200; Squibb Diagnostics, Princeton, New Jersey) for CT and normal saline for MR-DCG, in healthy normal volunteers, CT-DCG consistently better displayed the smaller components of the NLDS (e.g., the superior, inferior, and common canalicula) than MR-DCG. These structures were seen routinely on CT-DCG, while MR-DCG displayed the superior and inferior canulicular structures in approximately 50% and the common canaliculus in less than 20%.

While a variety of CT-DCG techniques allows personal preference and comfort, certain circumstances require techniques that are more specific. Routine placement of drops of contrast medium into the conjunctival cul-de-sac (tear lake) may offer inadequate visualization of the NLDS in those patients with known punctal or canalicular stenosis, other higher-grade stenoses, or conditions not favoring the flow of such contrast into or through the NLDS. For these patients, a less physiologic and more anatomic placement of contrast through cannulation is required. While some individuals may prefer the more pronounced attenuation of lipid-based contrast agents (e.g., Lipiodol ultrafluide; Guerbet, Villepinte, France), caution with the use of such agents is imperative. Their increased viscosity makes placement into the conjunctival sac impractical. Lipid-based contrast medium introduced through cannulation is more at risk for extravasation and related long-standing complications,[201] especially in the posttraumatic study or in assessing the patient with chronic inflammatory tissues of the NLDS. We routinely use water-soluble, low-osmolar contrast, with excellent results and increased safety. This approach provides excellent images. This CT-DCG technique better demonstrates the canaliculi of the upper drainage system (Fig. 10-19) than cannulation CT-DCG and offers further advantage when used with spiral (helical) CT and its volume data acquisition,[198–200] offering coronal and sagittal oblique reformations of superior quality along the axis of the NLDS. The extremely fast total data acquisition times (less than 20 to 30 seconds) ensures patient cooperation and almost no risk of movement, despite the acquisition of very thin (1 mm or less) overlapping axial scans through the area of interest. The high-quality reformations obviate the need for direct coronal imaging. Three-dimensional images of the NLDS can be reconstructed using a connectivity algorithm and viewed in relationship to adjacent orbital or facial skeletal structures. Patients may complain of slight dryness, burning, or irritation of the eye from the topical administration of water-soluble contrast material.[23, 199]

## Pediatrics

### Congenital Atresia

The nasolacrimal apparatus develops from a core of surface epithelium, the nasooptic fissure, trapped between the maxillary and frontonasal processes. Although canalization occurs uniformly throughout the length of the nasolacrimal drainage system, failure in this process is most common at the distal nasolacrimal canal. There is lack of perforation of the nasolacrimal canal at the inferior meatus (valve of Hasner), with a persistent layer of lacrimal and nasal epithelial cells, related to adhesions between the nasal mucosa and the nasolacrimal epithelium.[202] In some patients, a plug of epithelial cell debris causes obstruction.[203] Such distal obstruction may result in epiphora and mucoid discharge.[204]

Simple inspection allows diagnosis of congenital atresia of the lacrimal puncta. If only one punctum is involved, DCG should be performed through the opposite punctum to visualize the canaliculi. Retrograde filling of the canaliculus without reflux through the punctum indicates focal occlusion. If the canaliculus fails to visualize, there is atresia of the entire canaliculus.[88]

Congenital obstruction of the NLDS occurs commonly, but significant symptoms are relatively rare. Sevel[202] noted an incidence of NLDS obstruction in 30% of term fetuses and MacEwan and Young[205] noted such obstruction to be a common clinical problem, affecting as many as 20% of all infants, while Levy[206] noted epiphora occurring in only 6% of infants. Increased intraluminal pressure in the duct during initial respiratory efforts or crying at birth may rupture the distal membrane, forming the one-way valve of Hasner.[207, 208] These findings may partially explain the high proportion (85%) of spontaneous resolution of NLDS obstructions before the child reaches age 9 months.[209] The low rate of tear production during early infancy is also a factor in the low incidence of epiphora.

Rarely, concomitant obstruction is also present more proximally in the NLDS, creating a closed space that allows accumulation of fluid, causing a cystic swelling of the NLDS (Fig. 10-33). Such proximal obstruction occurs as the result of a valve-like unidirectional obstruction at the junction of the lacrimal canaliculi and sac (valve of Rosenmüller).[27] Cystic swelling may also result from some component of active intraluminal secretions. Berkowitz et al.[204] prefer the term *congenital nasolacrimal drainage system cyst* for this cyst, seen as a bluish mass below the medial canthal angle. The terms *mucocele, dacryocystocele,* and *amniotocele* are also applied to this entity. If a distended lacrimal sac is present at birth, without associated inflammatory changes, the cystic swelling is referred to as an *amniotocele containing sterile amniotic fluid.*[27] If the cyst is filled with epithelial debris and mucus generated by the NLDS, the term *mucocele* may be used.[208] Compression of the distended lacrimal sac does not tend to cause regurgitation through the puncta.[210] Conservative management is generally preferred. Probing may prevent dacryocystitis or pressure on the globes. Surgical intervention (usually probing only) is generally not recommended unless complications develop or obstruction persists after age 6 to 9 months. Complications of a congenital nasolacrimal cyst include epiphora, dacryocystitis, cellulitis, sepsis, and respiratory distress.

Cystic distention of the lacrimal sac expands the nasolacrimal fossa by pressure erosion, accentuating the posterior lacrimal crest. Nasal extension may cause respiratory distress. Probing of the nasolacrimal duct system, with relief of proximal and distal obstructions as initial treatment, may relieve respiratory distress.[211] However, intranasal marsupialization of the cyst is usually recommended if there is nasal airway compromise. Berkowitz et al.[204] suggest that NLDS cysts may be more common than was previously thought and that any neonate showing signs of NLDS obstruction should have a careful nasal examination to rule out an associated nasal mass. Obstruction to the NLDS may be an unrecognized cause of transient nasal mucosal congestion in the newborn.[204]

CT may help show the classic triad of a cystic medial canthal mass, dilation of the nasolacrimal duct, and a contiguous submucosal nasal cavity mass in the inferior meatus.[212, 213] Endoscopy may show this submucosal

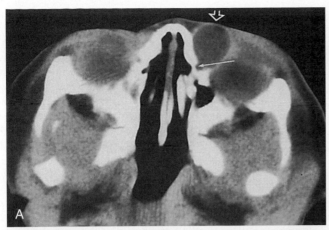

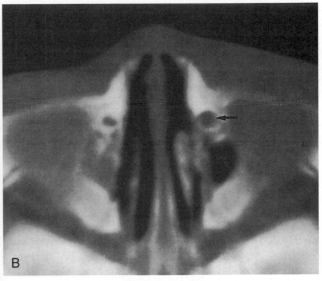

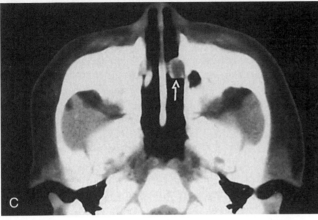

**FIGURE 10-33**   Congenital NLDS cyst (dacryocystocele) in a 10-day-old infant. **A**, Axial CT scan at the level of the inner canthus shows a low-density well-defined cystic mass (enlarged lacrimal sac) (*open arrow*) intimately associated with the left nasolacrimal fossa (*thin arrow*). **B**, Bone windows image at a level just inferior to the orbit floor shows a dilated left nasolacrimal canal (*arrow*). **C**, Soft-tissue axial image more inferiorly shows a well-defined soft-tissue mass (*arrow*) in the left nasal cavity. Classic triad of a cystic medial canthal mass, dilatation of the nasolacrimal duct, and contiguous submucosal nasal cavity mass in the inferior meatus. (Courtesy of Dr. Susan Blaser, Toronto, Canada.)

soft-tissue mass in the inferior meatus. Multiplanar MR imaging may better show the skull base and is useful in detecting findings that suggest other causes of medial nasoorbital mass lesions such as meningoceles, encephaloceles, and nasal gliomas. The presence of the classic triad suggests a congenital cyst or mucocele of the nasolacrimal duct, that is, a more distal duct obstruction. Obstructions that are more proximal tend to produce a lacrimal sac mucocele. However, mucoceles of the nasolacrimal duct system may extend either cranially or caudally; that is, mucoceles of the lacrimal sac may protrude downward into the nasolacrimal duct while mucoceles arising in the duct may extend upward to involve the lacrimal sac.[212] Mucoceles involving the lacrimal sac will have, as a clinical component, a mass in the medial canthus. Mucoceles of the distal nasolacrimal duct may present with cyst-like masses at the anteroinferior nasal cavity with a normal lacrimal sac and a superior nasolacrimal duct, because kinking of the thickened, inflamed mucosa in the upper portion of the mucocele prevents extension of secretions (or the mucocele) into the more proximal lacrimal apparatus.[212] The absence of a medial canthal mass therefore does not rule out obstruction of the NLDS or the diagnosis of a congenital NLDS cyst.

A variety of treatments have been described for congenital lacrimal system obstructions including massage (local), probing, irrigation, silicone intubation, and DCR. Although there is no consensus about the timing of or requirement for nasolacrimal probing, such probing is generally successful for treatment of nasolacrimal duct obstruction.[202, 214] However, the rate of failure of probing increases after the patient reaches 12 months of age. After 24 months of age, probing may fail in 67% of patients, and procedure-related complications increase significantly.[214, 215] Silicone intubation may be effective in those children in whom probing has failed; however, this technique also has associated complications such as laceration and erosion of the canaliculi, granuloma formation, corneal erosion, punctal injury, or premature intubation removal.[216] Formerly, DCR became the necessary procedure if silicone intubation failed. More recently, balloon dilation of the nasolacrimal system has been offered as a safe, effective alternative treatment for congenital nasolacrimal drainage obstruction, either as a primary procedure or after failure of probing or silicone intubation.[217, 218] Becker et al.[217] noted an overall postdilation patency rate of 95%, but the study had a limited follow-up period of 4 to 10 months.

Cho et al.[218] recently reported their hospital's treatment of 36 pediatric patients, older than 12 months of age, with congenital lacrimal system obstruction, 16 of whom had fluoroscopically guided balloon dilation (mean age, 33 months). Obstruction was most frequent at the valve of Hasner (15 eyes), with obstruction at the nasolacrimal duct in 2 eyes and at Krause's valve (junction of the lacrimal sac and duct) in 3 eyes; all but 2 eyes had complete obstruction. Seventy percent had had previous treatment with probing, irrigation, or silicone intubation (mean age, 34 months). The authors had a technical success rate (defined as free passage of contrast medium through the entire nasolacrimal system to the nasal cavity) in 95%, with clinical success (resolution of epiphora) in all patients in whom technical success was achieved (mean follow-up of 16 months). Becker et al. performed balloon dilation through the superior canaliculus in an antegrade method after puncturing the obstruction with a probe, while Cho et al. used a retrograde approach, to better avoid canalicular damage, after puncturing the obstruction with a relatively stiff ball-tip guidewire. For both groups of authors, the results of balloon dilation in congenital nasolacrimal system obstruction were far more successful than dilation in adult nasolacrimal obstruction.[219–221] This is probably explained by the differences in pathogenesis. The majority of congenital obstructions are related to developmental anomalies such as a thin, persistent layer of nasolacrimal and nasal epithelial cells at the valve of Hasner.[106, 202, 203, 218] Such anomalies respond well to balloon dilation, with a low incidence of reobstruction secondary to adhesions and fibrosis, in contrast to the epiphora in adults caused by acquired etiologies such as chronic infection and/or inflammation, chronic fibrosis, involutional stenosis, or constriction secondary to the aging process. The one technical failure in Cho et al.'s series was in a patient with obstruction proximal to the valve of Hasner and may have represented a more diffuse nasolacrimal duct stenosis. (See also the section on Dacryocystoplasty and Stent Placement.)

### Duplication

Canalicular duplication is usually asymptomatic. DCG will show the supernumerary duct as an opacified streak close to the superior or inferior canaliculus.[88]

## MAGNETIC RESONANCE DACRYOCYSTOGRAPHY

Routine MR imaging, with or without intravenous gadolinium, may show disease processes, whether inflammatory or neoplastic, invading the region of the nasolacrimal duct system (NLDS) and the medial canthus. MR imaging was not utilized to assess intrinsic abnormalities of the NLDS proper (canaliculi, lacrimal sac, or nasolacrimal duct), although it could detect significant dilatation of the lacrimal sac or nasolacrimal duct (Figs. 10-20, 10-26, and 10-30). Conventional NLDS contrast media for DCG, whether oil based or water soluble, tended to be viscous and were routinely introduced by cannulation. Although oil based contrast can be identified within the NLDS by its specific fat intensity signal on MR imaging, the inconvenience of cannulation, the increased viscosity and poor miscibility of such contrast agents with tear fluid, and the risks of granuloma formation if extravasation occurs limit the use of MR imaging for assessment of intrinsic nasolacrimal drainage pathology. MR imaging has maintained a complementary role to Digital Subtraction DCG (DS-DCG), with DS-DCG assessing the NLDS and MR/CT assessing the adjacent extraluminal soft tissues. The increased soft-tissue resolution of MR imaging and the anterior location of the NLDS allowing surface coil imaging favor the strengths of MR imaging. In 1993, Goldberg et al.[222] utilized gadolinium (gadopentetate dimeglumine [Magnevist]; Berlex Laboratories, Wayne, New Jersey) in a diluted state, either topically or by cannulation, to visualize directly the canaliculi, lacrimal sac, and nasolacrimal duct.

The gadolinium solution, initially diluted 10:1 in sterile saline, was further diluted 10:1 in a commercial liquid tear preparation such as methylcellulose. The prepared 1:100 solution represented a 0.5% concentration or 300 mOsm/L of gadolinium (from the initially commercial available 48.0% concentration). Used topically, the solution was introduced as an eyedrop into the conjunctival cul-de-sac, one drop per minute for 5 minutes immediately prior to scanning, with the patient in a supine position (Fig. 10-34). The authors recommended obtaining imaging within 5 to 10 minutes of introduction of the gadolinium solution. The contrast agent remains within the drainage system for approximately 20 minutes.

More recent studies[223] also suggest an interval of approximately 5 minutes between the final instillation of topical contrast into the conjunctival cul-de-sac and initial imaging to allow adequate passage of contrast through the NLDS (the time interval can be used for coil positioning, system tuning, localizer measurements, etc.). Blinking was encouraged between sequences since eyelid movements affect the lacrimal pump and tear transport.[141, 224] The required data acquisition of various sequences, including pre- and postintravenous contrast sequences, allows approximately 15 to 20 minutes for contrast medium distribution and visualization.

Rubin et al.[225] diluted gadolinium with sterile water to a 300 mOsm/L concentration for direct lacrimal sac infusion. Kirchhof et al.,[19] in an attempt to keep the viscosity of the eyedrops low, used saline instead of methylcellulose in the diluted gadolinium solution. They noted an accelerated passage of the eyedrops through the drainage system, making it difficult to trace the contrast agent in a patent nasolacrimal duct system.

Although topically applied gadolinium can assess functional outflow, canalicular injection of 1 ml of 0.5% gadolinium, using a lacrimal cannula, may be indicated in specific patients. The gadolinium solution in a 0.5% concentration is nonirritating to the ocular surface. MR-DCG has the potential to present information about the NLDS and the adjacent soft tissues, with superb soft-tissue resolution. DS-DCG, however, remains the gold standard for assessing the lacrimal drainage system. MR-DCG may be considered in patients with medial canthal masses or more complex tearing disorders, including congenital, postsurgical, or posttraumatic nasolacrimal obstruction or in those cases where a neoplastic process is suspected, either originating in the NLDS (lacrimal sac), adjacent paranasal sinuses, or orbit.[200, 222, 225] However, some suggest a role for MR-DCG in the assessment of the NLDS because DS-DCG fails to delineate the surrounding soft tissues and MR-DCG has increased sensitivity for detection of contrast more distally within the drainage system. MR-DCG does give detailed functional and morphologic information on the NLDS in a simple, noninvasive manner that does not use ionizing radiation. Newer MR-DCG techniques may be useful for depicting nasolacrimal obstruction, utilizing saline or water, without the use of chemical contrast media.[19, 199, 223, 226, 227]

In a study comparing DS-DCG and topical gadolinium-enhanced MR-DCG, Kirchhof et al.[19] found 100% sensitivity for demonstration of obstruction of the NLDS with either modality. The location of the obstruction was more precisely

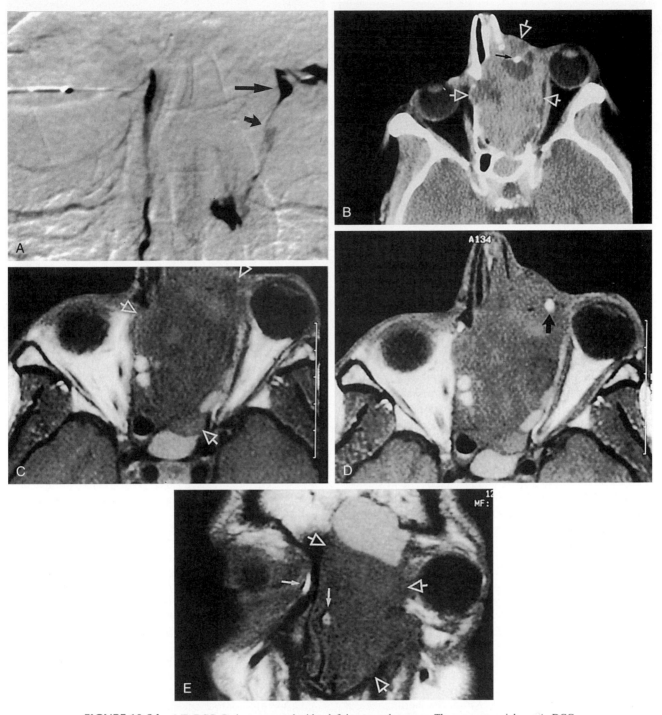

**FIGURE 10-34**   MR-DCG. Patient presented with a left inner canthus mass. There was no epiphora. **A,** DCG. Left lacrimal sac and canaliculi are displaced laterally (*large arrow*). Nasolacrimal duct courses inferomedially (*short arrow*) to drain into the nasal cavity. **B** to **E,** CT-DCG and MR-DCG performed to better show the relationship of the mass to the NLDS. **B,** Axial image of CT-DCG shows a large nasoethmoid mass (*open arrows*) invading the medial left orbit and inner canthus. NLDS with contrast medium (*thin arrow*) is seen coursing through the mass just anterior to the necrotic component of the mass. **C,** Axial T1-weighted pregadolinium image displays a large mass (*arrows*) within the nasal cavity and ethmoid sinuses, extending to the left inner canthus and displacing the left orbit contents laterally. **D,** Axial T1-weighted image with topical gadolinium (0.5% concentration) at the same level as **C** easily displays the left NLDS (*arrow*) surrounded by a mass. **E,** Coronal T1-weighted image shows a large left nasoethmoid mass (*open arrows*). Topical gadolinium is seen within the normal right lacrimal sac (*horizontal arrow*) and left nasal cavity (*vertical arrow*). Pathology: nasoethmoid squamous cell carcinoma.

*Illustration continued on following page*

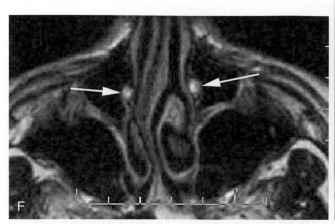

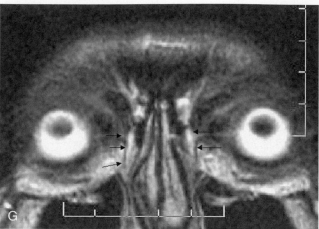

**FIGURE 10-34** *Continued.* **F** and **G,** Second patient. Topical saline used as contrast medium. One or 2 drops per minute instilled into the conjunctival sac for 4 to 5 minutes prior to scanning may better demonstrate the lumen of the NLDS (*arrows*) on axial (**F**) and coronal (**G**) T2-weighted sequences. The saline flows more quickly through the drainage system than topical gadolinium, especially if the gadolinium is partially diluted with artificial tear drops.

detected on MR-DCG, with the contrast material traced further distally with MR-DCG than with DS-DCG in 3 of the 11 patients. MR-DCG, however, like other imaging modalities, may also diagnose NLDS obstruction too proximal due to accumulation of thickened mucus within the duct system. This problem may be avoided by performing irrigation and careful expression of the lacrimal sac prior to any DCG-type, contrast-enhanced NLDS imaging study. In contrast to the increased signal of contrast medium, mucus was isointense with mucosa on T1-weighted images and slightly hypointense on T2-weighted images. A fluid-fluid level may be seen between the contrast agent and mucus on coronal T1-weighted images.[19] MR-DCG may better distinguish soft-tissue obstruction from bone obstruction, a factor in deciding whether dilatation of a stenosis (dacrycystoplasty) is feasible or whether a surgical procedure (DCR) will be needed.

MR-DCG may better assess the amount of lacrimal sac mucosa present and available for mucosal flap manipulation (lacrimal sac to nasal mucosa anastomoses needed for external DCR surgery), with normal sac mucosa well delineated on T2-weighted, fat-saturated sequences. Although both DS-DCG and MR-DCG displayed the obstruction of the lacrimal sac 1 year after DCR in one patient, only MR-DCG directly displayed the postoperative cicatricial scarring.[19] DS-DCG and MR-DCG were equivalent in assessing size and filling defects within the lacrimal sac, a factor of importance for endoscopic intranasal DCR considerations, since scarring and dacryolithiasis are significant prognostic factors and potential contraindications. DS-DCG was superior in only one patient in whom MR-DCG failed to delineate fistulas distal to the nasolacrimal sac.[19]

Fat-saturated MR imaging sequences were preferred, with T2-weighted images considered superior to T1-weighted and with the fat-saturated sequences allowing better visualization of the contrast agent. Coronal slices (obtained at 70° to the hard palate to be parallel to the course of the lacrimal sac–nasolacrimal duct) were considered more helpful. Axial images were complementary and were preferred for measurement of the lumen of the lacrimal sac or nasolacrimal duct.[19] Acknowledging the additional information about the surrounding soft tissues, Kirchof et al.[19] noted that both MR-DCG and DS-DCG reliably depicted obstructions of the NLDS, but because of the increased expense of MR-DCG and the limited experience in differentiating between obstruction and stenosis of the NLDS, DS-DCG should be the first imaging study. MR-DCG should function as a complementary study except in the pediatric age group. In epiphora patients under age 6, MR-DCG, noninvasive and free of radiation, can be performed with sedation only (in contrast to DS-DCG, which is performed under general anaesthesia) and should be the primary imaging modality for assessment.

In Caldemeyer et al.'s[199] study of CT-DCG and MR-DCG utilizing topical contrast material, CT-DCG, with iopamidol (Isovue 200; Squibb Diagnostics, Princeton, New Jersey) and MR-DCG with normal saline, respectively, placed into the conjunctival cul-de-sac of healthy normal volunteers, CT better displayed the finer drainage system components better than MR-DCG. CT also displayed the adjacent bone anatomy.

In a study comparing DS-DCG and MR-DCG, Yoshikawa et al.[226] concluded that topical contrast-enhanced MR-DCG by itself may not be sufficient when precise information, including the length of the stenosis and the degree of narrowing is necessary to plan for DCG or nasolacrimal stenting. MR-DCG findings were not compatible with DCG findings in half of the 14 patients. On initial phantom studies, all sequences could visualize ducts equal to or smaller than 0.7 mm in diameter filled with contrast material. The lower spatial resolution of MR-DCG (11 cm rounded receiving surface coil, body coil for transmission) compared to DS-DCG and the absence of pressure (topical application) may result in an overexpression of stenosis or in interpreting stenosis as an obstructive lesion.[226] Cannulation MR-DCG may help eliminate these limitations.

Hoffman et al.[223] noted difficulties in detecting contrast medium (diluted gadolinium topically placed) in the most distal part of the NLD in some patients with mild epiphora, yet there was filling of the lacrimal sac and proximal duct. They postulate a physiologic obstruction at the distal end of the nasolacrimal due to resistance of the valve of Hasner. Similar findings have been previously noted in DSG,[144] with long transport delays (30 minutes or longer) even in asymptomatic eyes. Circumstances causing increased production of tears or minimal narrowing of the nasolacrimal duct may contribute to epiphora. The marked variation in tear transport times limits the assessment of the functional MR-DCG exam and must be interpreted with clinical and other imaging findings. For these reasons, DCG remains the standard exam for assessing obstructions of the NLDS.[223]

Recent MR-DCG studies have assessed other solutions (with associated MR technique alterations) to augment or possibly replace gadolinium as a contrast agent.[199, 226, 227] Yoshikawa et al.[226] combined T1-weighted (transverse thin slice) spin-echo and 3D-T1 fast field echo (FFE) sequences utilizing a topical diluted gadolinium solution, (with reconstructed Maximum Intensity Projection (MIP) images projected in the anteroposterior direction for the 3D-FFE sequence) as well as two T2-weighted sequences. The T2-weighted sequences included a transverse thin-slice fast spin echo (FSE) sequence and a coronal thick-slice section T2-weighted projected image, with the coronal sequences utilizing a topical saline solution rather than the diluted gadolinium solution. MR-DCG diagnoses were made by combining the findings on the saline-enhanced T2-weighted and gadolinium solution-enhanced T1-weighted images. The transverse images confirmed the diagnosis from the projected images. If discrepancies were noted between the T2-weighted projected images on the FFE-MIP images, the narrowed site was determined by the gadolinium-enhanced FFE-MIP images. In a preliminary study of 10 normal volunteers, the lacrimal sacs and proximal portion of the nasolacrimal ducts were seen in all patients; however, the caudal aspects of the nasolacrimal ducts and the canaliculi were not visualized on most sequences in approximately half of the cases. The inability to visualize the caudal portions of nasolacrimal ducts in normal volunteers may be due to the relatively fast flow in the narrowing lumen of the caudal duct or to an increase in the viscosity of the intraluminal fluid. The long echo time of the T2-weighted projected images may need to be adjusted to each patient's circumstance and may limit the discrepancies seen between the T2-weighted projected images and the FFE-MIP images. In the clinical study, inconsistent findings were also noted between the T2-weighted projected images and the FFE-MIP images or with the DS-DCG findings.[226]

The lacrimal sac residual lumen volume and the condition of the mucosa were better seen on the T2-weighted sequences. Mucosal thickening, including low signal intensity mucosal fibrous thickening, was noted on T2-weighted sequences, with intravenous gadolinium-enhanced images offering further information if required. The T2-weighted sequences also displayed the residual caudal lumen of an obstructed or narrowed site, which may help predict the effectiveness of conservative treatments (e.g., irrigation therapy). Despite limitations, combined complementary T1- and T2-weighted sequences, with

respective diluted gadolinium or normal saline solutions as a less invasive study, may offer enough morphologic and functional information in the NLDS to have a screening role or potential to be the imaging examination of first choice for patients with lacrimal outflow disorders.[226]

Takehara et al.[227] have implemented MR-DCG techniques utilizing a less viscous combined normal saline–lidocaine hydrochloride solution as a contrast medium to emphasize the dynamic behavior of the fluid within the lacrimal pathway. The authors performed all studies via thin plastic lacrimal cannulas placed into the inferior lacrimal canaliculi bilaterally, with a Y-connector allowing bilateral simultaneous injection. Axial and coronal T2-weighted images were obtained using FSE or half Fourier single-shot FSE sequences without fat saturation. With the patient already in place within the gantry, the dynamic MR-DCG was performed while the patient injected the previously prepared combined saline-lidocaine solution by manual compression of the barrel of a single syringe. Thick-slice (20 to 30 mm), heavily T2-weighted images were repeatedly obtained during the injection. The section of study included the canaliculi, lacrimal sac, and nasolacrimal duct. Acquisition time for each image was less than 2 seconds. During the injection, imaging was repeated for 3 minutes with intervals of 4 to 5 seconds. Overall MR imaging time, including that for preliminary conventional T1- and T2-weighted sequences, was less than 20 minutes.

The solution's lower viscosity better filled the narrowed lumen of the NLDS. MR-DCG can be monitored and viewed during the course of the injection, so the patient can be directed to increase the injection rate if filling is incomplete or delayed. MR-DCG offers high temporal resolution, allows dynamic evaluation of fluid flow in the NLDS, and will not potentially miss the image that best demonstrates the obstructive segment. This concept parallels the advantages of DS-DCG compared to radiographic distention DCG and offers a dynamic capability superior to that of CT, without the radiation exposure. Such dynamic assessment, however, requires the facilitating solution to be introduced through lacrimal cannulas. Because of the decreased viscosity of the solution utilized, such cannulas, however, may be thinner and softer, allowing more comfortable, safer cannulation of the canaliculi.

In contrast to other MR-DCG techniques that are stationary or slow-flowing, this MR-DCG uses water injected into the lacrimal draining system as a substitute for other contrast media. The imaging strategy involves the acquisition of a series of heavily T2-weighted images since fluid-filled nasolacrimal ducts have long longitudinal and transverse relaxation times and will display high signal intensity on T2-weighted images. However, on these hydrographic images, everything looks black or white. The nasolacrimal abnormalities are evaluated indirectly using "all-or-nothing" images. The FSE sequence used was relatively immune to local magnetic field inhomogeneity (air in the maxillary sinus, dental prosthesis).[227] Dynamic MR-DCG, as a form of hydrographic imaging, does not reflect any soft-tissue contrast. Additional T1- and T2-weighted sequences are required for delineation of soft tissue (e.g., the presence of mucosal thickening or neoplasm). Half Fourier SS-FSE or FSE imaging using multiple thin slices provides static but detailed information. As also noted in more static MR-DCG studies with saline placed topically into the conjunctival cul-de-sac and imaged with heavily T2-weighted sequences, mucosal disease of the NLDS or adjacent paranasal sinuses can make visualization of the NLDS more difficult.[199] Comparison of images before and after contrast administration is important to distinguish mucosal thickening from normal flow of saline. Image subtraction may be feasible. This technique is probably limited in detecting dacryolithiasis. Further investigations are necessary to assess the true potential and capabilities of dynamic MR-DCG.

## DACRYOCYSTOPLASTY AND STENT PLACEMENT

### Balloon Dacryocystoplasty

See the previous section on Congenital Atresia for further comments on dacryocystoplasty and stents. A small-bore soft[228] or ball-tip[229] guidewire (0.018 inch diameter) is introduced into the superior punctum and guided under fluoroscopic control through the NLDS into the inferior meatus. With nasal endoscopic assistance or lacrimal instruments and lateral fluoroscopy, the guidewire, which prefers to pass toward the nasopharynx, is directed through the nares. A hook was devised to grasp the guidewire under fluoroscopic control, shortening the procedure time and eliminating the need for nasal endoscopy.[230] A deflated angioplasty balloon catheter is introduced in a retrograde direction over the guidewire (in contrast to Becker and Berry's[231] initial report of antegrade balloon dilation of the nasolacrimal duct's nasal ostium). Proper positioning and dilation are controlled by fluoroscopic guidance, with injection of radiographic contrast media to inflate the balloon catheter (Figs. 10-35 and 10-36). The tibial arterial balloon angioplasty catheter (Cook Inc., Bloomington, Indiana), which dilates to 3 to 4 mm in diameter, is useful for Dacryocytoplasty (DCP). Different methods of dilation have been described, with Munk et al.[228] and Janssen et al.[219] recommending two or three dilations of 20 to 30 seconds each, while Song et al.[220] recommended that each dilation last for 5 minutes. Lee et al.[229] found that the soft tip and lack of tapering of the Balt balloon (Montmorency, France) made it preferable for dilations. After the final dilation, the balloon is withdrawn inferiorly and the guidewire superiorly (to avoid having the stiff segment of the guidewire pass through the area of recent dilation). Song et al.[220] leave the guidewire in place and perform DCG via the inferior punctum to verify passage of contrast medium. Balloon catheters with gradually increasing calibers ranging from 3 to 5 mm may be used. An irrigation of the NLDS with sterile saline, with or without dexamethasone, through the dilation catheter and/or flushing through the superior canaliculus is performed at the end of the procedure. Dexamethasone and antibiotic (gentamycin) eyedrops may be prescribed for 1 week postdilation, as well as acetylcysteine eyedrops if abundant mucus was present in the NLDS.[219] Blood clot formation in the NLDS, especially the dilated lacrimal sac, during or after balloon dilation may be a cause of treatment failure. Song et al.[220] noted such filling defects in 3 of 36 eyes in

which DCG was performed immediately following dacryocystoplasty (DCP).

Janssen et al.[219] modified the Munk et al.[228] technique. In cases of complete obstruction in which reflux of contrast medium occurred through the opposite canaliculus, they recommend that DCG be repeated after occluding the noncannulated canaliculus by wedging within it a nonconducting lacrimal catheter. This may allow a small amount of contrast medium to outline an area of stenosis. For the DCP procedures, they favor a nontraumatizing 0.025 inch guidewire with a flexible curved tip (Terumo; Tokyo, Japan) to more easily negotiate the sharp curve between the common canaliculus and the lacrimal sac. Balloon catheter placement is restricted to the lacrimal sac or more caudally to prevent damage to the canaliculi. A balloon catheter with the balloon placed at the catheter tip allows dilation of stenoses high in the lacrimal sac and does not require the catheter tip to be passed into the common canaliculus.[221]

The study is performed under local anesthesia. Patients may experience some mild discomfort in the region of the medial canthus for 1 to 2 days after the procedure and a slightly blood-stained nasal discharge for 1 to 3 days. Evaluation of epiphora may be graded according to a subjective scale, as suggested by Munk et al.[228] This scale has proven useful in allowing comparisons in the epiphora patient population over time, as well as in comparing various patient groups and assessing degrees of success or benefits of treatment. In the system, Grade 0 is no epiphora; Grade 1 is occasional epiphora that requires drying or dabbing less than twice a day; Grade 2 is epiphora that requires drying 2 to 4 times a day; Grade 3 is epiphora that requires drying 5 to 10 times a day; Grade 4 is epiphora that requires drying more than 10 times a day; and Grade 5 is constant tear overflow. There is no standardized definition of success, with some results referring to Grade 0 or Grade 1 as a successful outcome posttreatment, while others may define an improvement of two or more grades as success. Still others may define Grade 2 to Grade 5 as poor outcomes despite improvement in the pretreatment status.

DCP may have a role in a defined patient population. Probing alone is frequently unsuccessful and has a greater risk of creating a false passage. In contrast to dilating probes, the use of balloon dilation offers radially directed dilating forces that are less likely to create severe tears. Fine guidewires of approximately one half the caliber of probes, with soft tips, especially when placed into a strictured or occluded NLDS, offer less risk of complication. Longitudinal shear forces by the larger catheters are reduced by the presence of a guidewire.

DCP is easily performed as an outpatient procedure, obviating the need for general anesthetic or controlled hypotension (used to control hemorrhage) and the relative invasiveness of DCR. More recent performance of DCR surgeries with local assisted anaesthesia and monitored sedation has improved operative field visibility and minimized blood loss while avoiding the hazards of general anaesthesia.[232] Still, the advantages of DCP, with diminished morbidity, cost, and operating room time, are obvious. No facial scarring or disfigurement occurs with DCP, and the procedure, if unsuccessful, does not preclude future DCR.

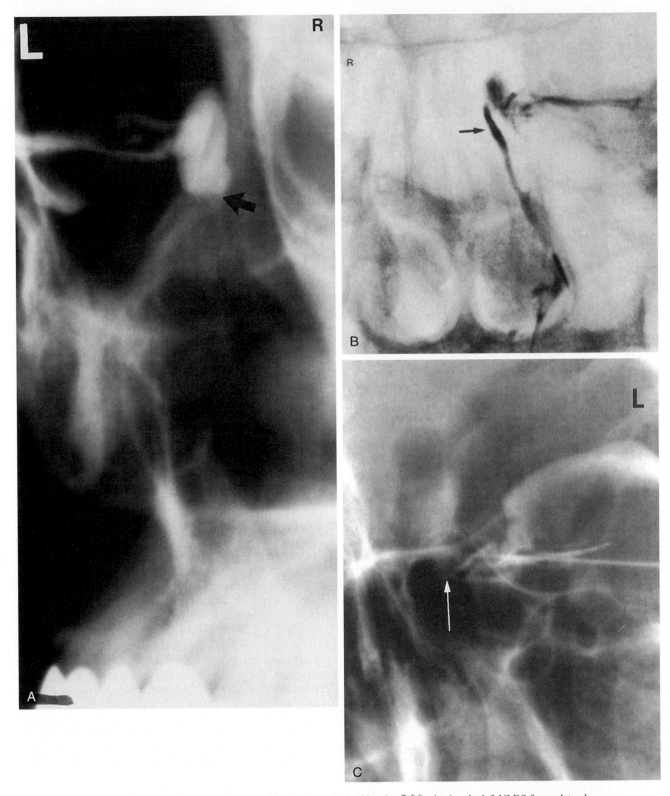

**FIGURE 10-35**   Balloon DCP. **A** and **B**, Case one. **A**, Predilatation DCG, viewing the left NLDS from a lateral oblique projection, shows a dilated lacrimal sac with complete obstruction (*arrow*) at the junction with nasolacrimal duct. **B**, Postdilatation DCG viewed anteriorly shows a normal-sized lacrimal sac (*arrow*) with spontaneous drainage through the nasolacrimal duct into the nasal cavity. **C** and **D**, Case two. **C**, Predilatation DCG (superior canaliculus injection) shows complete obstruction of the common canaliculus (*arrow*) with reflux into the inferior canaliculus and conjunctival sac.

*Illustration continued on following page*

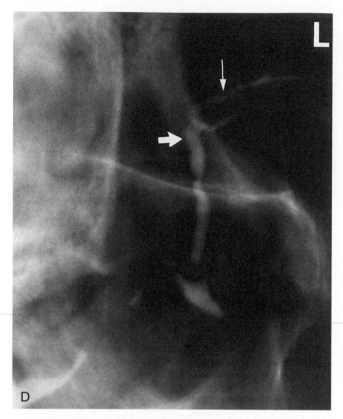

**FIGURE 10-35** *Continued.* **D,** Postdilatation film (superior canalicular injection) (*vertical arrow*) shows contrast material draining through the lacrimal sac (*horizontal arrow*) and nasolacrimal duct into the nasal cavity. (Courtesy of Dr. Peter Munk, Vancouver, Canada.)

The use of ionizing radiation for balloon DCP (versus surgical treatment of epiphora) is a disadvantage to be addressed and controlled, to offer minimal radiation exposure since the eye, including the radiosensitive lens, remains in the field of the primary x-ray beam. Mean radiation doses to the lens of the treated eye varied from 1.37 mGy[233, 234] to 4.6 mGy[235, 236] and from 5.43 mGy[233, 234] to 38.5 mGy[235, 236] for the contralateral eye. In both series, the treated eye was always closer to the image intensifier, with the higher mean radiation dose values to the contralateral lens, closer to the x-ray tube. The measured dose to the treated eye may be reduced by limiting the number of digital images obtained. The dose to both eyes, especially to the untreated eye, can be limited by tight collimation, restricted to the treated eye, especially in the posteroanterior images. Phantom studies measured the dose to the untreated lens as only 25% of that to the treated eye (lens) on such collimated posteroanterior images.[233, 234] Much of the DCP procedure is performed using lateral fluoroscopy and digital image acquisition, such that radiation to the contralateral lens cannot be avoided. Approximately 90% of the overall radiation dose to the lens of the untreated eye, closer to the x-ray tube, results from lateral projection versus 65% for the lens of the treated eye.[236] Restricting lateral imaging to fluoroscopy and abandoning such digital image acquisition, the major source of the higher lens dose, will further reduce the lens dose.[236] DCG performed before and after DCP, with the exception of complex cases, should similarly be restricted to posteroanterior projection images.

Although preliminary, Munk et al.[228] experienced very favorable DCP results, with DCPs being technically successful in 16 of 18 cases, with improved epiphora in 13 (complete resolution in 11) patients and no change in 3 patients. Follow-up, however, was limited to 6 months maximum post-DCP, and only four patients had follow-up DCG, all within 3 weeks of the initial procedure. No correlation between degree of epiphora and severity of stenosis on the preprocedure DCG was noted. In the cases of partial stenosis, no change was noted in the appearance of the postdilation DCG, and Munk et al. anticipated that reproducibility of the DCG would be difficult since the nasolacrimal duct, when patent, is an open system, decompressed from below. Munk et al. did not have trouble passing the guidewire in the two cases of complete obstruction. They felt, however, that tight stenosis of the common canaliculus may represent an absolute or relative contraindication to DCP.

Song et al.[220] also noted difficulty defining success (or failure) in interpreting the results. Full dilation of obstructed areas may be noted technically, with the epiphora not resolving. They postulate that placement of stents may be useful in such patients. Song et al.[220, 237, 238] and Lee et al.[229] have followed patients for a more extended period. In further follow-up of those initial successes (in 56% of dilations) assessed at 7 days, 45% showed recurrence of symptoms at 2 months.[220] Although Lee et al. achieved 71% and 51% initial technical and clinical success rates for partial and complete obstruction, respectively, the 2-year clinical patency rates fell to 20% and 25%, respectively. The grade of stenosis did not influence the duration of patency. In assessing their initial results, technical success but clinical failure was noted in 29% and 44% of patients with partial and complete obstruction, respectively, for a 40% overall clinical failure. These patients tended to have clinical improvement of epiphora for 2 to 3 days only. No technical failures were noted in the partial occlusion subgroup, while 5% of those with complete obstruction were technical failures. Dilations of common canaliculus obstructions were more technically difficult. The authors avoided dilation of the superior and inferior canaliculi lateral to the common canaliculus to avoid damage to the canaliculi. Patency rates for complete obstructions remained the same from 6 months to 2 years post-DCP follow-up, while those for partial occlusion decreased such that there was no significant difference between the long-term patency rates of occlusions and stenosis.[229]

Janssen et al.[219] reported 90% substantial success in DCP treatment of 21 nasolacrimal duct system (NLDS) with severe epiphora followed for 14 to 70 weeks. These authors speculate that the finer atraumatic, nonmetallic guidewire (Terumo) and a dilated balloon diameter not exceeding 3 mm (vs. 3 to 4 mm for Munk et al.[228]) and 4 to 5 mm for Song et al.[220] may explain the difference in results. In normal adults, the diameter of the membranous nasolacrimal duct is 4 to 6 mm. Therefore, a larger catheter whose caliber is greater than 3 mm may traumatize the nasolacrimal duct or the rich venous plexus between the membranous portion of the duct and the bony canal.[219]

Continued follow-up of fluoroscopically guided balloon

DCP for recanalization of obstructed NLDS, as a viable alternative to operative treatments, has led to further scrutiny of such procedures due to some disappointing longer-term results, despite its initial technical successes.[219, 220, 228, 229, 239–241]

Various hypotheses have been put forward to improve results. Primary placement of stents, initially in conjunction with balloon DCP[237, 238, 242] and subsequently obviating balloon DCP,[230] were suggested. Others have suggested technique alterations to navigate the difficulties presented by canalicular or upper lacrimal sac strictures. Suggestions have been made to address the challenges of recanalizing the

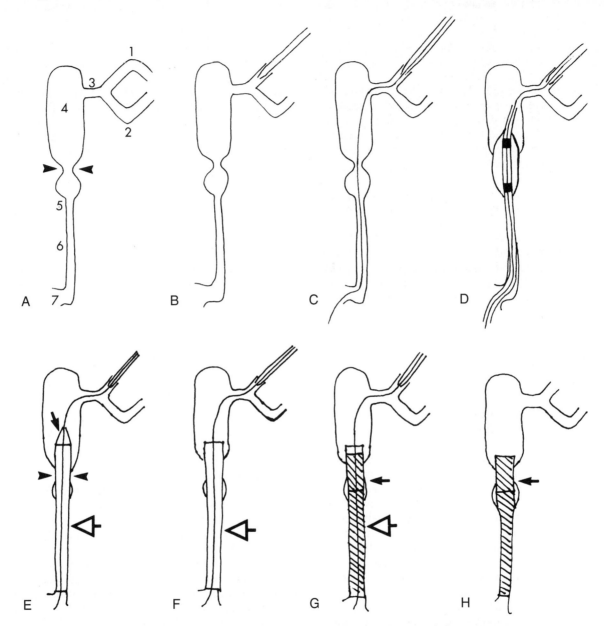

**FIGURE 10-36**  DCP technique. **A**, Normal NLDS. *1*, Superior canaliculus; *2*, inferior canaliculus; *3*, common canaliculus; *4*, lacrimal sac; *5*, junction of the lacrimal sac and nasolacrimal duct; *6*, nasolacrimal duct; *7*, valve of Hasner; *arrowheads*, stenosis in the lacrimal sac. **B** to **D**, Balloon DCP technique. **B**, Lacrimal catheter inserted into the superior canaliculus. **C**, Guidewire inserted through a lacrimal catheter in an antegrade manner and seen exiting through the valve of Hasner and manipulated through the nares. **D**, Balloon catheter inserted in a retrograde manner over a guidewire to an appropriate point to dilate the stenosis. (Modified from Janssen AG et al. Dacryocystoplasty: treatment of epiphora by means of balloon dilation of the obstructed nasolacrimal duct system. Radiology 1994;193:453–456.) **E** to **H**, Polyurethane stent technique. **E**, Steps **B** and **C** as above. No. 6 French sheath (*open arrow*) with dilator (*oblique arrow*) is passed retrograde over a guidewire through the lacrimal sac stenosis (*arrowheads*). **F**, Dilator removed from the sheath, which remains in place. **G**, Stent (*diagonal lines and horizontal arrow*) introduced retrograde over the guidewire into the sheath beyond the stenosis using a stent loader and pusher catheter (not shown). **H**, Sheath withdrawn while the stent is held in place by the pusher catheter. Once the stent is freed from the sheath, the pusher catheter is also withdrawn through the inferior nares, and the guidewire is withdrawn through the superior canaliculus. Stent extends inferiorly into the inferior meatus to ease retrieval if desired. (Modified from Song HY et al. Nonsurgical placement of a nasolacrimal polyurethane stent. Radiology 1995;194:233–237.)

more resistant occlusions extending the length of nasolacrimal duct. Such technical factors include flexible, steerable guidewires,[219, 221, 240, 243] hydrophilic-coated wires,[219, 221] nonmetal guidewires,[221] small-caliber catheters 2 to 3 mm in diameter,[221, 243] versus 3 to 4 mm catheters[228] or 4 to 5 mm catheters,[229, 240] decrease or absence of a catheter tip beyond the balloon,[221] shorter inflation period of 20 to 30 seconds,[228] 30 seconds,[221] 1 to 2 minutes,[243] versus 5 minutes,[229, 240] guiding cannulas,[221, 243] a Ritleng probe (through which guidewires may be passed),[224] and canalicular irrigation for flushing out or dislodging possible clots.[220, 221, 240, 245] The reason for consideration of the above factors is the desire to minimize ductal trauma as a factor in recurrence of epiphora, stenosis, or obstruction. Selection of the balloon catheter diameter and timing of inflation should be enough to tear the fibrotic component of the obstruction or stenosis, yet the catheter should be small enough in caliber or the duration of inflation should be short enough to prevent damage to the NLDS. The variety of options suggests that there is no universal solution. Personal preferences and individual choices are noted in the literature.

Strictures of the canaliculi and upper lacrimal sac can restrict the passage of steerable guidewires.[243] The floppy tip of the wire (of flexible systems) may become stuck or may coil in the small lumen of the lacrimal sac and not advance into the nasolacrimal duct. The relatively stiff ball-tip wire,[220] by elevating its handle superiorly, allows ease of manipulation of its tip into the lacrimal sac and the junction with the nasolacrimal duct but is more difficult to pass through stenotic lesions, increasing the risk of ductal wall damage or false passages.[243] Yet such stiff wires may be necessary to advance through the rigidity of complete obstructions of the nasolacrimal duct, where forceful advancement may be required.

Berkefeld et al.,[243] exploring beyond the technical issues in assessing their results in 85 patients treated with balloon DCP, looked at associated clinical factors that may predict reobstruction. They found recurrent episodes of active dacryocystitis; dacryolithiasis filling defects on initial DCG; posttraumatic strictures with bone canal narrowing; or long-segment rigid occlusions of the nasolacrimal duct, all factors in reobstruction, with 89% and 94% 12-month patency rates for focal stenoses or occlusions, respectively, if the above factors were not present. Otherwise, the reobstruction rate was 46% in patients with one of the above factors present.

In patients with active inflammatory changes, the potential benefit from removal of tight stenoses is limited to the short term, with active dacryocystitis involved with restenosis. Similarly, dacryolithiasis was seen to be a common cause of reobstruction after DCP, with filling defects seen on the preliminary DCG felt to be a contraindication to DCP. Posttraumatic stenoses frequently have bony narrowings that are too rigid for balloon dilation, with poor long-term outcomes and secondary inflammatory changes. Patients with multiple or diffuse stenoses or chronic (rigid) occlusions of the entire length of the nasolacrimal duct tend to have early reobstruction, probably secondary to the unavoidable trauma to the ductal wall and reactive mucosal overgrowth.[243] The high recurrence rates, between 45% and 80% in various series,[220, 229, 243] suggest a

limited value for balloon DCP. While stent placement may improve technical success rates and midterm patency rates, the long-term implantation of such stents has been associated with recurrence rates as high as 64%, depending on the location of the obstruction.[246] The operative treatment of postsaccal stenosis has consistently shown long-term success rates of 85% to 90%[30, 107–110] for external DCR and at least 75% for endonasal endoscopic DCR.[109] Results are independent of the cause or length of the stenotic lesion, suggesting that DCR, either external or endoscopic in approach, is the preferred approach to these patients with factors suggesting a high rate of reobstruction. For those patients with focal partial obstructions, either junctional (lacrimal sac–nasolacrimal duct) or within the nasolacrimal duct, or with short-distance occlusions of the distal nasolacrimal duct, clinical long-term success with balloon DCP may be realized (80% or more) as a treatment preferable to surgery or stent placement.[243]

Janssen et al.,[221] in noting the varying results of DCP obtained by different authors, felt that the differences may be due to different DCP techniques, as well as patient selection.[239] Lee et al.'s[229] results may have been negatively affected by the inclusion of posttrauma obstruction and possible deformations of the bony lacrimal canal, as well as the inclusion of patients with stenosis of the common canaliculus. Similarly, Ilgit et al.[240] included stenotic common canaliculi in their series. Janssen et al.[221] excluded patients with canalicular stenoses from their series and included patients with posttraumatic obstruction, but only after CT was utilized to evaluate the bony lacrimal canal. Other exclusion criteria included acute dacryocystitis, tumors, sarcoidosis, and Wegener's granulomatosis. No relationship was noted between the duration of epiphora (more or less than 1 year) and initial or long-term success.[221] More interestingly, and in contrast to the findings by Berkefeld et al.,[243] the length of obstruction (short obstruction limited to one level versus obstructions extending to two, three, or four levels) also showed no relationship to initial or long-term success.[221] However, patients with partial obstruction had greater initial and long-term success than patients with complete obstruction.[221] Others also noted these findings.[229, 240, 245]

The mechanism of DCP in the treatment of epiphora due to lacrimal obstruction is relatively unknown. The majority of treated patients have PANDO. As outlined by Linberg and McCormick,[161] the membranous nasolacrimal duct has a loose structure of connective tissue around the stratified columnar epithelium of the lacrimal duct. Within this loose tissue, a venous plexus, lymphocytes, and some fibrous tissue were found. In patients with acquired obstruction, they noted vascular congestion, lymphocytic infiltration, and edema causing compression of the duct, in its earlier phase by active chronic inflammation along the entire length of the narrowed nasolacrimal duct. Such stenosis leads to pooling of tears and infection, which, in turn, increases inflammatory edema and eventually gives rise to fibrosis. At the same time, infection may cause reflex hypersecretion of tears. Janssen et al.[221] postulate that the success of DCP (or DCR) does not necessarily mean long-term patency of the nasolacrimal duct, but rather the breaking of this cycle of obstruction and infection. Balloon dilation may resolve the obstruction but does not remedy the primary inflammatory process, which is likely to affect the recurrence of obstruction, with the dilatation crushing the mucosa of the duct at its stenotic segment, causing the development of a further inflammatory reaction and hemorrhage. Use of topical or systemic anti-inflammatory agents to reduce the early inflammatory reaction, flushing saline with or without antibiotics to dislodge clots, and intubation (or stents) to limit fibrosis and ensure patency have been attempted.

More recently, Kuchar and Steinkogler[247] have performed antegrade dilation of complete postsaccal stenosis patients, assessed by canalicular irrigation and transcanalicular endoscopy, using a Lacricath balloon catheter. Immediate postdilatation irrigation and endoscopy provided evidence of the reopened passage. Silicone intubation, for splinting the reopened stenoses, felt to be important for permanent patency during the initial scarring process, was performed immediately after the dilatation, with the tubes kept in place for 3 to 6 months. Such complementary postdilation silicone intubation, if consistently able to improve long-term patency rates, may offer an alternative to patients currently undergoing stenting. A 1 year patency rate of 73.3% was observed. Antegrade balloon dilatation, in conjunction with transcanalicular endoscopy, was felt to be easy and less expensive, without the need for more expensive imaging equipment the risks of radiation exposure.

The common canaliculus is second only to the lacrimal sac–nasolacrimal junction as the most common site for lacrimal drainage system obstruction.[47] In some patients, for canaliculodacryocystorhinostomy (with partial resection of the canalicular segment), silastic or rubber tubes are surgically placed for several months.[31] The standard surgical treatment of epiphora due to canalicular obstruction is conjunctival DCR, with a permanent bypass tube.[32, 248] Conjunctival DCR, indicated for obstructions at the canalicular level, forms a surgical tract between the conjunctiva and the internal anastomosis of the DCR. Glass (Pyrex) tubes are placed into the conjunctival tract as a permanent prosthesis, bypassing the canalicular obstruction. They require frequent, careful maintenance; may become dislodged or cause mild facial disfigurement; and require frequent cleaning and considerable patient commitment. Recurrent dacryocystitis, granuloma formation, eroded canaliculi, or, rarely, corneal irritation may result from the prolonged placement of such tubes. This surgery, in contrast to the standard DCR involving lacrimal sac or more distal obstructions, is more invasive and leads to a higher rate of recurrence at long-term follow-up. While these oculoplastic procedures have some patient compliance problems, which may suggest DCP as an alternative treatment, experience with DCP[220, 221, 228] suggests that such dilations of the NLDS should be limited to stenosis/obstructions of the distal lacrimal sac and nasolacrimal duct (i.e., the same patients for whom routine DCR is indicated).

Balloon catheter dilation of the canaliculi has been discouraged or considered contraindicated because of possible damage to the canaliculus or punctum.[51, 219, 221, 243] Recurrence rates of up to 60% to 70% were noted.[249] Stenosis in the canaliculi was not considered suitable for balloon dilation, and such dilation was limited to the diameter of the guidewire or lacrimal catheter. The risks of canalicular occlusion caused by laceration or recurrent

stenosis seemed high, and operative reconstruction may be difficult in such cases. Those performing DCP must avoid damaging the canaliculi, thereby creating the need for conjunctival DCR and a permanent glass prosthesis that otherwise may not have been necessary.[51]

Other investigators, in small series, reported balloon catheter dilation of the common canaliculus to be safe and effective.[220, 229, 240, 250] These initial series, as well as the surgical limitations of canalicular DCR, have encouraged Ko et al.[251] to develop further their techniques for evaluation of the safety and long-term effectiveness of balloon DCP in the treatment of common canalicular obstruction. In a study of 195 eyes with common canalicular obstruction (84 complete and 111 partial), the authors achieved initial technical success in 90% and 94%, respectively, of these patients. Patency rates were 51% at 6 months, 43% at 1 year, and 40% at 2 years, sparing this group of patients from an operative procedure. Their improved results may be related to the use of a slightly larger 3 mm balloon and better stabilization of the balloon catheter during inflation by passing it further retrograde along the guidewire such that the distal radiopaque marker, instead of the catheter tip, is advanced beyond the punctum, for a more efficient ballooning effect. Technical failures included seven patients with false passages and four patients in whom the obstructed canaliculus could not be negotiated with a guidewire. The recurrence of obstruction seemed related to ductal wall damage from guidewire or balloon catheter manipulation and resultant mucosal overgrowth, fibrosis, and recurrent episodes of active dacryocystitis.[243]

A previously designed polyurethane stent and a technique for lacrimal canalicular obstruction have had only limited experience.[252] The flexibility of the stent led to difficulty in advancing the tapered portion of the stent retrograde through the obstruction from the lacrimal sac. A high rate of stent occlusion occurred secondary to granulation tissue growth into the ballooned-out portion.[252] A more suitable introducer system, as well as a stent with no interstices at the ballooned-out portion, may offer greater success in the nonsurgical treatment of canalicular obstruction.[252]

## Stents

The tendency for obstructions to recur after dacryocystoplasty (DCP) may be due to the fibrotic nature of the stenosis/occlusion. Song et al.[238] addressed this problem in patients with obstruction of the nasolacrimal sac or duct with the placement of plastic stents immediately following balloon dilation. The plastic stent, with its distal tip left slightly protruding into the inferior meatus, may be easy to remove. This technique will not interfere with subsequent DCR. The firmness of these stents, however, led to patient discomfort and the need for a softer stent. Metallic stents, initially proposed for the creation of a larger, stable lumen, if blocked after placement, can only be removed surgically and may compromise subsequent DCR.[237, 238] Such metallic stents are also limited by a lack of longitudinal flexibility. Medium-type Palmaz balloon-expandable metallic stents offer greater longitudinal flexibility, with an articulated design for longer stenotic/occluded segments as well as a nonarticulated stent for more focal lesions. Although the balloon and stent could be dilated to 4 mm, stenosis of the stented lumen was noted on follow-up studies.[242] Mucosal-lined tracts do not tolerate metal well.[253, 254] Mucosal hyperplasia and a local inflammatory foreign tissue reaction to the metallic stent by the ductal wall, with tissue ingrowth through the metallic struts, are probable causes of stent stenosis and obstruction. Although tissue ingrowth may stabilize with time, the limited caliber of the NLDS lacks any reserve capacity to tolerate this initial tissue response. Metallic stents in the NLDS have been replaced by softer nonmetallic stents and are no longer used.

Song et al.[230] introduced a soft polyurethane stent that could be positioned with an introducer set (a stent loader, a No. 6 French sheath, a dilator, and a pusher catheter), obviating the need for balloon dilation of a stenotic or occluding segment. This method of DCP has the guidewire placed in an antegrade manner, with the dilator, sheath, and stent positioned in a retrograde fashion (Fig. 10-36,E-H). Fluoroscopic placement of the stent was technically successful in 50 of 51 attempts. Complete resolution of severe epiphora was noted in 47 and partial resolution in 3 of the 50 nasolacrimal systems treated. Treated stenoses were limited to the lacrimal sac, junction, and nasolacrimal duct. During limited follow-up of these patients, no stents migrated. Obstruction of one stent (probably caused by a blood clot) required lacrimal irrigation. It was hoped that this technique, as well as reducing costs, shortening procedure time, and improving patient tolerance, might offer better long-term results.

Song et al.[246] reviewed their long-term patency rate of polyurethane stent placement for the treatment of epiphora in 236 patients (283 obstructed lacrimal systems) with a follow-up period greater than 1 year. Stent placement was technically successful in 270 systems (95%). Assessment of these 270 systems 7 days after stent placement showed 87% with complete resolution of epiphora, 10% with partial resolution, and 3% with no resolution. In 77 patients (29.5%) with initial improvement, recurrence of epiphora occurred at a mean duration of 16 weeks poststenting due to obstruction of the stent. Recurrence rates of stent obstruction were correlated with levels of initial obstruction, with the highest recurrence rates (64%) for obstruction of the lacrimal sac, compared to only 26% for obstruction at the junction of the lacrimal sac–nasolacrimal duct and 15% at the nasolacrimal duct.

The causes of partial resolution of epiphora at 7 days were inadequate placement of the stent or partial obstruction of the stent by blood clot (excluding those patients who also had coexistent common canalicular obstruction). Stent placement was deemed inadequate when its mushroom tip was not placed in the dilated area. In the 3% of patients with no resolution, DCG at 7 days showed patency, and the cause of lack of improvement was not identified. Stent migration was noted in two patients in whom markedly dilated lacrimal systems were noted proximal to the obstruction. The stents were replaced with second stents with wider muchroom tips. Approximately one third of the obstructed stents were able to be recanalized by forceful irrigation with saline through the superior punctum, suggesting that the stents may have been impacted by mucus. Of the 56 obstructed stents removed, mucoid material was found in 26 and granulation tissue in 30. The incidence of mucus

plugging within the stent may be managed with acetylcys-teine eyedrops[219] or by reinterventions to maintain pa-tency.[246] The growth of granulation tissue into the stents may represent a foreign body reaction[255] and may be overcome by the use of stents without interstices in the ballooned-out portion or a coated drug-releasing stent.[246] Overgrowth of the proximal end of the stent by granulation tissue is a more serious complication.[246] Primary and secondary patency rates after DCP (with balloon dilatation) without stent placement have been higher than those for primary stent placement. In addition to obstruction of the stent, subclinical chronic infection from bacterial over-growth contributing to a cycle of infection, mucosal swelling, increased obstruction and stasis may result. Rapid restenosis frequently results despite removal of a dysfunc-tional stent.[239] Total obstruction of the lacrimal sac or common canaliculus may occur, with resultant impossibility of the classic operative DCR. Balloon dilation DCP by itself will not preclude future DCR.

Those patients with epiphora of traumatic etiology had a technical failure rate of 29% (in 34 systems) compared to a 1% technical failure in the larger group of patients with idiopathic epiphora (249 systems) of nontraumatic etiol-ogy.[246] Malalignment of the fractured bone is a relative contraindication to nonsurgical placement of a lacrimal stent. The overall patency rates 1 year poststenting of 85% and 74% for stenting of obstructive lesions at the nasolacrimal duct or at the junction between the lacrimal sec and nasolacrimal duct, respectively, are only slightly lower than the patency rates (87%) for DCR.[30, 107–110] Patency rates for stenting obstructive lesions at the contracted lacrimal sac (46%) were considerably lower than those obtained with DCR. Stent placement in the obstructed lacrimal system is most valuable as initial therapy for obstructions below the junction between the lacrimal sac and the nasolacrimal duct.

Berkefeld et al.[243] have expressed reservations about implantation of plastic prostheses (stents) for predominantly benign stenoses of a small-caliber, slow-flow ductal system. Complications may render operative reconstruction difficult. The authors suggest operative treatment for those patients not suitable for balloon DCP. Although placement of stents in the NLDS offers interesting possibilities for duct patency, chronic infection and fibrotic reactions may occur in the end, suggesting that the number of patients who receive a stent as initial treatment of lacrimal system obstruction and the indications for stent placement should be reconsidered.[221]

Assessment of the NLDS prior to placement of a stent may help prevent stent failure. A small, fibrotic lacrimal sac that does not have the capacity to receive the expanded mushroom tip will allow the stent to migrate and occlude. The size of the sac should allow proper placement of the stent below the internal punctum (sinus of Maier) with complete expansion of the mushroom tip. If the head of the stent is placed high in the sac, the stent may contact and block the internal punctum, blocking tear drainage and causing common canaliculus obstruction.[238] Accumulation of tears under the head of the stent may predispose the lacrimal sac to infection.[244] An incorrect length of the stent, with the distal tip contacting the nasal floor, may also lead to poor drainage. False passages are occasionally created, usually with the stent noted to be too medial in position, passing through the very thin bone of the medial wall of the inferior lacrimal sac fossa, during attempts to probe or pass the guidewire or stent through very tight obstructions. More recently, increased reporting of false passages during stent placement, either by the guidewire or by the stent, has been noted.[154, 156, 244] A site of relative weakness at the inferior medial aspect of the lacrimal sac, where Horner's muscle is incomplete or deficient, compared to the muscular envelope noted surrounding the remainder of the sac, was inferred to be a common site in four of five perforations.[154] The assistance of CT imaging, either routinely or if there is any concern about positioning of a guidewire or stent, during or after the procedure, may help identify malpositioned components.[154, 256]

Pabón et al.[256] noted that placement of the stent, confirmed in the proper anatomic tract, was a critical factor affecting long-term patency, with 73% of 61 such stents patent at 1 year compared to none of the 7 improperly positioned stents. Early stent blockage and the need for periodic irrigation may be indicative of malpositioning of the stent.

The presence of epiphora reflects abnormal drainage. The increased number of treatment options (probing, irrigation, intubation, external dacryocystorhinostomy (DCR), endocanalicular DCR, endoscopic DCR, dacryocystoplasty, stent placement) for the epiphora patient have led to a desire for increased functional and anatomic data from various imaging modalities to assist treatment decisions based on the site and nature of the obstruction or stenosis. For nasolacrimal duct obstruction, it is important to differentiate functional (incomplete or partial) from mechanical (complete) obstruction. If the stenosis is mild or incomplete and obstruction can be overcome during a pressure injection, then DCP or stent placement may be considered instead of DCR.[227] More static images, such as those obtained with CT-DCG or MR-DCG (especially if teardrop placement of contrast is used) or radiographic distention-DCG may not offer the required functional information.[227]

The role of CT-DCG immediately following DCG (with residual contrast in place) may assist patient selection for DCP for patients with posttraumatic obstruction,[189] patients with previous DCR failure,[194] or those in whom the guidewire cannot be passed with ease during DCP.[221] At the time of DCG, if imaging findings were suggestive of dacryocystitis, posttraumatic obstruction of the bony canal, tumors, sarcoidosis or Wegener's granulomatosis, these patients received CT for further assessment and possible exclusion from DCP consideration.[221] CT assessment of the nasolacrimal bony canal may reveal minimal diameters ranging from 2.5 to 4.0 mm,[221] in contrast to the assumed canal dimensions of 4 to 6 mm previously described.[158, 163]

Hurwitz[30] has outlined indications for DCR, including epiphora due to acquired obstruction within the nasolacrimal sac and duct; mucocele of the lacrimal sac; chronic dacryocystitis or conjunctivitis due to lacrimal sac obstruction; lacrimal sac infection that must be relieved before intraocular surgery; and congenital nasolacrimal duct obstruction that cannot be cured by probing. As noted by the recent number of articles on DCP or stenting,[246, 218, 221, 240] these are the same indications considered appropriate for DCP or stenting. Attempts to refine DCP techniques and

patient selection criteria, as well as controlled studies, may better define which procedure is best suited for specific patients. More stringent definitions of success, including minimum 2 year follow-up, resolution of the patient's presenting complaint, and 100% patency on syringing tests, would allow more appropriate evaluation of comparative treatments (J.J. Hurwitz, personal communication). DCR remains the treatment of choice for patients with posttraumatic or congenital obstruction of the bony nasolacrimal canal or obstruction of the nasolacrimal canal due to polyps or granuloma. Contraindications to DCR—acute dacryocystitis and tumors of the lacrimal sac,[30]—are also contraindications for dacryocystoplasty.[221]

## ENDOSCOPY OF THE LACRIMAL DRAINAGE SYSTEM

A prototype of a lacrimal canaliculoscope, develops in 1990, passed nicely into the canalicular system, was rigid, was less than 1 mm in external diameter—equivalent to a No. 0 lacrimal probe—and allowed direct visualization of the punctum and canaliculus.[257, 258] Newer-generation flexible endoscopes measure 0.3 to 0.5 mm in diameter and have good axial illumination and a 70° field of view, allowing direct visualization and excellent images of the canaliculi, lacrimal sac, nasolacrimal duct, and their mucous membranes[259] (Fig. 10-37). The endoscopic unit includes a Xenon light source, a video camera with an ocular attachment and a miniature camera system with a monitor and video camera. The above system can be combined with modified Jünemann probes, which have attachments for endoscopy and irrigation. Some probe models have a third attachment to couple a laser fiber.

Such procedures are performed in an outpatient setting with topical anaesthesia and a pericanalicular and perisaccal local anaesthetic. The punctum is dilated, and the endoscope is inserted and advanced during steady, gentle irrigation, which is necessary for good visibility. Patients experience discomfort similar to that of standard probing and irrigation.[259] Normal distention of the lacrimal system is seen as widening of the lumen and easy passage of the endoscope. Stenoses cannot be widened during irrigation and the endoscope meets with a degree of resistance, as in conventional probing. Mucosal characteristics can be identified and correlated with the type of obstruction. Normal lacrimal mucosa is smooth and pink; postinflammatory conditions show thickened reddish-gray mucosa with large papillae; stenosis (fibrotic plaque) presents as whitish-gray inelastic membranes; and submucosal folds are seen as thick gray strictures.[259] Heavy debris and secretions may be differentiated from complete stenosis by their clearance with irrigation. Partial obstruction may be visualized as a narrowed lumen, which widens during irrigation. Difficulties have been noted initially in the handling of the instruments, evaluation of the mucous membranes, or diagnosis of pathologic changes. There is improvement with experience and recognition of landmarks.[259] Endoscopy is currently utilized to visualize directly and localize more precisely obstructing lesions of the NLDS. Endoscopic examinations, combined with various types of lasers, may be utilized for treatment (endocanalicular laser-assisted DCR).

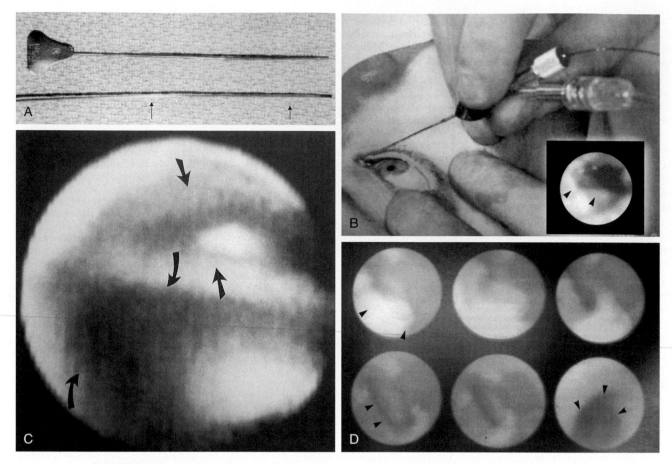

**FIGURE 10-37** Lacrimal endoscopy. **A,** Canaliculoscope (*arrows*), less than 1 mm in external diameter, is equivalent in external diameter to No. 0 lacrimal probe. Newer canaliculoscopes now measure 0.5 mm in diameter. **B,** Endoscope (with attachment for irrigation) positioned in the inferior canaliculus. Inset shows debris and submucosal folds (*arrowheads*). **C,** Canaliculoscope image shows the junction of the superior and inferior canaliculi (darker areas outlined by *arrows*) approaching the common canaliculus. **D,** Lower canaliculus. Top three pictures show mucus and debris (*arrowheads*) occluding the canaliculus. Bottom left and middle pictures show a very narrow lumen (*arrowheads*) after cleansing of the canaliculus. Bottom right picture shows widening of the lumen under pressure irrigation (*arrowheads*). (**A** and **C** Courtesy of Dr. Jeffrey J. Hurwitz, Toronto, Canada, from Ashenhurst ME, Hurwitz JJ. Lacrimal canaliculoscopy. Development of the instrument. Can J Ophthalmol 1991;26:306. **B** and **D** Courtesy of Dr. Klaus Müllner, Graz, Austria, with permission from Müllner K, Bodner E, Mannor G. Endoscopy of the lacrimal system. Br J Ophthalmol 1999;83:949–952.)

However, to date, bone penetration and osteotomy formation have been less successful than for external DCR.[39]

## SUMMARY

Epiphora is a common ophthalmologic complaint for which a number of imaging modalities are available. In our hands, intrinsic etiologies, based within or limited to the luminal component of the NLDS, remain routinely best assessed by digital subtraction (DS-DCG), with real-time images detailing the fine anatomic structures of the NLDS, including stenoses, obstructions (partial or complete), calculi, or morphologic abnormalities such as diverticulae or fistulae. CT and MR imaging display extrinsic lesions affecting the NLDS or mass lesions of the medial canthal and sinonasal-orbital regions. Without a proper index of suspicion, the lack of specificity of clinical signs in the epiphora patient may mask the opportunity to assess causal conditions arising within the wall, extramurally, extraorbit-

ally, within the adjacent paranasal sinuses or nasal cavity. CT offers the advantage of better overall assessment of both bone and soft-tissue detail and tends to be used more frequently, when craniofacial information is desired, as in face trauma or involvement by tumor of the adjacent bone structures. MR imaging offers excellent soft-tissue resolution, especially with orbital surface coils. To better visualize the NLDS on CT or MR imaging, these studies may be complemented by cannulation, with administration of DCG contrast medium, or contrast may be placed topically into the conjunctival cul-de-sac, as a less invasive test that may offer limited functional information. Specific MR-DCG techniques, to highlight fluids (e.g., water, saline) introduced within the NLDS, as a noncontrast medium-detectable substance, show promise but currently do not offer the anatomic detail seen with DS-DCG or the functional analysis seen with DSG. DSG remains an excellent modality for assessing the dynamics of the NLDS, including canalicular dynamics and the lacrimal pump, functional obstruction, and delays in transit. Data analysis and time-activity curves remain an important component of the study offering a quantitative picture of lacrimal drainage, and are especially useful in assessing those epiphora patients with no abnormality seen on DCG.

DCR remains the most consistent surgical treatment for epiphora secondary to an obstruction of the NLDS, with success rates approaching 90%. An alternative treatment, balloon DCP, is a less invasive, simple procedure performed under local anaesthetic on an outpatient basis. With careful patient selection, the most experienced clinicians have achieved encouraging results, approaching those for DCR. Stent placement may yet have a role, but it is no longer suggested as a primary alternative treatment. Knowledge of the criteria for patient selection for surgical procedures (external versus endoscopic DCR) or the alternative treatment, DCP, has led to greater awareness of NLDS factors and a more detailed analysis of lacrimal drainage imaging studies. Lacrimal endoscopy offers direct visualization of the NLDS membranes and precise localization of obstructing lesions. There is a learning curve. The exact role of lacrimal endoscopy, either as a diagnostic tool or in conjunction with surgical approaches such as laser DCR, has yet to be defined.

## Acknowledgments

The authors wish to express their appreciation to Chris Bobkowski and Salvatore Ceniti for their assistance in the preparation of this manuscript and to Jeff Hurwitz, MD. The authors acknowledge the close working relationship between the Departments of Ophthalmology and Medical Imaging and the stimulation of the radiologists' interest in the pathology of the NLDS by their clinical colleagues.

## REFERENCES

1. Ewing AE. Roentgen ray demonstration of the lacrimal abscess cavity. Am J Ophthalmol 1989;26:1–4.
2. Iba GB, Hanafee WN. Distension dacryocystography. Radiology 1968;90:1020–1022.
3. Campbell DM, Carter JM, Doub HP. Roentgen ray studies of the nasolacrimal passageways. Arch Ophthalmol 1922;51:462–470.
4. Hourn GE. X-ray visualization of the nasolacrimal duct. Ann Otol Rhinol Laryngol 1937;46:962–975.
5. Milder B, Demorest BH. Dacryocystography. I. The normal lacrimal apparatus. Arch Ophthalmol 1954;51:180–195.
6. Sargent EN, Ebersole C. Dacryocystography: the use of Sinografin for visualization of the nasolacrimal passages. AJR 1968;102:831–839.
7. Law FW. Dacryocystography. Trans Ophthalmol Soc UK 1967;87:395–407.
8. Munk FL, Burhenne LW, Buffam FV, et al. Dacryocystography: comparison of water-soluble and oil-based contrast agents. Radiology 1989;173:827–830.
9. Campbell W. The radiology of the lacrimal system. Br J Radiol 1964;37:1–26.
10. van der Plaat GF. X-ray enlargement technique. J Belg Radiol 1950;33:89.
11. Epstein E. Cine dacryocystography. Trans Ophthalmol Soc UK 1961;81:284–287.
12. Trokel SL, Potter GD. Kinetic dacryocystography. Am J Ophthalmol 1970;70:1010–1011.
13. Lloyd GAS, Jones BR, Welham RAN. Intubation macrodacryocystography. Br J Ophthalmol 1972;56:600–603.
14. Lloyd GAS, Welham RAN. Subtraction macrodacryocystography. Br J Radiol 1974;47:379–382.
15. El Gammal T, Brooks BS. Amipaque dacryocystography: biplane magnification and subtraction technique Radiology 1981;141:541–542.
16. Schatz CJ. Tear duct system. In: Som PM, Bergeron RT, eds. Head and Neck Imaging, 2nd ed. St. Louis: CV Mosby, 1991;813–827.
17. Galloway JE, Kavic TA, Raflo GT. Digital subtraction dacryocystography: a new method of lacrimal system imaging. Ophthalmology 1984;91:956–962.
18. King SJ, Haigh SF. Technical report: digital subtraction dacryocystography. Clin Radiol 1990;42:351–353.
19. Kirchhof K, Hähnel S, Jansen O, Zake S, Sartor K. Gadolinium-enhanced magnetic resonance dacryocystography in patients with epiphora. J Comput Assist Tomogr 2000;24:327–331.
20. Amanat LA, Hilditch TE, Kwok CS. Lacrimal scintigraphy. II. Its role in the diagnosis of epiphora. Br J Ophthalmol 1983;67:720–728.
21. Jackson A, Hardcastle MP, Shaw A, Gibbon WW. Reduction of ocular lens dosage in dacryocystography. Clin Radiol 1989;40:615–618.
22. Wearne MJ, Pitts J, Frank J, Rose GE. Comparison of dacryocystography and lacrimal scintigraphy in the diagnosis of functional nasolacrimal duct obstruction. Br J Ophthalmol 1999;83:1032–1035.
23. Zinreich SJ, Miller NR, Freeman LN, Glorioso LW, Rosenbaum AE. Computed tomographic dacryocystography using topical contrast media for lacrimal system visualization. Orbit 1990;9:79–87.
24. Hecht SD. Dacyocystorhinostomy. In: Hornblass A, Hanig CJ, eds. Oculoplastic, Orbital, and Reconstructive Surgery. Baltimore: Williams & Wilkins, 1990;1433–1440.
25. Nixon J. Birchall IWJ, Virjee J. The role of dacryocystography in the management of patients with epiphora. Br J Radiol 1990;63:337–339.
26. Hanna IT, MacEwan CJ, Kennedy N. Lacrimal scintigraphy in the diagnosis of epiphora. Nucl Med Commun 1992;13:416–420.
27. Jones LT, Wobig JL. Surgery of the Eyelids and Lacrimal System. Birmingham, Ala: Aesculapius, 1976;67, 141–151, 157–173.
28. Becker MH. The lacrimal drainage system. In: Gonzalez CF, Becker MH, Flanagan JC, eds. Diagnostic Imaging in Ophthalmology. New York: Springer-Verlag, 1986;88–91.
29. Mulligan NB, Ross CA, Francis IC, Moshegov CN. The valsalva DCR bubble test: a new method of assessing lacrimal patency after DCR surgery. Ophthal Plast Reconstr Surg 1994;10:121–123.
30. Hurwitz JJ. Dacryocystorhinostomy. In: Hurwitz JJ, ed. The Lacrimal System. Philadelphia: Lippincott-Raven, 1996;261–296.
31. Hurwitz JJ. Canaliculodacryocystorhinostomy. In: Hurwitz JJ, ed. The Lacrimal System. Philadelphia: Lippincott-Raven, 1996;267–302.
32. Hurwitz JJ. Lacrimal bypass surgery. In: Hurwitz JJ, ed. The Lacrimal System. Philadelphia: Lippincott-Raven, 1996;303–316.
33. Hurwitz JJ. Endonasal dacryocystorhinostomy. In: Hurwitz JJ, ed. The Lacrimal System. Philadelphia: Lippincott-Raven, 1996;317–321.
34. Whittet HB, Shun-Shin GA, Awdry P. Functional endoscopic transnasal dacryocystorhinostomy. Eye 1993;7:545–549.
35. Yung MW, Hardman-Lea S. Endoscopic inferior dacryocystorhinostomy. Clin Otolaryngol 1998;23:152–157.
36. Cokkeser Y, Evereklioglu C, Er H. Comparative external versus endoscopic dacryocystorhinostomy: results in 115 patients. Otolaryngol Head Neck Surg 2000;123:488–491.
37. Mannor GE, Millman AL. The prognostic value of preoperative dacryocystography in endoscopic intranasal dacryocystorhinostomy. Am J Opthalmol 1992;113:134–137.
38. Kong YT, Kim TI, Kong BW. A report of 131 cases of endoscopic laser lacrimal surgery. Ophthalmology 1994;101:1793–1800.
39. Levin PS, Stermogipson J. Endocanalicular laser assisted dacryocystorhinostomy. An anatomic study. Arch Ophthalmol 1992;110:1488–1490.
40. Pearlman SJ, Michalos P, Leib ML, Moazed KT. Translacrimal transnasal laser-assisted dacryocystorhinostomy. Laryngoscope 1997;107:1362–1365.
41. Woog JG, Metson R, Puliafito CA. Holmium:YAG endonasal laser dacryocystorhinostomy. Am J Ophthalmol 1993;116:1–10.
42. Wolff E. Anatomy of the Eye and Orbit, 7th ed., revised by R. Warwick. Philadelphia: WB Saunders, 1976;226–237.
43. Schaeffer JP. Variations in the anatomy of the nasolacrimal passages. Am Surg 1911;54:148–152.

44. Yazici B, Yazici Z. Frequency of the common canaliculus: a radiological study. Arch Ophthalmol 2000;118(10):1381–1385.

45. Gonnering RS, Bosniak SL. Recognition and management of acute non-infectious dacryocystic retention. Ophthal Plast Reconstr Surg 1989;5(1):27–33.

46. Tucker NA, Tucker SM, Linberg JV. The anatomy of the common canaliculus. Arch Ophthalmol 1996;114:1231–1234.

47. Malik SRK, Gupta AK, Chaterjee S, ct al. Dacryocystography of normal and pathological lacrimal passages. Br J Ophthalmol 1969;53:174–179.

48. Paulsen F, Thale A, Kohla G, Schauer R, Rochels R, Parwaresch R, Tillman B. Functional anatomy of human lacrimal duct epithelium. Anat Embryol 1998;198:1–12.

49. Thale A, Paulsen F, Rochels R, Tillmann B. Functional anatomy of the human efferent tear ducts: a new theory of tear outflow mechanism. Graefes Arch Clin Exp Ophthalmol 1998;236:674–678.

50. Paulsen FP, Thale AB, Hallmann UJ, Schaudig U, Tillmann BN. The cavernous body of the human efferent tear ducts: function in tear outflow mechanism. Invest Ophthalmol Vis Sci 2000;41:965–970.

51. Glatt HJ. Dacryocystoplasty: an oculoplastic surgeon's perspective (letter). Radiology 1991;180:289–290.

52. Blicker JA, Buffam FV. Lacrimal sac, conjunctival, and nasal culture results in dacryocystorhinostomy patients. Ophthal Plast Reconstr Surg 1993;9:43–46.

53. DeAngelis D, Hurwitz J, Mazzulli T. The role of bacteriologic infection in the etiology of nasolacrimal duct obstruction. Can J Ophthalmol 2001;36:134–139.

54. Buffam FV. Discussion in DeAngelis D, Hurwitz J, Mazzulli T. The role of bacteriologic infection in the etiology of nasolacrimal duct obstruction. Can J Ophthalmol 2001;36:139.

55. Hartikainen J, Lehtonen OF, Saari KM. Bacteriology of lacrimal duct obstruction in adults. Br J Ophthalmol 1997;81:37–40.

56. Boruchoff SA, Boruchoff SE. Infections of the lacrimal system. Infect Dis Clin North Am 1992;6:925–932.

57. Mauriello JA Jr, Wasserman BA. Acute dacryocystitis: an unusual cause of life-threatening orbital intracanal abscess with frozen globe. Ophthal Plast Reconstr Surg 1996;12:294–295.

58. Ntountas I, Morschbacher R, Pratt D, Patel BC, Anderson RL, McCann JD. An orbital abscess secondary to acute dacryocystitis. Ophthalmic Surg Lasers 1997;28:758–761.

59. Molgat YM, Hurwitz JJ. Orbital abscess due to acute dacryocystitis. Can J Ophthalmol 1993;28:181–182.

60. Janssen AG, Mansour K, Bos JJ, Manoliu RA, Castelijns JA. Abscess of the lacrimal sac due to chronic or subacute dacryocystitis: treatment with temporary stent placement in the nasolacrimal duct. Radiology 2000;215:300–304.

61. Hornblass A, Herschorn BJ, Stern K, Grimes C. Orbital abscess. Surv Ophthalmol 1984;29:169–178.

62. Weiss GH, Leib LM. Congenital dacryocystitis and retrobulbar abscess. J Pediatr Ophthalmol Strabismus 1993;30:271–272.

63. Remulla HD, Rubin PAD, Shore JW, Cunningham MJ. Pseudo-dacryocystitis arising from anterior ethmoiditis. Ophthal Plast Reconstr Surg 1995;11:165–168.

64. Duvoisin B, Schnyder P, Agrifoglio A. CT diagnosis of occult anterior ethmoid sinusitis in a case of lacrimal sac abscess. AJR 1988;151:837–838.

65. Stivero J, Hadar T, Feinmesser R. Fistulae in the inner canthus associated with ethmoiditis. J Laryngol Otol 1992;106:1076–1078.

66. Keast-Butler J, Lloyd GAS, Welham RAN. Analysis of intubation macrodacryocystography with surgical correlations. Trans Ophthalmol Soc UK 1973;93:593–596.

67. Welham RAN, Henderson PM. Results of dacryocystorhinostomy: analysis of cause of failure. Trans Ophthalmol Soc UK 1973;93:601–609.

68. Millman AL, Liebskind A, Putterman AM. Dacryocystography: the technique and its role in the practice of ophthalmology. Radiol Clin North Am 1987;25:781–786.

69. Welham RAN. Canalicular obstructions and the Lester Jones tubes. Trans Ophthalmol Soc UK 1973;93:623–632.

70. Spira R, Mondshine R. Demonstration of nasolacrimal duct carcinoma by computed tomography. Ophthal Plast Reconstr Surg 1986;2:159–161.

71. Agarwal ML. Dacryocystography in chronic dacryocystitis. Am J Ophthalmol l961;52:245–251.

72. Francois J, Bacskulin J. External congenital fistulae of the lacrimal sac. Ophthalmologica 1969;159:249–261.

73. Masi AV. Congenital fistula of the lacrimal sac. Arch Ophthalmol 1983;81:701–704.

74. Toda C, Imai K, Tsujiguchi K, Komune H, Enoki E, Nomachi T. Three different types of congenital lacrimal sac fistulas. Am Plast Surg 2000;45:651–653.

75. Howard R, Caldwell J. Congenital fistula of the lacrimal sac. Am J Ophthalmol 1969;67:931–934.

76. Welham RAN, Bergin DJ. Congenital lacrimal fistulas. Arch Ophthalmol 1985;103:545–548.

77. Tsibidas P, Roussos J. Supernumerary lacrimal canaliculi. Ann Ophthalmol 1979;11:265–267.

78. Epley KD, Karesh JW. Lacrimal sac diverticula associated with a patent lacrimal system. Ophthal Plast Reconstr Surg 1999;15:111–115.

79. Bullock JD, Goldberg SH. Lacrimal sac diverticula. Arch Ophthalmol 1989;107:756.

80. Polito E, Leccisotti A, Menicacci F, Motolese E, Addabbo G, Paterra N. Imaging techniques in the diagnosis of lacrimal sac diverticulum. Ophthalmologica 1999;209:228–232.

81. Hosal BM, Hurwitz JJ, Howarth DI. Orbital cyst of lacrimal sac derivation. Eur J Ophthalmol 1996;6:279–283.

82. Hornblass A, Gross ND. Lacrimal sac cyst. Ophthalmology 1987;94:706–708.

83. Berlin AJ, Rath R, Rich L. Lacrimal system dacryoliths. Ophthalmic Surg 1980;11:435–436.

84. Jones LT. Tear-sac foreign bodies. Am J Ophthalmol 1965;60:111–113.

85. Viers ER: Lacrimal Disorders in Diagnosis and Treatment. St. Louis: CV Mosby, 1976;54–59.

86. Wilkins RB, Pressly JP. Diagnosis and incidence of lacrimal calculi. Ophthalmic Surg 1980;11:787–789.

87. Hawes MJ. The dacryolithiasis syndrome. Ophthal Plast Reconstr Surg 1988;4:87–90.

88. Weber AL, Rodriguez-DeVelasquez A, Lucarelli MJ, Cheng HM. Normal anatomy and lesions of the lacrimal sac and duct: evaluated by dacryocystography, computed tomography, and MR imaging. Neuroimaging Clin North Am 1996;6:199–217.

89. Yazici B, Hammad AM, Meyer DR. Lacrimal sac dacryoliths: predictive factors and clinical characteristics. Ophthalmology 2001;108:1308–1312.

90. Maltzman BA, Favetta JR. Dacryolithiasis. Am Ophthalmol 1979;11:473–475.

91. Kaye-Wilson LG. Spontaneous passage of a dacryolith. Br J Ophthalmol 1991;75:564.

92. McCormick SA, Linberg JV. Pathology of nasolacrimal duct obstruction. Clinicopathologic correlates of lacrimal excretory system disease. Contemp Issue Ophthalmol 1988;5:169–202.

93. Jay JL, Lee WR. Dacryolith formation around an eyelash retained in the lacrimal sac. Br Ophthalmol 1976;60:722–725.

94. Baratz KH, Bartley GB, Campbell W, Garrity JA. An eyelash nidus for dacryoliths of the lacrimal excretory and secretory systems. Am J Ophthalmol 1991;111:624–627.

95. Herzig S, Hurwitz JJ. Lacrimal sac calculi. Can J Ophthalmol 1979;14(1):17–20.

96. Berlin AJ. Success rate of endoscopic laser-assisted dacryocystorhinostomy (letter). Ophthalmology 2000;107:4–5.

97. Richards W. Actinomycotic lacrimal caniculitis. Am J Ophthalmol 1973;75:155–157.

98. Wolter J, Stratford T, Harrell E. Cast-like fungus obstruction of the nasolacrimal duct. Arch Ophthalmol 1956;55:320–322.

99. Kristinsson JK, Sigurdsson H. Lacrimal sac plugging caused by *Aspergillus fumigatus*. Acta Ophthalmol Scand 1998;76:241–242.

100. Song HY, Jin YH, Lee HK, Sung KB. Non-operative management of dacryolithiasis. JVIR 1995;6:647–650.

101. Wilhelm KE, Hofer U, Textor HJ, Böker TH, Strunk HH. Dacryoliths; nonsurgical fluoroscopically-guided treatment during dacryocystoplasty. Radiology 1999;212:365–370.

102. von Graefe A. Koncretionen in unteren thraenenroerchen durch Pilzbildung. Arch Ophthalmol 1854;1:284–288.

103. Sathananthan N, Sullivan TJ, Rose GE, Moseley IF. Intubation dacryocystography in patients with a clinical diagnosis of chronic caniculitis ("streptothrix"). Br J Radiol 1993;66:389–393.

104. Francois J, Elewault-Ryssellaere M, De Vos E. Mycose et pseudo-mycoses des voies lacrymales. Ann Ocul 1966;199:1129–1142.

105. Bouzas AG. Virus aetiology of certain cases of lacrimal obstruction. Br J Ophthalmol 1973;57:849–851.

106. Hurwitz JJ, Welham RAN, Lloyd GAS. The role of intubation macrodacryocystography in management of problems of the lacrimal system. Can J Ophthalmol 1975;10:361–366.

107. McLachlan DL, Shannon GM, Flanagan JC. Results of dacryocystorhinostomy: analysis of the reoperations. Ophthalmic Surg 1980;11:427–430.

108. Tarbet KJ, Custer PL. External dacryocystorhinostomy. Surgical success, patient satisfaction, and economic cost. Ophthalmology 1995;102:1065–1070.

109. Hartikainen J, Antila J, Varpula M, Puukka P, Seppä H, Grénman R. Prospective randomized comparison of endonasal endoscopic dacryocystorhinostomy and external dacryocystorhinostomy. Laryngoscope 1998;108:1861–1866.

110. Allen K, Berlin AJ. Dacryocystorhinostomy failure: association with nasolacrimal silicone intubation. Ophthalmic Surg 1989;20:486–489.

111. Orcutt JC, Hillel A, Weymuller EA. Endoscopic repair of failed dacryocystorhinostomy. Ophthalmic Plast Reconst Surg 1990;6:197–202.

112. Welham RAN, Wulc AE. Management of unsuccessful lacrimal surgery. Br J Ophthalmol 1987;71:152–157.

113. Hurwitz JJ, Welham RAN, Maisey MN. Radiography in functional lacrimal testing. Br J Ophthalmol 1975;59:323–331.

114. Doucet TW, Hurwitz JJ. Canaliculodacryocystorhinostomy in the management of unsuccessful lacrimal surgery. Arch Ophthalmol 1982;100:619–621.

115. Esmaeli B, Valero V, Ahmadi MA, Booser D. Canalicular stenosis secondary to docetaxel (taxotere): a newly recognized side effect. Ophthalmology 2001;108:994–995.

116. Fezza JP, Wesley RE, Klippenstein KA. The treatment of punctual and canalicular stenosis in patients on systemic 5-FU. Ophthalmic Surg Lasers 1999;30:105–108.

117. Haidak DJ, Hurwitz BS, Yeung KY. Tear duct fibrosis (dacryostenosis) due to 5-fluorouracil. Ann Intern Med 1978;88:657.

118. Rossomondo RM, Carlton WH, Trueblood JH, Thomas RP. A new method of evaluating lacrimal drainage. Arch Ophthalmol 1972;88:523–525.

119. Brown M, El Gammal TA, Luxenberg MN, Eubig C. The value, limitations and applications of nuclear dacryocystography. Semin Nucl Med 1981;11:250–257.

120. Hilditch TE, Kwok CS, Amanat LA. Lacrimal scintigraphy. I. Compartmental analysis of data. Br J Ophthalmol 1983;67:713–719.

121. Hurwitz JJ, Maisey MN, Welham RAN. Quantitative lacrimal scintillography. I. Method and physiological application. Br J Ophthalmol 1975;59:308–312.

122. Hurwitz JJ, Maisey MN, Welham RAN. Quantitative lacrimal scintillography. II. Method and physiological application. Br J Ophthalmol 1975;59:313–322.

123. Hurwitz JJ, Welham RAN, Maisey MN. Intubation macrodacryocystography and quantitative scintillography: the "complete" lacrimal assessment. Trans Am Acad Ophthalmol Otolaryngol 1976;81:575–582.

124. Fraunfelder FT. Extraocular fluid dynamics: how best to apply topical ocular medication. Tr Am Ophthalmol Soc 1976;74:457–487.

125. Chavis RM, Welham RAN, Maisey MN. Quantitative lacrimal scintillography. Arch Ophthalmol 1978;96:2066–2068.

126. White WL, Glover AT, Buckner AB, Hartshorne MF. Relative canalicular tear flow as assessed by dacryoscintography. Ophthalmology 1989;96(2):167–169.

127. Rose JDG, Clayton CB. Scintigraphy and contrast radiography for epiphora. Br J Radiol 1985;58:1183–1186.

128. Rabinovitch J, Hurwitz JJ, Chin-Sang M. Quantitative evaluation of canalicular flow using lacrimal scintillography. Orbit 1984;3:263–266.

129. Robertson JS, Brown ML, Colvard DM. Radiation absorbed dose to the lens in dacryoscintigraphy with technetium 99m. Radiology 1979;133:747–750.

130. Rogers RT. Radiation dose to the skin in diagnostic radiology. Br J Radiol 1969;42:511–518.

131. Jones LT. An anatomical approach to problems of the eyelids and lacrimal apparatus. Arch Ophthalmol 1961;66:111–124.

132. Hill JC, Bethel W, Smirmaul HJ. Lacrimal drainage: a dynamic evaluation. Part I. Mechanics of tear transport. Can J Ophthalmol 1974;9:411–416.

133. Doane MG. Blinking and the mechanics of the lacrimal drainage system. Ophthalmology 1981;88:844–851.

134. Doane MG. Blinking and tear drainage. Adv Ophthalmic Plast Reconstr Surg 1984;3:39–52.

135. Hill JC, Bethel W, Smirmaul HJ. Lacrimal drainage: a dynamic evaluation. Part II. Clinical aspects. Can J Ophthalmol 1974;9:417–424.

136. Sorensen TB. Studies on tear physiology, pathophysiology and contact lenses by means of dynamic gamma camera and technetium. Acta Ophthalmol Suppl 1984;167:1–54.

137. White WL, Glover AT, Buckner AB. Effect of blinking on tear elimination as evaluated by dacryoscintigraphy. Ophthalmology 1991;98:367–369.

138. von Denffler HW, Dressler J, Pabst HW. Lacrimal dacryoscintigraphy. Semin Nucl Med 1984;14:8–15.

139. Daubert J, Nik N, Chandeyssoun PA, el-Choufi L. Tear flow analysis through the upper and lower systems. Ophthal Plast Reconstr Surg 1990;6:193–196.

140. Linberg JV, Moore CA. Symptoms of canalicular obstruction. Ophthalmology 1988;95(8):1077–1079.

141. Becker BB. Tricompartment model of the lacrimal pump mechanism. Ophthalmology 1992;99:1139–1145.

142. Rosengren B. On lacrimal drainage. Ophthalmologica 1972;164:409–421.

143. Amanat LA, Hilditch TE, Kwok CS. Lacrimal scintigraphy. I. Compartmental analysis of data. Br J Ophthalmol 1983;67:713–719.

144. Amanat LA, Hilditch TE, Kwok CS. Lacrimal scintigraphy. III. Physiological aspects of lacrimal drainage. Br J Ophthalmol 1983;67:729–732.

145. Francis IC, Kappagoda MB, Cole IE, Bank L, Dunn GD. Computed tomography of the lacrimal drainage system: retrospective study of 107 cases of dacryostenosis. Ophthal Plast Reconstr Surg 1999;15:217–226.

146. Bartley GB. Acquired lacrimal drainage obstruction: an etiologic classification system, case reports and a review of the literature. Part 1. Ophthal Plast Reconstr Surg 1992;8:237–242.

147. Bartley GB. Acquired lacrimal drainage obstruction: an etiologic classification system, case reports and a review of the literature. Part 2. Ophthal Plast Reconstr Surg 1992;8:243–249.

148. Bartley GB. Acquired lacrimal drainage obstruction: an etiologic classification system, case reports and a review of the literature. Part 3. Ophthal Plast Reconstr Surg 1992;9:11–26.

149. Zehavi C, Zadok J, Sacks D. The pitfalls of dacryostenosis. Ophthal Surg 1992;23:297–298.

150. Mauriello JA, Palydowycz S, DeLuca J. Clinicopathologic study of lacrimal sac and nasal mucosa in 44 patients with complete acquired nasolacrimal duct obstruction. Ophthal Plast Reconstr Surg 1992;8:13–21.

151. Hähnel S, Jansen O, Zake S, Sartor K. Ser wert der spiral-CT zur diagnose von stenosen der ableitenden Tranenwege. Röfo Fortschr Geb Röntgenstr Neuen Bildgeb Uerfahr 1995;163:210–214.

152. Friedman DP, Rao VM, Flanders AE. Lesions causing a mass in the medial canthus of the orbit: CT and MR features. AJR 1993;160:1095–1099.

153. Russell EJ, Czervionke L, Huckman M, Daniels D, McLachlan D. CT of the inferomedial orbit and lacrimal drainage apparatus: normal and pathologic anatomy. AJR 1985;145:1147–1154.

154. Pinto IT, Paul L, Grande C. Nasolacrimal polyurethane stent: complications with CT correlation. Cardiovasc Intervent Radiol 1998;21:450–453.

155. Hartikainen J, Aho HJ, Seppa H, Grenman R. Lacrimal bone thickness at the lacrimal sac fossa. Ophthalmic Surg Lasers 1996;27:679–684.

156. Yung MW, Logan BM. The anatomy of the lacrimal bone at the lateral wall of the nose: its significance to the lacrimal surgeon. Clin Otolaryngol 1999;24:262–265.

157. Dale DL. Embryology, anatomy, and physiology of the lacrimal drainage system. In: Stephensen CM, ed. Ophthalmic, Plastic, Reconstructive, and Orbital Surgery. Boston: Butterworth-Heinemann, 1997;19–30.

158. Whitnall SE. The Anatomy of the Human Orbit and Accessory Organ of Vision. H. Frowde, Hodder, Stoughton. Part 1. London: Oxford Medical Publication, 1921; chap. 5.

159. Janssen AG, Mansour K, Bos JJ, Castelijns JA. Diameter of the bony lacrimal canal: normal values and values bilateral to nasolacrimal duct obstruction. Assessment with CT. Am J Neuroradiol 2001;22:845–850.

160. Groessl SA, Sires BS, Lemke BN. An anatomic basis for primary acquired nasolacrimal duct obstruction. Arch Ophthalmol 1997;115:71–74.

161. Linberg JV, McCormick SA. Primary acquired nasolacrimal duct obstruction: a clinicopathologic report and biopsy technique. Ophthalmology 1986;93:1055–1063.

162. Well BA. Dacryocystitis. In: Viers ER, ed. The Lacrimal System. St. Louis; CV Mosby, 1971;118–119.

163. Duke-Elder S. Textbook of Ophthalmology. Vol. 1. The Development, Form, and Function of the Visual Apparatus. London: Kimpton, 1946;235.

164. Tucker N, Chow D, Stockl F, Codere F, Burnier M. Clinically suspected primary acquired nasolacrimal duct obstruction. Ophthalmology 1997;104:1882–1886.

165. Flanagan JC, Stokes DP. Lacrimal sac tumors. Ophthalmology 1978;85:1282–1287.

166. Loftus WK, Kew J, Metrewelic C. Nasolacrimal duct opacity on CT. Br J Radiol 1996;69:630–631.

167. Rheeman CH, Meyer DR. Enlargement of the nasolacrimal canal in the absence of neoplasia. Ophthalmology 1998;105:1498–1503.

168. Nasr AM, Huaman AM. Anterior orbital varix presenting as a lacrimal sac mucocele. Ophthal Plast Reconstr Surg 1998;14:193–197.

169. Mudgil AV, Meyer DR, Dipillo MA. Varix of the angular vein manifesting as a Medial canthal mass. Am J Ophthalmol 1993;116:245–246.

170. Stefanyszyn MA, Hidayat AA, Pe'er JJ, Flanagan JC. Lacrimal sac tumors. Ophthal Plast Reconstr Surg 1994;10:169–184.

171. Ryan SJ, Font RL. Primary epithelial neoplasms of the lacrimal sac. Am J Ophthalmol 1973;76:73–88.

172. Pe'er J, Hidayat AA, Ilsar M, Landau L, Stefanyszyn MA. Glandular tumors of the lacrimal sac. Their histopathologic patterns and possible origins. Ophthalmology 1996;103:1601–1605.

173. Powell JB. Nasolacrimal dysfunction. Laryngoscope 1983;93:498–515.

174. Ni C, D'Amico DJ, Fan CQ, Kuo PK. Tumors of the lacrimal sac: a clinicopathological analysis of 82 cases. Int Ophthalmol Clin 1982;22(1):121–140.

175. Jones IS. Tumors of the lacrimal sac. Am J Ophthalmol 1956;42:561–566.

176. Hornblass A, Jakobiec FA, Bosniak S, Flanagan JC. The diagnosis and management of epithelial tumors of the lacrimal sac. Ophthalmol 1980;87:476–490.

177. Erickson BA, Massaro BM, Mark LP, Harris GJ. Lacrimal collecting system lymphomas: integration of magnetic resonance imaging and therapeutic irradiation. Int J Radiat Oncol Biol Phys 1994;29:1095–1103.

178. Nakamura Y, Mashima Y, Kameyama K, Mukai M, Oguchi Y. Detection of human papillomavirus infection in squamous tumours of the conjunctiva and lacrimal sac by immunohistochemistry, in situ hybridisation, and polymerase chain reaction. Br J Ophthalmol 1997;81:308–313.

179. Pe'er JJ, Stefanyszyn M, Hidayat AA. Non-epithelial tumors of the lacrimal sac. Am J Ophthalmol 1994;118:650–658.

180. Milder B, Smith ME. Tumors of the lacrimal excretory system. In: Milder B, Weils BA, eds. The Lacrimal System. Norwalk, Conn: Appleton-Century-Crofts, 1983;145–152.

181. Mruthyunjaya P, Meyer DR. Juvenile xanthogranuloma of the lacrimal sac fossa. Am J Ophthalmol 1997;123:400–402.

182. Gruss JS, Hurwitz JJ, Nik NA, Kassel EE. The pattern and incidence of nasolacrimal injury in naso-orbital-ethmoid fractures: the role of delayed assessment and dacryocystorhinostomy. Br J Plast Surg 1985;38:116–121.

183. Gruss JS. Naso-ethmoid-orbital fractures: classification and role of primary bone grafting. Plast Reconstr Surg 1985;75:303–315.

184. Stranc MF. The pattern of lacrimal injuries in naso-ethmoid fractures. Br J Plast Surg 1971;24:339–346.

185. Nik NA, Hurwitz JJ, Gruss JS. Management of lacrimal injury after naso-orbito-ethmoid fractures. Adv Ophthalmic Plast Reconstr Surg 1984;3:307–317.

186. Balle VH, Andersen R, Slim C. Incidence of lacrimal obstruction following trauma to the facial skeleton. Ear, Nose, Throat J 1988;67:66–70.

187. Osguthorpe JD, Hoang G. Nasolacrimal injuries: evaluation and management. Otolaryngol Clin North Am 1991;24:59–78.

188. Unger JM. Fractures of the nasolacrimal fossa and canal: a CT study of appearance, associated injuries, and significance in 25 patients. AJR 1992;158:1321–1324.

189. Glatt HJ. Evaluation of lacrimal obstruction secondary to facial fractures using computed tomography or computed tomographic dacryocystography. Ophthal Plast Reconstr Surg 1996;12:284–293.

190. Hurwitz JJ, Archer KF, Gruss JS. Double stent intubation in difficult post-traumatic dacryocystorhinostomy. Ophthalmic Surg 1988;19:33–36.

191. Bolger WE, Bitzin CA, Parsons DS. Paranasal sinus bony anatomic variations and mucosal abnormalities: CT analysis for endoscopic sinus surgery. Laryngoscope 1991;101:56–64.

192. Blaylock WK, Moore CA, Linberg JV. Anterior ethmoid anatomy facilitates dacryocystorhinostomy. Arch Ophthalmol 1990;108:1774–1777.

193. Earwaker J. Anatomic variants in sinonasal CT. Radiographics 1993;13:381–415.

194. Glatt HJ, Chan AC, Barrett L. Evaluation of dacryocystorhinostomy failure with computed tomography and computed tomographic dacryocystography. Am J Ophthalmol 1991;112:431–436.

195. Gonnering RS, Lyon DB, Fisher JC. Endoscopic laser-assisted lacrimal surgery. Am J Ophthalmol 1991;111:152–157.

196. Linberg JV, Anderson RL, Bumsted RM, et al. Study of intranasal ostium external dacryocystorhinostomy. Arch Ophthalmol 1982;100:1758–1762.

197. Ashenhurst M, Jaffer N, Hurwitz JJ, Corrin SM. Combined computed tomography and dacryocystography for complex lacrimal problems. Can J Ophthalmol 1991;26(1):27–31.

198. Moran CC, Buckwalter K, Caldemeyer KS, Smith RR. Helical CT with topical water-soluble contrast media for imaging of the lacrimal drainage apparatus, AJR 1995;164:995–996.

199. Caldemeyer KS, Stockberger SM, Broderick LS. Topical contrast-enhanced CT and MR dacryocystography: imaging the lacrimal drainage apparatus of healthy volunteers. AJR 1998;171:1501–1504.

200. Kassel EE, Schatz CJ. Lacrimal apparatus. In: Som PM, Curtin HD, eds. Head and Neck Imaging, 3rd ed. St Louis: CV Mosby, 1996;1129–1183.

201. Mansfield DC, Zeki SM, MacKenzie JR. Case report: extravasation of lipiodol—a complication of dacryocystography. Clin Radiol 1994;49:217–218.

202. Sevel D. Development and congenital abnormalities of the nasolacrimal apparatus. J Pediatr Ophthalmol Strabismus 1981;18:13–19.

203. Busse HM, Müler KM, Kroll P. Radiological and histological findings of the lacrimal passages of newborns. Arch Ophthalmol 1980;98:528–532.

204. Berkowitz RG, Grundfast KM, Fitz C. Nasal obstruction of the newborn revisited: clinical and subclinical manifestations of congenital nasolacrimal duct obstruction presenting as a nasal mass. Otolaryngol Head Neck Surg 1990;103:468–471.

205. MacEwen CJ, Young JDH. Epiphora during the first year of life. Eye 1991;5:596–600.

206. Levy NS. Conservative management of congenital amnionotocele of the nasolacrimal duct. J Pediatr Ophthalmol Strabismus 1979;16:254–256.

207. Guerry D III, Kendig EJ Jr. Congenital impatency of the nasolacrimal duct. Arch Ophthalmol 1948;39:193–202.

208. Meyer JR, Quint DJ, Holmes JM, et al. Infected congenital mucocele of the nasolacrimal duct. AJNR 1993;14:1008–1010.

209. Petersen RA, Robb RM. The natural course of congenital obstruction of the nasolacrimal duct. J Pediatr Ophthalmol Strabismus 1978;15:246–250.

210. Harris GJ, DiClementi D. Congenital dacryocystocele. Arch Ophthalmol 1982;100:1763–1765.

211. Edmond JC, Keech RV. Congenital nasolacrimal mucocele associated with respiratory distress. J Pediatr Ophthalmol Strabismus 1991;28:287–289.

212. Castillo M, Merten DF, Weissler MC. Bilateral nasolacrimal duct mucocele, a rare cause of respiratory distress: CT findings in two newborns. AJNR 1993;14:1011–1013.
213. Rand PK, Ball WS, Kulwin DR. Congenital nasolacrimal mucoceles: CT evaluation. Radiology 1989;173:691–694.
214. Katowitz JR, Welsh MG. Timing of initial probing and irrigation in congenital nasolacrimal duct obstruction. Ophthalmology 1987;94: 698–709.
215. Young JDH, MacEwen CJ, Ogston SA. Congenital nasolacrimal duct obstruction in the second year of life: A multicenter trial of management. Eye 1996;10:485–491.
216. Migliori ME. Endoscopic evaluation and management of the lacrimal sump syndrome. Ophthal Plast Reconstr Surg 1997;13:281–284.
217. Becker BB, Berry FD, Koller H. Balloon catheter dilatation for treatment of congenital nasolacrimal duct obstruction. Am J Ophthalmol 1996;121:304–309.
218. Cho YS, Song HY, Ko GY, Yoon CH, Ahn HS, Yoon HK, Sung KB. Congenital lacrimal system obstruction: treatment with balloon dilation. JVIR 2000;11:1319–1324.
219. Janssen AG, Mansour K, Krabbe GJ, van der Veen S, Helder AH. Dacryocystoplasty: treatment of epiphora by means of balloon dilation of the obstructed nasolacrimal duct system. Radiology 1994;193:453–456.
220. Song HY, Ahn HS, Park CK, Kwon SH, Kim CS, Choi KC. Complete obstruction of the nasolacrimal system. I. Treatment with balloon dilatation. Radiology 1993;186:367–371.
221. Janssen AG, Mansour K, Bos JJ. Obstructed nasolacrimal duct system in epiphora: long-term results of dacryocystoplasty by means of balloon dilation. Radiology 1997;205(3):791–796.
222. Goldberg RA, Heinz GW, Chiu L. Gadolinium magnetic resonance imaging dacryocystography. Am J Ophthalmol 1993;115:738–741.
223. Hoffman KT, Hosten N, Anders N. High resolution conjunctival contrast enhanced MRI dacryocystography. Neuroradiology 1999;41: 208–213.
224. Reifler DM. Early descriptions of Horner's muscle and the lacrimal pump. Surv Ophthalmol 1996;41:127–134.
225. Rubin PAD, Bilyk JR, Shore JW, Sutula FC, Cheng HM. Magnetic resonance imaging of the lacrimal drainage system. Ophthalmology 1994;101:235–243.
226. Yoshikawa T, Hirota S, Sugimura K. Topical contrast-enhanced magnetic resonance dacryocystography. Radiat Med 2000;18(6): 355–362.
227. Takehara Y, Isoda H, Kurihashi K, Isogai S, Kodaira N, Masunaga H, Sugiyama M, Ozawa F, Takeda H, Nozaki A, Sakahara H. Dynamic MR dacryocystography: a new method for evaluating nasolacrimal duct obstructions. AJR 2000;175:469–473.
228. Munk PL, Lin DTC, Morris DC. Epiphora: treatment by means of dacryocystoplasty with balloon dilation of the nasolacrimal drainage apparatus. Radiology 1990;177:687–690.
229. Lee JM, Song HY, Han YM, Chung GH, Sohn MH, Kim CS, Choi KC. Balloon dacryocystoplasty: results in the treatment of complete and partial obstructions of the nasolacrimal system. Radiology 1994;192:503–508.
230. Song HY, Jin YH, Rim JH, Huh SJ, Kim YH, Kim TH, Sung KB. Non-surgical placement of a nasolacrimal polyurethane stent. Radiology 1995;194:233–237.
231. Becker BB, Berry FD. Balloon catheter dilatation in lacrimal surgery. Ophthalmic Surg 1989;20:193–198.
232. Kratky V, Hurwitz JJ, Ananthanarayan C, Avram DR. Dacryocystorhinostomy in elderly patients: regional anaesthesia without cocaine. Can J Ophthalmol 1994;29:13–16.
233. Wilhelm K, Kramer S, Ewen E, Schuller H, Schild H. Radiation dose to the ocular lens, parotid and thyroid glands in dacryocystography and fluoroscopically-guided dacryocystoplasty. ROFO Fortschr Geb Rontgenstr Neuen Bildgab Verfahr 1998;168:270–274 (German).
234. Wilhelm KE. Radiation dose in fluoroscopically-guided dacryocystoplasty (letter). Radiology 2001;219:577.
235. Ilgit ET, Meric N, Bor D, Öznur I, Konus Ö, Isik S. Lens of the eye: radiation dose in balloon dacryocystoplasty. Radiology 2000; 217:54–57.
236. Ilgit ET, Bor D, Meric N. (Reply). Radiation dose in fluoroscopically-guided dacryocystoplasty. Radiology 2001;219: 577–578.
237. Song HY, Ahn HS, Park CK, Kwon SH, Rim CS, Choi KC. Complete obstruction of the nasolacrimal system. II. Treatment with expandable metallic stents. Radiology 1993;186:372–376.
238. Song HY, Jin YH, Kim JH, Sung KB, Han YM, Cho NC. Nasolacrimal duct obstruction treated non-surgically with use of plastic stents. Radiology 1994;190:535–539.
239. Janssen AG. Imaging and interventional procedures for the lacrimal duct system. In: Mukherji SK, Castelijns JA, eds. Medical Radiology: Modern Head and Neck Imaging. Berlin: Springer, 2000;211–235.
240. Ilgit ET, Yüksel D, Ünal M, Akpek S, Isik S, Hsanreisoglu B. Transluminal balloon dilation of the lacrimal draining system for the treatment of epiphora. AJR 1995;165:1517–1524.
241. Kumar EN. Technical note: non-surgical treatment of epiphora by balloon dacryoplasty—the technique. Br J Radiol 1995;68:1116–1118.
242. Ilgit ET, Yüksel D, Ünal M, Akpek S, Isik S. Treatment of recurrent nasolacrimal duct obstructions with balloon-expandable metallic stents: results of early experience. AJNR 1996;17:657–663.
243. Berkefeld J, Kirchner J, Müller HM, Fries U, Kollath J. Balloon dacryocystoplasty: indications and contraindications. Radiology 1997;205:785–790.
244. Yazici B, Yazici Z, Parlak M. Treatment of nasolacrimal duct obstruction in adults with polyurethane stent. Am J Ophthalmol 2001;131:37–43.
245. Yazici Z, Yazici B, Parlak M, Erturk H, Savci G. Treatment of obstructive epiphora in adults by balloon dacryocystoplasty. Br J Ophthalmol 1999;83:692–696.
246. Song HY, Jin YH, Kim JH, Suh SW, Yoon HK, Kang SG, Sung KB. Nonsurgical placement of a nasolacrimal polyurethane stent: long-term effectiveness. Radiology 1996;200:759–763.
247. Kuchar A, Steinkogler FJ. Antegrade balloon dilatation of nasolacrimal duct obstruction in adults. Br J Ophthalmol 2001;85:200–204.
248. Steinsapin KD, Glatt HJ, Putterman AM. A 16-year study of conjunctival dacryocystorhinostomy. Am J Ophthalmol 1990;109: 387–393.
249. Goo DF, Song HY, Yoon H, Sung K. Lacrimal canalicular strictures: safety and effectiveness of balloon dilatation (abstract). Radiology 1996;201(P):411.
250. Song HY, Lee CO, Park S, Suh SW, Yoon HK, Kang SG, Sung KB. Lacrimal canalicular obstruction: safety and effectiveness of balloon dilation. JVIR 1996;7:929–934.
251. Ko YK, Lee DH, Ahn HS, Yoon HK, Sung KB, Song HY. Balloon catheter dilation in common canalicular obstruction of the lacrimal system: safety and long-term effectiveness. Radiology 2000;214: 781–786.
252. Song HY, Lee CO, Park S, Suh SW, Yoon HK, Kang SG, Sung KB. Lacrimal canaliculus obstruction: non-surgical treatment with a newly designed polyurethane stent. Radiology 1996;199:280–282.
253. Palmaz JC. Balloon-expandable intravascular stent. Am J Roentgenol 1988;150:1263–1269.
254. Palmaz JC. Intravascular stents: tissue–stent interaction and design considerations. Am J Roentgenol 1993;160:613–618.
255. Howes EL, Rao NA. Basic mechanisms in pathology. In: Spencer WH, ed. Ophthalmic Pathology. An Atlas and Textbook, 4th ed. Philadelphia: WB Saunders, 1996;2973.
256. Pabón IP, Díaz LP, Grande C, de la Cal López MA. Nasolacrimal polyurethane stent placement for epiphora: technical long-term results. JVIR 2001;12(1):67–71.
257. Hurwitz JJ. Endoscopy canaliculus. In Hurwitz JJ, ed. The Lacrimal System. Philadelphia: Lippincott-Raven, 1996;103–104.
258. Ashenhurst ME, Hurwitz JJ. Lacrimal canaliculoscopy: development of the instrument. Can J Ophthalmol 1991;26:306–308.
259. Müllner K, Bodner E, Mannor GE. Endoscopy of the lacrimal system. Br J Ophthalmol 1999;83:949–952.

# 11

# Visual Pathways

*Robert A. Zimmerman, Larissa T. Bilaniuk,*
*and Peter J. Savino*

The retrobulbar visual pathway (Fig. 11-1) includes all neural pathways involved in visual function from the point where the optic nerve originates in the posterior globe to the primary visual cortex lying within the medial aspects of the occipital lobes. The elements of the pathway can be affected by a variety of pathologic conditions, which, depending on their location, give rise to characteristic clusters of clinical symptomatology. The apparent symptoms therefore enable

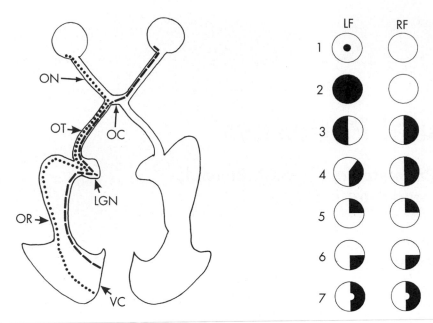

**FIGURE 11-1** **A,** Diagram of left visual pathway. *Dots,* The pathway that starts in the temporal portion of the retinas of the left eye and ends in the left occipital cortex; *dashes,* pathway from the nasal portion of the retinas of the right eye that crosses to the left in the optic chiasm and ends in the left occipital cortex; *ON,* optic nerve; *OC,* optic chiasm; *OT,* optic tract; *LGN,* lateral geniculate nucleus; *OR,* optic radiations; *VC,* visual cortex. **B,** Visual field defects that can occur with abnormalities involving the left visual pathway. Each visual field is represented separately; the figure on the left represents the patient's left visual field. *LF,* left field; *RF,* right field. Site of lesion: *ON—1.* Left central scotoma: *ON—2.* Complete blindness left visual field. *ON—3.* Bitemporal hemianopia. *OT, LGN—4.* Right incongruous homonymous hemianopia. *OR—5.* Right congruous upper quadrantic hemianopia. *OR—6.* Right congruous inferior quadrantic hemianopia. *VC—7.* Right congruous homonymous hemianopia with macular sparing.

the pathologic condition to be localized along the visual pathway with a high degree of certainty. For this reason, imaging techniques may be tailored to display the expected condition optimally. In the past, these imaging techniques included plain radiographs, orbital venography, pneumoencephalography, and complex motion tomography. However, during the past two decades, computed tomography (CT) and magnetic resonance (MR) imaging have become the mainstays of visual pathway imaging because they allow direct visualization of the elements of the pathway and the pathologic processes contained therein. Today, MR imaging is the procedure of choice.

This chapter defines the anatomy of the visual pathway, discusses the relevant embryology, delineates the role of CT and MR imaging, discusses the various pathologic entities that can affect the visual pathway and their clinical symptomatology, and illustrates the appearance of these pathologic conditions.

## EMBRYOLOGY OF THE RETROCHIASMATIC VISUAL PATHWAY

Embryologic development of the retrochiasmatic visual pathway is a complex process that occurs in a sequential, stepwise fashion. It involves the growth and development of both neural and vascular structures and is also affected by influences stemming from developing osseous structures.[1, 2] The embryology of the globe (discussed in Chapter 8) and optic nerve is described in general terms to place the development of the retrochiasmatic structures in perspective.

During the embryonic period of fetal life, specifically at 4 weeks of gestation, early vesicularization of the developing brain occurs.[1, 2] The optic pits appear on the surface of the rostral end of the developing embryo, and shortly thereafter, the optic vesicles evaginate from the prosencephalon, and the lens placode begins developing within the optic vesicle. By the end of 5 weeks of gestation, the optic vesicle has invaginated, forming the optic cup and the fetal fissure, a crease in the surface of the optic cup and stalk in which the hyaloid artery travels to vascularize the lens of the vesicle. Subsequently, early development of the various layers of the retina occurs. Within the developing retina, the axons of the ganglion cells begin to project into the optic stalk, giving rise to the first discernible structure of the optic nerve. By the end of 6 weeks of gestation, the lens capsule has formed around the lens vesicle, and progressive closure of the fetal fissure has begun.

The anlagen of the extraocular muscles begin to develop, arising from mesodermal tissues of the orbit, and by the end of 7 weeks of gestation, the fetal fissure has completely closed. At this time, the axons of the ganglion cells forming the optic nerve fibers reach the most proximal end of the optic stalk, with some crossing to form the chiasm. The lateral geniculate bodies begin to appear. The meningeal sheath surrounding the optic nerve forms and is contiguous with the dura covering the brain, as well as with the sclera enclosing the globe. Rods and cones begin to develop as a result of further retinal differentiation, and by the end of 8 weeks of gestation, retinal differentiation has progressed rapidly and the bony orbit has begun to develop. The optic stalk is entirely filled with nerve fibers, and as a result, the cavity of the optic vesicle no longer communicates with that of the forebrain. The optic chiasm is fully formed and separated from the floor of the third ventricle, with only the optic recess remaining as a remnant of the optic vesicle.

In the fetal period of intrauterine development, the optic pathway develops further, especially within the more central portions.[1, 2] By the end of 9 weeks of gestation, early differentiation of the occipital cortex is noted. At this point, the retina demonstrates a more mature, layered appearance, and by the end of 10 weeks of gestation, the optic tract has fully formed. The axons forming the optic nerve and tract reach the lateral geniculate bodies in the dorsolateral part of the mantle layer of the thalamus, and differentiation of the occipital cortex into marginal and mantle layers is completed by the end of 11 weeks of gestation, with full elaboration of the peripheral cortical layer. By the end of 16 weeks of gestation, the adult form of retinal vascularization is seen with entry of the central retinal artery via the optic nerve head, resulting from progressive atrophy of the hyaloid system.

Myelination of the optic tracts begins at the lateral geniculate nuclei at 20 weeks of gestation and proceeds peripherally in a direction opposite to that of axonal growth. The choroid now demonstrates three distinct layers. Myelination of the optic tract and chiasm continues from 24 to 28 weeks of gestation, and progressive enfolding of the calcarine cortex forming the calcarine fissure is noted. By the end of 32 weeks of gestation, all layers of the retina have been entirely formed, and the eyelids, which previously were fused, are now unfused. By the end of 36 weeks of gestation, the optic nerve has completed its myelination to the lamina cribrosa. Myelination of the optic radiations does not begin until approximately the time of birth. It then proceeds centrifugally over a 4-month period, beginning from the calcarine cortex toward the lateral geniculate bodies.

## ANATOMY OF THE VISUAL PATHWAYS

Light enters the globe via the cornea, passes through the aqueous humor, lens, and vitreous humor, and then strikes the retina, impinging on photoreceptor cells in the most posterior layer of its laminated structure. Depolarizations occur within the rods and cones, which transmit impulses to the bipolar cells in the intermediate layer of the retina. These bipolar cells are the primary afferent neurons of the visual system. Impulses are then transmitted to the ganglion cells, which lie in the more superficial anterior layer of the retina. The axons of the ganglion cells course upon the most anterior surface of the retina, converging on the posterior pole of the eye, where they initiate a 90° turn and pierce the sclera at the lamina cribrosa, coalescing to form the optic nerve. Myelination of the axons of the optic nerve occurs only within those axons that are outside the globe.[1] The axons anterior to the lamina cribrosa are not myelinated.

The optic nerves pass dorsomedially to the orbital apex, entering the skull via the optic canals.[3] They then combine at the optic chiasm, which is superior to the sella turcica in the suprasellar cistern at the base of the brain. Axons from the nasal half of the retina decussate to contribute to the contralateral optic tract, whereas axons from the temporal half of the retina remain uncrossed.

Each visual field projects on parts of both retinas, with the right visual field projected on the nasal half of the right retina and the temporal half of the left retina. A monocular crescent of the most peripheral area of the right visual field is projected only onto the nasal half of the right retina because of anatomic asymmetry, with the nasal retina being longer than the temporal retina. Fibers from both retinas, which carry information about the right visual field, combine at the optic chiasm, forming the left optic tract. Therefore the whole right visual field projects to the left hemisphere.[1]

The optic tract courses dorsolaterally around the hypothalamus and the rostral part of the cerebral peduncle within the perimesencephalic cistern, synapsing with cells of the lateral geniculate bodies (Fig. 11-1). A small number of fibers, the pupillary motor fibers, project in a medial caudal direction, forming the brachium of the superior colliculus, a projection to the superior colliculus and pretectal areas. The lateral geniculate nucleus lies in the dorsolateral aspect of the thalamus, ventral to the pulvinar and lateral to the medial geniculate body and cerebral peduncle. It is a precisely ordered six-layered structure. The contralateral half of the binocular visual field is represented in all layers of the lateral geniculate body. However, crossed and uncrossed fibers end in different layers. Crossed fibers project to layers 1, 4, and 6, whereas uncrossed fibers project to layers 2, 3, and 5.

Cell bodies of the lateral geniculate nucleus give rise to the optic radiations (geniculocalcarian tracts), which pass to the ipsilateral primary visual cortex lying on the medial aspect of the occipital lobes surrounding the calcarian sulcus (Fig. 11-1). Fibers of the optic radiations first pass through the retrolenticular part of the internal capsule (the most posterior part of the posterior limb of the internal capsule). They then arch laterally around the lateral ventricles and sweep posteromedially to synapse with cell bodies in the calcarine cortex. Fibers from the ventrolateral aspect of the lateral geniculate nucleus, carrying information from the inferior quadrant of the retina (superior visual field), sweep ventrally into the temporal lobe, pass laterally over the inferior horn of the lateral ventricle forming the so-called Myer's loop, and turn posteriorly to proceed to the calcarine cortex, inferior to the calcarine sulcus. Fibers from the dorsomedial aspect of the lateral geniculate nucleus, carrying information from the superior quadrant of the retina (inferior visual field), follow a more direct posterior course to the calcarine cortex, superior to the calcarine sulcus.

The calcarine cortex is topographically ordered in an anterior to posterior direction, as well as in a superior to inferior one.[1] The most posterior area receives information from the central (macular) visual field, the middle third receives binocular information from the contralateral visual field, and the most anterior third receives monocular information from the contralateral visual field. From the cell bodies lying within the calcarine cortex, axons project to the visual association cortex in surrounding areas.

As a result of precise topographic localization of the visual fields at each part of the visual pathway, discrete lesions can be localized clinically with a high degree of accuracy. Lesions causing interruption of the optic nerve result in monocular blindness (Fig. 11-2). Lesions interrupting the decussating fibers at the optic chiasm cause bitemporal hemianopsia (Fig. 11-3). Partial interruption of the retrochiasmal portion of the visual pathway results in incomplete hemianopsias that are localizing. With complete interruption and total homonymous hemianopsia, there is no localizing information. Interruption of the pathway at the optic tract causes contralateral homonymous hemianopsia. If the optic radiations are interrupted within the temporal lobe, a contralateral superior quadrantanopsia results (Fig. 11-4). Cortical lesions (Fig. 11-5) superior to the calcarine sulcus result in an inferior quadrantanopsia, whereas lesions inferior to the calcarine sulcus (Fig. 11-6) cause a superior quadrantanopsia. Lesions of the occipital pole result in central macular hemianopic deficits.

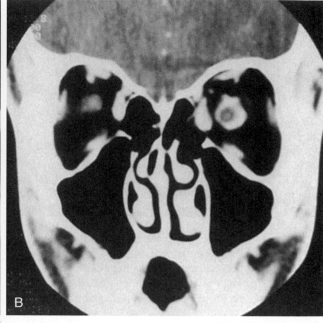

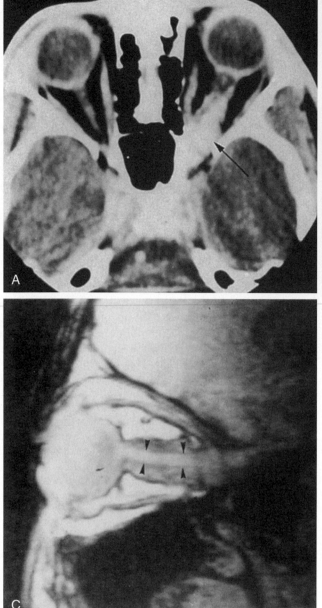

**FIGURE 11-2** Left perioptic meningioma. **A**, Axial contrast-enhanced CT scan shows a hyperdense mass (*arrow*) enlarging the optic nerve complex on the left. Note that the optic nerve appears less dense and the surrounding mass seems more dense. **B**, Coronal CT scan after injection of contrast medium shows a mass encasing the optic nerve. The mass is thicker on the lateral aspect than on the medial aspect. The patient is a 16-year-old male with neurofibromatosis. **C**, Sagittal T1-weighted image shows the optic nerve centrally (*arrowheads*), surrounded by an irregular tumor mass that extends back toward the optic foramen.

## IMAGING TECHNIQUES

The indications for imaging of the optic pathways are based on clinical findings and symptomatology, which include some form of visual loss. The rapidity of onset of visual loss suggests the type of pathologic condition responsible, whereas the specific visual field deficit suggests the location of the pathologic process within the visual pathway. In a patient under 45 years of age, sudden onset of monocular blindness, when associated with pain, suggests an optic nerve neuritis. Gradually progressive monocular blindness, especially if associated with proptosis, suggests a mass lesion such as perioptic meningioma involving the optic nerve sheath (Fig. 11-2) as one of the likely causes. The ophthalmoscopic findings of disk edema or optic atrophy are frequently associated with neoplasia and mass effect or an inflammatory process. If the finding is unilateral, the optic nerve is the likely site of involvement. However, if bilateral disk edema or optic atrophy is present, an intracranial cause is more likely. For example, papilledema is bilateral disk swelling due to increased intracranial pressure. Bitemporal hemianopsia is most commonly caused by a disease involving the optic chiasm; the most common disease is a pituitary adenoma (Fig. 11-3) that causes compression of the decussating fibers of the optic pathway. Other conditions with similar clinical findings include lesions that cause extrinsic compression of the chiasm (e.g., craniopharyngioma, meningioma, or carotid artery aneurysm) or intrinsic lesions of the chiasm, such as a chiasmatic glioma. Inflammatory conditions such as sarcoidosis, Langerhans' histiocytosis X, or tuberculosis may also involve the optic chiasm. Homonymous hemianopsia suggests a disease

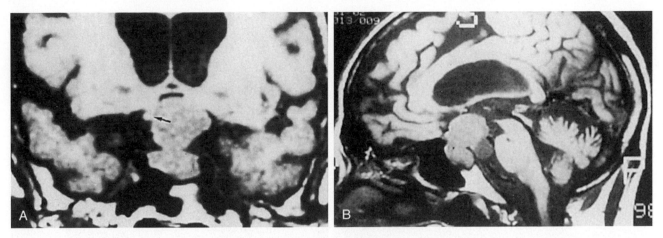

**FIGURE 11-3**   Pituitary adenoma with chiasmal compression in a 70-year-old male with bitemporal hemianopsia. **A**, Coronal T1-weighted image shows an isointense mass within the sella, expanding it to the left and extending through the diaphragma sella (site of the waist) into the suprasellar cistern. Note the compression of the right optic nerve (*arrow*). **B**, Sagittal T1-weighted image shows an intrasellar tumor mass. The optic chiasm is not distinguishable in this view.

process involving the retrochiasmatic portion of the visual pathway. Sudden onset of this visual field deficit suggests a vascular cause, whereas more gradual development suggests a mass lesion as the cause. If the deficit is incomplete and congruent (equally involving the superior and inferior quadrants of the contralateral visual field), the lesion is likely to lie within the calcarine cortex of the occipital lobe (Fig. 11-5). If the deficit is incomplete and incongruous, the lesion is likely to involve optic tracts, or it may lie either in the temporal lobe involving Meyer's loop (superior quadrantinopsia) (Fig. 11-4) or in the parietal lobe (inferior quadrantinopsia) (Fig. 11-7).

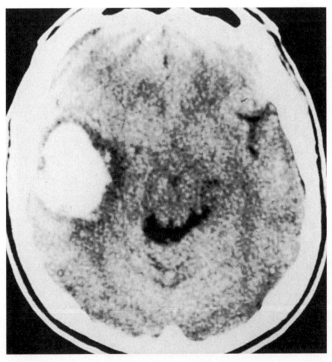

**FIGURE 11-4**   Temporal lobe hematoma. Axial CT image shows a hyperdense mass in the anterior aspect of the right temporal lobe.

CT evaluation of the visual pathway should be obtained with intravenous contrast enhancement unless the patient has experienced recent trauma or has a history of severe contrast reaction, or unless a foreign body, hemorrhage, or infarction along the course of the visual pathway is suspected. Axially oriented 5-mm-thick, contiguous CT sections should be obtained from the foramen magnum to the orbital floor; then 2-mm-thick sections should be obtained from the orbital floor to the orbital roof.[4] The remainder of the head can be imaged with contiguous 5-mm-thick scans. Coronal contiguous images 2 mm thick should be obtained with the patient's neck in maximally tolerated extension. The anatomic region included should extend from the dorsum of the sella to the anterior aspect of the globe and should include the sella turcica and the orbit.[5] A 20-cm field of view should be used for the axial images, with subsequent magnification of the orbital region to maximally display any pathology in the area. The coronal images should be obtained with a 12- to 15-cm field of view.

In general, MR imaging is the modality of choice for visualization of the elements of the visual pathway, except in patients with a history of trauma or when a fracture or foreign body with unknown ferromagnetic properties is suspected.[6-9] Once a modality for imaging has been chosen, the imaging protocol may be specifically altered to visualize optimally the region of the optic pathway most likely to contain the pathologic condition.

MR imaging of the elements of the optic pathway involves the use of a head coil. A dedicated orbit surface coil can be utilized to evaluate intraorbital lesions. Using the head coil, axial and coronal images with a TR of 500 to 800 msec and a TE of 20 msec should be obtained. Scans 3 mm thick, with no interscan space, one excitation, a 256 × 256 matrix, and a 14-cm field of view optimally display the structures of the orbit.[6, 10] The remainder of the intracranial optic pathway may be imaged using a sagittal TR 600, TE 20 spin-echo sequence with 5-mm-thick images, a 22-cm field of view, two excitations, and a 256 × 256 matrix. This should be followed by an axial study using a TR of 6000 and a TE of 100 msec, 5-mm-thick slices, one or two excitations,

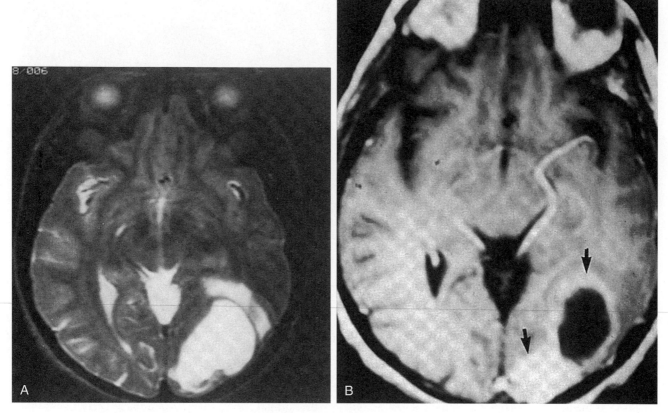

**FIGURE 11-5**   Occipital lobe metastasis from carcinoma of the lung. **A**, Axial T2-weighted image shows hyperintense mass in the left temporal occipital region; a point of separation exists between the most posterior portion of the mass and the anterior segment of high signal intensity edema in adjacent white matter. **B**, Axial T1-weighted image after injection of contrast medium shows tumor enhancement (*arrows*).

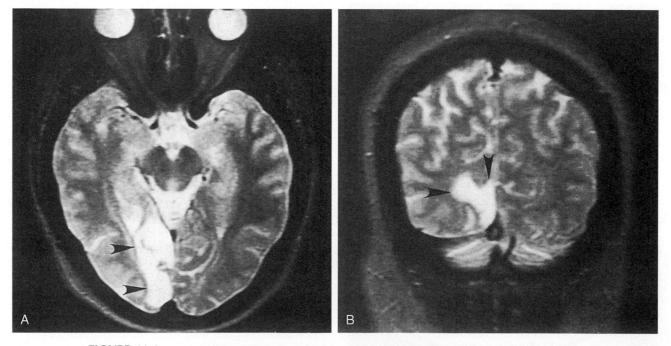

**FIGURE 11-6**   **A**, Axial T2-weighted image shows a high signal intensity occipital infarct (*arrowheads*). **B**, Coronal T2-weighted image. The infarct (*arrowheads*) lies below the calcarine fissure.

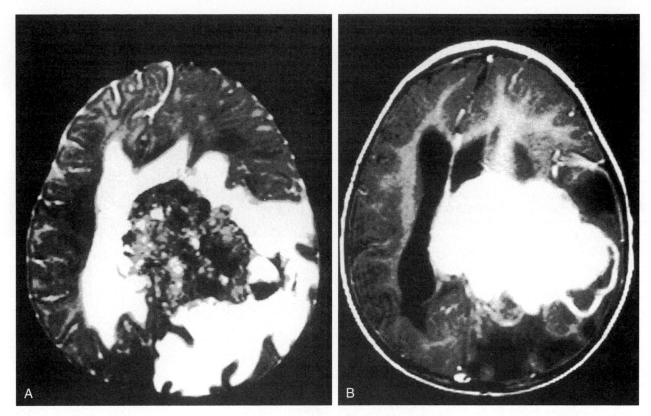

**FIGURE 11-7**   Choroid plexus carcinoma. Lateral ventricle, left side, invading the brain and producing right inferior quadrantic hemianopsia. **A**, Axial T2-weighted image shows a mass that is predominantly low in signal intensity, on its lateral margin is surrounded by vasogenic edema within the left cerebral hemisphere, and on its medial margin is within the displaced body of the left lateral ventricle. **B**, Axial T1-weighted image after gadolinium injection shows marked enhancement of the tumor mass.

a 512 × 512 matrix, and a 20-cm field of view.[8, 11] Techniques designed to suppress the signal from the orbital fat make pathologic conditions involving the optic nerve more visible and may be useful when subtle lesions are suspected.[12, 13] One such sequence involves the use of inversion recovery imaging (STIR).[14] Such a technique uses a TR of 2500, a TE of between 30 and 60, a TI of 150, two excitations, a 256 × 256 matrix, 3-mm-thick images, and a 1-mm interscan space. Fat suppressed, T2-weighted spin-echo images with a 256 × 256 matrix and a 2-mm slice thickness in the axial and coronal planes are also useful. In fluid attenuated inversion recovery imaging (FLAIR) the high signal of cerebrospinal fluid (CSF) is suppressed, while showing the abnormal high signal of increased water in pathologic tissue such as plaques of multiple sclerosis or areas of acute infarction.[15] FLAIR imaging can be obtained with turbo sequences in 3 minutes with a 256 × 256 matrix, one acquisition, and a 5-mm slice thickness. A typical pulse sequence uses a TR of 9000 msec, a TE of 120 msec, and a TI of 2200 msec. Contrast enhancement achieved with intravenous administration of gadolinium diethylenetri-aminepentaacetic acid (DTPA) in a dose of 1 mmol/kg has demonstrated clinical utility in diagnosing both intraorbital and intracranial pathologic conditions, including neoplasms and inflammatory or infectious conditions. The use of fat-saturated, T1-weighted images with gadolinium enhancement in the axial (Fig. 11-8) and coronal (Fig. 11-9) planes is currently the procedure of choice for detecting

abnormal enhancement of the optic nerve or surrounding tissues.

## NORMAL CT AND MR IMAGING ANATOMY

The normal intraorbital optic nerve/sheath complex is well visualized on axial and coronal CT because of the natural contrast between it and the surrounding retrobulbar adipose tissue.[14] The normal optic nerves appear symmetric and homogeneous. The normal diameter of the nerve is 3 to 5 mm (average, 4.5 mm) on axial scans and 4 to 6 mm (average, 5 mm) on coronal scans.[4, 16] The intracanalicular portion of the optic nerve is poorly visualized with CT because of beam-hardening artifact from the surrounding bony canal. Unless intrathecal contrast material is used,[5, 17] the intracranial portion of the nerve, as well as the optic chiasm and optic tract, are poorly visualized on CT because of inadequate contrast between the CSF and the neural tissues.[5] Without contrast material in the CSF, the location of the intracranial portion of the nerve, the optic chiasm, and the optic tract is inferred on the basis of knowledge of their anatomic location relative to adjacent structures such as the suprasellar cistern, hypothalamus, medial aspect of the temporal lobes, and lateral aspect of the midbrain. The position of the lateral geniculate nucleus (LGN) is inferred by localizing the pulvinar of the thalamus, since the LGN is not directly visualized on CT. The optic radiations also are not directly seen, but their expected location may be inferred by observing the appropriate area of the temporal lobe adjacent to the temporal horn of the lateral ventricle and the parietal lobe adjacent to the atrium of the lateral ventricle. The most distal portion of the optic radiation can also be inferred by its position relative to the occipital horns of the lateral ventricles. The calcarine cortex is directly visualized along the medial aspect of the occipital lobes.

On MR imaging, using spin-echo short TR/TE (600/20) and long TR/short TE (3000/30) sequences, the intraorbital optic nerve demonstrates signal intensity similar to that of cerebral white matter.[5] It is of low signal intensity relative to the high signal intensity of the retrobulbar adipose tissue. On spin-echo long TR/long TE (3000/90) images, the optic nerve has a signal intensity similar to that of orbital fat; however, often a small amount of high signal intensity CSF can be visualized in the subarachnoid space between the nerve sheath and the optic nerve. On turbo spin-echo long TR/long TE (6000/1000) images, the high signal intensity CSF outlines the optic nerve. The intracanalicular portion of the optic nerve is well visualized on MR imaging because of the absence of signal from the cortical bone forming the optic canal.[6] Short TR/short TE imaging sequences, particularly in the coronal projection, display the intracranial portion of the optic nerve as a relatively higher signal intensity structure within the lower signal intensity CSF of the suprasellar cistern.[18] The optic chiasm and optic tracts demonstrate similar characteristics and are best visualized in either the coronal or sagittal plane.[19] The LGN occasionally may be seen on long TR/long TE images as a high signal intensity nuclear aggregation. More commonly, the LGN is seen as a contour arising from the diencephalon and protruding into the ambiens cistern adjacent to the thalamus. The optic radiation may be seen as cerebral white matter intensity structures within the temporoparietal and occipital lobes; their course is inferred by knowledge of the anatomic location of this portion of the optic pathway. The calcarine cortex may be directly observed on either coronal, axial, or sagittal short or long TR images. The two gyri making up the

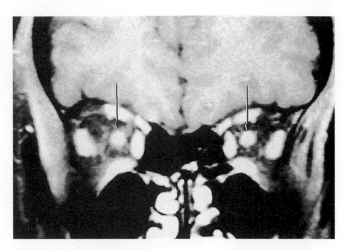

**FIGURE 11-9** Multiple sclerosis in a 16-year-old female with bilateral scotomata and evidence of acute optic neuritis on fundoscopic examination. Coronal fat-suppressed, gadolinium-enhanced, T1-weighted MR image shows bilateral enlargement and enhancement of the intraorbital optic nerves (*arrows*).

primary visual cortex may be positively identified, since they are easily seen flanking the calcarine sulcus.

## PATHOLOGIC CONDITIONS

### Optic Nerve Visual Pathway Glioma

Gliomas of the optic nerve or visual pathway are relatively uncommon low-grade neoplasms that can involve various portions of the retrobulbar visual pathway, including the optic nerve, chiasm, optic tracts, and radiations. These tumors appear most frequently during the first decade of life, and there is a slight female preponderance. There is also an association between optic nerve gliomas and intracranial visual pathway gliomas and neurofibromatosis type 1.

#### *Clinical Findings*

Optic nerve gliomas constitute approximately 3% of all orbital tumors; they outnumber perioptic meningiomas by approximately 4 to 1.[10] Optic nerve gliomas occur most frequently in the first decade of life (median age, 5 years); however, they may be present at birth and have been reported in patients as old as 60 years of age.[20, 21] They may occur at any point in the retrobulbar visual pathway, including the optic nerve, chiasm, or optic tract, lateral geniculate bodies, and optic radiations.[20–22] Involvement of the optic chiasm coexistent with gliomas of both optic nerves is more common than involvement of a single optic nerve.[20] Bilateral optic nerve gliomas imply neurofibromatosis type 1. Invasion of the globe by the tumor, although extremely rare, has been observed.[21]

Approximately 15% or more of patients with optic nerve gliomas demonstrate the findings of neurofibromatosis at the time of diagnosis (range, 12% to 38%).[20, 21] Visual pathway gliomas appear early in life, often before the clinical stigmata of neurofibromatosis become evident.

The clinical picture of patients with optic nerve gliomas depends on whether the primary involvement is orbital or intracranial. Intraorbital gliomas usually appear early, with

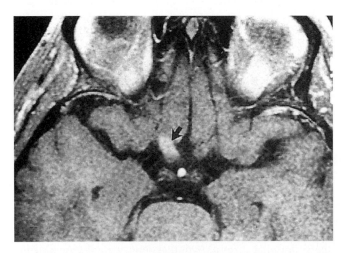

**FIGURE 11-8** Multiple sclerosis in a 34-year-old woman with monocular visual loss of the right eye of recent origin. Axial fat-suppressed, gadolinium-enhanced, T1-weighted image shows enhancement of the enlarged right intracranial optic nerve (*arrow*).

painless proptosis. Globe motility usually is not restricted. Optic atrophy is the most frequent ophthalmoscopic finding, with occasional disc edema.[20] Loss of or decreased vision occurs and may progress to total loss of vision. Occasionally, peripheral visual constriction may be observed. Clinically, intraobital optic nerve glioma and meningioma are difficult to differentiate.[21]

Intracranial visual pathway gliomas generally appear with symptoms related to the portion of the brain that is involved. These symptoms include seizures, nystagmus, hydrocephalus, and changes in mental status. Loss of vision is the most common initial symptom.[20] The presence of nystagmus is highly suspicious for chiasmal involvement.

### Pathologic Findings

The cell of origin for optic nerve gliomas has not been definitively elucidated; thus, these neoplasms are included in the general classification as gliomas. Specifically, they are usually classified as grade I astrocytomas (juvenile pilocytic astrocytomas).[20, 22] The tumors are slow-growing, with no tendency to metastasize. Malignant transformation does not occur in childhood gliomas. Development of optic nerve gliomas is observed to occur in stages, from generalized hyperplasia of the glial cells within the nerve to complete disorganization with loss of landmarks within the nerve and the nerve sheath. The tumor usually causes smooth fusiform enlargement of the optic nerve (Fig. 11-10), although it may be somewhat asymmetric with respect to the nerve. A reactive meningeal hyperplasia may be incited, which extends beyond the position of the tumor itself, making it difficult to differentiate it from a perioptic meningioma.[22] Microscopically, the tumor is composed of round, spindle-shaped cells similar in appearance to those of the normal optic nerve. Because no mitoses are present, the tumors do not enlarge by cell division, but rather by hyperplasia of adjacent glial connective tissue and meninges, with

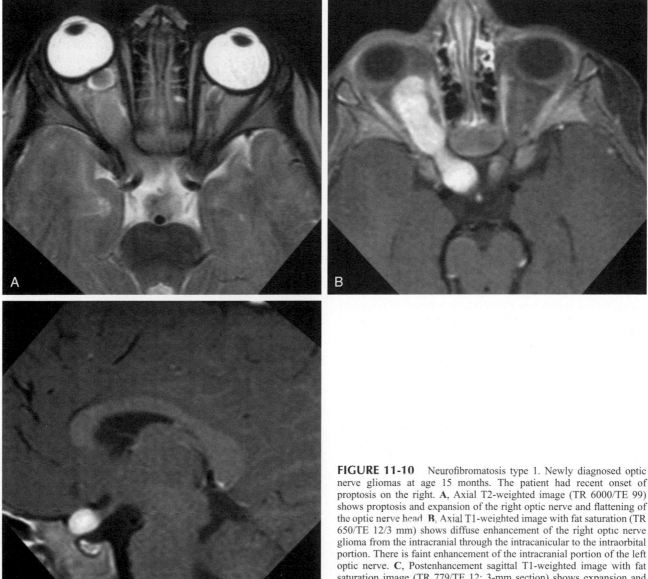

**FIGURE 11-10**   Neurofibromatosis type 1. Newly diagnosed optic nerve gliomas at age 15 months. The patient had recent onset of proptosis on the right. **A,** Axial T2-weighted image (TR 6000/TE 99) shows proptosis and expansion of the right optic nerve and flattening of the optic nerve head. **B,** Axial T1-weighted image with fat saturation (TR 650/TE 12/3 mm) shows diffuse enhancement of the right optic nerve glioma from the intracranial through the intracanicular to the intraorbital portion. There is faint enhancement of the intracranial portion of the left optic nerve. **C,** Postenhancement sagittal T1-weighted image with fat saturation image (TR 779/TE 12; 3-mm section) shows expansion and enhancement of the intracranial optic nerve just proximal to the optic canal. The chiasm is uninvolved.

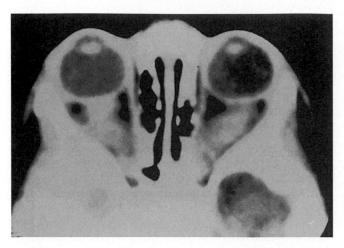

**FIGURE 11-11** Bilateral optic gliomas with neurofibromatosis. Axial contrast CT scan shows bilateral enlargement and enhancement of optic nerve gliomas.

production of intracellular and extracellular mucopolysaccharides.

### CT Appearance

Optic nerve gliomas may be unilateral or bilateral.[23] Unenhanced CT of these tumors typically demonstrates a marked diffuse, often fusiform, enlargement of an optic nerve, often with a characteristic kinking or buckling.[21, 24] Within the tumor, areas of lucency caused by mucinous or cystic changes may be observed, but calcification is not found in unirradiated optic nerve gliomas. Following administration of a contrast medium, a moderate to intense enhancement of the tumor is often observed, frequently containing irregular parenchymal lucencies.[21, 24] Bilateral optic nerve gliomas are thought to be characteristic of neurofibromatosis type 1 (Figs. 11-10 and 11-11).[24] Extension of the tumor through the optic foramen commonly results in enlargement of the optic canal. When the epicenter of the tumor involves the optic chiasm, both anterior and posterior components of the glioma may be seen. Such involvement is helpful in differentiating among lesions of the chiasm. Whatever imaging study is done, it must adequately evaluate the entire visual pathway, because frequently not only the optic nerve and chiasm but also the retrochiasmatic visual pathways are involved.[6]

### MR Imaging Appearance

When evaluating the visual pathways (specifically the optic nerves) for optic nerve glioma, thin sections (3 mm or less) should be obtained, because excessive slice thickness may make lesions inapparent as a result of volume averaging.[23, 25] Precise anatomic definition of optic nerve gliomas is generally superior on MR imaging compared with CT, especially where the lesion passes through the optic canal (Figs. 11-10 and 11-12).[22] Sagittal MR imaging may give information not available with standard axial or coronal CT scanning techniques. In addition, the sensitivity of MR imaging to extensive visual pathway gliomas with involvement of the chiasm, optic tracts, lateral geniculate bodies, and optic radiations is much greater than that of CT (Fig. 11-12).[26] On MR imaging, a lesion involving the optic nerve

is generally well defined, showing enlargement of the nerve (Fig. 11-10). On short TR/TE images, optic nerve gliomas are usually isointense to cortex and hypointense to white matter. Invariably they are hypointense to orbital fat. On long TR/TE images, the lesions demonstrate a mixed to homogeneous appearance that is hyperintense to white matter, cortex, and orbital fat.[27] Following administration of gadolinium contrast material, increased signal intensity on short TR/TE images is often seen (Figs. 11-10 and 11-12). The MR appearance of optic glioma is somewhat variable, depending on whether the tumor grows within the optic nerve (Fig. 11-12) or grows around the optic nerve into the perineural space. In the latter case, when the perineural portion enhances, it may mimic the perioptic meningioma and may be misdiagnosed, especially in the adolescent or adult patient. Intrinsic masses within the optic nerve, such as occult vascular malformations (Fig. 11-13), can be differentiated from intrinsic optic glioma by the presence of blood products on long TR images.

## Perioptic Meningioma

Perioptic meningiomas are benign tumors arising from the meningoendothelial cells of the arachnoid. The rests from which these cells arise occur in a variety of locations within both the orbit and the cranial vault. Intraorbital meningiomas occur at the orbital apex, along the course of the optic nerve sheath, or unrelated to the optic nerve, usually in the extraconal space from the periosteum of the orbital wall.[21] Meningiomas make up approximately 5% to 7% of all primary orbital tumors, are more common in females than in males (4 to 1), and appear most frequently in the fourth and fifth decades of life (median age, 38 years).[28] They may occur in children (25% in the first decade), and they are much more frequent in patients with neurofibromatosis type 2 than in the general population.

### Clinical Findings

The symptoms the patient displays depend on the size of the tumor and its location within the orbit. Small intracanalicular perioptic meningiomas may be difficult to detect and yet may cause significant visual symptomatology. Proptosis and visual loss are the usual symptoms in patients with perioptic meningiomas.[29] Disk elevation, optic atrophy with central or peripheral scotomata, or both are commonly seen because of the tumor's proximity to the optic nerve. Tumors that occur within the optic canal frequently appear with central scotomata, often without other symptoms.[29]

### Pathologic Findings

Of the various histologic types of meningioma, the meningothelial variety is the most common within the orbit. Microscopically, the tumor consists of solid sheets of distinctively central vacuolated cells, with rare mitoses. Within the orbit, other histologic types of meningioma such as fibroblastic, transitional, syncytial, psammomatous, and angioblastic varieties are much less common. The rare orbital angioblastic meningioma is difficult to differentiate from hemangioblastoma and hemangiopericytoma.[24] Regardless of the histology, perioptic meningiomas in children tend to be more aggressive than those in adults. These

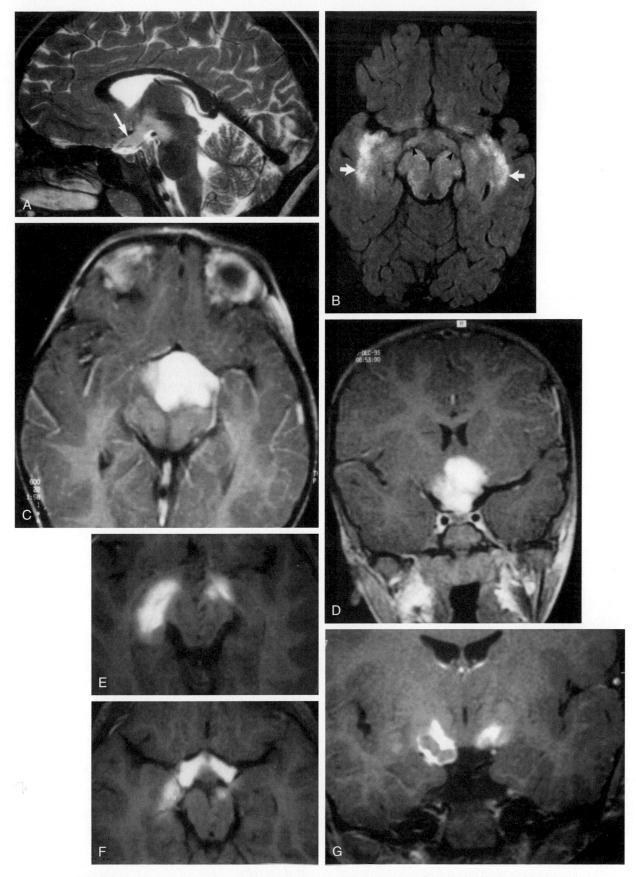

**FIGURE 11-12**   Visual pathway gliomas. **A**, Sagittal T2-weighted image in a 6-year-old male shows high signal intensity of an enlarged optic chiasm (*arrow*). Tumor extends posteriorly up against the brainstem and superiorly into the hypothalamus. **B**, FLAIR image in a 3-year-old female with neurofibromatosis type 1, shows involvement of the optic chiasm and optic tracts (*arrowheads*), as well as the brainstem and both medial temporal lobes (Meyer's loops) (*arrows*). **C** and **D**, Chiasmatic hypothalamic astrocytoma; **C**, T1-weighted axial image after contrast injection shows diffuse enhancement of the mass, as does the coronal image in **D**. **E** to **G**, Optic tract extension of chiasmatic glioma in a 6-year-old male with neurofibromatosis type 1. **E** and **F**, Axial T1-weighted, fat-suppressed images show contrast-enhanced tumor extending posteriorly from the chiasm into both optic tracts. Coronal T1-weighted, fat-suppressed image shows the right optic tract to be more involved than the left.

childhood tumors are often only partially encapsulated and have a propensity to grow by infiltration, breaking through the dura and involving other orbital structures. Orbital meningiomas, when adjacent to the bony wall, may induce a reactive hyperostosis, whereas those at or near the orbital apex may cause demineralization with enlargement of the optic canal.[28] Optic atrophy with a decrease in the number of axons within the nerve results from compression of the nerve by the tumor. The tumor grows either as an eccentric mass along one side of the optic nerve or as a circumferential lesion. Intratumoral psammomatous calcifications may be present, particularly within highly cellular areas of the tumor.

### CT Appearance

On CT, perioptic meningiomas (Fig. 11-2) appear either as a localized eccentric mass at the orbital apex[14] or as a well-defined tubular thickening (64%) or fusiform enlargement (23%) of the optic nerve sheath complex.[21, 30–32] Stippled calcification within the tumor is common (Fig. 11-2), helping to differentiate it from the optic nerve glioma. Secondary enlargement of the optic canal, with bony hyperostosis, may be seen if the tumor is located in the appropriate position.[21, 24] Because the detection of calcification and bony change is helpful in making the diagnosis of perioptic meningioma, a noncontrast-enhanced CT scan with very thin sections (1 mm) may be considered superior to nonenhanced MR imaging in evaluating small perioptic lesions.[26] After administration of a contrast medium with CT, moderate to marked enhancement of the tumor is seen. The so-called tram-track sign of perioptic meningioma is caused by uniform enhancement of a circumferential meningioma (Fig. 11-3). This may simulate dural inflammation, a finding that may be present in cases of optic neuritis and idiopathic inflammatory pseudotumor.

### MR Imaging Appearance

MR imaging displays the tumor as an abnormally enlarged optic nerve silhouette. Signal characteristics depend on the pulse sequence. On short as well as long TR/TE scans, perioptic meningiomas show diminished signal intensity relative to normal brain tissue.[21] Relative to orbital fat, on short TR/TE images the lesions are hypointense, whereas on long TR/TE images they are isointense. The calcifications within the tumor may be visualized as regions of signal void on MR imaging; however, most frequently intratumoral calcification is not seen. MR imaging may show meningiomatous bone involvement as a region of absence of the expected signal void within an area of cortical bone.[33] Chemical shift artifact, resulting in a dark line on one side of the optic nerve, may mimic calcification. Similarly, the subarachnoid space within the optic nerve sheath may appear dark on appropriate pulse sequences, mimicking circumferential calcification. This may be ruled out by using an appropriate pulse sequence designed to increase the signal intensity of CSF.[6] Gadolinium has become critical (Fig. 11-14B)[33] in the diagnosis of small perioptic tumors. Fat suppression is necessary with thin (2- to 3-mm) T1-weighted images in order to separate the enhancing tumor from the intraconal fat (Fig. 11-15).

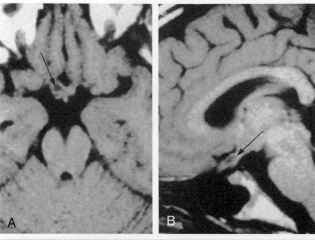

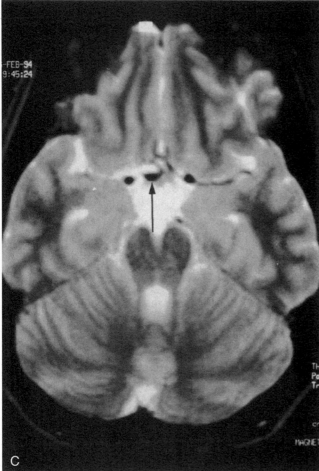

**FIGURE 11-13**   Occult vascular malformation of the right optic nerve in an 18-year-old female with monocular visual loss in the right eye for more than 1 year. The patient was referred with the diagnosis of right optic glioma. **A** and **B**, Axial and sagittal T1-weighted images without gadolinium enhancement show a hypointense, cystic expansion (*arrow*) of the intracranial portion of the optic nerve. **C**, Axial T2-weighted image shows hypointense blood (*arrow*), dependent within the cyst, the supernatant within the cyst being hyperintense. The findings are consistent with an occult vascular malformation. The same findings were present 1 year before this examination.

## Sarcoidosis

Sarcoidosis is a granulomatous disease of unknown cause that involves several organ systems, most commonly

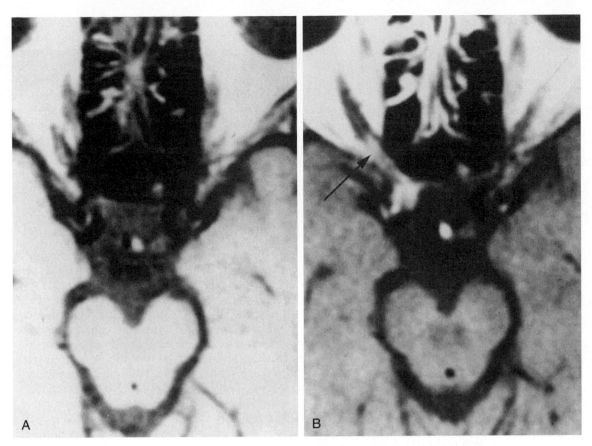

**FIGURE 11-14**   Perioptic meningioma. **A**, Axial T1-weighted image before administration of gadolinium shows no specific abnormality. **B**, Axial T1-weighted image after intravenous administration of gadolinium shows enhancement of tumor (*arrow*) that extends from the region of the anterior clinoid process on the right, through the optic canal, and along the optic nerve. Surgery revealed a perioptic meningioma.

mediastinal and peripheral lymph nodes, lungs, liver, spleen, skin, eyes, and lacrimal glands.[28, 34, 35] Pathologically, it is characterized by noncaseating granulomas, which may occur in any tissue or organ of the body. Ophthalmic changes caused by sarcoidosis occur in up to 60% of cases.[34] The most frequently involved area within the orbit is the lacrimal gland; however, infiltration may be seen in any orbital structure.[33, 36]

### Clinical Findings

Two clinical presentations of sarcoidosis are noted. The subacute form generally occurs in patients under 30 years of age, particularly in women of Swedish, Puerto Rican, and Irish descent, and is characterized by rapid appearance of erythema nodosum, possibly with accompanying polyarthritis in association with bilateral hilar adenopathy. The second form is a chronic disease that affects patients over 30 years of age; the pulmonary parenchyma is involved, and the disease spreads beyond the thorax.[28] In general, the disease is seen predominantly in African Americans 20 to 40 years of age.[34] Patients with subacute sarcoidosis tend to exhibit peripheral and cranial nerve involvement, with the seventh cranial nerve most commonly involved and the optic nerve next most commonly affected. Involvement of the third, fourth, or sixth cranial nerves may produce extraocular muscle palsies. In the chronic form of sarcoidosis, CNS involvement is more common than peripheral nerve involvement, and the optic nerve is much more frequently

affected than in the subacute form (recall that the optic nerve is an extension of a central brain tract and not a peripheral nerve). Optic nerve sarcoidosis may occur intracranially, with chiasmal involvement, or in the intracanalicular or intraorbital portions, and optic nerve involvement in this form of the disease may lead to optic atrophy.

Anterior uveitis, the most frequent sign of sarcoidosis, is characteristic of the subacute form of sarcoidosis, whereas a nonspecific granulomatous uveitis occasionally accompanied by cataract or secondary glaucoma is more indicative of the chronic form. Intracranial sarcoidosis is clinically evident in 5% of the cases, whereas 15% of autopsy cases demonstrate CNS involvement.[2] These patients may exhibit papilledema, disk edema secondary to increased intracranial pressure. Optic atrophy may be present as a result of inflammation of the optic nerve, compression by sarcoid granuloma, infarction due to sarcoid vasculitis, or glaucoma caused by intraocular inflammation.

### Pathologic Findings

The basic lesion of sarcoidosis is a noncaseating epithelioid cell tubercle. Langerhans' giant cells are seen interspersed within the epithelioid cells centrally, and a thin rim of lymphocytes rings the individual tubercles. Inclusion bodies are characteristically seen within the giant cells in the tubercle. Although, as part of their natural course, the sarcoid granulomas may disappear without any evidence of scarring, they usually heal with sclerosis at the margins of the tubercles, and calcification does not occur during the healing process.[28]

Intracranial involvement by sarcoidosis generally occurs in one of two patterns. The most common one is granulomatous leptomeningitis with involvement of the leptomeninges, including those investing the optic nerves. The second pattern is that of coalescence of sarcoid nodules into distinct parenchymal brain masses.[37] In the leptomeninges, the cranial nerves, pituitary gland, third ventricle, hypothalamus, and (in rare cases) pineal gland are involved.[33, 38] Hydrocephalus may result from sarcoid lesions of the aqueduct, fourth ventricular outlet foramina, or basal meninges, occasionally resulting in vessel obstruction with subsequent infarction.[39]

### CT Appearance

Diffuse infiltration of the leptomeninges is the most common CT finding. On the unenhanced study, areas of diffuse, irregularly increased attenuation along the leptomeninges may be seen. However, a normal study is the most frequent finding.[34, 40, 41] With orbital involvement the lacrimal gland may be enlarged, and irregular thickening of the meninges of the optic nerve may be present. Brain parenchymal involvement produces discrete nodules that, on an unenhanced CT scan, may be isodense or slightly hyperdense to the surrounding normal parenchyma. The nodules may be multiple or singular or may even form large, discrete masses upon coalescence. Surrounding edema is usually not present. Following administration of a contrast medium, diffuse, irregular enhancement along the basal cisterns can be seen. The borders of the cortical sulci may enhance similarly as a result of leptomeningeal spread within the perivascular spaces of Virchow-Robin.[34] Homogeneous enhancement of parenchymal nodules also occurs after administration of the contrast medium.[34, 39, 42] Obstructive hydrocephalus may be seen when structures adjacent to the third ventricle or the aqueduct or the outlet foramina of the fourth ventricle are involved. Cranial nerve involvement generally produces fusiform or irregular enlargement of the nerve with homogeneous enhancement after administration of contrast medium.[34] Compression or direct invasion of the cranial nerves may occur as a consequence of infiltration of the basal meninges. Calcification is not a feature of sarcoidosis.[38]

### MR Imaging Appearance

Orbital sarcoidosis is evaluated well with MR imaging, which demonstrates a high degree of anatomic detail not seen with CT, particularly in areas where image degradation occurs on CT caused by beam-hardening artifact (i.e., in the intracanalicular and intracranial portions of the optic nerve).[43–47] MR imaging demonstrates sarcoid involvement of the optic nerve as diffuse enlargement of the optic nerve sheath complex of a variable signal intensity that is usually isointense to extraocular muscle on short TR/TE images and minimally hyperintense to orbital fat on long TR/TE images (Fig. 11-16).[33, 36, 48] Lacrimal gland involvement by sarcoid is generally seen as diffuse enlargement of the gland with a signal intensity pattern that may be either low or high on long TR/TE images.[33, 36] The two major pathologic changes of intracranial sarcoid are well demonstrated by MR imaging. They consist of abnormal tissue involving the meninges (Figs. 11-17 and 11-18) and the brain parenchyma (Fig. 11-16) in addition to

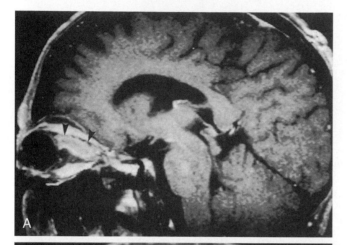

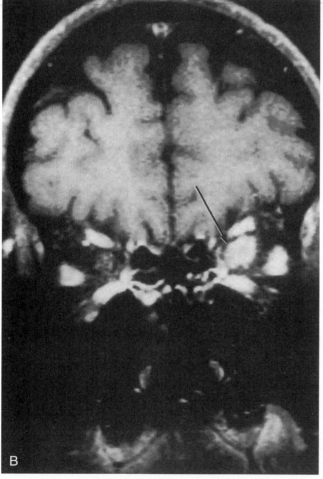

**FIGURE 11-15** Perioptic meningioma in a 53-year-old male with left monocular visual loss and evidence of optic atrophy on fundoscopic examination. Symptoms had been progressive over a number of years. **A,** Oblique sagittal, fat-suppressed, gadolinium-enhanced T1-weighted MR image shows a mass (*arrowheads*) surrounding the optic nerve, extending from the globe back to the optic canal. **B,** Coronal fat-suppressed, T1-weighted, gadolinium-enhanced MR image shows that the left optic nerve (complex) is enlarged and enhancing (*arrow*).

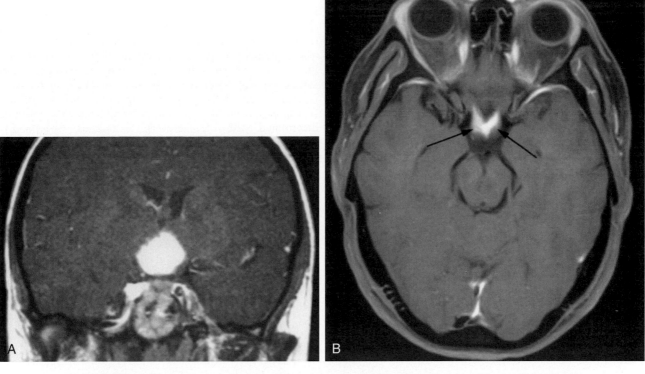

**FIGURE 11-16**    Sarcoidosis involving the hypothalamus and/or the optic chiasm. **A**, A 16-year-old female with hypothalamic dysfunction and visual impairment. Contrast-enhanced, T1-weighted coronal image shows a large enhancing mass. **B**, A 26-year-old female with chiasmatic and bilateral intracranial optic nerve involvement by sarcoid. Fat-suppressed, axial T1-weighted image after contrast injection shows enhancement of the areas of involvement (*arrows*).

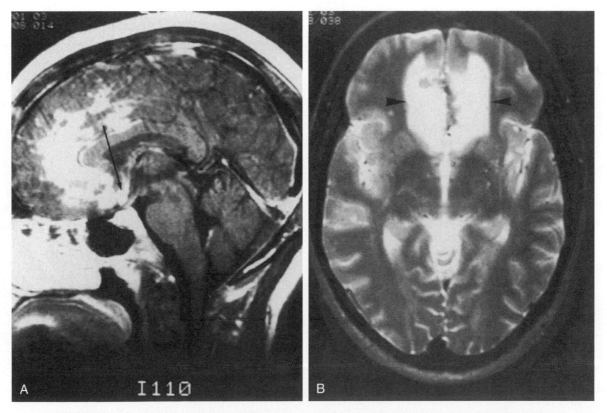

**FIGURE 11-17**    Leptomeningeal sarcoidosis. **A**, Sagittal T1-weighted image after injection of contrast material shows marked enhancement of leptomeninges between the frontal lobes, extending along the corpus callosum, and down onto the surface of the optic chiasm (*arrow*). **B**, Axial T2-weighted image shows bifrontal edema (*arrowheads*) within the cortex and white matter of the frontal lobes at the site of leptomeningeal involvement by sarcoid.

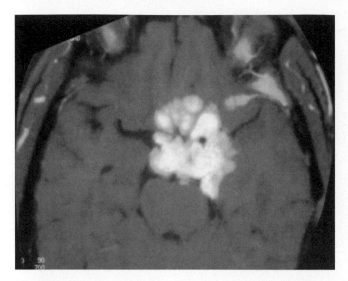

**FIGURE 11-18** Leptomeningeal sarcoidosis presenting as a mass in a 45-year-old female with encasement of the chiasm and optic nerves. T1-weighted axial, fat-suppressed image after gadolinium injection. Except for the nodularity of the mass, its appearance mimicked a meningioma of the lesser wing of the sphenoid.

intensity and is also a common location for visualization of abnormal sarcoid tissue. The parenchymal regions of sarcoidosis also have similar signal characteristics. MR imaging has greater sensitivity than CT for detecting regions of sarcoidosis, [45, 50] and the hydrocephalus associated with sarcoid involvement of the CSF pathway is clearly identified with MR imaging. The site of obstruction responsible for the hydrocephalus may also be determined with MR imaging techniques. Specifically, the absence of a flow void sign within the aqueduct or within the foramina of Magendie or Luschka may indicate these to be the primary sites of obstruction.[51] The use of gadolinium in evaluating sarcoid has proven helpful in demonstrating the extent of meningeal involvement (Figs. 11-17 and 11-18). However, the MR appearance of leptomeningeal sarcoid is not specific; a similar picture may be seen with tuberculosis and other bacterial meningitides such as pneumococcal meningitis (Figs. 11-19 and 11-20). In these circumstances, the clinical picture as well as CSF laboratory studies are important in the differential diagnosis.

hydrocephalus and small areas of infarction.[49] Meningeal involvement by sarcoid tissue is most commonly seen in the region of the basal cisterns as focal areas of high signal intensity tissue on long TR/TE images (Fig. 11-17B). However, the signal intensity characteristics may vary, and the tissue occasionally may be hypointense to normal brain parenchyma on long TR/TE images. Periventricular involvement demonstrates similar signal

## Lyme Disease

Lyme disease is a worldwide tick-transmitted spirochetosis with endemic foci in North America and Europe. The spirochete is *Borrelia burgdorferi*, and the ticks that transmit the disease infect both deer and white-footed mice.

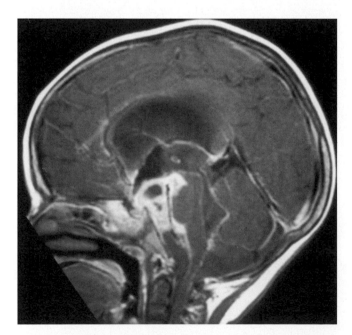

**FIGURE 11-19** Tuberculous meningitis. Infant with hydrocephalus and cranial nerve palsies. Sagittal T1-weighted image after gadolinium injection shows a contrast-enhancing suprasellar subarachnoid collection encasing the chiasm and anterior brainstem. Findings are consistent with granulomatous meningitis at the base of the brain.

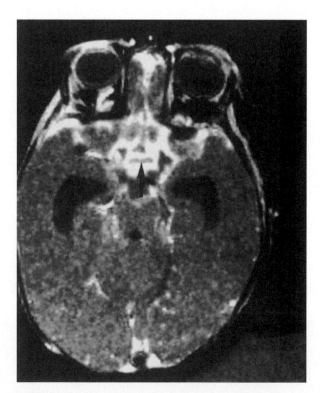

**FIGURE 11-20** Pneumococcal meningitis in a comatose 1-year-old infant with hydrocephalus. Axial thin-section, postgadolinium injection, T1-weighted scan shows that the optic chiasm (*arrow*) is coated by a contrast-enhancing subarachnoid infiltrate. Note that the temporal horns are markedly dilated secondary to hydrocephalus.

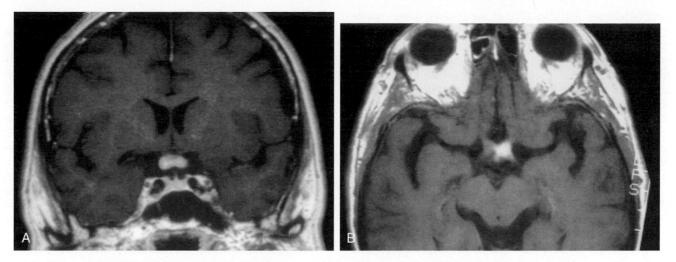

**FIGURE 11-21**   Lyme disease involving the optic chiasm in a 66-year-old female. Coronal (**A**) and axial (**B**) T1-weighted images after contrast injection show enhancement and enlargement of the optic chiasm. **A** is before treatment and **B** is 1 week after the beginning of treatment, showing some response to antibiotic therapy.

## Clinical Findings

A bite by an infected tick can result in Lyme disease, causing a variety of manifestations, including arthritis, rash, cardiac manifestations and CNS involvement in 15% to 20% of cases.[52] In the CNS, cranial neuropathies (facial palsy, 80%), meningitis, headache, and cerebral parenchymal involvement resulting in mental changes can occur. [52]

## Pathologic Findings

Lymphoplasmacytic perivascular and meningitic infiltration has been recognized in association with a CSF lymphomonocytic pleocytosis. Beyond these manifestations the CNS findings have not been well described pathologically.

## CT Appearance

The CT findings that have been recognized are those occurring in the white matter as areas of hypodensity mimicking the lesions of multiple sclerosis. CT is not reliable in recognizing the cranial nerve findings seen on MR imaging as focal enlargement and contrast enhancement.

## MR Imaging Appearance

The MR imaging findings most often consist of cranial nerve enhancement after gadolinium injection, with the seventh cranial nerve(s) most frequently involved.[53] However, high signal intensity lesions in the white matter can occur that mimic the lesions of multiple sclerosis.[54] Involvement of the optic nerves and/or chiasm (Fig. 11-21) is seen as swelling with high signal on T2-weighted scans and FLAIR and as contrast enhancement after gadolinium injection.[54] A positive serologic test should be followed by a full course of antibiotics. MR imaging can be used to follow the response to treatment.

## Craniopharyngioma

Craniopharyngioma is a benign tumor that arises from remnants of Rathke's pouch. These tumors occur most commonly in a suprasellar location, as well as within the sella turcica. They represent 1% to 3% of intracranial tumors and are found most frequently in children. However, they have two other age peaks, one in young adulthood and one in the fifth decade.[55]

## Clinical Findings

Patients with craniopharyngioma most frequently complain of a headache and visual disturbances occur commonly, related to impingement of the tumor on the optic pathway at the level of the chiasm or optic tracts.[56] Hypothalamic and pituitary dysfunction may be seen, and when the tumor occurs in a child, growth failure may result.[57]

## Pathologic Findings

Craniopharyngiomas originate from squamous cell epithelial rests arising from Rathke's pouch. They are benign, slow-growing tumors. Grossly, the tumor is well encapsulated and adherent to (and possibly superficially invasive into) the surrounding tissues. As the tumor enlarges, the adjacent structures are compressed, including the optic chiasm anteriorly, the pituitary gland inferiorly, the hypothalamus superiorly, and the elements of the circle of Willis peripherally.[55] The tumor is usually cystic, with interspersed solid areas. The cystic region contains either a liquid or semisolid dark brown, greasy material composed of cholesterol crystals, keratin, and calcified debris. Microscopically, the solid portions of the tumor consist of nests of stratified squamous or columnar epithelium within a fibrous stroma similar to that of the enamel organ of the tooth. For this reason, these tumors are considered to have an adamantinomatous histologic pattern.[57] Approximately 75% of craniopharyngiomas contain significant amounts of calcium.

## CT Appearance

On CT, craniopharyngiomas usually appear as rounded, lobulated, or irregularly marginated masses occupying the suprasellar cistern (85% of the time) and occasionally involving the sella turcica (20% of the time).[58] Cystic components are noted in 85% of the lesions. These cystic regions demonstrate a variable attenuation ranging from markedly hypodense to isodense relative to CSF (Fig. 11-22). The attenuation probably depends on the cholesterol content. Calcification is present in approximately 75% of the cases, varying from 70% to 90% in craniopharyngiomas occurring in children to 35% to 50% in those occurring in adults. The character of the calcification is generally conglomerate, although rim-like calcifications may occur about the cystic portions of the lesion (Fig. 11-22). After administration of a contrast medium, the solid portions of the tumor usually enhance markedly.

### MR Imaging Appearance

Because of its multiplanar imaging capabilities, MR imaging displays very well the anatomic configuration of the lesion relative to adjacent brain structures.[57] On short TR/TE images, the tumor generally has increased to intermediate signal intensity as a result of T1 shortening (Fig. 11-23A). This is most likely the result of increased protein concentration (greater than 9000 mg/100 ml), the presence of free methemoglobin, or both.[59] In rare cases the signal intensity is diminished, particularly if the lesion is predominantly cystic (Fig. 11-23C), with a low protein concentration within the cyst fluid. Focal areas of diminished signal intensity on short TR/TE and long TR/TE images may be secondary either to elevated keratin content within the cystic portions of the tumor or to calcification within the solid portions. As a rule, hyperintense signal is seen on long TR/TE images as a result of T2 prolongation.[57, 60] Comparison of CT and MR imaging shows CT's greater sensitivity in displaying calcification; this makes it a more specific radiologic procedure for craniopharyngioma identification, particularly when used in conjunction with the clinical history. MR imaging, on the other hand, is more sensitive to the presence of a tumor and gives a more accurate preoperative demonstration of the extent and location of the tumor, which is important in planning the surgical approach.[57, 60, 61] It has been shown that the craniopharyngioma's wall and solid portions enhance after administration of gadolinium (Fig. 11-24B). Thus, gadolinium increases the sensitivity of MR imaging in the evaluation of craniopharyngiomas, particularly in regard to tumor residual and recurrence after surgical excision.

MR proton spectroscopy has proven useful in differentiating craniopharyngiomas from hypothalamic astrocytomas and pituitary adenomas in children and adolescents.[62] Craniopharyngiomas show a peak in the lipid, lactate part of the scale (1 to 2 ppm), while hypothalamic astrocytomas show elevated choline to Naa ratios (e.g., 2.6 vs. a normal ratio of 0.75) and pituitary adenomas show no metabolites.[62]

## Rathke's Cleft Cyst

Rathke's cleft cyst is a benign lesion consisting of a cystic remnant of Rathke's pouch that occurs within the anterior portion of the sella turcica or the anterior aspect of the suprasellar cistern.

### Clinical Findings

Rathke's cleft cysts usually are small and without discernible clinical symptoms. If they are symptomatic, patients may have hypopituitarism, diabetes insipidus, headache, or visual disturbances related to impingement on the visual pathway at the level of the optic chiasm or the optic tracts; however, only 60 symptomatic cases have been reported in the world literature.[63]

### Pathologic Findings

The anterior lobe of the pituitary, the pars tuberalis and the pars intermedia, are derived from Rathke's pouch, which is also the origin of the Rathke's cleft cyst. The cyst is generally a simple structure lying primarily within the anterior portion of the sella turcica, occasionally with protrusions into the suprasellar cistern region, forming a dumbbell-shaped lesion. Microscopically, the wall of the cyst in the intrasellar portion is lined by a simple cuboidal epithelium, which may be ciliated, whereas the suprasellar portion may be lined by stratified squamous epithelium.[55] The single-cell layer forming the wall of the cyst often contains goblet cells, and the cystic contents usually have a serous or mucoid consistency, with varying amounts of cellular debris. This variable protein content probably accounts for the variable appearance of the cystic portion of the lesion on CT and MR imaging.

### CT Appearance

Rathke's cleft cyst usually appears as a well-circumscribed cystic structure that has a mass effect, lies

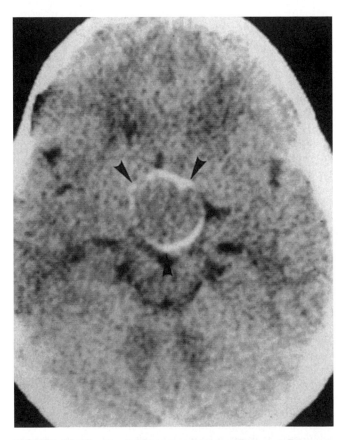

**FIGURE 11-22**   Craniopharyngioma. Axial nonenhanced CT image shows a suprasellar tumor with a peripheral rim of calcification (*arrowheads*) and a central region that is isodense to brain.

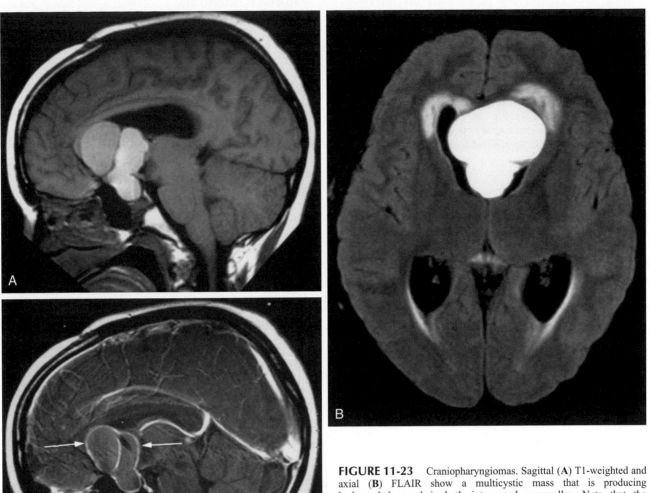

**FIGURE 11-23**   Craniopharyngiomas. Sagittal (**A**) T1-weighted and axial (**B**) FLAIR show a multicystic mass that is producing hydrocephalus and is both intra- and suprasellar. Note that the loculations are hyperintense and variable in signal intensity on the T1-weighted image. The chiasm is compressed. **C**, Sagittal T1-weighted postgadolinium injection image shows the same mass after initial surgical drainage. The contents of the mass are less intense. There is a peripheral rim of contrast enhancement (*arrows*).

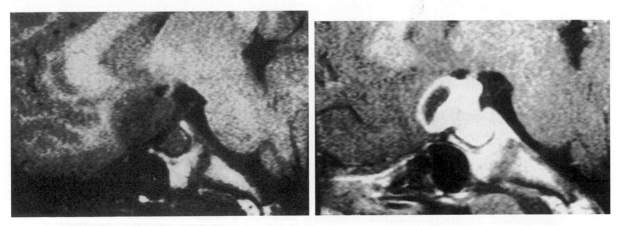

**FIGURE 11-24**   Craniopharyngioma in a 10-year-old male with evidence of clinical involvement of the left optic tract in the form of an incongruous homonymous hemianopsia. **A**, Sagittal T1-weighted MR image before gadolinium enhancement shows a soft-tissue mass both within and above the sella turcica; the mass abuts on the optic tract. **B**, T1-weighted MR image following gadolinium injection shows enhancement of the partially cystic mass.

within the sella turcica, and occasionally has suprasellar extension.[64] The wall of the cyst is generally thin, and the cyst contents usually are similar to CSF, although they may appear hypodense. The rim of tissue may enhance after administration of a contrast medium, and it occasionally contains small amounts of calcium. More complex cysts display a slightly increased density, with septa partitioning the cystic portion.[63] Differential considerations for the simple form of Rathke's cleft cyst include arachnoid cyst and cystic pituitary adenoma, whereas the more complex cysts may be impossible to differentiate from craniopharyngioma.

### MR Imaging Appearance

Simple cysts generally have signal intensity characteristics similar to those of CSF; that is, they usually appear hypointense to brain parenchyma on short TR/TE images and hyperintense to brain parenchyma on long TR/TE pulsing sequences. If the cyst fluid contains significant amounts of cholesterol, increased signal intensity is noted on short TR/TE images, with diminishing intensity on progressively longer TR/TE images. Complex cysts, which represent a transitional form between a simple Rathke's cleft cyst and a craniopharyngioma, demonstrate signal heterogeneity on long TR/TE images, with an isointense to hyperintense signal on short TR/TE images (Fig. 11-25). MR imaging better displays the relationship of the Rathke's cleft cyst to adjacent structures, particularly the optic chiasm and hypothalamus (Fig. 11-26).

## Pituitary Adenoma

Pituitary adenomas are benign neoplasms arising within the substance of the pituitary gland. They occur with equivalent frequency in males and females between 20 and 50 years of age. MR imaging has become the procedure of choice for evaluating tumors of the pituitary gland.

### Clinical Findings

Adenomas of the pituitary gland can be separated into microadenomas (less than 1 cm in diameter) and macroadenomas (greater than 1 cm in diameter). The microadenomas typically appear with endocrine abnormalities, the specific findings depending on which hormone is being elaborated by the adenoma. Macroadenomas, on the other hand, appear more often with symptoms caused by mass effect, such as those resulting from chiasmatic compression or pituitary insufficiency.

Lateral extension of the pituitary adenoma into the cavernous sinus can involve cranial nerves III, IV, and VI. This can produce motility disturbances on the basis of isolated or combined cranial neuropathies. If there is an acute increase in the size of the adenoma, such as can occur with pituitary apoplexy, there can be rapid lateral expansion and the patient can suffer rapid onset of an ocular motility disturbance, with or without a sudden decrease in vision.

### Pathologic Findings

Pituitary adenomas are usually unencapsulated solid tumors that may penetrate adjacent structures.[65] The tumors

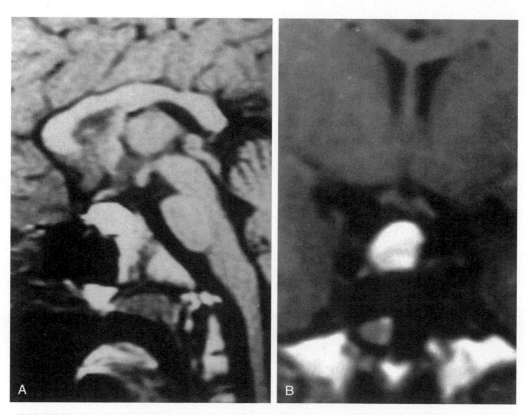

**FIGURE 11-25** Cyst of Rathke's pouch. **A,** Sagittal T1-weighted image shows a hyperintense intrasellar mass bowing upward into the chiasmatic cistern just below the optic chiasm. **B,** Coronal T1-weighted image shows an intrasellar mass with suprasellar extension; note that chiasm is not compressed.

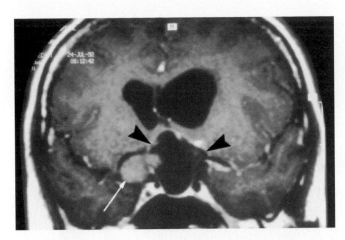

**FIGURE 11-26**   Cyst of Rathke's pouch. Contrast-enhanced coronal T1-weighted image shows a multilobulated intra- and suprasellar cystic mass (*arrowheads*) with one component (*arrow*) isointense to brain. There is no enhancement of the mass. The chiasm was compressed. Hydrocephalus is present.

can contain necrotic, cystic, or hemorrhagic regions and rarely contain calcification.[66] Of these adenomas, 25% to 30% are nonfunctional, 25% are prolactin-secreting tumors, 20% elaborate growth hormone, and 10% secrete adrenocorticotropic hormone (ACTH).[66] Microscopically, the adenomas are composed of sheets and cords of cells with a delicate stroma, and the functional adenomas usually contain highly granulated cells indicative of their cytochemical activity. Ischemia with consequent necrosis and hemorrhage may occur secondary to compromise of the blood supply, which results from compression at the diaphragma sellae. This eventually may cause a rapidly expanding sellar mass, with consequent optic nerve compression, headache, and occasional meningeal irritation. The incidence of malignant degeneration among pituitary adenomas is exceedingly small.

### CT Appearance

The specific findings associated with pituitary adenoma vary, depending on the size of the lesion.[67, 68, 69] Microadenomas typically are seen as focal hypodense areas within the surrounding pituitary gland, causing convexity of the upper surface of the gland and an increase in the height of the gland greater than 9 mm. Associated displacement of the infundibulum away from the side of the lesion may be seen, and thinning of the ipsilateral sellar floor may be present. These findings are more often found in lesions elaborating prolactin. Lesions elaborating growth hormone or ACTH may be more difficult to visualize because they tend to be less well defined. Also, the ACTH-producing adenomas may be very small. After administration of a contrast medium, microadenomas tend to be hypodense relative to the surrounding normally enhancing pituitary gland.

Macroadenomas display findings that depend on the size of the lesion (Fig. 11-27). They tend to enlarge the sella, causing sloping of the sellar floor, with possible extension into the sphenoid sinus. Depending on the degree of suprasellar extension, macroadenomas may displace the chiasm, the temporal lobes, and even the third ventricle.[68] After administration of a contrast medium, the macroad-

enomas generally appear isodense to slightly hypodense compared with the cavernous sinuses. If the lesion is solid, homogeneous enhancement occurs (Fig. 11-28A), whereas cystic or necrotic areas within a lesion tend to remain less dense relative to the remainder of the lesion. Macroadenomas may contain calcification, either homogeneously distributed throughout the tumor or deposited in a rim. If infarction of the tumor occurs, a hypodense area secondary to edema may be seen; alternatively, a hyperdense area secondary to hemorrhage may be seen (Fig. 11-29A). However, these findings are often difficult to delineate on CT.[62]

### MR Imaging Appearance

MR imaging usually allows accurate delineation of pituitary adenomas greater than 3 mm.[63] Smaller adenomas may also be diagnosed, but with less reliability.[70] A more specific diagnosis of a sellar mass may be achieved with MR imaging than with CT, and MR imaging is clearly better able to characterize subacute hemorrhage within the tumor.[61, 63, 71] Overall anatomic definition is more accurate with MR imaging than with CT (Figs. 11-29B, 11-30 and 11-31). Equivalent demonstration of sellar or dorsum sellae erosion is noted with the two imaging modalities,[72] but CT is better able than MR imaging to demonstrate intratumoral calcification.

Findings of a pituitary adenoma on MR imaging are similar to those noted on CT. Specifically, the primary findings are an upward bulge on the superior surface of the pituitary gland, with contralateral deviation of the infundibulum and sloping of the ipsilateral sellar floor (Fig. 11-31).[63] On short TR/TE images the adenomas tend to be slightly hypointense to the surrounding normal pituitary gland and may or may not be associated with a mass effect.[63] Occasionally pituitary adenomas may be isointense to the

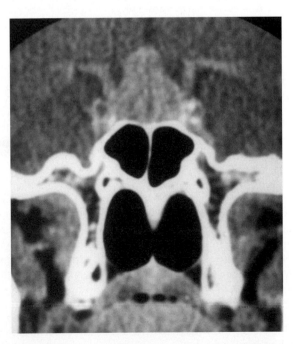

**FIGURE 11-27**   Pituitary adenoma; coronal contrast-enhanced CT image shows upward enlargement of the pituitary gland. The optic chiasm is affected.

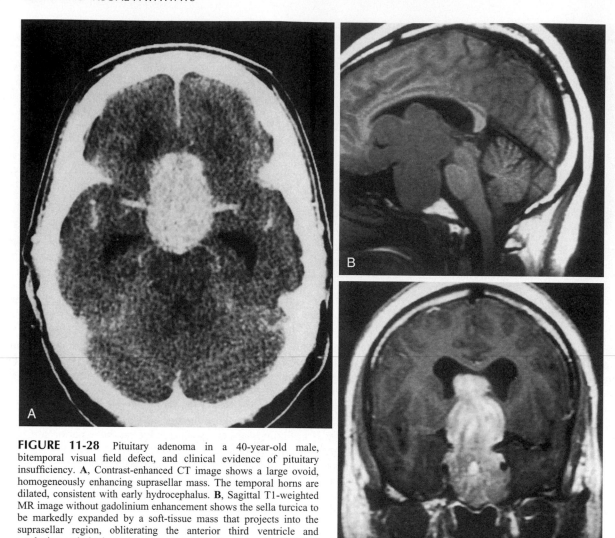

**FIGURE 11-28** Pituitary adenoma in a 40-year-old male, bitemporal visual field defect, and clinical evidence of pituitary insufficiency. **A,** Contrast-enhanced CT image shows a large ovoid, homogeneously enhancing suprasellar mass. The temporal horns are dilated, consistent with early hydrocephalus. **B,** Sagittal T1-weighted MR image without gadolinium enhancement shows the sella turcica to be markedly expanded by a soft-tissue mass that projects into the suprasellar region, obliterating the anterior third ventricle and producing early hydrocephalus by obstructing the foramen of Monro. **C,** Coronal postcontrast-enhanced, T1-weighted MR image shows enhancement throughout the solid tumor.

surrounding normal pituitary tissue.[72] On long TR/TE images the appearance of the adenomas varies,[63] but they may be moderately hyperintense relative to surrounding pituitary tissue.[72] Pituitary adenomas usually demonstrate homogeneous signal intensity; however, occasionally they are of mixed intensity due to necrosis, hemorrhage, or cyst formations.[72]

Suprasellar extension with impingement on and displacement of the optic chiasm is best demonstrated on coronal and sagittal sections (Fig. 11-30).[61, 68] Coronal sections are also better for demonstrating tumor extension into the cavernous sinuses (Fig. 11-32).[73] Demonstration of extension into the cavernous sinuses is often difficult with MR imaging because the medial wall of the cavernous sinus is very thin, and violation of this tissue plane may be difficult to see. However, when the tumor extends around the intracavernous carotid artery, displacing it medially, or is found above it, displacing it downward, invasion of the cavernous sinus can be diagnosed.

There is no evidence of a difference in signal intensity between secretory and nonsecretory pituitary adenomas.[63]

Cystic pituitary adenomas characteristically display high signal intensity on long TR/TE images and low signal intensity on short TR/TE images at the site of the cyst (Fig. 11-31). Subacutely hemorrhagic pituitary adenomas display high signal intensity on short TR/TE images because of the paramagnetic effect of methemoglobin (Fig. 11-33).[74] On short TR/TE images, after administration of a paramagnetic contrast agent such as gadolinium, a pituitary microadenoma is shown as a focal area of hypointensity relative to the surrounding enhancing normal pituitary tissue.[75, 76] This is true only if the images are acquired very early after administration of the contrast medium.[53] Dynamic scanning during contrast injection in the coronal plane through one thin section aids in diagnosis. On images obtained late after administration of the contrast medium, the microadenoma enhances and may not be distinguished from the normal pituitary gland. Macroadenomas show contrast enhancement.

Following performance of a transsphenoidal hypophysectomy, one possible complication is herniation of the optic chiasm, of the intracranial portion of the optic nerve, and/or

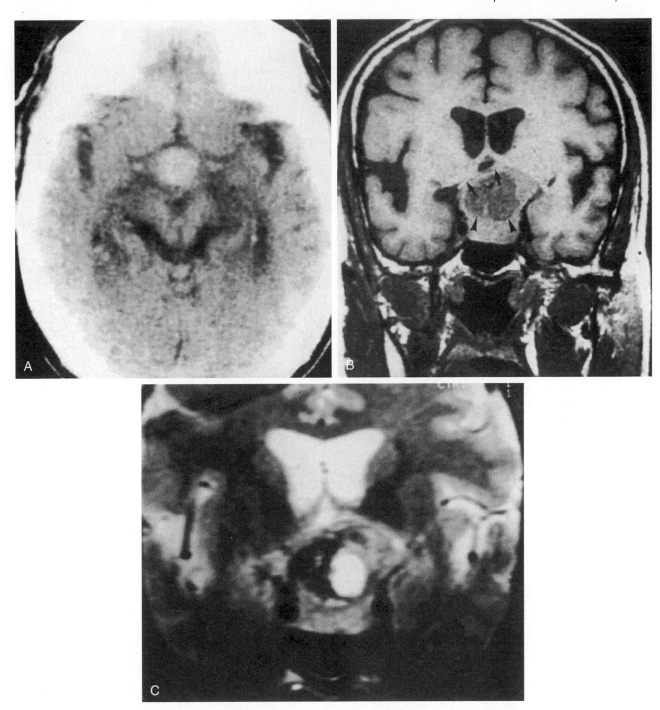

**FIGURE 11-29**   Pituitary apoplexy. **A**, Axial CT image without contrast medium shows a hyperdense suprasellar mass consistent with either bleeding or calcification. **B**, Coronal T1-weighted image shows an intrasellar and suprasellar mass extending slightly more to the left. The chiasm is displaced and compressed from below (*arrows*). The mass contains a slightly less intense zone (*arrowheads*) consistent with deoxyhemoglobin. **C**, Coronal T2-weighted image shows that the same area of hypointensity within the pituitary adenoma seen in **B** is of both high and low signal intensity. High signal intensity more to the left of the midline represents an area of cystic necrosis, whereas low signal intensity represents deoxyhemoglobin.

of the proximal aspect of the optic tracts into the surgically created empty sella. The herniation of the suprasellar visual system is well delineated with MR imaging. A visual deficit may or may not be present. The degree of deficit bears no relationship to the severity of herniation as seen on MR imaging.[77]

## Aneurysms

Aneurysms may be responsible for visual symptoms if they impinge directly on the visual pathway.[78, 79] The most common aneurysms to do this arise from the internal carotid artery at the origin of the ophthalmic artery. Aneurysms

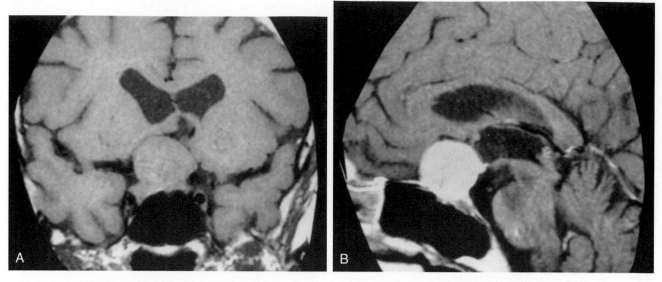

**FIGURE 11-30**   Pituitary adenoma in a 40-year-old male with bitemporal hemianopsia. **A,** Coronal T1-weighted image shows a large intra- and suprasellar mass stretching the chiasm from below. **B,** Sagittal T1-weighted image shows the adenoma enhancing. Note that the tumor did not expand into the aerated sphenoid sinus but upward, indicating an open diaphragma sellae.

occurring in this location compress either the optic chiasm, the intracranial portion of the optic nerve, or the proximal portion of the optic tract.

### Clinical Findings

Aneurysms arising from the internal carotid artery at the origin of the ophthalmic artery most often appear in patients between 50 and 70 years of age, and most patients are female. Of the aneurysms in this location, 75% are discovered at the time of angiographic evaluation for subarachnoid hemorrhage that has originated from another

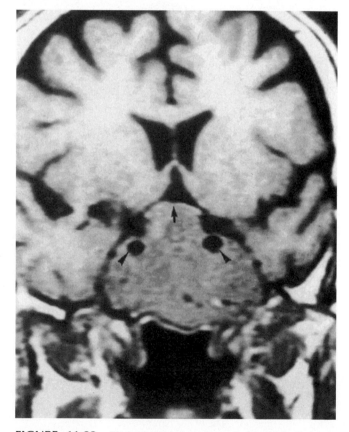

**FIGURE 11-32**   Pituitary adenoma. Coronal T1-weighted image shows a large pituitary adenoma elevating and compressing the optic chiasm (*arrow*). Both cavernous sinuses are invaded, and the tumor has extended lateral to the flow void of intracavernous internal carotid arteries (*arrowheads*). Note the outward convexity of the lateral margin of the cavernous sinuses.

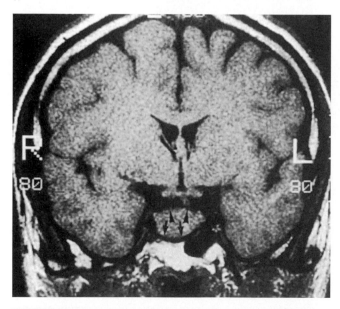

**FIGURE 11-31**   Pituitary adenoma. Coronal T1-weighted image shows downward bowing of an enlarged sella (*arrows*), upward convexity of the gland (*arrowheads*), and displacement of the infundibular stalk to the left.

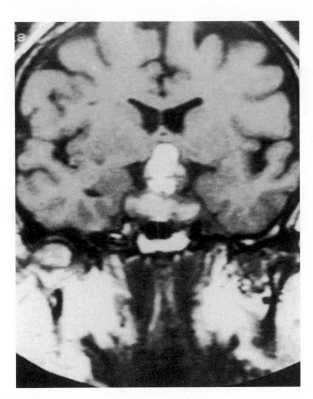

**FIGURE 11-33** Pituitary adenoma with intratumoral hemorrhage. Coronal T1-weighted image shows an intrasellar and suprasellar mass of mixed signal intensity, which is caused by the presence of methemoglobin. Note that the mass extends laterally and compresses both cavernous sinus regions.

aneurysm. However, in approximately 25% of patients with these aneurysms, the presentation is solely because of visual symptoms. The aneurysms associated with visual symptoms are often found to be large (greater than 2.5 cm in diameter).[80, 81] Also, more than half of the patients with these aneurysms have at least one other intracranial aneurysm, and the most common site of the additional aneurysm is the same site on the contralateral side.[82]

A diverse range of visual abnormalities is encountered, but visual acuity is nearly always impaired. This usually begins on the side of the aneurysm and may progress over months or years, leading eventually to blindness. Visual field abnormalities are also diverse because of the variety of ways in which the optic nerves and chiasm can be displaced by the aneurysm. Most commonly, unilateral or bilateral temporal field defects are seen, and the clinical presentation of aneurysms in this location can mimic that of pituitary tumors.

### Pathologic Findings

Grossly, these aneurysms tend to be saccular ones arising from the upper surface of the internal carotid artery at the origin of the ophthalmic artery.[83] Microscopically, within the aneurysm dome, there is fragmentation of the interna of the vessel with degeneration of the smooth muscle wall. Frequently the dome of the aneurysm contains layers of adherent thrombus of varying ages.

### CT Appearance

Although aneurysms at the internal carotid-ophthalmic artery junction that cause visual pathway symptoms are usually intact, they are most frequently discovered when the patient seeks help for symptoms of a subarachnoid hemorrhage. Therefore, the CT findings of an aneurysm in this location often coincide with the findings of subarachnoid hemorrhage, which most commonly consist of high-density material lying within the sulci and cisternal spaces. Depending on the location of the ruptured aneurysm, high-density material reflecting hemorrhage may be seen within the ventricular system or within the brain parenchyma itself.

The appearance of the aneurysm causing visual pathway symptoms depends on whether there is partial thrombosis within the aneurysmal dome. If no thrombus is present, the aneurysm usually appears as a rounded area of slightly increased density lying cephalad to the cavernous sinus adjacent to the optic chiasm. The structures in the region may be displaced. After injection of a contrast medium, there is homogeneous enhancement of the aneurysm (Fig. 11-34), and rim calcification may or may not be present (Fig. 11-35). A partially thrombosed aneurysm appears on an unenhanced CT scan as a well-circumscribed mass with an isodense periphery and central hyperdensity. The hyperdense central patent lumen enhances upon administration of contrast medium, and a peripheral rim of enhancement may occur because of increased vascularity within the aneurysm wall. If the aneurysm is completely thrombosed, only isodense thrombotic material may be seen within its central portion.[84] Three-dimensional (3D) CT angiography is emerging as a useful technique for evaluation of intracranial aneurysms. Utilizing a continuous peripheral intravenous infusion of contrast material (1 ml/sec for a total dose of 2 ml/kg), rapid dynamic thin-section CT images are obtained through the circle of Willis. Surface-rendering 3D reconstruction algorithm software is then used to produce images of the circle of Willis, the cavernous and supraclinoid internal carotid arteries, and any associated aneurysms. Rotational evaluation of the produced images is then performed. This technique provides additional information regarding the position of an aneurysm relative to adjacent vascular and bony structures and, by inference, to adjacent neural structures, without the use of more contrast or imaging time than is required for a routine contrast-enhanced head CT scan.[85]

### MR Imaging Appearance

Compared with CT, MR imaging more precisely characterizes giant aneurysms and defines their location relative to that of adjacent anatomic structures. However, MR imaging is much less sensitive than CT for detecting acute subarachnoid hemorrhage. Fluid-attenuated inversion recovery imaging is useful in showing subarachnoid hemorrhage on MR imaging as high signal intensity within cisterns and sulci between 3 to 45 days after the bleed.[86] Therefore, in the setting of symptoms suggesting acute subarachnoid hemorrhage, CT is the imaging modality of choice. However, MR angiography (MRA) is being used as a screening technique for detection and delineation of intracranial aneurysms in asymptomatic high-risk patient groups, and aneurysms as small as 3 to 4 mm in diameter can be visualized. The sensitivity of MRA for detection of intracranial aneurysms varies between 70% and 95% (Fig. 11-36). Conventional contrast angiography remains the most sensitive modality for detecting intracranial aneurysms.[87, 88, 89] Nevertheless, this modality is limited by its ability to demonstrate only the patent portions of the lumen of the aneurysm, and because many aneurysms contain thrombus, which partially or completely obliterates the lumen, the full extent of the lesion often cannot be defined by conventional angiography.

The characteristic appearance of a partially thrombosed aneurysm on MR imaging has been well described.[84, 88, 90, 91] On spin-echo imaging, partially thrombosed aneurysms demonstrate a flow phenomenon, usually a flow void, within the patent portion of the lumen. The laminated thrombus along the margins of the aneurysm dome exhibits mixed signal intensities, reflecting the various stages of clot formation. A periluminal rim of hyperintensity is usually seen, reflecting methemoglobin surrounding the patent portion of the lumen (Fig. 11-34B). The parent vessel (i.e., the internal carotid artery) shows a signal void because of high-velocity flow. Gradient echo acquisition images, which display high-velocity flow as regions of high signal intensity, demonstrate blood flow within the lumen of the parent vessel and within the patent portion of the lumen of the aneurysm. On spin-echo images, aneurysms with no thrombus formation appear as areas of signal void (Figs. 11-37 and 11-38) and on gradient echo acquisition images as areas of high signal intensity. If the aneurysm is completely thrombosed, mixed signal intensity caused by various stages of clot formation is seen within the aneurysmal mass on spin-echo images (Fig. 11-38).

The relationship of the aneurysm to the elements of the visual pathway is delineated with MR imaging. The coronal plane is helpful in showing the relationship of the aneurysm to the optic chiasm, nerve, and tract, as well as the aneurysm's relationship to the structures of the sella turcica and the cavernous sinus. Additionally, mass lesions (other than aneurysms) impinging on the optic chiasm are well delineated with coronal MR imaging.[92, 93]

## Infarction

Cerebral infarction, a localized area of tissue necrosis produced by circulatory insufficiency, is the most common

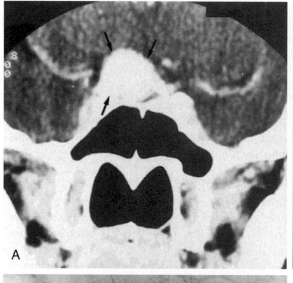

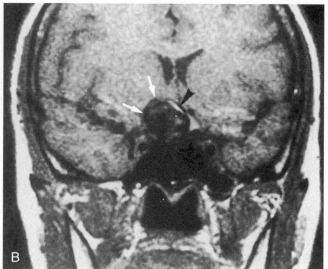

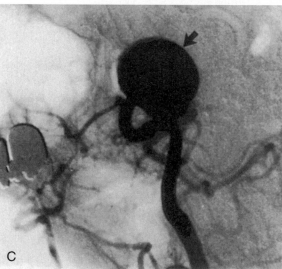

**FIGURE 11-34** Intrasellar projection of an ophthalmic artery aneurysm. **A,** Coronal CT image after injection of contrast medium shows a mass in the suprasellar space (*arrows*) lying partly within the sella. **B,** Coronal T1-weighted image shows a hypointense flow void of blood within the lumen of the intrasellar and suprasellar aneurysm (*arrows*). The small area of hyperintensity in the superior margin may represent laminar clot (*arrowhead*). Note the irregular hyperintensity extending across the Sylvian fissures bilaterally at the same level as the aneurysm, representing flow artifacts in the phase-encoding direction. **C,** Internal carotid arteriogram subtraction film shows an ophthalmic artery aneurysm (*arrow*).

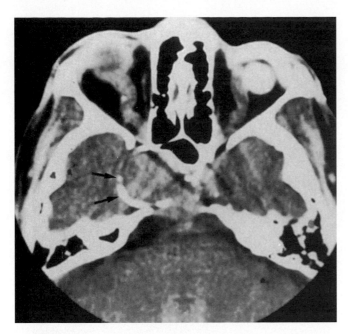

**FIGURE 11-35**   Intracavernous aneurysm. Plain axial CT image shows a mass with peripheral calcification (*arrows*) that is eroding the sphenoid bone and sella turcica.

pathologic disorder affecting the CNS. Cerebral infarctions may be further subdivided into ischemic and hemorrhagic forms. They may be due to arteriosclerosis, which may or may not be associated with thrombosis, emboli, or venoocclusive disease.

### Clinical Findings

Circulatory insufficiency may be caused by involvement of the anterior cerebral circulation (internal carotid arteries and their branches) or the posterior cerebral circulation (the vertebral basilar system). Amaurosis fugax, or transient loss of vision in one eye, is the most common ocular symptom of internal carotid artery ischemia. Specific findings vary from altitudinal or arcuate visual field defects to complete loss of light perception in the affected eye. Vision may return after a few minutes, but permanent visual loss because of central retinal artery occlusion can and often does occur. Cholesterol emboli may be found in association with amaurosis fugax, and ophthalmoscopic evaluation reveals these emboli within the retinal arterioles as characteristic bright yellowish-orange plaques. Because the internal carotid artery and its branches supply the frontal lobes, parietal lobes, portions of the temporal lobes, the corpus striatum, and the internal capsule, an occlusion may produce a variety of contralateral motor and sensory dysfunctions in addition to the visual findings.

Insufficiency of the circulation of the vertebral basilar system causes transient ischemic attack or infarction with complex and diverse neurologic symptoms. In addition to ocular symptoms, vertigo and nausea may be present if the cochlear vestibular system is involved. Involvement of the auditory system may produce tinnitus or partial deafness. Headache, dysphagia, dysarthria, and hiccuping may also occur. The ocular symptoms include transient or permanent homonymous hemianopsia and possibly blurred vision with

diplopia. The homonymous hemianopsia arises as a result of infarction of the occipital lobe's visual cortex, which is fed by branches of the posterior cerebral artery. Diplopia occurs because vascular insufficiency produces infarction in the fasciculi connecting the brainstem nuclei or in the brainstem nuclei of the third, fourth, and sixth cranial nerves. Internuclear ophthalmoplegia may occur as a result of interruption of the vascular supply to the medial longitudinal fasciculus (Figs. 11-39 and 11-40), but this does not usually manifest as diplopia.

### Pathologic Findings

Infarcts may be divided into two basic categories, depending on the amount of hemorrhage that occurs in the involved tissue. Infarction caused by thrombotic events generally produces an anemic or nonhemorrhagic infarction, whereas infarctions of embolic cause often are associated with a variable degree of hemorrhage into the interstitial space.[47, 56] Infarctions affecting the elements of the visual pathway are not dissimilar to infarctions in other regions of the brain, showing no discernible histologic differences. Their distinguishing factor is their position relative to the various portions of the visual pathway. The mechanism of infarction, whether hemorrhagic or anemic, is the same: deprivation of blood supply to a given area. In hemorrhagic infarctions, transitory occlusion of a vessel results in ischemic change of the brain tissue and the involved blood vessel's walls. When the blood supply is reestablished, blood elements penetrate the damaged vascular wall into the interstitial space, creating parenchymal hemorrhage.

The earliest grossly visible change in the evolution of an ischemic infarction is a slight discoloration and softening of the affected tissue, which occurs approximately 6 to 8 hours after occlusion of the vessel. Histologically, at this point there is diffuse swelling of the neurons, with resultant

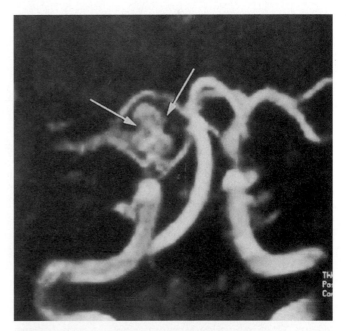

**FIGURE 11-36**   Aneurysm of the ophthalmic artery in a 53-year-old woman with right monocular visual loss; 3D time-of-flight MR angiography shows an aneurysm (*arrows*) arising from the internal carotid artery at the site of origin of the ophthalmic artery.

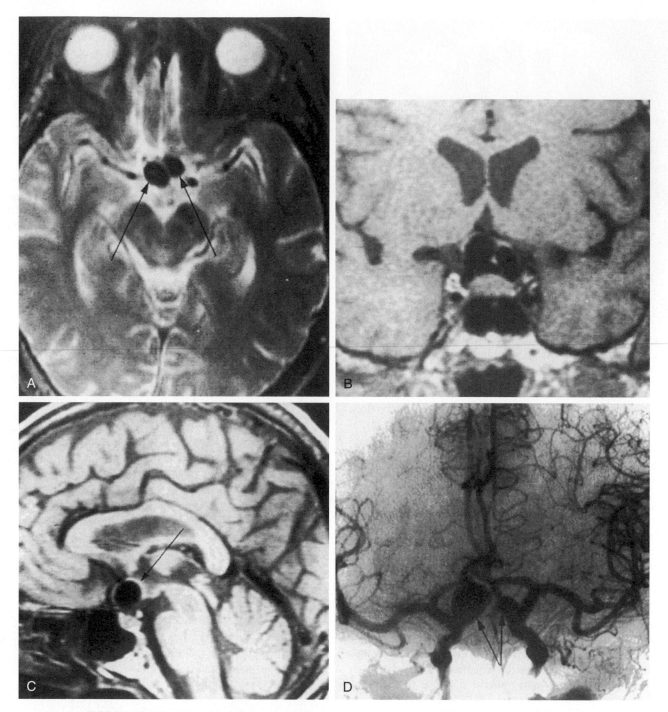

**FIGURE 11-37** Bilateral ophthalmic artery aneurysms presenting with bitemporal hemianopsia. **A**, Axial T2-weighted image shows two areas of hypointensity (*arrows*) in the suprasellar cistern consistent with aneurysms. **B**, Coronal T1-weighted image shows two hypointense lumens of aneurysms projecting medially from the region of the internal carotid arteries and compressing the optic chiasm bilaterally. **C**, Sagittal T1-weighted image shows a larger aneurysm as a hypointense flow void and depicts the aneurysm's relationship to the chiasm (*arrow*), which is compressed from below. **D**, AP right and left carotid arteriogram subtraction films superimposed to show the relationships of both ophthalmic artery aneurysms, which project medially (*arrows*).

cytotoxic edema.[94] At 48 to 72 hours after occlusion of the vessel, tissue integrity is lost in the affected region and the surrounding tissue displays diffuse vasogenic edema. The combination of cytotoxic and vasogenic edema, with the resultant mass effect, may produce cerebral herniations that, depending on their site of occurrence, may damage neural transmission along the visual pathway (e.g.,

optic tract with temporal lobe herniation). Eventually, if the area of infarction is large enough, there is liquefaction and cyst formation surrounded by firm glial tissue. Histologically, in the final stages of evolution of an anemic infarction, gliosis both replaces and surrounds the necrotic region. Infarct evolution may take weeks to many months.[56] In addition to being associated with emboli, hemorrhagic

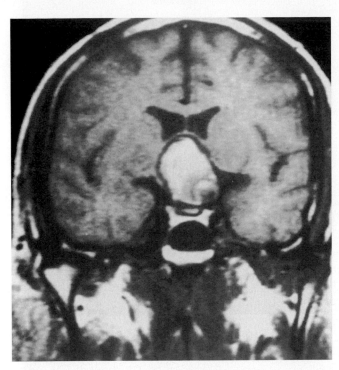

**FIGURE 11-38**  Thrombosed aneurysm. Coronal T1-weighted image shows a suprasellar mass composed of high signal intensity methemoglobin.

infarction may be seen in association with hypertension and venous occlusion (Fig. 11-40), bleeding dyscrasias, or anticoagulant administration.[95] After extravasation of blood into the interstitial tissue, significant mass effect may occur, resulting in herniation. In fact, hemorrhagic infarction may result from a herniation that caused temporary compression of a trapped blood vessel. With reperfusion of the vessel on reduction of the herniation, blood suffuses through the damaged vascular wall into the infarcted brain.

### CT Appearance

The effects of an ischemic infarction may be visible as early as 3 to 6 hours after the ictus (Fig. 11-41A).[96] Occasionally, a thromboembolism within the vessel serving the area of infarction may be visualized on a CT scan as a region of hyperdensity in the vessel lumen before development of subsequent parenchymal changes (Fig. 11-42A).[97, 98] This finding is not, however, a reliable indicator of vessel occlusion or subsequent infarction, as it may be due to increased hematocrit or calcification within the vessel walls, as can occur with diabetes or hypertension.[99] However, changes may be seen more reliably between 8 and 24 hours after the onset of ischemia. These changes are regions of hypodensity in the involved vascular distribution, including both white and gray matter (Fig. 11-40A). The region of hypodensity, which represents intracellular (cytotoxic) edema, becomes more sharply defined over the next several days. Cytotoxic edema and tissue necrosis reach their maximum between the third and fifth days after the ictus, producing variable amounts of mass effect. In occipital lobe infarctions or infarctions involving the optic radiations, this may be perceived as effacement of the adjacent sulci and/or atrium and occipital horn of the lateral ventricle. Larger infarctions may cause marked mass effect and result in descending transtentorial herniation with occlusion of the posterior cerebral artery when it is trapped on the tentorial edge. Occlusion of the posterior cerebral artery results in infarction of the posterior temporal and occipital lobes.

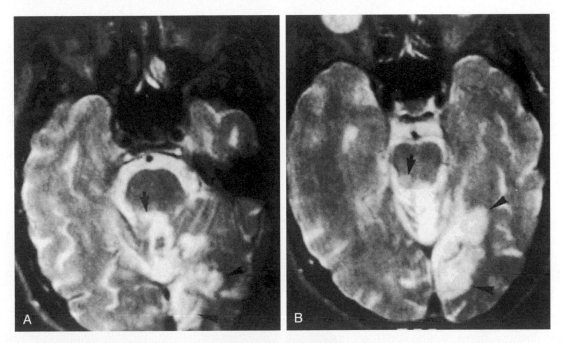

**FIGURE 11-39**  Left occipital lobe, midbrain, and upper brainstem infarction. **A,** Axial T2-weighted image shows hyperintense signal intensity at the site of the left occipital lobe infarct (*arrowheads*). Note the hyperintense focus of infarction in the periaqueductal region of the upper pons (*arrow*). **B,** Slightly higher axial T2-weighted image shows the further superior extent of a hyperintense infarct involving the left occipital and medial temporal lobes (*arrowheads*). A high signal intensity focus is present in the dorsal aspect of the right midbrain (*arrow*).

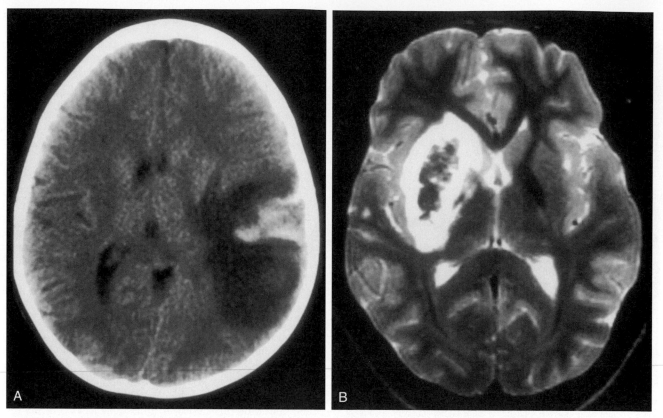

**FIGURE 11-40** Hemorrhagic infarction. **A,** A 7-year-old female with cortical vein and transverse sinus thrombosis. Axial plain CT image shows a hypodense region in the left hemisphere with a central hyperdense hemorrhagic component. This hemorrhagic infarct causes a mass effect and a shift of midline structures to the right. **B,** A 15-year-old female with an embolic event. Axial T2-weighted MR image shows a right basal ganglionic region of both low (hemorrhage) and high (edema) signal intensity with mass effect.

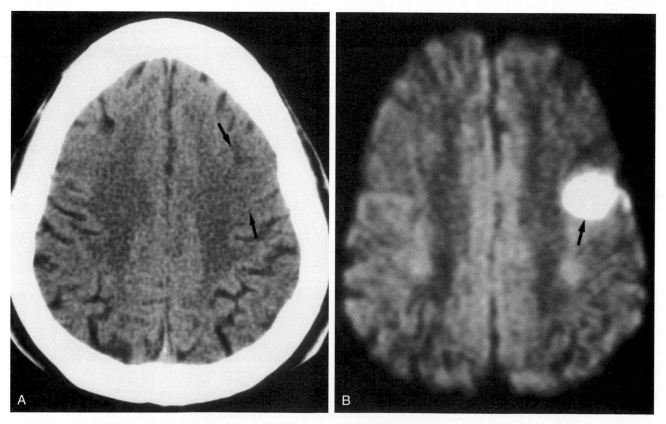

**FIGURE 11-41** Acute embolic ischemic infarction in a 17-year-old female. **A,** CT image without contrast shows subtle posterior frontal cortical and subcortical hypodensity (*arrows*). **B,** Diffusion-weighted image shows acute infarction as high signal intensity (*arrow*).

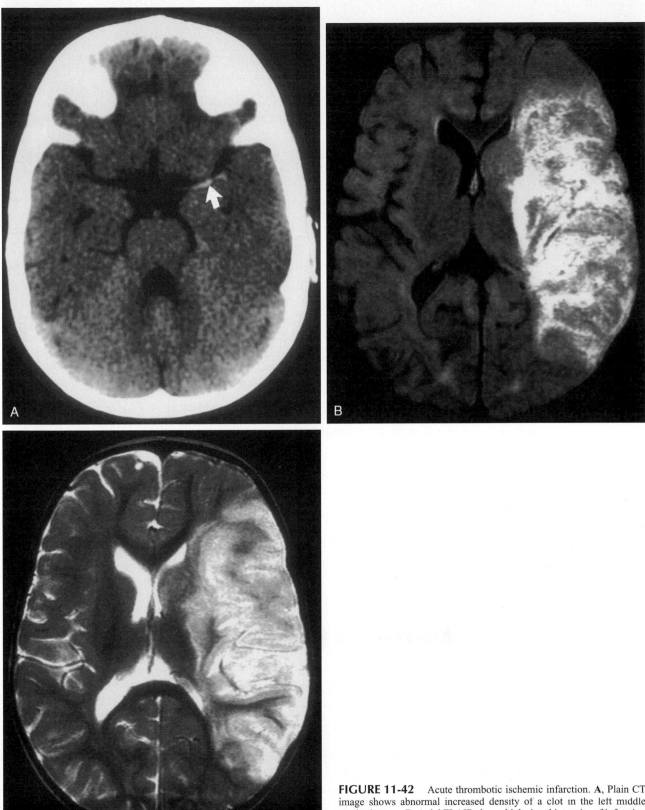

**FIGURE 11-42** Acute thrombotic ischemic infarction. **A**, Plain CT image shows abnormal increased density of a clot in the left middle cerebral artery. **B**, Axial FLAIR shows high signal intensity of infarction within the left middle cerebral artery territory. **C**, T2-weighted axial image shows an infarct with mass effect.

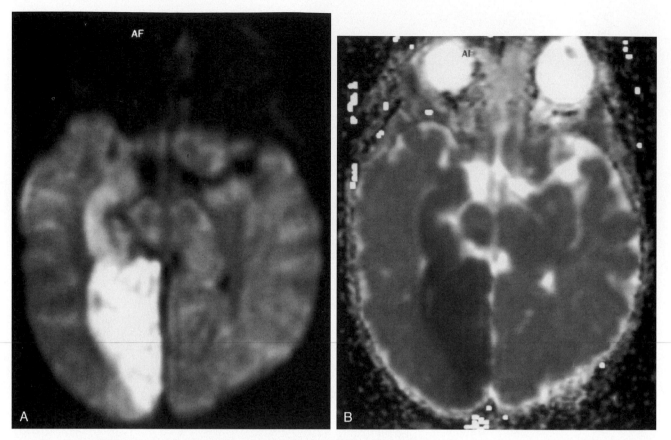

**FIGURE 11-43**  Acute embolic occlusion of the right posterior cerebral artery with ischemic infarction. **A,** Axial diffusion-weighted image shows high signal intensity indicating cytotoxic edema at the site of infarction. **B,** Axial ADC map shows low signal. Calculations of ADC measurements showed one-half normal values consistent with infarction.

Vasogenic (interstitial) edema is seen more often with embolic infarction. This follows reperfusion of the affected area, usually occurs 2 to 14 days after the acute event, and is responsible for a significant degree of mass effect. Approximately 1 month after the ictus, cystic cavitation in the infarcted region occurs pathologically and is responsible for increasingly sharp definition of the region of the infarct. The infarcted region also becomes smaller because of progression of gliosis, and there is resultant increase in the depth of the adjacent sulci and enlargement of the adjacent ventricle. Hemorrhagic infarctions, which result from embolic phenomena, overall are less frequent, representing only 20% of cases. The hemorrhage, when visible, is seen on an unenhanced CT scan as a region of high density involving the cortex or the deep white matter.

### MR Imaging Appearance

MR imaging is the most valuable imaging tool in the evaluation of cerebral infarction because of its high sensitivity to increased tissue water content. The sensitivity of MR imaging in the early detection of infarction is much higher than that of CT.[100–103] Experimentally, infarctions may be detected with MR imaging 1 to 2 hours after the onset of ischemia.[104, 105] The earliest detectable changes are vascular flow-related abnormalities including absence of the flow void normally seen within the cerebral vessels. Also, on administration of gadolinium DTPA, enhancement of the arterial wall may occur, and these findings may be seen within minutes of onset. Early brain swelling can be detected on short TR/short TE images without associated parenchymal signal intensity changes on T2-weighted images.[105, 106] Diffusion weighted MR imaging, which evaluates local water mobility in vivo, can detect alterations in the involved brain parenchyma before the appearance of signal intensity changes on conventional T1-weighted and T2-weighted spin-echo images (Figs. 11-41A and 11-43).[94, 101, 102, 107, 108] The earliest parenchymal signal changes visible are caused by a prolongation of both T1 and T2 relaxation times, with resultant high signal intensity in the region of infarction on long TR/long TE images (Figs. 11-42C and 11-44A) and low signal intensity in the same region on short TR/short TE sequences (Fig. 11-45B).[109] This is frequently visible 6 to 12 hours after the onset of symptoms and is attributable to the development of cytotoxic edema. With further evolution of the infarction, absolute T1 and T2 prolongation becomes somewhat diminished, and only a slight alteration of signal intensity results in the affected area.[110] The mass effect produced by the region of infarction is clearly identified with MR imaging, with greater anatomic delineation of affected structures than is seen on CT. Contrast enhancement of the region may be demonstrated as early as 16 to 18 hours after the ictus and may be exaggerated in character.[105, 106, 111] Again, the region of enhancement correlates with areas of breakdown in the blood-brain barrier.[111, 112] Interestingly, as

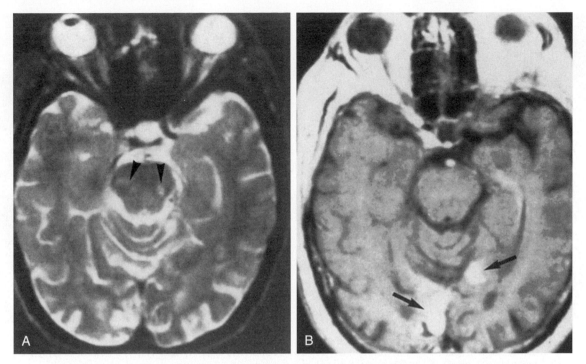

**FIGURE 11-44**   Multiple infarcts. **A,** Axial T2-weighted image shows several high-intensity foci in the upper pons (*arrowheads*) that are consistent with small infarcts. **B,** Axial T1-weighted image after injection of contrast medium shows enhancement of the right occipital lobe and left medial temporal lobe infarcts (*arrows*) not seen on the T2-weighted image.

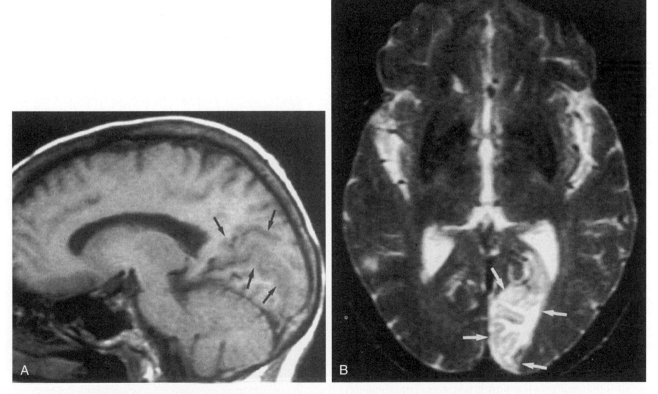

**FIGURE 11-45**   Left occipital infarct in a 50-year-old male with abrupt onset of right homonymous hemianopsia. **A,** Sagittal T1-weighted MR image without contrast injection shows decreased signal intensity involving the cortex (*arrows*) above and below the calcarine fissure. **B,** Axial T2-weighted MR image shows high signal intensity involving the cortex and subjacent white matter (*arrows*) in the left temporooccipital region including the calcarine cortex.

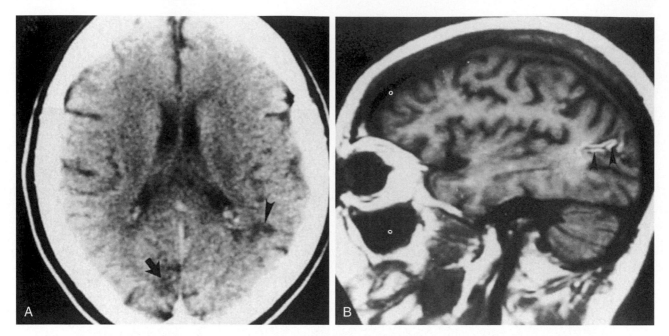

**FIGURE 11-46** Hemorrhagic infarcts of the parietal and occipital lobes. **A,** Axial CT image without contrast shows a vague hypodensity in the right occipital lobe (*arrow*) and another vague hypodensity (*arrowhead*) in the left parietal lobe. **B,** Sagittal T1-weighted image shows hyperintense methemoglobin (*arrowheads*) in the cortex.

edema and mass effect develop, the rapidity with which enhancement occurs declines, presumably as a result of compression of the microvasculature. The regions of enhancement following administration of gadolinium are seen as areas of increased signal intensity on short TR/TE images (Fig. 11-44B). Brain parenchymal change secondary to ischemia caused by vasculitis shows the same basic characteristics with regard to signal intensity as ischemia from either embolic or thrombotic phenomena. However, there is a difference in distribution in that the regions of ischemia are more diffuse throughout the brain, tending to occur in the regions of gray and white matter interface.

Hemorrhagic infarction may be demonstrated as areas of high signal intensity on short TR/TE images (Fig. 11-46B) within the cortex or deep gray matter structures once deoxyhemoglobin within the extravasated blood has been oxidized to methemoglobin.[9] As evolution of the infarction proceeds and cystic encephalomalacia develops, the associated parenchymal volume loss is clearly delineated with MR imaging. Gliosis and demyelination within white matter tracts result in T2 prolongation and, consequently, high signal intensity in the affected areas on long TR/long TE images. Both deoxyhemoglobin and intracellular methemoglobin, as well as hemosiderin, produce loss of signal on T2-weighted images (Figs. 11-40B and 11-47).

## Demyelinating Disease

The most common form of demyelinating disease to affect the optic pathway is multiple sclerosis. The characteristic changes seen in demyelination are caused by both plaque formation and gliosis, with resultant alteration in the appearance of the involved parenchyma. The neurophysiologic consequences of the loss of myelin are based on impaired transmission of neural impulses passing through the affected area.

### Clinical Findings

Multiple sclerosis has a wide variety of signs and symptoms, which characteristically localize to at least two different anatomic areas within the CNS and occur with a series of relapses and remissions, separated by at least 1

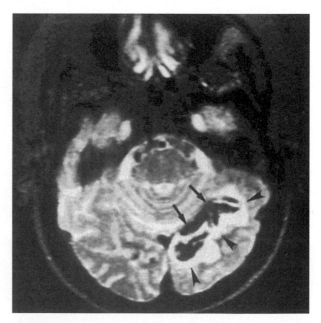

**FIGURE 11-47** Hemorrhagic infarct. Axial T2-weighted image shows marked hypointensity of deoxyhemoglobin (*arrows*) in the cortex of portions of a hemorrhagic infarction. Surrounding hyperintensity is present (*arrowheads*).

month.[113] Initially the diagnosis may be difficult to confirm, since the presentation may be caused by a single lesion, or the course may be slowly progressive and not intermittent. Multiple sclerosis most characteristically affects patients between 10 and 50 years of age who reside in northern Europe or the northern United States, and females are affected more frequently than males in a ratio of 1.4 to 1.[114]

Approximately half of patients with multiple sclerosis show clinical signs of optic nerve involvement. Visual evoked responses and electrophysiologic tests of optic nerve and pathway function are positive in approximately 90% of patients with multiple sclerosis. However, only 20% of patients show isolated optic neuritis as their initial clinical symptom.[19] Visual involvement, when present, is typically unilateral, with dense regions of visual loss within the visual fields. Impaired color perception, ocular muscle palsies, and nystagmus are common, and internuclear ophthalmoplegia occasionally is present. Adrenal leukodystrophy (ADL) and Krabbe's disease are examples of dysmyelinating diseases that may cause visual symptoms and involve the visual pathway. ADL usually appears during childhood, with progressive ataxia and loss of hearing and sight. Patients with Krabbe's disease may show symptoms of developmental delay, irritability, and spasticity, often beginning at 3 to 6 months of age.

### Pathologic Findings

In multiple sclerosis, the areas of demyelination are seen as focal lesions with well-circumscribed margins. Successive histologic changes occur, consisting of demyelination, a microglial reaction, and then astrocytic proliferation.[22] In the initial stages, oligodendrocytes and the myelin sheaths degenerate, without change in the axon. At this time, an associated vascular congestion with perivascular lymphocytic and plasma cell infiltrates is present. As a result, swelling is present in the acute stage of the inflammation. Later, microglia phagocytize the myelin debris, and this debris stimulates an intense gliosis that forms a firm glial scar in the late stage. Schilder's disease is characterized by large, symmetric zones of demyelination, with degeneration of neural fibers and gliosis. These zones occur throughout the CNS, including the optic nerve and optic radiation.[22] Histopathologically, the lesions are identical to those seen in multiple sclerosis.[115] Krabbe's disease, or globoid cell leukodystrophy, is caused by a deficiency of galactocerebroside beta-galactosidase, which leads to abnormal accumulation of galactoside and its derivative psychosine, which is toxic to oligodendroglial cells. As a consequence, multinucleated globoid cells (macrophages) accumulate in the white matter and are associated with extensive demyelination and astrogliosis.[116]

### CT Appearance

The plaques of multiple sclerosis are sometimes detectable by nonenhanced CT as hypodense lesions within the periventricular white matter (Fig. 11-48). Occasionally, the plaques are large and demonstrate mass effect. However, they usually are less than 1.5 cm in greatest dimension. In approximately 5% of cases, multiple sclerosis plaques may be seen within the cortical gray matter or deep gray matter of the cerebral hemispheres.[117] After administration of a contrast medium, plaques in the acute phase may demon-

strate enhancement. However, enhancement patterns vary, with none being characteristic of multiple sclerosis. High doses of contrast media have been used to increase the sensitivity of CT in the detection of multiple sclerosis plaques.[118] Steroid administration, however, suppresses the enhancement of acute multiple sclerosis plaques because of stabilization of the blood-brain barrier. With chronic multiple sclerosis, generalized cerebral atrophy may be seen as a result of extensive gliosis.

In adolescents with MS, the lesions observed tend to be more numerous and often confluent with a greater likelihood of infratentorial involvement and a decreased incidence of cortical atrophy.[119] The appearance of Schilder's disease on CT has been described as large, confluent areas of hypodensity within the deep cerebral hemispheric white matter, particularly the centrum semiovale. These areas may show peripheral contrast enhancement. CT scans of patients with Krabbe's disease typically demonstrate areas of low density in the cerebellum deep white matter, medial and lateral to the dentate nuclei. Interestingly, areas of increased density are noted symmetrically involving the thalami and subthalami, with extension to the corona radiata.[116, 120]

### MR Imaging Appearance

Because MR imaging is the most sensitive method of evaluation for patients with multiple sclerosis, it has replaced CT in the diagnosis and follow-up of patients with this disease.[113, 114, 121–126]

Multiple sclerosis lesions characteristically demonstrate T2 prolongation, with consequent high signal intensity of the affected areas on long TR/TE scanning sequences (Fig. 11-48).[127] The plaques usually are located within the periventricular white matter (Fig. 11-49). The finger-like extensions radiating away from the lateral angle of the lateral ventricle have been labeled *Dawson's fingers*.[125] These are well seen on FLAIR images.[125] However, because of the sensitivity of MR imaging, increasingly, more plaques have been detected within the white matter of the cerebellum, brainstem, and spinal cord.[128–130] The activity of the plaques is difficult to ascertain. With intravenous administration of gadolinium, enhancement may be seen at the site of acute demyelination, with breakdown of the blood-brain barrier.[131–133] Additionally, enhancement of the leptomeninges may be seen as an inconstant occurrence. The cause and significance of plaque enhancement are in dispute; consequently, they cannot be taken as unequivocal supportive evidence of the presence or absence of MS or as an indicator of the activity of the disease process.[133–135] MR proton spectroscopy is able to differentiate areas of demyelination from regions of disrupted blood-brain barrier and consequent edema, both of which may exhibit enhancement following gadolinium DTPA administration. Proton spectroscopy (MRS) appears to be a more sensitive indicator of the true time course of demyelination in MS.[131] Short inversion time (inversion recovery sequences [STIR]), as well as other fat-suppressed MR techniques, are useful for evaluating the optic nerve in patients with clinically diagnosed optic neuritis[136] by demonstrating the plaque responsible for the observed clinical findings (Fig. 11-50B).[137, 138] However, visual potentials remain more sensitive than MR imaging for detection of optic nerve lesions. The MR imaging findings in Krabbe's disease appear to be

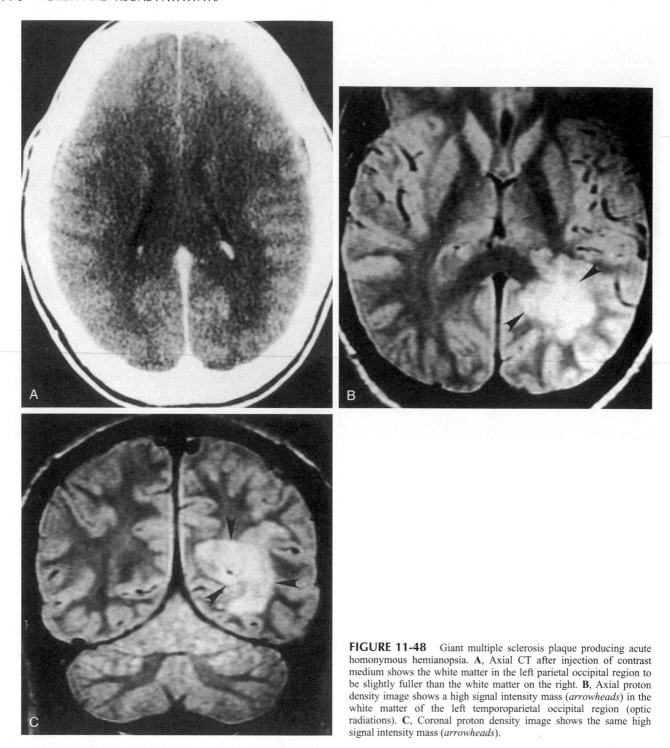

**FIGURE 11-48**   Giant multiple sclerosis plaque producing acute homonymous hemianopsia. **A,** Axial CT after injection of contrast medium shows the white matter in the left parietal occipital region to be slightly fuller than the white matter on the right. **B,** Axial proton density image shows a high signal intensity mass (*arrowheads*) in the white matter of the left temporoparietal occipital region (optic radiations). **C,** Coronal proton density image shows the same high signal intensity mass (*arrowheads*).

variable but usually consist of high signal intensity within the cerebral deep white matter on long TR/TE images. There does not appear to be a reproducible correlation between the areas of high density in the deep gray matter and deep white matter in the supratentorial brain demonstrated on CT and the alterations in these areas on MRS. Consequently, CT is used to demonstrate the characteristic changes in this disease.[116]

## Cerebral Neoplastic Disease

Intracranial tumors affect the visual pathway either by disruption of the neural connections or by exertion of a mass effect, which causes distortion and subsequently impairs the functioning of the visual pathway. An extensive variety of neoplasms may involve the supratentorial brain and consequently the visual pathway.

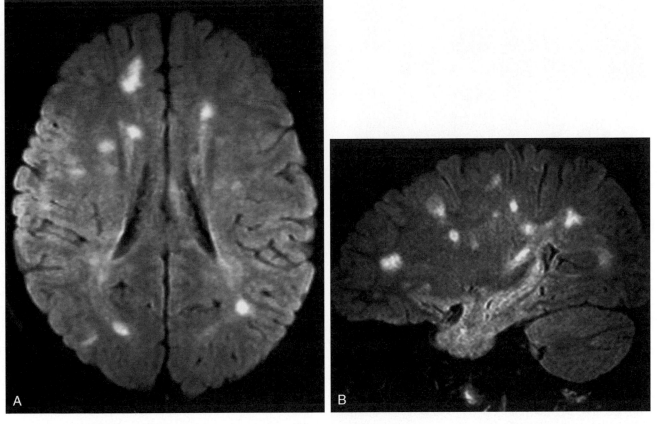

**FIGURE 11-49**   Multiple sclerosis. **A** and **B**, Axial and sagittal FLAIR images show multiple high-intensity multiple sclerosis plaques.

### Clinical Findings

The location of a particular neoplasm within the brain often can be determined by clinical signs and symptoms. Large tumors that raise intracranial pressure result in papilledema. Hemiplegia is present if the tumor involves the primary motor cortex. Neoplasms within the parietal lobe often result in visual field defects, particularly those involving the superior parietal optic radiations and thus affecting the inferior quadrant of the contralateral visual field. If the neoplasm involves the angular gyrus of the dominant hemisphere, there may be an inability to recognize printed words (alexia) and an inability to write (agraphia).

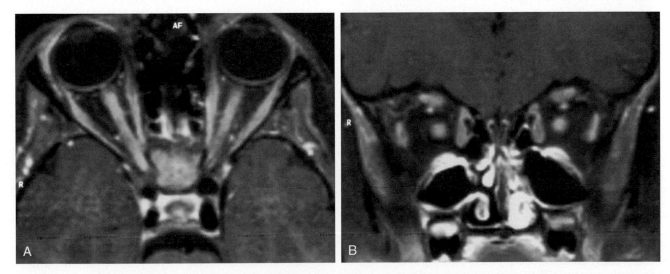

**FIGURE 11-50**   Multiple sclerosis. Bilateral optic neuritis. **A** and **B**, Axial and coronal T1-weighted images with fat suppression after gadolinium injection show symmetric enhancement of the intraorbital optic nerves.

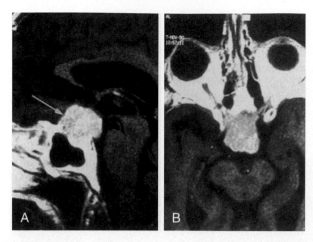

**FIGURE 11-51** Suprasellar meningioma arising from the planum sphenoidale and diaphragma sellae in a 55-year-old female with bitemporal hemianianopsia. **A**, Sagittal T1-weighted MR image following gadolinium injection shows enhancement of a suprasellar mass (*arrows*) that compresses the optic chiasm. **B**, Axial T1-weighted MR image after gadolinium injection shows the anterioposterior and lateral extent of the mass.

Within the temporal lobe, neoplasms can produce superior homonymous quadrantinopsia. If the tumor occurs at the confluence of the dominant frontal, temporal, and parietal lobes, an expressive aphasia frequently is present. Tumors occupying the occipital lobe often cause a congruous contralateral homonymous hemianopsia. If the tumor occupies the association areas of the occipital lobe, the patient may be unable to recognize familiar people (pragmatagnosia). Other clinical findings with intracranial neoplasm include morning headache, nausea, lethargy, and impaired consciousness, depending on the size and location of the tumor. Papilledema may be observed in patients with tumors anywhere in the supratentorial brain.

### Pathologic Findings

A wide variety of different tumor types may involve the supratentorial brain and thus the visual pathway.[139] In general terms, the tissue types may be derived from the neural glia, which includes the astrocytes and oligodendrocytes, from the ependyma and its homologues, neurons, primitive undifferentiated cells, and meninges. The tumors may also be metastatic from other regions of the body. Tumors derived from astrocytes include astrocytomas, juvenile pilocytic astrocytomas, and oligodendrogliomas. Astrocytomas range from well-differentiated, histologically benign lesions to highly aggressive anaplastic forms such as glioblastoma multiforme. Intracranial meningiomas arise from the dura, impairing the visual pathway by exertion of a mass effect (Fig. 11-51). Epidermoid tumors arise from cell rests within the suprasellar cistern, enlarging to produce masses that can compress the optic chiasm (Fig. 11-52). FLAIR shows higher signal intensity in the epidermoid tumors than in arachnoid cysts, aiding in their diagnosis (Fig. 11-52).[140–142] Metastatic deposits to the brain from distant primary tumors are responsible for 20% to 25% of all intracranial tumors. The most frequent cell types are bronchogenic and breast carcinomas (Fig. 11-53). Metastatic foci usually are multiple and are found most frequently at the junction of the gray and white matter. The brain tissue surrounding the metastatic focus may show a high degree of vasogenic edema. Microscopically, the metastatic foci are usually identical to the primary neoplasm.

### CT Appearance

On CT, intracranial neoplasms are most often identified as mass lesions with or without contrast enhancement and with or without varying degrees of peritumoral edema. Depending on the tumor's location, there may be associated hydrocephalus or other physical distortion of the neuraxis. Astrocytomas are usually isodense to hypodense to normal brain parenchyma on an unenhanced CT scan. The amount of peritumoral edema frequently reflects the grade of the tumor, as does the degree of enhancement after administration of a contrast medium. More aggressive tumor types, in general, demonstrate a greater degree of enhancement and more peritumoral vasogenic edema. Glioblastoma multiforme often demonstrates intense enhancement in a mixed or ring enhancing pattern and may have a markedly irregular margin (Fig. 11-54). Oligodendrogliomas tend to be of high density before administration of a contrast medium and to contain calcification in more than 90% of cases except in the pediatric population, in which calcification is seen in approximately 40% of cases (Fig. 11-55).[143, 144] On plain CT, meningiomas are usually hyperdense relative to normal brain parenchyma. Calcification is found in approximately 20% of cases. Peritumoral edema may be present, and enhancement is usually homogeneous and intense. Metastatic lesions may be either single or multiple and vary in size.[145] From 3% to 14% of metastatic deposits contain intratumoral hemorrhage.[146] The metastatic lesions on an unenhanced scan are hypodense to surrounding brain unless they contain intratumoral hemorrhage, and edema is almost always present to some degree. Enhancement characteristics vary, but enhancement is almost always present (97%).[145]

### MR Imaging Appearance

In general, MR imaging demonstrates greater sensitivity in tumor detection than does CT.[147] With the exception of the demonstration of calcification and bone abnormalities associated with intracranial tumors, MR better characterizes a tumor once it is detected. With its lack of beam-hardening artifacts, direct multiplanar imaging, and greater contrast sensitivity, MR imaging better depicts the anatomic extent of a tumor than does CT. Acquisition of gadolinium-DTPA–enhanced images of brain neoplasms helps to define the integrity of the blood-brain barrier within the lesion and thus helps to characterize the tumor more completely and limit the differential diagnosis.[148, 149] The appearance of the various tumor types on MR imaging is a function of many factors, including variations in water content; the presence or absence of hemorrhage, fat, calcification, or paramagnetic material such as melanin; and the degree of vascularity of the tumor.[150]

Astrocytomas appear as mass lesions of high signal intensity on long TR/TE images (Fig. 11-56). Peritumoral edema may be seen on long TR/TE images as an area of high signal intensity spreading through the adjacent white matter. It is difficult to differentiate edema from tumor extension solely on the basis of spin-echo images (Figs. 11-56 and 11-57).[60] With increasing grade of the tumor, the tumor

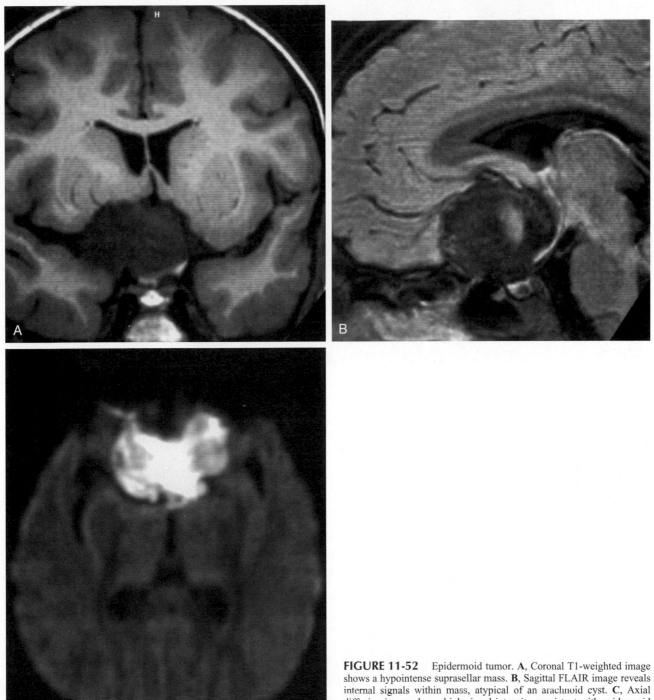

**FIGURE 11-52**   Epidermoid tumor. **A**, Coronal T1-weighted image shows a hypointense suprasellar mass. **B**, Sagittal FLAIR image reveals internal signals within mass, atypical of an arachnoid cyst. **C**, Axial diffusion image shows high signal intensity consistent with epidermoid tumor rather than arachnoid cyst.

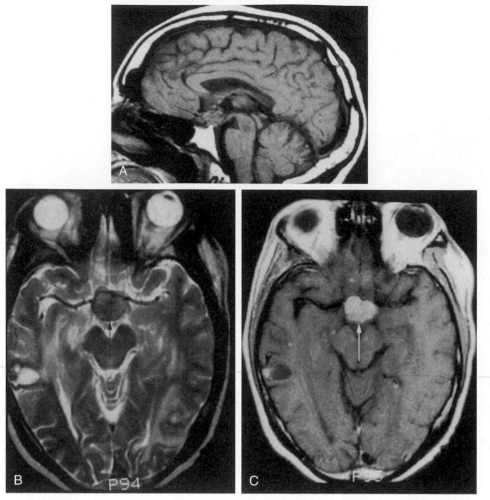

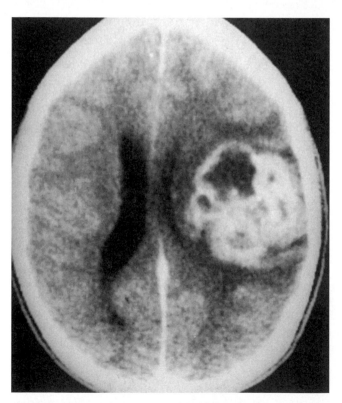

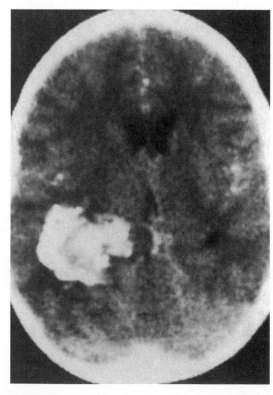

FIGURE 11-53 Metastatic carcinoma of the breast in a 60-year-old female with known carcinoma of the breast presenting with visual loss. **A,** Sagittal T1-weighted MR image shows an irregular mass (*arrow*) involving the optic chiasm. **B,** Axial T2-weighted image shows metastasis (*arrow*) to the optic chiasm to be hypointense, with a hypointense metastasis in the right temporal lobe surrounded by hyperintense vasogenic edema. There is a diffuse increase in signal intensity throughout the white matter secondary to prior radiation therapy. **C,** Axial T1-weighted MR image after gadolinium injection shows enhancement of both the chiasmatic mass (*arrow*) and the right temporal tumor (*arrowhead*).

FIGURE 11-54 Glioblastoma multiforme. Axial CT image after injection of contrast medium shows marked enhancement of an irregular mass in the left frontal parietal region. The body of the left lateral ventricle is compressed.

FIGURE 11-55 Oligodendroglioma. Axial CT image after enhancement shows a dense (calcified) right temporal lobe-thalamic mass.

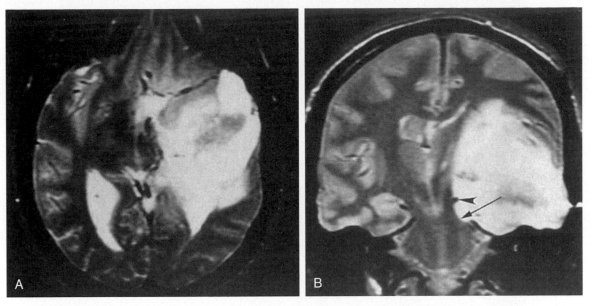

**FIGURE 11-56**   A 43-year-old-male with malignant degeneration of a low-grade astrocytoma of the temporal lobe. **A,** Axial T2-weighted image shows a hyperintense mass involving the left temporal lobe. Edema and tumor are not separable. **B,** Coronal proton density image shows the mass involving the temporal lobe on the left to have high signal intensity. The mass extends superiorly and medially. The tumor mass herniates (*arrow*) over the free edge of the tentorium and displaces medially the basilar vein of Rosenthal (*arrowhead*) against the mesencephalon. The optic tract is compressed.

margins tend to be more irregular. Glioblastoma multiforme, which is the most anaplastic form of astrocytoma, appears on long TR/TE images as a markedly hyperintense, irregularly bordered mass lesion. Also, with increasing tumor grade, there is progressive disruption of the blood-brain barrier, which, after intravenous administration of gadolinium, results in a progressively intense T1 shortening that is seen as increased signal intensity on short

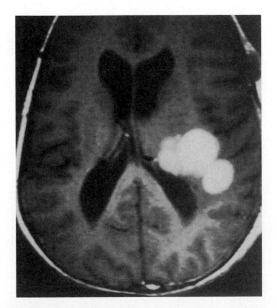

**FIGURE 11-57**   Anaplastic astrocytoma of optic radiations. Axial T1-weighted image after administration of gadolinium shows an enhancing tumor mass involving the left optic radiations.

TR/TE images (Fig. 11-58). In pediatric patients, contrast enhancement can be seen in low-grade astrocytomas as well (Fig. 11-58). Oligodendrogliomas typically show hypointensity on short TR/TE images, with increased signal intensity on long TR/TE scans with signal void in areas of intratumoral calcification. Vasogenic peritumoral edema is infrequently seen, and enhancement following gadolinium-DTPA administration occurs in less than half of the cases.[143, 144]

Meningiomas demonstrate signal characteristics that reflect the amount of calcification, vascularity, and interstitial fluid present within the mass.[151] In general, on short and long TR/TE images, meningiomas are isointense to hypointense to surrounding normal brain parenchyma (Fig. 11-59). As a result of the decreased conspicuity of meningiomas on MR imaging, detection is based on the displacement of normal structures of the neuraxis, including the white matter and vascular structures. On long TR/long TE images, surrounding edema, if present, helps to demarcate isointense meningiomas (Fig. 11-60). Intravenous administration of gadolinium delineates meningiomas much more clearly, because there is usually moderate to marked homogeneous enhancement.

Intracranial metastases display a variety of appearances on MR imaging. Characteristically, they appear on long TR/TE images as foci of increased signal intensity at the gray matter–white matter interface. Peritumoral edema is often present and may be difficult to distinguish from the tumor itself. Subtle differences in T1 and T2 relaxation time between the edema and the tumors may help in the differentiation. However, intravenous administration of gadolinium produces a clearer delineation (Fig. 11-61). The sensitivity for detection of single or multiple metastatic foci is increased with the use of gadolinium, thereby increasing

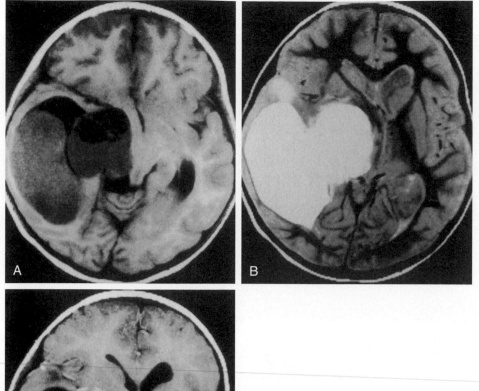

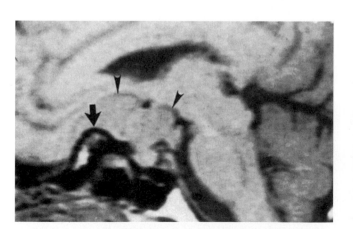

FIGURE 11-58 Pilocytic astrocytoma involving the temporal lobe and basal ganglia in an 18-month-old female with weakness of the left side and a left homonymous visual field defect. **A**, Axial T1-weighted MR image without contrast injection shows a mass that is both cystic and solid in the right temporal lobe and basal ganglia, extending into and displacing the upper brainstem. **B**, Proton density MR image shows the cystic and solid components to be hyperintense. **C**, Axial T1-weighted MR image following gadolinium injection shows enhancement of the more medial solid portion of the tumor.

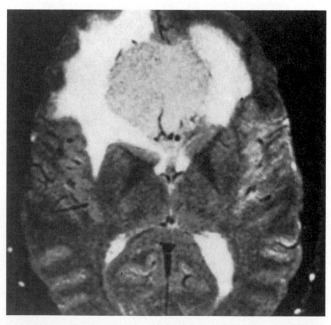

FIGURE 11-59 Suprasellar planum sphenoidal meningioma. Sagittal T1-weighted image shows a slightly hypointense suprasellar mass (*arrowheads*). Hyperostosis of the planum is present (*arrow*).

FIGURE 11-60 Olfactory groove meningioma. Axial T2-weighted image shows an isointense mass between the frontal lobes surrounded by high signal intensity edema.

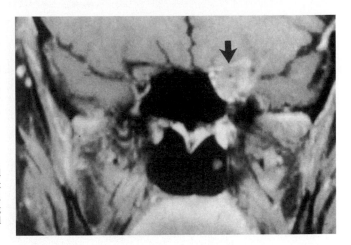

**FIGURE 11-61** Metastatic breast carcinoma to the anterior clinoid process and optic canal in a 67-year-old female with a history of breast carcinoma presenting with visual loss in the left eye. Coronal T1-weighted, fat-suppressed, gadolinium-enhanced MR image shows a contrast-enhancing mass (*arrow*) involving the region of the left optic canal and anterior clinoid process.

the certainty of the diagnosis of a metastatic cause (Fig. 11-50).[152] In metastatic lesions to the wall of the orbit, fat-suppressed, gadolinium-enhanced images are important in demonstrating the disease (Fig. 11-58). In fact, in cases in which multiplicity of lesions is uncertain with the standard dose of 1.0 mmole/kg gadolinium-DTPA, doubling or

tripling the dose has been shown to increase the likelihood that additional lesions will be detected.[153–155]

Aggressive infectious disease processes affecting immunocompromised patients, such as those with HIV, may mimic the appearance of metastatic lesions (Figs. 11-62 and 11-63).

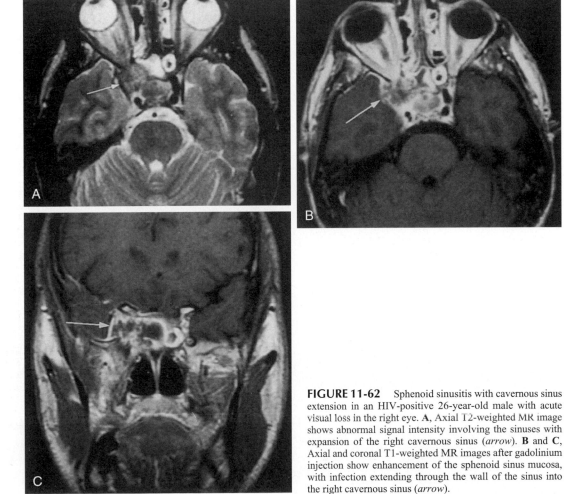

**FIGURE 11-62** Sphenoid sinusitis with cavernous sinus extension in an HIV-positive 26-year-old male with acute visual loss in the right eye. **A,** Axial T2-weighted MR image shows abnormal signal intensity involving the sinuses with expansion of the right cavernous sinus (*arrow*). **B** and **C,** Axial and coronal T1-weighted MR images after gadolinium injection show enhancement of the sphenoid sinus mucosa, with infection extending through the wall of the sinus into the right cavernous sinus (*arrow*).

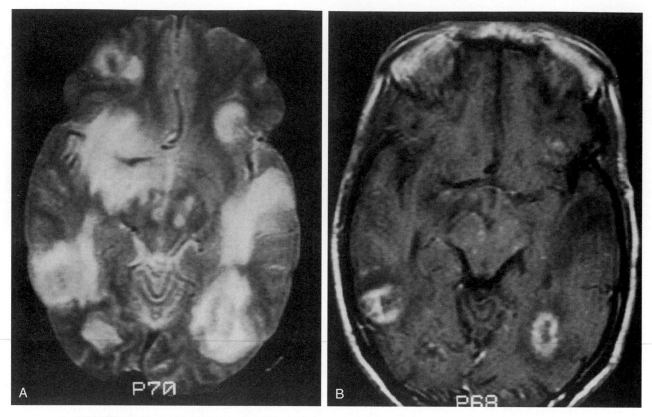

**FIGURE 11-63**   Toxoplasmosis abscesses in an HIV-positive 30-year-old male. **A,** Axial T2-weighted MR image shows multiple high signal intensity masses at the gray matter–white matter junctions and within the brainstem. **B,** Axial T1-weighted MR image after gadolinium injection shows enhancing masses with central necrosis.

# REFERENCES

1. Duke-Elder, ed. System of Ophthalmology. London: Henry Kimpton, 1963.
2. Newell F, ed. Ophthalmology: Principles and Concepts. St. Louis: C.V. Mosby.
3. Gray H, ed. Anatomy of the Human Body. 29th ed. Philadelphia: Lea & Febiger, 1985.
4. Unsold R, DeGroot J, Newton TH. Images of the optic nerve: anatomic CT correlation. AJR 1980;135:767–773.
5. Daniels DL, Haughton VM, Williams AL, Gager WE. Computed tomography of the optic chiasm. Radiology 1980;137:123–127.
6. Bilaniuk LT, Atlas SW, Zimmerman RA. Magnetic resonance imaging of the orbit. Radiol Clin North Am 1987;25:509–528.
7. Azar-Kia B, et al. MR imaging evaluation of optic nerve (abstract). AJNR 1987;8:967.
8. Albert A, Lee BC, Saint-Louis L, et al. MRI of optic chiasm and optic pathways. AJNR 1986;7:255–258.
9. Hendrix LE, Kneeland JB, Haughton VM, et al. MR imaging of optic nerve lesions: value of gadopentetate dimeglumine and fat suppression technique. AJNR 1990;849–854.
10. Hershey BL, Peyster RG. Imaging of cranial nerve. II. Semin Ultrasound CT MR 1987;8(3):164.
11. Daniels DL, Herfkins R, Gager WE, et al. Magnetic resonance imaging of the optic nerves and chiasm. Radiology 1984;152:79–83.
12. Simon J, Szumowski J, Totterman S, et al. Fat suppression MR imaging of the orbit. AJNR 1988;9:961–968.
13. Jackson A, Sheppard S, Johnson AC. Combined fat and water suppressed MRI imaging of orbital tumors. AJNR 1999;20:1963.
14. Atlas SW, Grossman RI, Hackney DB, et al. STIR MR imaging of the orbit. AJR 1988;51:1025–1030.
15. Bastianello S, Bozzao A, Paolillo A, et al. Fast spin-echo and fast fluid-attenuated inversion-recovery versus conventional spin-echo sequences for MR quantification of multiple sclerosis lesions. AJNR 1997;18:699.
16. Ozgen A, Aydingoz U. Normative measurements of orbital structures using MRI. J Comput Assist Tomogr 2000;24:493.
17. Daniels DL, Pech P, Kay MC, et al. Orbital apex: correlative anatomic and CT study. AJR 1985;145:1141–1146.
18. Doyle AJ. Optic chiasm position on MR images. AJNR 1990;11:553–555.
19. el Gammal TE. MR of normal optic chiasm. AJNR 1991;12:584.
20. Eggers H, Jakobiec FA, Jones IS. Optic nerve gliomas. In: Jones IS, Jakobiec FA, eds. Diseases of the Orbit. New York: Harper & Row, 1979;417–433.
21. Azar-Kia B, Naheedy MH, Elias DA, et al. Optic nerve tumors: role of magnetic resonance imaging and computed tomography. Radiol Clin North Am 1987;25:561–581.
22. Naumann GOH, Atle DJ. Optic nerve. In: Naumann GOH, Atle DJ, eds. Pathology of the Eye. New York: Springer-Verlag, 1987;723–770.
23. Davis PC, Hopkins KL. Imaging of pediatric orbit and visual pathways: computed tomography and magnetic resonance imaging. Neuroimaging Clin North Am 1999;9:93.
24. Mafee MF, Putterman A, Valvassori GE, et al. Orbital space occupying lesion: role of computed tomography and magnetic resonance imaging. Radiol Clin North Am 1987;25:529–559.
25. Sobel DF, Kelly W, Kjos BO, et al. MR imaging of orbital and ocular disease. AJNR 1985;6:259–264.
26. Atlas SW, Bilaniuk LT, Zimmerman RA, et al. Orbit: initial experience with surface coil spin-echo MR imaging at 1.5T. Radiology 1987;164:501–509.
27. Haik BG, Saint-Louis L, Bierly J, et al. Magnetic resonance imaging in the evaluation of optic nerve gliomas. Ophthalmology 1987;94:709–717.
28. Jones IS, Jacobiec FA, eds. Diseases of the Orbit. New York: Harper & Row, 1979.

29. Sibony PA, Krauss HR, Kennerdell JS, et al. Optic nerve sheath meningiomas: clinical manifestations. Ophthalmology 1984;11:1313–1326.

30. Hart WM, et al. Bilateral optic nerve meningiomas. AJNR 1980;1:375.

31. Daniels DL, Williams AL, Syvertsen A, et al. CT recognition of optic nerve sheath meningioma: abnormal sheath visualization. AJNR 1982;3:181–183.

32. Samples JR, Robertson DM, Taylor JZ, et al. Optic nerve meningioma. Ophthalmology 1983;90:1591–1594.

33. Atlas SW. Magnetic resonance imaging of the orbit: current status. Magn Resn Q 1989;5:39–96.

34. Hovda E, Wall M, Numaguchi Y, et al. Neurosarcoidosis involving optic nerves and leptomeninges: computed tomography findings. J Comput Assist Tomogr 1986;10:129–133.

35. Beardsley TL, et al. Eleven cases of sarcoidosis of the optic nerve (abstract). AJNR 1985;6:133.

36. Atlas SW, Grossman RI, Savino PJ, et al. Surface coil MR of orbital pseudotumor. AJR 148:803–808.

37. Urbach H, Kristof R, Zentner J, et al. Sarcoidosis presenting as an intra- or extra-axial cranial mass: report of two cases. Neuroradiology 1997;39:516.

38. Wall MJ, Peyster RG, Finkelstein SD, et al. A unique case of neural sarcoidosis with pineal and suprasellar involvement: CT and pathological demonstration. J Comput Assist Tomogr 1985;9:381–383.

39. Mirfakhraee M, Crofford MJ, Guinto FC Jr, et al. Virchow-Robin space: a path of spread in neurosarcoidosis. Radiology 1986;158:715–720.

40. Post MJD, Quencer RM, Tabei SZ, et al. CT demonstration of sarcoidosis of the optic nerve, frontal lobes and falx cerebri: a case report and literature review. AJNR 1982;3:523–526.

41. Hayes WS, Sherman JL, Stern BJ, et al. MR and CT evaluation of intracranial sarcoidosis. AJR 1987;149:1043–1049.

42. Clark WC, Acker JD, Dohan FC, et al. Presentation of central nervous system sarcoidosis as intracranial tumors. J Neurosurg 1985;63:851–856.

43. Walker FO, McLean WT Jr, Elster A, et al. Chiasmal sarcoidosis. AJNR 1990;11:1205–1207.

44. Engleken JD, Yuh WT, Carter KD, et al. Optic nerve sarcoidosis: MR findings. AJNR 1992;12:228–230.

45. Sherman JL, et al. MR evaluation of intracranial sarcoidosis: comparison with CT. AJNR 1987;8:940.

46. Sherman JL, Stern BJ, Sarcoidosis of the CNS: comparison of unenhanced and enhanced MR images. AJNR 1990;11:915–923.

47. Seltzer S, Mark AS, Atlas SW. CNS sarcoidosis: evaluation with contrast enhanced MR imaging. AJNR 1991;12:1227–1233.

48. Cooper SD, Brady MB, Williams JP, et al. Neurosarcoidosis: evaluation using computed tomography and magnetic resonance imaging. J Comput Assist Tomogr 1988;12:96–99.

49. Miller DH, Kendall BE, Barter S, et al. Magnetic resonance imaging in central nervous system sarcoidosis. Neurology 1988;38:378–383.

50. Ketonen L, Oksanen V, Kuuliaha I. Preliminary experience of magnetic resonance imaging in neurosarcoidosis. Neuroradiology 1987;29:127–129.

51. Hayes WS, Sherman JL, Stern BJ, et al. MR and CT evaluation of intracranial sarcoidosis. AJR 1987;49:1043–1049.

52. Packner AR, Duray P, Steere AC. Central nervous system manifestations of Lyme disease. Arch Neurol 1989;46:790–795.

53. Vanzieleghem B, Lemmerling M, Carton D. Lyme disease presenting with bilateral facial nerve palsy: MRI findings and review of the literature. Neuroradiology 1998;40:739.

54. Fernandez RE, Rothberg Ferencz G, Wujack D. Lyme disease of the CNS; MR imaging findings in 14 cases. AJNR 1990;11:479–481.

55. Kissane JM, Anderson WAD, eds. Anderson's Pathology. 9th ed. St. Louis: C.V. Mosby, 1989.

56. Crane TB, Yee RD, Hepler RS, et al. Clinical manifestations and radiologic findings in craniopharyngiomas in adults. Am J Ophthalmol 1982;94:220–228.

57. Pusey E, Kortman KE, Flannigan BD, et al. MR of craniopharyngiomas: tumor delineation and characterization. AJR 1987;149:383–388.

58. Price AC, et al. Craniopharyngioma: correlation of high resolution CT and MRI (abstract). AJNR 1985;6:465.

59. Ahmadi J, Destian S, Apuzzo ML, et al. Cystic fluid in craniopharyngiomas: MR imaging and quantitative analysis. Radiology 1992;182:783–785.

60. Lee BCP, Deck MF. Sellar and juxtasellar lesion: detection with MR. Radiology 1985;157:143–147.

61. Donovan JL, Nesbit GM. Distinction of masses involving the sella and suprasellar space: specificity of imaging features. AJR 1996;167:597.

62. Sutton LN, Wang ZJ, Wehrli SL, et al. Proton spectroscopy of suprasellar tumors in pediatric patients. Neurosurgery 1997;41:388–394.

63. Kucharczyk W, Peck WW, Kelly WM, et al. Rathke cleft cysts. CT, MR imaging and pathologic features. Radiology 1987;165:491–495.

64. Nagasaka S, et al. Rathke's cleft cyst (abstract). AJNR 1982;3:360.

65. Johnson CE, et al. Correlation of MR signal intensity, surgical findings and pathologic features of large pituitary adenomas: differentiation of soft cellular and firm fibrotic tumors (abstract). AJNR 1988;9:1013.

66. Robbins SL, Cotran RS, Kumar L, eds. Pathologic Basis of Disease. 3rd ed. Philadelphia: W.B. Saunders, 1984.

67. Taylor S. High resolution direct coronal CT of the sella and parasellar region (abstract). AJNR 1980;1:364.

68. Majos C, Coll S, Aguilera C. Imaging of giant pituitary adenomas. Neuroradiology 1998;40:651.

69. Davis PC, Hoffman JC Jr, Tindall GT, et al. CT surgical correlation in pituitary adenomas: evaluation of ••• in 113 patients. AJNR 1985;6:711–716.

70. Davis PC, Hoffman JC Jr, Spencer T, et al. MR imaging of pituitary adenoma: CT, clinical, and surgical correlation. AJR 1987;1797–1802.

71. Kunhara N, Takashi S, Hugano S. Hemorrhage in pituitary adenoma: correlation of MR imaging with operative findings. Eur Radiol 1998;8:971.

72. Karnaze MG, Sartor K, Winthrop JD, et al. Suprasellar lesions: evaluation with MR imaging. Radiology 1986;161:77–82.

73. Cottier J-P, Destrieux C, Brunereau L, et al. Cavernous sinus invasion by pituitary adenoma: MR imaging. Radiology 2000;215:463–469.

74. Ostrov SG, Quencer RM, Hoffman JC, et al. Hemorrhage within pituitary adenomas: how often associated with pituitary apoplexy syndrome? AJR 1989;153:153–160.

75. Davis PC, et al. DTPA and MR imaging of the pituitary gland: preliminary report. AJNR 1987;8:817.

76. Newton DR, Dillon WP, Normal D, et al. Gadolinium DTPA enhanced MR imaging of pituitary adenomas. AJNR 1989;10:949–954.

77. Kaufman B, et al. Herniation of the suprasellar visual system and third ventricle into empty sellae: morphologic and clinical considerations. AJNR 1989;10:65.

78. Bull J. Massive aneurysms at the base of the brain. Brain 1969;92:535–570.

79. Vinuela F, Fox A, Chang JK, et al. Clinico-radiological spectrum of giant super elinoid internal carotid artery aneurysms. Neuroradiology 1984;26:93–99.

80. Ferguson GG. Carotid ophthalmic artery aneurysms. In: Wilkins RH, Regarchary SS, eds. Neurosurgery. New York: McGraw-Hill, 1986;•••.

81. Banna M, Lasjaunias P. Intracavernous carotid aneurysm associated with proptosis in a 13 month old girl. AJNR 1991;12:969–970.

82. Deeb ZL, Schimel S, Rothfus WE, et al. Diagnosis of bilateral intracavernous carotid artery aneurysms by computed tomography. J Comput Assist Tomogr 1986;10:121–127.

83. Rhoton AL. Microsurgical anatomy of saccular aneurysms. In: Wilkins R, Rengarchary S, eds. Neurosurgery. New York: McGraw-Hill, 1986;•••.

84. Atlas SW, Grossman RI, Goldberg HI, et al. Partially thrombosed giant intracranial aneurysms: correlation of MR and pathologic findings. Radiology 1987;162:111–114.

85. Aoki S, Sasaki Y, Machida T, et al. Cerebral aneurysms: detection and delineation using 3D CT angiography. AJNR 1992;13:1115–1120.

86. Noguchi K, Ogawa T, Seto H, et al. Subacute and chronic subarachoid hemorrhage: diagnosis with fluid-attenuated inversion-recovery imaging. Radiology 1997;203:257–262.

87. Ross JS, Masaryk TJ, Modic MT, et al. Intracranial aneurysms: evaluation by MR angiography. AJNR 1990;11:449–455.

88. Hirsch W, et al. MRI in evaluation of parasellar aneurysms (abstract). AJNR 1987;8:957.

89. Pinto RS, Kricheff II, Butler AR. Correlation of computed tomographic, angiographic and neuropathological changes in giant cerebral aneurysms. Radiology 1979;132:85–92.

90. Olsen WL, Brant-Zawadzki M, Hodes J, et al. Giant intracranial aneurysms: MR imaging. Radiology 1987;163:431–435.

91. Becker RD, et al. MR appearance of intracranial aneurysms (abstract). AJNR 1987;8:964.

92. Slavin ML, Lam BL, Decker RE, et al. Chiasmal compression from fat packing after transsphenoidal resection of intrasellar tumor in two patients. Am J Ophthalmol 1993;115:368–371.

93. Cohen MM, Lessell S. Chiasm as syndrome due to metastasis. Arch Neurol 1979;36:565–567.

94. Beauchamp NJ Jr, Ulug AM, Passe TJ, van Zijl PCM. MR diffusion imaging in stroke: review and controversies. RadioGraphics 1998;18:1269.

95. Drake ME, et al. Conversion of ischemic to hemorrhagic infarction by anticoagulant administration: report of 2 cases with evidence from serial CT brain scans (abstract). Arch Neurol 1983;40:44–46.

96. Von Kummer R, Allen KL, Holle R, et al. Acute stroke: usefulness of early CT findings before thrombolytic therapy. Radiology 1997;205:327.

97. Tomsick TA, Brott TG, Chambers AA, et al. Hyperdense middle cerebral artery sign on CT: efficacy in detecting middle cerebral artery thrombosis. AJNR 1990;11:473–477.

98. Tomsick TA, Brott T, Barsan W, et al. Prognostic value of the hyperdense middle cerebral artery sign and stroke scale score before ultraearly thrombolytic therapy. AJNR 1996;17:79.

99. Rauch RA, Bazan C III, Larsson EM. Hyperdense middle cerebral arteries identified on CT as a false sign of vascular occlusion. AJNR 1993;14:669–673.

100. Drayer B. Imaging of cerebral infarction and intracerebral hematoma using MR, CT and SPECT (abstract). AJNR 1985;6:464.

101. Moseley ME, Kucharczyk J, Mintorovitch J, et al. Diffusion weighted MR imaging of acute stroke: correlation with T2 weighted and magnetic susceptibility-enhanced MR imaging in cats. AJNR 1990;11:423–429.

102. Fisher M, et al. Diffusion weighted MR imaging and ischemic stroke. AJNR 1992;13:1103.

103. Bryan RN, Levy LM, Whitlow WD, et al. Diagnosis of acute cerebral infarction: comparison of CT and MR imaging. AJNR 1991;12:611–620.

104. Unger EC, Gado MH, Fulling KF, et al. Acute cerebral infarction in monkeys: an experimental study using MR imaging. Radiology 1987;162:789–795.

105. Yuh WTC, Crane MR, Loes DJ, et al. MR imaging of cerebral ischemia: findings in the first 24 hours. AJNR 1991;12:621–629.

106. Mueller DP, Yuh WT, Fisher DJ. Arterial enhancement in acute cerebral ischemia: clinical and angiographic correlation. AJNR 1993;14:661–668.

107. Chien D, Kwong KK, Gress DR, et al. MR diffusion imaging of cerebral infarction in humans. AJNR 1992;13:1097–1102.

108. Maier SE, Gudbjartsson H, Patz S, et al. Line scan diffusion imaging: characterization in healthy subjects and stroke patients. AJR 1998;171:85.

109. Marshal VG, Bradley WG Jr, Marshall CE, et al. Deep white matter infarction: correlation of MR imaging and histopathologic findings. Radiology 1988;167:517–522.

110. Brant-Zawadzki M, Pereira B, Weinstein P, et al. MRI of acute experimental ischemia in cats. Am J Neuroradiol 1985;7:7–11.

111. Elster AD. MR contrast enhancement in brainstem and deep cerebral infarction. AJNR 1991;12:1127–1132.

112. Virasponge C, Mancuso H, Quisling R. Human brain infarcts: Gd-DTPA–enhanced MR imaging. Radiology 1986;161:785–794.

113. Sheldon JJ, Siddharthan R, Tobias J, et al. MR imaging of multiple sclerosis: comparison with clinical and CT examinations in 74 patients. AJR 1985;145:957–964.

114. Uhlenbrock D, Seidel D, Gehlen W, et al. MR imaging in multiple sclerosis: comparison with clinical CSF and visually evoking potential findings. AJNR 1988;9:59–67.

115. Poser CM, Goutieres F, Carpentier MA, et al. Schilder's myelinoclastic diffuse sclerosis. Pediatrics 1986;77:107–112.

116. Choi S, Enzmann. Infantile Krabbe disease: complementary CT and MR findings. AJNR 1993;14:1164–1166.

117. Mikol F, et al. Computed tomography in multiple sclerosis. Rev Neurol 1980;136:481.

118. Spiegel SM, Vinuela F, Fox AJ, et al. CT of multiple sclerosis: reassessment of delayed scanning with high doses of contrast material. AJR 1985;145:497–500.

119. Osborn AG, Harnsberger HR, Smoker WR, et al. Multiple sclerosis in adolescents: CT and MR findings. AJR 1990;155:385–390.

120. Mehler MF, Rabinowich L. Inflammatory myelinoclastic diffuse sclerosis (Schilders disease): neuroradiologic findings. AJNR 1989;10:176–180.

121. Paty DW, Oger JJ, Kastrukoff LF, et al. MRI in the diagnosis of MS: a prospective study with comparison of clinical evaluation, evoking potentials, oligoclonal banding and CT. Neurology 1988;38:180–185.

122. Gebarski SS, Garbrielsen TO, Gilman S. The initial diagnosis of multiple sclerosis: clinical impact of magnetic resonance imaging. Ann Neurol 1985;17:469–474.

123. Johnson MA, Li DK, Bryant DJ, et al. Magnetic resonance imaging: serial observations in multiple sclerosis. AJNR 1984;5:495–499.

124. Ebner F, Millner MM, Justich E. Multiple sclerosis in children: value of serial MR studies to monitor patients. AJNR 1990;11:1023–1027.

125. Yhousry TA, Filippi M, Becker C, et al. Comparison of MR pulse sequences in the detection of multiple sclerosis lesions. AJNR 1997;18:959.

126. Kurihara N, Takahashi S, Furuta A, et al. MR imaging of multiple sclerosis simulating brain tumor. Clin Imag 1996;20:171.

127. Nowell MA, Grossman RI, Hackney DB, et al. MR imaging of white matter disease in children. AJR 1988;151:359–365.

128. De La Paz RL, et al. High field MR imaging of spinal cord multiple sclerosis (abstract). AJNR 1987;8:949.

129. Rosenblatt MA, Behrens MM, Zweifach PH, et al. Magnetic resonance imaging of optic tract involvement in multiple sclerosis. Am J Ophthalmol 1987;104:74–79.

130. Edwards MK, Farlow MR, Stevens JC. Cranial MR in spinal cord MS: diagnosing patients with isolated spinal cord symptoms. AJNR 1986;7:1003–1005.

131. Grossman RI, Lenkinski RE, Ramer KN, et al. MR proton spectroscopy in multiple sclerosis. AJNR 1992;13:1535–1543.

132. Larsson EM, Holtas S, Nilsson O. Gd DTPA enhanced MR of suspected spinal multiple sclerosis. AJNR 1989;10:1071–1076.

133. Simon JH. Contrast-enhanced MR imaging in the evaluation of treatment response and prediction of outcome in multiple sclerosis. J Magn Reson Imag 1997;7:29.

134. Grossman RI. Meningeal enhancement in multiple sclerosis: truth or coincidence. AJNR 1992;13:401–402.

135. Barkhoff F, Valk J, Hommes OR, et al. Meningeal Gd-DTPA enhancement in multiple sclerosis. AJNR 1992;13:397–400.

136. Merandi SF, Kudryk BT, Murtagh FR, et al. Contrast enhanced MR imaging of optic nerve lesions in patients with acute optic neuritis. AJNR 1991;12:923–926.

137. Jackson A, Sheppard S, Laitt RD, et al. Optic neuritis: MR imaging with combined fat- and water-suppression techniques. Radiology 1998;206:57.

138. Edwards MK, et al. Clinical utility of inversion recovery MR in the diagnosis of MS (abstract). AJNR 1989;10:898.

139. Hart MN, Earle KM. Primitive neuroectodermal tumors of the brain in children. Cancer 1973;32:890–897.

140. Ikushima I, Korogi Y, Hirai T, et al. MR of epidermoids with a variety of pulse sequences. AJNR 1997;18:1359–1363.

141. Lang ADP, Mitchell PJ, Wallace D. Diffusion weighted magnetic resonance imaging of intracranial epidermoid tumors. Australas Radiol 1999;43:16.

142. Kallmes DF, Provenzale JM, Cloft HJ, et al. Typical and atypical MR imaging features of intracranial epidermoid tumors. AJR 1997;169:883.

143. Lee YY, Van Tassel P. Intracranial oligodendrogliomas: imaging findings in 35 untreated cases. AJR 1989;152:361–369.

144. Tice H, Barnes PD, Goumnerova L, et al. Pediatric and adolescent oligodendrogliomas. AJNR 1993;14:1293.

145. Pechova-Peterova V, Kalvach P. CT findings in cerebral metastases. Neuroradiology 1986;28:254–258.

146. Atlas SW, Grossman RI, Gomori JM, et al. Hemorrhagic intracranial malignant neoplasm: spin-echo MR imaging. Radiology 1987;164:71–77.

147. Lee BCP, Kneeland JB, Cahill PT, et al. MR recognition of supratentorial tumors. AJNR 1985;6:871–878.

148. Haustein J, Landiado M, Niendorf HP, et al. Administration of gadopentitate dimeglumine in MR imaging of intracranial tumors: dosage and field strength. AJNR 1992;13:1199–1206.

149. Nägele T, Petersen D, Klose U, et al. Dynamic contrast enhancement of intracranial tumors with snapshot-FLASH imaging. AJNR 1993;14:89–98.

150. Spoto GP, Press GA, Hesselink JR, et al. Intracranial ependymoma and subependymoma: MR manifestations. AJNR 1990;11:83–91.

151. Sheporaitis LA, Osborn AG, Smirniotopoulos JG, et al. Intracranial mcningioma. AJNR 1992;13:29–37.

152. Healy ME, Hesselink JR, Press GA, et al. Increased detection of intracranial metastases with intravenous Gd-DTPA. Radiology 1987;165:619–624.

153. Yuh WTC, Engelken JD, Muhonen MG, et al. Experience with high dose gadolinium MR imaging in the evaluation of brain metastasis. AJNR 1992;13:335–345.

154. Davis PC, Hudgins PA, Peterman SB, et al. Diagnosis of cerebral metastases: double dose delayed CT vs. contrast enhanced MR imaging. AJNR 1991;12:293–300.

155. Sze G, Milano E, Johnson C, et al. Detection of brain metastases: comparison of contrast enhanced MR with unenhanced MR and enhanced CT. AJNR 1990;11:785–791.

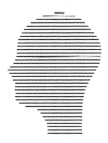

# Central Skull Base

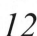

*12*

# Central Skull Base: Embryology, Anatomy, and Pathology

*Hugh D. Curtin, James D. Rabinov, and
Peter M. Som*

## INTRODUCTION

Advances in the techniques of skull base surgery could not have been realized without the developments made in modern imaging. The precise preoperative mapping of a lesion and the demonstration of its relationship to vital neural and vascular structures have allowed surgeons to plan an approach maximizing the chance for resection while minimizing morbidity. Before the CT and MR imaging era, the extent of a tumor was determined at the time of surgery, and the morbidity of the extensive approaches needed to stage a tumor was considered unwarranted in many cases. Today the surgeon can differentiate a tumor that has a possibility of complete resection from one where cure is unlikely and removal would cause unacceptably high morbidity.

The field of skull base surgery is still evolving, with many questions yet to be answered. Certainly there is controversy regarding what procedures are reasonable and appropriate. Thus, although technically a skull base lesion can be accurately mapped and surgically extirpated, it remains for further analysis to determine when a treatment represents a significant advantage to a patient.

Surgeons from several disciplines combine their skills to achieve approaches that, though extensive, are designed to keep manipulation of the crucial and fragile neurovascular structures to a minimum. The tenet of these procedures is to move bone, not brain.

Other therapeutic options such as proton and neutron beams, gamma knife radiosurgery, and various other focused beam radiotherapeutic technologies all require precise imaging definition of tumor boundaries if the lesion is to be treated and crucial radiosensitive structures spared.

The skull base can be divided into several regions—anterior, central, and posterior or posterolateral. The anterior skull base consists of the floor of the anterior cranial fossa and the frontal sinus, including the roof of the ethmoid sinuses, nasal cavity, and orbits. This topic is covered in Chapters 1 to 7. The posterolateral skull base is the temporal bone, and this topic is covered in Chapters 19 to 26. The present chapter covers the central skull base.

The primary component of the central basicranium is the sphenoid bone, with a smaller contribution from the basiocciput. In addition, the soft tissues immediately contiguous to these bony structures form an integral part of the central skull base, and such structures as the cavernous sinus, the pterygopalatine fossa, and the soft tissues adjacent to the foramen ovale and the superior orbital fissure are also discussed in this chapter.

## EMBRYOLOGY

The basicranium develops primarily from cartilage precursors, with a small component from membranous bone. A review of certain details of basicranium development is important in understanding some of the normal and abnormal imaging findings.

The primordial embryonic germ disk is composed of the two primary germ layers, the epiblast and the hypoblast. The epiblast, which will evolve into the ectoderm, develops from the floor of the amniotic cavity, while the hypoblast develops from the roof of the yolk sac. At the fourteenth day of embryonic life, demarcation at the anterior pole of the embryonic disk occurs, and a thickening, the prechordal plate, arises in the future midcephalic region. This prechordal plate prefaces the development of the oropharyngeal region and eventually gives rise to the endodermal layer of the oropharyngeal membrane. In the third week of gestation, the mesoderm proliferates in all directions between the two primary layers of the embryo, adding thickness to the embryonic disk.[1] These mesodermal cells are derived from the primitive streak at the caudal end of the ectodermal side of the embryo. Within the mesoderm, as a result of proliferation and differentiation, a more condensed core of cells, the notochord, stretches from the cranial end of the primitive streak toward the cranial end of the embryo and the prechordal plate. The notochord acts as an axial skeleton for the embryo and has a profound effect on the later development of the spine and the skull base. The notochord induces the formation of the neural plate in the overlying ectoderm (neural ectoderm).

Embryonic differentiation continues, and the formation of the primitive brain and cranial nerves begins. Only after the positions of these neural primordia are established does the skull base itself begin to form. Condensations of the mesenchyme along the notochord (paraxial mesoderm) and contributions from the neural crest progress from the occipital level cranially. This process forms the basal condensation referred to as the *desmocranium*. This mesenchymal blastema extends beyond the level of the tip of the notochord into the prechordal area. It is within this desmocranium that chondrification eventually occurs.[2, 3]

The notochord is contained within the basal condensation of mesoderm and maintains a close relationship to the developing brain and primitive pharynx (Fig. 12-1). The terminus of the notochord is close to the oropharyngeal membrane, separating the ectoderm of the stomatodeum from the endoderm of the primitive pharynx. The formation of Rathke's (hypophyseal) pouch, from the mucosa of the stomatodeum (ectoderm), is thought to be influenced by the notochord. This pouch, which will generate the anterior pituitary gland, passes through the basal mesoderm just cephalad to the tip of the notochord on the way to meet the diverticulum of the diencephalon, which will pass downward, forming the posterior pituitary.[4] Rathke's pouch and tract pass through the mesoderm before chondrification occurs.

Before reaching the prechordal plate, the notochord comes into contact with the endoderm of the primitive pharynx, close to the position of Rathke's pouch, but on the endodermal side of the oropharyngeal membrane. It is at this level that a small outpouching from the pharyngeal mucosa develops, apparently drawn cranially by the notochord. This is the pouch of Luschka, and its position is identified by the pharyngeal bursa, a midline evagination from the nasopharyngeal wall.[5]

Chondrification centers appear within the basal mesodermal condensation. Those centers forming around the distal notochord are the parachordal cartilages. The cartilages from the occipital sclerotomes (from the four occipital somites) are incorporated into the basal cartilaginous plate. Together the parachordal- and sclerotome-derived cartilages are responsible for the formation of the basiocciput.[6]

At about the same time and slightly more cephalad, the prechordal cartilage centers are forming.[3, 6] The hypophyseal ossification centers form on either side of the hypophysis and fuse together (Fig. 12-2), completely obliterating the remnant of Rathke's duct.[3] The fused hypophyseal cartilages represent the precursors of the basisphenoid, forming most of the body of that bone. The paired presphenoid (or trabecular) cartilages fuse to become the precursor of the most anterior part of the sphenoid bone (anterior to the tuberculum sella) and give rise to the mesethmoid cartilage. The mesethmoid cartilage, in turn, develops into the perpendicular plate of the ethmoid and the crista galli.

The sphenoid bone is completed by a group of more laterally placed cartilages also developing from the basal mesoderm.[6] The orbitosphenoid cartilage forms the lesser wing of the sphenoid and contributes to the optic foramen, and the alisphenoid cartilage center produces the medial part

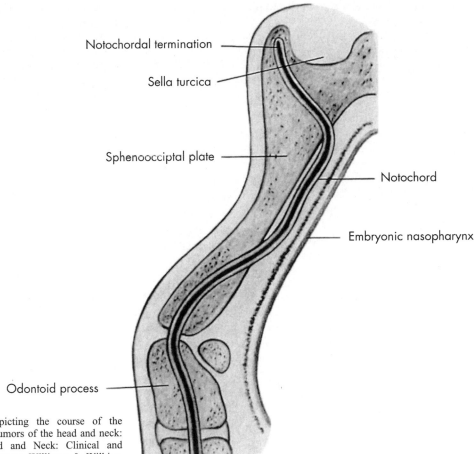

Notochordal termination

Sella turcica

Sphenoocciptal plate

Notochord

Embryonic nasopharynx

Odontoid process

**FIGURE 12-1**  Midsagittal section depicting the course of the notochord. (From Batsakis JG. Soft tissue tumors of the head and neck: unusual forms. In: Tumors of the Head and Neck: Clinical and Pathological Considerations. 2nd ed. Baltimore: Williams & Wilkins, 1979; 353.)

of the greater sphenoid wing. The more lateral wing forms from condensed mesenchyme (intramembranous bone) rather than having a cartilaginous precursor.

The basiocciput and the various cartilage centers representing the sphenoid bone fuse into a cartilaginous continuum called the basal cartilaginous plate. The various foramina of the final basicranium are present within this primitive cartilaginous formation because the nerves and vessels have developed before chondrification begins and the cartilage is forced to develop around them. The bilateral otic capsule chondrifications also fuse to the parachordal cartilages and thus are joined with the basal plate.

Ossification centers now form within the cartilaginous precursor centers. This mechanism produces the presphenoid and postsphenoid as well as the lesser and greater wings. The pterygoid plates and portions of the greater wings form by intramembranous ossification. The small hamulus of the pterygoid develops endochondrally from a small chondroid center.

As ossification progresses, most of the cartilage between the centers is obliterated. Remaining cartilage can be found in various synchondroses, which persist into adult life. The most prominent ones are in the foramen lacerum and petroclival junction. The presphenoid and postsphenoid bones usually fuse by birth, but occasionally the separation persists in the newborn.[7] The bones of Bertin are two small, paired ossification centers that quickly fuse with the anterior sphenoid. It is here that pneumatization of the sphenoid bone begins. Thus, the initial air cells are formed in the

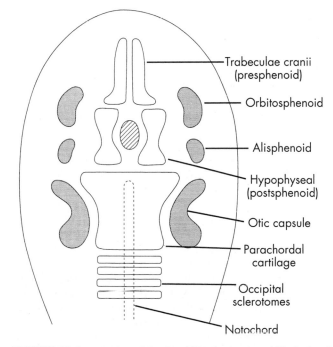

Trabeculae cranii (presphenoid)

Orbitosphenoid

Alisphenoid

Hypophyseal (postsphenoid)

Otic capsule

Parachordal cartilage

Occipital sclerotomes

Notochord

**FIGURE 12-2**  Diagram of the chondrification centers within the basal mesodermal condensation. The hypophyseal centers form on either side of the hypophysis and eventually fuse to form the sella and obliterate the pharyngohypophyseal canal. The postsphenoid is formed from these cartilage centers. The presphenoid forms more anteriorly. The orbitosphenoid and alisphenoid will contribute to the greater and lesser wings respectively.

presphenoid and progress into the more posterior and lateral ossification centers.

## ANATOMY

The sphenoid bone is rightfully the focus of any discussion of the central skull base (Fig. 12-3).[8–11] The anterior basiocciput, articulating with the posterior inferior aspect of the sphenoid bone, also makes an important contribution to the central skull base. Equally crucial to imaging evaluation of the central skull base is an understanding of the contiguous soft tissues.

### Bone

The sphenoid bone consists of a body, the greater and lesser wings, and the pterygoid processes (Fig. 12-4). The term *sphenoid* is derived from the Greek word for "wedge," perhaps referring to its shape or its position between the basiocciput and the anterior skull base. The bone itself has been likened to the appearance of a diving horned owl when viewed from the anterior.

The central part of the sphenoid bone is a block-like structure variably hollowed out by the sphenoid sinus and bordered by many perforations, allowing passage of nerves and vessels. The great wings of the sphenoid sweep laterally, reaching and contributing to the lateral surface of the calvarium, just anterior to the squamous part of the temporal bone. Here the sphenoid bone articulates with the frontal bone, temporal bone, and parietal bone. The lesser wings are more medial in position and form the superior margin of the superior orbital fissure. The anterior clinoid is the posterior margin of the lesser wing. The pterygoid processes, with medial and lateral plates, drop inferiorly from the junction of the body and the greater wing.

Although much of the surface anatomy of the sphenoid bone, such as the sella turcica, the anterior and posterior clinoid processes, and the pterygoid plates, is familiar to the reader, other, slightly more obscure landmarks may be helpful in analyzing some of the imaging findings.

The superior surface of the sphenoid bone forms part of the floor of the anterior cranial fossa (Fig. 12-4B). Just posterior to the cribriform plate of the ethmoid bone, the ethmoid process of the sphenoid bone makes up the most anterior part of the planum sphenoidale. The planum is a flat region separating the cribriform area anteriorly from the chiasmatic sulcus, or groove, posteriorly. The planum is contiguous laterally with the flat superior surface of each lesser sphenoid wing.

The chiasmatic sulcus is a small, linear, transversely oriented depression just posterior to the planum (Fig. 12-4B-D). The anterior rim of the sulcus is referred to as the limbus and represents the most posterior ossification of the presphenoid ossification center. The posterior rim of the chiasmatic sulcus is the tuberculum, which represents the anterior ossification of the postsphenoid ossification center. The sulcus itself is thus the region that remains between these two ossification centers and is not the expected location of the optic chiasm, as its name implies.

The turberculum separates the sulcus from the sella turcica. The optic canals enter the intracranial compartment at the level of the lateral margins of the chiasmatic sulcus.

The dorsum sella is a roughly rectangular plate of bone forming the posterior wall of the sella. The posterior surface of the dorsum is continuous with the posterior surface of the body of the sphenoid and basiocciput. This sloping surface is called the clivus.

On each side, the sphenoid bone is separated from the petrous apex of the temporal bone by the large foramen lacerum. The foramen lacerum is continuous with the smaller, more posterior petrooccipital fissure (petroclival synchondrosis). Both of these are filled with plates of cartilage.

The carotid artery exits the tip of the petrous apex and passes along the lateral aspect of the sphenoid body, causing a groove that reaches almost to the anterior clinoid process. This groove may cause an indentation on the lateral wall of the sphenoid sinus when viewed from within the sinus (Fig. 12-5).

The inferior surface of the sphenoid is very irregular, with many grooves and spurs (Fig. 12-4E,F). The pterygoid processes have already been mentioned. The free margin of the upper posterior edge of the medial pterygoid plate splits to form a shallow groove called the scaphoid fossa. The fossa extends posterolaterally toward the spine of the sphenoid. The tensor veli palatini muscle attaches to the scaphoid fossa and to the sphenoid spine. The sphenomandibular ligament also attaches to this spine.

More medially, the body of the sphenoid forms the roof of the nasopharynx. The rostrum of the sphenoid is in the midline and articulates with the vomer. More superiorly, on the anterior surface of the body, the midline ethmoid crest of the sphenoid articulates with the perpendicular plate of the ethmoid. The orifices to the sphenoid sinus are just lateral to this crest.

An understanding of the various perforations, foramina, and fissures of the sphenoid bone can be achieved best by studying cross-sectional images along with the pictures of specimens (Figs. 12-6 to 12-9).

In the axial plane (Fig. 12-7), the optic foramina (canals) converge toward the sella and optic chiasm and are almost perpendicular to one another. The cross-sectional shape of the optic canal changes from its intracranial to its extracranial margins. The intracranial margin of each optic canal has a slightly oval shape with the long axis horizontal. The midportion of the canal is circular and the intraorbital margin of the canal has an oval shape with the long axis vertical. The superior orbital fissure is a curving cleft when viewed from the front. When viewed in the axial plane, the fissure is directed toward the anterior cavernous sinus rather than toward the region of the sella. In the majority of cases a small amount of the orbital fat extends through the fissure to abut the cavernous sinus.

Just caudal to the superior orbital fissure, the foramen rotundum and the Vidian canal (pterygoid canal) pass from posterior to anterior through the skull base. The foramen rotundum is shorter, wider, and fairly straight, and it is found immediately inferior to the superior orbital fissure. In some individuals the foramen is extremely short, appearing only as a gap in the bone on axial images. The foramen rotundum passes from the cavernous sinus region to the pterygopal-

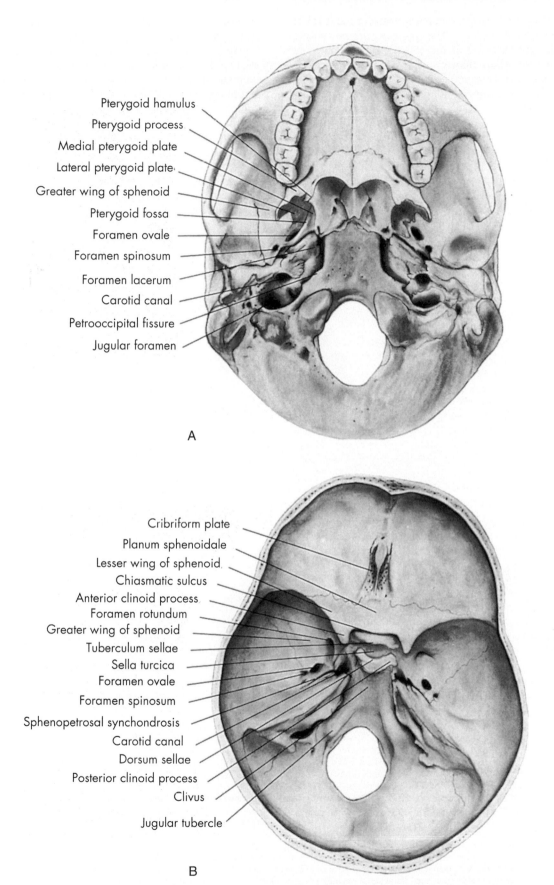

**FIGURE 12-3**   **A,** Exocranial view of the skull base. **B,** Endocranial view of the skull base.

atine fossa (Fig. 12-7D) and enters the fossa at the level of the inferior orbital fissure. The inferior orbital fissure separates the greater wing of the sphenoid from the more anteriorly located orbital floor.

The Vidian canal (pterygoid canal) (Fig. 12-7F) has its ventral margin more medial than its dorsal end, and its dorsal aspect points toward the carotid canal (petrous portion) rather than toward the cavernous sinus, as does the foramen rotundum. The Vidian canal is more inferior, slightly medial, longer, and narrower than the foramen rotundum. The anterior opening of the Vidian canal flairs (Vidian's trumpet) into the pterygopalatine fossa at the level of the sphenopalatine foramen. This foramen communicates between the pterygopalatine fossa and the posterior nasal cavity and nasopharynx.

The foramina ovale and spinosum (Fig. 12-7F) also

extend through the sphenoid bone at the junction of the body and greater wing. They transmit the third division of the trigeminal nerve and the middle meningeal artery, respectively. The foramen ovale is anterior and medial to the foramen spinosum. The foramen ovale angles somewhat anteriorly and slightly laterally toward its extracranial opening. The foramen of Vesalius (emissary sphenoidal foramen) is an inconstant channel that passes anterior and slightly medial to the foramen ovale, carrying a small vein from the cavernous sinus. Other canals occasionally can be seen passing close to the foramen ovale through the medial greater wing of the sphenoid and root of the pterygoid. These are believed to carry venous connections from the cavernous sinus to the pterygoid plexus.[12]

The same anatomic landmarks also can be appreciated in the coronal plane (Figs. 12-8 and 12-9). Now the foramen

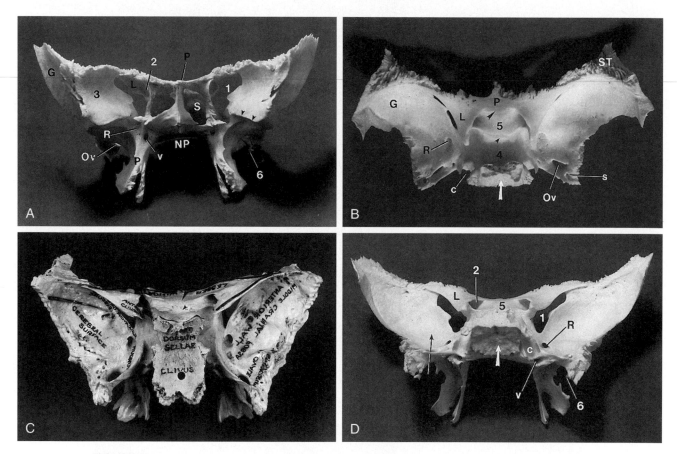

**FIGURE 12-4**   **A,** Anterior view of the sphenoid shows the superior orbital fissure (*1*), which can be followed down to the foramen rotundum (*R*). *G,* Greater wing; *L,* lesser wing of the sphenoid; *3,* orbital surface of the greater wing; *2,* optic canal; *V,* Vidian canal; *Ov,* foramen ovale; *6,* spine of the sphenoid; *NP,* nasopharyngeal area; *P,* planum sphenoidale; *S,* sphenoid sinus. The arrowheads are placed along the margin of the inferior orbital fissure. **B,** View from above. *G,* Greater wing; *L,* lesser wing of the sphenoid; *R,* foramen rotundum; *P,* planum sphenoidale; *Ov,* foramen ovale; *S,* foramen spinosum; *4,* sella turcica. The chiasmatic sulcus (*5*) can be followed out laterally to the intracranial end of the optic canal. *Large arrowhead,* limbus; *small arrowhead,* tuberculum sella; *large arrow,* sphenoid portion of the clivus; *C,* notch in the sphenoid bone through which passes the carotid artery. The dorsum sella has been broken off in this picture. **C,** View from posteriorly. (Courtesy Dr. Lewis E. Etter collection.) Posterior view of the clivus and dorsum sella with the clinoids intact. The relationship of the superior orbital fissure and foramen rotundum can be identified. The foramen ovale is seen further posteriorly. The tuberculum sella (*small arrowhead*) and the limbus (*larger arrowhead*) form the boundaries of the chiasmatic groove. **D,** View from posteriorly (the dorsum sella has been removed). The superior orbital fissure (*1*) can be followed toward the foramen rotundum (*R*). Optic canal intracranial opening (*2*) passing toward the chiasmatic sulcus (*5*). *L,* Lesser wing of the sphenoid; *C,* groove for the carotid artery; *v,* intracranial opening of the Vidian canal; *6,* spine of the sphenoid. The large white arrow shows the junctional surface of the basisphenoid at the sphenooccipital suture. The small black arrow passes through the foramen ovale.

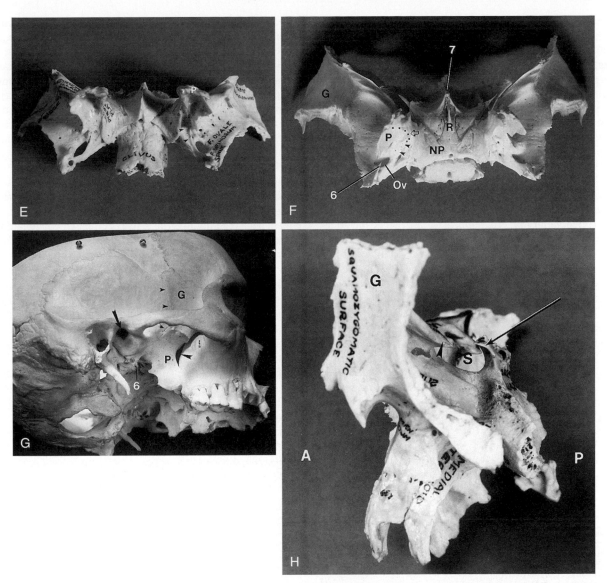

**FIGURE 12-4**    *Continued.* **E**, View from inferiorly showing the nasopharyngeal surface of the sphenoid bone. The pterygoid process (*P*) projects toward us. The scaphoid groove (*arrowheads*) is the attachment of the tensor veli palatini. The foramen ovale and foramen spinosum can be identified. **F**, View from inferiorly shows the rostrum (*R*) of the sphenoid, the sphenoid crest (*7*), the nasopharyngeal surface (*NP*), the greater wing of the sphenoid (*G*), and the pterygoid process (P). The letter P is on the lateral plate. The dotted line curves onto the medial plate indicated by the open arrow. The scaphoid fossa (*small arrowheads*) is the origin of the tensor veli palatini. The foramen ovale (*Ov*) and foramen spinosum (unlabeled) are partially obscured by the spine (*6*) of the sphenoid. **G**, Lateral view of the skull shows the pterygoid process (*P*) and the lateral surface of the greater wing (*G*) of the sphenoid. The large arrowhead indicates the pterygopalatine fossa. The small arrowheads are seen along the suture between the greater wing of the sphenoid and the squamosa of the temporal bone. The arrow indicates the glenoid fossa of the temporomandibular joint. *6*, Spine of the sphenoid. **H**, Lateral view of the sphenoid bone disarticulated. (Courtesy Dr. Lewis E. Etter collection.) Lateral view shows the greater wing of the sphenoid (*G*) and the pterygoid plates. More centrally, the posterior clinoid (*arrow*) is seen at the top of the dorsum sella. *Arrowhead*, Anterior clinoid; *S*, sella.

rotundum and the Vidian canal are seen in cross section, while the foramina ovale and spinosum are seen in longitudinal section. More posteriorly, Meckel's cave and the cavernous sinus structures are seen well in the coronal cross section.

At imaging, the normal appearance of the sphenoid bone depends on the degree of sinus development (Figs. 12-6 and 12-10) and the type of marrow present in the bone. The medullary space of the infant is predominantly red marrow.

This is gradually replaced by fat of inactive yellow marrow.[13] This change begins in early childhood and progresses into adolescence. Usually by the late teens, the sphenoid medullary cavity is completely replaced by fat, giving a characteristic appearance at CT and MR imaging. For example, the medullary space of the basicranium in most infants less than 1 year of age has a uniformly low signal intensity on T1-weighted images. Areas of high signal intensity, representing fat, rapidly appear, and by the age of

7, some fatty marrow is present in virtually all people. Frequently, there are patches of both high and low signal intensity, giving an irregular MR pattern.[14, 15] By the age of 15, a uniformly fatty marrow with high signal intensity on T1-weighted images is present in most people, although some red marrow with lower T1-weighted signal intensity can persist into adulthood.

In the adult, fat is usually evenly distributed throughout the medullary space, interspersed around the remaining trabeculae. Some areas may be devoid of trabeculae, suggesting a cystic cavity such as a mucocele. However, the typical MR imaging signal intensities of fat or the typically low CT density allow the radiologist to make this differentiation (Figs. 12-11 and 12-12).

The sphenooccipital synchondrosis represents the junction of the occipital and sphenoid bones. This often can be seen on sagittal MR imaging or even on plain films in infants. It fuses in most children by the age of 8 years. The synchondrosis is a linear cleft that passes from the intracranial clivus to the pharyngeal surface of the basicranium. Sometimes the synchondrosis between the anterior and posterior ossification centers of the sphenoid can be seen in the infant (Fig. 12-13). This more ventral synchondrosis passes from the tuberculum or the anterior wall of the sella to the pharyngeal side of the sphenoid.[16, 17] This structure is anterior to the course of Rathke's pouch and tract and should not be confused with that embryonic structure.

Sphenoid sinus air cell development begins at birth. Initial air cell development is in the presphenoid region anteriorly, and further enlargement proceeds posteriorly to invade the basisphenoid.[18] Sinus development is slow for the first several years and then accelerates, so that by about the age of 7 or 8 years, the dorsal margin of the sinus has reached the anterior sella turcica.[13, 18] Expansion then continues in all directions, with sinus aeration frequently extending into the dorsum sella and anterior clinoids. Large sinuses can appear to extend down well into the basiocciput. Laterally, the air cells can extend between the foramen rotundum and the Vidian canal into the root of the pterygoid or even into the greater wing. If there is development of these lateral air cells, the space between the foramen rotundum and the Vidian canal is wider than if these air cells are not present. This increased separation should not be considered pathologic.[19]

The position of the septations within the sphenoid sinus varies considerably. Many of these septations pass from anterior to posterior. They can attach to the roof of the sphenoid (the floor of the sella). Some can curve laterally to attach to the bony wall separating the carotid artery from the sphenoid sinus. In this case, a fracture at the carotid groove is of concern if the septation is manipulated at surgery. The foramen rotundum may project into the lower lateral sinus wall, usually as a curved ridge. The Vidian canal may be in the sphenoid bone below the floor of the sphenoid sinus or it may be on a septum just above the sinus floor. A final normal variation of the architecture of the sphenoid bone is the formation of arachnoid granulations along the inner surface of the greater wing of the sphenoid, where the bone forms the anterior wall of the middle cranial fossa (Fig. 12-14). These "pits" can be visualized frequently on CT and should not be considered pathologic. In cases of nontraumatic CSF leaks these pits have been implicated as a causal factor. It has been suggested that the thin bone separating one of these pits from another may break, creating a communication with an air cell in the greater wing of the sphenoid.[20]

The occipital bone forms the margin of the foramen magnum and extends up to meet the basisphenoid at the sphenooccipital synchondrosis (Fig. 12-15). This synchondrosis is usually about one third up the length of the posterior surface of the clivus. It is the basilar part of the occipital bone that forms the region anterior to the foramen magnum. The lateral part of the occipital bone forms the lateral margin of the foramen magnum and includes the large occipital condyles, prominent landmarks on the caudal aspect of the skull. The jugular process of the occipital bone juts laterally and has a rounded prominence called the jugular tubercle along its superior margin. The hypoglossal canal passes just above the occipital condyle and just below the jugular tubercle. Posterior to the condyle is the condyloid canal, which enters this fossa carrying an emissary vein.[21, 22]

## Bordering Soft Tissues

The evaluation of the soft tissues that border the skull base can be crucial in the analysis of disease. Just as lesions arising in the skull base itself can expand into these areas, lesions arising above or below the skull base can invade it. Importantly, the imaging demonstration of normal soft tissues between the skull base and a tumor is reassuring evidence that the skull base has not been invaded.

### Extracranial Soft Tissues

The extracranial openings of the fissures and foramina of the skull base are bordered by soft tissues primarily

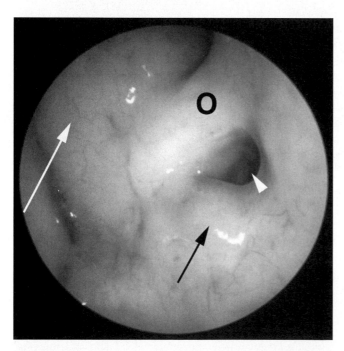

**FIGURE 12-5** Endoscopic view of the sphenoid sinus. Note that the image is slightly rotated from the vertical plane due to the obliquity of the approach. Note the small recess (*arrowhead*) between the optic canal impression (*O*) and the bulge from the carotid artery (*black arrow*). The white arrow indicates the impression of the sella.

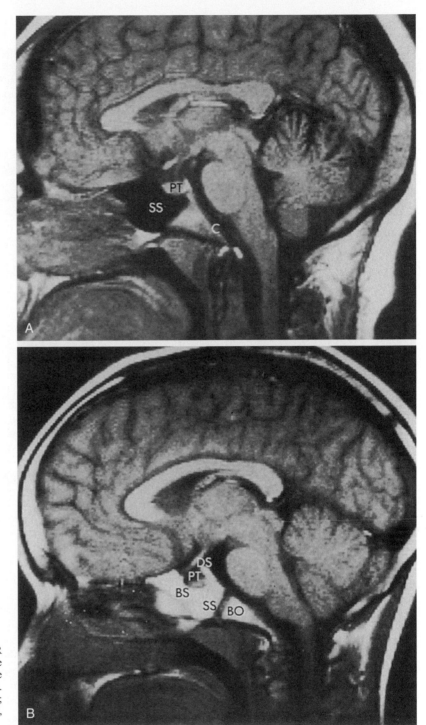

**FIGURE 12-6   A**, Midline sagittal T1-weighted MR image of the skull base in an adult. *PT*, Pituitary within the sella turcica; *SS*, sphenoid sinus; *C*, clivus. **B**, Midline sagittal T1-weighted MR image of the skull base in a child. *DS*, Dorsum sellae; *PT*, pituitary within the sella turcica; *BS*, basisphenoid; *SS*, sphenooccipital synchondrosis; *BO*, basiocciput.

containing fat, and just as in the remainder of the head and neck, this fat is important in the imaging analysis of the skull base. Because fat has a very characteristic appearance on CT and MR imaging, excellent contrast is afforded between normal tissue and most lesions, particularly cellular tumors. Thus, for instance, as a tumor approaches the base of the skull, the progressive obliteration of the fat planes allows detection of tumor infiltration.

The optic canal and the superior orbital fissure open into the orbit (Fig. 12-7), and although the optic nerve and the extraocular muscles occupy space in the orbital apex, there is still sufficient fat to allow detection of most lesions. Indeed, as mentioned, the orbital fat normally protrudes slightly through the superior orbital fissure into the region of the anterior cavernous sinus.

The foramen rotundum and the Vidian canal open into the pterygopalatine fossa. The fossa is filled almost entirely by fat (Figs. 12-7 and 12-8). This narrow cleft (Fig. 12-4G) behind the medial posterior wall of the maxillary sinus takes its name from the bones that make up the walls of this space. The pterygoid process of the sphenoid forms the posterior wall (Fig. 12-16), while the superiorly projecting orbital process of the palatine bone makes up the anterior wall. The pterygopalatine fossa connects with five spaces: the central skull base and middle cranial fossa via the Vidian canal and the foramen rotundum, the orbit via the inferior orbital fissure, the infratemporal fossa via the retromaxillary or pterygomaxillary fissure, the nasal cavity via the sphenopalatine foramen, and the oral cavity via the pterygopalatine canals in which run the greater and lesser palatine nerves (Figs. 12-17 to 12-19). In addition, the second division of the trigeminal nerve branches in the pterygopalatine fossa before carrying sensory innervation to the face and to the mucosa of the palate (Fig. 12-17), and these nerves can be the pathway of tumor spread. Thus, the pterygopalatine fossa is an important landmark in staging of head and neck tumors.

*Text continued on p. 797*

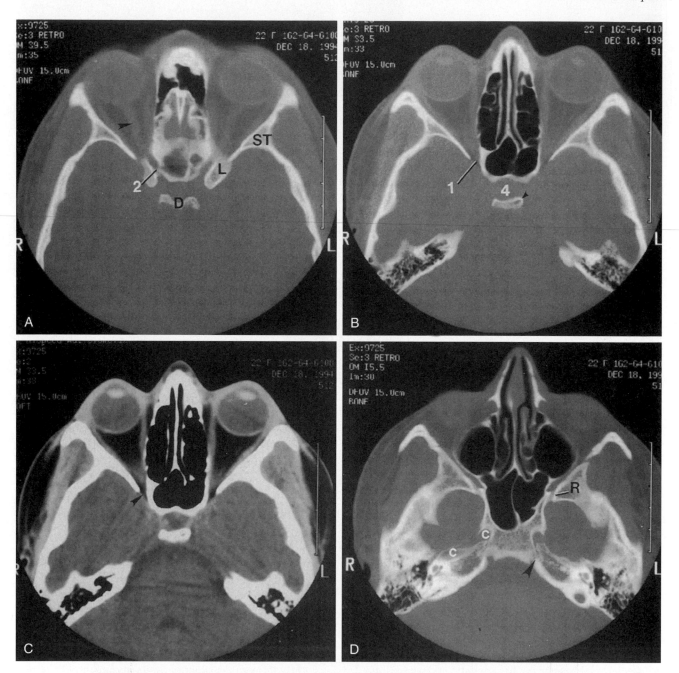

**FIGURE 12-7**    Axial CT scan of the skull base from superior to inferior. **A,** Level of the optic canal. *2,* Optic canal; *L,* lesser wing of the sphenoid; *D,* dorsum sella; *ST,* position of the "sphenoid triangle." Note how the optic nerve (*arrowhead*) converges toward the optic canal. **B,** Level of the superior orbital fissure. *1,* Superior orbital fissure; *4,* sella turcica. The arrowhead indicates the posterior clinoid at the lateral aspect of the dorsum sella. Note how the superior orbital fissure is oriented anteriorly to posteriorly rather than converging toward the optic chiasm. **C,** Soft-tissue algorithm at the same level. Note how a small amount of fat (*arrowhead*) protrudes through the superior orbital fissure. **D,** Level of the foramen rotundum. The foramen rotundum (*R*) passes from the pterygopalatine fossa to the middle cranial fossa. *C,* Carotid canal. The medial *C* is immediately above the foramen lacerum. The medial *C* is in a small notch as the artery turns superiorly along the lateral aspect of the sphenoid bone. The petrooccipital (or petroclival) fissure is indicated by the arrowhead.

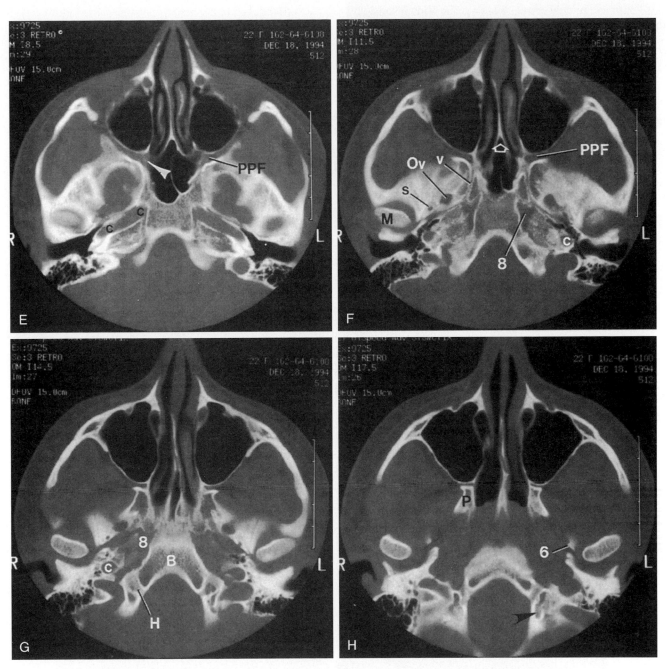

**FIGURE 12-7**   *Continued.* **E**, Level of the pterygopalatine fossa. The pterygopalatine fossa (*PPF*) is situated between the maxillary sinus anteriorly and the sphenoid bone posteriorly. The arrowhead indicates the sphenopalatine foramen, which connects the pterygopalatine fossa with the posterior nasal cavity and nasopharynx. *C*, Carotid canal. The more medial C is immediately above the foramen lacerum. **F**, Level of Vidian canal. *v*, Vidian canal; *Ov*, foramen ovale; *S*, foramen spinosum; *M*, mandible; *8*, foramen lacerum; *C*, inferior portion of the carotid canal; *PPF*, pterygopalatine fossa. The line indicating the PPF passes from the infratemporal fossa through the pterygomaxillary fissure into the pterygopalatine fossa. The open arrowhead indicates pneumatization extending into the rostrum of the sphenoid. Note how the Vidian canal passes from the pterygopalatine fossa posteriorly to the region close to the foramen lacerum rather than into the middle cranial fossa. **G**, Below the level of the Vidian canal. *B*, Basiocciput; *H*, hypoglossal canal; *8*, foramen lacerum; *C*, cross section of the lower vertical segment of the carotid canal. **H**, Through the level of the spine of the sphenoid. *6*, spine of the sphenoid. The small lucency just anterior to this point is the lower foramen spinosum. The arrowhead indicates the condyloid canal carrying an emissary vein. *P*, Pterygoid process.

*Illustration continued on following page*

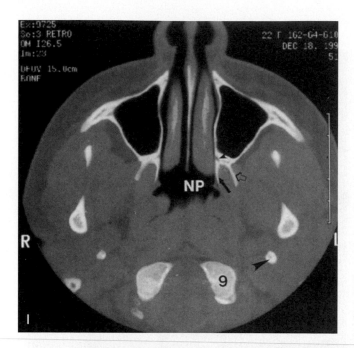

**FIGURE 12-7**   *Continued.* **I,** Level of the occipital condyle. *9,* Occipital condyle; *large black arrowhead,* styloid process; *black arrow,* medial pterygoid plate; *open arrow,* lateral pterygoid plate; *small arrowhead,* pterygopalatine canal extending toward the palatine foramen; *NP,* nasopharynx.

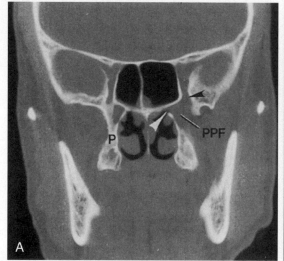

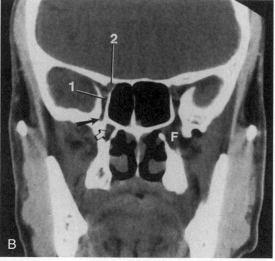

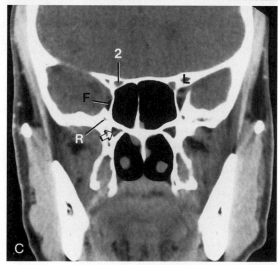

**FIGURE 12-8**   Coronal CT image through the sphenoid. **A,** Level of the pterygopalatine fossa. The pterygopalatine fossa (*PPF*) is seen as a lucent area containing fat. The line indicating the PPF extends through the pterygomaxillary fissure from the infratemporal fossa. The black arrowhead indicates the junction of the pterygopalatine fossa with the orbital apex. The inferior orbital fissure also converges to this point. The white arrowhead indicates the sphenopalatine foramen, whereby the pterygopalatine fossa communicates with the posterior nasal cavity. *P,* Pterygoid process. **B,** Soft-tissue algorithm at the same level shows the fat (*F*) in the pterygopalatine fossa. The fat in the fossa tapers toward the trumpet-shaped entrance (*open arrow*) of the Vidian canal on the right side. The black arrow indicates the anterior opening of the foramen rotundum. The superior orbital fissure (*1*) notably contains fat. *2,* Exocranial entrance of the optic canal. **C,** Slightly posteriorly. The open arrow shows the further tapering of the fat toward the anterior entrance of the Vidian canal. *R,* Foramen rotundum; *F,* small amount of fat that protrudes more posteriorly than the lateral bony wall of the superior orbital fissure; *2,* optic canal; *L,* lesser wing of the sphenoid.

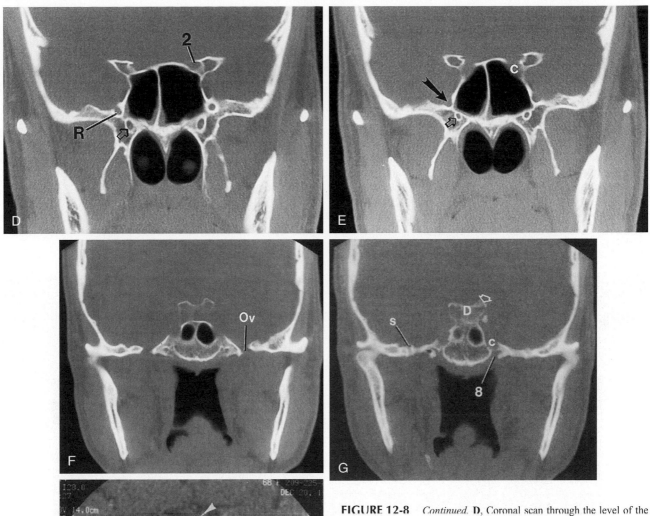

**FIGURE 12-8**   *Continued.* **D,** Coronal scan through the level of the foramen rotundum shows the relationship of the foramen rotundum (*R*) to the Vidian canal (*open arrow*) in the body of the sphenoid. The optic canal (*2*) is seen just medial to the anterior clinoid. **E,** Slightly posterior scan shows the foramen rotundum opening (*arrow*) into the middle cranial fossa. The Vidian canal (*open arrow*) continues dorsally. The carotid artery (*C*) makes a groove in the lateral wall of the sphenoid sinus. **F,** Level of the foramen ovale (*Ov*). Note that the extracranial opening is slightly more laterally positioned than is the intracranial opening. The foramina converge toward the cavernous sinus. **G,** Level of the foramen spinosum. *S,* Foramen spinosum; *8,* foramen lacerum; *C,* lower carotid artery. Note the groove in the sphenoid bone just above the foramen lacerum. A calcification is seen in the more superior aspect of the carotid artery. *D,* Dorsum sella; *open white arrow,* posterior clinoid. **H,** Coronal soft tissue algorithm shows the foramen lacerum (*8*). *C,* Carotid canal; *MC,* Meckel's cave; *white arrow,* optic chiasm.

Within the fat of the pterygopalatine fossa are the branches of the maxillary nerve, the pterygopalatine ganglion, and small vessels. Though a small amount of soft tissue can be identified in the fossa, the predominant imaging finding is fat, which serves as an important imaging landmark when evaluating potential tumor spread.

The foramen ovale opens into the masticator space below the skull base. As the third division of the trigeminal nerve exits the skull via this foramen, the nerve emerges into fat along the medial margin of the lateral pterygoid muscle.[23] The nerve passes just superficial (lateral) to the sphenomandibular ligament and the fusion of fascial layers that form the

medial boundary of the masticator space. The tensor veli palatini muscle takes its origin along a line from the scaphoid fossa to the spine of the sphenoid bone. This small, thin muscle plays an important role in the fascial organization of the parapharyngeal spaces.

### Intracranial Soft Tissues

Intracranially, most of the foramina converge to the region of the cavernous sinus and Meckel's cave (Figs. 12-7 and 12-8). The optic canals open into the suprasellar cistern. The cavernous sinus is a venous sinusoid structure situated between the layers of the dura, bordering the pituitary fossa and the body of the sphenoid (Fig. 12-20). The cavernous sinus forms much of the medial wall of the middle cranial fossa.

The dural organization at Meckel's cave and the cavernous sinus is derived from the dural coverings of the contiguous inner surfaces of the skull. Two layers can be appreciated. The outer (peripheral) layer of the dura follows the bone of the skull base. The inner layer is reflected upward, forming the lateral wall of Meckel's cave and the cavernous sinus before attaching to the clinoids. This inner layer of dura has a secondary reflection that passes anteriorly from posteriorly, forming Meckel's cave. This cave can be thought of as a very loose root sleeve around the trigeminal nerve and ganglion.

The cavernous sinus is located at the superomedial aspect of Meckel's cave and extends anteriorly from that point. The cavernous sinus contains several nerves. The ophthalmic division of the trigeminal nerve passes into the cavernous sinus on the way to the superior orbital fissure. The maxillary division of the trigeminal nerve has a shorter course within the cavernous sinus before entering the foramen rotundum. The third division of the trigeminal nerve exits almost directly from Meckel's cave and does not truly enter the cavernous sinus. The semilunar or Gasserian ganglion, the convergence of the divisions of the nerve, lies along the lateral wall of Meckel's cave. The oculomotor, trochlear, and abducens nerves traverse the entire anteroposterior length of the cavernous sinus before exiting the skull at the superior orbital fissure.

The internal carotid artery also traverses the cavernous sinus. The artery curves superiorly immediately after exiting the petrous carotid canal. This brings the artery into the

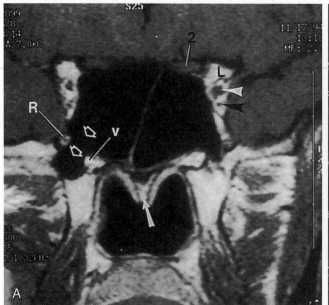

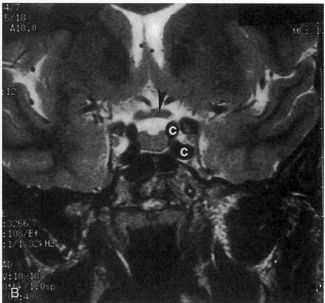

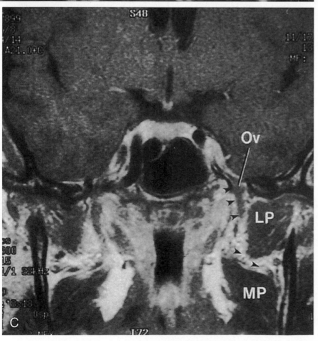

**FIGURE 12-9** Coronal high-resolution MR image. **A,** T1-weighted image through the level of the foramen rotundum. *R,* V$_2$ in the foramen rotundum; *v,* Vidian canal. Note how the air cell from the sphenoid sinus squeezes between (*open arrows*) the foramen rotundum and the Vidian canal. *L,* Lesser wing of the sphenoid; *2,* optic nerve in the optic canal; *white arrowhead,* cranial nerve III; *black arrowhead,* cranial nerve IV; *white arrow,* rostrum of the sphenoid. **B,** Coronal T2-weighted image shows the carotid artery (*c*) and the optic chiasm (*black arrowhead*). Cranial nerves again can be visualized within the cavernous sinus. **C,** Through the foramen ovale. V$_3$ (*small arrowheads*) can be followed through the foramen ovale (*Ov*). The nerve passes medial to the lateral pterygoid (*LP*). The course of the nerve then passes between the lateral pterygoid and medial pterygoid (*MP*) toward the entrance of the nerve into the mandible.

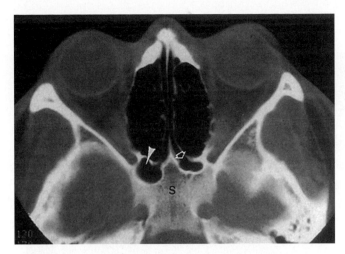

**FIGURE 12-10**   Normal but poorly pneumatized sphenoid. Small air cells (*arrowhead*) form in the anterior part of the sphenoid bone (*S*). The ostium (*open arrow*) can be followed into the sinus on the left side.

cavernous sinus between Meckel's cave and the lateral wall of the sphenoid sinus. The artery then curves anteriorly, making a short bend before passing through the dura just below the optic nerve.

## IMAGING

Plain film investigation of the skull base has given way to CT and MR imaging. However, the skull base is ever present on any projectional image of the skull or of the sinuses. Indeed, a major factor in the development of the different views used in plain film radiography of the temporal bone and sinuses was an attempt to project the area of interest away from the confusing densities of the skull base. Although plain films are seldom used when skull base

pathology is suspected, skull base problems can mimic various types of facial and sinus pathology. Thus, familiarity with the normal projectional anatomy is appropriate. This is discussed in Chapter 2.

CT can be performed in the axial and coronal planes. Other slice orientations and three-dimensional (3D) images can be reformatted. The advent of multidetector scanners with slice thicknesses approaching the dimensions of the pixel allows high-quality reformatting in any plane. This imaging advance is lessening, and in many cases eliminating, the need to perform direct coronal imaging. In turn, this eliminates the imaging-degrading beam-hardening artifacts from dental restorations so common on direct coronal CT. A slice thickness of no greater than 3 mm should be used, with thinner scans used to answer specific diagnostic questions regarding some of the smaller skull base foramina. The optimal slice thickness may change as more experience with the multidetector scanners is gathered.

Contrast is used whenever the cavernous sinus is examined or intracranial tumor is suspected. Bone algorithms are utilized to optimally visualize the thin cortices around the various foramina, and soft-tissue algorithms allow evaluation of the soft tissues adjacent to the skull base.

Although MR imaging can be performed in any plane, the routine examination should include the sagittal, axial, and coronal views, particularly in tumor cases. Gadolinium is used routinely to evaluate the cavernous sinus and potential intracranial tumor. Because some enhancing tumors can be as bright as fat, the interface between the lesion and the fat planes below the skull base can be lost unless either a precontrast sequence is obtained or fat suppression is used. One must be careful when fat suppression is employed, because the interface between the sphenoid sinus air and its wall often results in a significant susceptibility effect. This "blooming" can void the signal from important structures such as the cavernous sinus and the foramen rotundum (Fig. 12-21). The radiologist must be confident that the foramen

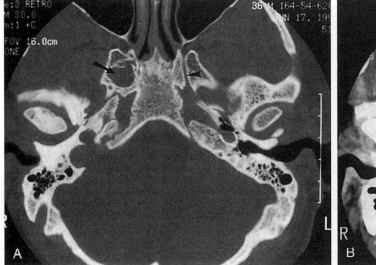
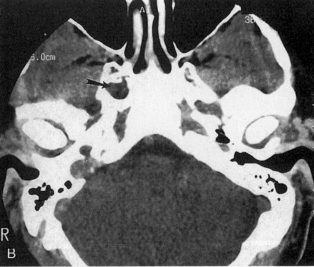

**FIGURE 12-11**   Normal variant in the sphenoid. **A,** Axial CT bone algorithm shows what appears to be a dilated cystic structure in the pterygoid process (*arrow*). The normal pterygoid (Vidian) canal is seen (*arrowhead*) on the opposite side. **B,** Soft-tissue algorithm shows that the area within this cystic structure contains fat, indicating that this represents a variation in ossification rather than obstructed secretions.

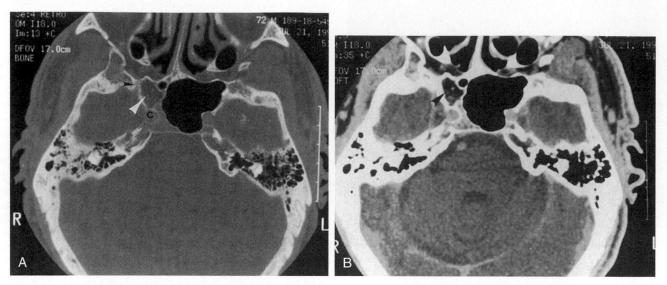

**FIGURE 12-12** **A**, Normal nonpneumatized CT bone algorithm. An area (*white arrowhead*) in the right sphenoid initially can be confused with an obstructed sinus. However, on careful inspection, there appear to be trabeculae within the area. The foramen rotundum (*black arrowhead*) is seen just lateral to the area in question. **B**, On the soft-tissue algorithm at the same level, the area of concern shows a fatty density (*arrowhead*), indicating that this indeed represents normal fatty marrow.

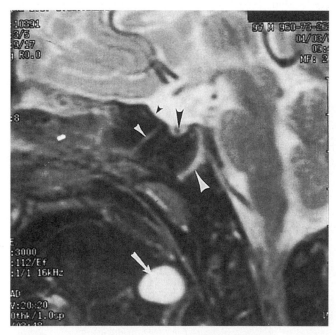

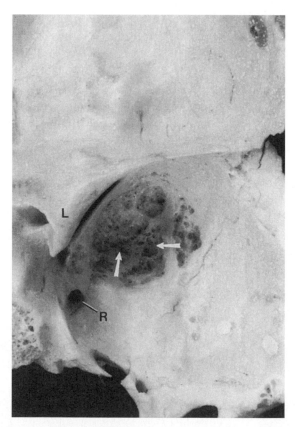

**FIGURE 12-13** Normal clivus in a child evaluated for thyroglossal duct remnant or cyst. T2-weighted image shows the thyroglossal abnormality in the tongue base (*white arrow*). The synchondrosis (*small white arrowhead*) between the pre- and postsphenoid ossification centers is easily identified, as is the synchondrosis between the sphenoid and occipital bones. *Large black arrowhead*, pituitary fossa; *small black arrowhead*, chiasmatic groove.

**FIGURE 12-14** Arachnoid granulations extending into the sphenoid bone. Viewed from above, the arachnoid granulations extend through the intracranial cortex of the greater wing of the sphenoid, leaving rather extensive pitted perforations (*arrows*) of the cortex. The position of the small pits would put the granulations in close proximity to a laterally extending sphenoid air cell. *L*, Lesser wing of the sphenoid; *R*, foramen rotundum.

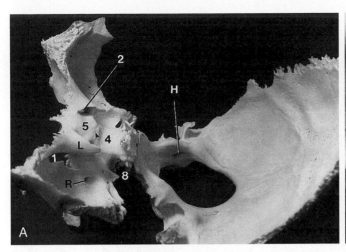

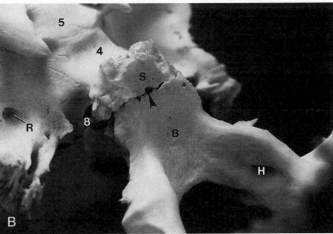

FIGURE 12-15    **A,** View from above and laterally of the sphenoid and occipital bones. *1,* Superior orbital fissure; *2,* optic canal; *4,* sella turcica; *5,* chiasmatic sulcus; *L,* lesser wing of the sphenoid; *R,* foramen rotundum; *H,* hypoglossal canal; *small arrowhead,* tuberculum sella; *8,* approximate position of the foramen lacerum at the tip of the temporal bone. **B,** Close-up of the sphenooccipital synchondrosis from above, laterally and slightly posteriorly. *8,* Approximate position of the foramen lacerum. The notch immediately above the 8 would hold the carotid artery. *R,* Foramen rotundum; *B,* basiocciput; *S,* posterior sphenoid; *4,* sella turcica; *5,* chiasmatic groove; *H,* hypoglossal canal; *arrowhead,* sphenooccipital structure.

has been adequately visualized either with or without fat suppression. Frequently, a subtle vascular plexus can be identified around the nerve within the foramen. Because of these plexes, symmetric slight enhancement of the cranial nerves as they exit the skull base may be seen routinely. It is only when there is asymmetric enhancement that pathology should be suspected. On the other hand, the Gasserian ganglion has sparse vascularity, and thus this ganglion should not enhance routinely on contrast MR sequences. If enhancement is seen within a Gasserian ganglion, it should be considered pathologic.

Fat suppression is often used with the newer fast spin-echo, T2-weighted sequences. On conventional spin-echo images, fat has a high T1-weighted and a low T2-weighted signal intensity. However, on fast spin-echo imaging, fat has a high signal intensity on both T1-weighted and T2-weighted images. Thus, on the T2-weighted fast spin-echo images, fat suppression can give an imaging appearance similar to that of the conventional spin-echo

images. Again, the susceptibility effect of air and tissue can present imaging problems.

If the areas of the central skull base, cavernous sinuses, and sphenoid sinus are to be evaluated, a suggested protocol for the routine case includes T1-weighted sequences with and without gadolinium and T2-weighted scans; 3-mm-thick sections are used for the T1-weighted sequences, and 4- to 5-mm-thick sections are used for the T2-weighted scans.

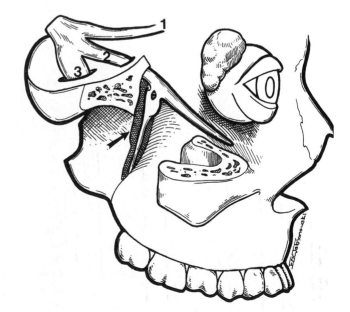

FIGURE 12-17    Branching of the trigeminal nerve. The trigeminal nerve forms three divisions in the region of Meckel's cave. The ophthalmic nerve (*1*) extends through the superior orbital fissure. The maxillary nerve (*2*) extends through the foramen rotundum into the pterygopalatine fossa (*arrow*). Here it branches into the infraorbital and palatine branches extending to the more superficial regions of the face and palate. The mandibular nerve (*3*) exits through the foramen ovale.

FIGURE 12-16    Anterior view of the sphenoid. The approximate projection of the pterygopalatine fossa is seen in the dotted outline. The foramen rotundum (*arrow*) and the Vidian canal (*open arrow*) enter the pterygopalatine fossa. *S,* Superior orbital fissure.

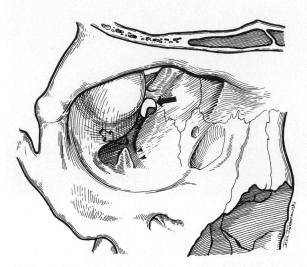

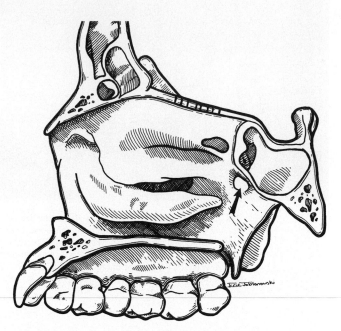

**FIGURE 12-18**   View of the foramen rotundum looking through the orbit. The foramen rotundum (*arrow*) barely can be seen poking up behind the inferior orbital fissure. The inferior orbital fissure (*open arrow*) extends between the orbital surface of the greater wing of the sphenoid and the orbit. The pterygopalatine fossa extends straight inferiorly from the point where the inferior orbital fissure appears to meet the foramen rotundum. The infraorbital canal (*arrowheads*) passes anteriorly from the inferior orbital fissure.

**FIGURE 12-19**   Medial view of the nasal cavity shows the position of the sphenopalatine foramen (*arrow*). Though covered by mucosa, this represents a passageway through the osseous structures between the posterior nasal cavity and the pterygopalatine fossa.

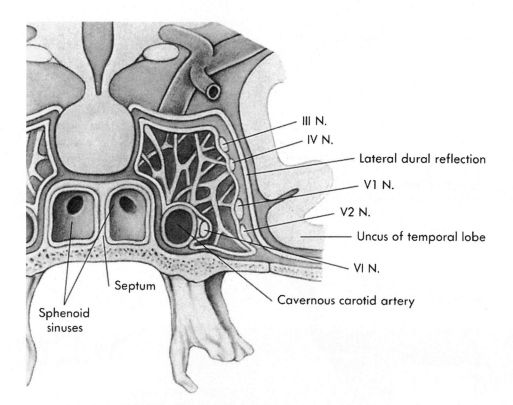

**FIGURE 12-20**   Coronal view of the cavernous sinus region.

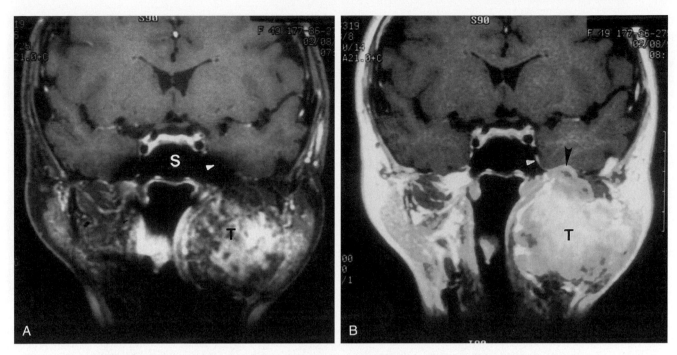

**FIGURE 12-21**    Very large benign tumor of the parotid gland extending through the floor of the middle cranial fossa. **A**, Coronal T1-weighted MR image with fat suppression after gadolinium administration. The tumor (*T*) can be readily visualized. The sphenoid sinus (*S*) is filled with air. The air causes "blooming" of the sinus laterally (*arrowhead*), obscuring the lower cavernous sinus in the region of the foramen ovale. This is due to the susceptibility effect. **B**, Without fat suppression, on a T1-weighted image after gadolinium administration, the lateral margin of the sphenoid sinus (*arrowhead*) is much better seen, as is the lower cavernous sinus. A small amount of tumor obscured with the previous image is well seen (*arrowhead*) protruding into the middle cranial fossa. *T*, Tumor.

Usually, high resolution (high matrix, low field of view) is included in the plane most likely to visualize a key structure.

In cases where a CSF leak is of concern or determination of the precise margin of the brain must be demonstrated relative to a defect in the skull base, either a high-resolution, T2-weighted sequence or a true inversion recovery sequence may be added.

## NONNEOPLASTIC DISORDERS

### Congenital and Developmental Anomalies

There are many normal variations in the sphenoid bone, most notably the degree of sinus pneumatization and the rate and final extent of replacement of red marrow by fatty yellow marrow. These variations were discussed previously under normal imaging appearance of the sphenoid bone.

Congenital or developmental abnormalities may represent either actual developmental problems of the sphenoid bone itself or reactions of the sphenoid bone to problems occurring elsewhere. For example, a cephalocele can occur through an actual deficiency in the sphenoid bone, whereas the distortion of the greater wing of the sphenoid that occurs in a patient with premature closure of the coronal suture represents an attempt of a normal sphenoid bone to compensate for an abnormality elsewhere. Although various dysplasias could be included in this section, they are discussed in this chapter and in Chapter 24.

## Cephaloceles

A cephalocele is a protrusion of intracranial contents through a defect in the skull. The dura may be thinned or actually dehiscent. If the protrusion is composed of only the meninges and the subarachnoid space containing CSF, the term meningocele is used. If the sac also contains brain, the appropriate term is encephalocele. Though meningoceles can occur anywhere in the skull, most are found in the midline.

Cephaloceles occur sporadically, approximately once in 4000 births.[24] Most involve the cranial vault, with only about 20% of encephaloceles involving the anterior or central skull base. Of these, most are anterior in location (sincipital encephaloceles) and are considered to represent failures of neural tube fusion at the level of the anterior neuropore. A different mechanism must be postulated for those cephaloceles that pass through the region of the sphenoid.

Some authors have attributed the passage of encephaloceles through the sphenoid bone to persistence of the craniopharyngeal canal.[25] However, other authors question this concept, indicating that the adenohypophysis ascends too early, well before there is significant organization of the developing basicranium.[26] These authors have attributed the small canal occasionally identified traversing the sphenoid, between its pharyngeal surface and the pituitary fossa, to small blood vessels present in the embryo.

A second proposed theory is that these basal cephaloceles are herniations through defects related to problems with fusion of the many ossification centers participating in formation of the skull base. These authors indicate that the route taken by most of these encephaloceles through the sphenoid bone conforms most closely to the synchondrosis between the presphenoid and postsphenoid ossification centers. This course passes from the region of either the tuberculum sella or the anterior wall of the sella, anteriorly and inferiorly toward the pharynx (Fig. 12-13). This theory also explains the occurrence of lateral basal encephaloceles that pass between the nonunited ossification centers of the postsphenoid and alisphenoid, precursors of the body and greater sphenoid wing, respectively.[27] Some encephaloceles appear to pass directly through the more lateral greater wing of the sphenoid.[28] This structure is formed by membranous bone, and perhaps in these cases a defect in formation of the bone itself can be implicated. This type of defect is seen in neurofibromatosis but can occur as an isolated abnormality as well.

The outer covering of the cephalocele is determined by the tissues found adjacent to the defect.[29] This may be a derivative of skin or mucous membrane, depending on the location. Most of the basal encephaloceles pass into the nose or nasopharynx and are covered by mucosa. By comparison, those cephaloceles that pass laterally into the infratemporal fossa have a fibrous wall derived from the dura and from the myofascial elements found in that location. Basal encephaloceles have been categorized depending on their point of passage through the skull base and on their final destination.[25, 28, 30] One system includes the following types: (1) transethmoidal, (2) sphenoethmoidal, (3) sphenorbital, (4) transsphenoidal, and (5) sphenomaxillary. Perhaps it is easiest to group the abnormalities into midline basal and lateral basal encephaloceles.

The transsphenoidal, sphenoethmoidal, and transethmoidal varieties occur in the midline (Figs. 12-22 and 12-23). The sphenoethmoidal passes through the sphenoethmoid area into the posterior nasal cavity or anterior nasopharynx. If the abnormality extends into the sphenoid sinus but does not perforate the floor to reach the nasopharynx, the term transsphenoidal is used. As the name suggests, transethmoidal encephaloceles are more anterior in location, passing through the anterior ethmoid and cribriform plate into the more anterior sinonasal system. Another term that may be encountered is sphenopharyngeal encephalocele. This type extends through the sphenoethmoid region into the nasopharynx and can be included in the sphenoethmoid group.

Lateral basal encephaloceles include the sphenorbital and sphenomaxillary types. The sphenorbital encephalocele passes through the region of the superior orbital fissure into the orbit, causing proptosis, often pulsatile proptosis. This type is commonly associated with neurofibromatosis and is considered to be an expression of the mesodermal component of this disease (Fig. 12-24) because the greater wing and often the lesser wing of the sphenoid do not develop normally and have defective ossification.[31] This gives the characteristic plain film appearance of a bare or empty orbit (Fig. 12-25).

The sphenomaxillary encephalocele is extremely rare, and few documented examples exist (Fig. 12-26).[27, 32–35] These lesions may squeeze into the pterygopalatine fossa and then pass laterally into the infratemporal fossa, presenting as a mass in the cheek. The more lateral transalar encephaloceles do not fit well into either the sphenomaxil-

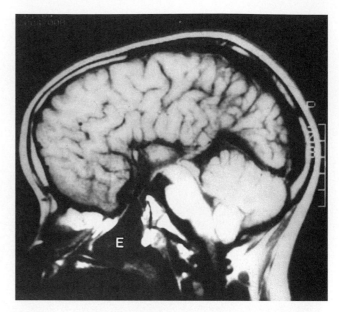

**FIGURE 12-22** Sphenoethmoidal encephalocele. Sagittal T1-weighted MR image shows the encephalocele (*E*) extending into the nasal cavity, resting on the hard palate. The connection can be followed through the anterior sella and anterior sphenoid. This would be the approximate position of the fusion line of pre- and postsphenoids. The cystic abnormality did contain brain tissue along the wall and therefore qualifies as an encephalocele.

lary or sphenorbital groups, but they certainly could be included in the category of lateral basal encephalocele.

Patients with basal encephaloceles frequently have other anomalies. Most involve the midface. Hypertelorism is common, particularly with the more anterior varieties of encephaloceles. Cleft lip and cleft palate are also frequently associated findings, as is agenesis of the corpus callosum.[36]

The clinical presentation of cephaloceles varies; a submucosal mass in the nasal cavity or nasopharynx may present with airway obstruction, CSF leaks or recurrent meningitis may result from the weakened barrier between the sinonasal tract and the intracranial contents, and symptoms relating to involved central nervous system components can also be found. Herniations of the optic pathways, hypothalamus, or portions of the frontal lobes occur with midline defects. When the temporal lobe protrudes into the defect, the patient may present with seizures.

When imaging cephaloceles, the bony defect is better seen on CT than MR imaging. Usually there is a smooth cortical margin surrounding the tract, and the soft-tissue mass is identified passing into the extracranial region. Three-dimensional reformatted images can be used to show the relationship of the defect to the remaining basicranium.

Although MR imaging does not show the bony anatomy quite as well as CT, it better characterizes the contents of the herniated soft tissues and any related intracranial abnormalities.

## Altered Ossification

If the presphenoid ossification extends further dorsally than normal, the postsphenoid ossification bone is correspondingly shorter than normal. This results in the limbus, chiasmatic sulcus, and tuberculum being vertically oriented, elongating the anterior wall of the sella turcica. The resulting sella configuration is J-shaped, and this type of altered ossification occurs in such conditions as Turner's syndrome, achondroplasia, and the mucopolysaccharidoses. This represents a developmental J-shaped sella rather than one that occurs due to erosion of the dorsum sellae by a hypothalamic mass.

## Vascular Variants

There are many minor variations of the arterial and venous vessels in and around the central skull base. Many represent normal variations of origin or course. The course of the carotid artery in the region of the cavernous sinus is quite constant; however, the artery can curve more medially than normal, pushing into the sphenoid sinus. The

lateral sinus wall bone covering the medial aspect of the artery can be dehiscent, putting the vessel at risk during surgical procedures involving the sphenoid sinus (Fig. 12-27). Even when the artery is in a normal position, the bone separating the carotid artery from the sphenoid sinus may be quite thin. If a septation of the sphenoid sinus curves to attach to this thin bone, there is concern that manipulation of the septation may fracture the bony wall, injuring the vessel.

The persistent trigeminal artery is a large arterial variant that represents an abnormal persistent communication between the carotid artery and the basilar circulation (Figs. 12-28 and 12-29). This vessel is seen easily on arteriography and may be large enough to be visualized on CT or MR imaging. The vessel passes from the proximal cavernous carotid artery posteriorly to connect with the basilar artery.

The effect of the variations of venous passages through the skull base is thought to account for at least some of the

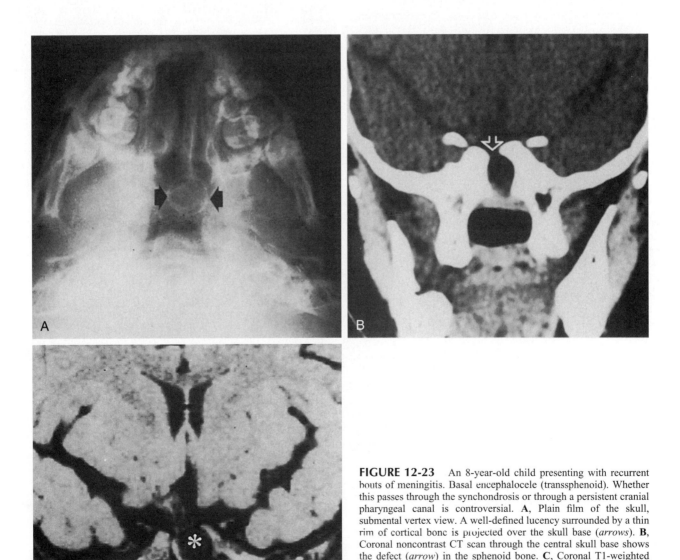

**FIGURE 12-23**  An 8-year-old child presenting with recurrent bouts of meningitis. Basal encephalocele (transsphenoid). Whether this passes through the synchondrosis or through a persistent cranial pharyngeal canal is controversial. **A,** Plain film of the skull, submental vertex view. A well-defined lucency surrounded by a thin rim of cortical bone is projected over the skull base (*arrows*). **B,** Coronal noncontrast CT scan through the central skull base shows the defect (*arrow*) in the sphenoid bone. **C,** Coronal T1-weighted image through the central skull base demonstrates herniation of the pituitary gland (*asterisk*) into the defect. Note the proximity of the pituitary gland to the roof of the nasopharynx. (Courtesy Dr. Das Narla.)

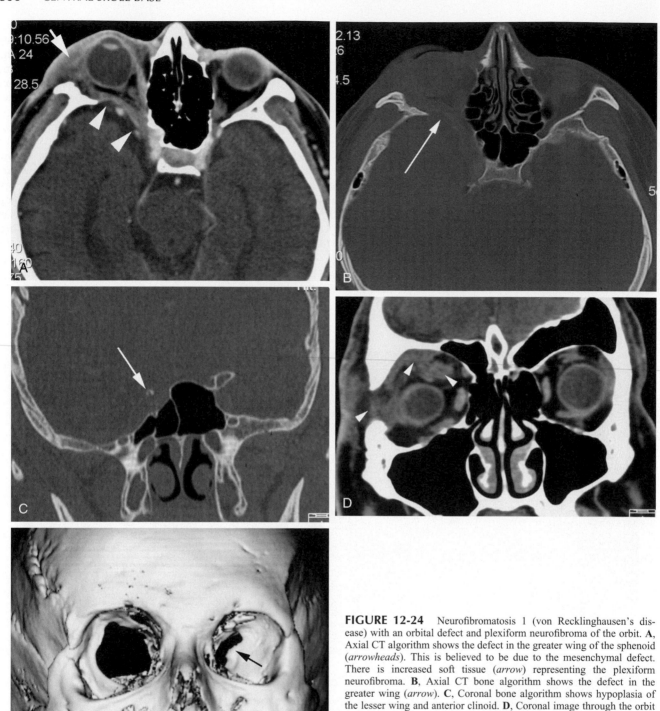

**FIGURE 12-24**    Neurofibromatosis 1 (von Recklinghausen's disease) with an orbital defect and plexiform neurofibroma of the orbit. **A,** Axial CT algorithm shows the defect in the greater wing of the sphenoid (*arrowheads*). This is believed to be due to the mesenchymal defect. There is increased soft tissue (*arrow*) representing the plexiform neurofibroma. **B,** Axial CT bone algorithm shows the defect in the greater wing (*arrow*). **C,** Coronal bone algorithm shows hypoplasia of the lesser wing and anterior clinoid. **D,** Coronal image through the orbit shows increased soft tissue along the upper muscle complex and the lateral orbits (*arrowheads*) representing the plexiform neurofibroma. **E,** Three-dimensional reformat of axial CT data shows the defect in the greater wing of the sphenoid on the right side. Compare this with the superior orbital fissure (*arrow*) on the normal side.

channels and foramina seen in the region of the foramen ovale. The best known of these variable channels is the foramen of Vesalius just anterior and medial to the foramen ovale. Ginsberg et al. used the term lateral rotundal canal to describe a channel passing vertically just lateral to the foramen rotundum.[12] They are thought to be channels connecting the cavernous sinus with the pterygoid plexus.

## Developmental Changes Caused by Extrinsic Factors

The skull base develops in a complex environment, and the growth patterns of the sphenoid bone are modified by abnormalities occurring in the adjacent region. Craniosynostosis, or premature closure of a suture, prevents normal growth of a particular segment of the skull. The remaining bones of the skull also become distorted as they attempt to make room for the growing brain (Fig. 12-30). The skull base has a limited ability to respond in these situations, but some characteristic changes are seen. Thus, coronal synostosis limits the ability of the calvarium to add to its length, yielding a brachiocephalic skull that is foreshortened from front to back and may be larger than normal in its vertical dimension. The greater wing of the sphenoid bone displaces anteriorly, as does the petrous bone, and the orbit is pushed forward and is somewhat shortened. These changes can occur on one or both sides, depending on the extent of sutural involvement.

Abnormalities in the contiguous soft tissues and CSF spaces also can have an effect on the shape, thickness, and position of the sphenoid bone. Primary or congenital arachnoid cysts are abnormal arachnoid or collagen-lined cavities that characteristically do not communicate with the ventricular system. They account for 1% of intracranial space-occupying lesions and usually appear in the first five decades of life.[37, 38] Men are more commonly affected than women. Although these abnormalities abut the skull base, they are developmental abnormalities of the subarachnoid space rather than of the skull base itself. In the early embryo

there are no subarachnoid spaces around the brain. The forming brain is surrounded by loose mesenchyme, and all CSF is contained within the ventricles. It is hypothesized that as pulsations of the CSF force fluid into the subarachnoid space during normal development, some of the CSF becomes trapped between the developing pia and the arachnoid.[39] These cysts can occur in many locations; the middle cranial fossa is a frequent site. The cysts can expand progressively during antenatal development. The exact mechanism of this enlargement is unknown, although many theories have been proposed.[39] At imaging, the wings of the sphenoid can be remodeled. The greater wing is frequently thinned and pushed forward, and the lesser wing may be elevated. The cyst itself has a characteristic appearance on the imaging following the appearance of CSF on either CT or MR imaging. These cysts are dark (no restricted diffusion) on diffusion-weighted imaging, helping to differentiate them from an epidermoid in questionable cases.

Another congenital abnormality that has a secondary effect on the skull base is the Arnold-Chiari malformation. The inferiorly displaced brainstem can appear to cause a pressure effect on the clivus, giving it a scalloped, more vertical appearance. This is an incidental finding because the changes in the brain itself are far more obvious.

## Cartilage Dysplasias

Because most of the sphenoid bone develops from cartilaginous precursors, various cartilage dysplasias will have an effect on the growth of the sphenoid bone. These are discussed later in this chapter.

## Inflammation and Obstruction

A variety of inflammatory processes can involve the central skull base. Chief among them is sphenoid sinus infection. Infection can spread to the bone and to the cavernous sinus, causing cavernous sinus thrombosis.

Inflammatory changes in the sphenoid sinus have the same imaging appearance as sinusitis in other sinuses (Fig. 12-31) (see Chapter 5). Mucosal thickening and fluid can be identified, and chronic sinusitis can lead to sclerosis of the bony walls (Fig. 12-32). Fungal infections can invade the wall, reaching the cavernous sinus (Figs. 12-32 and 12-33), and thrombosis of the carotid artery and cavernous sinus can occur. Thrombosis can be identified on imaging as filling defects replacing the normal enhancement of the cavernous sinus (Fig. 12-34).[40] Venous channels leading to and from the cavernous sinus may be thrombosed. The inflammatory tissue does enhance and may blend with the enhancing sinus mucosa on CT. The cavernous sinus may bulge laterally, and the dura may enhance. Eventually, narrowing of the carotid artery can be seen within the sinus.

Necrotizing (malignant) otitis is an invasive pseudomonal infection that occurs almost exclusively in elderly diabetics and starts in the external auditory canal.[41–44] The infection can then spread across the soft tissues beneath the skull base and can even cross the midline. Invasion of the petroclival fissure or the central basicranium can occur in

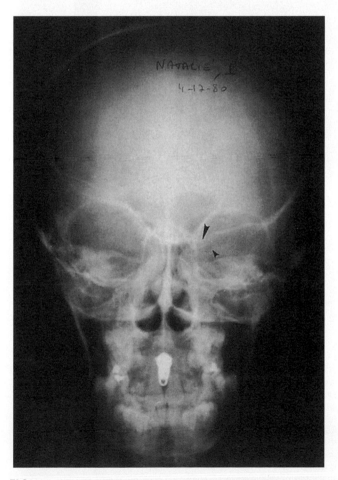

**FIGURE 12-25** Neurofibromatosis with congenital defect of the sphenoid. The lesser wing of the sphenoid (*large black arrowhead*) and the superior orbital fissure (*small black arrowhead*) can be identified on the normal side. These two structures are not visualized on the abnormal side because of the maldevelopment of the lesser and greater wings of the sphenoid.

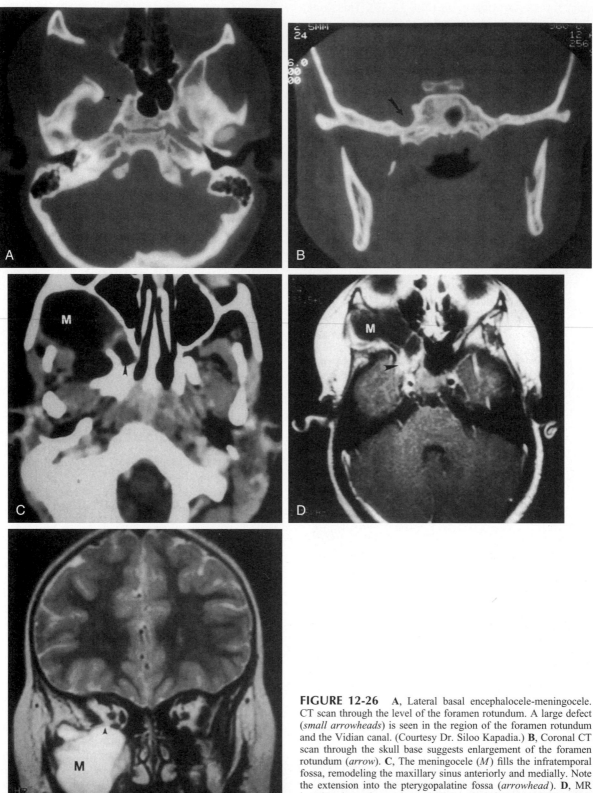

**FIGURE 12-26** **A,** Lateral basal encephalocele-meningocele. CT scan through the level of the foramen rotundum. A large defect (*small arrowheads*) is seen in the region of the foramen rotundum and the Vidian canal. (Courtesy Dr. Siloo Kapadia.) **B,** Coronal CT scan through the skull base suggests enlargement of the foramen rotundum (*arrow*). **C,** The meningocele (*M*) fills the infratemporal fossa, remodeling the maxillary sinus anteriorly and medially. Note the extension into the pterygopalatine fossa (*arrowhead*). **D,** MR imaging shows the meningocele (*M*) in the infratemporal fossa. This area contains CSF. Some glial tissue was seen in the wall. Note the small area of enhancement (*arrowhead*) near the cavernous sinus at the neck of the abnormality. **E,** Coronal T2-weighted image through the meningocele. The abnormality bulges (*arrowhead*) into the superior orbital fissure. The orbital contents, though displaced, are fairly normal.

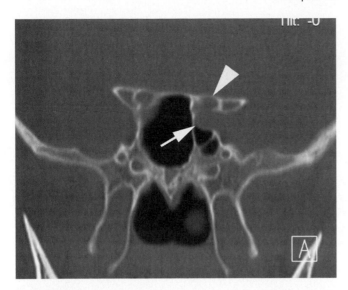

**FIGURE 12-27**   Medially positioned carotid artery impressing into the sphenoid sinus. The carotid artery (*arrow*) bulges into the sphenoid sinus. The bony plate separating the artery from the sinus may be thin or dehiscent. Optic canal (*arrowhead*).

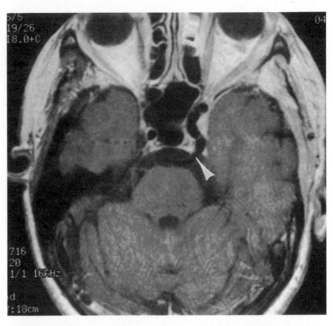

**FIGURE 12-29**   Persistent trigeminal artery. The postcontrast T1-weighted MR image shows the flow void connecting the intracavernous carotid artery with the basilar artery. *Arrowhead*, trigeminal artery.

later stages, and MR imaging can show obliteration of the clival fat.[45–47]

The Tolosa-Hunt syndrome is a presumed idiopathic inflammatory condition involving the orbital apex, superior orbital fissure, and cavernous sinus. This is discussed in Chapter 9.

Obstruction of the sphenoid sinus can result from the sequelae of inflammatory disease or rarely from tumor. Early in the process, the obstructed sinus secretions have a low (10 to 25 HU) CT attenuation. If the secretions become desiccated, their attenuation increases. *Aspergillus* colonization of the obstructed sinus cavity may add to the density as well. Eventually, the sinus may become very dense, mimicking the appearance of enhancement on nonenhanced scans. On MR imaging the signal intensities vary with the protein concentration of the obstructed secretions (Fig.

12-35).[48–50] With extreme desiccation, particularly when combined with *Aspergillus* colonization, the appearance may be "black" on all sequences. This topic is discussed in Chapter 5.

A mucocele is the final result of sinus obstruction, with the pressures within the sinus eventually remodeling the bone outward. Sphenoid sinus mucoceles are discussed in the next section.

## TUMORS AND TUMOR-LIKE CONDITIONS

Tumors can arise from the skull base itself or from any of the tissues adjacent to or passing through it.[51–54] The

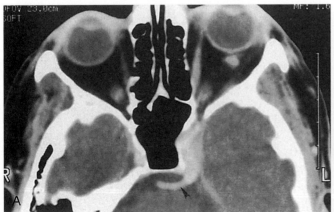
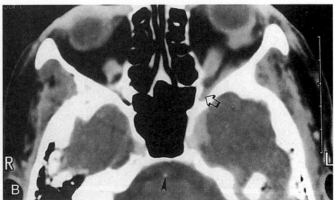

**FIGURE 12-28**   **A**, Persistent trigeminal artery shows the embryonic connection (*arrowhead*) between the carotid artery in the cavernous sinus and the basilar artery. **B**, Lower scan shows a very small basilar artery (*arrowhead*). Also note the obscuration of the fat at the junction of the upper pterygopalatine fossa and inferior orbital fissure (*open arrow*). This is a patient with perineural tumor extension along the branches of the trigeminal nerve. Adenoid cystic carcinoma.

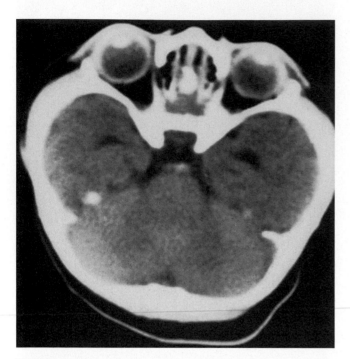

**FIGURE 12-30** Bilateral coronal synostosis. Axial CT scan through the skull base in a 2-year-old child shows the changes typical of coronal synostosis, including bilateral calvarial bulging of the region of the sphenozygomatic suture and fullness of both middle cranial fossae.

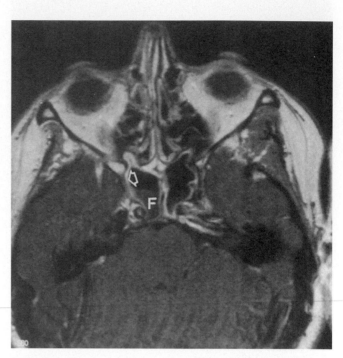

**FIGURE 12-31** Sphenoid sinusitis and T1-weighted image after gadolinium administration. The patient has an air-fluid level in the sphenoid. *F*, Fluid; *open arrow*, enhancing mucosa.

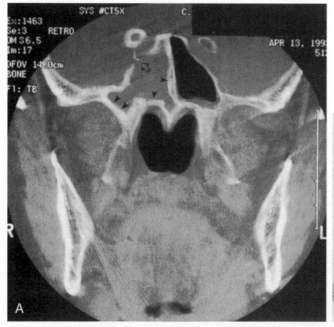

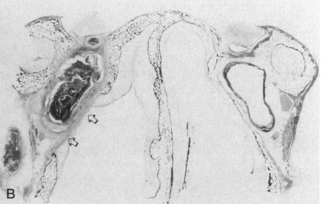

**FIGURE 12-32** **A**, Chronic sphenoid sinusitis with fungus (*Aspergillus*) extending into the cavernous sinus. The sclerotic change (*black arrowheads*) along the margin of the sphenoid sinus indicates chronicity. Note the defect (*open arrow*) in the upper lateral cortex of the sphenoid sinus. The calcification just lateral to this point of erosion represents a calcification in the carotid artery. **B**, Autopsy section shows the bony defect (*open arrows*) between the cavernous sinus and the sphenoid sinus. Note the thrombosis in the carotid artery. (Courtesy of Dr. Berrylin J. Ferguson.)

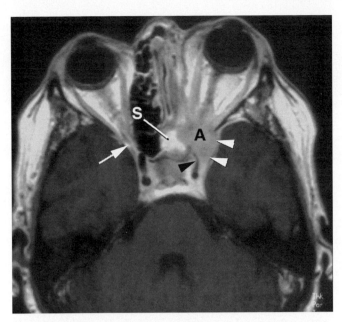

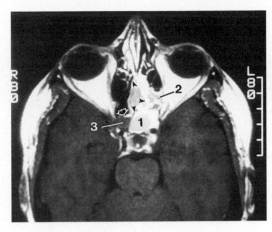

FIGURE 12-35   Esthesioneuroblastoma. The small tumor shows intermediate enhancement and causes the region of the nasal septum to bulge in all directions (*small black arrowheads*). The sinuses show various signal intensities reflecting various protein concentrations. The bright signal in the left sphenoid (*1*) could be due to a fairly high protein concentration or to hemorrhage. The intermediate signal intensity in the posterior left ethmoid (*2*) shows a lower protein concentration than in the left sphenoid. The low signal in the right sphenoid (*3*) is typical of relatively recent obstruction with high water and low protein concentrations. The enhancement of the mucosal margin (*open arrow*) also helps differentiate the obstructed sinus from the tumor.

FIGURE 12-33   *Aspergillus* of the sphenoid sinus extending into the orbital apex and cavernous sinus. Axial postcontrast T1-weighted image shows the *Aspergillus* (*A*) with moderate enhancement. The lesion was intermediate to slightly dark on T2-weighted images. There is expansion of the anterior cavernous sinus (*white arrowheads*), with narrowing of the carotid artery (*black arrowhead*). There are retained secretions in the more medial sphenoid sinus (*S*). Note how the bright fat protruding through the superior orbital fissure is obliterated on the left side. Compare this to the normal fat on the right side (*white arrow*).

apparent site of origin of a primary tumor is a helpful indicator of the lesion's histology, and subtle differences in location can cause the radiologist to favor one diagnosis over another.

Tumors develop according to the tissues present in a particular region. Hence, based on the anatomy, the skull base can be organized into three general regions (Fig.

12-36). In the midline, the sphenoid is a block of bone perforated by a sinus and covered by dura. Two important embryologic structures, the notochord and Rathke's pouch, pass through this part of the bone. Any of these tissues can contribute to pathology. Hence, in the midline, there can be chordomas (notochord), meningiomas, bone and sinus tumors, and rare lesions related to Rathke's pouch remnants.

Just off the midline in the sagittal plane of the fissures and formina, one still finds meningeal lesions. The lateral recess of the sphenoid sinus can extend into this area, so that pathology related to the sinus as well as rare bone lesions

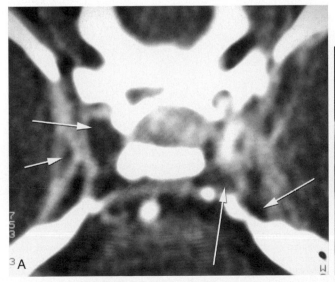

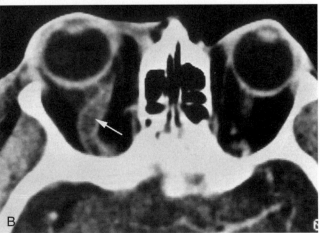

FIGURE 12-34   Thrombosis of the cavernous sinus. Postcontrast axial CT scan. **A,** There are filling defects (*arrows*) in places normally opacified in the cavernous sinus. **B,** There is a defect (*arrow*) filling the superior ophthalmic vein. (Courtesy of Bernard Schuknecht, Zurich.)

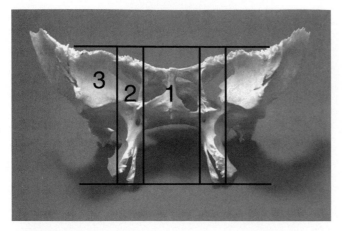

**FIGURE 12-36** The sphenoid bone can be divided into three basic regions. In zone 1, the central sphenoid, lesions are predominantly related to bone, dura, sella, or the sphenoid sinus. Lesions arising in zone 2 may arise from dura but also arise from nerves and vessels. The lesions in zone 3 are usually related to the bone or dura. Metastases and meningiomas are common here.

can present here. Chondroid lesions are common here because the foramen lacerum and petrooccipital fissure contain cartilage. The various foramina carry nerves and vessels, so that nerve sheath tumors and aneurysms can arise

here. Further laterally in the greater wing of the sphenoid, there are no fissures and foramina. This region is simply a bone covered by dura, and the lesions arising here reflect this simplicity. Most lesions are meningiomas or bone-related tumors. In this region, osseous metastases are also common. Certainly there is overlap in the anatomy and in the resultant pathology that occurs in these areas. However, analysis based on these general regions of the bone can be a helpful beginning to diagnosis.

## Chordomas

Chordomas are malignant neoplasms arising from remnants of the embryonic notochord. More than one-third of these tumors arise in the skull base.[55–57] The terminus of the notochord is in the sphenoid bone just inferior to the sella turcica and the dorsum sella, and thus the skull base chordomas arise in the region of the clivus. Thirty-five percent of chordomas occur in the skull base compared with 50% in the sacrococcygeal region and 15% in the spine.[58]

Histologically, the lesion has a characteristic cell, the physaliphorous cell, with large vacuoles containing mucin and glycogen and with a "bubbly" appearance of the cytoplasm (Fig. 12-37).[58, 59] The cells tend to clump

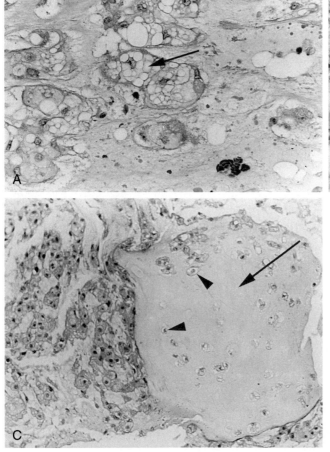

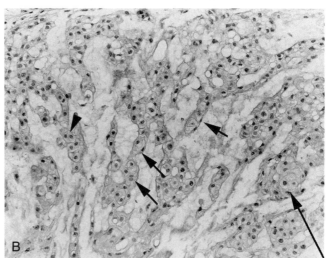

**FIGURE 12-37** Chordoma histology. **A**, Classic chordoma. Typical physaliphorous cell with "bubbly" (*arrow*) cytoplasm. **B**, Classic chordoma. The cells are arranged in cords (*short arrows*) and clumps (*long arrow*). The cords may be several cells thick. The cells abut one another over large areas. Some cells (*arrowhead*) appear to partially surround others. **C**, Chondroid chordoma shows a hyaline-like matrix (*arrow*) with small apparent lacunae containing cells (*arrowheads*). The cells within these small spaces, however, are cytokeratin positive and are not chondrocytes. Note the more typical area of classic chordoma immediately to the left of the "chondroid" section. (Courtesy of Dr. Andrew Rosenberg.)

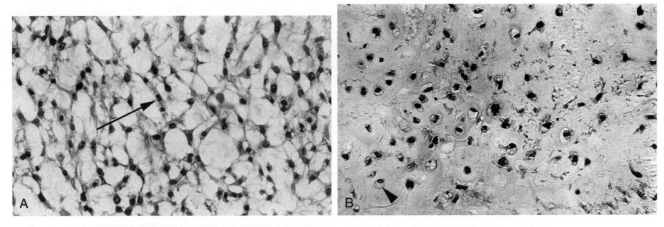

**FIGURE 12-38**   Chondrosarcoma histopathology. **A**, Myxoid chondrosarcoma. The cells (*arrow*) are true chondrocytes. They are negative for various epithelial markers including cytokeratin. Note how the cells abut one another end to end but do not form true cords. There are only small areas of contact between ends of cells. The cells are within a myxoid matrix. **B**, Hyaline-type chondrosarcoma. The cells are found within true hyalin matrix. The cells (*arrowheads*) are within small lacunae. These cells do not stain for various epithelial markers and are true chondrocytes. (Courtesy of Dr. Andrew Rosenberg.)

together into nests or chords (Fig. 12-37B), and adjacent cells have large segments of contact, at times partially wrapping around one another. The myxoid matrix surrounding the cells gives the tumor a gray, translucent appearance at gross examination. Small dystrophic calcifications and hemorrhages can also be seen.

A variant of chordoma has been described based on the histologic appearance (Fig. 12-37C), as regions within this variant resemble the hyaline type of chondrosarcoma (Fig. 12-38). This lesion was referred to as a "chondroid chordoma" by Heffelfinger et al. in 1973.[58] Small cells resembling chondrocytes are found in a matrix that resembles the hyaline matrix of the hyaline type of chondrosarcoma (see below). This tumor was thought to be a chordoma with cartilaginous differentiation. The variations in the designation received significant attention in the literature because of perceived differences in prognosis between classic chordoma and chondroid chordoma. However, immunohistochemical techniques have indicated that neither the cell nor the matrix of the "chondroid" portion of this variant is of true chondroid derivation. The cells in these regions stain positive for cytokeratin and for other epithelial markers such as epithelial membrane antigen and carcinoembryonic antigen. Such epithelial markers, particularly cytokeratin, are almost always negative in a true chondroid lesion but are positive in cells of classic chordoma and in notochordal tissue.[59] The term "chondroid" in chondroid chordoma, therefore, refers only to a histologic mimic. The lesion does not contain true cartilage or tissue of cartilage origin and thus is not a dimorphic tumor. Notably, both the original descriptions by Heffelfinger et al. and the cases labeled immunohistochemically as "chondroid" chordomas more recently by Rosenberg et al. contained not only regions of "pseudocartilage," but also areas of the typical classic chordoma.[58, 59] The controversy regarding separation of chordoma and chondrosarcoma is further described later in this chapter under "Chondrosarcoma."

A final type of chordoma is the dedifferentiated chordoma. This type usually arises in the sacrococcygeal region rather than in the skull base. The dedifferentiated component is usually malignant fibrous histiocytoma or occasionally osteosarcoma. These tend to be very aggressive tumors with a poor prognosis.

Skull base chordomas arise within the basiocciput basisphenoid. Rarely, a chordoma can arise in the nasopharynx or can be completely intracranial in location. These locations are explained by the tortuous course of the notochord. Though most of the pathway of the notochord is within the osseous basicranium, short segments of the course transiently pass out of the bone into the soft tissue of the nasopharynx and into the posterior fossa. The passage of the notochord into the posterior fossa also explains a normal variant found in the dura or subarachnoid space of the midline posterior fossa at the level of the pons. A small amount of notochordal tissue occasionally can be present and is referred to as ecchordosis physaliphora. This tissue is also positive for cytokeratin and other epithelial immunohistochemical markers. Though usually small, this benign tissue occasionally can be fairly large. The descent of the notochord into the nasopharynx is believed to be related to the development of the pharyngeal bursa and therefore Thornwaldt's cyst. This is discussed in Chapter 28.

Chordomas can occur at any age, but in the craniovertebral area most cases are diagnosed between the ages of 30 and 50 years. This contrasts with the sacrococcygeal chordomas, which have a peak incidence in the 40- to 60-year age group. Men are more commonly affected than women. There have been cases reported of apparent familial lineage of chordoma.[60, 61] Cytogenetic analysis has been done in a few cases, with variable results.[60–62]

Common presenting symptoms of craniovertebral chordomas include orbitofrontal headaches and visual disturbances. The headache may result from involvement or stretching of the dura. Visual problems or ophthalmoplegia can result when the optic nerves and neural contents of the cavernous sinus are involved. Tumors can involve the trigeminal nerve and eventually can affect cranial nerves VII and VIII as the lesion approaches the internal auditory canal.

More inferiorly, cranial nerves IX through XII can be affected. Tumors can also cause symptoms by growing into the pituitary gland or by pushing the brainstem. Lesions extending into the nasopharynx can cause problems with breathing.

On CT, the chordoma is usually a midline clival lesion with both bone destruction and a soft-tissue mass. The margin between the tumor and normal bone is not sclerotic.[63] Radiodensities are frequently present and tend to be fairly large (Fig. 12-39). These densities are not calcifications and are thought to represent remaining fragments of the destroyed bone rather than new matrix formation.[64] Specifically, these tumors do not tend to show

the small, calcified ringlets that may be present in chondrosarcomas. The expanding tumor may cross the petrooccipital fissure to reach the petrous bone or may extend intracranially, pushing the pons and brainstem posteriorly. Those rare tumors that occur outside of the bone, either intracranially or in the soft tissues of the nasopharynx, may or may not erode bone. At least part of the soft-tissue component of the tumor will enhance after intravenous contrast, but frequently there are regions that do not enhance and remain of relatively low density (Fig. 12-39). Cystic areas commonly are seen within the tumor.

The MR imaging appearance is quite variable. Usually there is a hypointense to isointense soft-tissue mass on

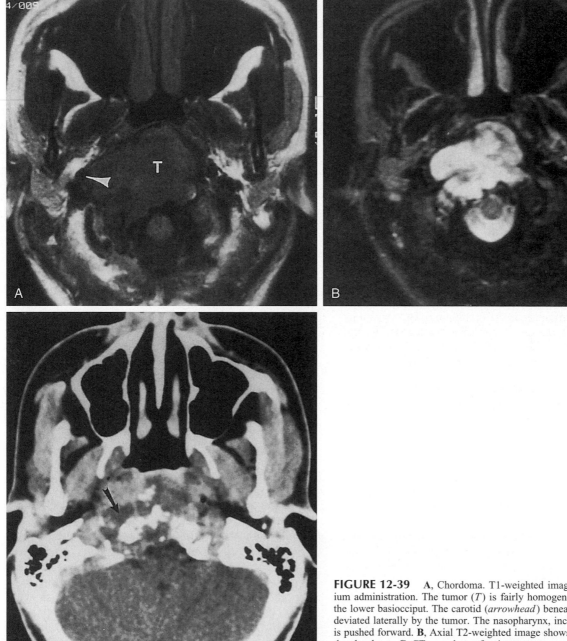

**FIGURE 12-39** **A,** Chordoma. T1-weighted image without gadolinium administration. The tumor (*T*) is fairly homogeneous in the area of the lower basiocciput. The carotid (*arrowhead*) beneath the skull base is deviated laterally by the tumor. The nasopharynx, including the mucosa, is pushed forward. **B,** Axial T2-weighted image shows the high signal of the chordoma. **C,** CT scan done after intravenous contrast administration shows areas of low density (*arrow*) and fairly large "calcifications" representing residual bone from the destruction of the lower clivus.

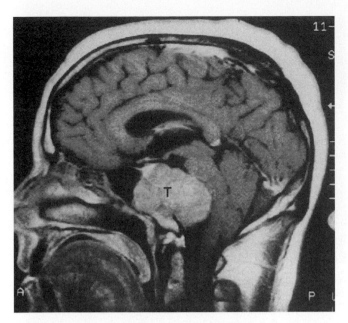

**FIGURE 12-40** Chordoma. T1-weighted image after contrast administration shows the tumor (*T*), with fairly homogeneous intermediate enhancement without cystic areas.

T1-weighted images (Figs. 12-39 and 12-40).[65, 66] Cystic areas, large or small, containing hemorrhage or mucoid material, are frequently present and can be bright on T1-weighted images (Fig. 12-41). Occasionally, a remaining piece of bone is large enough to cause a signal void. On T2-weighted images, the tumors characteristically have a high signal intensity.[67] Old hemorrhage may be seen as dark

areas on T2-weighted sequences (Fig. 12-42). MR imaging is excellent for detecting the margin of the lesion close to the cavernous sinus and for determining the relationship of the tumor to the brainstem.

Angiography shows a relatively avascular lesion without large intratumoral blood vessels. The normal vessels in and around the basicranium are frequently displaced by the tumor.

Chordomas grow slowly, and metastasis is quite rare. However, even after radical surgery, local recurrence is frequent.[68] Seeding along the surgical entrance pathway can also occur (Fig. 12-43).[69] "Drop" metastasis seeding the subarachnoid space of the spine has been reported but is uncommon.[70] The tumor's location within the clivus and its proximity to both carotid arteries and multiple cranial nerves make complete resection almost impossible in many cases. Treatment is frequently a combination of surgery and radiation therapy.[71] Chordomas are resistant to conventional radiotherapy, but success has been achieved with proton beam therapy, focused radiation therapy, and radiosurgery.[72–75] Often the tumor is partially resected to diminish the volume or to move the tumor away from critical structures prior to proton beam therapy.[76]

After radiation therapy, the lesion is not expected to disappear. Rather, control is considered if there is lack of growth and progression of symptoms. The indicated 5-year control rate after proton beam therapy has been 55% to 70%. A poorer prognosis has been described in women, in patients whose tumors show necrosis on imaging, and in patients who have tumors with measured volumes greater than 70 ml.[77, 78] Of note, a recent study indicated that chondroid chordoma (keratin positive) had the same prognosis as standard chordoma and did not share the better prognosis of

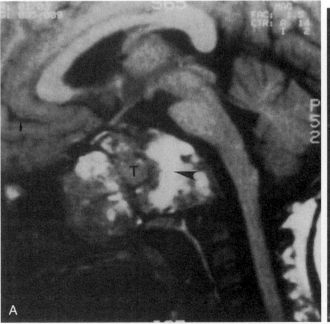

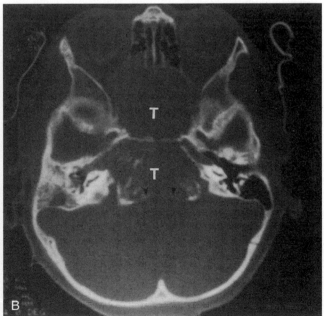

**FIGURE 12-41** **A**, Chordoma of the skull base. Sagittal image shows the tumor replacing the sphenoid sinus. The tumor (*T*) has both intermediate and high (*large black arrowhead*) areas of signal intensity. Chordomas can have a variety of appearances, including areas of high signal representing either cystic areas or hemorrhage. **B**, Axial CT image shows the tumor with both anterior and posterior components (*T*). The expansion of the clival surface (*arrowheads*) is seen posteriorly.

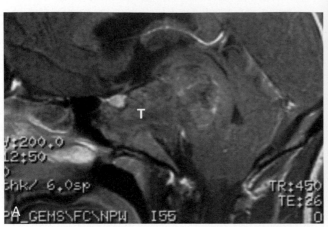

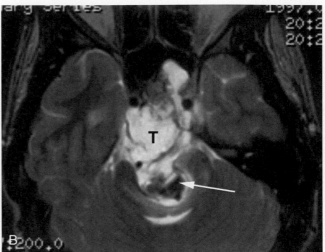

**FIGURE 12-42**    Chordoma of the basisphenoid. **A,** Postcontrast sagittal T1 image shows low enhancement of the tumor (*T*). Note how the lesion pushes posteriorly into the pons. **B,** Axial T2-weighted image shows the general high signal of the tumor (*T*), but there is an area of low signal representing hemosiderin from previous hemorrhage (*arrow*).

chondrosarcoma (see below).[79] Complications of radiation therapy, including proton beam therapy, include radiation optic neuritis and necrosis. Radiation change is frequently seen in the temporal lobes, where edema, gliosis, or even radiation necrosis can be present (Fig. 12-44).

## Chondrosarcomas

Chondrosarcomas can arise from bone, cartilage, or even tissues without a cartilaginous component, and 6.5% of these tumors arise in the head and neck region.[80–82] In the skull base, chondrosarcomas are most commonly found in the region of the various synchondroses that remain after

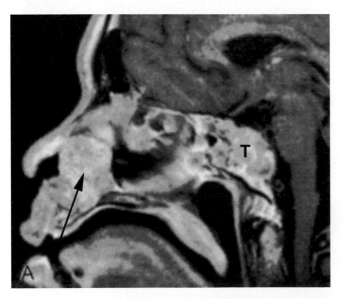

**FIGURE 12-43**    Recurrence of chordoma after the transsphenoidal approach to partial resection. Much of the tumor (*T*) remains in the upper basicranium. Note the recurrence (*arrow*) in the anterior part of the nasal septum.

ossification replaces the embryonic chondroid basal plate. These tumors have a particular propensity for the petro-occipital (petroclival) synchondrosis or fissure (Figs. 12-45 to 12-47), and thus chondroid tumors in the deep skull base region tend to be off midline. The junction of the nasal septum and the rostrum of the sphenoid is another location where these tumors tend to arise (Fig. 12-48).[83] Chondrosarcoma can arise in the midline basisphenoid/basiocciput, presumably related to the sphenooccipital synchondrosis.

Chondrosarcoma invades locally but seldom metastasizes.[84] Tumors spread away from the petrooccipital fissure, involve the clivus and petrous portion of the temporal bone, and bulge into the subarachnoid space cisterns or into the soft tissues beneath the skull base.

Chondrosarcomas vary in histologic type. Conventional chondrosarcoma includes the hyaline and myxoid types or a combination of the two (Fig. 12-38). Other types of chondrosarcoma include clear cell, dedifferentiated, and mesenchymal. Virtually all skull base chondrosarcomas are of the conventional type. A recent series of 200 cases showed the combination of hyaline and myxoid types to be most common, occurring in 63% of cases.[79] The relatively pure hyaline type accounted for 7.5% of cases, and the myxoid type accounted for 29.5% of cases. Both histologic patterns include true chondrocytes, but the surrounding matrix differs. The matrix in the hyaline type is more solid compared to the more mucinous or gelatinous matrix seen in the myxoid type. The hyaline matrix can mineralize, giving the characteristic ringlet calcification appearance on CT.

Conventional chondrosarcomas can be graded, reflecting degrees of differentiation. Almost all chondrosarcomas of the central skull base are well or moderately differentiated. Most are slow growing.

Chondrosarcomas can occur at almost any age, but most occur in middle age. The presentation depends on the location and local extension, and headaches or various cranial nerve palsies often cause the patient to seek medical attention.

Treatment may combine surgery with various types of

focused beam or particle radiation or may consist of radiation alone.[72, 85] Complete surgical removal is usually impossible due to the location of the lesion and its proximity to neural and vascular structures. These tumors grow slowly, and the prognosis is generally good.

On CT, chondrosarcomas have a varied appearance, depending on the amount of chondroid matrix present.[86] There is usually a significant soft-tissue component that has a dense appearance on noncontrast studies and enhances to some degree after contrast administration. Calcification of the tumor matrix is characteristic but is not always present. Thus, the degree of calcification is quite variable, with some chondrosarcomas having almost no calcification, while others, particularly the low-grade tumors, having extensive, even dense, calcification (Figs. 12-47 and 12-49). The calcifications tend to be small ringlets or incomplete rings, suggesting the cartilaginous nature of the matrix. Frequently, the margin between tumor and normal bone is fairly abrupt, and although this transition zone is fairly narrow, the tumor margin is not sclerotic.

On MR imaging, these tumors usually have an intermediate T1-weighted and a fairly high T2-weighted signal intensity. After gadolinium administration there is detectable enhancement, but the signal change is not profound (Fig. 12-50). Heavy calcifications may be detectable on MR imaging, but smaller ones cannot be seen. Indeed, even if there is fairly extensive calcification, this may not be evident on MR imaging. Therefore, there may be a significant difference between the amount of calcification seen on CT and the size of any MR signal voids that suggest the presence of calcifications.

Chondrosarcoma usually occurs as an isolated tumor, but it can occur as multiple tumors. Chondrosarcoma can occur in Ollier's disease (multiple enchondromatosis) and Maffucci syndrome (multiple enchondromas with associated cutaneous hemangiomas).[87, 88] Chondrosarcoma can also complicate Paget's disease.

## Chordoma Versus Chondrosarcoma

Significant controversy surrounds the separation of some chordomas and chondrosarcomas of the central skull base. There is a significant overlap of the histologic patterns of these two tumors, potentially leading to ambiguity in diagnosis. This ambiguity can create problems in planning therapy and determining prognosis.

In the central skull base, there are two histologic types of chordoma and two histologic types of chondrosarcoma. Chordomas are either classic chordoma or chondroid chordoma (Fig. 12-37). Chondrosarcomas are either hyaline or myxoid (Fig. 12-38).[59, 79] The majority of chondrosarcomas are a mixture of myxoid and hyaline histologic types, and virtually all chondroid chordomas also contain regions of classic chordoma histology. There are histologic similarities between the "chondroid" part of the chondroid chordoma and hyaline chondrosarcoma and between the classic pattern of chordoma and the myxoid pattern of chondrosarcoma.

As mentioned previously, the term "chondroid" in chondroid chordoma refers to a histologic mimic rather than to true chondroid matrix. In the original descriptions of the chondroid chordoma, Heffelfinger et al. referred to a lesion that had areas of classic chordoma as well as regions that histologically resembled hyaline cartilage.[58] The lesion was thought to have cartilage differentiation within a chordoma. The so-called chondroid part of the chondroid chordoma resembles the hyaline-type chondrosarcoma, but the cells are actually typed immunohistochemically as epithelially derived cells rather than chondrocytes. Since the "chondroid" component of chordoma resembles hyaline-type chondrosarcoma, one would expect the controversy to be related to this overlapping appearance. However, most of the confusion has actually been between myxoid chondrosarcoma and classic chordoma.

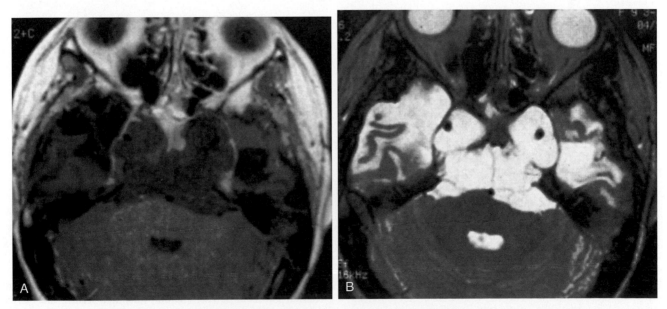

**FIGURE 12-44**    Chordoma after treatment. **A,** The expansile lesion of the basicranium shows very little enhancement. Note the changes in the contiguous temporal tips from radiation therapy. **B,** Axial T2-weighted image shows the typical high signal within the lesion and abnormal signal in the temporal lobes.

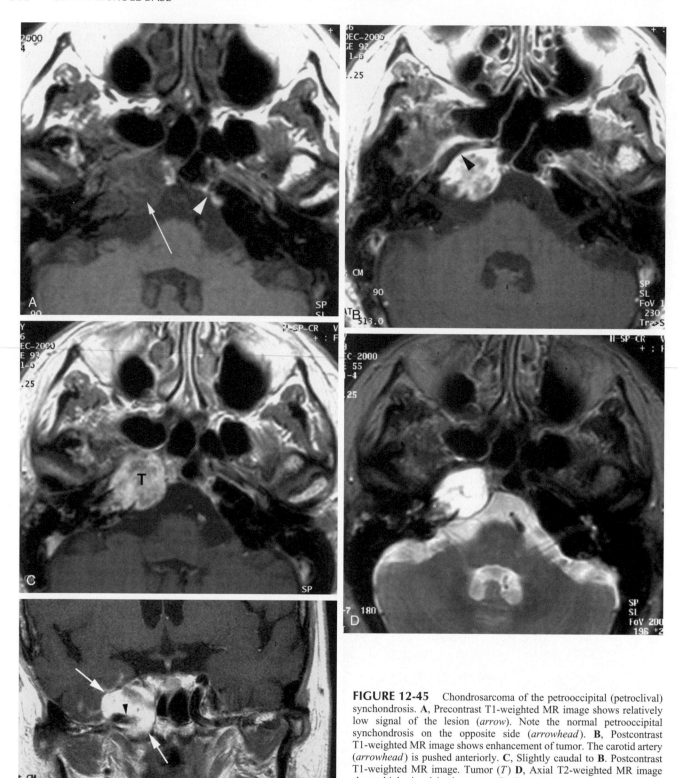

**FIGURE 12-45**   Chondrosarcoma of the petrooccipital (petroclival) synchondrosis. **A**, Precontrast T1-weighted MR image shows relatively low signal of the lesion (*arrow*). Note the normal petrooccipital synchondrosis on the opposite side (*arrowhead*). **B**, Postcontrast T1-weighted MR image shows enhancement of tumor. The carotid artery (*arrowhead*) is pushed anteriorly. **C**, Slightly caudal to **B**. Postcontrast T1-weighted MR image. Tumor (*T*) **D**, Axial T2-weighted MR image shows high signal in the tumor. **E**, Coronal postcontrast T1-weighted MR image shows the tumor (between arrows) extending through the fissure. The flow void is seen in the displaced carotid artery (*arrowhead*).

The myxoid type of chondrosarcoma also has some similarities to the chordoma. The myxoid matrix surrounding cells is similar to that seen in the classic pattern of chordoma. Cells can be found in strands resembling the chord pattern in chordoma. Vacuoles present in some chondrocytes give an appearance resembling the physaliphorous cell of the chordoma. These similarities lead to misdiagnosis of many myxoid chondrosarcomas as chordomas. However, differentiation can be made using the microscopic appearance and immunohistochemical staining.[79]

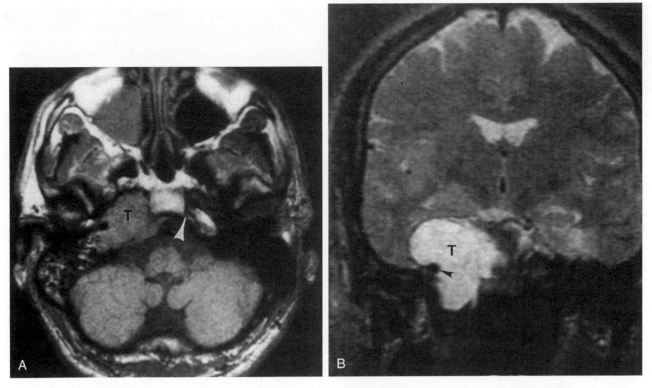

**FIGURE 12-46** **A,** Chondrosarcoma of the petrooccipital synchondrosis. The tumor (*T*) shows an intermediate signal intensity on this T1-weighted image without contrast. Compare the position of this chondrosarcoma with the normal petrooccipital synchondrosis on the normal side (*arrowhead*). **B,** T2-weighted coronal image shows the tumor (*T*) extending inferiorly through the region of the petrooccipital synchondrosis and the foramen lacerum. The carotid artery (*arrowhead*) is pushed laterally.

In the myxoid chondrosarcoma, the cells tend to abut one another in only a small area at the end of each cell and thus they form chains or strands of cells. In the classic chordoma, cells abut along larger areas, forming larger groups of cells arranged into sheets, nests, and chords, a pattern not found in the chondrosarcoma. Cells may almost completely surround one another. In other words, the "chord" is differentiated from the strands found in the CSA by the greater length of cell contact. Chords tend to be more than one cell thick compared to the single-cell strands of cells in the CSA.

The most conclusive evidence, however, comes from immunohistochemical examination.[59, 79] The cells of chon-

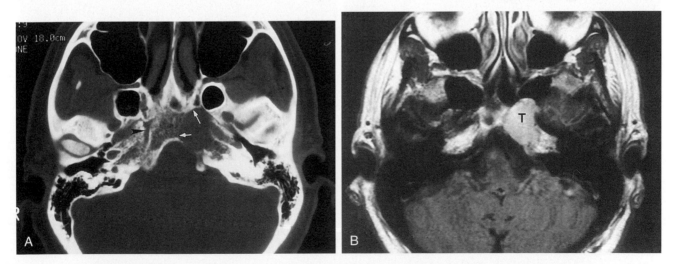

**FIGURE 12-47** Chondrosarcoma arising in the foramen lacerum and petroclival fissure. **A,** CT bone scan algorithm shows a fairly smooth margin (*arrows*) of tumor arising in the region of the foramen lacerum. Note the normal foramen lacerum (*black arrowhead*) on the opposite side. **B,** T1-weighted postcontrast image. The tumor shows intermediate enhancement. The abnormality had a lower signal intensity on the T1-weighted precontrast image and relatively high signal intensity on the T2-weighted images (not shown).

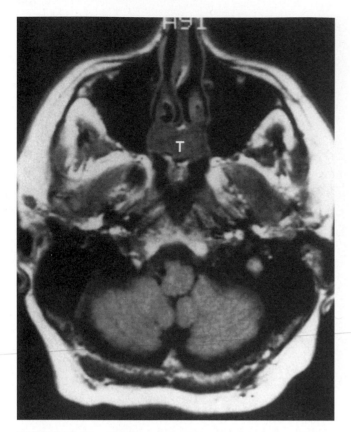

**FIGURE 12-48** Chondrosarcoma of the nasal septum. The tumor (*T*) is seen in the posterior part of the nasal septum. Chondrosarcoma is a likely diagnosis for the rare tumor arising in this region.

drosarcoma (myxoid or hyaline) are true chondrocytes and do not stain for cytokeratin or other epithelial markers. This is true for chondroid lesions throughout the body. In the chordoma (classic and "chondroid") the cells do stain for these epithelial markers, reflecting their origin from the notochord. Notochordal tissue shows the same immunohistochemical profile as the chordoma.

Distinguishing the CSA from the chordoma is important, as the prognosis is quite different. In general, chordomas, including the "chondroid" variants, do more poorly than CSA. Although results vary, in a recent report of a large series of tumors treated with a combination of surgery and proton beam therapy, the 5-year control rate was about 51% for chordoma compared to over 90% for CSA.[79]

In the final analysis, one can say that chordoma virtually always arises in the midline and that a lesion arising in the region of the petroclival (petrooccipital) synchondrosis is very unlikely to be a chordoma, but rather is a chondrosarcoma. Chondrosarcomas, however, can arise in the midline related to either the sphenooccipital synchondrosis or the posterior nasal septum. Although the degree and appearance of calcification may give a clue to the identity of a lesion when the site of origin is ambiguous, the location of the tumor's origin is the dominant diagnostic indicator.

## Other Chondroid Tumors

Other chondroid tumors of the skull base include chondromas, chondromyxoid fibroma, and, very rarely, chondroblastoma (Fig. 12-51). Truly benign chondromas are

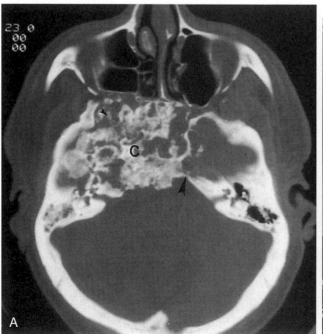
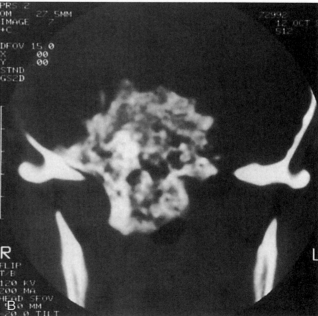

**FIGURE 12-49** Chondrosarcoma of the skull base. **A,** The chondrosarcoma (*C*) replaces much of the body of the sphenoid and the right greater wing. Although the lesion definitely involves and extends across the midline, the center point of the tumor is close to the foramen lacerum. The petrooccipital fissure on the opposite side (*black arrowhead*) is normal. Small ringlets of calcification (*small black arrowhead*) are visualized within the tumor. **B,** Very heavy calcification is seen in this tumor.

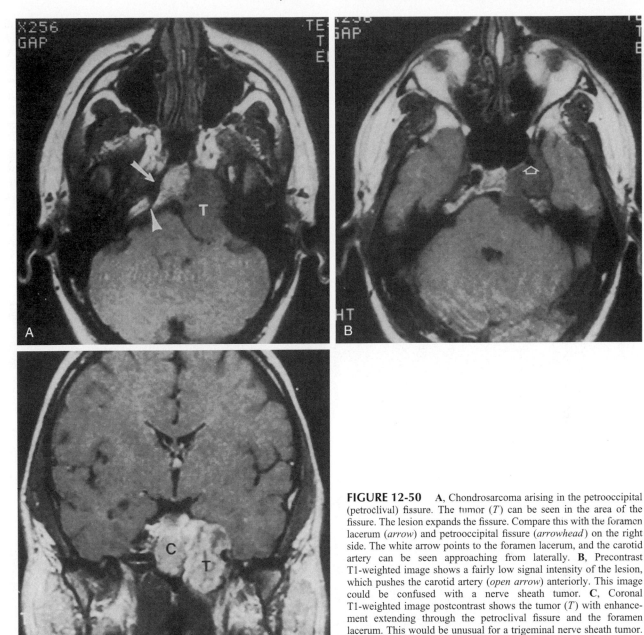

**FIGURE 12-50** **A,** Chondrosarcoma arising in the petrooccipital (petroclival) fissure. The tumor (*T*) can be seen in the area of the fissure. The lesion expands the fissure. Compare this with the foramen lacerum (*arrow*) and petrooccipital fissure (*arrowhead*) on the right side. The white arrow points to the foramen lacerum, and the carotid artery can be seen approaching from laterally. **B,** Precontrast T1-weighted image shows a fairly low signal intensity of the lesion, which pushes the carotid artery (*open arrow*) anteriorly. This image could be confused with a nerve sheath tumor. **C,** Coronal T1-weighted image postcontrast shows the tumor (*T*) with enhancement extending through the petroclival fissure and the foramen lacerum. This would be unusual for a trigeminal nerve sheath tumor. The enhancement of the tumor should not be confused with a normal high signal in the clivus and body of the sphenoid (*C*).

sharply defined and may be calcified. Most are probably more appropriately considered low-grade chondrosarcomas. Rarely, chondromas of the skull base (in addition to the more common chondrosarcomas already mentioned) can be found in patients with Ollier's disease (multiple enchondromatosis) and the Maffucci syndrome (Fig. 12-52) (multiple enchondromas associated with subcutaneous hemangiomas).[87, 88] Several cases were reported in the region of the petrooccipital synchondroses, and astrocytomas can also occur in these conditions.

Chondromyxoid fibroma has been reported as an expansile mass in the skull base.[89, 90] The lesion is not infiltrating and is considered to be less destructive than chordoma, but it may overlap with chondrosarcoma in imaging appearance.

## Meningiomas

Meningiomas are benign tumors that arise from the arachnoidal cells of the meninges.[91, 92] The peak incidence is between the ages of 20 and 60 years. Most meningiomas are found either along the convexities or parasagittally. A skull base origin is less common. Meningiomas can arise along almost any part of the sphenoid, including the greater wing, the planum sphenoidale, the tuberculum sella, and the wall of the cavernous sinus. From the initial site of origin, the tumor extends along the dural surfaces or intraosseously, and once it penetrates through the bone, a substantial extracranial mass can develop.

The clinical presentation depends on the site of origin, but headaches can be present with any of these tumors.

Meningioma of the planum sphenoidale may cause olfactory symptoms, and tumors closer to the chiasmatic sulcus can cause visual problems. Ophthalmoplegia can result as the nerves in the cavernous sinus are compromised.

The classification of meningiomas of the greater wing of the sphenoid is based on the location of the tumor. If the sphenoid wing is separated into thirds, both the degree of difficulty of resection and the likelihood of cranial neuropathy increase from laterally to medially. Tumors of the medial third, referred to as sphenocavernous meningiomas, are most likely to cause cranial neuropathies and represent the greatest surgical challenge. Recent surgical technical developments have improved surgical access to these difficult tumors, and if such surgery is planned, great precision in the imaging evaluation is required because of the close proximity of the lesion to critical neurovascular structures.

Meningiomas arising from the more lateral portion of the greater wing of the sphenoid may be fairly silent clinically because the cranial nerves are not directly involved. Although some of these meningiomas are globular in shape, many lesions in this location can be classified as hyperostosing en plaque meningiomas. Tumor growth can progress in any direction. As the tumor extends into the orbit, painless proptosis may occur. Inferior growth may cause a mass effect in the infratemporal fossa, presenting as a mass in the cheek or as problems with mastication. Lateral extension growth may displace the temporalis muscle. Medial growth can affect the trigeminal nerve, particularly the third division. Tumors from any location around the sphenoid bone can compress the brain, and seizures may be the presenting symptom.

Because arachnoid cells accompany the cranial nerves, it

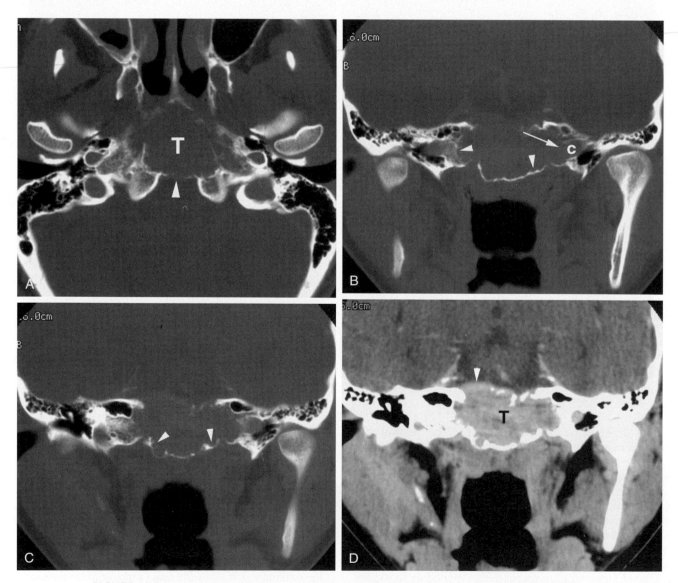

**FIGURE 12-51**    Chondromyxoid fibroma. **A**, Axial CT bone algorithm shows a tumor (*T*) bulging slightly through the posterior plate of the clivus (*arrowhead*). **B**, Coronal bone algorithm shows slight curvilinear scallops (*arrowheads*) along the margin. The bony wall (*arrow*) of the carotid canal (*C*) is eroded. **C**, Coronal bone algorithm shows slight scalloped areas (*arrowheads*). **D**, Coronal postcontrast soft-tissue window shows the tumor (*T*) bulging (*arrowhead*) into the posterior fossa.

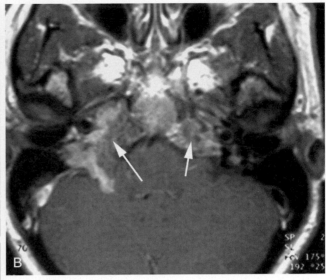

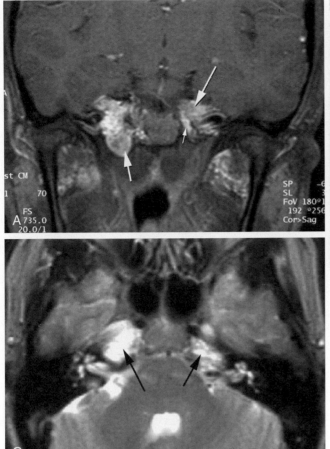

**FIGURE 12-52**    Bilateral chondrosarcomas in Maffucci's syndrome. **A,** Coronal postgadolinium T1-weighted image. Bilateral lesions (*large arrows*) are seen in the petrooccipital synchondroses. Note that a small part of the synchondrosis (*small arrow*) remains on the left. **B,** Axial T1-weighted postgadolinium image shows the irregular enhancement of the tumors (*arrows*). **C,** Axial T2-weighted image. The lesions (*arrows*) have high signal.

is not surprising that meningiomas can be found adjacent to and traversing various neural foramina.[93] These tumors can cause enlargement or erosion of these foramina, simulating a nerve sheath tumor. Gross destruction of the skull base can simulate malignancy.

On CT, there is enhancement of the soft-tissue component of the tumor. Calcifications may be detectable, and hyperostosis may be seen as thickening of the involved cortex or the trabeculae within the bone. Alternatively, as the meningioma extends through the skull base, a permeative bone pattern rather than a destructive or sclerotic pattern can be seen, often appearing on CT as a "washed-out" bone. Meningiomas arising from the planum sphenoidale may show characteristic sclerosis or upward "blistering" of the bone (Fig. 12-53). Both plain films and CT can demonstrate this finding.

Pneumosinus dilatans refers to enlargement of an air-filled sinus (Fig. 12-54). Pneumosinus dilatans of the sphenoid can occur either in isolation or in association with meningioma.[94-96] There is some controversy regarding terminology, as there are physicians who use the term "pneumosinus dilatans" only when referring to a dilated aerated sinus seen with adjacent tumor. Other people use the term to indicate any expanded air-filled sinus. When occurring with meningioma, the enlargement of the sinus may be focal or diffuse, depending on the position of the tumor, and focal hyperostosis may or may not be present.

The enlarged sinus is not opacified unless there is additional inflammatory/obstructive pathology in the sinus itself. The cortex is usually intact, though a focal dehiscence may occur. Pneumosinus dilatans has been described with meningioma arising within the optic canal as well as on the intracranial surface of the sphenoid bone (Fig. 12-55).[97, 98] Apparent enlargement of the sinus can also occur in acromegaly, in fibrous dysplasia, and in Sturge-Weber and Klippel-Trenaunay-Weber syndromes.[99]

On MR imaging, meningiomas are usually isointense to brain parenchyma (Fig. 12-56). After the administration of gadolinium, these lesions enhance intensely (Fig. 12-57). A "dural tail" frequently can be seen extending along the dura at the margin of the tumor (Fig. 12-58). Hyperostosis is more difficult to visualize on MR imaging, but sometimes it can be appreciated as an enlargement of the signal void or as a low-signal area representing the cortical bone (Fig. 12-59).

Imaging is particularly important with those tumors in the sphenocavernous region, and the relationship of the tumor to the vital structures of the cavernous sinus is better defined on MR imaging than on CT.[100] Because the normal cavernous sinus often enhances slightly more intensely than the tumor, the interface between tumor and normal structures can be defined. The enlarging tumor often impinges on and may obliterate the CSF signal in Meckel's cave. Tumor also may extend through the bony medial wall of the cavernous sinus

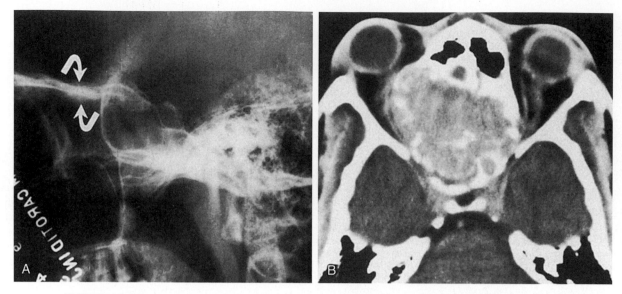

**FIGURE 12-53** Meningioma in a 52-year-old female presenting with headache and altered mental status. **A,** Lateral plain film of the skull demonstrating hyperostosis in the region of the planum sphenoidale (*curved arrows*). **B,** Axial contrast-enhanced CT slice through the region of the planum demonstrating a large, expansile mass occupying the floor of the anterior cranial fossa emanating from the planum sphenoidale. Irregular enhancement and bony destruction are apparent.

to appear as an enhancing mass within the sphenoid sinus. Here there can be difficulty distinguishing the tumor from any inflammatory mucosal disease or primary malignancy within the sinus.

One of the most important relationships to note is the effect of the tumor on the internal carotid artery, as meningiomas can surround and frequently will narrow this vessel (Figs. 12-56 and 12-57).[101] A more superior tumor extent can involve the middle cerebral artery. Meningiomas also have been described following the carotid artery inferiorly into the petrous carotid canal.

## Craniopharyngiomas and Rathke's Pouch Cysts

The craniopharyngioma arises from remnants of the pharyngohypophyseal (Rathke's) pouch, and most of these benign tumors are found in the sella or in the suprasellar cistern. Those lesions arising in the sellar or suprasellar region can grow into the sphenoid bone. Rarely, a craniopharyngioma occurs completely within the sphenoid bone, presumably developing from remnants of the pharyngohypophyseal duct trapped within the bone (Fig. 12-60).[102–104]

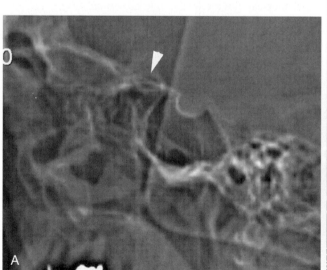
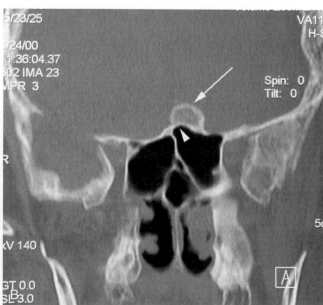

**FIGURE 12-54** Pneumosinus dilatans adjacent to probable meningioma. **A,** Lateral skull view shows the expansion or "blistering" of the planum (*arrowhead*) just anterior to the limbus. **B,** A heavily calcified lesion (*arrow*) is seen adjacent to the upward expansion (*arrowhead*) of the sinus.

Although craniopharyngiomas are described in Chapter 11, they are included here because of the very rare intraosseous occurrence of the tumor. Though these lesions occur predominantly in the first two decades of life, they can occur at any age; indeed, several of those reported in sphenoid bone have occurred in older patients. Those that are predominantly in the sphenoid bone can extend upward into the pituitary fossa and result in decreased pituitary function. Optic nerve abnormalities are not common with these ''intraosseous'' tumors unless there is further extension into the suprasellar cistern or involvement of the optic canals.

The craniopharyngioma is very similar histologically to some odontogenic lesions, as the pharyngohypophyseal pouch is an ectodermal evagination from the embryonic oral cavity, anterior to the buccopharyngeal membrane, and may develop oral ectoderm-related histopathology.[105, 106] The similarity of the craniopharyngioma to the ameloblastoma has given rise to the term adamantinomatous craniopharyngioma. According to some authors, some of the histologic features of craniopharyngioma more closely approximate the keratinizing and calcifying odontogenic cysts than they do the ameloblastoma.[105]

Histologically, the adamantinomatous craniopharyngioma contains epithelial lobules with palisading nuclei along the periphery. Cystic spaces are filled with fluid or debris, and the so-called wet keratin is considered characteristic of this form of craniopharyngioma.[107] Wet keratin is a conglomeration of large, keratinized cells with ''ghost'' nuclei reflecting the necrobiotic nature of these cells. Calcifications are frequently seen within the lesion, and an inflammatory response along the periphery of the tumor can stimulate bone formation. This is the type of histology that accounts for the typical imaging appearance of the craniopharyngioma with cyst formation and calcification. Reports of infrasellar craniopharyngiomas are rare, but some of the findings that are characteristic of the suprasellar type are found in these infrasellar lesions. The tumor may have a

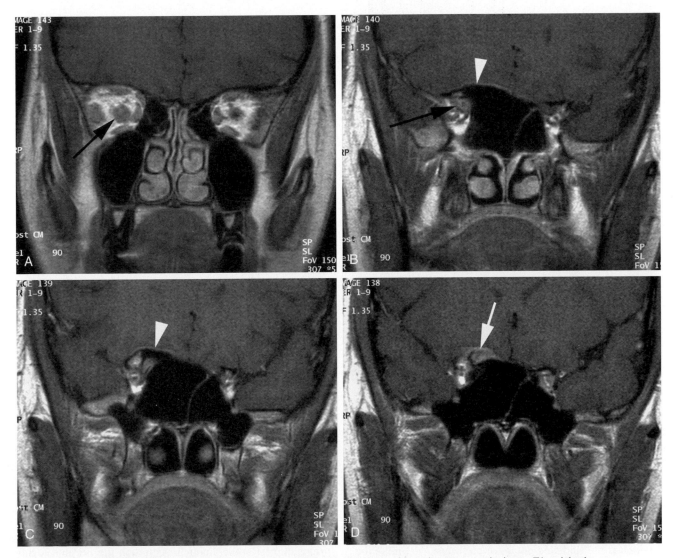

**FIGURE 12-55**   Pneumosinus dilatans of the sphenoid sinus with optic nerve meningioma. T1-weighted postgadolinium coronal images. **A**, Meningioma of the optic nerve sheath (*arrow*). **B**, Anterior to the optic foramen; enlargement of the nerve sheath (*black arrow*) and enlargement of the sphenoid sinus (*arrowhead*). **C**, Dilation of the air cell (*arrowhead*) extending into the anterior clinoid. **D**, The meningioma (*arrow*) extends intracranially at the opening of the optic canal.

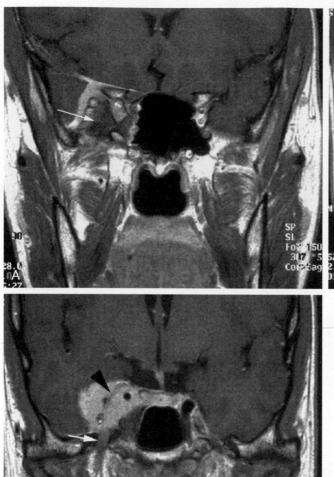

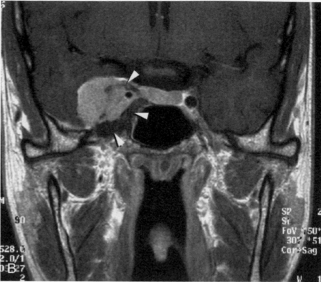

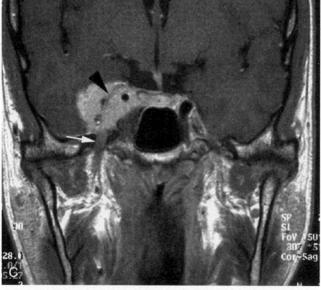

**FIGURE 12-56** Meningioma of the sphenocavernous region. Coronal MR poscontrast images. **A,** Coronal image through the level of the superior orbital fissure shows the intermediately enhancing tumor as well as the hyperostosis (*arrow*), shown as the thickening of the low signal bone. Note the intermediate signal in the foramen rotundum and superior orbital fissure. **B,** Slightly posteriorly, the hyperostosis (*arrowheads*) is noted, with narrowing of the carotid artery. **C,** Just above the foramen ovale, the lesion is seen on either side of the residual dural leaflet (*arrowhead*). Note the normal third division of the trigeminal nerve in the foramen ovale (*arrow*).

soft-tissue component that can extend downward into the nasopharynx or anteriorly into the nasal cavity. Cyst formation and calcification can be found within the tumor or at its margin. Sclerotic changes within the sphenoid bone may reflect the inflammatory component of the lesion.[102]

A rare form of the tumor is the papillary or papillary-squamous craniopharyngioma, considered a distinct variant.[108–110] This tumor type is seen in adults and is frequently located in the region of the floor of the third ventricle. This entity is more cellular, typically lacks calcification, and appears to be more solid at imaging. Cystic components are less common than in the more common adamantinomatous type.

A second type of lesion related to the pharyngohypophyseal pouch is the Rathke's pouch or cleft cyst.[111] Unlike the craniopharyngioma, this cyst is lined by a single layer of epithelial cells, which may be cuboidal or columnar. Goblet cells also can be found frequently. Imaging shows a cystic mass, usually in the sella or suprasellar cistern, with no

significant soft-tissue component and smooth, sharp margins. MR imaging can show a low or high T1-weighted signal intensity, depending on the protein content of the cyst fluid. T2-weighted images usually have high signal intensity.

Rathke's cleft cysts also can be found completely within the sphenoid bone (Fig. 12-61). In these cases, differentiation from a mucocele may be impossible. The MR imaging signal intensities are the same, and at biopsy the wall is very similar to that of a mucocele. The cyst contents may be helpful in this regard because the fluid of a Rathke's cleft cyst tends to be yellow and clear, with a low mucoid content.

Such a cyst within the sphenoid bone arises from the remnant of Rathke's pouch. Although the original location of this structure is within the body of the sphenoid, just below the floor of the sella, the variability of formation of the sphenoid sinus may "push" the cyst dorsally or superiorly, giving the cyst an eccentric location.

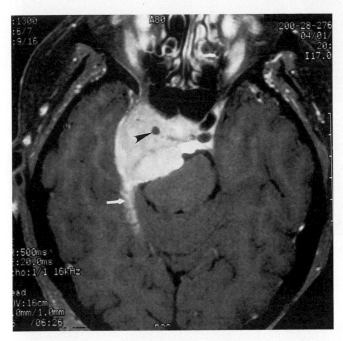

**FIGURE 12-57** Meningioma. The tumor fills the region of the cavernous sinus. The carotid artery is narrowed (*black arrowhead*), and there is enhancement extending along the tentorium (*arrow*). Note that although the tumor enhances, one can still separate the margin of the lesion from the enhancement in the venous structures.

## Juvenile Angiofibromas

The juvenile angiofibroma is a benign tumor arising adjacent to the sphenopalatine foramen. Almost all of these tumors occur in adolescent males, and nasal obstruction and epistaxis are the most common presenting symptoms. The

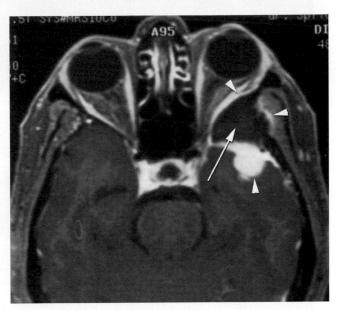

**FIGURE 12-59** Meningioma of the sphenoid triangle (greater wing). There is hyperostosis, with an increase in the size of the bone of the sphenoid triangle (*arrow*). There is enhancement in the temporalis fossa, orbit, and middle cranial fossa (*arrowheads*). Note the globular appearance of the intracranial component.

tumor is very vascular and thus has a characteristic appearance at imaging (Fig. 12-62). On CT and MR imaging the tumor enhances intensely, and on MR imaging there are flow voids representing the larger high-flow vessels. The location and routes of extension are characteristic and can be seen on either modality. On MR imaging, the tumor tends to have an intermediate signal intensity on T1-weighted

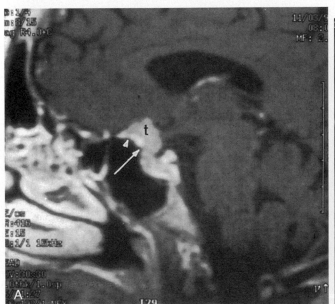

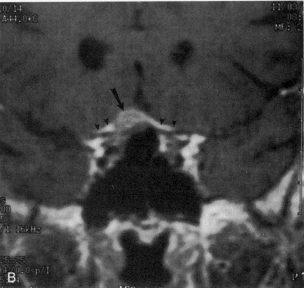

**FIGURE 12-58** Meningioma of the chiasmatic groove and planium. **A,** Postgadolinium sagittal T1-weighted image shows the tumor (*t*) extending along the chiasmatic groove and onto the planium sphenoidale. The arrow indicates the position of the tuberculum sella, and the small white arrowhead indicates the limbus separating the chiasmatic groove from the planium. Note how the tumor spills over into the sella turcica. **B,** Coronal T1-weighted postcontrast image shows the tumor (*arrow*) with intermediate enhancement. Notice the enhancement of the dural tails (*small black arrowheads*) extending in either direction from the main tumor.

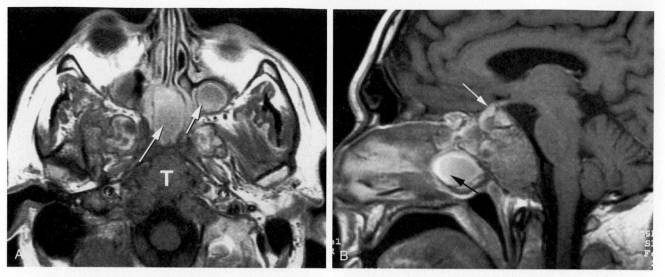

**FIGURE 12-60** Craniopharyngioma. Predominantly infrasellar. **A,** Axial image shows the expansile lesion (*T*) extending into the nasal septum and the maxillary sinus (*arrows*). Note the small fluid levels of the cystic cavities within the anterior part of the tumor. **B,** Sagittal postcontrast image shows the lesion extending superiorly along the anterior pituitary stalk (*white arrow*). Fluid-fluid level (*black arrow*).

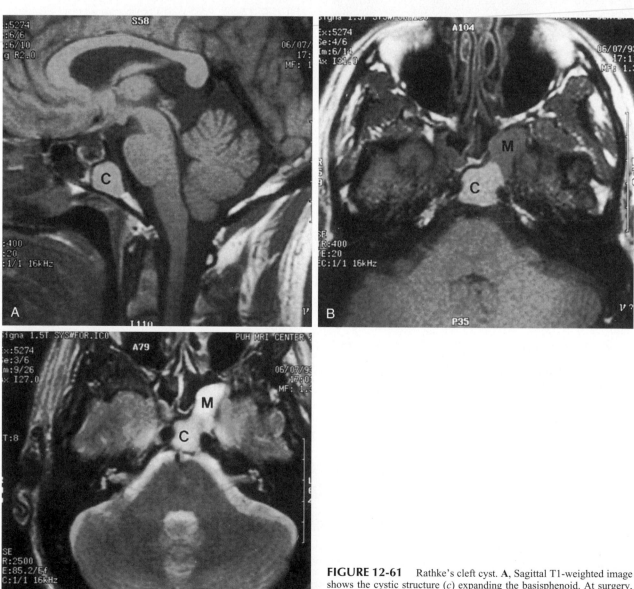

**FIGURE 12-61** Rathke's cleft cyst. **A,** Sagittal T1-weighted image shows the cystic structure (*c*) expanding the basisphenoid. At surgery, this structure did not contain mucous secretions but rather a watery yellow fluid. **B,** The cystic structure (*c*) is seen in the posterior sphenoid. More anterior and lateral sphenoid was filled with trapped mucus (*m*). **C,** T2-weighted image shows high signal intensity both within the cyst and from the mucous retention.

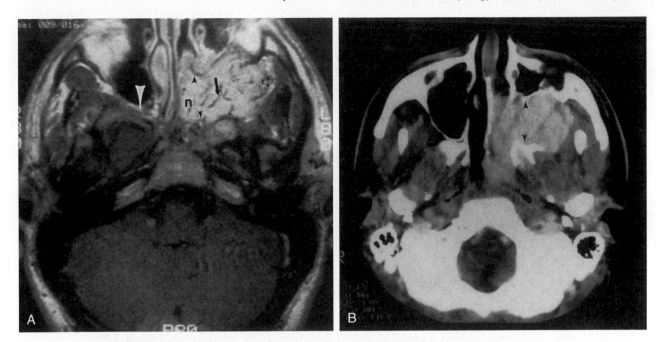

**FIGURE 12-62**   **A,** Juvenile angiofibroma expanding the pterygopalatine fossa. The T1-weighted postgadolinium MR image shows enhancing tumor in the region of the pterygopalatine fossa. It expands laterally (*open arrow*) into the infratemporal fossa, and medially the tumor passes through the region of the sphenopalatine foramen (*small black arrowheads*) into the posterior nasal cavity (*n*) and nasopharynx. Compare this with the normal pterygopalatine fossa (*white arrowhead*) on the opposite side. Flow voids representing large vessels (*black arrow*) can be seen within the tumor. **B,** CT scan shows the enlargement of the pterygopalatine fossa (*small black arrowheads*) by the enhancing mass. There is remodeling of the posterior wall of the maxillary sinus anteriorly. The pterygoid plates are pushed slightly posteriorly.

images and a relatively high signal intensity on T2-weighted sequences.

The tumor is locally invasive. In almost every case, tumor extends into the pterygopalatine fossa via the sphenopalatine foramen. The fossa is widened and its normal fat content obliterated. As the tumor grows, the posterior wall of the maxillary sinus is pushed anteriorly and the pterygoid plates are remodeled posteriorly. Actual bone erosion can occur at any margin but is frequently seen at the anterior surface of the upper pterygoid process. From this point the tumor can erode into the sphenoid sinus or posteriorly and superiorly through the more central skull base. As the tumor approaches the cavernous sinus and the middle cranial fossa, the dura remains intact initially. As the tumor continues to grow, the outer dural layer may be elevated so that, even if there is apparent tumor extension into the anterior cavernous sinus at imaging, the tumor still remains epidural in location at surgery. Once near the cavernous sinus, the tumor usually parasitizes intracranial vessels (Fig. 12-63). Eventually, though rare, larger tumors can break through the dural barrier and can even invade the brain.

The tumor can also grow laterally from the pterygopalatine fossa into the infratemporal fossa via the pterygomaxillary fissure. Anterior extension initially pushes the posterior antral wall anteriorly, but eventually the tumor can break through and expand into the sinus. Similarly, tumor in the pterygopalatine fossa can break through the pterygoid process or extend superiorly through the inferior orbital fissure into the orbit. Further extension through the superior orbital fissure is a common route of intracranial extension.

Although the tumor extent is mapped anatomically by CT and MR imaging, angiography is done to delineate the blood supply, often as a prelude to embolization. The primary blood supply is almost always from the terminal branches of the internal maxillary or the ascending pharyngeal arteries. Preoperative embolization effectively reduces intraoperative bleeding. Other arteries frequently may supply the tumor. Of particular concern are those coming from the internal carotid circulation. The arteries of the Vidian canal and the foramen rotundum usually fed from the termination of the sphenomaxillary artery can reverse the flow and carry the blood supply from the internal carotid artery to feed the tumor (Fig. 12-64). A blood supply from branches of the ophthalmic artery also has been demonstrated.

## Pituitary Adenomas

Pituitary adenomas are discussed in Chapter 11. However, they are mentioned in this section because of their intimate relationship with the skull base. Two types are particularly pertinent to this discussion—the invasive pituitary adenoma and the infrasellar adenoma.

The invasive pituitary adenoma has its site of origin within the pituitary fossa.[112] As most pituitary adenomas enlarge, they extend superiorly through the diaphragm sella into the suprasellar cistern and toward the optic chiasm. Inferior enlargement displaces the sella floor downward. When a tumor actually breaks through the sella floor or grows laterally into the cavernous sinuses, it is considered an invasive pituitary adenoma (Fig. 12-65). The lesion can be

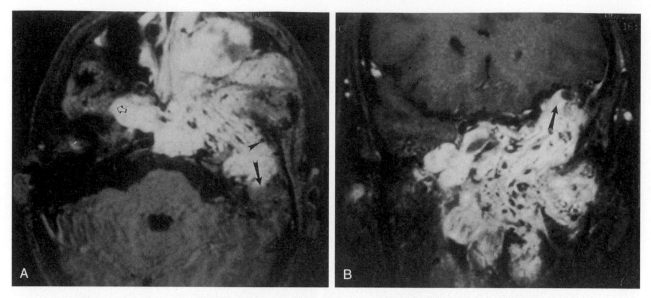

**FIGURE 12-63** Juvenile angiofibroma. **A,** Axial postgadolinium T1-weighted image with fat suppression. This extensive tumor extends across the midline into the opposite infratemporal fossa (*open arrow*). There is extensive tumor (*black arrow*) extending intracranially. Flow voids (*arrowheads*) are seen within the tumor. **B,** Coronal postgadolinium T1-weighted image with fat suppression shows extensive intracranial tumor (*black arrow*) protruding superiorly. The lesion parasitized branches of the middle cerebral artery.

very large and destructive, at times reaching the nasopharynx or nasal cavity. In these cases, the imaging differentiation from a malignancy such as nasopharyngeal carcinoma can be quite difficult.[113] One differentiating point is that when a nasopharyngeal tumor invades the cavernous sinuses, it usually encases and narrows the carotid artery.

However, when an invasive adenoma invades the cavernous sinuses, these arteries are surrounded but not narrowed. The lesion appears to squeeze around the vessel.

An extremely rare occurrence is a tumor of pituitary histology that is completely within the body of the sphenoid bone (Fig. 12-66).[114, 115] In these cases, the floor of the sella turcica has been reported to be intact. These extremely unusual tumors presumably arise from remnants of the

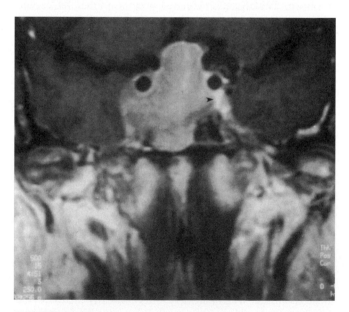

**FIGURE 12-64** Lateral subtraction view of an internal carotid artery angiogram shows the presence of supply to this juvenile angiofibroma via dural branches of the cavernous carotid artery (*arrows*), consistent with tumor invasion of the cavernous sinus.

**FIGURE 12-65** Invasive pituitary adenoma. Coronal postcontrast T1-weighted MR image. The adenoma shows intermediate enhancement, but the margin (*arrowhead*) between the adenoma and the normal cavernous sinus can be easily appreciated on the left-hand side. On the right side the adenoma extends further into the cavernous sinus, wrapping partially around the carotid artery. There is also inferior extension into the sphenoid body.

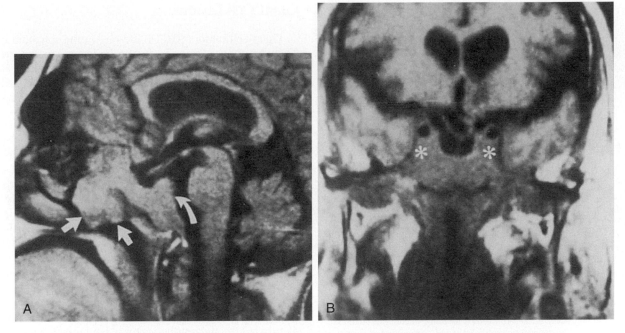

**FIGURE 12-66**   Intrasphenoid pituitary adenoma in a 38-year-old female presenting with amenorrhea, galactorrhea, and hyperprolactinemia. Midsagittal (**A**) and coronal (**B**) T1-weighted images show the presence of a mass involving the body of the sphenoid bone. The mass is relatively isointense to brain and extends inferiorly to the nasal fossa and nasopharynx (**A**, *straight arrows*), posteriorly to involve the clivus (**A**, *curved arrow*). It invades both cavernous sinuses (**B**, *asterisk*). A sphenoid sinus malignancy or chordoma also would be in the differential diagnosis.

pharyngohypophyseal pouch trapped by the closing ossification centers of the developing embryo. Another possibility is that the floor of the sella is not intact. In this case, the lesion invades the floor of the sella turcica and pushes or extrudes into the sphenoid sinus. The pulsation of the CSF transmitted through an incomplete diaphragm sella may help push the lesion down. As the lesion is pushed out of the sella, the appearance of an empty sella may be present.

## Neurogenic Tumors

The numerous foramina of the sphenoid bone transmit several major cranial nerves and a variety of smaller nerves. Tumors can arise from these nerves.

Schwannomas (nerve sheath tumors) arise from the nerve sheath. Although the tumor can arise from virtually any nerve, the nerve most commonly affected in the central skull base is the trigeminal nerve. Hypoglossal nerve schwannomas are rare, as are lesions arising from cranial nerves III, IV, and VI in the region of the cavernous sinus. Schwannomas of cranial nerves IX, X, and XI arise at the margin of the basicranium in the medial jugular foramen.

The trigeminal schwannoma can arise in Meckel's cave or in the cistern along the course of the nerve (Fig. 12-67). Extension may occur through the foramen ovale, the foramen rotundum, or the superior orbital fissure (Figs. 12-68 and 12-69). When near the petrous apex, these schwannomas frequently have a dumbbell shape, with the anterior component enlarging the cavernous sinus and impinging on the middle cranial fossa, while the posterior component protrudes into the posterior fossa beneath the

tentorium (Fig. 12-70). Other trigeminal schwannomas can remain isolated in either the posterior or the middle cranial fossae (Fig. 12-71). Rarely, a schwannoma can arise below the skull base in the masticator space or the pterygopalatine fossa. These tumors can protrude cranially, enlarging the foramen rotundum or the foramen ovale.

Like schwannomas elsewhere, trigeminal schwannomas can be solid or they can have a variable cystic component.

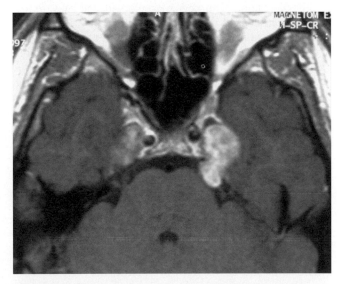

**FIGURE 12-67**   Schwannoma of Meckel's cave. The lesion on the left fills Meckel's cave and protrudes into the posterior fossa, giving it a dumbbell appearance.

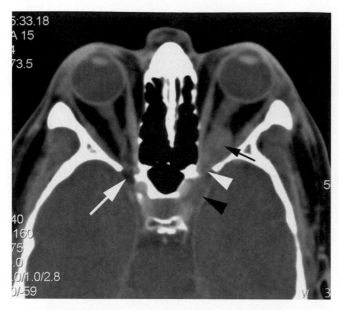

**FIGURE 12-68**   Schwannoma extending through the superior orbital fissure. Note the lesion in the orbit (*black arrow*) extending through and obliterating the fat of the superior orbital fissure (*white arrowhead*) as the lesion extends into the anterior cavernous sinus (*black arrowhead*). Compare the obliteration of the fat on the left with the intact superior orbital fissure fat on the right (*white arrow*).

The smooth bony margin of an expanded foramen, if present, is best appreciated on CT. The cortex is usually maintained. These tumors enhance with contrast on either CT or MR imaging. On MR imaging, these tumors tend to have intermediate T1-weighted signal intensity. Cystic components can have low or high T1-weighted signal intensity. On T2-weighted images, these tumors have a fairly high signal intensity that is slightly higher than that of brain but is not as high as that of CSF.

Neurofibromas can affect the cranial nerves in neurofibromatosis type I (von Recklinghausen's disease). These lesions are made up of Schwann cells as well as perineural-like and fibroblastic cells.[116] Axons may be seen incorporated within the tumor. The nerve is enlarged and may follow through and expand the foramina (Figs. 12-72 and 12-73).

The plexiform neurofibroma is associated with neurofibromatosis type I. This abnormality is a more diffuse neurofibroma and is more infiltrative than either the localized neurofibroma or a classic schwannoma (Fig. 12-74). The tumor can follow and diffusely enlarge a branching nerve or plexus or can be a major component of a massive soft-tissue neurofibroma, a form of neurofibroma infiltrating diffusely through the soft tissues. Calcifications can sometimes be seen within these tumors on CT scans. The distribution of the trigeminal nerve can be affected, and when the tumor involves the orbit it often can be seen, with its irregular margins, extending into the orbital fat and around the orbital muscles. The plexiform neurofibroma may be associated with enlargement of the superior orbital fissure and with underdevelopment of the greater wing of the sphenoid, findings characteristic of neurofibromatosis I (Figs. 12-24 and 12-75). However, either the bony defect or the plexiform tumor can occur as an isolated lesion. Plexiform neurofibroma can also undergo malignant change. Primary malignant nerve sheath tumors are rare.

## Giant Cell Lesions

Giant cell tumors (GCTs) are rare in the sphenoid bone. They have been reported in the body and in the greater sphenoid wing (Fig. 12-76). As in other areas of the body, the GCT of the sphenoid tends to occur in young adults. Most occur in the third or fourth decade of life but can occur at almost any age.[117, 118] A recent report described a series of pediatric patients with the lesion.[118] There is a slight female predominance.

The lesion expands the cortex of the bone but frequently leaves small gaps, producing an interrupted bony shell along the outer margin. There can be marginal sclerosis. With MR imaging, the lesion is described as having relatively low signal intensity on both T1-weighted and T2-weighted sequences. These lesions enhance moderately. Although cysts and fluid-fluid levels with areas of high signal intensity have been described, many GCTs are relatively homogeneous solid tumors.

The tumors may present with headache or cranial nerve palsies. Biopsy shows oval or plump spindle-shaped mononuclear cells and multinucleated giant cells evenly distributed throughout the lesion.[53] Each giant cell can have as many as 50 to 100 nuclei; most have 20 to 30. Reactive bone formation, hemorrhage, and cyst formation have also been described.

The GCT is one of the lesions considered to be a potential precursor of the aneurysmal bone cysts. Cysts can occur in part of the lesion or may replace the entire tumor. GCT can be primary or secondary. Secondary lesions can develop in pagetoid bone.

The giant cell granuloma (giant cell reparative granuloma, central giant cell granuloma) is most common in the mandible and maxilla but has been reported in the skull base, including the temporal bone and sphenoid.[119–123] The word "central" in the name central giant cell granuloma refers to a lesion whose origin is in bone rather than within the soft tissues of the oral cavity. Thus, a lesion arising in the gingiva is referred to as a peripheral giant cell granuloma. The giant cell granuloma is considered to be reactive rather than a true neoplasm. Trauma or hemorrhage have been suggested as inciting stimuli, but these are not definable in every case. There is a slight female predominance and the lesions occur at slightly younger ages than GCTs, typically between the ages of 10 and 25 years.[53]

The lesions are lytic and expansile and can have a sharp margin. The cortex is expanded, and the lesion is surrounded by a thin rim of bone. The cortex is frequently interrupted in some segments, and new bone formation has been reported.[123] On MR imaging, the giant cell granuloma tends to have low signal intensity on T1-weighted and T2-weighted sequences and the lesion enhances. There also can be significant hemorrhage into the lesion with cyst formation.

Histology shows giant cells, but they are not as evenly distributed throughout the lesion as in the GCT.[53] Each giant cell has fewer nuclei than the true GCT. In addition to the giant cells there are spindle-shaped fibroblasts, chronic inflammatory cells, and hemosiderin-laden macrophages, as well as collagen formation.

Brown tumors are indistinguishable histologically or radiologically from giant cell granuloma. They tend to occur later, in the fourth and fifth decades of life, and are seen in patients with hyperparathyroidism.[120] They are more common in primary than secondary hyperparathyroidism, though they have been found in patients undergoing long-term dialysis. The serum calcium level is high, and the phosphorus level is low.

## Aneurysmal Bone Cysts

Aneurysmal bone cysts (ABCs) occasionally are found in the sphenoid bone. On imaging, they appear as expansile masses with multiple cystic spaces. They have hemorrhage with large, blood-filled cavities, and fluid-fluid levels are characteristic. The patients are almost always less than 20 years old.

Several types of bone lesions have been considered to be precursors to ABCs. GCT, chondroblastoma, osteoblastoma, benign fibroosseous lesions, giant cell granuloma, chondromyxoid fibroma, bone cysts, eosinophilic granuloma, and hemangioma have all been mentioned.[53] Occasionally, an ABC can form within a malignancy. The ABC can have solid regions that mimic giant cell granuloma, with giant cells, fibroblasts, and hemorrhage.

## Langerhans Cell Histiocytosis

Langerhans cell histiocytosis (LCH) is a proliferation of histiocytic and histiocytic like cells.[53] The typical histiocyte like cell is the Langerhans cell. The common histio-

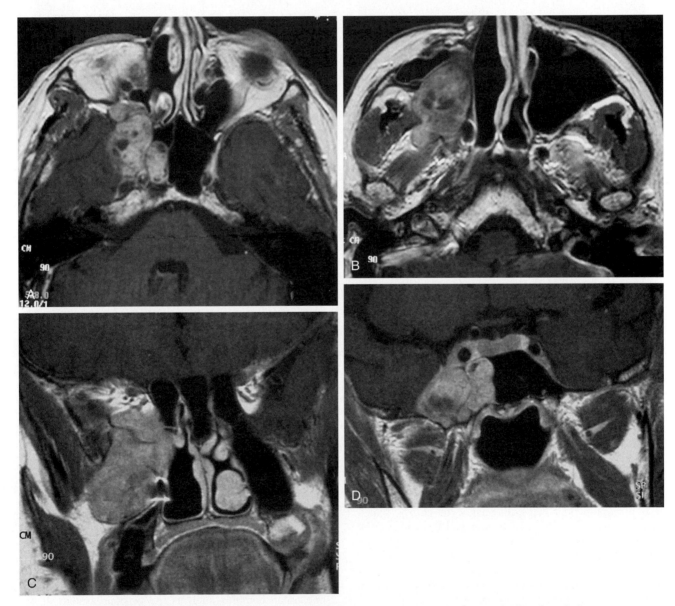

**FIGURE 12-69**   Schwannoma at $V_2$. **A**, Axial postcontrast image shows the tumor extending through the foramen rotundum into the upper pterygopalatine fossa. The lesion also extends into the sphenoid sinus. **B**, Image slightly caudal to **A** shows the tumor in the pterygopalatine fossa bowing the posterior wall of the maxillary sinus anteriorly. **C**, Coronal image shows the mass at the level of the pterygopalatine fossa extending up to the orbital fat. **D**, Coronal image at the level of the anterior cavernous sinus.

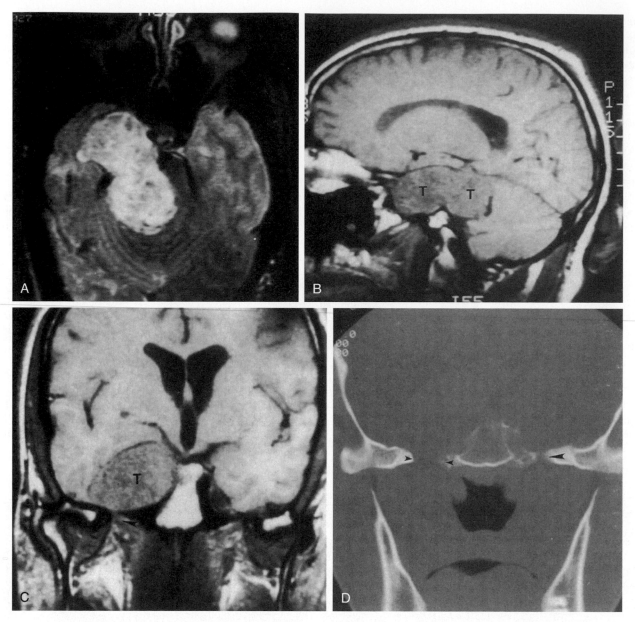

**FIGURE 12-70** Nerve sheath tumor of the trigeminal nerve (schwannoma). The tumor (*T*) has both a middle cranial fossa and a posterior fossa component. Note that the carotid artery is pushed medially. **A,** The T2-weighted image shows relatively high signal but areas of intermediate signal as well. **B,** Sagittal image shows the dumbbell configuration of the tumor, with components both above and below the tentorium. The constriction is at the position of the tentorium. **C,** Coronal image shows the tumor expanding the region of the cavernous sinus and obscuring Meckel's cave. A small amount of fat (*arrowhead*) is seen just beneath the foramen ovale, indicating that the tumor did not spread by this route. **D,** Coronal bone algorithm. The foramen ovale between the small black arrowheads is enlarged even though the tumor did not extend through this foramen. Compare with the foramen ovale opposite (*large black arrowhead*).

cyte is a mononuclear cell with phagocytic ability, which contains many intracellular inclusions and lysosomes. The Langerhans cell has fewer lysosomes and less phagocytic ability than the usual histiocyte. The characteristic feature of the Langerhans cell is a folded large nucleus having a kidney or coffee bean shape. The lesion in LCH contains varying numbers of Langerhans cells mixed with eosinophils and more typical histiocytes.

The group of diseases included under the name Langerhans cell histiocytosis includes eosinophilic granuloma, Hand-Schuller-Christian (HSC), disease and Letterer-Siwe disease. These diseases, though related by histopathology, behave very differently. Eosinophilic granuloma (EG) usually has only one lesion at presentation and in such cases behaves clinically like a benign disease. If multiple lesions are present, a less benign course may be present. HSC disease is a chronic disease that is predominantly isolated to one organ complex such as the osseous system. It has a prognosis between those of EG and Letterer-Siwe disease. Letterer-Siwe disease is a multisystem, more acute disease that can be rapidly fatal. The classification is not exact, and there is often overlap. In general, the younger the patient, the more severe the disease. Letterer-Siwe disease almost always presents in the first 3 years of life. HSC usually presents between 3 and 5 years of age and infrequently in slightly older persons. EG usually presents between the ages of 5 and 20 years.

The disease can involve almost any bone. LCH frequently involves the cranial vault and, less commonly, the skull base. The localized lesion of EG is the most likely variant to present as an isolated diagnostic problem in the skull base. Lesions can have a characteristic "punched-out," sharply defined margin or can be more irregular, with a sclerotic margin. In the cranial vault, the lesion classically has a sharp margin with a beveled edge. A "button sequestrum" lesion is a lytic lesion in which residual bone remains. In the skull, most lesions are lytic, with or without sclerosis.

At radiography or CT scanning, the lesion may present as a "punched-out" abnormality, with a sharp margin and no sclerosis (Fig. 12-77). Alternatively, the lesion may have a more irregular sclerotic margin.[124, 125] On MR imaging, the lesion is seen as a solid mass, often obliterating the signal void of the cortex. The lesion usually has a high T2-weighted signal intensity but occasionally can have a fairly low signal intensity.[126] There is moderate enhancement. High signal intensity can be seen in contiguous soft tissues on T2-weighted images, reflecting the inflammatory nature of the lesion.[125]

Lesions involving the skull base can give cranial nerve palsies or present with pain and inflammatory symptoms. In the temporal bone, the lesion can mimic otitis media; however, there is no improvement on antibiotics. Systemic symptoms and peripheral eosinophilia are occasionally present. Lesions may be treated by curettage or by radiation therapy, depending on accessibility and proximity to crucial structures.

## Miscellaneous Tumors and Lesions of the Sphenoid Bone

Though rare, osteosarcomas, Ewing's sarcoma, hemangiomas, and other miscellaneous tumors occasionally can be identified in the skull base. Similarly, lymphoma is uncommon, usually extending into the bone from contiguous soft-tissue disease. The rarity of these lesions precludes definitive statements about their imaging characteristics. However, anecdotal experience has shown that osteosarcoma can occur in the body or wing of the sphenoid.[127, 128] Imaging diagnosis relies on the identification of an osteoid matrix, seen best on CT. Lymphoma is very cellular and has a relatively low T2-weighted signal intensity. The primary mass is usually in the nasopharynx, but lymphoma can occasionally arise within the bone.

Plasmacytoma can affect the skull base and usually has a lytic, fairly homogeneous appearance on CT. On MR imaging, presumably because of cellularity, the tumor usually has an intermediate signal intensity on both T1-weighted and T2-weighted images. The lesion enhances

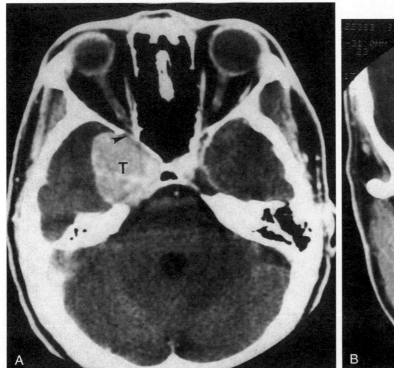
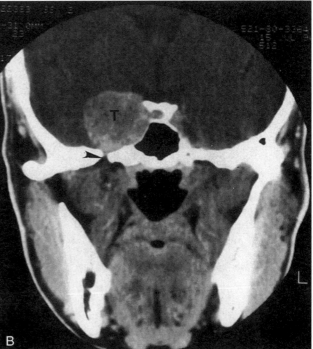

**FIGURE 12-71**   Neuroma of the cavernous sinus area. CT scan with contrast enhancement. **A,** Axial scan. The tumor (*T*) is seen at the level of the superior orbital fissure. The tumor bulges into and compresses the fat in the superior orbital fissure (*black arrowhead*) but does not protrude into the orbit. **B,** Coronal scan shows the tumor (*T*) scalloping and eroding the sphenoid sinus and dorsum sella. Again, it extends to but not through the foramen ovale. Note the maintenance of the normal fat (*black arrowhead*) just beneath foramen ovale.

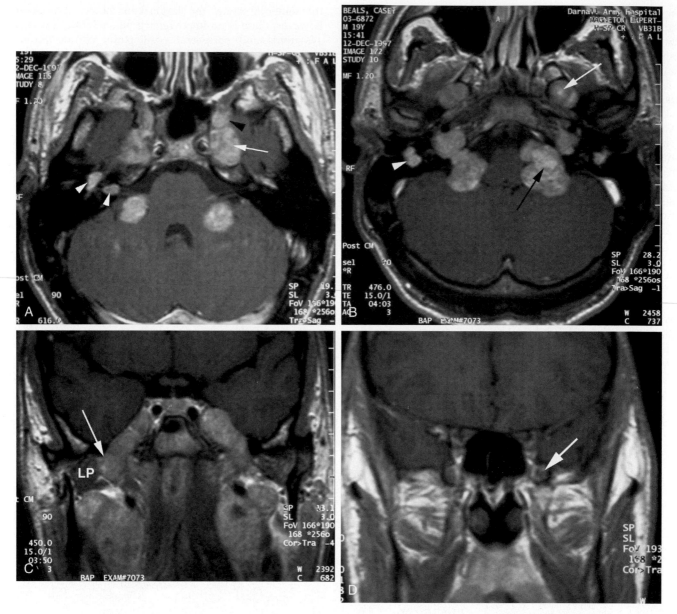

**FIGURE 12-72** Neurofibromatosis 1 (von Recklinghausen's disease). Multiple neurofibromas involving multiple cranial nerves bilaterally. **A,** Axial postgadolinium image at the level of Meckel's cave shows bilateral lesions of the trigeminal nerve (*arrow*) as well as a lesion of the internal auditory canal following the facial nerve (*arrowheads*). The lesions of the trigeminal nerve follow the course of the foramen rotundum (*black arrowhead*). **B,** Axial postgadolinium scan slightly caudal to **A.** The neurofibroma extending through the foramen ovale is situated just medial to the lateral pterygoid muscle (*white arrow*). Lesion of the pars nervosa (*black arrow*) and lesion of the vertical facial nerve canal (*white arrowhead*). **C,** Coronal image shows the extension through the foramen ovale. Note how the lesion (*arrow*) just beneath the foramen ovale is situated just medial to the lateral pterygoid muscle (*LP*). Lesions are also seen lower in the neck. **D,** Coronal image through the region of the foramen rotundum shows the enlargement of the actual nerve (*arrow*) within the foramen surrounded by the small venous plexus.

on either CT or MR imaging. Although plasmacytoma can occur as an isolated lesion, many of these patients eventually develop multiple myeloma.

Carcinoma occasionally arises from the mucosal elements contained within the sphenoid sinus (Fig. 12-78). The tumor has an appearance similar to that of any invasive malignancy, and the diagnosis may be suggested by the relationship of the tumor to the sinus and surrounding structures.

Vascular lesions are rare in the skull base, and they may be benign or malignant.[129, 130] Benign lesions include hemangiomas or various vascular malformations. Hemangiomas have high T2-weighted signal intensity, may expand the bone, and enhance significantly. The bone may soften, and basilar invagination can result. Vascular malignancies potentially involving the skull base include angiosarcoma, hemangioendothelioma, hemangiopericytoma, and Kaposi's sarcoma.[53, 129]

Gorham's disease (massive osteolysis, disappearing bone disease, vanishing bone disease, phantom bone disease) is believed to develop from a vascular lesion.[4, 53, 131–137] Both hemangioma and lymphangioma have been mentioned as underlying lesions. This lesion at biopsy has a mixture of small-caliber blood vessels and fibrosis, with only a few osteoblasts. Both the skull and the skull base can be involved. At imaging, the bone is replaced by soft tissue, and there is a loss of bone volume (Fig. 12-79). The bone "disappears" or collapses. Malignancy, infection, and metabolic causes of bone loss must be excluded before the diagnosis is considered. The lesion may stop progressing spontaneously. Both surgery and radiotherapy have been attempted as curative therapies. The final diagnosis of many

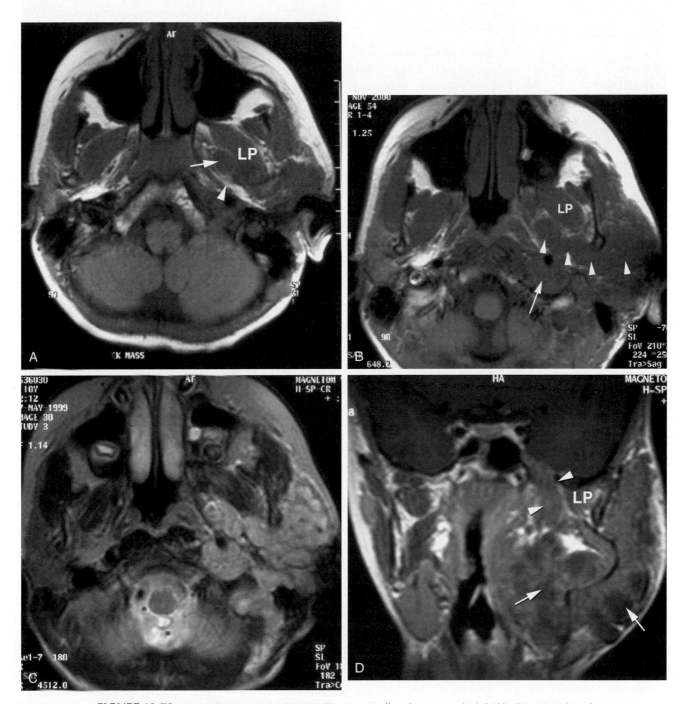

**FIGURE 12-73**    Neurofibromatosis 1 with neurofibroma extending along V₃ on the left side. Demonstration of the pathway of the auriculotemporal nerve. **A,** Axial T1-weighted precontrast image shows the tumor (*arrow*) just beneath foramen ovale along the medial margin of the lateral pterygoid muscle (*LP*). Note the fat (*arrowhead*) just beneath the skull base. **B,** The enlarged nerve can be followed along the course of the auriculotemporal nerve (*arrowheads*) extending posteriorly and laterally, just posterior to the upper mandible. *LP,* Lateral pterygoid muscle (*arrow*). A second lesion extends posterior to the carotid (*arrow*). **C,** T2-weighted image shows the relatively high signal of the lesions. **D,** Coronal T1-weighted postcontrast image shows the lesion extending up to and through the foramen ovale (*arrowheads*) just medial to the lateral pterygoid (*LP*). Lesions lower in the neck (*arrows*).

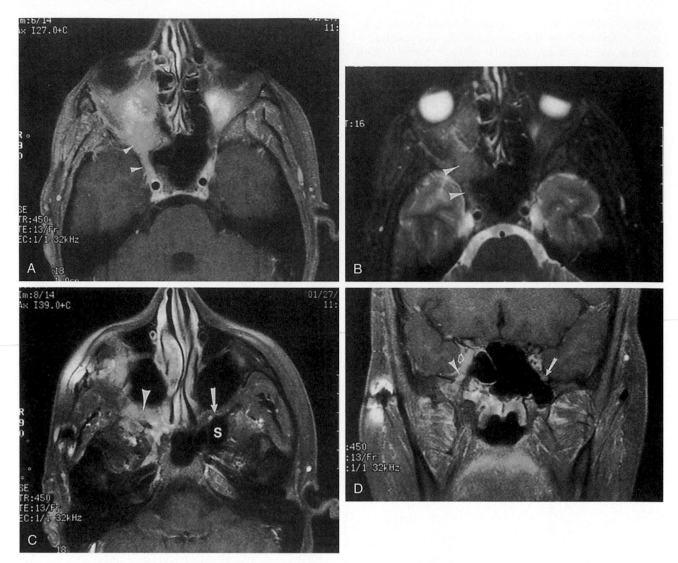

**FIGURE 12-74** Diffuse neurofibroma extending along branches of the trigeminal nerve. **A**, Axial T1-weighted postcontrast image with fat suppression shows the tumor (*white arrowheads*) extending from the cavernous sinus anteriorly into the orbital apex and upper pterygopalatine fossa. **B**, T2-weighted image again shows the tumor (*arrowheads*), which has a fairly low signal intensity. **C**, Scan inferior to **A** shows the tumor (*white arrowhead*) filling and expanding the pterygopalatine fossa. Compare this with the normal pterygopalatine fossa (*arrow*) on the opposite side. In this fat-suppressed image, the signal within the normal pterygopalatine fossa is low. A laterally extending air cell from the sphenoid sinus (*S*) is seen extending into the attachment of the pterygoid plate. **D**, The tumor is seen in the anterior cavernous sinus and posterior superior orbital fissure (*open arrow*). The arrowhead indicates the approximate position of the foramen rotundum. The normal foramen rotundum on the opposite side (*arrow*) is identified. Again, note that the expanding sphenoid air cell on the normal side extends between the foramen rotundum and the Vidian canal. (Courtesy of Dr. Norman Leeds.)

of these rare tumors is made at biopsy, and usually the role of imaging is to accurately map the lesion.

## Mucoceles

Obstruction of the sphenoid sinus ostium can result in a mucocele. The term mucocele is used by radiologists to indicate an airless, "mucus-filled" sinus, with an enlarged sinus cavity. Mucoceles can occur as isolated lesions or in association with polyps or other inflammatory disease. Any part of the sinus can be expanded. The anterior clinoid process is frequently pneumatized and thus can be enlarged

by a mucocele (Fig. 12-80). If a mucocele forms near the root of the pterygoid process, where the air cells pass between the foramen rotundum and the Vidian canal, this bone can be enlarged. However, the separation of the Vidian and rotundum canals varies with the degree of air cell development and extension of air cells into the pterygoid process.[19] Thus, asymmetric separation of the foramina alone does not indicate mucocele. As the mucocele enlarges, it can erode or thin the bony cortex of the sphenoid sinus wall or the cortex of one of these foramina. When present, this erosion or scalloping is a reliable indicator of actual sinus expansion. As discussed in Chapter 5, the signal intensities on MR imaging can vary in relation to the protein

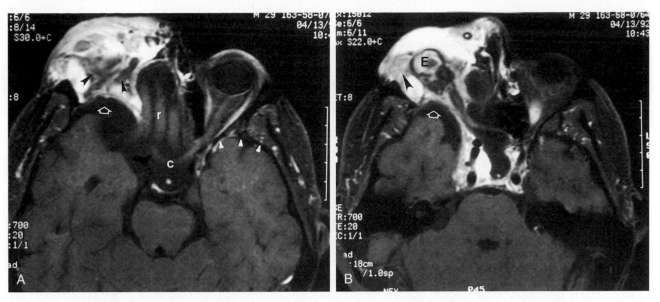

**FIGURE 12-75** **A,** Neurofibromatosis with an orbital encephalocele and a plexiform neurofibroma. The abnormal neurofibroma (*arrowheads*) is seen within the malformed orbit. There is also a defect in the sphenoid bone, with herniation of the CSF space (*open arrow*) into the posterior orbit. *r,* Gyrus rectus; *c,* chiasm. Note the normal position of the anterior wall of the middle cranial fossa (*small white arrowheads*) on the opposite side. **B,** Axial postcontrast T1-weighted images after fat suppression. A plexiform neurofibroma (*arrowhead*) is seen within the malformed orbit. A small residual eye (*E*) can be identified. At this level, the temporal lobe can be seen following the CSF space (*open arrow*) into the posterior orbit.

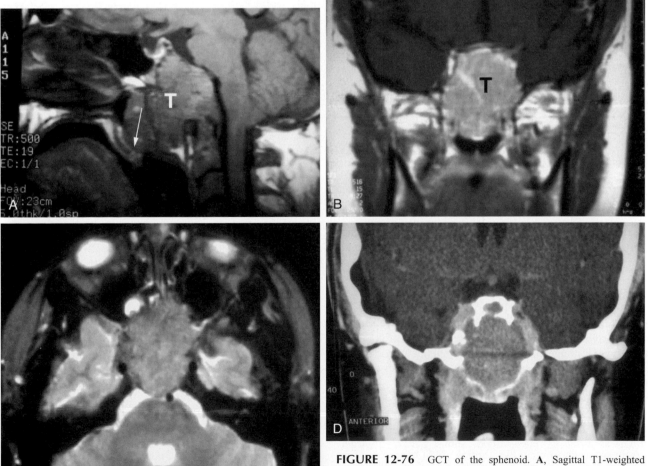

**FIGURE 12-76** GCT of the sphenoid. **A,** Sagittal T1-weighted image shows the tumor (*T*) in the skull base extending into and occluding the nasopharynx (*arrow*). **B,** Coronal postcontrast T1-weighted image shows moderate enhancement of the tumor (*T*). **C,** Axial T2-weighted image shows intermediate to low signal. **D,** Coronal CT image. The lesion extends to the cavernous sinuses on either side.

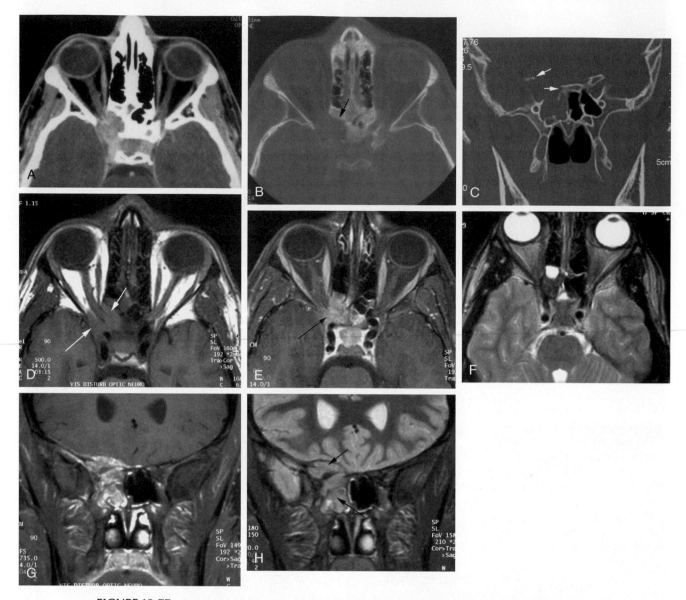

**FIGURE 12-77**    Langerhans histiocytosis (eosinophilic granuloma). **A**, Axial postcontrast CT algorithm shows a lesion in the orbital apex and lateral sphenoid with slight enhancement. **B**, Axial CT bone algorithm shows the lesion with a sharp margin (*arrow*). Note the demineralization around the optic nerve canal. **C**, Coronal bone algorithm shows a sharp nonsclerotic margin (*arrows*). **D**, T1-weighted MR image shows intermediate signal intensity of the lesion (*arrows*). **E**, Postgadolinium image shows moderate enhancement (*arrow*). **F**, Axial T2-weighted image shows the lesion to be relatively dark. **G**, Coronal postcontrast image shows the lesion bulging the dura superiorly and involving the apex as well as the lateral sphenoid. **H**, Coronal STIR (Short Tau Inversion Recovery) lesion (*arrows*).

concentration of the retained secretions (Fig. 12-81) and the presence of *Aspergillus* or other mycetomas. On contrast-enhanced MR images, a thin line of enhancing mucosa along the wall of the sinus identifies the obstructed nature of the sinus.[138]

## Aneurysms

Aneurysms involving the central skull base can arise from the intracavernous portion of the carotid artery or extend from the petrous portion of the carotid, and though most aneurysms occur spontaneously, some occur after trauma (Figs. 12-82 to 12-86).[139] Despite the fact that transsphenoidal approaches to the pituitary gland, endoscopic explorations of the sphenoid, and various skull base approaches to the cavernous sinus put the artery at risk, postsurgical aneurysms (or pseudoaneurysms) are rare. Sphenoid sinus inflammatory disease, especially fungal disease, can extend into the cavernous sinus and cause an aneurysm.

Aneurysms can present with headache. Pressure on the nerves in the cavernous sinus can lead to ophthalmoplegia (with or without headache) or to facial pain. Hemorrhage is unusual. A small aneurysm confined to the cavernous sinus is unlikely to bleed, but larger ones occasionally can rupture.

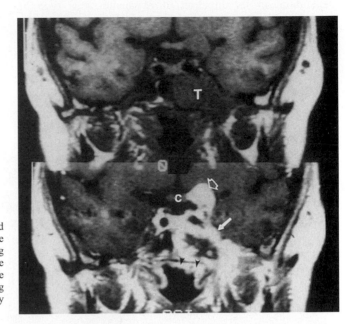

**FIGURE 12-78**   Carcinoma of the sphenoid sinus. Coronal T1-weighted MR images. The upper image shows the tumor (*T*) in the lateral sphenoid. The lower image (postcontrast) shows the enhancement (*white arrow*) extending into the cavernous sinus, with a fairly low signal in the central part of the tumor. A nodule of tumor (*open arrow*) is seen against the chiasm (*C*). The lower enhancement (*small black arrowheads*) represents the enhancing mucosa rather than the tumor itself. The mucosa is displaced slightly inferiorly by the tumor in the submucosal location.

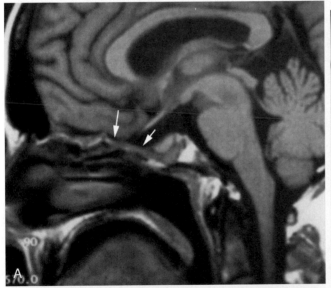

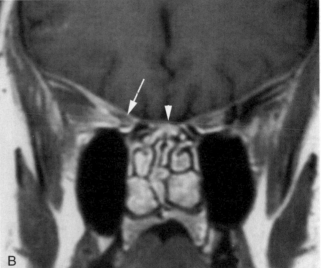

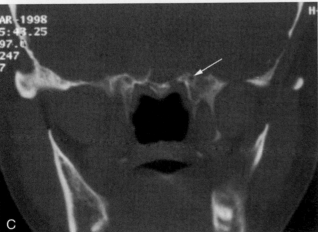

**FIGURE 12-79**   Gorham's disease (presumed). The patient presented with bilateral disturbance and ophthalmoplegia. No evidence of malignancy or an infectious process was found at presentation. **A,** Sagittal T1-weighted image shows collapse of the anterior sphenoid and posterior ethmoid (*arrows*). **B,** Coronal postcontrast image shows collapse of the bone of the orbital apex (*arrow*) compressing the neural and muscular structures. Note the loss of vertical height of the sphenoethmoid junction (*arrowhead*). **C,** Coronal CT scan shows collapse of the upper sphenoid. There has been bone loss of the lateral wall and roof of the sphenoid. The bone around the foramen rotundum has "dissolved." Vidian canal (*arrow*) remains.

Depending on its direction of expansion, this type of aneurysm can rupture into the sphenoid sinus or into the subarachnoid space. The rupture can also be into the cavernous sinus, resulting in a carotid cavernous sinus fistula rather than a frank hemorrhage. If the aneurysm contains thrombosis, embolization to more distal arteries can lead to a central neurologic presentation.

An aneurysm of the cavernous portion of the internal carotid artery will enlarge the cavernous sinus; however, a small aneurysm may be undetectable. Usually, an aneurysm bows the lateral cavernous sinus wall laterally. The bony lateral sphenoid sinus wall may be bowed medially into the sinus. Small aneurysms are quite difficult to detect on planar imaging because of the normal tortuosity of the carotid artery. Careful examination of imaging done in multiple planes will lessen the likelihood of overlooking such an

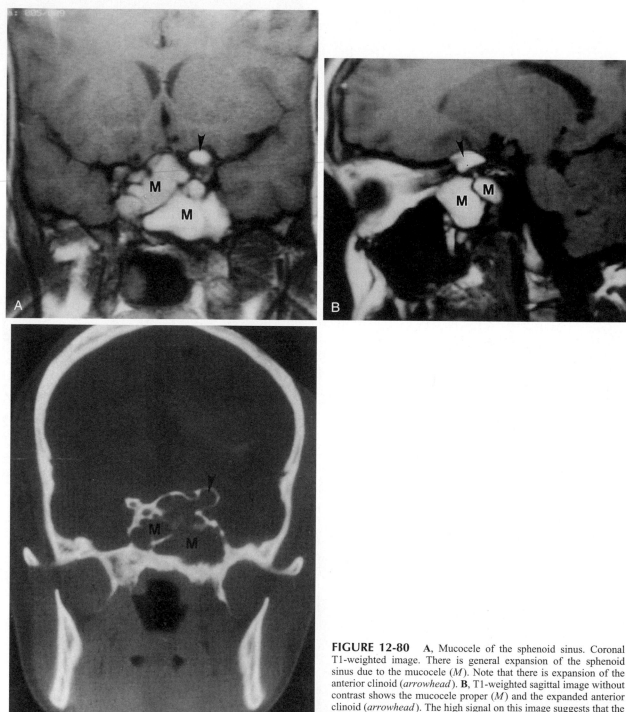

**FIGURE 12-80** **A,** Mucocele of the sphenoid sinus. Coronal T1-weighted image. There is general expansion of the sphenoid sinus due to the mucocele (*M*). Note that there is expansion of the anterior clinoid (*arrowhead*). **B,** T1-weighted sagittal image without contrast shows the mucocele proper (*M*) and the expanded anterior clinoid (*arrowhead*). The high signal on this image suggests that the mucocele has been present long enough to have a higher protein concentration. **C,** Bone window CT image of the mucocele shows the generalized expansion (*M*) and the more localized expansion of the anterior clinoid (*arrowhead*).

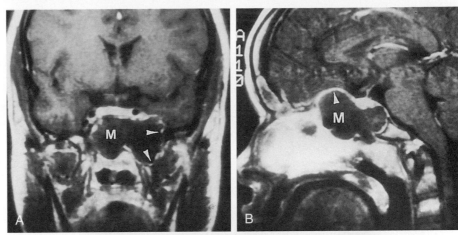

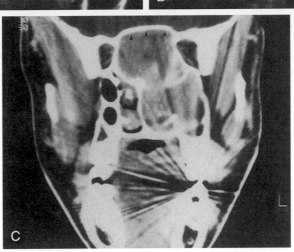

FIGURE 12-81 A, Mucocele of the sphenoid sinus. Coronal image shows the mucocele (*M*). There is expansion laterally (*white arrowheads*) in the position that would be typical of a lateral sphenoid air cell. The low signal on this postcontrast T1-weighted image is thought to be caused by very high protein content and desiccation. It might also be due to *Aspergillus*, which would give a very low signal. B, Postcontrast T1-weighted sagittal image shows the mucocele with upward expansion in the region of the planum (*white arrowhead*). Again, note the low signal and lack of enhancement in the mucocele cavity. C, Coronal CT image. The mucocele expands the planum and the cortex superiorly (*small arrowheads*).

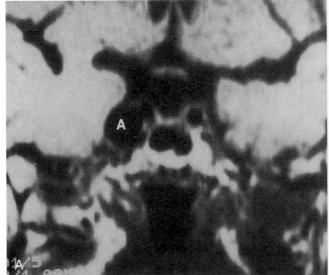

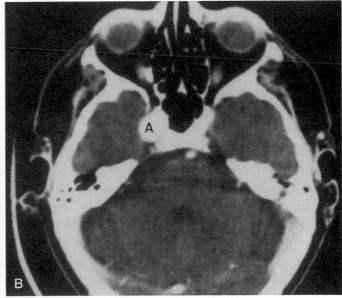

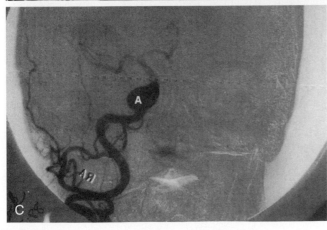

FIGURE 12-82 Aneurysm. A, T1-weighted image without contrast. The aneurysm (*A*) causes the wall of the cavernous sinus to bulge laterally and is seen as a flow void in the region of the cavernous sinus. B, Axial scan again shows the aneurysm (*A*). It impinges posteriorly on the anterior part of Meckel's cave. The fat in the superior orbital fissure is maintained. C, Anteroposterior view of the aneurysm during injection arteriography. The aneurysm (*A*) can be seen in the cavernous segment of the carotid artery.

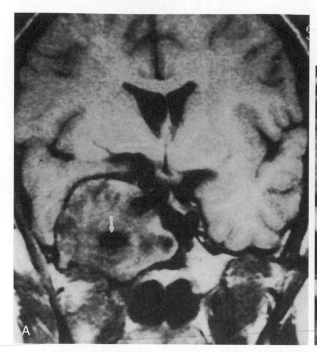
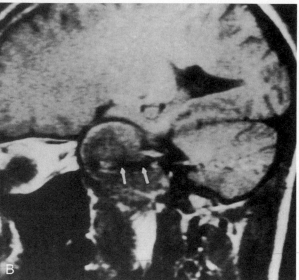

**FIGURE 12-83** **A**, Coronal T1-weighted MR image. Partially thrombosed aneurysm of the petrous and cavernous carotid arteries. The flow void (*arrow*) is seen in the central part of the aneurysm. Most of the "mass" is filled with thrombus of varying signal intensities. **B**, Sagittal T1-weighted image without contrast again shows the flow void of the central lumen (*arrows*) within the larger mass, which is partially thrombosed.

aneurysm. If the lumen is patent, MRA or CT angiography may demonstrate the aneurysm. Catheter arteriography is not usually necessary for evaluation of a potential intracavernous aneurysm.

The imaging appearance of a large aneurysm is varied and depends on the patency of the lumen and the presence of partial thrombosis. If little thrombus is present, the lumen may completely opacify on enhanced CT, blending with and "disappearing" into the enhancing cavernous sinus. A dynamic CT scan's arterial phase may help separate the aneurysm from the normal cavernous sinus. If, on the other hand, thrombus fills part of the aneurysm, the lesion usually has a low density with an enhancing rim. A channel of opacification, representing residual lumen, occasionally can be seen. Calcification sometimes can be present in the aneurysm's wall.

On MR imaging, the appearance of an aneurysm also varies, depending on the presence or absence of partial thrombosis (Fig. 12-83). The lumen of a small aneurysm still may be detected if there is rapid blood flow causing a signal flow void. Larger aneurysms may be free of thrombus and appear as a large, rounded flow void. However, the flow in the aneurysm may be turbulent, giving a variety of signal intensities. The movement of the blood usually can be defined with various flow-sensitive sequences.

Thrombus, which partially or completely fills the lumen of an aneurysm, has a variable appearance on MR imaging. Layers of thrombus of varying age may be identified, and the appearance reflects the evolution of the blood products within the thrombus.[140] Thrombus of intermediate age is often bright on T1-weighted and T2-weighted images, reflecting concentrations of methemoglobin. This signal is seen most commonly bordering the residual lumen. Low

signal areas, usually seen at the periphery of the aneurysm, reflect the presence of hemosiderin.

On rare occasions, these aneurysms, when large, can erode through the skull base, usually in the floor of the middle cranial fossa.[141]

Treatment of the aneurysm depends on its size, its location, and the presenting symptoms. Small aneurysms may be followed, but larger ones are usually treated. Alternatives to surgery include endovascular occlusion of the parent vessel or placement of balloons or coils within the aneurysm.

## SECONDARY TUMOR INVOLVEMENT OF THE SKULL BASE

The skull base is frequently the site of tumor spread, involved most commonly by direct invasion from an adjacent primary neoplasm. Hematogenous metastasis from distant primary tumors also occurs. An important route of extension of primary head and neck tumors is perineural spread along the cranial nerves to and through the various skull base foramina.

### Direct Encroachment

Tumors that arise close to the skull base frequently invade the bone because the fascial planes of the infratemporal fossa and nasopharynx preferentially direct the spread of neoplasm toward the skull base.[142] Nasopharyngeal cancer characteristically invades the midline skull base.[143] The strong pharyngobasilar fascia wrapping around the posterior

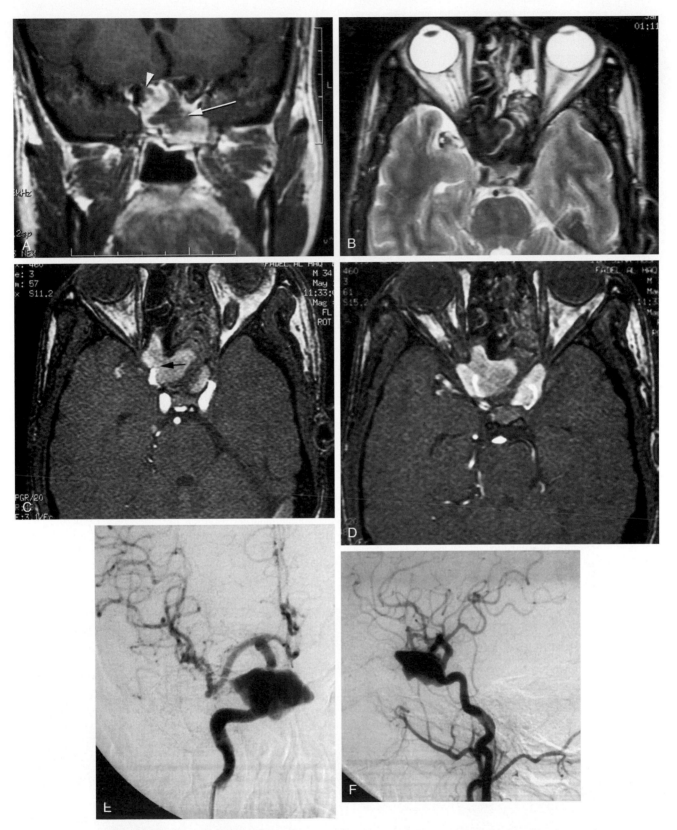

**FIGURE 12-84**    Carotid aneurysm (possible pseudoaneurysm) extending into the sphenoid sinus. **A,** Coronal T1-weighted image shows variable signal intensity (*arrow*) within an expanded sphenoid sinus. The enhancement along the margin might suggest mucocele. There is slight irregularity (*arrowhead*) adjacent to the right carotid artery. **B,** Axial T2-weighted image shows low signal within the sphenoid. **C,** SPGR image shows the proximity of the carotid artery (*arrow*) to the sphenoid sinus. **D,** Axial SPGR image slightly cephalad to **C** shows the expansion of the sinus. **E** and **F,** AP and lateral internal carotid injection and lateral common carotid injection shows the aneurysm filling the sphenoid sinus. (Courtesy of Dr. Mohammad Radwan, Ibn Sina Hospital, Kuwait.)

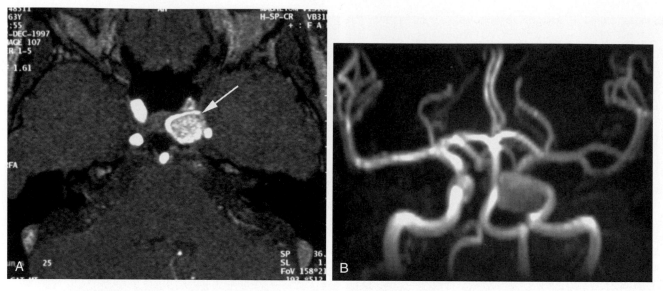

**FIGURE 12-85** Aneurysm of the cavernous carotid extending into the sella. **A,** Axial gradient echo image shows high signal representing flow (*arrow*) within the aneurysm. **B,** MRA 3D time-of-flight shows the aneurysm extending medially from the cavernous carotid.

and lateral walls of the nasopharynx can limit lateral tumor growth, directing tumor growth superiorly toward the roof of the nasopharynx. Here the skull base, the undersurface of the sphenoid bone, is unprotected by any fascial layer, and thus the sphenoid bone is frequently eroded by nasopharyngeal carcinoma. Because many of these malignancies arise off midline in the region of the fossa of Rosenmuller, the foramen lacerum and the petrooccipital fissure immediately above this part of the nasopharynx are frequently invaded. Tumor spreading through this cleft, along the lateral aspect of the sphenoid body and basiocciput, can reach the cavernous sinus, middle cranial fossa, or posterior fossa. Such tumors encounter the carotid artery as soon as the foramen lacerum is breached. Erosion may extend through

the cortex of the sphenoid bone proper to reach the clival marrow. Although erosion of the cortex is appreciated more easily on CT, high-resolution MR imaging better shows the presence and degree of marrow invasion (Fig. 12-87). Lateral tumor extension may pass over the pharyngobasilar fascia to reach the soft tissues in the upper masticator space, immediately below the foramen ovale. Tumor can then pass upward to reach the middle cranial fossa. Lateral extension also can occur along the eustachian tube toward the middle ear. Tumor can spread to the pterygoid process or through the sphenopalatine foramen into the pterygopalatine fossa. Here there is access to the Vidian canal and foramen rotundum. Usually the Vidian canal and the foramen rotundum are involved by direct tumor extension as tumor

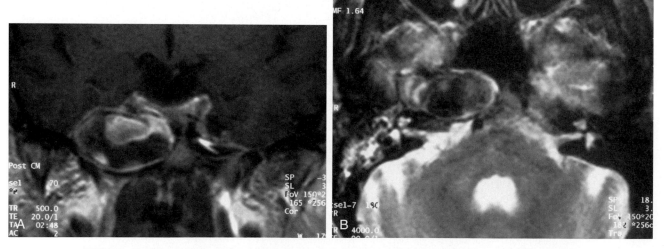

**FIGURE 12-86** Petrous carotid aneurysm. **A,** Coronal T1-weighted postcontrast image shows partial thrombosis of the enlarged aneurysm of the petrous apex. Areas of bright signal represent enhancement indicating flow. **B,** Axial T2-weighted image shows the low signal of hemosiderin within portions of the aneurysm. Note the fluid in the middle ear and mastoid due to obstruction of the eustachian tube.

invades directly through the bone at the junction of the pterygoid process and body of sphenoid rather than by true perineural spread, where tumor follows the nerve selectively as a conduit.

Sarcomas, lymphomas, and other malignancies also invade directly into the skull base (Fig. 12-88).[144] Tumors can arise in the infratemporal fossa and erode into the greater wing of the sphenoid bone. The foramen ovale may represent the line of least resistance as a tumor expands within the masticator space.

## Perineural Spread

Tumor can selectively follow a nerve or the sheath of a nerve to reach and ultimately pass through a foramen of the skull base.[145–148] Adenoid cystic carcinoma has a strong propensity for this type of spread. Other malignancies such as lymphoma, melanoma, and even squamous cell carcinoma have shown this type of tumor extension. The trigeminal nerve and its branches travel from the brainstem to many areas of the face, sinuses, and oral cavity, and this nerve is a primary route for perineural spread of tumors of the head and neck. The auriculotemporal nerve, a branch of the third division ($V_3$), can carry tumor from the parotid gland to the main trigeminal nerve and through the foramen ovale to reach the cavernous sinus.[149] Tumors from the palate, sinuses, and face can follow the second division ($V_2$) to the pterygopalatine fossa and then through the foramen rotundum.[150] Perineural spread along the first division ($V_1$) is less common, but occasionally a lacrimal gland or skin malignancy can extend along this nerve through the superior orbital fissure. As tumor follows the nerve, the nerve and foramen usually enlarge (Figs. 12-89 and 12-90). Less

commonly, tumor may extend along a nerve without causing enlargement, and skip areas of tumor along the nerve can occur with adenoid cystic carcinoma.[151]

Enhancement of a normal-sized nerve on a gadolinium-enhanced MR image is considered suggestive of perineural tumor spread. However, neuritis or secondary edema also may cause nerve enhancement. Usually, once the tumor has passed intracranially through a neural foramen, the tumor enlarges, now free from the restriction of the canal.

A key concept in assessment of possible perineural extension relates to the presence of fat at the extracranial opening of the various neural foramina.[152] Each of the major neural trunks or branches that may serve as a pathway for perineural spread emerges from the skull base into a variable amount of fat, and effacement or obliteration of this fat suggests the presence of tumor. Conversely, if the fat at the appropriate location is normal, the presumption is that the tumor has not reached the skull base. This can be an important factor in planning potential surgery.

One of the most important perineural pathways to and through the central skull base is the second division of the trigeminal nerve (Fig. 12-17). The maxillary division of the trigeminal nerve passes through the foramen rotundum to reach the pterygopalatine fossa. Here the main trunk divides into the infraorbital, palatine, and superior alveolar branches, traveling to the anterior face, posterior hard palate, maxillary sinus, and maxillary teeth, respectively. The palatine nerves are particularly important because the mucosa covering the posterior hard palate contains a large concentration of minor salivary glands. Adenoid cystic carcinoma, with its propensity to spread along nerves, is a common occurrence in this location. If tumor follows the palatine nerves to the pterygopalatine fossa, the fat within the fossa is obliterated (Figs. 12-89, 12-91, and 12-92).

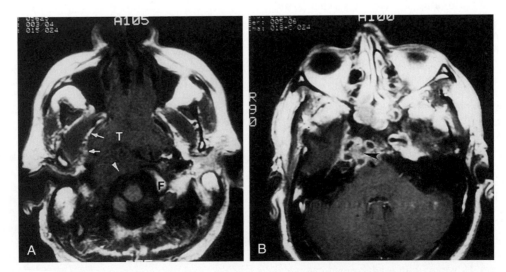

**FIGURE 12-87**   Nasopharyngeal carcinoma invading the basiocciput. **A,** The tumor (*T*) expands outward. There is a smooth expansion (*arrowheads*) of the wall of the nasopharynx without extension into the parapharyngeal fat. This demonstrates the strength of the fascial layers. Even though the tumor did not extend through the fascia, there is invasion of the bone (*arrowhead*), and there is obliteration of the fat within the medullary cavity and absence of the cortex. Compare this with the fat (*F*) in the occipital condyle on the normal side. MR imaging is very sensitive to tumor extension through the medullary fat. Small cortical erosions, however, can be missed. **B,** Postgadolinium image shows tumor extension (*arrowhead*) through the petrooccipital fissure at the lateral aspect of the sphenoid bone. Although enhancement can obscure the margins of the tumor below the skull base, it is helpful in demonstrating the tumor extent relative to the cavernous sinus and dural margin.

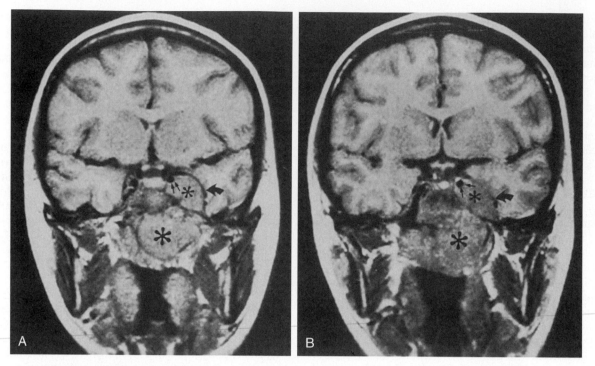

**FIGURE 12-88** A 12-year-old male presents with restriction of ocular motion and nasal stuffiness. Rhabdomyosarcoma of the nasopharynx with extension through the skull base. Coronal T1-weighted image shows the presence of a mass within the nasopharynx (*large asterisk*), with skull base destruction and invasion of the left cavernous sinus (*small asterisk*). Note the lateral deviation of the lateral dural reflection of the cavernous sinus (*curved arrow*). The mass abuts the cavernous internal carotid artery (*small arrows*). (From Braun IF. MRI of the nasopharynx. Radiol Clin North Am 1989;27(2):315.)

From this fossa, tumor can follow nerves through the foramen rotundum and Vidian canal to the region of the cavernous sinus.

The trigeminal nerve exiting the foramen ovale passes into a small amount of fat in the upper masticator space just medial to the lateral pterygoid muscle (Fig. 12-73). If tumor follows the auriculotemporal nerve from the parotid gland to the foramen ovale, this fat is obliterated. This pathway is a significant problem, as the tumor may not yet be palpable and the finding can be quite subtle. The patient typically presents with facial pain, as the sensory branches of the trigeminal nerve are involved.

Tumor following branches of the trigeminal nerve may reach the lower lateral aspect of Meckel's cave in the region of the Gasserian ganglion. Normally, there is slight enhancement of the periganglionic venous plexus, giving the appearance of a thin V. The V appears to thicken as tumor enlarges (Fig. 12-89).[153] Finally, the tumor can grow posteriorly from the cavernous sinus, following the preganglionic fibers of the trigeminal nerve toward the brainstem.

Typically, perineural spread occurs in a retrograde manner, toward the brain. However, antegrade spread can occur from branch points. For example, a tumor of the hard palate with retrograde perineural extension can reach the pterygopalatine fossa. From there, the malignancy can spread in an antegrade manner along the infraorbital nerve and spread in a retrograde pathway through the foramen rotundum. Similarly, once tumor has reached Meckel's cave, it can pass back out of the skull in an antegrade fashion through the fo-

ramen ovale into the masticator space. The topic of perineural tumor spread is also covered in Chapter 13.

## Hematogenous Metastasis

Hematogenous metastasis can reach the basicranium from primary tumors in the lung, kidney, breast, prostate, and a variety of other, more rare locations. The imaging findings are usually those of lytic destruction. Apparent bone expansion rarely can occur in tumors originating in the thyroid or the kidney. Sclerotic changes may be present in prostate metastasis and rarely with squamous cell carcinomas, giving an appearance much like that of a meningioma. Any part of the sphenoid bone may be involved. If the greater wing of the sphenoid is affected, the metastasis tends to grow outward in all directions. Thus, tumor is seen along the lateral wall of the orbit, along the dura of the middle cranial fossa, and elevating the temporalis muscle away from the destroyed calvarium (Fig. 12-93). A meningioma can give a similar appearance.

## TRAUMA

Though the sphenoid and basiocciput are substantial bones, fractures are not uncommon.[154-157] Such fractures are almost always associated with other severe facial bone, cranial vault, and skull base fractures. Of the various elements of the skull base, the orbital roofs, temporal bones, and posterior basiocciput are more likely to be fractured than the more central basicranium.[156] Any of these fractures should be carefully followed to determine if they extend into the more central skull base. Of particular concern are fractures of the temporal bone, as they frequently extend

obliquely into the lateral wall of the cavernous sinus, where they can injure the carotid artery.

Fractures of the central basicranium can compromise the numerous neurovascular structures traversing the bone (Fig. 12-94). In addition, muscles of ocular motion, mastication, and eustachian tube function attach to the sphenoid bone,

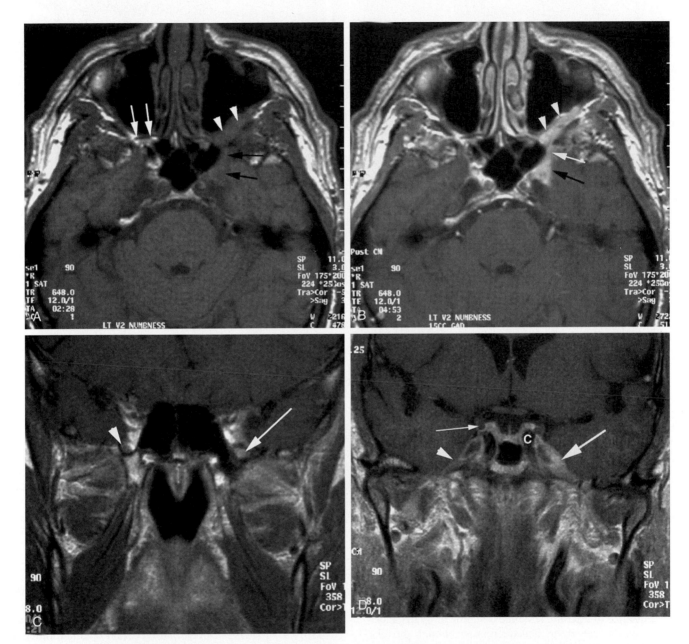

**FIGURE 12-89**   Perineural tumor from the hard palate extending through the pterygopalatine fossa and foramen rotundum into the region of the Gasserian ganglion. **A,** Axial precontrast T1-weighted image through the pterygopalatine fossa. There is obliteration of the fat as the tumor fills the pterygopalatine fossa (*arrowheads*). The lesion extends along the foramen rotundum into the anterior cavernous sinus (*black arrows*). Compare the appearance of the pterygopalatine fossa on the normal side (*white arrows*). **B,** Axial postcontrast image. There is enhancement of the tumor in the pterygopalatine fossa (*arrowheads*). It does not enhance to the signal intensity of fat. Again, the lesion is seen in the foramen rotundum (*white arrow*) and the anterior cavernous sinus (*black arrow*). **C,** Coronal postcontrast T1-weighted image. Note visualization of the actual enlargement of the nerve within the foramen rotundum (*arrow*). Compare this with the normal nerve on the opposite side (*arrowhead*) surrounded by a small, enhancing venous plexus. **D,** Coronal image through the involved region of the Gasserian ganglion. There is intermediate enhancement and thickening of the V (*arrow*) representing the region of the Gasserian ganglion. Note the normal venous plexus showing slight enhancement around the Gasserian ganglion (*arrowhead*) on the normal side. Third nerve (*small arrow*). *C,* carotid.

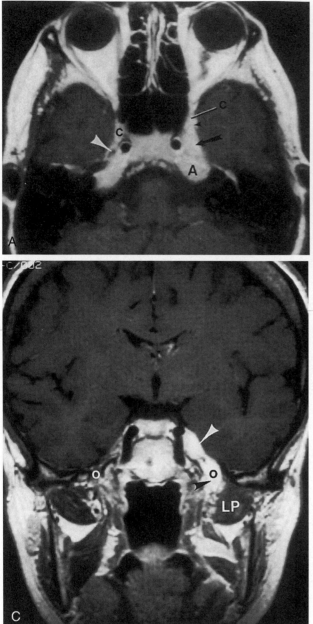

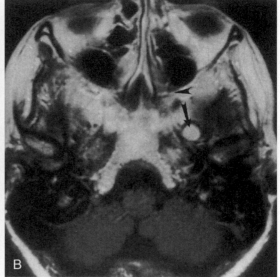

**FIGURE 12-90** **A,** Melanoma extending along the branches of the trigeminal nerve. MR postcontrast T1-weighted image. The tumor (*black arrow*) is seen in the region of Meckel's cave and the posterior cavernous sinus. Its junction with the normal enhancing cavernous sinus (*small black arrowhead*) can be identified anterior to the tumor. Similarly, the tumor should not be confused with the fat in the petrous apex (*A*). (*C*), Normal cavernous sinus; normal Meckel's cave (*white arrowhead*). **B,** More inferior scan just beneath the foramen ovale shows the nerve enlargement (*black arrow*) caused by the perineural extension. The pterygopalatine fossa (*black arrowhead*) is normal. **C,** Coronal T1-weighted postgadolinium image shows the perineural extension at the level of the cavernous sinus (*white arrowhead*), the foramen ovale (black *O*), and beneath the foramen ovale (*black arrowhead*). Note that the enlarged nerve is just at the medial margin of the lateral pterygoid (*LP*). The normal appearance of the foramen ovale is shown on the opposite side (white *O*).

and separation of the attachments of these muscles can result in functional deficits. The thinner plates of bone such as the greater wing of the sphenoid and the pterygoid plates offer less resistance to fracture, and unless significantly displaced, these fractures can be inconsequential. Although dysfunction of the attached muscles can cause problems in mastication, frequently the patients are asymptomatic. Significant inward displacement of a fracture of the greater wing can tear the dura and traumatize the brain.

The pterygoid processes of the sphenoid bone represent the posterior supporting strut of the facial skeleton. As such, the pterygoid plates are involved in the Le Forte fractures, separating the facial bones from the skull base. These fractures are discussed in Chapter 7. Fractures that do involve the sphenoid body and basiocciput place the numerous traversing neurovascular structures at risk, be-

cause the various neural foramina represent weak points in the bone, and the nerve within may be crushed, contused, or lacerated. A displaced bone fragment may also impinge upon the nerve.

Any of the nerves can be involved, and ophthalmoplegia or paresthesias can be the sequelae. Severe trauma can result in the superior orbital fissure syndrome, including a dilated pupil, ptosis, and extraocular muscle dysfunction. The optic nerve is of particular concern, and in a patient with vision loss after trauma, the optic canal must be carefully examined (Fig. 12-95). Any fracture of the orbital roof or of the lamina papyracea should prompt careful analysis of the optic canal. A displaced fragment may put pressure on the nerve, and if it is not quickly corrected, permanent visual loss will result. Immediate loss of vision can represent either actual nerve injury or nerve compression.[158] On the other hand, a delayed

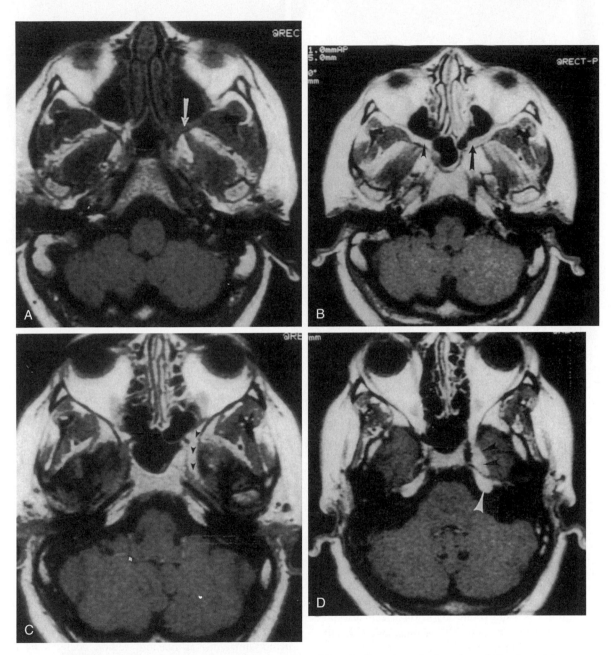

**FIGURE 12-91**    Adenoid cystic carcinoma of the palate extending along the branches of $V_2$. **A,** Axial T1-weighted image through the pterygopalatine fossa shows obliteration (*white arrow*) of the fat within the pterygopalatine fossa. Compare this with the normal fossa on the opposite side. Fat normally should be identified in this narrow structure. **B,** Postgadolinium T1-weighted image. Now the tumor enhances (*black arrow*). Without fat suppression (compare with the noncontrast study), this appearance might be considered normal. Compare it with the high signal of the fat in the normal pterygopalatine fossa on the opposite side. **C,** Postgadolinium T1-weighted image (slightly higher) shows enhancement of the tumor within the foramen rotundum (*black arrowheads*) leading toward Meckel's cave. **D,** Slightly higher postcontrast enhancement T1-weighted image shows the enhancement in the lower cavernous sinus (*black arrowheads*) obscuring Meckel's cave. The high signal of the fat in the petrous apex (*white arrowhead*) should not be confused with tumor.

*Illustration continued on following page*

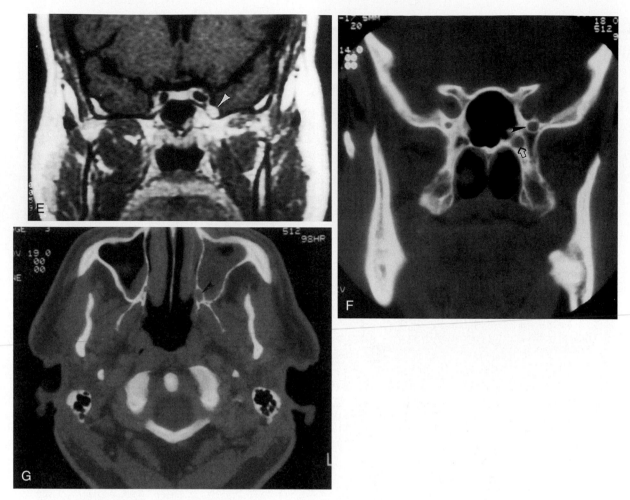

**FIGURE 12-91** *Continued.* **E,** Coronal MR T1-weighted postgadolinium image shows the enlargement of the second division of the trigeminal nerve just posterior (*white arrowhead*) to the foramen rotundum. The nerve is enlarged and enhances, indicating tumor involvement. **F,** Coronal bone algorithm shows enlargement of the foramen rotundum (*black arrowhead*) and the Vidian canal (*open black arrow*). This indicates tumor extension along both nerves. **G,** Enlargement of the lower pterygopalatine canal (*black arrowhead*), which connects the pterygopalatine fossa with the hard palate.

onset or progressive loss of vision usually represents an accumulating hematoma or edema. The optic nerve and optic canal can be visualized by axial and coronal CT. Identification of small fracture lines requires high-resolution, thin slices using bone algorithms. Because an orbital hematoma also can affect the optic nerve, the soft tissues should be carefully examined.

Fractures crossing the course of the carotid artery and involving the bone contiguous to the artery may or may not injure the wall of this vessel. These fractures can affect the thin, bony wall of the lateral sphenoid sinus at the indentation caused by the segment of the artery entering the cavernous sinus or they can be associated with fractures of the area of the anterior clinoid. Significant tears can result in death or in a carotid cavernous (CC) fistula (Fig. 12-96). In CC fistula, CT and MR imaging may show enlargement of the venous structures extending away from the cavernous sinus. Streaky reticulation of the orbital fat due to edema is usually seen, as well as the enlargement of the venous structures.

A fracture of the sphenoid bone can create a connection between the CSF spaces and the sphenoid sinus, resulting in a CSF leak, demonstrable by cisternography (Fig. 12-97). Such a communication can lead to meningitis, which is often delayed in onset. As stated, fractures of the sphenoid are often associated with other fractures of the skull or the skull base. Anosmia, periorbital ecchymosis ("raccoon eyes"), hemotympanum, or mastoid region ecchymosis (Battle's sign) may be seen in conjunction with findings related to the central skull base.

## MISCELLANEOUS CONDITIONS

### Dysplasias

The basicranium develops primarily through enchondral bone formation. As such, the central skull base can be involved by any generalized disorder that affects cartilaginous bone formation. Many of the findings are incidental. However, bony enlargement, characteristic of some dysplasias, and bone softening, characteristic of others, can lead to

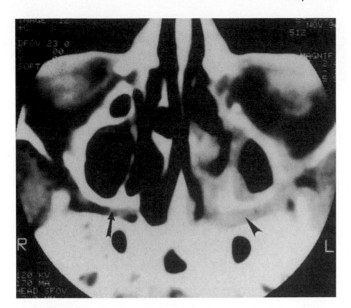

**FIGURE 12-92**   Axial CT image showing adenoid cystic carcinoma following the second division of the trigeminal nerve. The tumor (*black arrowhead*) obliterates the fat in the pterygopalatine fossa. Compare this with the fat (*arrow*) on the normal side.

significant problems resulting from compression of various cranial nerves or even of the brainstem and spinal cord. The base of the skull also is affected by generalized metabolic and hematologic diseases in which there are diffuse changes throughout the bony skeleton. Many of these entities cause softening of the bone, leading to a lack of support for the cranium. This can result in a protrusion of the upper spine into the foramen magnum or in a flattening of the skull base itself. These phenomena are referred to respectively as basilar invagination and platybasia.

## Platybasia Versus Basilar Invagination

Platybasia and basilar invagination are terms used to characterize certain findings in patients with abnormal bony architecture of the basicranium. Although platybasia and basilar invagination may occur together, they represent different changes in the skull base. Platybasia is a flattening of the skull base. The basal angle of Weneke is the angle formed between a line drawn from the nasion to the center of the sella turcica and a line drawn from the center of the sella turcica down along the posterior aspect of the clivus. The normal adult basal angle is about 140°. If this angle is significantly increased, platybasia is present.

More frequently, the skull base softens and the upper cervical spine appears to push up into the base of the skull. Actually, the skull base is settling down around the focal pressure of the spine. This is true basilar invagination. There are several reference lines, developed to assess possible basilar invagination on plain films, that can be applied easily to midline sagittal MR imaging.

Chamberlain's line extends from the posterior margin of the hard palate to the posterior margin of the foramen magnum. If the tip of the odontoid is 5 mm or more above this line, basilar invagination is present. At times, the lip of the occipital bone, which makes up the posterior margin of the foramen magnum, is difficult to visualize on the lateral radiograph. To deal with this problem, McGregor's line was developed, extending from the posterior margin of the hard palate to the most inferior point on the cortex of the occipital bone posterior to the foramen magnum. This point is much easier to see on the lateral radiograph. Using this system, basilar invagination is considered to be present if the tip of the odontoid is 7 mm above the line or if more than one third of the height of the

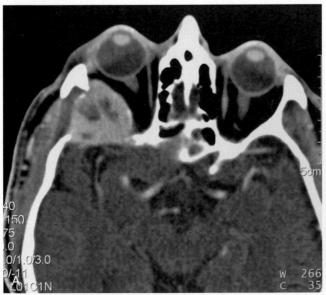

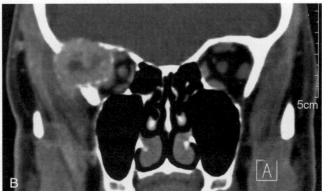

**FIGURE 12-93**   Metastatic renal carcinoma to the sphenoid triangle (greater wing of the sphenoid). **A,** The tumor is seen replacing the bone of the sphenoid triangle and extending into the orbit, temporalis fossa, and middle cranial fossa. **B,** Coronal CT postcontrast image.

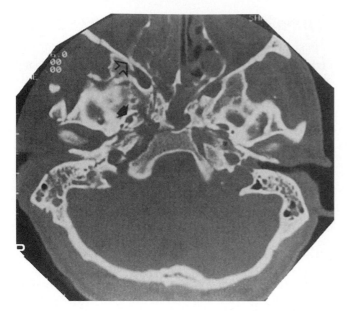

**FIGURE 12-94** A 23-year-old male following an automobile accident presents with superior orbital fissure syndrome and multiple cranial nerve deficits. Multiple skull base fractures. Axial CT scan through the skull base shows the presence of multiple fractures associated with fluid in the ethmoid and sphenoid sinuses. Multiple fractures causing narrowing of the orbital apex and inferior orbital fissure (*open arrow*) are appreciated, as well as a fracture involving the foramen ovale (*black arrow*).

Although platybasia can occur in many situations, the findings are characteristic of abnormalities such as Paget's disease, osteogenesis imperfecta, and osteomalacia. These abnormalities are all associated with softened abnormal bone incapable of supporting the weight of the skull. On the other hand, basilar invagination has been reported in achondroplasia, ankylosing spondylitis, Arnold-Chiari malformation, atlantoaxial dislocation, cleidocranial dysplasia, congenital craniovertebral junction abnormalities, Crouzon's syndrome, Down's syndrome, familial primary basilar impression, fibrous dysplasia, Haju-Cherney syndrome, histiocytosis, chronic hydrocephalus, hyperparathyroidism, hypophosphatasia, Klippel-Feil syndrome, mucopolysaccharidosis, occipital craniotomy in a child, osteogenesis imperfecta, osteomalacia, osteomyelitis, osteopetrosis, osteoporosis, Paget's disease, pyknodysostosis, rheumatoid arthritis, rickets, and an unfused posterior arch of the atlas.[159]

odontoid process is above this line. Because on a sagittal MR image both the posterior lip of the foramen magnum and the lowest point on the occiput can be easily identified, either system can be used.

## Fibrous Dysplasia

Fibrous dysplasia is an abnormality of the bone with abnormal development of the fibroblasts and abnormal mineralization.[160–163] The bone is enlarged, and on CT, the cortex tends to be maintained and the enlarged medullary space can have a variety of appearances, depending on the amount of fibrous and osteoid matrix present. The appearance on CT varies from a fairly lucent medullary space to a densely calcified one. Some cases have a mixture of dense and sclerotic changes sometimes referred to as pagetoid. The

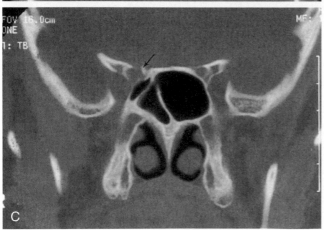

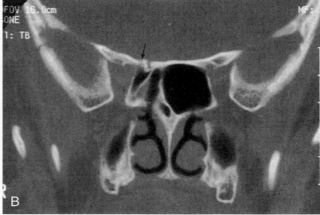

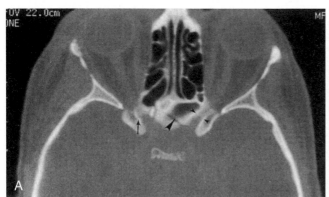

**FIGURE 12-95** **A,** Fracture of the sphenoid bone extending through the optic canal. Axial CT image shows the fracture line (*large black arrowhead*) extending across the sphenoid. The lucency of one of the fracture lines (*black arrow*) extends across the optic canal itself. Compare this with the normal intact cortices of the optic canal on the left side (*small black arrowhead*). **B,** Coronal CT bone algorithm shows the fracture (*arrow*) as a lucency extending along the region of the optic canal. The lesser wing of the sphenoid may be slightly displaced. **C,** A small bony fragment (*arrow*) is seen within the medial aspect of the optic canal itself. A displaced fragment impinging on the nerve can significantly compromise the visual pathway.

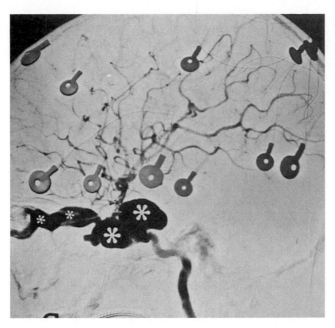

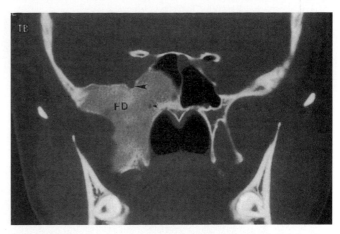

**FIGURE 12-98**   Fibrous dysplasia (*FD*) shows a typical "ground glass" appearance. The Vidian canal (*small black arrowhead*) and the groove for the second division of the trigeminal (*large black arrowhead*), just posterior to the foramen rotundum, have been incorporated or displaced by the expanding abnormality.

**FIGURE 12-96**   A 23-year-old male who presents with pulsatile exophthalmos and decreased visual acuity following a motorcycle accident. Skull base fracture with resultant cavernous carotid fistula. Lateral subtraction view of an internal carotid artery angiogram shows findings typical of a carotid cavernous fistula. Contrast from the arterial system has extravasated into the cavernous sinus (*large asterisks*) and subsequently into the superior ophthalmic vein (*small asterisks*). Arterial pressure transmitted to the venous system in the superior ophthalmic vein causes the pulsatile exophthalmos.

classic CT and plain film appearance is the "ground glass" medullary space surrounded by intact cortices (Fig. 12-98).

On MR imaging, the lesion has fairly low T1-weighted and T2-weighted signal intensity (Fig. 12-99). The internal matrix enhances with gadolinium, a phenomenon not as easily appreciated on CT. Although the classic appearance is one of a fairly homogeneous internal density on CT or signal intensity on MR imaging, inhomogeneous areas can be

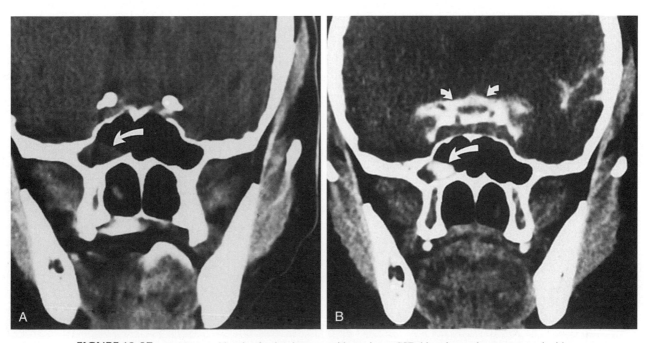

**FIGURE 12-97**   A 25-year-old male after head trauma with persistent CSF rhinorrhea and recurrent meningitis. Traumatic CSF fistula demonstrated by water-soluble contrast cisternography. Coronal CT scan through the sphenoid sinus obtained. Before **A** and following **B**, the intrathecal instillation of water-soluble contrast material. A soft-tissue density is appreciated involving the right lateral floor of the sphenoid sinus (*curved arrow*), as seen on the study before the instillation of contrast material. Following the instillation of contrast, increased density is appreciated in this region, consistent with the accumulation of contrast, documenting the presence of a CSF fistula. Also noted is the presence of contrast material within the suprasellar cistern (*small curved arrows*) outlining the chiasm and vascular structures. The fracture site was not identified.

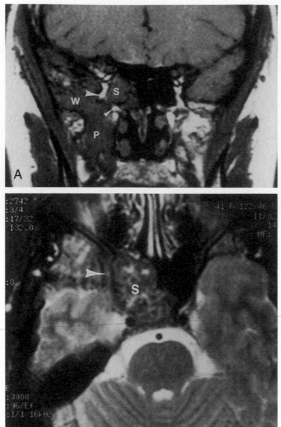

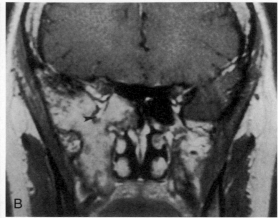

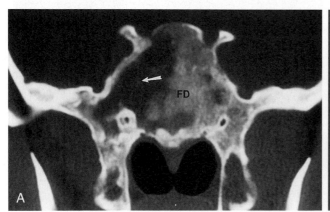

**FIGURE 12-99** Fibrous dysplasia of the sphenoid. **A,** Coronal T1-weighted image without contrast shows the abnormal bone involving the greater wing (*W*), pterygoid process (*P*), and body (*S*) of the sphenoid. The high signal represents fat at the extracranial opening of the foramen rotundum (*large white arrowhead*) and the Vidian canal (*small white arrowhead*) as the fibrous dysplasia impinges on the pterygopalatine fossa. **B,** Postcontrast enhancement T1-weighted image shows the enhancement of the fibrous dysplasia. Again, note the fat at the anterior end of the foramen rotundum (*arrowhead*). **C,** Axial T2-weighted image shows the fibrous dysplasia in the body of the sphenoid (*S*). The foramen rotundum (*arrowhead*) can be seen extending along the upper edge of the abnormality. In this image, the abnormality might be confused with a more significant tumor.

present.[164] Some areas may be predominantly fibrous tissue with the appropriate CT and MR imaging findings. Some areas may represent hemorrhage and cyst formation. In the central skull base, parts of the sphenoid sinus may become isolated and obstructed. The trapped secretions can give signal intensities similar to those of the inhomogeneities of the fibrous dysplasia itself (Fig. 12-100). This can be of

concern if the patient is evaluated for pain, as early mucocele formation cannot be differentiated from a static cystic region in fibrous dysplasia. Increasing size suggests mucocele formation. Most of the mineralized matrix is considered to be immature woven bone. Occasionally, small amounts of cartilage formation can occur, but this is unusual (Fig. 12-101).

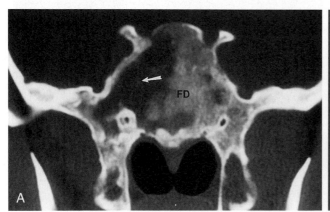

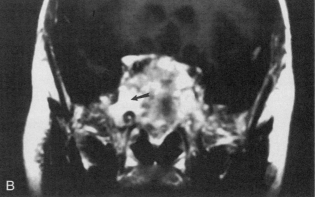

**FIGURE 12-100** Fibrous dysplasia **A,** Fibrous dysplasia with low-density area on CT. The fibrous dysplasia (*FD*) fills and expands most of the body of the sphenoid. There are areas of low density (*arrow*), which could represent either cystic components of the fibrous dysplasia or areas of obstructed secretions because of the sinus mucosa. **B,** Coronal T1-weighted MR image shows high signal intensity consistent with the cystic portion of the fibrous dysplasia. However, note that this area extends between the Vidian canal and the foramen rotundum, which would be the usual position of a laterally extending air cell.

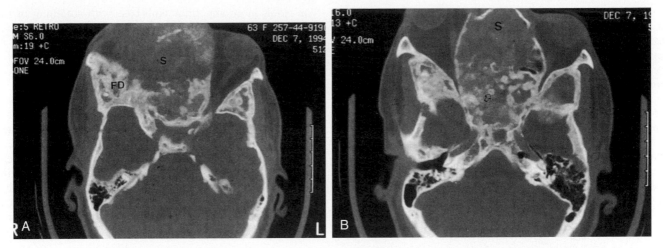

**FIGURE 12-101**   **A,** Fibrous dysplasia with secondary osteosarcoma. Fibrous dysplasia (*FD*) involves the greater wing of the sphenoid, extending into the sphenoid bone and including the lesser wing. It is bilateral. The sarcoma (*S*) is seen in the region of the nasal cavity extending into the orbit. **B,** More inferior scan shows the sarcoma (*S*) in the anterior nasal cavity. This fibrous dysplasia has small areas of cartilage formation histologically. This is shown as small rings of calcification (*open arrow*) on the CT scan.

## Paget's Disease

Paget's disease is a process of unknown cause in which osteoclastic activity is abnormal.[165] The normal osseous structure is replaced by an abnormal matrix that is more vascular than normal. The osteoblasts continue to respond to this abnormal situation and lay down a thicker, more sclerotic, but softer bone. This bone involves the cortex and the trabeculae within the medullary cavity, and there is poor corticomedullary differentiation. There is more bone than usual, and the bone can be dense or lucent (Fig. 12-102). The findings in the temporal bone appear to be primarily lytic because they involve and demineralize the otic capsule. Again, because the bone is softer than normal, basilar invagination is frequently present. In this disease, the remodeling of the softened bone may be so extensive that there is true platybasia and basilar invagination. Secondary sarcoma can occur.[166]

## Bone Dysplasias, Mucopolysaccharidosis, and Metabolic Diseases

Many of the bone dysplasias cause abnormal density and shape of the skull base.[167, 168] Terminology varies, but this group of lesions includes the various osteochondrodysplasias, dysostoses, and osteopetroses.[160] Basilar invagination, though occurring occasionally, is not a typical finding in many of these bone disorders because the abnormal bone is not particularly soft. The distribution and appearance of the findings in the long bones and the craniofacial skeleton are used to establish the diagnosis. Thickening of the bone may take place at the expense of the neural foramina (Fig. 12-103), and cranial nerve palsies can result.[169, 170] Involvement of the sphenoid bone can lead to blindness or various ophthalmoplegias. Temporal bone involvement can lead to deafness and facial nerve paralysis.

Achondroplasia is an abnormality that affects the development of enchondral bone, and thus the skull base is predictably involved. The failure of growth at the sphenooccipital synchondrosis leads to a short clivus and a smaller sphenoid bone. The floor of the posterior fossa is higher and more horizontal than normal, with variable narrowing of the foramen magnum. If pronounced, this can lead to severe neurologic problems. A typical J-shaped sella is an incidental finding. Platybasia occurs because of maldevelopment of the occipital vertebral junction.

Osteogenesis imperfecta causes a deficient, weakened

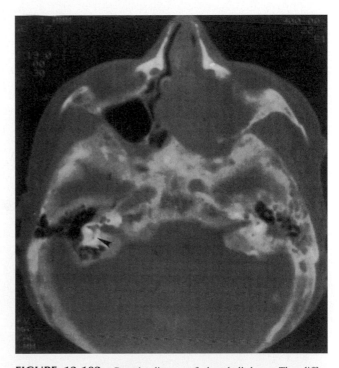

**FIGURE 12-102**   Paget's disease of the skull base. The diffuse, abnormally mineralized bone is seen in the temporal bone and sphenoid. There is relative sparing but some demineralization of the otic capsule (*arrowhead*). The patient had a sarcoma in the region of the maxillary sinus and nasal cavity.

bone structure, and basilar invagination occurs. The severity is quite variable in the tarda form. Wormian bones and narrowing of the foramen magnum also are present. The temporal bone can be involved with what appears to be extensive otosclerosis and production of undermineralized bone around the labyrinth.

The mucopolysaccharidoses (Morquio's, Hurler's, Hunter's, Maroteaux-Lamy, etc.) are lysosomal storage diseases. The skull base shows abnormal growth, and again, a J-shaped sella is present. The bone of the skull base may be thicker than usual, but because the bone is abnormal, basilar invagination can be present. Associated craniovertebral anomalies, with atlantoaxial instability, are considered more significant problems and can lead to severe neurologic deficits.

Hyperparathyroidism and other metabolic diseases also can result in an abnormal skull base with softening of the normal bone. However, the diagnosis usually is known or is made by evaluation of other parameters.

## CEREBROSPINAL FLUID LEAK

A CSF leak may either be related to trauma, with a fracture creating the communication between the CSF space and the sinonasal cavities (Fig. 12-97), or may occur spontaneously.[171] The patient may present with clear rhinorrhea that is evident when the patient bends forward. Alternatively, the patient may swallow the CSF. Meningitis or intracranial abscesses may occur because the communication becomes an entrance pathway for microorganisms found in the sinonasal tract. The most common site of CSF

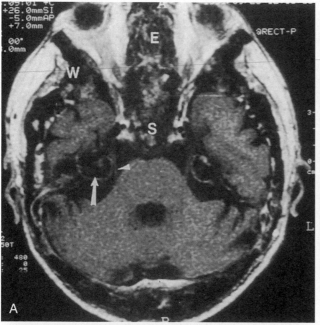

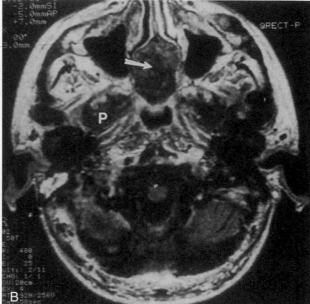

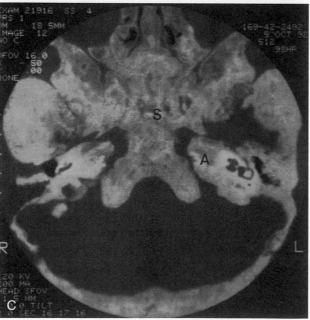

**FIGURE 12-103** Engelmann's disease (progressive diaphyseal dysplasia). This dysplasia of the skull base shows considerable thickening and sclerosis of the bone. **A,** Axial T1-weighted postcontrast MR image shows the abnormal bone in the body (*S*) of the sphenoid and ethmoid (*E*) and the greater wing of the sphenoid. There is also enlargement of the petrous apex (*white arrow*). Note the position of the preganglionic segment and trigeminal nerve (*arrowhead*). **B,** More inferior scan shows the expansion of the nasal septum (*arrow*) and the enlarged, dysplastic bone replacing the pterygoid process (*P*). **C,** CT bone algorithm shows the dysplastic sclerotic bone in the sphenoid (*S*) and the apex of the temporal bone (*A*). The patient had bilateral facial paralysis, multiple cranial nerve palsies, and hearing and vision loss.

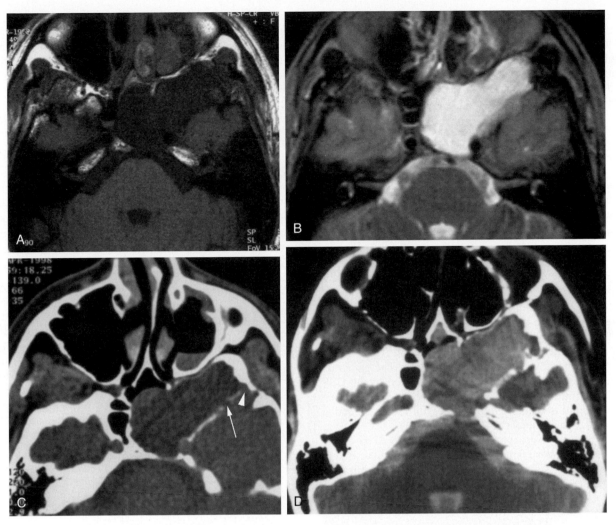

**FIGURE 12-104**   CSF leak into an enlarged sphenoid sinus. **A,** Axial T1-weighted image shows low signal equivalent to CSF in an expanded sphenoid sinus. The lateral extent of the sinus extends into the medial greater wing at the attachment of the pterygoid process. **B,** Axial T2-weighted image shows high signal compatible with CSF. **C,** Axial CT image prior to injection of intrathecal contrast shows a small pit (*arrow*) along the anterior wall of the middle cranial fossa. A small defect (*arrowhead*) appears to extend into the cystic cavity. This may represent extension of arachnoid granulations or a small fracture at that site. **D,** Postintrathecal contrast image shows filling of the cystic cavity as well as the prepontine cistern and fourth ventricle.

breech is anteriorly through the region of the cribriform plate or ethmoid roof. The second most common site is the temporal bone, where fractures may be associated with a CSF leak. If the tympanic membrane is ruptured, the fluid passes out into the external auditory canal as otorrhea. If the membrane is intact, the fluid passes through the eustachian tube into the nasopharynx and posterior nasal cavity. The patient can present with rhinorrhea, mimicking a fracture of the anterior skull base, and sphenoid sinus fluid levels, suggesting a fracture of the sphenoid sinus walls. CSF leaks through fractures of the sphenoid bone, communicating with the sphenoid sinus, are uncommon but do occur. The fracture must connect the sphenoid sinus and the CSF space, and so the location is usually over a lateral air cell at the root of the pterygoid process or in the floor of the middle cranial fossa. Here the cavernous sinus does not cover and ''protect'' the sinus. Of course, fractures through the sinus roof, especially if there is also an ''empty'' sella, can cause a CSF leak.

Tumors, especially those arising in the pituitary gland, can cause a nonsurgical CSF leak. Encephaloceles and congenital anomalies also rarely are responsible for CSF rhinorrhea. Spontaneous CSF rhinorrhea can pass along a communication through the anterior wall of the middle cranial fossa into a lateral air cell in the root of the pterygoid process or greater wing of the sphenoid.

Arachnoid granulations frequently are found in the anterior wall of the middle cranial fossa. A small defect in the dura can complete the communication through the thin bone. The communication is typically from the CSF space into the lateral or pterygoid air cell of the sphenoid sinus. This is the air cell protruding laterally between Vidian's canal and the foramen rotundum into the attachment of the pterygoid process. The CSF flows out through the sphenoid ostium into the posterior nasal cavity. Due to the pulsatile pressure of the CSF, an affected air cell may expand, mimicking a mucocele (Fig. 12-104).

CSF fistulas may be seen after skull base surgery.

Considerable effort is put into preventing this complication. One of the primary goals of reconstructive flap design is isolation of the CSF and the intracranial structures from the external world, particularly the sinonasal tract, with its plethora of potential pathogens. However, the pulsating pressure of the CSF works against the surgeon, and leaks occasionally occur. Because of the distorted postoperative anatomy, collections within the soft tissues or grafts may occur. These pseudomeningoceles may be clinically inconsequential if small, but they must be surgically corrected if large. The radiologic evaluation is done with CT or MR imaging. In the postoperative case, the area of primary concern is obvious, but the identification of the defect in the skull base often is not specifically useful because large defects are routine. Very useful is the identification of a fluid collection in the contiguous soft tissues or an intracranial air bubble near the site of the leak.

In the nonoperated patient, high-resolution CT is performed with a bone algorithm to look for a bony dehiscence.[172] Even if a defect is not seen, a collection of fluid within a sinus may suggest the location of the leak. Because the middle ear and mastoid are potential sites for the CSF leak, these areas must be carefully examined. In either the operated or the nonoperated patient, if the leak is not obvious, intrathecal contrast can be used. The patient is placed in the position that clinically is related to the CSF leak, and further CT imaging is done.[172, 173] Contrast cisternography is unlikely to be successful unless an active leak exists at the time of the study.

Radionuclide cisternography is considered to be more sensitive than these studies, but it does not accurately localize the leak site. The radionuclide is injected intrathe-

cally, and pledgets are placed in the areas most likely to detect a leak (i.e., the pledgets may be placed high in the nasal cavity by the otolaryngologist). Later, the pledgets are retrieved and measured for radioactivity. Although this procedure can be done to confirm that a leak is present, it requires an active leaking at the time of the study. Recently, clinicians have been better able to verify that the rhinorrhea fluid is indeed CSF by testing the fluid for beta 2-transferrin, which is present in CSF but not in sinonasal secretions.

## RHIZOTOMY INJECTIONS

In order to control pain, alcohol may be injected into the Gasserian ganglion. Radiopaque material is often mixed with the injected alcohol. This appearance is characteristic and should not be confused with a calcified neoplasm (Fig. 12-105). The material is injected via the foramen ovale and can follow the nerve or can track along the dura.

## REFERENCES

1. Sperber GH. Early embryonic development. In: Sperber GH ed. Craniofacial Embryology. 4th ed. London: Wright, 1989;7–30.
2. Burdi AR. Early development of the human basicranium: its morphogenic controls, growth patterns, and relations. In: Bosma JF ed. Symposium on Development of the Basicranium. DHEW Pub. No. (NIH) 76–989. Bethesda, Md: U.S. Dept. of Health, Education, and Welfare, Public Health Service National Institutes of Health, 1976;81–92.
3. Gasser RF. Early formation of the basicranium in man. In: Bosma JF ed. Symposium on Development of the Basicranium DHEW Pub. No. (NIH) 76–989. Bethesda, Md: U.S. Dept. of Health Education and Welfare Public Health Service National Institutes of Health, 1976; 29–43.
4. Romanoff AL. The Avian Embryo: Structural and Functional Development. New York: Macmillan, 1960.
5. Beltramello A, Puppini G, El-Dalati G, et al. Fossa navicularis magna. AJNR 1998;19(9):1796–1798.
6. Sperber GH. The cranial base. In: Sperber GH ed. Craniofacial Embryology. 4th ed. London: Wright, 1989;101–118.
7. Bosma JF. Introduction to the symposium on development of the basicranium. In: Bosma JF ed. Symposium on Development of the Basicranium. DHEW Pub. No. (NIH) 76–989. Bethesda, Md: U.S. Dept. of Health Education and Welfare Public Health Service National Institutes of Health, 1976;3–29.
8. Gray H, Williams PL, Bannister LH. Gray's Anatomy: The Anatomical Basis of Medicine and Surgery. 38th ed. New York: Churchill Livingstone, 1995.
9. McMinn RMH, Hutchings RT, Logan BM. Color Atlas of Head and Neck Anatomy. 2nd ed. London and Baltimore: Mosby-Wolfe, 1994.
10. Pernkopf E, Platzer W. Pernkopf Anatomy: Atlas of Topographic and Applied Human Anatomy. Vol. 1: Head and Neck. 3rd ed. Baltimore: Urban & Schwarzenberg, 1989.
11. Romrell LJ. Sectional Anatomy of the Head and Neck with Correlative Diagnostic Imaging. Philadelphia: Lea & Febiger, 1994.
12. Ginsberg LE, Pruett SW, Chen MY, Elster AD. Skull-base foramina of the middle cranial fossa: reassessment of normal variation with high-resolution CT. AJNR 1994;15(2):283–291.
13. Aoki S, Dillon WP, Barkovich AJ, Norman D. Marrow conversion before pneumatization of the sphenoid sinus: assessment with MR imaging. Radiology 1989;172(2):373–375.
14. Applegate GR, Hirsch WL, Applegate LJ, Curtin HD. Variability in the enhancement of the normal central skull base in children. Neuroradiology 1992;34(3):217–221.
15. Okada Y, Aoki S, Barkovich AJ, et al. Cranial bone marrow in children: assessment of normal development with MR imaging. Radiology 1989;171(1):161–164.

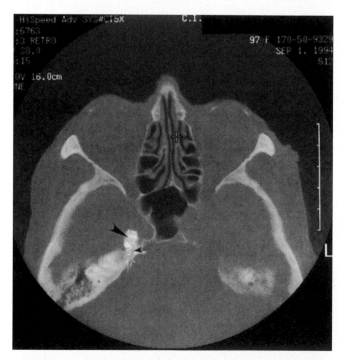

**FIGURE 12-105**   Radiopaque foreign body from glycerol rhizotomy. The radiopaque material (*large black arrowhead*) was added to the alcohol, which was injected into the area of Meckel's cave in the hope of relieving facial pain. The nerve (*small black arrowhead*) can be seen surrounded by this contrast.

16. Shopfner CE, Wolfe TW, O'Kell RT. The intersphenoid synchondrosis. Am J Roentgenol Radium Ther Nucl Med 1968;104(1): 184–193.
17. Kier EL, Rothman SLG. Radiologically significant anatomic variations of the developing sphenoid in humans. In: Bosma JF ed. Symposium on Development of the Basicranium. DHEW Pub. No. (NIH) 76–989. Bethesda, Md: U.S. Dept. of Health Education and Welfare Public Health Service National Institutes of Health, 1976; 107–140.
18. Fujioka M, Young LW. The sphenoidal sinuses: radiographic patterns of normal development and abnormal findings in infants and children. Radiology 1978;129(1):133.
19. Lewin JS, Curtin HD, Eelkema E, Obuchowski N. Benign expansile lesions of the sphenoid sinus: differentiation from normal asymmetry of the lateral recesses. AJNR 1999;20(3):461–466.
20. Kaufman B, Yonas H, White RJ, Miller CF. Acquired middle cranial fossa fistulas: normal pressure and nontraumatic in origin. Neurosurgery 1979;5(4):466–472.
21. Ginsberg LE. The posterior condylar canal. AJNR 1994;15(5): 969–972.
22. Weissman JL. Condylar canal vein: unfamiliar normal structure as seen at CT and MR imaging. Radiology 1994;190(1):81–84.
23. Curtin HD. Separation of the masticator space from the parapharyngeal space. Radiology 1987;163(1):195–204.
24. James HE. Encephalocele, dermoid sinus, and arachnoid cyst. In: McLaurin RL ed. Pediatric Neurosurgery. 2nd ed. Philadelphia: WB Saunders, 1989;97–105.
25. Pollock JA, Newton TH, Hoyt WF. Transsphenoidal and transethmoidal encephaloceles. A review of clinical and roentgen features in 8 cases. Radiology 1968;90(3):442–453.
26. Silverman FN. Some features of developmental changes observed clinically in the sphenoid and basicranium. In: Bosma JF ed. Symposium on Development of the Basicranium. DHEW Pub. No. (NIH) 76–989. Bethesda, Md: U.S. Dept. of Health Education and Welfare Public Health Service National Institutes of Health, 1976; 319–345.
27. Kapadia SB, Janecka IP, Fernandes S, et al. Lateral basal encephalocele of the infratemporal fossa. Otolaryngol Head Neck Surg 1996;114(1):116–119.
28. Elster AD, Branch CL Jr. Transalar sphenoidal encephaloceles: clinical and radiologic findings. Radiology 1989;170(1 Pt 1): 245–247.
29. Nager GT. Cephaloceles. Laryngoscope 1987;97(1):77–84.
30. David DJ, Proudman TW. Cephaloceles: classification, pathology, and management. World J Surg 1989;13(4):349–357.
31. Kapadia SB, Janecka IP, Curtin HD, Johnson BL. Diffuse neurofibroma of the orbit associated with temporal meningocele and neurofibromatosis-1. Otolaryngol Head Neck Surg 1998;119(6): 652–655.
32. Leblanc R, Tampieri D, Robitaille Y, et al. Developmental anterobasal temporal encephalocele and temporal lobe epilepsy. J Neurosurg 1991;74(6):933–939.
33. Muller H, Slootweg PJ, Troost J. An encephalocele of the sphenomaxillary type. Case report. J Maxillofac Surg 1981;9(3):180–184.
34. Morris WM, Losken HW, le Roux PA. Spheno-maxillary meningoencephalocele. A case report. J Craniomaxillofac Surg 1989;17(8): 359–362.
35. Chapman PH, Curtin HD, Cunningham MJ. An unusual pterygopalatine meningocele associated with neurofibromatosis type 1. Case report. J Neurosurg 2000;93(3):480–483.
36. Sadeh M, Goldhammer Y, Shacked I, et al. Basal encephalocele associated with suprasellar epidermoid cyst. Arch Neurol 1982;39(4): 250–252.
37. Meche FGA, van der Braakman R. Arachnoid cysts in the middle cranial fossa: cause and treatment of progressive and nonprogressive symptoms. J Neurol Neurosurg Psychiatry 1983;46(12):1102–1107.
38. Sato K, Shimoji T, Yaguchi K, et al. Middle fossa arachnoid cyst: clinical, neuroradiological, and surgical features. Childs Brain 1983;10(5):301–316.
39. Naidich TP, McLone DG, Radkowski MA. Intracranial arachnoid cysts. Pediatr Neurosci 1985;12(2):112–122.
40. Schuknecht B, Simmen D, Yuksel C, Valavanis A: Tributary venosinus occlusion and septic cavernous sinus thrombosis: CT and MR findings. AJNR 1998;19(4):617–626.
41. Chandler JR. Malignant external otitis: further considerations. Ann Otol Rhinol Laryngol 1977;86(4 Pt 1):417–428.
42. Chandler JR. Malignant external otitis. Laryngoscope 1968;78(8): 1257–1294.
43. Nadol JB Jr. Histopathology of *Pseudomonas* osteomyelitis of the temporal bone starting as malignant external otitis. Am J Otolaryngol 1980;1(5):359–371.
44. Damiani J, Damiani K, SE K. Malignant external otitis with multiple cranial nerve involvement. Am J Otol 1979;1:115–120.
45. Curtin HD, Wolfe P, May M. Malignant external otitis: CT evaluation. Radiology 1982;145(2):383–388.
46. Grandis JR, Curtin HD, Yu VL. Necrotizing (malignant) external otitis: prospective comparison of CT and MR imaging in diagnosis and follow-up. Radiology 1995;196(2):499–504.
47. Rubin J, Curtin HD, Yu VL, Kamerer DB. Malignant external otitis: utility of CT in diagnosis and follow-up. Radiology 1990;174(2): 391–394.
48. Dillon WP, Som PM, Fullerton GD. Hypointense MR signal in chronically inspissated sinonasal secretions. Radiology 1990;174(1): 73–78.
49. Som PM, Dillon WP, Fullerton GD, et al. Chronically obstructed sinonasal secretions: observations on T1 and T2 shortening. Radiology 1989;172(2):515–520.
50. Zinreich SJ, Kennedy DW, Malat J, et al. Fungal sinusitis: diagnosis with CT and MR imaging. Radiology 1988;169(2):439–444.
51. Barnes L, Kapadia SB. The biology and pathology of selected skull base tumors. J Neurooncol 1994;20(3):213–240.
52. Batsakis JG. Vasoformative tumors. In: Batsakis JG ed. Tumors of the Head and Neck: Clinical and Pathological Considerations. 2nd ed. Baltimore: Williams & Wilkins, 1979;297–327.
53. Dorfman HD, Czerniak B. Bone Tumors. St. Louis: CV Mosby, 1998.
54. Campanacci M. Bone and Soft Tissue Tumors: Clinical Features, Imaging, Pathology, and Treatment. 2nd rev. ed. Padova, Vienna, New York: Piccin Nuova Libraria and Springer-Verlag, 1999.
55. Batsakis J, Kittleson A. Chordomas: otorhinolaryngologic presentation and diagnosis. Arch Otolaryngol 1963;78:168–172.
56. Burger PC, Scheithauer BW, Armed Forces Institute of Pathology (U.S.), Universities Associated for Research and Education in Pathology. Tumors of the Central Nervous System. Washington, DC: Armed Forces Institute of Pathology. 1994 Atlas of tumor pathology. Third series, fasc. 10.
57. Mabrey R. Chordoma: a study of 150 cases. Am J Cancer 1935;25:501–506.
58. Heffelfinger MJ, Dahlin DC, MacCarty CS, Beabout JW. Chordomas and cartilaginous tumors at the skull base. Cancer 1973;32(2): 410–420.
59. Rosenberg AE, Brown GA, Bhan AK, Lee JM. Chondroid chordoma—a variant of chordoma. A morphologic and immunohistochemical study. Am J Clin Pathol 1994;101(1):36–41.
60. Dalpra L, Malgara R, Miozzo M, et al. First cytogenetic study of a recurrent familial chordoma of the clivus. Int J Cancer 1999;81(1): 24–30.
61. Miozzo M, Dalpra L, Riva P, et al. A tumor suppressor locus in familial and sporadic chordoma maps to 1p36. Int J Cancer 2000;87(1): 68–72.
62. Buonamici L, Roncaroli F, Fioravanti A, et al. Cytogenetic investigation of chordomas of the skull. Cancer Genet Cytogenet 1999;112(1):49–52.
63. Weber A, Liebsch N, Sanchez R, et al. Chordomas of the skull base: radiological and clinical evaluation. Neuroimaging Clin North Am 1994;4(3):515–527.
64. Firooznia H, Pinto R, Lin J, et al. Chordoma: radiologic evaluation of 20 cases. AJR 1976;127:797–799.
65. Sze G, Uichanco LI, Brant-Zawadzki M, et al. Chordomas: MR imaging. Radiology 1988;166:187–191.
66. Meyers S, Hirsch WJ, Curtin H, et al. Chordomas of the skull base: MR features. AJNR 1992;13:1627–1636.
67. Oot R, Melville G, New P, et al. The role of MR and CT in evaluating clival chordomas and chondrosarcomas. AJNR 1988;9: 715–723.
68. Batsakis JG. Soft tissue tumors of the head and neck: unusual forms. In: Batsakis JG ed. Tumors of the Head and Neck: Clinical and Pathological Considerations. 2nd ed. Baltimore: Williams & Wilkins, 1979;353–385.

69. Fischbein NJ, Kaplan MJ, Holliday RA, Dillon WP. Recurrence of clival chordoma along the surgical pathway. AJNR 2000;21(3):578–583.

70. Uggowitzer MM, Kugler C, Groell R, et al. Drop metastases in a patient with a chondroid chordoma of the clivus. Neuroradiology 1999;41(7):504–507.

71. al-Mefty O, Borba LA. Skull base chordomas: a management challenge. J Neurosurg 1997;86(2):182–189.

72. Debus J, Schulz-Ertner D, Schad L, et al. Stereotactic fractionated radiotherapy for chordomas and chondrosarcomas of the skull base. Int J Radiat Oncol Biol Phys 2000;47(3):591–596.

73. Hug EB, Loredo LN, Slater JD, et al. Proton radiation therapy for chordomas and chondrosarcomas of the skull base. J Neurosurg 1999;91(3):432–439.

74. Kondziolka D, Lunsford LD, Flickinger JC. The role of radiosurgery in the management of chordoma and chondrosarcoma of the cranial base. Neurosurgery 1991;29(1):38–45; discussion 45–46.

75. Sims E, Doughty D, Macaulay E, et al. Stereotactically delivered cranial radiation therapy: a ten-year experience of linac-based radiosurgery in the UK. Clin Oncol 1999;11(5):303–320.

76. Crockard A, Macaulay E, Plowman PN. Stereotactic radiosurgery. VI. Posterior displacement of the brainstem facilitates safer high dose radiosurgery for clival chordoma. Br J Neurosurg 1999;13(1):65–70.

77. O'Connell JX, Renard LG, Liebsch NJ, et al. Base of skull chordoma. A correlative study of histologic and clinical features of 62 cases. Cancer 1994;74(8):2261–2267.

78. Terahara A, Niemierko A, Goitein M, et al. Analysis of the relationship between tumor dose inhomogeneity and local control in patients with skull base chordoma. Int J Radiat Oncol Biol Phys 1999;45(2):351–358.

79. Rosenberg AE, Nielsen GP, Keel SB, et al. Chondrosarcoma of the base of the skull: a clinicopathologic study of 200 cases with emphasis on its distinction from chordoma. Am J Surg Pathol 1999;23(11):1370–1378.

80. Pritchard D, Lunke R, Taylor W, et al. Chondrosarcoma: a clinicopathologic and statistical analysis. Cancer 1980;45:149–152.

81. Jones H. Cartilaginous tumors of the head and neck. J Laryngol Otol 1973;87:135–138.

82. Lee Y, Van Tassel P. Craniofacial chondrosarcomas: imaging findings in 15 untreated cases. AJNR 1989;10:165–171.

83. Rassekh CH, Nuss DW, Kapadia SB, et al. Chondrosarcoma of the nasal septum: skull base imaging and clinicopathologic correlation. Otolaryngol Head Neck Surg 1996;115(1):29–37.

84. Guccion J, Font R, Enziger F, et al. Extraskeletal mesenchymal chondrosarcoma. Arch Pathol 1973;95:336–337.

85. Weber AL, Brown EW, Hug EB, Liebsch NJ. Cartilaginous tumors and chordomas of the cranial base. Otolaryngol Clin North Am 1995;28(3):453–471.

86. Brown E, Hug E, Weber A. Chondrosarcoma of the skull base. Neuroimaging Clin North Am 1994;4(3):529–541.

87. Ramina R, Coelho Neto M, Meneses MS, Pedrozo AA. Maffucci's syndrome associated with a cranial base chondrosarcoma: case report and literature review [see comments]. Neurosurgery 1997;41(1):269–272.

88. Balcer LJ, Galetta SL, Cornblath WT, Liu GT. Neuro-ophthalmologic manifestations of Maffucci's syndrome and Ollier's disease. J Neuroophthalmol 1999;19(1):62–66.

89. Keel SB, Bhan AK, Liebsch NJ, Rosenberg AE. Chondromyxoid fibroma of the skull base: a tumor which may be confused with chordoma and chondrosarcoma. A report of three cases and review of the literature. Am J Surg Pathol 1997;21(5):577–582.

90. Shek TW, Peh WC, Leung G. Chondromyxoid fibroma of skull base: a tumor prone to local recurrence. J Laryngol Otol 1999;113(4):380–385.

91. Ojemann R. Meningiomas: clinical features and surgical management. In: Wilkins R, Rengachary S, eds. Neurosurgery. New York: McGraw-Hill, 1985;635–654.

92. Cushing H. The meningiomas (dural endothelioma): their source and favoured seats of origin. Brain 1922;45:282–289.

93. Batsakis J. Other neuroectodermal tumors and related lesions of the head and neck. In: Batsakis J ed. Tumors of the Head and Neck: Clinical and Pathological Considerations. 2nd ed. Baltimore: Williams & Wilkins, 1979;348–352.

94. Miller NR, Golnik KC, Zeidman SM, North RB. Pneumosinus dilatans: a sign of intracranial meningioma. Surg Neurol 1996;46(5):471–474.

95. Skolnick CA, Mafee MF, Goodwin JA. Pneumosinus dilatans of the sphenoid sinus presenting with visual loss. J Neuroophthalmol 2000;20(4):259–263.

96. Reicher MA, Bentson JR, Halbach VV, et al. Pneumosinus dilatans of the sphenoid sinus. AJNR 1986;7(5):865–868.

97. Hirst LW, Miller NR, Allen GS. Sphenoidal pneumosinus dilatans with bilateral optic nerve meningiomas. Case report. J Neurosurg 1979;51(3):402–407.

98. Hirst LW, Miller NR, Hodges FJ, et al. Sphenoid pneumosinus dilatans. A sign of meningioma originating in the optic canal. Neuroradiology 1982;22(4):207–210.

99. Spoor TC, Kennerdell JS, Maroon JC, et al. Pneumosinus dilatans, Klippel-Trenaunay-Weber syndrome, and progressive visual loss. Ann Ophthalmol 1981;13(1):105–108.

100. Hirsch WL Jr, Hryshko FG, Sekhar LN, et al. Comparison of MR imaging, CT, and angiography in the evaluation of the enlarged cavernous sinus. AJR 1988;151(5):1015–1023.

101. Young S, Grossman R, Goldberg H, et al. MR of vascular encasement in parasellar masses: comparison with angiography and CT. AJNR 1988;9(1):35–38.

102. Bret P, Beziat JL. [Sphenoido-nasopharyngeal craniopharyngioma. A case with radical excision by Le Fort I-type maxillotomy]. Neurochirurgie 1993;39(4):235–240.

103. Chakrabarty A, Mitchell P, Bridges LR. Craniopharyngioma invading the nasal and paranasal spaces, and presenting as nasal obstruction. Br J Neurosurg 1998;12(4):361–363.

104. Hillman TH, Peyster RG, Hoover ED, et al. Infrasellar craniopharyngioma: CT and MR studies. JCAT 1988;12(4):702–704.

105. Bernstein M, Buchino J. The histology similarity between craniopharyngioma and odontogenic lesions: a reappraisal. Oral Pathol 1983;56(5):502–511.

106. Alvarez-Garijo J, Froufe A, Taboada D, et al. Successful surgical treatment of an odontogenic ossified craniopharyngioma. J Neurosurg 1981;55:832–835.

107. Burger P, Scheihauer B. Craniopharyngiomas. In: Burger P, Scheihauer B, eds. Atlas of Tumor Pathology: Tumors of the Central Nervous System. Washington, DC: Armed Forces Institute of Pathology, 1994;349–354.

108. Lopez-Carreira M, Dominguez-Franjo P, Madero S, et al. Suprasellar papillary squamous craniopharyngioma. A case report. J Neurosurg Sci 1997;41(2):175–178.

109. Sartoretti-Schefer S, Wichmann W, Aguzzi A, Valavanis A. MR differentiation of adamantinous and squamous-papillary craniopharyngiomas. AJNR 1997;18(1):77–87.

110. Crotty TB, Scheithauer BW, Young WF Jr, et al. Papillary craniopharyngioma: a clinicopathological study of 48 cases. J Neurosurg 1995;83(2):206–214.

111. Hanna E, Weissman J, Janecka IP. Sphenoclival Rathke's cleft cysts: embryology, clinical appearance and management. Ear Nose Throat J 1998;77(5):396–399, 403.

112. Murphy F, Vesely D, Jordan R, et al. Giant invasive prolactinomas. Am J Med 1987;83(7):995–1002.

113. Hoffman JJ. Radiology of sellar and parasellar lesions. In: Wilkins R, Rengachary S, eds. Neurosurgery. New York: McGraw-Hill, 1985;822–834.

114. Slonin S, Haykal H, Cushing GW, et al. MRI appearance of an ectopic pituitary adenoma: a case report and review of the literature. Neuroradiology 1993;35:546–548.

115. Tovi F, Hirsch M, Sacks M, Leiberman A. Ectopic pituitary adenoma of the sphenoid sinus: report of a case and review of the literature. Head Neck 1990;12(3):264–268.

116. Scheithauer BW, Woodruff JM, Erlandson RA, Universities Associated for Research and Education in Pathology: Tumors of the peripheral nervous system. Washington, DC: Armed Forces Institute of Pathology, 1999. (Universities Associated for Research, Education in Pathology, eds. Atlas of tumor pathology. Third series; fasc. 24.)

117. Kioumehr F, Rooholamini SA, Yaghmai I, et al. Giant-cell tumor of the sphenoid bone: case report and review of the literature. Can Assoc Radiol J 1990;41(3):155–157.

118. Weber AL, Hug EB, Muenter MW, Curtin HD. Giant-cell tumors of the sphenoid bone in four children: radiological, clinical, and pathological findings. Skull Base Surg 1997;4:163–173.

119. Rhea JT, Weber AL. Giant-cell granuloma of the sinuses. Radiology 1983;147(1):135–137.

120. Som PM, Lawson W, Cohen BA. Giant-cell lesions of the facial bones. Radiology 1983;147(1):129–134.

121. Rogers LF, Mikhael M, Christ M, Wolff A. Case report 276. Giant cell (reparative) granuloma of the sphenoid bone. Skeletal Radiol 1984;12(1):48–53.
122. Lewis ML, Weber AL, McKenna MJ. Reparative cell granuloma of the temporal bone. Ann Otol Rhinol Laryngol 1994;103(10):826–828.
123. Nemoto Y, Inoue Y, Tashiro T, et al. Central giant cell granuloma of the temporal bone. AJNR 1995;16(Suppl4):982–985.
124. Sampson JH, Rossitch E, Young JN, et al. Solitary eosinophilic granuloma. Neurosurgery 1992;31:755.
125. Hermans R, DeFoer B, Smet MH, et al. Eosinophilic granuloma of the head and neck. Pediatr Radiol 1994;24:33.
126. Brisman, Feldstein, Tarbell, et al. Eosinophilic granuloma of the clivus. Neurosurgery 1997;41:273–279.
127. Ashkan K, Pollock J, D'Arrigo C, Kitchen ND. Intracranial osteosarcomas: report of four cases and review of the literature [see comments]. J Neurooncol 1998;40(1):87–96.
128. Whitehead RE, Melhem ER, Kasznica J, Eustace S. Telangiectatic osteosarcoma of the skull base. AJNR 1998;19(4):754–757.
129. Rushing EJ, White JA, D'Alise MD, et al. Primary epithelioid hemangioendothelioma of the clivus. Clin Neuropathol 1998;17(2):110–114.
130. Rajshekhar V, Chandy MJ. Haemangioma of the skull base producing basilar impression. Br J Neurosurg 1989;3(2):229–233.
131. Anavi Y, Sabes WR, Mintz S. Gorham's disease affecting the maxillofacial skeleton. Head Neck 1989;11(6):550–557.
132. Frankel DG, Lewin JS, Cohen B. Massive osteolysis of the skull base. Pediatr Radiol 1997;27(3):265–267.
133. Gorham LW, Wright AW, Schultz HH, Maxon FC. Disappearing bones: a rare form of massive osteolysis. Am J Med 1954;17(5):674–682.
134. Heffez L, Doku HC, Carter BL, Feeney JE. Perspectives on massive osteolysis. Report of a case and review of the literature. Oral Surg Oral Med Oral Pathol 1983;55(4):331–343.
135. Jackson JBS. A boneless arm. Boston Med Surg J 1838;10:368–369.
136. Mawk JR, Obukhov SK, Nichols WD, et al. Successful conservative management of Gorham disease of the skull base and cervical spine. Childs Nerv Syst 1997;13(11–12):622–625.
137. Murphy JB, Doku HC, Carter BL. Massive osteolysis: phantom bone disease. J Oral Surg 1978;36(4):318–322.
138. Lanzieri CF, Shah M, Krauss D, Lavertu P. Use of gadolinium-enhanced MR imaging for differentiating mucoceles from neoplasms in the paranasal sinuses. Radiology 1991;178(2):425–428.
139. Chambers E, Rosenbaum A, Norman O, et al. Traumatic aneurysm of cavernous internal carotid artery, secondary epistaxis. AJNR 1981;2:405–409.
140. Atlas S, Grossman R, Goldberg H, et al. Partially thrombosed giant intracranial aneurysm: correlation of MR and pathologic findings. Radiology 1987;162:111–114.
141. Fisher A, Som P, Mosesson R, et al. Giant intracranial aneurysms with skull base erosion and extracranial masses: CT and MR findings. JCAT 1994;18:939–942.
142. Lederman M. Cancer of the Nasopharynx: Its Natural History and Treatment. Springfield, Ill: Charles C Thomas, 1961.
143. Chong VF, Mukherji SK, Ng SH, et al. Nasopharyngeal carcinoma: review of how imaging affects staging. JCAT 1999;23(6):984–993.
144. Malogolowkin M, Ortega J. Rhabdomyosarcoma of childhood. Pediatr Ann 1988;17(4):251–257.
145. Ballantyne A, McCarten A, Ibanez M. The extension of cancer of the head and neck through peripheral nerves. Am J Surg 1963;106:651–654.
146. Conley J, Dingman DL. Adenoid cystic carcinoma in the head and neck (cylindroma). Arch Otolaryngol 1974;100(2):81–90.
147. Dodd G, Dolan P, Ballantyne A, et al. The dissemination of tumors of the head and neck via the cranial nerves. Radiol Clin North Am 1970;8(3):445–453.
148. Spiro R, Huvos A, Strong E. Adenoid cystic carcinoma of salivary origin: a clinicopathologic study of 242 cases. Am J Surg 1974;128:512–520.
149. Laine F, Braun I, Jensen M, et al. Perineural tumor extension through the foramen ovale: evaluation with MR imaging. Radiology 1990;174:65–71.
150. Curtin H, Williams R, Johnson J. CT of perineural tumor extension: pterygopalatine fossa. AJNR 1984;5:731–737.
151. Nemzek WR, Hecht S, Gandour-Edwards R, et al. Perineural spread of head and neck tumors: how accurate is MR imaging? AJNR 1998;19(4):701–706.
152. Curtin HD. Detection of perineural spread: fat is a friend [editorial; comment]. AJNR 1998;19(8):1385–1386.
153. Williams LS. Advanced concepts in the imaging of perineural spread of tumor to the trigeminal nerve. Top Magn Reson Imaging 1999;10(6):376–383.
154. Ghobrial W, Amstutz S, Mathog R. Fractures of the sphenoid bone. Head Neck Surg 1986;8:447–451.
155. Gurdjian E, Webster J. Head Injuries: Mechanism, Diagnosis, and Management. Boston: Little, Brown, 1958.
156. McLaurin R, McLennan J. Diagnosis and treatment of head injury in children. In: Youmans J, ed. Neurological Surgery. 2nd ed. Philadelphia: WB Saunders, 1982;2084–2136.
157. Thomas L. Skull fractures. In: Wilkins R, Rengachary S, eds. Neurosurgery. New York: McGraw-Hill, 1985;1623–1626.
158. Manfredi S, Raji M, Sprinkle P, et al. Computerized tomographic scan findings in facial fractures associated with blindness. Plast Reconstr Surg 1981;68:479–482.
159. Taybi H, Lachman RS. Radiology of Syndromes, Metabolic Disorders, and Skeletal Dysplasias. 4th ed. St. Louis: CV Mosby, 1996.
160. Resnick D. Diagnosis of Bone and Joint Disorders. 3rd ed. Philadelphia: WB Saunders, 1995.
161. Daffner R, Kirks D, Gehweiler JJ, et al. Computed tomography of fibrous dysplasia. AJR 1982;139:943–946.
162. Fries J. The roentgen features of fibrous dysplasia of the skull and facial bones. AJR 1957;77:71–75.
163. Leeds N, Seaman W. Fibrous dysplasia of the skull and its differential diagnosis. Radiology 1962;78:570–578.
164. Casselman J, DeJonge I, Neyt L, et al. MRI in craniofacial fibrous dysplasia. Neuroradiology 1993;35:234–237.
165. Olmsted WW. Some skeletogenic lesions with common calvarial manifestations. Radiol Clin North Am 1981;19(4):703–713.
166. Smith J, Botet JF, Yeh SD. Bone sarcomas in Paget disease: a study of 85 patients. Radiology 1984;152(3):583–590.
167. Beighton P, Durr L, Hamersma H. Clinical features of sclerosteosis: a review of the manifestations in 25 affected individuals. Ann Intern Med 1976;84:393–397.
168. Beighton P, Hamersma H, Horan F. Craniometaphyseal dysplasia: variability of expression within a large family. Clin Genet 1979;15:252–258.
169. Hamersma H. Facial nerve paralysis in the osteopetroses. In: Fisch V, ed. Proceedings of the 3rd Symposium on Facial Nerve Surgery. Zurich: 1976;555–576.
170. Applegate L, Applegate G, Kemp S. MR of multiple cranial neuropathies in a patient with Camurati-Engelmann disease: case report. AJNR 1991;12:557–559.
171. Shetty PG, Shroff MM, Fatterpekar GM, et al. A retrospective analysis of spontaneous sphenoid sinus fistula: MR and CT findings. AJNR 2000;21(2):337–342.
172. Stone JA, Castillo M, Neelon B, Mukherji SK. Evaluation of CSF leaks: high-resolution CT compared with contrast-enhanced CT and radionuclide cisternography. AJNR 1999;20(4):706–712.
173. Drayer B, Wilkins R, Boehnke M, et al. Cerebrospinal fluid rhinorrhea demonstrated by metrizamide CT cisternography. AJR 1977;129:149–152.

— *13* —

# Imaging of Perineural Tumor Spread in Head and Neck Cancer

*Lawrence E. Ginsberg*

## INTRODUCTION

In malignancies of the head and neck, tumor may spread along the neural sheath (via the endoneurium, perineurium, or perineural lymphatics) by a process known as perineural tumor spread (PNS). PNS most commonly occurs in a retrograde direction, toward the central nervous system, but also can occur in an antegrade manner. Early in the twentieth century there were scattered reports of this phenomenon.[1] The first comprehensive report on PNS was the frequently referenced work by A.J. Ballantyne et al., while in the imaging literature, the landmark article was by Dodd et al., who reported the plain film imaging findings in 40 patients.[2, 3] Despite the fact that PNS is well known, it remains a vexing clinical problem because it may be clinically silent and because it is often missed at imaging.

## PERINEURAL INVASION VERSUS PERINEURAL SPREAD

It is important to distinguish between perineural invasion and perineural spread, as there is some confusion in the literature concerning the use of the term *perineural*. Perineural *invasion* is the microscopic finding of tumor cells surrounding very small nerve branches, and as such it cannot be seen on imaging.[4] It is an ominous prognostic sign associated with an increased local recurrence rate and decreased survival.[5, 6] This chapter is concerned with macroscopic or large nerve PNS, in which there is gross tumor spread, sometimes over a considerable length of the nerve.

Since PNS may be asymptomatic, it is critical that radiologists be vigilant in their efforts to detect it prior to the institution of therapy. The finding of PNS may convert a lesion thought to be resectable into a nonresectable one. The presence of PNS may also mean that radiation fields need to be expanded to encompass the tumor spread. In the case of a parotid tumor, the finding of PNS may indicate that a temporal bone resection with a partial facial nerve resection may be needed to ensure a tumor-free margin along the facial nerve.

As mentioned, failure to diagnose PNS may have grave implications, particularly if the mode of therapy fails to address the disease extension along the nerve. Such failure virtually guarantees a tumor recurrence, which actually represents a progression of undetected residual disease. Furthermore, failure to recognize PNS on imaging studies is a not infrequent cause of legal action against radiologists. Reasons for failing to diagnose PNS include lack of familiarity with the types of cancers that commonly are associated with it, lack of familiarity with the common routes and imaging appearance of PNS, and inadequate imaging.

## THE MOST COMMON ANATOMIC LOCATIONS AND TUMOR HISTOLOGIES ASSOCIATED WITH PNS

Though virtually any head and neck malignancy may be associated with PNS, certain primary sites and cancer types are clearly more likely to spread along the perineural route. Cutaneous malignancies, particularly squamous cell carcinomas and desmoplastic melanomas, tend to be associated with PNS, and such tumor spread is often associated with a recurrence of skin cancer.[6–10] Although these tumors may occur anywhere on the face, there is a predilection for the side of the nose and the lower lip, areas supplied by the maxillary division of the trigeminal nerve ($V_2$).[11, 12]

Mucosal primaries such as squamous cell carcinoma and especially minor salivary gland cancers such as adenoid cystic carcinoma are also associated with PNS.[13–16] In particular, primary tumors in the palate may gain direct access to the palatine nerves that innervate these mucosal surfaces, while nasopharyngeal tumors may spread to $V_2$ via extension into the pterygopalatine fossa (PPF) or to $V_3$ via extension into the masticator space.[13, 14, 17]

Virtually any salivary gland cancer, especially those arising in the parotid gland, may be associated with PNS. In such cases, although the facial nerve is at greatest risk for PNS, the auriculotemporal branch of the mandibular nerve may also provide a route for PNS.[13, 18] Another clinical setting involving the parotid gland that may result in PNS is either direct tumor extension or intraparotid metastases from an adjacent primary or recurrent skin cancer.[13, 19]

In addition to the cancers just mentioned, other malignancies, regardless of their histology or primary location, may also be associated with PNS if they involve anatomic sites such as the masticator space, PPF, or cavernous sinus/ Meckel's cave.[13] For reasons that are unclear, cancers in certain locations do not often spread along perineural pathways. These sites include the submandibular gland, tongue, buccal mucosa, tonsil, larynx, pharynx, and floor of the mouth. Exceptions at these locations may occur, particularly if the tumor has extended to one of the areas mentioned that are associated with PNS.

## SIGNS AND SYMPTOMS ASSOCIATED WITH PNS

The signs and symptoms most commonly associated with PNS include pain, paresthesias, numbness, formication (the sensation of ants and worms under the skin), and motor denervation weakness. The last is most often encountered as either facial paralysis or masticator muscle weakness when the facial nerve and $V_3$, respectively, are involved.[13, 19] Although microscopic perineural invasion may have similar symptoms, PNS should be considered when the neurologic symptoms suggest broader involvement than would be expected based on the location of the lesion (e.g., a small facial skin cancer with multiple divisions of the affected trigeminal nerve). Multiple cranial neuropathies are also an ominous finding, suggesting either PNS proximal to the cavernous sinus, tumor spread from one cranial nerve to another, or leptomeningeal disease.[7, 11] While the above-mentioned symptoms may suggest PNS, up to 40% of patients with PNS have either nonspecific symptoms or are asymptomatic.[7, 19, 20–22]

## COMMON CLINICAL SETTINGS ASSOCIATED WITH PNS

In addition to the presence of a primary tumor in a high-risk location, there are postoperative clinical settings that are associated with PNS. These include the development of a cranial neuropathy in a patient who has had a previously resected tumor, with or without an obvious local recurrence.[7, 10, 11, 22] A typical history is that of a previous resection of a skin lesion thought either to be benign or malignant (often the specimen is no longer available for review, and occasionally the patient may not remember the surgery) associated with a new neurologic deficit along the corresponding branch of the trigeminal nerve or a more generalized trigeminal neuropathy.[10] Another common scenario is the development of a facial nerve paralysis in a patient who has had a prior resection of a parotid mass. Such histories should prompt a careful imaging search for PNS, and it is important that these patients not simply be diagnosed as having ''Bell's palsy'' or ''trigeminal neuralgia'' until more sinister causes are excluded.[10]

Unfortunately, the radiologist may not be aware that a lesion was previously resected, and the appropriate history must be specifically sought. On the other hand, if a neurologic deficit was caused by therapy or the initial presentation of the primary lesion, the patient may not report any new symptoms. Thus, if parotidectomy resulted in a facial nerve palsy, postoperative imaging may be the only way to establish the presence of PNS prior to the onset of additional cranial neuropathies.

Lastly, though rare, evidence of PNS may present clinically prior to detection of the associated primary cancer.[23] This might occur with an asymptomatic, submucosal, slow-growing tumor such as an adenoid cystic carcinoma. Several such tumors arising in the palate with PNS to the cavernous sinus have been reported.[23] Thus, an important corollary in the setting of no known primary tumor is that any patient who presents with a mass in one of the common proximal locations associated with PNS (the PPF, Meckel's cave, or the cavernous sinus) should have a careful clinical and radiologic evaluation for a primary clinically silent head and neck malignancy.

## ANATOMIC NEUROLOGIC CONSIDERATIONS

The cranial nerves most often involved in PNS from head and neck cancer are the trigeminal and facial nerves.[13, 15] Rarely, spinal nerve branches may be affected. In order to recognize PNS when it is visible on imaging studies, the radiologist must be familiar with the cranial nerve anatomy, including the branches that innervate a particular head and neck location and the proximal course of those nerves.

### Ophthalmic Division of the Trigeminal Nerve (V₁)

The ophthalmic division of the trigeminal nerve (V₁) is uncommonly affected by PNS.[24–26] This nerve provides purely sensory innervation to the eye, lacrimal gland, conjunctiva, part of the nasal mucosa, and skin of the nose, eyelids, forehead, and scalp.[27] Figure 13-1 depicts the anatomy of the ophthalmic nerve. After emerging from the Gasserian ganglion in Meckel's cave, the ophthalmic nerve courses through the cavernous sinus, passes through the superior orbital fissure to enter the orbit, and then divides into the nasociliary, lacrimal, and frontal nerves (Fig. 13-1).

The frontal nerve is the largest branch; it divides into a smaller supratrochlear branch and a larger supraorbital branch (Fig. 13-1). The supratrochlear nerve runs anteromedially and exits the orbit to provide cutaneous innervation to the medial supraorbital region and the lower forehead near the midline. Cutaneous cancers in this region may have PNS along the supratrochlear nerve (Fig. 13-2). The supraorbital nerve courses anteriorly between the levator palpebrae and the orbital roof and then exits the orbit, where it divides into medial and lateral branches (Fig. 13-1). These branches provides sensory innervation to the scalp in the immediate supraorbital region and as far back as the lambdoidal suture.[27] Small branches also supply innervation to the frontal sinus mucosa and the pericranium. The supraorbital nerve is also at risk for PNS when a skin cancer arises in its region of innervation.

The lacrimal nerve provides innervation to the lacrimal gland, having first received a twig from the zygomaticotemporal nerve, which is a small branch of V₂ (containing postganglionic parasympathetic innervation from the pterygopalatine ganglion, originating in the greater superficial petrosal nerve, a branch of the facial nerve).[27] The nasociliary nerve provides small branches that innervate the frontal dura and the nasoethmoid mucosa. While it is theoretically possible that cancers along the distribution of these nerves (lacrimal gland, nasoethmoid, etc.) could be associated with retrograde PNS, such cases have not been reported.

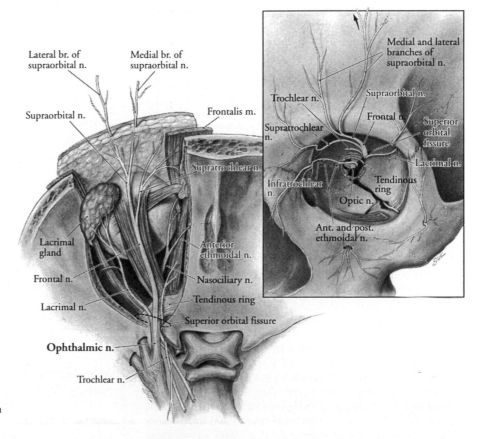

**FIGURE 13-1**   Diagrammatic representation of ophthalmic nerve (V₁) anatomy.

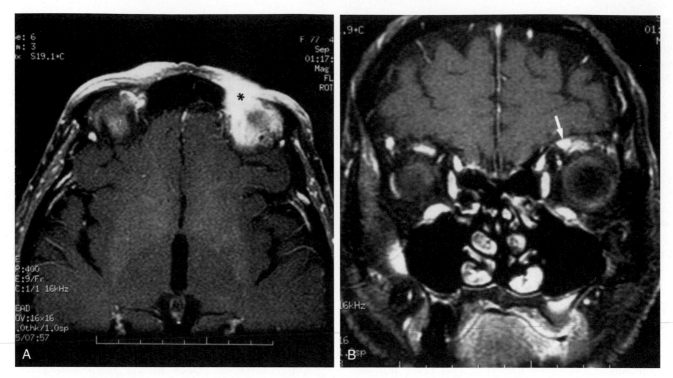

**FIGURE 13-2** Squamous cell carcinoma in the left medial supraorbital region with PNS along the supratrochlear branch of the ophthalmic nerve. **A,** Contrast-enhanced axial T1-weighted MR image with fat suppression shows enhancing tumor in the left supraorbital region (*asterisk*). **B,** Contrast-enhanced coronal T1-weighted MR image with fat suppression shows thickening and abnormal enhancement of the supratrochlear branch of the ophthalmic nerve (*arrow*) just medial to the normally enhancing superior muscle complex.

## Maxillary Division of the Trigeminal Nerve ($V_2$)

The maxillary division of the trigeminal nerve ($V_2$) provides sensory innervation to the skin of the midface, the mucosa of the palate, sinonasal region, and maxillary gingiva, and the maxillary teeth. Figure 13-3 depicts the anatomy of the maxillary nerve. The maxillary nerve courses through the cavernous sinus and then through the foramen rotundum to enter the PPF. Within the PPF, the maxillary nerve gives rise to several palatine branches as well as the zygomatic nerve. The palatine nerves course inferiorly through the greater and lesser palatine foramina to innervate the hard and soft palates, respectively.[14] The zygomatic nerve enters the orbit through the inferior orbital fissure, runs along the lateral orbital wall, and divides into the zygomaticofacial and zygomaticotemporal branches.[27] The zygomaticotemporal nerve sends a small twig to the lacrimal nerve, as mentioned earlier. Both the zygomaticotemporal and zygomaticofacial nerves exit the orbit through its lateral wall and supply innervation to the skin of the temporal region and lateral cheek (Fig. 13-3).[27] Also within the PPF, the maxillary nerve gives off the posterior superior alveolar nerve to the maxillary sinus.

More distally, the maxillary nerve enters the infraorbital canal as the infraorbital nerve and gives off the anterior and middle superior alveolar nerves to the maxillary teeth and gingiva. The infraorbital nerve then emerges from the infraorbital foramen and divides into its terminal branches, supplying the skin of the midfacial region and lateral nose (Fig. 13-3). Proximal or retrograde PNS from any of these

innervated sites can occur along the respective distal branches of $V_2$, generally eventually involving the PPF.[28] Thus, tumors arising in the cheek are at particularly high risk of PNS along the infraorbital nerve, often with tumor in the PPF (Figs. 13-4, 13-5).[6, 8, 10, 13, 22, 28]

Skin cancers in the temporal region and upper lateral face may spread to the orbit via the zygomatic nerve (Fig. 13-5). A palate lesion can spread along the palatine nerves and then to the PPF (Figs. 13-6, 13-7).[14] Maxillary sinus tumors may have PNS along the superior alveolar nerves to enter the PPF.[28] If a nasopharyngeal carcinoma has extended into the nasal cavity, it may spread laterally through the sphenopalatine foramen to enter the PPF (Fig. 13-8).[13, 17] Once in the PPF, retrograde PNS can occur along the main trunk of $V_2$ through the foramen rotundum, with subsequent involvement of the cavernous sinus and Meckel's cave or even the more proximal main trigeminal nerve trunk (Figs. 13-7, 13-8).[13, 15, 28]

Once tumor is in the PPF, PNS may also occur along the vidian nerve (or nerve of the pterygoid canal) (Fig. 13-9).[13, 14, 29, 30] Antegrade PNS may occur once the PPF is involved. Commonly this occurs along branches of $V_2$, especially the infraorbital nerve (Fig. 13-7C).[3, 13, 15, 28] Once tumor has spread into Meckel's cave, antegrade PNS may also occur along $V_3$ (Fig. 13-7D).

## Mandibular Division of the Trigeminal Nerve ($V_3$)

The mandibular division of the trigeminal nerve ($V_3$) provides sensory innervation to the skin of the lower face

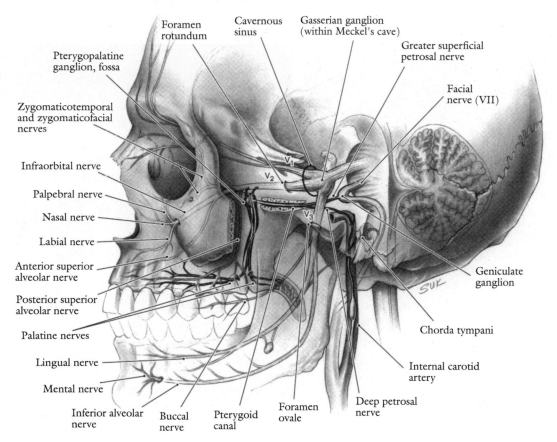

**FIGURE 13-3** Diagrammatic representation of $V_2$ and $V_3$ anatomy. (From Ginsberg LE. Imaging of perineural tumor spread in head and neck cancer. Semin Ultrasound CT MR 1999;2:175–186.)

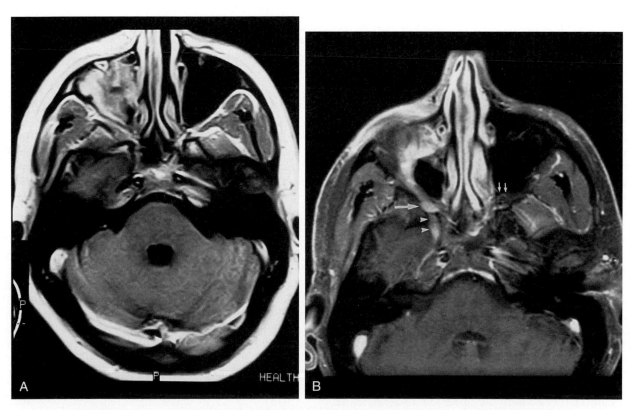

**FIGURE 13-4** Squamous cell carcinoma in the right infraorbital region with PNS along the infraorbital branch of the maxillary nerve ($V_2$). **A,** Axial contrast-enhanced MR image without fat suppression. It is almost impossible to identify tumor within the right PPF. This scan was performed at an outside institution, and there was no precontrast T1-weighted imaging to help evaluate the PPF. **B,** Axial contrast-enhanced MR image with fat suppression allows visualization of excessive enhancement representing PNS in the right PPF (*long arrow*). Note the lack of significant enhancement in the normal left PPF (*short arrows*). On the right side, there is continued posterior or retrograde PNS within the foramen rotundum (*arrowheads*).

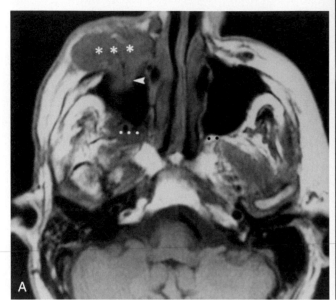
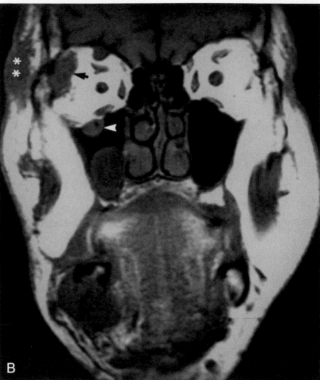

**FIGURE 13-5**   Recurrent desmoplastic melanoma in multiple facial locations with PNS along the zygomatic and infraorbital branches of the maxillary nerve (V₂). **A,** Axial T1-weighted MR image shows large right-sided cheek recurrence (*asterisks*) spreading posteriorly along the infraorbital nerve (*arrowhead*). Tumor can be seen widening and replacing the expected hyperintense fat within the right PPF (*white dots*). Note the normal hyperintense fat in the left PPF (*black dots*). **B,** Coronal T1-weighted MR image shows a grossly enlarged right infraorbital nerve representing perineural spread (*arrowhead*). Note the right-sided tumor recurrence in the temporal region (*asterisks*). The lateral intraorbital mass (*arrow*) likely represents PNS along the zygomaticotemporal/ zygomaticofacial branches of V₂ (see Fig. 13-3). (From Ginsberg LE. Imaging of perineural tumor spread in head and neck cancer. Semin Ultrasound CT MR 1999;2:175–186.)

and the preauricular/temporal region, the mandibular teeth, and the mucosa of the mandibular gingiva, floor of the mouth, the tongue (anterior two thirds), and the buccal mucosa.[27] The mandibular nerve also provides motor innervation to the muscles of mastication and the mylohyoid and anterior belly of the digastric muscles. Figures 13-3 and 13-10 depict the anatomy of V₃. Exiting Meckel's cave, the mandibular nerve avoids the cavernous sinus and courses inferiorly through the foramen ovale to enter the masticator space, where it divides into anterior and posterior trunks. The anterior trunk primarily gives rise to motor branches (for the masseter, temporalis, and pterygoid muscles). The posterior trunk gives rise to the auriculotemporal and inferior alveolar nerves, branches commonly associated with PNS, and the lingual nerve, which is seldom associated with PNS.

The auriculotemporal nerve, depicted in Figure 13-10, arises just below the foramen ovale and provides cutaneous innervation to a broad area of the lateral and upper face. It also provides postganglionic parasympathetic innervation to the parotid gland though the fibers that originate in the facial and glossopharyngeal nerves as the lesser superficial petrosal nerve.[27, 31] The lesser superficial petrosal nerve has a very complicated course, but ultimately it synapses in the otic ganglion just beneath the foramen ovale and then uses

the auriculotemporal nerve as a conduit to reach the parotid gland.[31]

The inferior alveolar nerve enters the mandible via the mandibular foramen on the medial surface of the mandibular ramus and provides sensory innervation to the mandibular teeth and gingiva. It terminates as the mental nerve, which exits the mental foramen in the anterior mandibular body and provides cutaneous innervation to the lower lip and chin.

Tumors in any anatomic location supplied by V₃ can have retrograde PNS, ultimately involving the main trunk of the mandibular nerve within the masticator space. Tumor may then spread upward through the foramen ovale to eventually affect Meckel's cave.[13, 15, 18, 20] Thus, a skin cancer of the lower lip or chin can spread along the mental nerve to involve the inferior alveolar branch of V₃ and the main trunk of V₃, and ultimately extend through the foramen ovale (Figs. 13-11, 13-12).[11, 13] Parotid or lateral facial tumors can spread along the auriculotemporal branch of V₃ and thus gain access to the main trunk of the mandibular nerve (Fig. 13-13).[13, 15, 18] Any tumor originating within or spreading to the masticator space may have PNS along the mandibular nerve and extend through the foramen ovale (Figs. 13-14, 13-15). As mentioned, once tumor affects Meckel's cave, it can spread posteriorly along the main trigeminal trunk (Figs.

13-12, 13-15). Antegrade PNS may also occur from Meckel's cave to involve the cavernous sinus and subsequently $V_2$ (Fig. 13-12) or $V_3$ (Fig. 13-7D).

## Facial Nerve

The anatomy of the facial nerve is complicated and need not be covered here in its entirety (see Chapters 19, 20, and 21). Diagrammatic representations of the facial nerve can be found in Figures 13-3, 13-17, and 13-20. Almost always, PNS involving the facial nerve occurs with malignancies that arise in the parotid origin or with nearby skin cancers that secondarily invade or metastasize to the parotid gland. These lesions may have PNS along the distal facial nerve (Fig. 13-16).[3, 13, 15] Tumor may then spread along the facial nerve to involve the posterior genu, horizontal or tympanic segment, geniculate ganglion, labyrinthine segment, or ultimately the intracanalicular portion within the internal auditory canal (Fig. 13-16). Less commonly, PNS may

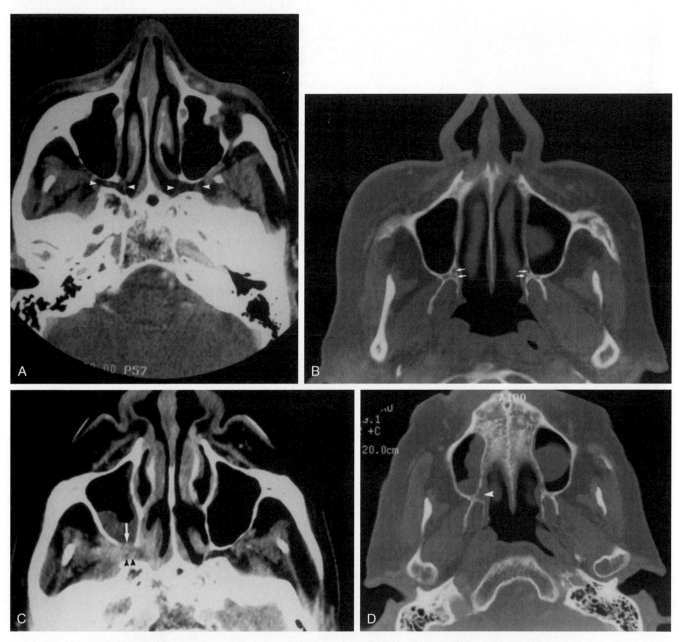

**FIGURE 13 6**    Squamous cell carcinoma of the right soft palate with development of perineural spread along the palatine nerves. Axial contrast-enhanced soft-tissue (**A**) and bone window (**B**) CT scans at the time of diagnosis of the palate lesion. The PPFs (*arrowheads*) are normal. On the bone window images through the pterygoid plates, the palatine foramen are normal (*arrows*). The palatine branches of $V_2$ traverse these foramina en route to/from the palate and PPF. Axial contrast-enhanced soft-tissue (**C**) and bone window (**D**) CT scans at levels similar to those of **A** and **B** obtained 3 months later. There is abnormal widening and enhancement representing PNS within the right PPF (*arrowheads*). The posterior wall of the right maxillary sinus is destroyed (*arrow*). On the bone windows, the right palatine foramina are now destroyed (*arrowhead*). Compare with **B**. (From Ginsberg LE, DeMonte F. Imaging of perineural tumor spread from palatal carcinoma. AJNR 1998;19: 1417–1422.)

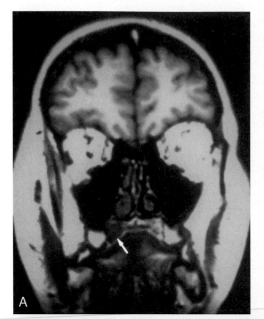

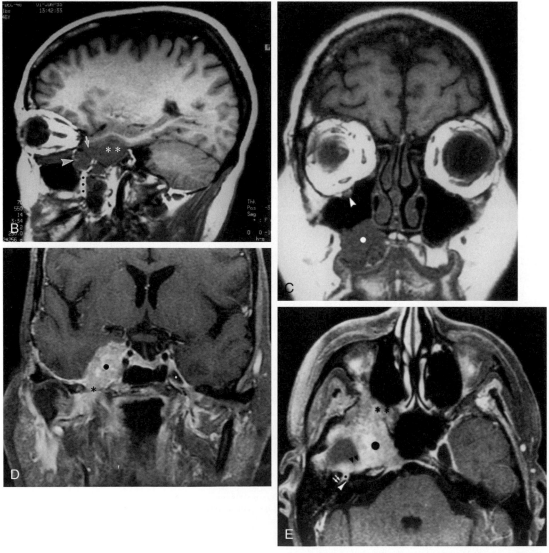

**FIGURE 13-7** Adenoid cystic carcinoma of the right hard palate initially presenting with multiple cranial nerve palsies secondary to PNS to the cavernous sinus. **A,** Coronal T1-weighted MR image from brain MR imaging at the time of initial presentation shows a subtle submucosal mass in the right hard palate (*arrow*). This lesion was not appreciated clinically or radiographically. **B,** Sagittal T1-weighted MR image from the same study as **A** shows a large mass in the cavernous sinus (*asterisks*), in the foramen rotundum (*arrow*), and in the upper aspect of the PPF (*arrowhead*). Note that the fat in the lower PPF is normal (*black dots*), indicating a skip lesion from the palatal primary. Because the primary lesion went unnoticed, radiotherapy to the cavernous sinus was the sole therapy. **C to E,** MR images obtained 2 years after presentation. The patient now had recurrence of cranial neuropathies including a new right facial nerve paralysis. **C,** Coronal T1-weighted MR image shows that the right palatal primary lesion is much larger (*white dot*). Note the enlargement of the right infraorbital nerve, indicating antegrade perineural tumor spread. **D,** Coronal contrast-enhanced, fat-suppressed MR image shows massive tumor in Meckel's cave (*black dot*) with downward antegrade PNS through a widened foramen ovale (*asterisk*). Note the normal Meckel's cave on the left side (*white dot*) with peripheral but not central enhancement. **E,** Axial contrast-enhanced, fat-suppressed MR image shows massive tumor in the cavernous sinus and Meckel's cave (*large black dot*) and the PPF (*asterisks*). Tumor is also extending posterolaterally along the greater superficial petrosal nerve (*black arrowheads*), through the facial hiatus, and into the geniculate ganglion (*small black dot*). There is further tumor spread involving the labyrinthine (*white arrowhead*) and horizontal or tympanic segment (*white arrows*) of the right facial nerve. This latter finding accounts for the patient's facial nerve paralysis. (A, B, and D from Ginsberg LE, DeMonte F. Imaging of perineural tumor spread from palatal carcinoma. AJNR 1998;19:1417–1422. From Ginsberg LE, DeMonte F. Palatal adenoid cystic carcinoma presenting as perineural spread to the cavernous sinus. Skull Base Surg 1998;8(1):39–43.)

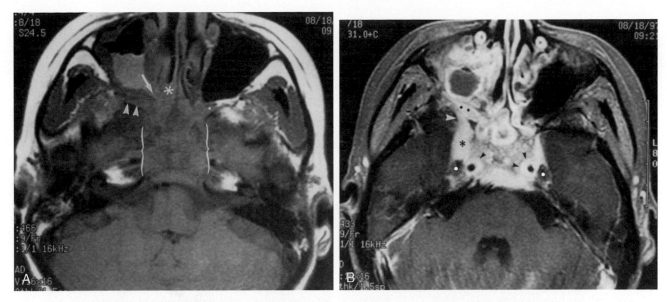

**FIGURE 13-8**   Nasopharyngeal carcinoma with $V_2$ perineural spread. **A**, Axial T1-weighted MR image shows tumor in the right nasal cavity (*asterisk*) with lateral extension through a widened sphenopalatine foramen (*arrow*) involving the right PPF (*arrowheads*). To a lesser extent, the left PPF is similarly affected (*white dot*). Note that the central skull base is diffusely infiltrated by tumor (*brackets*). **B**, Axial contrast-enhanced, fat-suppressed T1-weighted MR image shows enhancement of all tumor components including the right PPF (*black dots*). Tumor is extending posteriorly along the right maxillary nerve through the foramen rotundum (*white arrowhead*) to involve the cavernous sinus (*asterisk*). The left cavernous sinus is also infiltrated by tumor, which could have arrived there along the internal carotid artery, a common route of spread in nasopharyngeal cancer. Note the subtle abnormal enhancement surrounding the cavernous segment of both internal carotid arteries (*black arrowheads*). Bilaterally, Meckel's caves remain intact, with CSF signal intensity and no enhancement centrally (*white dots*). (From Ginsberg LE. Imaging of perineural tumor spread in head and neck cancer. Semin Ultrasound CT MR 1999;2:175–186.)

involve the facial nerve from a small facial nerve branch, the greater superficial petrosal nerve.

## Interconnections Between the Trigeminal and Other Cranial Nerves

As alluded to earlier, small distal branches of the trigeminal nerve serve as terminal conduits for branches of other cranial nerves, primarily the facial nerve. This relationship has implications for PNS, and many of these interconnections are depicted in Figure 13-17. The most important of these connections involves the greater superficial petrosal nerve (GSPN). This nerve is a branch of the facial nerve that provides parasympathetic innervation to the lacrimal gland, palate, nasal cavity, and nasopharynx.[27, 30] The anatomy of the GSPN is depicted in Figures 13-3, 13-17, and 13-18. Facial nerve fibers, originating in the nervus intermedius, leave the geniculate ganglion as the GSPN. Exiting from the superior surface of the temporal bone through a small foramen known as the facial hiatus (Fig. 13-19), the intracranial segment of the GSPN courses medially and anteroinferiorly along the surface of the petrous bone to the foramen lacerum. There it joins the deep petrosal nerve of the sympathetic carotid plexus to enter the vidian or pterygoid canal as the vidian nerve or nerve of the pterygoid canal (Fig. 13-3).[30] Upon exiting the vidian canal, this nerve enters the PPF, where the preganglionic fibers synapse in the sphenopalatine (pterygopalatine) ganglion. In the PPF, some of the postganglionic fibers join the palatine

nerves (branches of $V_2$) and course inferiorly to the hard and soft palates (Fig. 13-17).[14] Other postganglionic parasympathetic fibers from the sphenopalatine ganglion supply secretomotor and vasomotor innervation to the nasal cavity and lacrimal gland via other branches of $V_2$ (Fig. 13-17).[30]

While it is theoretically possible that a lacrimal malignancy could spread via the fibers that connect it to the GSPN, this has not been reported. In practical terms, PNS along the GSPN usually occurs after any tumor reaches the PPF. Via PNS, the tumor gains access to the vidian nerve, and then spreads in a retrograde manner along the GSPN and into the geniculate ganglion (Fig. 13-9).[30] Also, as can be seen from Figure 13-18, the GSPN lies immediately beneath Meckel's cave, and as a result of this anatomic relationship, tumor within Meckel's cave may spread to the GSPN and then continue in a retrograde manner (Figs. 13-7, 13-12).[13] In Figure 13-12, a squamous cell carcinoma of the lower lip first spread along the mental and inferior alveolar branches of $V_3$, up through the foramen ovale into Meckel's cave, and then ultimately into the temporal bone and geniculate ganglion via the GSPN (Fig. 13-12).

## Spinal Nerves

In the head and neck, PNS generally involves branches of cranial nerves. However, cutaneous innervation to much of the neck, as well as parts of the face, is provided by branches of the superficial cervical plexus, derived from the ventral divisions of the first four cervical spinal nerves (Fig.

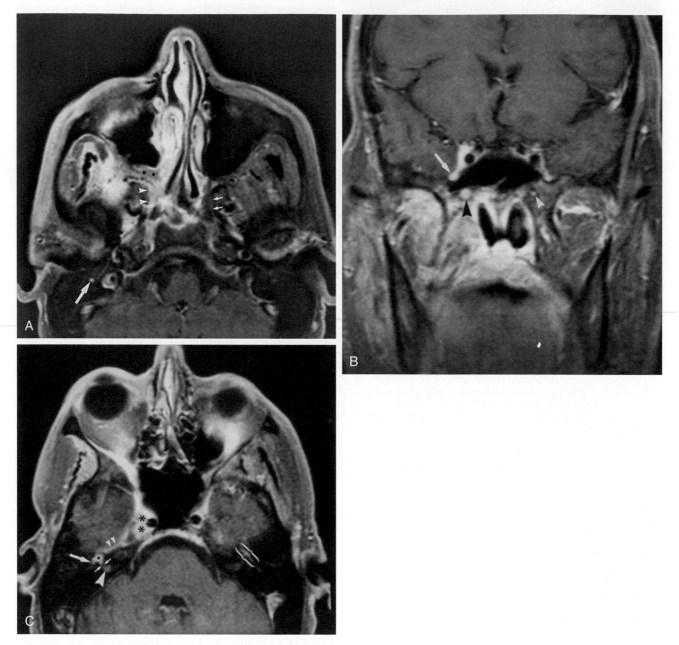

**FIGURE 13-9** Palatal adenoid cystic carcinoma with extensive PNS. This patient was initially believed to have trigeminal neuralgia because of facial pain. A cavernous sinus/Meckel's cave mass was subsequently discovered on MR imaging. The palatal primary was not discovered until much later, and the patient ultimately developed a right-sided facial palsy. **A,** Axial contrast-enhanced, fat-suppressed T1-weighted MR image shows tumor enhancement in the right PPF (*black dots*). There is enlargement and excessive enhancement in the right vidian canal (*arrowheads*) indicating PNS along the vidian nerve. The normal left vidian canal is only faintly seen (*short arrows*). There is probably abnormal enhancement in the descending segment of the right facial nerve (*long arrow*). **B,** Coronal contrast-enhanced, fat-suppressed MR image shows enlargement and excessive enhancement representing PNS in both the right foramen rotundum (*arrow*) and the right vidian canal (*black arrowhead*). The cavernous sinus looks abnormal as well. The left vidian canal shows normal enhancement (*white arrowhead*). **C,** Axial contrast-enhanced, fat-suppressed MR image shows tumor involvement of the right cavernous sinus and the anterior aspect of Meckel's cave (*asterisks*). The greater superficial petrosal nerve courses directly beneath this area, as shown in Figure 13-18. There is abnormal enhancement indicating PNS along the greater superficial petrosal nerve (*small arrowheads*). The geniculate ganglion enhances brightly and is grossly enlarged (*black dot*). There is abnormal enhancement representing continued tumor spread to involve the labyrinthine (*small arrows*), intracanalicular (*large arrowhead*), and proximal tympanic (*large arrow*) segments of the right facial nerve. On the left side, the geniculate ganglion is of normal size (and enhances normally), and only the proximal GSPN and the proximal tympanic segment of the facial nerve enhance (*brackets*). (From Ginsberg LE, DeMonte F, Gillenwater AM. Greater superficial petrosal nerve: anatomy and MR findings in perineural tumor spread. AJNR 1996;17:389–393.)

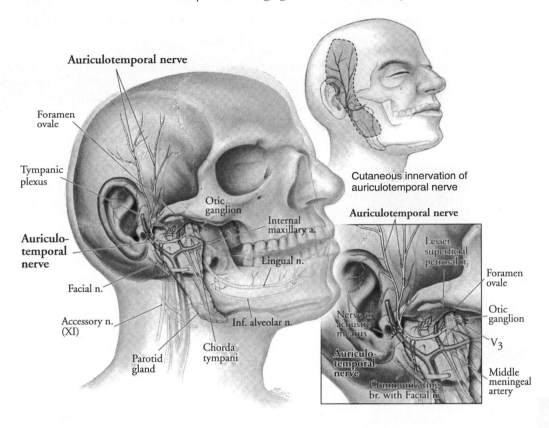

**FIGURE 13-10**    Diagrammatic representation of the auriculotemporal branch of V₃.

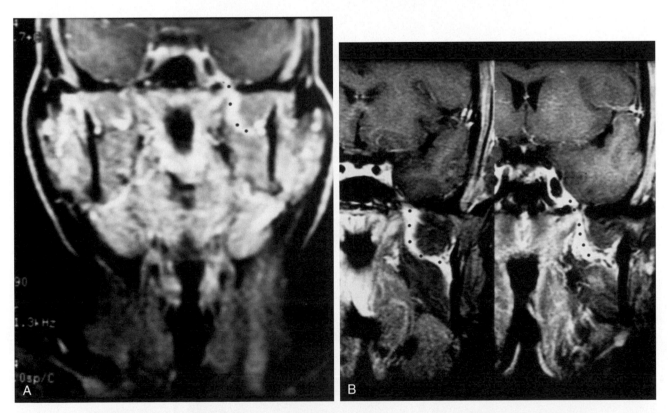

**FIGURE 13-11**    Squamous cell carcinoma of the left lower lip with PNS along the inferior alveolar branch of V₃. **A,** Coronal contrast-enhanced T1-weighted MR image without fat suppression obtained at an outside institution. Though visible, the perineural tumor along the proximal mandibular nerve and foramen ovale is hard to see (*black dots*). **B,** Repeat imaging with fat suppression; the tumor enhancement is far more conspicuous (*black dots*).

13-20).[27, 32] A case of PNS along the great auricular nerve, a branch of this plexus, secondary to a recurrent skin carcinoma in the lower parotid region has been reported (Fig. 13-21).[32] It is possible that cutaneous malignancies in other locations may spread along other branches of the superficial cervical plexus, such as the lesser occipital or transverse cutaneous nerves, and even spread intraspinally.

## IMAGING OF PERINEURAL TUMOR SPREAD

Little is known about the sensitivity and specificity of imaging of PNS, as there are few studies that directly address this issue. Nemzek et al. reported a detection rate of 95% but found that the mapping of the entire extent of PNS

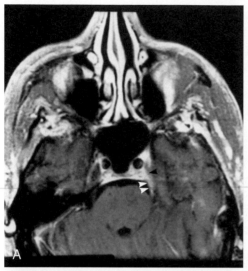

**FIGURE 13-12**    Squamous cell carcinoma of the left lower lip with extensive PNS. The patient had had a lesion resected from his lip 11 months earlier. At the time of recent presentation, the patient not only had neuropathy of the entire trigeminal distribution, but a facial nerve paralysis as well. No local recurrence was clinically apparent. **A,** Axial contrast-enhanced, fat-suppressed MR image at the time of recent presentation shows tumor in Meckel's cave (*black arrow*) and extension of tumor posteriorly along the main trunk of the left trigeminal nerve (*arrowheads*). These findings explain the patient's complete trigeminal neuropathy. However, the facial palsy could not be explained. Although perineural involvement of the greater superficial petrosal nerve and geniculate ganglion was suspected, the imaging was equivocal. Axial T2-weighted (**B**) and contrast-enhanced, fat-suppressed T1-weighted (**C**) MR images show hyperintense signal and abnormal enhancement, respectively, in the left masticator muscles (*arrowheads*). These muscles were not atrophic; this represents subacute denervation secondary to tumor involvement of the proximal mandibular nerve, not tumor within the masticator space. The patient had no trismus, only weakness in opening the mouth. **D** and **E,** Axial contrast-enhanced, fat-suppressed T1-weighted images obtained 3 months after images **A** to **C. D,** Progression of the main trigeminal trunk disease, now directly invading the pons (*arrowhead*), is seen. In **E,** there is tumor involvement of the geniculate ganglion (*black arrow*), proximal tympanic (*arrowhead*), and labyrinthine segments (*white arrow*) of the left facial nerve. This was not visible 3 months previously and helped explain the patient's facial palsy. This facial nerve disease was presumably a skip lesion along the left greater superficial petrosal nerve. In both **D** and **E,** there is probably antegrade PNS to involve the PPF (*black dots*). (From Ginsberg LE. Imaging of perineural tumor spread in head and neck cancer. Semin Ultrasound CT MR 1999;2:175–186.)

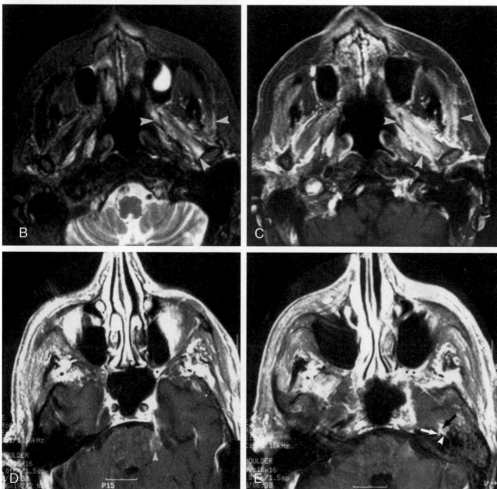

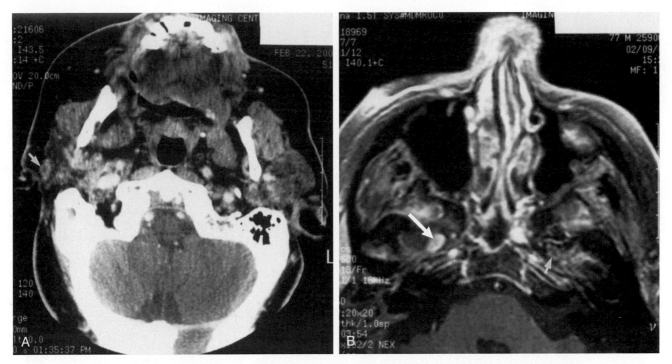

**FIGURE 13-13**   Recurrent preauricular cutaneous squamous cell carcinoma with parotid invasion and PNS along the auriculotemporal branch of $V_3$. **A**, Axial contrast-enhanced CT scan shows tumor in the superficial lobe of the right parotid gland (*arrow*). There was no bulky tumor extending into the masticator space. **B**, Axial contrast-enhanced, fat-suppressed T1-weighted image shows excessive enhancement representing tumor in the foramen ovale (*large arrow*). From the parotid gland, the only way tumor could spread to the foramen ovale is along the auriculotemporal nerve. Note that there is a small amount of normal enhancement in the normal left foramen ovale (*small arrow*).

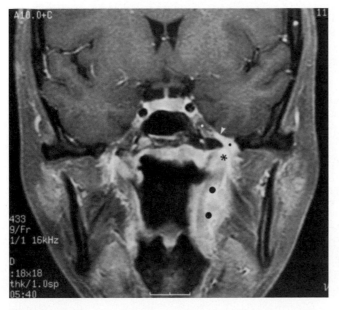

**FIGURE 13-14**   Nasopharyngeal carcinoma with lateral extension to the masticator space and mandibular nerve via PNS. Coronal contrast-enhanced, fat-suppressed T1-weighted image shows the left nasopharyngeal lesion (*large black dots*) with lateral extension to involve the upper masticator space (*asterisk*). Tumor is extending perineurally through the widened foramen ovale (*small black dot*). Although there is tumor in the most proximal aspect of the mandibular nerve (*arrowhead*), Meckel's cave (*white dot*) appears to be spared. (From Ginsberg LE. Imaging of perineural tumor spread in head and neck cancer. Semin Ultrasound CT MR 1999;2:175–186.)

was only 65% accurate.[21] The latter number might have been higher if fat suppression had been employed on the postcontrast sequences used in that study. For the imaging of PNS, sensitivity and specificity are difficult to measure with certainty because, in many cases, the imaging is so suggestive of PNS that biopsy is not performed.

Another factor limiting the imaging sensitivity and specificity for PNS is the imaging technique. Even in the presence of definite PNS, inadequate technique (or artifact, patient motion, etc.) can result in the disease being inconspicuous on the images and therefore not diagnosed. If proper imaging technique is adhered to, the overwhelming majority of PNS can be detected prior to initiating therapy.

## Technical Considerations

One of the most important technical considerations is a knowledge of the indications for the imaging study prior to the examination. This allows the study to be tailored to the specific problem. Often, a CT or MR examination has been performed as a routine brain study with a 23 cm field of view (FOV). In this setting, detection of PNS is compromised, as the FOV is excessive and the images are too small to reveal fine neural structures. Whether the examination is a CT or an MR imaging study, the FOV should be no greater than 18 cm and preferably only 16 cm. Thin slices, 3 to 5 mm, should be obtained. For CT, high-resolution bone algorithm

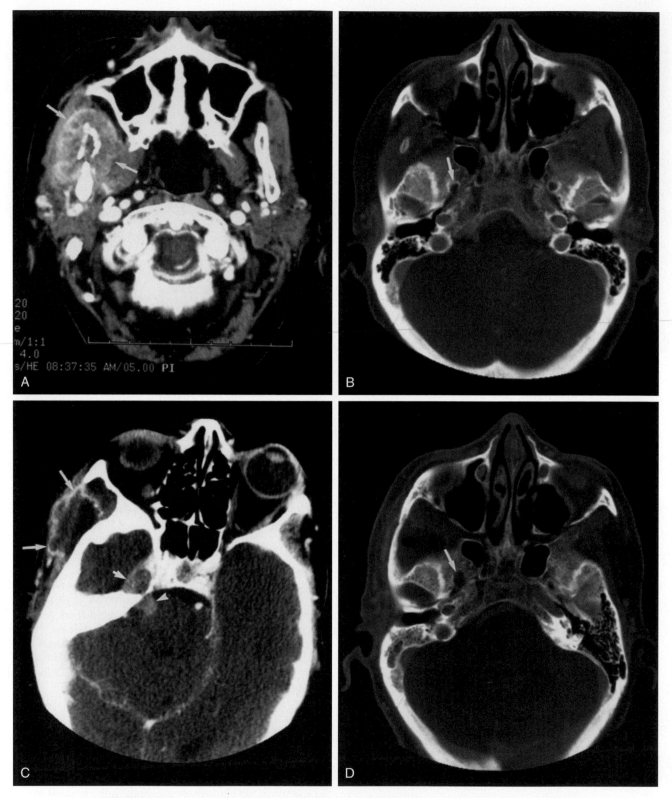

**FIGURE 13-15** Squamous cell carcinoma of the right retromolar trigone with extension into the masticator space and subsequent PNS along $V_3$. Axial contrast-enhanced CT soft-tissue (**A**) and bone window (**B**) images at presentation show extensive tumor involvement of the right mandibular ramus and adjacent musculature (*arrows* in **A**). Note that the foramen ovale is normal, with intact cortical margins (*arrow* in **B**). No intracranial abnormality was visible on higher images at this time. Axial contrast-enhanced CT soft-tissue window (**C**) and bone window (**D**) images obtained 6 months after **A** and **B**. Despite surgery and radiotherapy, the patient had a large recurrence (*long arrows* in **C**). Note the enlargement and loss of the cortical margin in the right foramen ovale, suggesting PNS (*arrow* in **D**; compare this with the appearance of the foramen ovale in **B**). The soft-tissue window image shows enlargement and central enhancement indicating tumor in Meckel's cave (*short arrow* in **C**) with continued spread to involve the main right trigeminal trunk (*arrowhead*).

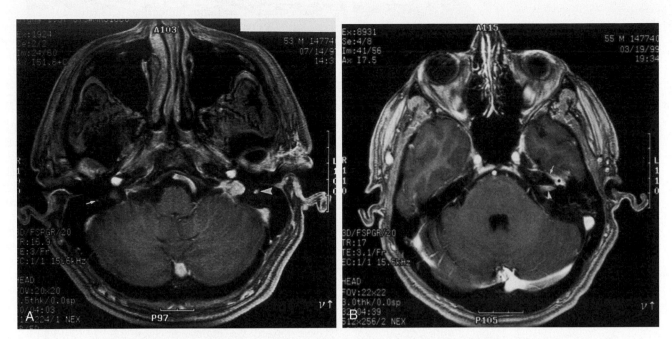

**FIGURE 13-16**   Adenocarcinoma of the left parotid gland with PNS along the facial nerve. **A,** Axial contrast-enhanced SPGR MR image obtained at an outside facility 1 month after left parotidectomy. The facial nerve was paralyzed postoperatively. This study was read as postoperative changes only; no mention was made of the abnormal enhancement and enlargement of the left descending facial nerve segment (*arrowhead*). The right descending facial nerve is normal (*arrow*). The tympanic and more anterior aspects of the left facial nerve are normal. Postoperatively, the patient had radiotherapy to the parotid region. **B,** Axial contrast-enhanced SPGR MR image obtained at an outside facility 20 months after **A,** by which time the patient had developed left-sided hearing loss. There is tumor in the geniculate ganglion (*black dot*), proximal greater superficial petrosal nerve (*arrow*), and internal auditory canal (*arrowhead*). This case demonstrates progression of PNS with initial failure to diagnose. The patient ultimately developed widespread leptomeningeal disease.

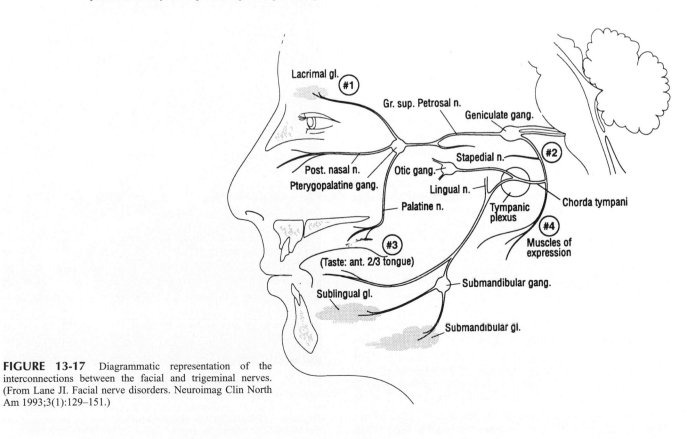

**FIGURE 13-17**   Diagrammatic representation of the interconnections between the facial and trigeminal nerves. (From Lane JI. Facial nerve disorders. Neuroimag Clin North Am 1993;3(1):129–151.)

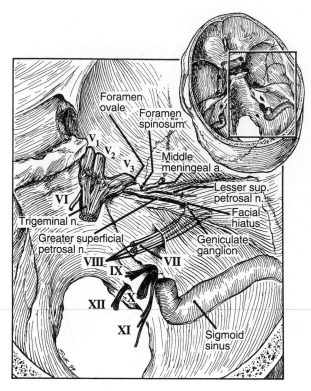

**FIGURE 13-18**   Diagrammatic representation of the greater superficial petrosal nerve. (From Ginsberg LE, DeMonte F, Gillenwater AM. Greater superficial petrosal nerve: anatomy and MR findings in perineural tumor spread. AJNR 1996;17:389–393.)

images should also be generated for evaluation of subtle bone erosion.

When MR imaging is performed, it is crucial to obtain axial T1-weighted images prior to the administration of contrast. This is necessary because the normal hyperintense signal intensity of fat in the PPF and foraminal areas is best assessed on this sequence. The presence of PNS has been overlooked, in part, because this sequence was omitted (Fig. 13-4). Although there is some controversy in the literature as to whether postcontrast MR imaging should be fat suppressed, it is generally agreed that in the evaluation of PNS, fat suppression should be used.[32] Though this technique is sometimes prone to artifact, there are numerous cases in which the lack of fat suppression has made PNS either difficult to see or completely inconspicuous (Figs. 13-4, 13-11). Postcontrast axial and coronal MR images should be obtained routinely.

## Imaging Diagnosis of PNS

On CT, imaging findings suggestive of PNS include widening or destruction of neural foramina/canals, excessive enhancement within neural foramina/canals, or excessive enhancement or widening of the cavernous sinus, PPF, or Meckel's cave. In addition, the loss of fat planes immediately adjacent to neural foramina or within the PPF, even in the absence of abnormal enhancement, widening, or bone destruction, are highly suggestive findings of PNS (Figs. 13-6, 13-15).[13, 18, 28, 34–36] Caution should be used when

interpreting bone destruction on CT, as it may simply be the direct effect of the tumor rather than PNS (Fig. 13-22).

On MR imaging, findings suggestive of PNS include any of the following: excessive enhancement of a cranial nerve branch (either within the cisternal portion or within a canal or foramen), loss of the normal fat pad adjacent to a foramen,[34, 35] or widening/excessive enhancement within the PPF, Meckel's cave, or the cavernous sinus (Figs. 13-2, 13-4, 13-5, 13-7 to 13-9, 13-11, 13-14, 13-16, 13-23). Again, loss of the normal T1-hyperintense fat in the PPF should be regarded as highly suspicious for PNS (Figs. 13-5, 13-8).

With regard to Meckel's cave, the site of the gasserian (trigeminal) ganglion, this space is filled primarily with CSF. As such, it should be of fluid density on CT and of fluid signal intensity on MR imaging. The ganglion has only some peripheral vascularity, and as such, there normally should be no central enhancement within Meckel's cave. Such enhancement is a strong indicator of the presence of disease (Figs. 13-7, 13-9, 13-12, 13-13, 13-15, 13-23).[13] In severe cases of PNS affecting the trigeminal nerve, it may be possible to observe thickening and abnormal enhancement of the main trigeminal trunk extending back from Meckel's cave toward the brainstem (Figs. 13-12, 13-13, 13-23). Although MR imaging is better at detecting PNS in the main trigeminal trunk, it can sometimes be seen with CT (Fig. 13-15).

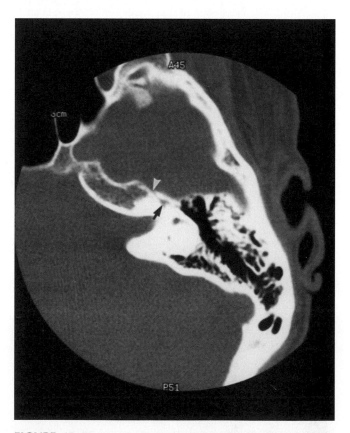

**FIGURE 13-19**   Axial CT bone window demonstrating the facial hiatus (*arrowhead*) for the greater superficial petrosal nerve, extending anteriorly from the geniculate ganglion (*arrow*). (From Ginsberg LE, DeMonte F, Gillenwater AM. Greater superficial petrosal nerve: anatomy and MR findings in perineural tumor spread. AJNR 1996;17:389–393.)

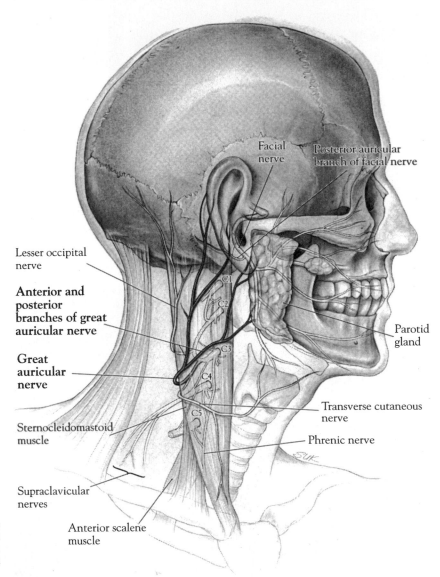

**FIGURE 13-20**    Diagrammatic representation of the cervical plexus and great auricular nerve. (From Ginsberg LE, Eicher SA. Great auricular nerve: anatomy and imaging of perineural tumor spread. AJNR 2000;21:568–571.)

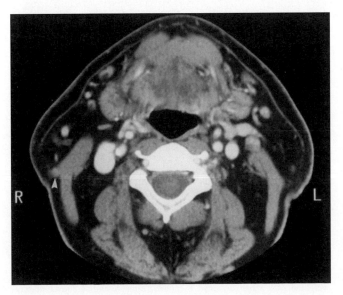

**FIGURE 13-21**    Recurrent cutaneous squamous cell carcinoma in the right lower parotid region with PNS along the great auricular nerve. Axial contrast-enhanced CT scan shows a subtly enhancing mass lateral to the right sternocleidomastoid muscle (*arrowhead*) representing PNS along the course of the great auricular nerve. (From Ginsberg LE, Eicher SA. Great auricular nerve: anatomy and imaging of perineural tumor spread. AJNR 2000;21:568–571.)

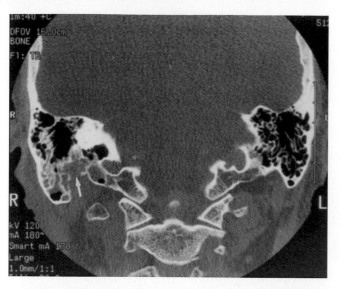

**FIGURE 13-22** Squamous cell carcinoma of the right parotid gland with CT bone findings suggesting PNS along the descending facial nerve and stylomastoid foramen. The coronal CT bone window shows bone destruction at the stylomastoid foramen (*arrow*). The facial nerve canal was explored at surgery, and the nerve was found to be normal. These bone changes, though consistent with PNS, were secondary to the direct effects of the primary tumor.

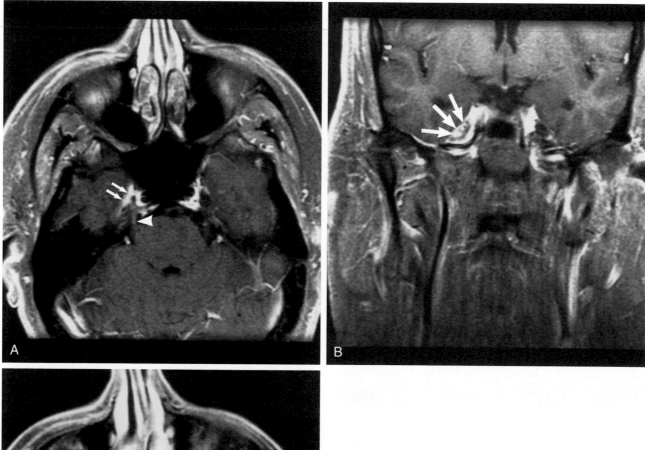

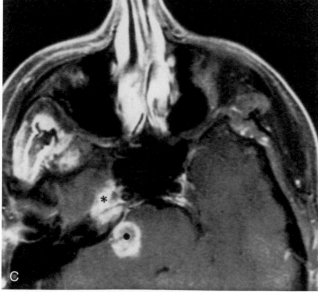

**FIGURE 13-23** Squamous cell carcinoma of the right forehead with very subtle PNS along the ophthalmic nerve ($V_1$). One year after excision of the primary skin cancer, the patient developed sensory neuropathy in the entire right trigeminal distribution. Axial (**A**) and coronal (**B**) contrast-enhanced, fat-suppressed T1-weighted MR images show very subtle abnormal enhancement within Meckel's cave on the right (*arrows* in **A** and **B**) and even subtler enhancement of the main trigeminal trunk (*arrowhead* in **A**). Biopsy of the right supraorbital region confirmed perineural infiltration of the supraorbital branch of $V_1$. The abnormal enhancement was presumed to represent a skip lesion originating on $V_1$, as there was no imaging evidence of tumor in the orbit, superior orbital fissure, or cavernous sinus. The patient received radiotherapy, as the disease was deemed inoperable. **C**, Axial contrast-enhanced, fat-suppressed T1-weighted MR image obtained 8 months after **A** and **B** shows massive disease recurrence/progression with bulky tumor in Meckel's cave (*asterisk*) and the pons (*black dot*).

The radiologist should also be alert to the potential for *skip lesions*, segments of normal intervening nerve between regions of PNS (Figs. 13-12, 13-23).[7, 10, 33, 37] In the literature, skip lesions have also been referred to as *resurfacing*. As previously mentioned, the radiologist should also be aware of the presence of antegrade PNS (Fig. 13-7).

## Secondary Imaging Findings

The presence of secondary findings associated with PNS may either lend support to a case of suspected PNS or alert the radiologist to the presence of undiagnosed PNS. These findings chiefly are those of denervation of the mandibular division of the trigeminal nerve, whose branches innervate the muscles of mastication as well as the anterior belly of the digastric and mylohyoid muscles.[18, 38] In the chronic stages (more than 20 months following denervation), these muscles undergo fatty infiltration and/or atrophy, findings readily seen on CT or MR imaging (Fig. 13-24).[18, 38]

However, in the acute (less than 1 month) and subacute (1 to 20 months) stages of muscular denervation, there are findings that are seen only on MR imaging. These findings include increased T2-weighted signal intensity and abnormal enhancement within the affected muscles (Fig. 13-12).[38, 39] Although these imaging findings may suggest tumor involvement, particularly if the primary tumor is nearby, there are ways to differentiate tumor from denervation. On imaging, subacutely denervated muscle retains its internal striations, which are generally lost in the presence of

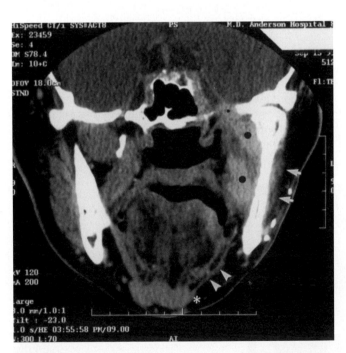

**FIGURE 13-24**   Oral cavity squamous cell carcinoma with spread to the masticator space, V₃ PNS, and chronic denervation of the V₃-innervated musculature. Coronal contrast-enhanced CT scan shows tumor in the left pterygoid musculature (*large black dots*) and within the foramen ovale (*small black dot*). Note the atrophy of the mylohyoid (*arrowheads*), anterior belly of the digastric (*asterisk*), and masseter muscles (*arrows*) on the left side.

tumor.[40] Clinically, a patient with tumor in the masticator muscles usually has trismus, whereas a patient with denervation has weakness of the masticator musculature.

## IMAGING PITFALLS

Various pitfalls exist in the imaging of PNS. Alone or in concert, they may result in PNS either not being diagnosed or being overdiagnosed.

## Technique

As previously mentioned, if proper imaging technique is not employed, it is easy to overlook the diagnosis of PNS. The use of an excessively large FOV, the lack of a T1-weighted axial MR image to evaluate the PPF, and the lack of fat suppression on postcontrast MR imaging (Figs. 13-4, 13-11) are all problems that may contribute to the missed diagnosis of PNS.

## Questionable PNS

In the early stages of PNS, the imaging findings can be extremely subtle. In some cases the findings are subtle but definite (Fig. 13-23), while in other cases the findings are so subtle as to be questionable. In the latter case, the radiologist must inform the surgeon of the possibility of PNS so that either a surgical exploration is performed to prove or disprove the presence of PNS or early follow-up imaging is obtained to evaluate the possible progression of PNS.

## Asymmetric Foraminal Enhancement

All of the neural foramina and canals of the skull base normally contain emissary veins.[31] Slow-flowing blood within these veins usually results in some degree of enhancement after contrast administration, particularly on fat-suppressed MR images (Figs. 13-13B, 13-25).[41] Although most of the skull base foramina are quite symmetric, some normal asymmetry can occur.[31] If the patient is scanned with a slightly tilted or rotated scan angle, any asymmetry of these foramina should be viewed with caution prior to diagnosing an abnormality. That is, the radiologist should be certain that any asymmetry in the size of these foramina or in the degree of enhancement is truly caused by disease and not by asymmetric scanning of the patient.

## PERSISTENT POSTTREATMENT IMAGING ABNORMALITIES

Following treatment for proven or strongly suspected PNS, the imaging findings may remain abnormal for an indefinite period of time. The imaging findings may rival the original appearance of PNS despite the lack of clinical evidence of persistent or progressive disease.[42] Obviously, on a given imaging study, it is impossible to exclude active

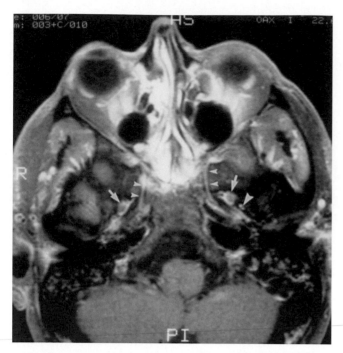

**FIGURE 13-25**   Normal foraminal enhancement on MR imaging. Axial contrast-enhanced, fat-suppressed T1-weighted MR image shows normal enhancement of both vidian canals (*small arrowheads*), both foramina ovale (*arrows*), and the left foramen spinosum (*large arrowhead*).

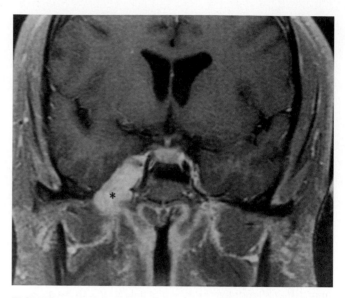

**FIGURE 13-27**   Right cavernous sinus/Meckel's cave schwannoma with extension through the foramen ovale. Coronal contrast-enhanced, fat-suppressed T1-weighted MR image shows an enhancing mass extending inferiorly through a grossly widened foramen ovale (*asterisk*). For Figures 13-26 and 13-27, prior to establishing the diagnosis, the possibility of PNS from a head and neck cancer should at least be considered and sought radiographically. (From Ginsberg LE. Imaging of perineural tumor spread in head and neck cancer. Semin Ultrasound CT MR 1999;2:175–186.)

disease in the face of findings that suggest PNS. However, one should be aware that imaging findings of PNS may not revert to normal even if the disease has been successfully treated.

It has been shown that once the PPF is violated surgically, images of this structure will appear abnormal indefinitely.[43] The persistent imaging findings consist of loss of the normal high T1-weighted fat signal intensity and the presence of excessive enhancement on contrast-enhanced images. Unfortunately, these findings are identical to those seen with PNS. Therefore, following surgery of the PPF, imaging studies should be interpreted with caution to avoid overdiagnosing PNS or local recurrence.[43] The best way

to evaluate PPF is to compare serial follow-up imaging studies.

## MIMICS OF PNS

The radiologist should be aware that there are other diseases that may have imaging and clinical findings identical to those of PNS. While there may be adjunctive clinical or radiologic signs that point to such a diagnosis, any given case may nonetheless present a diagnostic challenge. Thus, meningioma, occurring near a neural foramen, may extend through that foramen and mimic PNS (Fig. 13-26).[13]

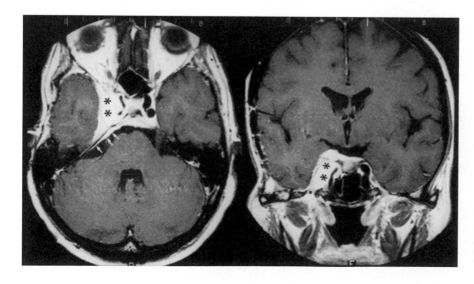

**FIGURE 13-26**   Cavernous sinus/Meckel's cave meningioma with extension through the foramen ovale. Left (axial) and right (coronal) contrast-enhanced T1-weighted MR images without fat suppression show a characteristic right cavernous sinus/Meckel's cave meningioma (*asterisks*). Note the dural tail extending posteriorly along the right petrous ridge (*arrows*). The lesion is seen on the coronal image to be extending inferiorly through a widened foramen ovale (*black dot*). (From Ginsberg LE. Imaging of perineural tumor spread in head and neck cancer. Semin Ultrasound CT MR 1999;2:175–186.)

Occasionally a schwannoma, particularly when it involves the trigeminal or facial nerves, may mimic PNS (Fig. 13-27). Finally, though uncommon and probably clinically obvious, advanced rhinocerebral mucormycosis may spread along cranial nerve branches and appear quite similar on imaging to PNS.[44]

## CONCLUSION

It is clear that PNS is a serious complication and a major diagnostic challenge. Only by learning more about the relevant neuroanatomy and by obtaining a thorough clinical history of the head and neck cancer patient can the radiologist properly perform and interpret imaging studies so as to ensure that PNS is accurately diagnosed.

## REFERENCES

1. Peet MM. Tumors of the gasserian ganglion. Surg Gynecol Obstet 1927;44:202–207.
2. Ballantyne AJ, McCarten AB, Ibanex ML. The extension of cancer of the head and neck through peripheral nerves. Am J Surg 1963;106: 651–667.
3. Dodd GD, Dolan PA, Ballantyne AJ, et al. The dissemination of tumors of the head and neck via the cranial nerves. Radiol Clin North Am 1970;8:445–461.
4. Batsakis JG. Pathology consultation: nerves and neurotropic carcinomas. Ann Otol Rhinol Laryngol 1985;94:426–427.
5. Soo KC, Carter RL, O'Brien CJ, et al. Prognostic implications of perineural spread of squamous carcinomas of the head and neck. Laryngoscope 1986;96:1145–1148.
6. Goepfert H, Dichtel WJ, Medina JE, et al. Perineural invasion in squamous cell skin carcinoma of the head and neck. Am J Surg 1984;148:542–547.
7. Woddruff WW, Yeates AE, McLendon RE. Perineural tumor extension to the cavernous sinus from superficial facial carcinoma: CT manifestations. Radiology 1986;161:395–399.
8. Majoie CB, Hullsmans FJH, Casteljins JA, et al. Perineural tumor extension of facial malignant melanoma: CT and MRI. J Comput Assist Tomogr 1993;17(6):973–975.
9. Batsakis JG, Raymond AK. Pathology consultation: desmoplastic melanoma. Ann Otol Rhinol Laryngol 1994;103:77–79.
10. Catalano PJ, Chandranath S, Biller HF. Cranial neuropathy secondary to perineural spread of cutaneous malignancy. Am J Otol 1995;16: 772–777.
11. Banerjee TK, Gottschalk PG. Unusual manifestations of multiple cranial nerve palsies and mandibular metastasis in a patient with squamous cell carcinoma of the lip. Cancer 1984;53:346–348.
12. Anderson CA, Krutchkoff D, Ludwig M. Carcinoma of the lower lip with perineural extension to the middle cranial fossa. Oral Surg Oral Med Oral Pathol 1990;69:614–618.
13. Ginsberg LE. Imaging of perineural tumor spread in head and neck cancer. Semin Ultrasound CT MR 1999;2:175–186.
14. Ginsberg LE, DeMonte F. Imaging of perineural tumor spread from palatal carcinoma. AJNR 1998;19:1417–1422.
15. Parker GD, Harnsberger HR. Clinical-radiologic issues in perineural tumor spread of malignant diseases of the extracranial head and neck. RadioGraphics 1991;11:383–399.
16. Dodd GD, Jing BS. Radiographic findings in adenoid cystic carcinoma of the head and neck. Ann Otol Rhinol Laryngol 1972;81:591–598.
17. Chong VFH, Fan YF, Khoo JBK. Nasopharyngeal carcinoma with intracranial spread: CT and MR characteristics. J Comput Assist Tomogr 1996;20(4):563–569.
18. Laine FJ, Braun IF, Jensen ME, et al. Perineural tumor extension through the foramen ovale: evaluation with MR imaging. Radiology 1990;174:65–71.
19. Mendenhall WM, Parsons JT, Mendenhall NP, et al. Carcinoma of the skin of the head and neck with perineural invasion. Head Neck 1989;11:301–308.
20. Caldemeyer KS, Mathews VP, Righi RR, et al. Imaging features and clinical significance of perineural spread or extension of head and neck tumors. RadioGraphics 1998;18:97–110.
21. Nemzek WR, Hecht S, Gandour-Edwards R, et al. Perineural spread of head and neck tumors: how accurate is MR imaging? AJNR 1998;19:701–706.
22. Arcas A, Bescos S, Raspall G, et al. Perineural spread of epidermoid carcinoma in the infraorbital nerve: case report. J Oral Maxillofac Surg 1996;54:520–522.
23. Ginsberg LE, DeMonte F. Palatal adenoid cystic carcinoma presenting as perineural spread to the cavernous sinus. Skull Base Surg 1998;8(1):39–43.
24. McNab AA, Francis AC, Benger R, et al. Perineural spread of cutaneous squamous cell carcinoma via the orbit. Ophthalmology 1997;104:1457–1462.
25. Alonso PE, Bescansa E, Salas J, et al. Perineural spread of cutaneous squamous cell carcinoma manifesting as ptosis and ophthalmoplegia (orbital apex syndrome). Br J Plast Surg 1995;48:564–568.
26. Esmaeli B, Ginsberg LE, Goepfert H, et al. Squamous cell carcinoma with perineural invasion presenting as a Tolosa-Hunt-like syndrome: a potential pitfall in diagnosis. Ophthal Plast Reconstr Surg 2000;16(6): 450–452.
27. Berry M, Bannister LH, Stranding SM. Nervous system. In: Bannister LH, Berry MM, Collins P, Dyson M, Dussek JE, Ferguson MWJ, eds. Gray's Anatomy, 38th ed. New York: Churchill Livingston, 1995;901–1937.
28. Curtin HD, Williams R, Johnson J. CT of perineural tumor extension: pterygopalatine fossa. AJNR 1984;5:731–737.
29. Pandolfo I, Gaeta M, Blandino A, et al. Case report: MR imaging of perineural metastasis along the vidian nerve. J Comput Assist Tomogr 1989;13:498–500.
30. Ginsberg LE, DeMonte F, Gillenwater AM. Greater superficial petrosal nerve: anatomy and MR findings in perineural tumor spread. AJNR 1996;17:389–393.
31. Ginsberg LE, Pruett SW, Chen MY, et al. Skull-base foramina of the middle cranial fossa: reassessment of normal variation with high-resolutioon CT. AJNR 1994;15:283–291.
32. Ginsberg LE, Eicher SA. Great auricular nerve: anatomy and imaging of perineural tumor spread. AJNR 2000;21:568–571.
33. Barakos JA, Dillon WP, Chew WM. Orbit, skull base, and pharynx: contrast-enhanced fat suppression MR imaging. Radiology 1991;179: 191–198.
34. Matzko J, Becker DG, Phillips CD. Obliteration of fat planes by perineural spread of squamous cell carcinoma along the inferior alveolar nerve. AJNR 1994;15:1843–1845.
35. Curtin HD. Detection of perineural spread: fat is a friend. Editorial. AJNR 1998;19(8):1385–1386.
36. Curtin HD, Williams R. Computed tomographic anatomy of the pterygopalatine fossa. RadioGraphics 1985;5(3):429–440.
37. Lee YY, Castillo M, Nauert C. Intracranial perineural metastasis of adenoid cystic carcinoma of head and neck. J Comput Assist Tomogr 1985;9:219–223.
38. Russo CP, Smoker WRK, Weissman JL. MR appearance of trigeminal and hypoglossal motor denervation. AJNR 1997;18:1375–1383.
39. Davis SB, Mathews VP, Williams DW. Masticator muscle enhancement in subacute denervation atrophy. AJNR 1995;16:1292–1294.
40. Chong J, Chan LL, Langstein HN, Ginsberg LE. MR imaging of the muscular component of myocutaneous flaps in the head and neck. AJNR 2001;22(1):170–174.
41. Ginsberg LE. The posterior condylar canal. AJNR 1994;15:969–972.
42. Sohn-Williams L, Mancuso AA, Menhenhall W. Perineural spread of skin carcinoma: clinical significance and natural history of the MR and CT findings following radiation therapy. Presented at the 84th annual meeting of the Radiological Society of North America, Chicago, December 1, 1998.
43. Chan LL, Chong J, Gillenwater AM, Ginsberg LE. The pterygopalatine fossa: postsurgical MR imaging appearance. AJNR 2000;21: 1315–1319.
44. McLean FM, Ginsberg LE, Stanton CA. Perineural spread of rhinocerebral mucormycosis. AJNR 1996;17:114–116.

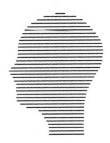

# Jaws and Temporomandibular Joints

## *14*

# Embryology and Anatomy of the Jaw and Dentition

### *James J. Abrahams, Reuben Rock, and Michael W. Hayt*

## EMBRYOLOGY OF THE JAWS

Embryologically, the maxilla, mandible, and facial soft tissues arise from a number of structures early in the fourth week of development. These structures are the central unpaired frontonasal prominence, the paired nasomedial processes, and the paired maxillary and mandibular prominences. The last three of these arise from the first branchial arch. These all surround a ventral depression, the stomodeum, which will later become the mouth. These structures arise from neural crest tissues (Fig. 14-1) and are also described in detail in Chapter 1.[1–4]

As the embryo develops, the nasomedial and maxillary processes become more prominent and fuse to form the upper lip and upper jaw. The two nasomedial processes fuse to form the intermaxillary segment that is the precursor for the philtrum of the upper lip, the primary palate, and the premaxillary component of the upper jaw. These structures merge by intermingling of the underlying mesenchyme and disintegration of the overlying epithelia. The frontonasal prominence is displaced as the nasomedial processes merge, and it does not contribute significantly to the upper jaw.[1,4]

The mandible forms from the enlargement and fusion of the bilateral mandibular prominences. The mandibular skeleton develops from a cartilaginous derivative of the first branchial arch called *Meckel's cartilage.* When the maxillary and mandibular processes fuse laterally, they form the corners of the lips, or commissures.

As these facial structures are formed, mesenchymal cells of the first and second branchial arches invade them and form the muscles of mastication (first branchial arch, supplied by cranial nerve V, the trigeminal nerve) and the muscles of facial expression (second branchial arch, supplied by cranial nerve VII, the facial nerve).

Most of the differential jaw and facial growth occurs between 4 and 8 weeks, but changes occur in the different regions at different rates throughout fetal development and the early neonatal period. Relative to the adult, the neonatal face is small due to the fact that the jaws are still rudimentary at birth, the teeth undeveloped and unerupted, and the paranasal sinuses small.

As mentioned above, the various components forming the jaws fuse and mesenchymal merging occurs, leaving only the two nostrils and mouth as normal openings. If there is any interference with this process, a number of anomalies can occur, resulting in cleft lip, cleft chin, cleft anterior palate, and clefts at the corners of the mouth. If the commissures do not form correctly, a large mouth or macrostomia can occur (also see Chapter 1).

## EMBRYOLOGY OF THE DENTITION

The process by which the teeth form is called odontogenesis. Humans have two sets of teeth: the primary dentition (deciduous) and the secondary dentition (permanent). The presence of teeth in the maxilla and mandible contributes to the formation of the jaws and to the final shape of the face. There are 20 deciduous teeth and 32 permanent teeth.

Each tooth develops from ectoderm and ectomesenchyme (mesenchyme of the head). The enamel arises from the ectoderm, while the other tissues (dentin, cementum, periodontal ligament, and pulp contents) arise from the mesenchyme. The mesenchyme (ectomesenchyme) represents a migration of neural crest cells into the developing arches of the mandible and maxilla. Tooth development begins with the formation of the primary dental lamina invaginating into that mesenchyme. This dental lamina is a thickening of the oral epithelium overlying the jaws. These cells migrate into the primitive jaws in the sixth week of development. In 10 places in each of the mandibular and maxillary arches, cells of this dental lamina start to multiply faster than the surrounding cells and condense to form the tooth buds or tooth germs.[1-4]

Each tooth will develop and erupt at a specific time, but the overall pattern of odontogenesis is common to all teeth. The tooth germs of the permanent succedaneous teeth (the permanent teeth replacing deciduous teeth) arise from the secondary dental lamina and appear lingual to each deciduous tooth germ. These permanent succedaneous teeth are the permanent central and lateral incisors, canines, and first and second premolars. The premolars arise from the secondary lamina associated with deciduous (primary) molars and erupt into their corresponding positions. The permanent first, second, and third molars arise from the primary dental lamina posterior to the primary second molar. All the tooth buds except for the second and third permanent molars are present and start developing before birth.

As the tooth bud grows, it develops into a cap shape by invagination of mesenchyme (Fig. 14-2). The ectodermal component forms the enamel organ, which is composed of the outer enamel epithelium, the stellate reticulum, and the

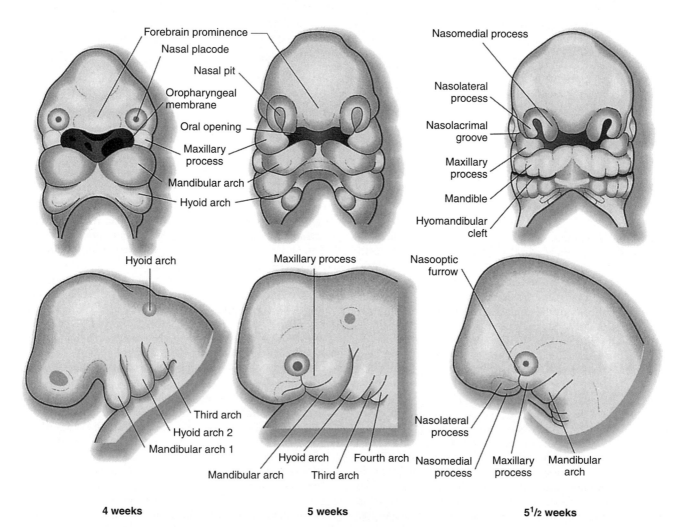

**FIGURE 14-1**  Frontal and lateral views of heads of human embryos from 4 to 8 weeks of age. (From Carlson BM. Human Embryology and Developmental Biology. St. Louis: CV Mosby, 1994.)

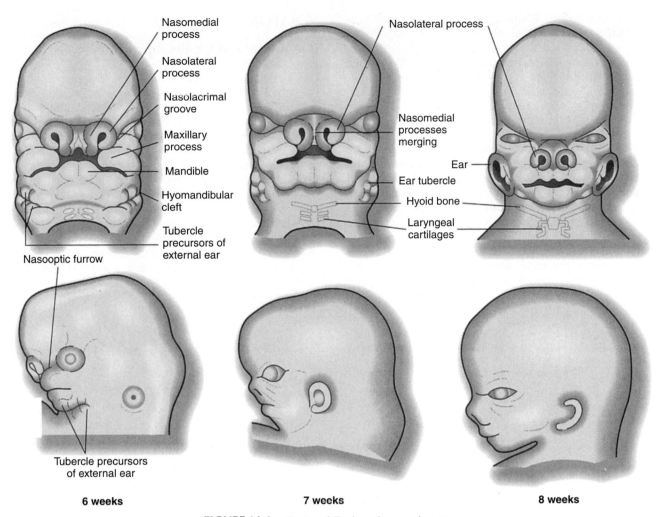

**FIGURE 14-1** *Continued.* For legend see previous page.

inner enamel epithelium. A layer of more condensed cells develops from the stellate reticulum along the inner enamel epithelium, called the stratum intermedium. The enamel forms from the inner enamel epithelium, whose cells elongate into ameloblasts. Ameloblasts form the enamel of the tooth (Fig. 14-3).[2,3]

The invaginating mesenchyme forms the dental papilla. The peripheral cells of the dental papilla take on a columnar form and become known as *odontoblasts*. These cells will form the dentin of the tooth. The ameloblast and odontoblast layers are separated by a basement membrane. The future dentinoenamel junction is demarcated by the basement membrane. The dental papilla will later form the dental pulp, which is the soft tissue inside the root chamber of the tooth and contains nerves, vessels, and connective tissue.

At this stage, the tooth bud is starting to take on the shape of a bell and is called the *bell stage*. Later in the bell stage, the ameloblasts and odontoblasts start to produce the precursors of enamel and dentin. This starts to occur at about the fifth fetal month. The enamel is formed in a matrix in the shape of rods or a prism, but only after predentin is formed next to the inner enamel epithelium. In other words, enamel formation (amelogenesis) is induced by the production of dentin (dentinogenesis) (Fig. 14-4). Predentin later calcifies into dentin as the tooth develops. Both amelogenesis and dentinogenesis begin at the cusp or top of the tooth, and these processes continue toward the future apex or root. Enamel formation occurs only in the preeruptive tooth, while dentin deposition occurs throughout life. Enamel formation terminates with the development of an organic layer, the enamel cuticle. After this forms, the inner and outer enamel epithelia and the remains of the stratum intermedium form the reduced enamel epithelium, which fuses with the overlying oral epithelium to induce eruption of the teeth (movement of the tooth into the oral cavity).[2,3]

The dental laminae (primary and secondary) start to disintegrate at this stage. The cells of the dental lamina can disappear completely or can remain as groups of epithelial cells. These remnants may later give rise to lesions such as odontogenic (of tooth origin) cysts. As this occurs, further condensation of the mesenchyme around the tooth bud occurs, forming the dental sac. Also, the tooth buds become surrounded by islands of bone matrix that are developing in the jaws. Cells of the dental sac will produce other components of the teeth, such as cementum and the periodontal ligament. These will anchor the tooth in the bony socket (alveolus) of the jaws. As the teeth form, they start to migrate toward the surface of the jaws. Usually, no teeth are seen in the mouth at birth, but natal teeth can occasionally be seen. Teeth erupt at different times during life in a fairly predictable pattern (Table 14-1).[3]

A number of anomalies of tooth development can occur.[5] These anomalies include too many teeth (supernumerary), too few teeth (hypodontia), the total lack of teeth (anodontia), or abnormal tooth shape and size, which may involve either the crown or the roots. Included are conditions such as fused teeth, enlarged teeth (macrodontia), or small teeth (microdontia); development of dentin and enamel can be faulty, resulting in conditions such as amelogenesis and dentinogenesis imperfecta. In these cases, the teeth are soft and prone to caries (dental decay), as well as to fracture from minor trauma, and anomalies of eruption, which include ectopia (tooth found in an abnormal position), impaction (impedance of eruption by bone or another tooth), ankylosis (the tooth is attached directly to bone, with no periodontal ligament), and delayed and premature eruption.

## ANATOMY

### Dentition and General Considerations

The teeth of the mandible and maxilla are each embedded in a horseshoe-shaped bony ridge called the alveolar process. Each process divides the oral cavity into two compartments: a more central one adjacent to the tongue called the oral cavity proper and a more peripheral one adjacent to the cheeks and lips called the oral vestibule. A horseshoe-shaped furrow formed where the mucous membrane of the lip and cheek reflect up onto the alveolar process is termed the fornix vestibuli. In the midline, vertically oriented folds of mucosa, the labial frenula, help connect the upper and lower lips to the alveolar process. The lingual frenum, or frenulum, is a similar structure in the midline on the undersurface of the tongue.

When fully dentured, the adult jaw contains 32 teeth—16

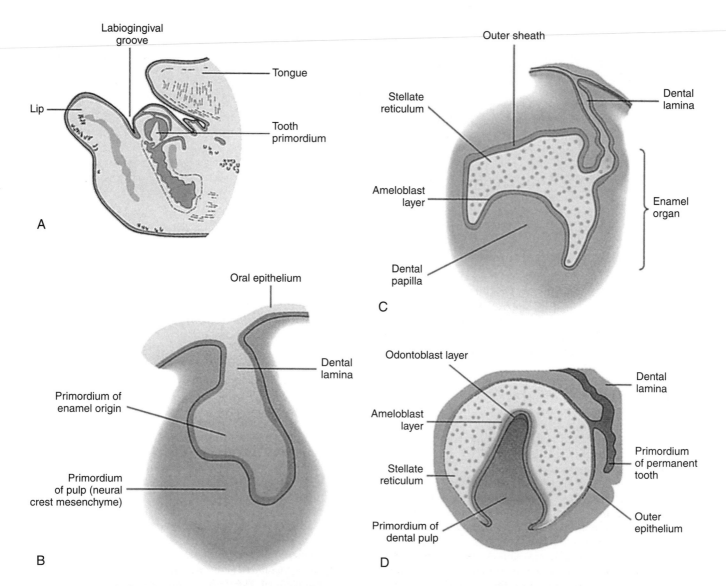

**FIGURE 14-2**  The development of a deciduous tooth. **A**, Parasagittal section through the lower jaw of a 14-week-old human embryo showing the relative location of the tooth primordium. **B**, Tooth primordium in a 9-week-old embryo. **C**, Tooth primordium at the cap stage in an 11-week-old embryo, showing the enamel organ. **D**, Central incisor primordium at the bell stage in a 14-week-old embryo before deposition of enamel or dentin.

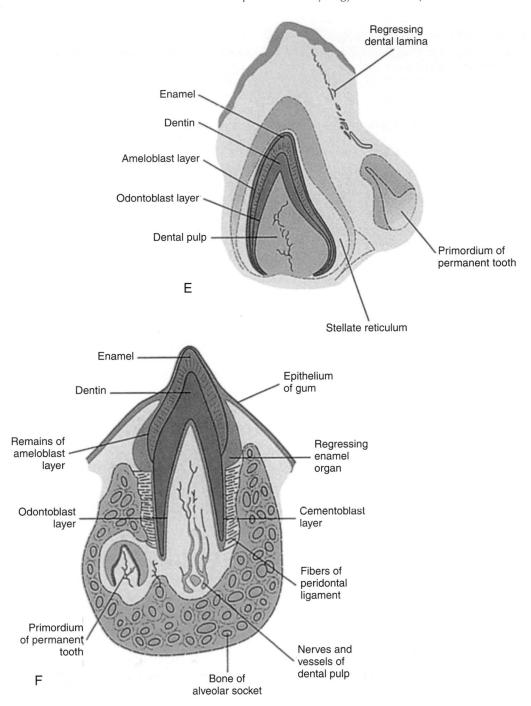

**FIGURE 14-2**   *Continued.* **E,** Unerupted incisor tooth in a term fetus. **F,** Partially erupted incisor tooth showing the primordium of a permanent tooth near one of its roots. (From Carlson BM. Human Embryology and Developmental Biology. St. Louis: CV Mosby, 1994.)

in the maxilla and 16 in the mandible. The teeth can be referred to by number or by name (Fig. 14-5). They are numbered sequentially, starting in the posterior right maxilla with tooth number 1 and continuing to number 16 in the posterior left maxilla. In the mandible they continue with tooth number 17 in the posterior left and end with tooth number 32 in the posterior right. The teeth are named beginning in the midline and moving distally on either side as follows: the central incisor, the lateral incisor, the canine,

the first premolar, the second premolar, the first molar, the second molar, and the third molar.

The dentition of the pediatric jaw is different than that of the adult jaw. When fully dentured, it contains 20 teeth, 10 in the maxilla and 10 in the mandible, instead of the 32 teeth in the adult. Children lack the premolars and third molars. Instead of numbers, the teeth can be referred to by letter or by name (Fig. 14-5). They are lettered sequentially starting in the posterior right maxilla with tooth letter A (maxillary

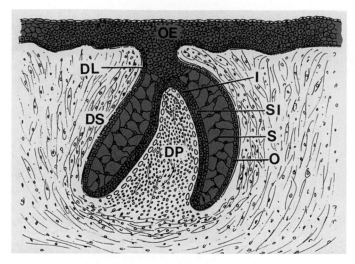

**FIGURE 14-3** Illustration of a tooth germ. The four epithelial cell layers of the enamel organ (bell stage) are indicated as (*I*) inner, (*SI*) stratum intermedium, (*S*) stellate reticulum, and (*O*) outer. The dental papilla (*DP*) is enclosed within the four cell layers of the enamel organ and is continuous with the dental sac (*DS*), which surrounds the outer surface of the enamel organ. The dental lamina (*DL*) connects the enamel organ to the oral epithelium (*OE*). (From Melfi RC. Permar's Oral Embryology and Microscopic Anatomy. Philadelphia: Lea & Febiger, 1994.)

right second molar) and continuing to letter K (maxillary left second molar) in the posterior left maxilla. In the mandible, they continue with tooth letter L (mandibular left second molar) in the posterior left and end with letter U (mandibular right second molar) in the posterior right mandible. The teeth are named beginning in the midline and moving distally (posteriorly) on either side as follows: the central incisor, the lateral incisor, the canine, the first molar, and the second molar.

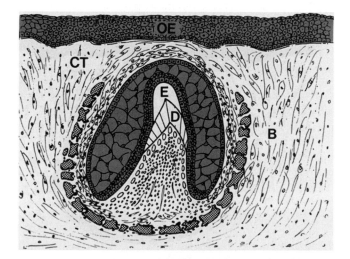

**FIGURE 14-4** Illustration of an advanced tooth germ with enamel (*E*) and dentin (*D*) present in the coronalmost part. Ameloblasts are present around the enamel, whereas cervically the inner epithelial cells have not yet differentiated into ameloblasts. The dental sac surrounds the enamel organ and is continuous with the dental papilla. Developing bone (*B*) of the jaw is present, and the developing tooth is separated from the oral epithelium (*OE*) by connective tissue (*CT*). (From Melfi RC. Permar's Oral Embryology and Microscopic Anatomy. Philadelphia: Lea & Febiger, 1994.)

The portion of the tooth exposed in the oral cavity is called the anatomic crown (arrowheads in Fig. 14-6C), and the portion of the tooth embedded in the bony socket is referred to as the root (Fig. 14-7B). Most of the tooth is composed of dentine; however, the outer surface of the crown is covered by the smooth, dense enamel, and the outer surface of the root is covered by dense cementum, a tissue very similar to bone. A constriction where the crown and root meet is referred to as either the cervical constriction or the cementoenamel junction (Cc in Fig. 14-7B).

On CT, particularly in young people, the dense enamel appears separate from the dentine and looks like a dense band covering the crown of the tooth (E in Fig. 14-7B). With age, receding gingiva and bone cause portions of the root to be exposed in the oral cavity. The crown now differs from the original anatomic crown (that portion covered with enamel) and should be referred to as the functional crown. The arrows in Figure 14-6C point to the functional crown, and the arrowheads point to the anatomic crown.

The neurovascular bundle of the tooth enters the root apex via the apical foramen and travels through the root canal and into an expanded pulp chamber in the crown. The root canal and pulp chamber are seen on CT as a relatively radiolucent area in the center of the root and crown (Fig. 14-7B). Accessory apical foramina along the side of the root, rather than the apex of the root, may occasionally exist.

Each crown has five free surfaces.[6] The biting surface, or the surface where the upper and lower teeth oppose each other, is referred to as the occlusal surface (Figs. 14-6A and 14-7B). The surface facing toward the inside, or toward the oral cavity, is called the lingual surface in the mandible and the palatal surface in the maxilla (Fig. 14-6A). The outer surface of the tooth facing toward the lip and cheek is termed the labial surface for the incisors and canines and the buccal surface for the premolars and molars (Fig. 14-6C). This surface may more simply be referred to as the facial surface for all the teeth. The other tooth surfaces are the contact surfaces where one tooth contacts a neighboring tooth. Of

**Table 14-1**
**THE USUAL TIMES OF ERUPTION AND SHEDDING OF DECIDUOUS AND PERMANENT TEETH**

| Teeth | Eruption | Shedding |
|---|---|---|
| **Deciduous** | | |
| Central incisors | 6–8 mo | 6–7 yr |
| Lateral incisors | 7–10 mo | 7–8 yr |
| Canines | 14–18 mo | 10–12 yr |
| First molars | 12–16 mo | 9–11 yr |
| Second molars | 20–24 mo | 10–12 yr |
| **Permanent** | | |
| Central incisors | 7–8 yr | |
| Lateral incisors | 8–9 yr | |
| Canines | 12–13 yr | |
| First premolars | 10–11 yr | |
| Second premolars | 11–12 yr | |
| First molars | 6–7 yr | |
| Second molars | 12–13 yr | |
| Third molars | 15–25 yr | |

Source: Carlson BM. Human Embryology and Developmental Biology. St. Louis: CV Mosby, 1994;292.

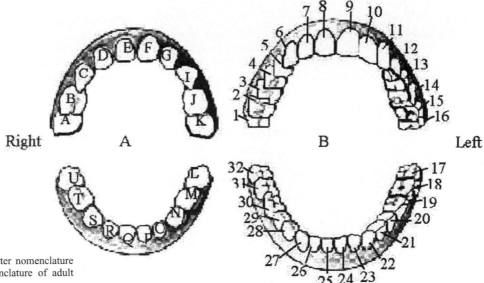

**FIGURE 14-5** Illustration showing letter nomenclature of pediatric teeth (*A*) and number nomenclature of adult teeth (*B*).

these two surfaces, the one closest to the midline is referred to as the mesial surface, and the other is referred to as the distal surface (Figs. 14-6C and 14-7B). The mesial surface in the incisors and canines may also be called the medial surface, but in the premolars and molars it is termed the anterior surface. Likewise the distal surface in the incisors and canines may be called the lateral surface and in the premolars and molars the posterior surface.

Direction also can be described with this terminology. For example, toward the midline would be referred to as mesial, or anterior, and moving in the direction of the molars would be referred to as distal, or posterior. When referring to the crown of the tooth, one may move in the occlusal direction (toward the opposing tooth) or in the cervical direction (toward the cervical constriction), and when referring to the root, one may move in the cervical or apical direction. The use of this terminology is nicely exemplified by naming the roots of the teeth. For example, the first mandibular molar contains three roots, two buccal and one lingual. Of the two buccal roots, one is termed the mesiobuccal and the other is termed the distobuccal (Fig. 14-7B). The lingual one is simply called the lingual root.

The teeth are held in the bony socket by a highly specialized periodontal ligament that provides the teeth with small degrees of motion or "give" within the socket. On plain films, the ligament appears as a radiolucency between the cementum of the root and the lamina dura of the bony socket. The periodontal space normally measures between 0.1 and 0.2 mm and is therefore not typically identified on CT. Figure 14-7A, however, does show the lamina dura and to a lesser degree the periodontal space. A radiolucency seen on CT between the tooth root and the alveolar bone may represent a pathologic state such as periodontal disease, which is discussed later. In the cervical portion of the tooth, the fibers of the periodontal ligament radiate from the cementum of the root into the gingiva and serve to attach the gingiva to the tooth.

## MANDIBLE

The anatomy of the mandible is described on the anatomic specimen in Figure 14-6 and on the illustrations of the neurovascular and muscular structures in Figures 14-8 and 14-9.[6-15] This anatomy is then labeled on the cross-sectional, axial, and panoramic CT images in Figure 14-10.[16]

### Anatomic Specimen

#### Lingual Surface

The mandibular nerve, the third division of the trigeminal nerve, and the mandibular artery (Fig. 14-8A), enter the lingual surface of the mandible through the mandibular foramen (Mf in Fig. 14-6A). The foramen is situated in the center of the ramus, 1 to 2 cm posterior to the third molar at the craniocaudal level of the crowns of the teeth. The nerve and artery then travel anteriorly in the inferior alveolar canal (mandibular canal) (Fig. 14-8A). The canal typically hugs the lingual aspect of the mandible until it curves labially to exit the mandible at the mental foramen (M in Fig. 14-6C; Fig. 14-8A), which on the labial surface of the mandible is between the first and second premolars at the level of the roots. As the neurovascular bundle travels through the mandible, small nutrient canals extend coronally to supply the teeth (Fig. 14-8A, *arrow*). At the mental foramen the main trunk of the mandibular nerve exits as the mental nerve and supplies sensory fibers to the skin overlying the mandible and lower lip (Fig. 14-8A). A smaller branch, the incisive nerve, continues toward the midline within the mandible in the incisive canal (Fig. 14-11). It is accompanied by the incisive artery. This nerve innervates the canine and lateral incisor teeth, and the artery exits through the lingual foramen, which is located in the midline, inferiorly on the lingual aspect of the mandible (Lf in Figs. 14-6B and 14-11C). After exiting the mandible, this artery anastomosis with the lingual artery of the tongue (Fig. 14-9A).

The mylohyoid nerve, a small branch of the mandibular nerve, rather than entering the mandibular foramen with the rest of the nerve, travels anteriorly in the mylohyoid groove on the lingual surface of the mandible (Mg in Fig. 14-6A). The mylohyoid nerve supplies the mylohyoid muscle (Fig. 14-9A,C,D), which fans out like a sling to form the functional floor of the oral cavity. This muscle inserts on the mandible along a bony ridge, the mylohyoid line (Ml in Fig. 14-6A). This line acts as a landmark, separating the oral cavity from the suprahyoid portion of the neck. Inferior to the mylohyoid muscle is the submandibular fossa (S in Fig. 14-6A), a slight concavity in the mandible for the submandibular gland. A small portion of the gland wraps around the posterior aspect of the mylohyoid muscle to enter the sublingual space (Fig. 14-9A). Superior to the mylohyoid line and muscle is the sublingual fossa (Sl in Fig. 14-6A), in which is situated the sublingual gland (Fig. 14-9A).

Also above the mylohyoid muscle are the geniohyoid and genioglossus muscles, which insert on a midline bony protuberance called the genial tubercle (Gt in Figs. 14-6B and 14-11C). It has four bony spines, two superior ones for the right and left genioglossus muscles and two inferior ones for the right and left geniohyoid muscles (Figs. 14-9C,D and

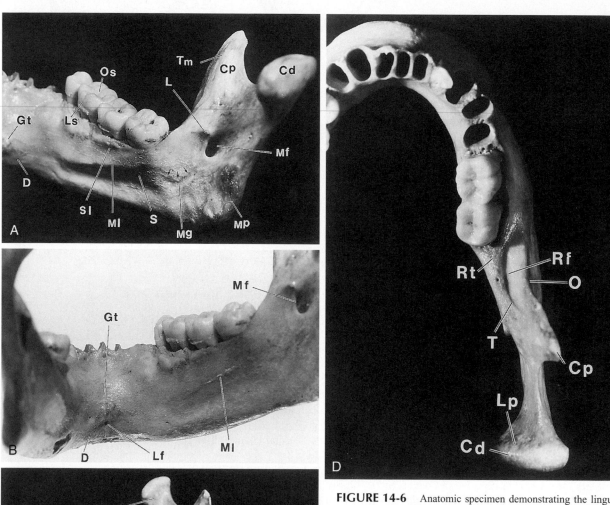

**FIGURE 14-6**   Anatomic specimen demonstrating the lingual (**A** and **B**), buccal (**C**), and superior (**D**) aspects of the mandible. *A* indicates alveolar process; *B*, buccinator muscle insertion; *Bs*, buccal surface; *Cd*, condyle; *Ce*, cemento enamel junction; *Cp*, coronoid process; *D*, digastric fossa; *Ds*, distal surface; *Gt*, genial tubercle; *L*, lingula; *Lf*, lingual foramen; *Lp*, lateral pterygoid muscle insertion; *Ls*, lingual surface; *M*, mental foramen; *Mf*, mandibular foramen; *Mg*, mylohyoid groove; *Ml*, mylohyoid lines; *Mm*, masseter muscle insertion; *Mn*, mandibular notch; *Mp*, medial pterygoid insertion; *Ms*, mesial surface; *O*, oblique line; *Os*, occlusal surface; *Rf*, retromolar fossa; *Rt*, retromolar triangle; *S*, submandibular fossa; *Sl*, sublingual fossa; *T*, temporal crest; *Tm*, temporalis muscle insertion; *arrowheads*, anatomic crown; *black and white arrows*, functional crown; *small black arrows*, mylohyoid groove. (From Abrahams JJ. Anatomy of the jaw revisited with a dental CT software program: pictorial essay. AJNR 1993;14:979–990.)

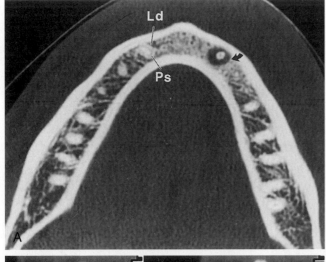

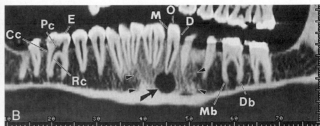

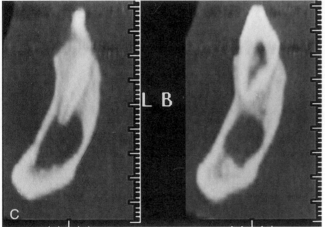

**FIGURE 14-7**   Mandibular DentaScan demonstrating a radicular cyst surrounding the root apex of the left canine. **A,** Axial view demonstrating the radicular cyst (*black arrow*). The periodontal space (*Ps*) typically not seen on CT can be visualized in this patient between the lamina dura (*Ld*) and the tooth. **B,** Panoramic view illustrating an area of sclerotic osteitis condensans (*arrowheads*) surrounding the radicular cyst (*black arrow*). The cervical constriction (*Cc*), pulp chamber (*Pc*), root canal (*Rc*), and dense enamel (*E*) are nicely demonstrated on the right first molar. The mesial (*M*), occlusal (*O*), and distal (*D*) surfaces of the left canine are demonstrated, as well as the mesiobuccal (*Mb*) and distobuccal (*Db*) roots of the left first molar. The lingual root of the left first molar is not seen in this plane. **C,** Cross-sectional views demonstrating the radicular cyst surrounding the root apex.

14-11C). Inferior to the mylohyoid muscle and to either side of the genial tubercle are the digastric fossae (D in Fig. 14-6A,B), each for the origin of the anterior belly of the digastric muscle (Fig. 14-9A).

The temporalis muscle (Fig. 14-9B) inserts on the coronoid process, the most superoanterior extension of the mandibular ramus (Cp in Fig. 14-6A,C). From here this muscle runs deep to the zygomatic arch to flare out over the lateral surface of the calvarium. Its function is to elevate the mandible, thus closing the jaw. Between the coronoid process and the more posterior articular condyle is the mandibular notch (Mn in Fig. 14-6C). The lateral pterygoid muscle (Fig. 14-9B) inserts on the anterior aspect of the condyle (Lp in Fig. 14-6C; Fig. 14-9D) and depresses, protrudes, and moves the jaw from side to side. The medial pterygoid (Fig. 14-9B) inserts more inferiorly on the angle of the mandible near the junction of the body and ramus (Mp in Fig. 14-6A; Fig. 14-9D) and serves to close the mandible along with the temporalis muscle.

### Buccal Surface

On the buccal surface a bony ridge, the oblique line (O in Fig. 14-6C), is formed where the coronoid process (Cp in Fig. 14-6C) merges with the body of the mandible. The buccinator muscle (Fig. 14-9B), which compresses the cheeks to hold food between the teeth, inserts between the oblique line and the more medially (lingually) situated alveolar process (B in Fig. 14-6C; Fig. 14-9D). The deep and superficial portions of the masseter muscle (Fig. 14-9B,D) insert on the buccal surface of the ramus (Mm in Fig. 14-6C; Fig. 14-9D), having originated from the inferior and medial aspect of the zygomatic arch. This muscle acts to close the jaw along with the medial pterygoid and temporalis muscles. Portions of the platysma muscle also insert on the buccal aspect of the mandible along a line that runs inferiorly from the region of the molars to the mental protuberance (Fig. 14-9D). Anteriorly, between the first and second premolar teeth, the mental foramen is identified (M in Fig. 14-6C).

### Superior Surface

The alveolar process, which houses the teeth, forms the most superior portion of the mandibular body. Its curved, or horseshoe, configuration is more acute than that of the body itself. This causes the alveolar process in its posterior (distal) aspect to be medially (lingually) positioned in relation to the mandibular body (Fig. 14-6D). The cross-sectional Denta-Scan images nicely illustrate how the alveolar process is situated on the lingual aspect of the mandible in image 10 (lower right) of Figure 14-10D.

Posterior to the teeth, the alveolar process tapers to form the retromolar triangle (Rt in Fig. 14-6D) that merges with the lingual aspect of the ramus to form the temporal crest (T in Fig. 14-6D). Buccal to this, the anterior portion of the coronoid process (Cp in Fig. 14-6D) merges with the body of the mandible to form the oblique line (O in Fig. 14-6D). Between the oblique line and the temporal crest lies the retromolar fossa (Rf in Fig. 14-6D). The lateral pterygoid muscle inserts on the anterior lingual aspect of the condyle (Lp in Fig. 14-6D).

## CT Images: Cross-Sectional View

### Lingual Surface

Cross-sectional images 1 through 5 in Figure 14-10 are through the distal aspect of the right mandible, near the junction of the ramus and body. The mandibular foramen (Mf), the lingula (L), and the mylohyoid groove (Mg) are clearly seen on these images. More anteriorly (images 9

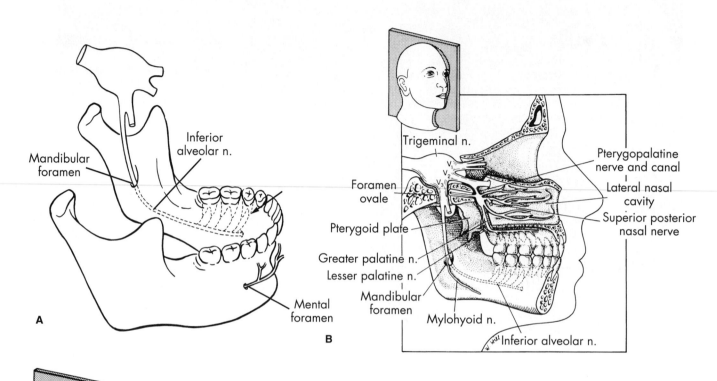

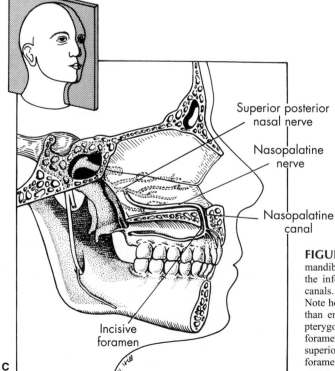

**FIGURE 14-8** Neurovascular structures. **A,** View of the mandible illustrating the mandibular foramen, the mental foramen, and the nutrient canals, which extend from the inferior alveolar canal toward the teeth. *n* indicates nerve and arrow nutrient canals. **B,** Parasagittal view through the trigeminal nerve and the lateral nasal cavity. Note how the myelohyoid nerve travels on the lingual surface of the mandible rather than entering the mandibular foramen. The greater palatine nerve arises from the pterygopalatine nerve, a branch of V2. **C,** Midsagittal view through the incisive foramen and the nasal septum. Note how the nasopalatine nerve, a branch of the superior-posterior nasal nerve, travels along the nasal septum and through the incisive foramen. (From Abrahams JJ. Anatomy of the jaw revisited with a dental CT software program: pictorial essay. AJNR 1993;14:979–990.)

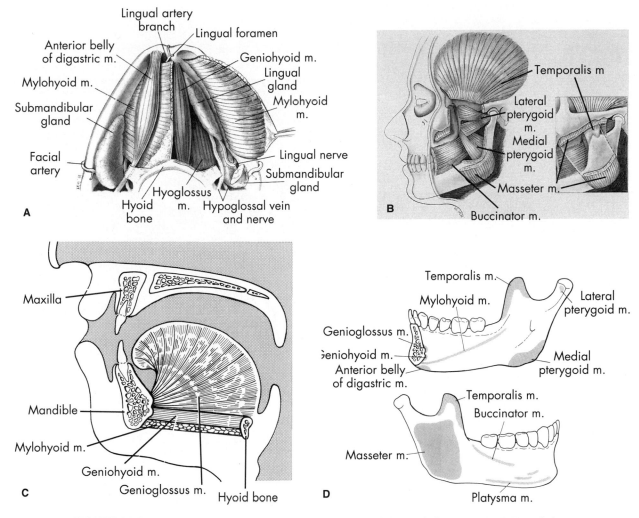

**FIGURE 14-9**   Muscles and insertions. **A,** Mandible viewed from below. *m* indicates muscle. **B,** Lateral view with zygomatic arch and coronoid process removed. **C,** Midline sagittal view through the genial tubercle. **D,** Muscle insertions. Lingual surface (*upper figure*). Buccal surface (*lower figure*). (From Abrahams JJ. Anatomy of the jaw revisited with a dental CT software program: pictorial essay. AJNR 1993;14:979–990.)

through 11 in Fig. 14-10D,E), the mylohyoid line (Ml), the submandibular fossa (S), and the sublingual fossa (Sl) are identified. In the region of the midline (images 27 and 28 in Fig. 14-10F), the genial tubercle (Gt) and the digastric fossa (D) can be seen. The superior (Gt-g) and inferior (Gt-h) processes of the genial tubercle, where the genioglossus and geniohyoid muscles insert, are better visualized in Figure 14-11C. This figure also demonstrates the lingual foramen (Lf) just below the genial tubercle.

### Buccal Surface

The oblique line (O) that is formed where the coronoid process (Cp) merges with the body of the mandible is seen in the posterior images (images 4 through 7 in Fig. 14-10D). More anteriorly (image 20 in Fig. 14-10E), the mental foramen (M) can be seen in cross section. The course of the neurovascular bundle can be clearly traced on the cross-sectional images as it enters the mandibular foramen on the lingual surface, travels through the inferior alveolar canal (I), and finally exits the mental foramen on the buccal surface.

### Superior Surface

On the buccal aspect of the superior surface, the coronoid process (Cp) is again visualized on the more distal images in Figure 14-10D. On more anterior images, the coronoid process merges with the mandible to form the oblique line (O) seen in image 7 of Figure 14-10D. On the lingual aspect of the superior surface, the temporal crest (T) is visualized on the more distal images (image 6 in Fig. 14-10D). More anteriorly the temporal crest becomes the retromolar triangle (Rt in image 8, Fig. 14-10D), and finally the alveolar process (A in image 10, Fig. 14-10D). The molars, which are normally seen in the alveolar process at this point, are absent in this edentulous patient. In the posterior mandible the alveolar process assumes a more lingual position in relation to the body of the mandible. This can be appreciated by comparing the position of the alveolar process to that of the mandible in image 10 (Fig. 14-10D) and image 17 (Fig. 14-10E). The retromolar fossa (Rf in Fig. 14-10D) is identified between the oblique line and the temporal crest.

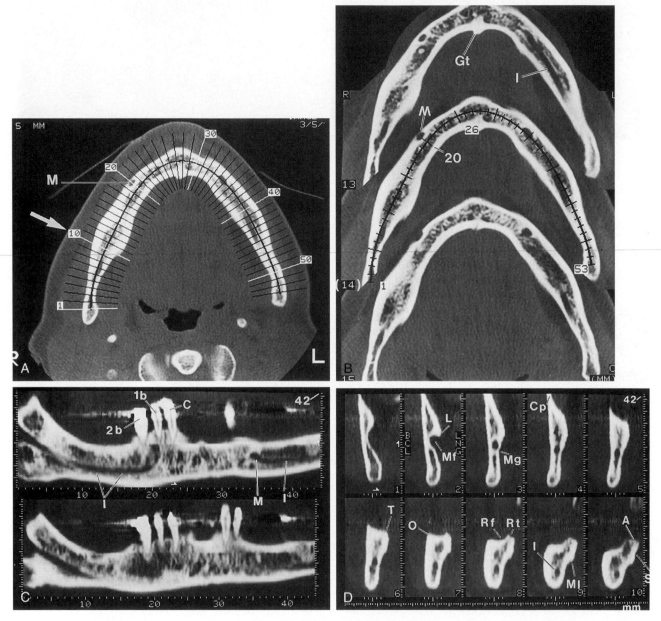

**FIGURE 14-10**   CT (DentaScan) image of mandible. The anatomy identified on the mandibular anatomic specimen in Figure 15-6 is now identified on these CT images. **A,** Axial image of mandible with superimposed curve. The curve defines the plane and location in which the panoramic images in **C** are reformatted. Numbered lines drawn perpendicular to this curve (*arrow*) define the plane and location in which the cross-sectional images viewed in **D** through **F** are reformatted. Mental foramen (*M*). **B,** Axial images illustrating the inferior alveolar canal (*I*), the mental foramen (*M*), and the genial tubercle (*Gt*). The numbers along the left side of the figure refer to the particular number of the axial image. Note that the mental foramen, which is seen on axial image number 14 at the twentieth perpendicular line, is also seen in **E** on cross-sectional image 20 (lower right) at the level of the fourteenth tick mark on the side of the image. The tick marks and numbers allow images to be correlated with one another. **C,** Panoramic views. The numbered tick marks along the bottom of the images correspond to the numbered perpendicular lines displayed on the axial image in **A.** The tick marks along the side of the image correspond to the axial images that were used to reformat these images. Note that there were 42 axial images acquired and thus 42 tick marks along the side of this image. Inferior alveolar canal (*I*), mental foramen (*M*), second bicuspid (*2b*), first bicuspid (*1b*), and cuspid (*C*). **D** through **F,** Cross-sectional views. Images 1 through 10 (**D**) are through the posterior right mandible (see perpendicular lines 1 through 10 in **A**).

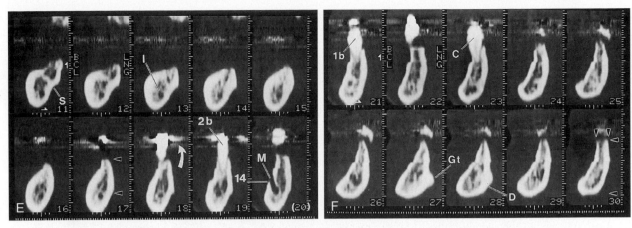

**FIGURE 14-10** *Continued.* Images 11 through 20 (**E**) are more anterior. Images 21 through 30 (**F**) extend to the midline. The images of the left half of the mandible are not shown. Arrowheads in image 17 (**E**) indicate that the height of the mandible distal to the mental foramen is measured from the top of the alveolar process to the top of the mandibular canal, and mesial to the foramen it is measured from the top of the alveolar process to the bottom of the mandible (*arrowheads* in **F**, image 30). Measurement of the width is also demonstrated in image 30 (**F**). *mm* at the bottom of **D** indicates the millimeter scale. Note how streak artifact from dental restoration (*curved arrow* in **E**) does not degrade visualization of the bone. *A* indicates alveolar process; *C*, cuspid; *Cp*, coronoid process; *D*, digastric fossa; *Gt*, genial tubercle; *I*, inferior alveolar canal; *M*, mental foramen; *Mf* mandibular foramen; *Mg*, mylohyoid groove; *Ml* mylohyoid line; *O*, oblique line; *Rf*, retromolar fossa; *Rt*, retromolar triangle; *S*, submandibular fossa; *Sl*, sublingual fossa; *T*, temporal crest; *1b*, first bicuspid; and *2b*, second bicuspid. (From Abrahams JJ. Anatomy of the jaw revisited with a dental CT software program: pictorial essay. AJNR 1993;14:979–990.)

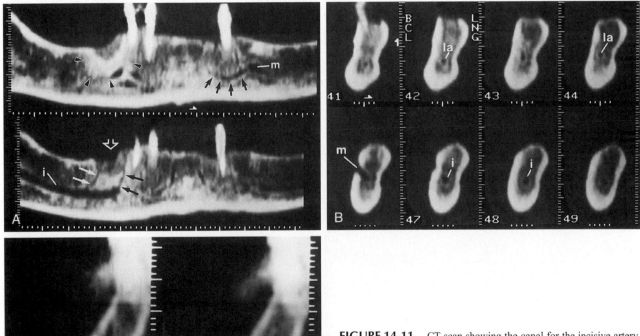

**FIGURE 14-11** CT scan showing the canal for the incisive artery. **A,** This panoramic view of the mandible demonstrates a small canal for the incisive artery (*black arrows*). Note how it extends medial to the mental foramen (*m*) and toward the midline. Also seen are several small nutrient canals (*black and white arrows*) extending from the inferior alveolar canal (*i*) on either side of an extraction socket (*open arrow*). An area of osteitis condensans surrounds the extraction socket (*arrowheads*). **B,** Cross-sectional views of the mandible demonstrate the left inferior alveolar canal (*i*) distal to the mental foramen (*m*) and the canal for the incisive artery (*Ia*) medial to it. On the cross-sectional images, care should be taken not to confuse the inferior alveolar canal with the incisive artery canal. **C,** Midline cross-sectional images in another patient. The incisive artery exits in the midline through the lingual foramen (*Lf*) and an anastomosis with the lingual artery. *Gt-h* indicates genial tubercle (geniohyoid insertion) and *Gt-g* genial tubercle (genioglossus insertion). (From Abrahams JJ. Anatomy of the jaw revisited with a dental CT software program: pictorial essay. AJNR 1993;14:979–990.)

## Internal Anatomy

Internally the inferior alveolar canal (I) is seen from its origin at the mandibular foramen to its termination at the mental foramen (M). From the region of the mental foramen, a smaller canal, the canal for the incisive artery (Ia), can be seen extending toward the midline (Fig. 14-11B). On the cross-sectional images, the canal distal to the mental foramen is the inferior alveolar canal and the canal mesial to the mental foramen is the canal for the incisive artery (Fig. 14-11A,B). In the midline, the canal for the incisive artery exits the lingual foramen (Lf in Fig. 14-11C) to anastomose with the lingual artery.

### Axial View

On the axial view, the genial tubercle (Gt), mental foramen (M), and inferior alveolar canal (I) are identified in Figure 14-10A,B.

### Panoramic View

On the panoramic view, the course of the inferior alveolar canal (I in Fig. 14-10C and i in Fig. 14-11A) can be traced to its exit point, the mental foramen (M). The canal for the incisive artery (Ia) is visualized extending from the mental foramen toward the midline in Figure 14-11A. Also in Figure 14-11A, nutrient canals (black and white arrows) can be seen extending cephalad from the inferior alveolar canal (i) toward the teeth.

## MAXILLA

The anatomy of the maxilla is described first on the anatomic specimen in Figure 14-12 and then on the illustrations of the neurovascular structures in Figure 14-8.[7–15] This anatomy is then identified on the axial,

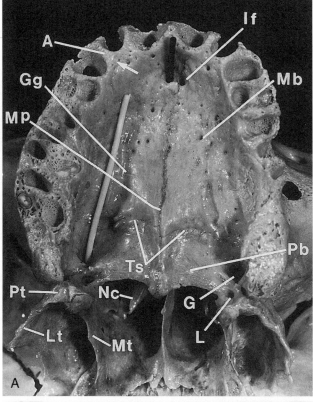

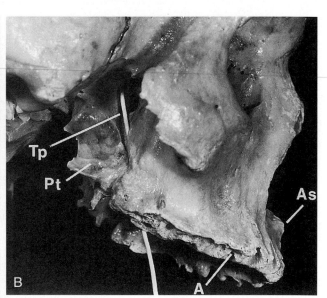

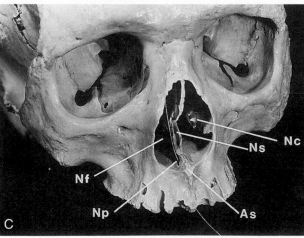

**FIGURE 14-12** Anatomic specimen demonstrating the inferior (**A**), lateral (**B**), and anterior (**C**) aspects of the maxilla. The white probe demonstrates the course of the greater palatine nerve; the black probe demonstrates the course of the nasopalatine nerve. *A* indicates alveolar process; *As*, anterior nasal spine; *G*, greater palatine foramen; *Gg*, groove for greater palatine nerve; *If*, incisive foramen; *L*, lesser palatine foramen; *Lt*, lateral pterygoid plate; *Mb*, maxillary bone, palatine process; *Mp*, median palatine suture; *Mt*, medial pterygoid; *Nc*, nasal concha; *Nf*, nasal fossa; *Np*, nasopalatine canal; *Ns*, nasal septum; *Pb*, palatine bone, horizontal plate; *Pt*, pterygoid process; *Tp*, pterygopalatine fossa; and *Ts*, transverse suture. (From Abrahams JJ. Anatomy of the jaw revisited with a dental CT software program: pictorial essay. AJNR 1993;14:979–990.)

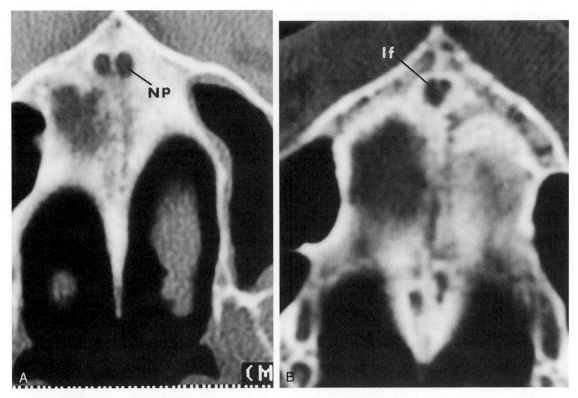

**FIGURE 14-13**   Axial views of the nasopalatine canal and the incisive foramen. **A,** The more superior axial image demonstrates the two nasopalatine canals (*Np*). **B,** The inferior slice demonstrates their common opening, the incisive foramen (*If*). (From Abrahams JJ. Anatomy of the jaw revisited with a dental CT software program: pictorial essay. AJNR 1993;14:979–990.)

panoramic, and cross-sectional CT images in Figures 14-13 and 14-14.[17]

## Anatomic Specimen

The hard palate is composed of several bones delineated by sutures. The transverse suture (coronally oriented Ts in Fig. 14-12A) separates the horizontal plate of the palatine bone (Pb in Fig. 14-12A) from the palatine process of the maxillary bone (Mb in Fig. 14-12A). The median palatine suture (Mp in Fig. 14-12A), which runs in an anteroposterior (sagittal) direction, divides the palate into right and left halves. The pterygoid process of the sphenoid bone (Pt in Fig. 14-12A) is just posterior to the alveolar process. In younger patients, a coronally oriented suture also separates the premaxilla from the maxilla. This suture extends from the incisive foramen (If in Fig. 14-12A) to the lateral incisor-cuspid region (arrow in Fig. 14-12A).

As in the mandible, the teeth are housed in the alveolar process (A in Fig. 14-12A), a horseshoe-shaped bony process in the periphery of the anterior and lateral aspects of the hard palate. Cephalad to the alveolar process are the maxillary sinuses posteriorly and the nasal fossa anteriorly (Nf in Fig. 14-12C). Within the nasal fossa the nasal conchae (Nc in Fig. 14-12C) and nasal septum (Ns in Fig. 14-12C) are seen. A bony protuberance, the anterior maxillary spine (As in Fig. 14-12B,C), is situated just below the nasal fossae in the midline.

Posterior to the maxillary sinus and between it and the pterygoid process (Pt in Fig. 14-12A,B) lies the pterygopalatine fossa (Tp in Figs. 14-12B and 14-14C). The maxillary branch (V2) of the trigeminal nerve enters the pterygopalatine fossa after exiting the skull base through the foramen rotundum. From here a branch, the pterygopalatine nerve (Fig. 14-8B), travels inferiorly through the pterygopalatine canal to exit the greater (G in Fig. 14-12A) and lesser (L in Fig. 14-12B) palatine foramina as the greater and lesser palatine nerves. In Figure 14-12A, a white probe, representing the greater palatine nerve, is seen exiting the greater palatine foramen. After exiting, this nerve changes from a craniocaudal direction to run anteromedially (and horizontally) in a groove (Gg in Fig. 14-12A) in the hard palate. As it travels in the groove, sensory fibers are given off to supply the posterior two-thirds of the hard palate and teeth. The pterygopalatine nerve, represented by the other end of the white probe in Figure 14-12B, can be traced back into the pterygopalatine fossa (Tp in Fig. 14-12B).

Another branch of the pterygopalatine nerve, the superior posterior nasal nerve (Fig. 14-8B,C), enters the posterior nasal cavity through the sphenopalatine foramen. From here it gives off the nasopalatine nerve, a medial branch that runs anteroinferiorly along the nasal septum to enter the nasopalatine canal and incisive foramen (Figs. 14-8C and 14-12C). The incisive foramen is readily seen as a small, round opening in the hard palate just posterior to the central incisors (If in Fig. 14-12A). Sensory fibers supply the anterior hard palate and, along with the anterior superior alveolar nerve (a branch of the infraorbital nerve), supply the central teeth. The terminal portions of the nasopalatine nerve anastomose with the terminal portion of the greater palatine nerve. In Fig. 14-12A,C, the black probe represents the course of the nasopalatine nerve. Note how the black probe enters the incisive foramen (If in Fig. 14-12A), travels through the nasopalatine canal (Np in Fig. 14-12C), and then along the nasal septum (Ns in Fig. 14-12C) to merge with the superior posterior nasal nerve (Fig. 14-8C). The right and left nasopalatine canals are situated in the anteroinferior nasal fossa on either side of the nasal septum.

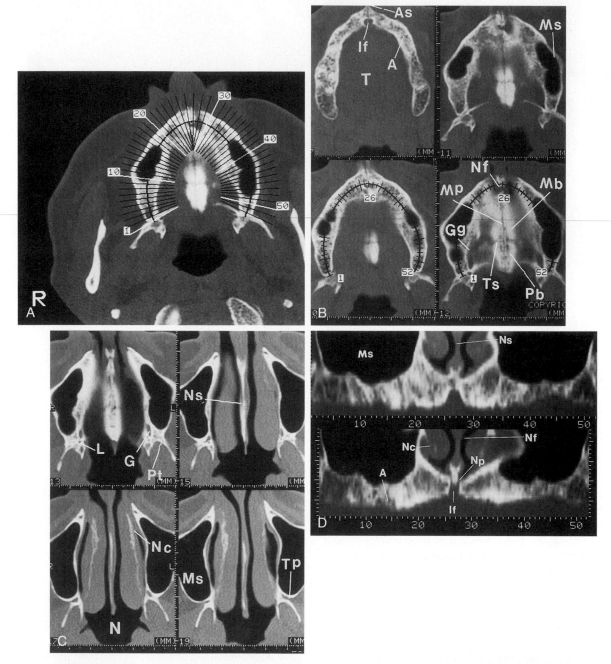

**FIGURE 14-14** CT (DentaScan) image of maxilla. The anatomy identified on the maxillary anatomic specimen is now identified on these CT images. **A,** Axial image with superimposed curve. The curve defines the plane and location in which the panoramic images seen in **D** are reformatted. Numbered lines drawn perpendicular to this curve define the plane and location in which the cross-sectional images viewed in **E** and **F** are reformatted. **B,** Axial views through the alveolar ridge and hard palate. *A* indicates alveolar process; *As,* inferior nasal spine; *Gg,* groove for greater palatine nerve; *If,* incisive foramen; *Mb,* maxillary bone—palatine process; *Mp,* median palatine suture; *Ms,* maxillary sinus; *Nf,* nasal fossa; *Pb,* palatine bone—horizontal plate; *Ts,* transverse suture; and *T,* tongue. **C,** Axial views through the maxillary sinuses and the pterygopalatine fossa. *G* indicates greater palatine foramen; *L,* lesser palatine foramen; *Ms,* maxillary sinus; *Nc,* nasal concha; *Ns,* nasal septum; *Pt,* pterygoid process; and *Tp,* pterygopalatine fossa. **D,** Panoramic views. *A* indicates alveolar process; *If,* incisive foramen; *Ms,* maxillary sinus; *Nc,* nasal concha; *Nf,* nasal fossa; *Np,* nasopalatine canal; and *Ns,* nasal septum.

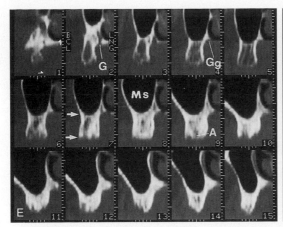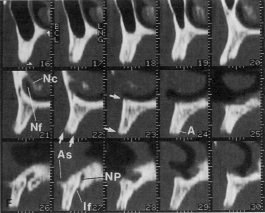

**FIGURE 14-14**   *Continued.* **E** and **F**, Cross-sectional views. Images 1 through 15 (**E**) are through the posterior right maxilla (see perpendicular lines 1 through 15 in **A**); images 16 through 30 (**F**) are more anterior on the right and extend to the midline (see perpendicular lines 16 through 30 in **A**). The arrows in image 7 (**E**) indicate how the height of the distal alveolar process is measured from the floor of the maxillary sinus to the top of the alveolar process and the mesial alveolar process (**F** in image 23) is measured from the floor of the nasal fossa to the top of the alveolar process (*arrows* in image 23). The arrows in image 22 (**F**) indicate how the width of the alveolar process is measured. *A* indicates alveolar process; *As*, anterior maxillary spine; *G*, greater palatine foramen; *Gg*, groove for greater palatine nerve; *If*, incisive foramen; *Ms*, maxillary sinus; *Nc*, nasal concha; *Nf*, nasal fossa; and *Np*, nasopalatine canal. (From Abrahams JJ. Anatomy of the jaw revisited with a dental CT software program: pictorial essay. AJNR 1993;14:979–990.)

## CT Images

### Axial View

The more caudal axial images in Figure 14-14B demonstrate the alveolar process (A), incisive foramen (If), and anterior maxillary spine (As). The teeth, which are normally visualized in the alveolar process at this level, are not seen in this edentulous patient. In the more cranial images the maxillary sinus (Ms) is visible cephalad to the posterior aspect of the alveolar ridge, and the nasal fossa (Nf) is seen cephalad to the anterior aspect of this ridge (Fig. 14-14B). The nasal septum (Ns), nasal concha (Nc), and nasopharynx (N) are visualized in Figure 14-14C. Figure 14-13 illustrates how the right and left nasopalatine canals appear as two separate openings on the more superior cuts but fuse to form a common opening, the incisive foramen, on the inferior images. This is also readily seen on the panoramic view (Fig. 14-14D).

The sutures are identified at the level of the hard palate (Fig. 14-14B). The maxillary bone (Mb) is separated from the palatine bone (Pb) by the transverse suture (Ts). The median palatine suture (MP) separates the right and left halves of the palatine bones. Also seen at the level of the hard palate is the groove for the greater palatine nerve (Gg). Just cephalad to the hard palate (Fig. 14-14C) the greater (G) and lesser (L) palatine foramina are seen.

If the greater palatine foramen is followed cephalad, it merges with the pterygopalatine fossa (Tp) (Fig. 14-14C), which is situated between the posterior wall of the maxillary sinus and the pterygoid process.

### Panoramic View

The panoramic view in Figure 14-14D illustrates the position of the maxillary sinuses (Ms) and nasal fossae (Nf) just cephalad to the alveolar process (A). On either side of the nasal septum (Ns), the right and left nasal palatine canals

(Np) are clearly visualized merging with the more inferior incisive foramen (If).

### Cross-Sectional View

In Figure 14-14E,F, images 1 through 25 correspond to the right half of the maxilla, images 26 and 27 represent the midline with the incisive foramen, and images 28 through 30 represent the more medial aspect of the left maxilla. This may be more readily appreciated by looking at perpendicular lines 1 through 30, which are superimposed on the axial image in Fig. 14-14A. In the right posterior maxilla (Fig. 14-14E), the greater palatine foramen is visualized (G in image 2). As one moves toward the midline, the most proximal portion of the groove (Gg) for the greater palatine nerve can be seen in images 3 through 5. The maxillary sinuses (Ms) are visualized cephalad to the alveolar process on the more posterior images, and the nasal fossae (Nf) are visualized cephalad to the alveolar process on the more anterior images (21 to 23 in Fig. 14-14F). In the midline (images 26 and 27, Fig. 14-14F), the nasopalatine canal (Np), incisive foramen (If), and anterior maxillary spine (As) are seen.

## REFERENCES

1. Sperber GH. Craniofacial Embryology 4th ed. London: Wright, 1989.
2. Melfi RC. Permar's Oral Embryology and Microscopic Anatomy: a textbook. Philadelphia: Lea & Febiger, 1994.
3. Carlson BM. Human Embryology and Developmental Biology. St. Louis: Mosby, 1994.
4. Moore KL, Persaud TVN. The Developing Human. Philadelphia: WB Saunders, 1988.
5. Farman AG, Nortjé CJ, Wood RE. Oral and Maxillofacial Diagnostic Imaging. St. Louis: CV Mosby, 1993.
6. Sicher H. The viscera of the head and neck. In: Sicher H. Oral Anatomy. 4th ed. St. Louis: CV Mosby, 1965;191–324.

7. Wishan M, Bahat O, Krane M. Computed tomography as an adjunct in dental implant surgery. Int J Periodont Restor Dentistry 1988; 8:30–47.

8. Ennis LM, Harrison MB Jr, Phillips JE. Normal anatomical landmarks of the teeth and jaws as seen in the roentgenogram. In: Ennis LM. Dental Roentgenology. 6th ed. Philadelphia: Lea & Febiger, 1967;334–407.

9. Gray H. Osteology. In: Gray H. Anatomy of the Human Body. 28th ed. Philadelphia: Lea & Febiger, 1969;107–293.

10. Gray H. The peripheral nervous system. In: Gray H. Anatomy of the Human Body. 28th ed. Philadelphia: Lea & Febiger, 1969;907–1042.

11. Gray H. The digestive system. In: Gray H. Anatomy of the Human Body. 28th ed. Philadelphia: Lea & Febiger, 1969;1161–1263.

12. Gray H. Arteries of the head and neck. In: Gray H. Anatomy of the Human Body. 28th ed. Philadelphia: Lea & Febiger, 1969;1161–1263.

13. Meschan I. The skull. In: Meschan I. An Atlas of Anatomy Basic to Radiology. Philadelphia: WB Saunders, 1975;209–287.

14. Sicher H. The skull. In: Sicher H. Oral Anatomy. 4th ed. St. Louis: CV Mosby, 1965;23–140.

15. Sicher H. The nerves of the head and neck. In: Sicher H. Oral Anatomy. 4th ed. St. Louis: CV Mosby, 1965;364–398.

16. Abrahams JJ. Anatomy of the jaw revisited with a dental CT software program: pictorial essay. AJNR 1993;14:979–990.

17. Abrahams JJ. The role of diagnostic imaging in dental implantology. Radiol Clin North Am 1993;31(1):163–180.

## 15

# Dental CT Reformatting Programs and Dental Imaging

*James J. Abrahams, Michael W. Hayt,*
*and Reuben Rock*

Edentulism is present in almost half of the population that is between 45 and 74 years of age.[1] Traditionally, edentulism has been treated with removable dentures; however, not all patients are candidates for dentures, and many have continued difficulty with speech, oral function, and reduced self-esteem. In response to these problems, dentists developed nonremovable bridges that are attached to oral implants, metal posts surgically embedded in the jaw (Fig. 15-1). During the past decade, it has been determined that CT, with a dental reformatting program, is the method of choice for the preoperative assessment of these patients, and as a result of this work, new dialogues and interactions have been created between the radiologist and the dentist and oral surgeon. This, in turn, has brought new territories and unfamiliar diseases to the radiologist's attention. Radiologists now evaluate the dental aspects of the oral cavity, including implants, periodontal disease, odontogenic tumors, and other lesions of the jaw.[2–8] The goal of this chapter is to present a comprehensive discussion of dental imaging, including dental CT reformatting programs, and orthopantomographic and intraoral films.

## DENTAL CT PROGRAMS

Dental CT programs use thin, 1-mm axial CT images of the maxilla and mandible to reformat a series of multiple cross-sectional and panoramic images of the jaw. The orientation of the cross-sectional images, which can be confusing, is illustrated in Figure 15-2. The cross-sectional and panoramic images are illustrated in Figure 15-1. After the patient is scanned and the axial images have been acquired, the reformatting program is run to produce the panoramic and cross-sectional views described below.

## Scan Parameters

The thin axial images are obtained in the following fashion. First, the patient is placed supine in the gantry, using a head holder, chin strap, and sponges on either side of the head to prevent motion. The patient is then instructed to remain motionless. A lateral digital scout view is first obtained to define the upper and lower limits of the study and to determine if the scan plane is parallel to the alveolar ridge. Because the DentaScan program does not permit angulation of the gantry, if the scan plane is not correctly positioned the patient should be repositioned and a repeat lateral digital scout scan performed. Once the scan plane is correct, 1-mm contiguous scans are obtained using a bone algorithm, dynamic mode, 15-cm field of view, 512 × 512 matrix, 140 kV and 70 mA. If both the mandible and maxilla are being studied, a separate run should be performed for

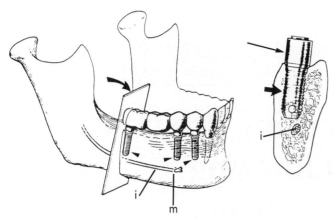

**FIGURE 15-1** View of the mandible illustrating the plane of orientation of the cross-sectional DentaScan images. The top of the plane (*curved arrow*) corresponds to one of the numbered perpendicular lines on the axial image in Figure 15-2A. Note how the height and width of the alveolar process and the location of the mandibular canal can be readily determined on the cross-sectional image. Three root form implants are seen (*arrowheads*) supporting a four-tooth prosthesis. The abutment (*thin arrow*) attached to the fixture (*broad arrow*) raises it above the surface of the bone and gingiva and into the oral cavity. Inferior alveolar canal (*i*), mental foramen (*m*). (From Langer B, Sullivan D. Osseointegration: its impact on the relationship of periodontics and restorative dentistry. Part 1. Int J Periodont Res 1989;9:86.)

each because the scan angle of the mandible is slightly different than that of the maxilla.

## Running the Dental Program

Once the axial images are acquired, they are processed with the dental CT reformatting program. Programs may vary slightly from manufacturer to manufacturer; however, the following guidelines generally apply. An axial image that nicely shows the curve of the mandible or maxilla at the level of the roots of the teeth is selected by the technologist and a curved line, along the midportion of the alveolus, is superimposed on the axial image (Figs. 15-2A and 15-3A) by depositing the cursor on approximately six different points along the curve of the jaw. The program then automatically connects these points to produce a smooth curve that will be superimposed on the jaw. This curved line defines the plane and location of the reformatted panoramic images (Figs. 15-2C and 15-3D). Several images are then reformatted both buccally and lingually to this curve.

The reformatted cross-sectional images (Figs. 15-2D–F and 15-3E,F) are defined by multiple numbered lines that the program automatically deposits perpendicular to the curved line (Figs. 15-2A and 15-3A). Figure 15-2A shows the plane and orientation of the cross-sectional images and the distance between the numbered perpendicular lines. The distance between the cross-sectional images can be varied. In general, a 2-mm spacing is used. If a stent with radiographic markers is utilized, 1-mm slices may be necessary to visualize the markers. The mandibular canal (neurovascular bundle) is easily visualized on the cross-sectional images, and the width and contour of the jaw can be readily assessed (Fig. 15-2D–F). Streak artifact, which degrades visualization of bone on direct coronal images, does not degrade the

reformatted cross-sectional images because the artifact is projected at the level of the crowns of the teeth and not over the bony alveolus (curved arrow in Fig. 15-2E).

When the program is completed, three types of images are displayed: axial, cross-sectional, and panoramic. Typically there are approximately 30 to 50 axial images, 40 to 100 cross-sectional images, and 5 panoramic images. It is important to film these images in a consistent fashion to avoid confusing the referring dentist. Life-size (one to one magnification) cross-sectional and panoramic images are preferred. This can usually be accomplished with most programs by filming four images on a 14 × 17-inch x-ray film. If this cannot be accomplished, the manufacturer of the program should be consulted. A millimeter scale displayed on the films (mm at the bottom of Fig. 15-2D) is used to verify the degree of magnification and to obtain accurate measurements. One can place calipers on the bone image to be measured and transfer this caliper setting to the millimeter scale. Any minification or magnification of the images equally minifies or magnifies the scale and thus does not affect the measurements.

Optimally, filming is done on a laser printer. Most often the axial images are filmed with 12 images per film, while the cross-sectional and panoramic images are filmed with 4 images per film. Each cross-sectional and panoramic image actually contains multiple images (see Fig. 15-2). The images are typically photographed at a width (window) of 3000 to 4000 and a level (center) of 300 to 500 (Figs. 15-2 and 15-3).

## Interpretation of Dental CT Program Images and Measurements

An understanding of the anatomy and pathology of the jaw is necessary to appropriately interpret the images displayed by the dental CT programs. It should first be noted that each CT view can be related to the others by a series of scale marks that appear on the films. The marks that run along the side of the cross-sectional and panoramic images (Fig. 15-2C,D) correspond to the direct axial slices that were used to reformat the images. For example, in Figure 15-2, 42 axial images were obtained to reformat the images; thus there are 42 scale marks along the side of the reformatted cross-sectional (Fig. 15-2D) and panoramic (Fig. 15-2C) images. The marks along the bottom of the panoramic images (Fig. 15-2C) correspond to the numbered cross-sectional images. The numbered scale lines correspond to the numbered lines drawn perpendicular to the curve superimposed on the axial image in Figure 15-2A. They therefore also correspond to the numbered cross-sectional images in Figure 15-2D–F. To illustrate how one view can be related to another, note how the right mental foramen (M) in Figure 15-2E, which is seen on cross-sectional image 20 (lower right) at the level of the fourteenth scale mark on the side of the image, is also seen in Figure 15-2B on axial image 14 at the twentieth perpendicular line. The same process can be applied to the panoramic view.

When the scan is performed as part of the preoperative workup of a dental implant patient, the status of the dentition and the proposed implant sites must be established. It should be stated whether the patient is completely or partially edentulous and, if partially edentulous, where the teeth are absent. In the partially edentulous patient, it is presumed that the implants will be placed in the edentulous segments; thus measurements are obtained in these regions. The measure-

ments are obtained from the cross-sectional images at about 10-mm intervals. If the cross-sectional images are 2 mm apart, then measurements are made on every fifth cross-sectional image. If the cross-sectional images are 1 mm apart, measurements are provided for every tenth image. The

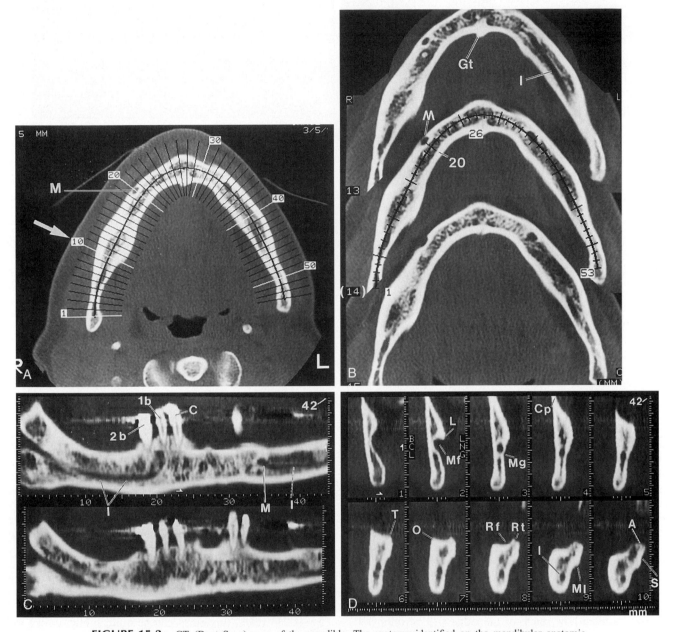

**FIGURE 15-2**   CT (DentaScan) scan of the mandible. The anatomy identified on the mandibular anatomic specimen in Figure 14-6 is now identified on these CT images. **A**, Axial image of mandible with a superimposed curve. The curve defines the plane and location in which the panoramic images in **C** are reformatted. Numbered lines drawn perpendicular to this curve (*arrow*) define the plane and location in which the cross-sectional images viewed in **D** through **F** are reformatted. Mental foramen (*M*). **B**, Axial images illustrating the inferior alveolar canal (*I*), the mental foramen (*M*), and the genial tubercle (*Gt*). The numbers along the left side of the figure refer to the particular number of the axial image. Note that the mental foramen, which is seen on axial image number 14 at the twentieth perpendicular line, is also seen in **E** on cross-sectional image 20 (lower right) at the level of the fourteenth tick mark on the side of the image. The tick marks and numbers allow images to be correlated with one another. **C**, Panoramic views. The numbered tick marks along the bottom of the images correspond to the numbered perpendicular lines displayed on the axial image in **A**. The tick marks along the side of the image correspond to the axial images that were used to reformat these images. Note that there were 42 axial images acquired and thus 42 tick marks along the side of this image. Inferior alveolar canal (*I*), mental foramen (*M*), second bicuspid (*2b*), first bicuspid (*1b*), and cuspid (*C*). **D** through **F**, Cross-sectional views. Images 1 through 10 (**D**) are through the posterior right mandible (see perpendicular lines 1 through 10 in **A**).

*Illustration continued on following page*

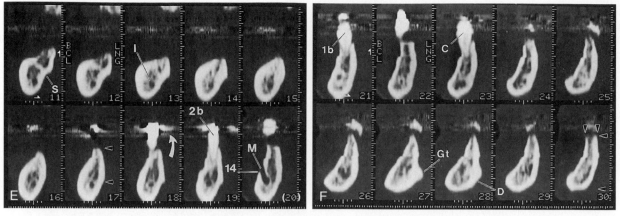

**FIGURE 15-2**  *Continued.* Images 11 through 20 (**E**) are more anterior. Images 21 through 30 (**F**) extend to the midline. The images of the left half of the mandible are not shown. Arrowheads in image 17 (**E**) indicate that the height of the mandible distal to the mental foramen is measured from the top of the alveolar process to the top of the mandibular canal, and mesial to the foramen it is measured from the top of the alveolar process to the bottom of the mandible (*arrowheads* in **F**, image 30). Measurement of the width is also demonstrated in image 30 (**F**). *mm* at the bottom of **D** indicates the millimeter scale. Note how streak artifact from the dental restoration (*curved arrow* in **E**) does not degrade visualization of the bone. *A* indicates alveolar process; *C,* cuspid; *Cp,* coronoid process; *D,* digastric fossa; *Gt,* genial tubercle; *I,* inferior alveolar canal; *M,* mental foramen; *Mf,* mandibular foramen; *Mg,* mylohyoid groove; *Ml,* mylohyoid line; *O,* oblique line; *Rf,* retromolar fossa; *Rt,* retromolar triangle; *S,* submandibular fossa; *Sl,* sublingual fossa; *T,* temporal crest; *1b,* first bicuspid; and *2b,* second bicuspid. (From Abrahams JJ. Anatomy of the jaw revisited with a dental CT software program: pictorial essay. AJNR 1993;14:979–990.)

height and width of the alveolar process are measured as described in the following paragraph.

In the mandible, the height in the region distal (posterior) to the mental foramen is measured from the top of the alveolar process to the top to the mandibular canal (Fig. 15-2E, arrowheads in image 17). Methods of locating the mandibular canal, if it is not initially visualized on the cross-sectional images, are discussed later. In the region mesial (anterior) to the mental foramen, the full height of the mandible is obtained because the mandibular canal ends at the mental foramen and thus it is not present mesial to the foramen. Measurements in this area are provided from the top of the alveolar ridge to the bottom of the mandible (Fig. 15-2F, arrowheads in image 30). The width is measured near the top of the alveolar process (Fig. 15-2F, arrowheads in image 30). Occasionally, if the alveolar process comes to a point secondary to atrophy, it may be difficult to obtain a measurement. In this situation the surgeon may choose to remove the top pointed portion of the ridge (alveoloplasty), providing a broad base for an implant. This obviously affects the height of the alveolar ridge, and it is best to let the surgeon estimate how much of the ridge will be removed. Often under these circumstances, one simply states that the ridge is pointed, and a measurement for the width is not provided.

In the maxilla, the height in the distal (posterior) aspect is measured from the top (inferior surface) of the alveolar process to the floor of the maxillary sinus (Fig. 15-3E, arrows in image 7). More mesially (anteriorly), the height is usually not limited by the maxillary sinuses and is measured from the alveolar ridge to the nasal fossa floor (Fig. 15-3F, arrows in image 23). The width is measured in the same manner as that described for the mandible (Fig. 15-3F, arrows in image 22). In the completely edentulous patient, it is more desirable to place the implants centrally because the

height of the alveolar process is not limited by the more distal mandibular canal or the maxillary sinuses.

## Identifying the Mandibular Canal

It is extremely important to identify the mandibular canal on cross-sectional images and to provide the measurement from the top of the alveolar ridge to the top of this canal. If the canal is not properly identified, its injury during implant surgery can be quite debilitating for the patient, resulting in permanent paresthesia and hypesthesia of the face. Typically the canal is readily seen on cross-sectional images. However, there are times when portions of the canal or even the entire canal may be hard to visualize on the cross-sectional images. In this situation the following methods may be helpful in locating the canal.

The first method involves the cortical niche sign, which refers to an indentation along the inner or medullary margin on the lingual cortex of the mandible. This niche is created by the mandibular nerve as it traverses the mandible (Fig. 15-4). However, this niche can be quite subtle, unlike that shown in Figure 15-4, and it is not identified in all patients. When present, it is a good way to identify the canal. Care should be taken not to confuse other cortical irregularities with the cortical niche sign. The cortical niche is a continuous defect seen on multiple cross-sectional images. Other cortical irregularities are randomly situated and are not seen consecutively on multiple images. When the canal is identified with the cortical niche sign, its location should be confirmed with the other methods.

The next method, referred to as triangulation, utilizes the scale marks on the films to relate an anatomic structure well seen on one view to its location on another view. With this method, the panoramic and axial views can be utilized to identify the canal on the cross-sectional views. For example, in Figure 15-5A, it is difficult to see the canal on the cross-sectional images, but the canal is readily seen in the panoramic view (Fig. 15-5B). The information from the panoramic view can be used to triangulate the location of the canal on the cross-sectional image, as shown in Figure 15-5.

To locate the canal on cross-sectional image 14 (Fig. 15-5A), first refer to the fourteenth scale mark along the bottom of the panoramic view (Fig. 15-5B). A vertical line from this point is then drawn up to the bottom of the canal and extended across in a perpendicular direction toward the scale marks on the left side of the panoramic image. Note

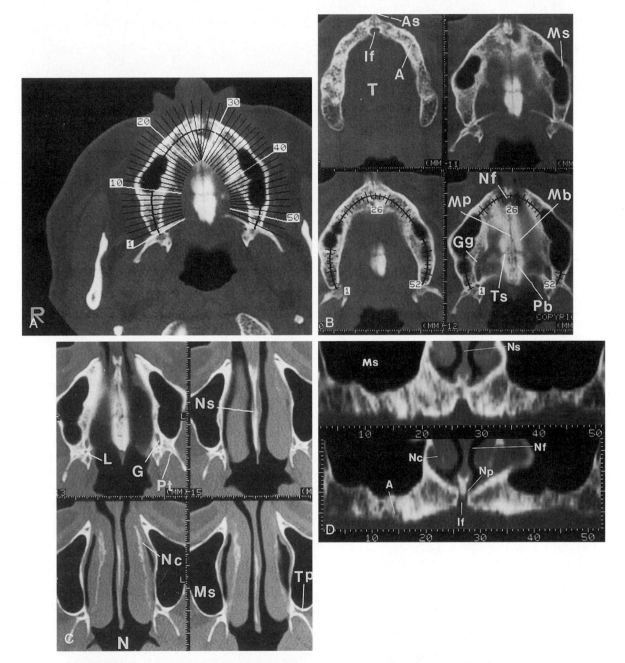

**FIGURE 15-3**   CT (DentaScan) scan of maxilla. The anatomy identified on the maxillary anatomic specimen in Figure 15-12 is now identified on these CT images. **A,** Axial image with superimposed curve. The curve defines the plane and location in which the panoramic images seen in **D** are reformatted. Numbered lines drawn perpendicular to this curve define the plane and location in which the cross-sectional images viewed in **E** and **F** are reformatted. **B,** Axial views through the alveolar ridge and hard palate. *A* indicates alveolar process; *As,* inferior nasal spine; *Gg,* groove for greater palatine nerve; *If,* incisive foramen; *Mb,* maxillary bone—palatine process; *Mp,* median palatine suture; *Ms,* maxillary sinus; *Nf,* nasal fossa; *Pb,* palatine bone—horizontal plate; *Ts,* transverse suture; and *T,* tongue. **C,** Axial views through the maxillary sinuses and the pterygopalatine fossa. *G* indicates greater palatine foramen; *L,* lesser palatine foramen; *Ms,* maxillary sinus; *Nc,* nasal concha; *Ns,* nasal septum; *Pt,* pterygoid process; and *Tp,* pterygopalatine fossa. **D,** Panoramic views. *A* indicates alveolar process; *If,* incisive foramen; *Ms,* maxillary sinus; *Nc,* nasal concha; *Nf,* nasal fossa; *Np,* nasopalatine canal; and *Ns,* nasal septum.

*Illustration continued on following page*

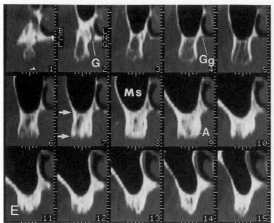
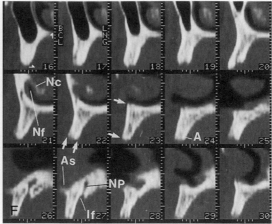

**FIGURE 15-3** *Continued.* **E** and **F**, Cross-sectional views. Images 1 through 15 (**E**) are through the posterior right maxilla (see perpendicular lines 1 through 15 in **A**); images 16 through 30 (**F**) are more anterior on the right and extend to the midline (see perpendicular lines 16 through 30 in **A**). The arrows in image 7 (**E**) indicate how the height of the distal alveolar process is measured from the floor of the maxillary sinus to the top of the alveolar process and the mesial alveolar process (*F* in image 23) is measured from the floor of the nasal fossa to the top of the alveolar process (*arrows* in image 23). The arrows in image 22 (**F**) indicate how the width of the alveolar process is measured. *A* indicates alveolar process; *As,* anterior maxillary spine; *G,* greater palatine foramen; *Gg,* groove for greater palatine nerve; *If,* incisive foramen; *Ms,* maxilllary sinus; *Nc,* nasal concha; *Nf,* nasal fossa; and *Np,* nasopalatine canal. (From Abrahams JJ. Anatomy of the jaw revisited with a dental CT software program: pictorial essay. AJNR 1993;14:979–990.)

that this line intersects the twenty-first scale mark along the left side of the image. The level of the canal in cross-sectional image 14 can then be identified by counting up 21 scale marks along the side of the image (Fig. 15-5A). This same process can also be utilized with the axial images.

Finally, if a canal is identified on some cross-sectional images but not on others, the images on which it is identified can be utilized to estimate the position of the canal on the other images. This can be done because the distance from the bottom of the mandible to the bottom of the canal tends to be relatively constant. The only region where the distance is not constant is immediately adjacent to the mandibular foramen and the mental foramen. It is the distance from the top of the canal to the top of the alveolar process that varies secondary to atrophic changes. With this knowledge, one can extrapolate the location of the canal from the images in which it is visualized. For example, in Figure 15-2E, the distance from the bottom of the canal to the bottom of the mandible in image 11 is 5 mm, and in image 15 it is also 5 mm. Therefore, if the canal was not visualized in image 15, its location could be estimated by utilizing the position of the canal that was visible on image 11. Usually the right and left hemimandibles are symmetric, and the distance from the bottom of the mandible to the bottom of the canal on the right side at a particular point is approximately the same as the distance measured at that same point on the left. Thus, if the canal is identified on the cross-sectional images of the right half of the mandible, but not on the left side, this information can be used to estimate the position of the canal on the left side. It is recommended that one use several of these methods to confirm the location of the canal rather than relying on only one method.

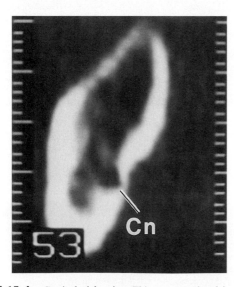

**FIGURE 15-4** Cortical niche sign. This cross-sectional image of the mandible demonstrates an indentation on the lingual cortex of the mandible called the cortical niche sign (*Cn*), which is created by the mandibular nerve as it traverses the mandible. This sign, which is often more subtle than this, can be helpful in identifying the location of the mandibular canal. (From Abrahams JJ. CT assessment of dental implant planning. Oral Maxillofac Surg Clin North Am 1992;4:1–18.)

## Dictated Report

A complete and comprehensive report should be provided for the referring dentist or oral surgeon. First, the report usually provides a discussion of the density and general health of the jaw. Also described are the presence of such conditions as maxillary sinus disease, periodontal disease, root canal procedures, extraction sockets, retained roots, atrophy, cysts, osteitis condensans, contour irregularities, surgical changes, and anomalies such as torus palatinus or mandibularus. Next, the status of the dentition is discussed. State whether the patient is partially or completely edentulous. If the patient is partially edentulous, state whether the edentulous area is central or distally on the right or left.

If the scan is being performed for dental implants, then measurements of the alveolar ridge are provided of the edentulous regions where the implants are likely to be placed. The measurements are taken from the cross-sectional images at about 10-mm intervals, as described above, and reported in a tabular fashion. The location of the mental foramina and incisive foramen are identified as a reference point and for easier interpretation. For example, the following measurements were obtained from Figure 15-2E,F:

Image 17:   Height 14 mm, width 4 mm
Image 20:   Left mental foramen
Image 25:   Height 26 mm, width 4 mm

If a stent with radiopaque markers is utilized, then the markers on the images are numbered with a wax pencil, measurements are obtained on the cross-sectional images where the markers appear, and the image number is provided in the report. In Figure 15-6, the measurements at the markers are as follows:

Marker 4 (Image 21):   Height 13 mm, width 6 mm
Marker 5 (Image 27):   Height 12 mm, width 5 mm

If the scan was performed to evaluate a lesion rather than implant placements, the alveolar measurements are not needed. Instead, a description of the lesion is provided. Is there expansion of the jaw or destruction of the cortex? Is the lesion lytic or opaque? Is it diffuse or focal? Are the roots of the teeth displaced or eroded?

Finally, the report should end with a brief impression, describing any pertinent pathology and the degree of atrophy of the alveolar process in the case of dental implants. One should also state that "all measurements should be verified prior to surgery." This statement is included because the surgeon may choose to place the implant at a somewhat different angle than that measured by the radiologist and because, when the report is transcribed, it is possible for numbers to be typed incorrectly, and this may be difficult for the radiologist to notice.

## ORTHOPANTOMOGRAPHIC (PANOREX) RADIOGRAPHY

Panoramic radiography is usually performed in a dentist's office. The typical use of this modality is to provide an overview for evaluating the jaws and dentition in a single radiograph (Fig. 15-7). This technique demonstrates the relationship of the teeth to the surrounding structures. It is extremely valuable before exodontia (removal of teeth) and for evaluating mandibular fractures. Since it shows the relationships of the teeth to the other teeth and surrounding structures, it is useful in orthodontic treatment planning and for demonstrating orthodontic movement of teeth. Other situations, such as abnormally erupted teeth, extractions, relationship of tumors to teeth, and so on, can also be assessed (Fig. 15-7).

Panoramic radiography of the jaws helps overcome limitations of conventional intraoral radiography. The radiation dose to the patient is 10 times less than that of the full-mouth intraoral radiography survey. Further, it allows overall coverage of the entire dental arches and associated structures on one radiograph. There can, however, be up to 25% distortion, and measurements may therefore be difficult. This is a relatively fast and painless procedure. It is also very useful when a patient cannot open the mouth due to trismus or trauma. The mandibular ramus, styloid process, temporo-

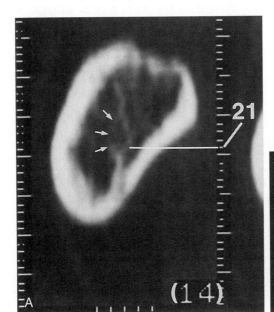
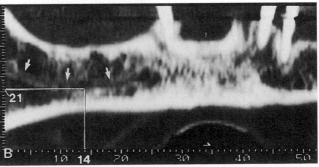

**FIGURE 15-5**   Triangulation. When the inferior alveolar canal is not initially seen on the cross-sectional images, as in this case (**A**), its location can be determined by triangulating from the panoramic (**B**) or axial image, as described in the section of text on "Identifying the Mandibular Canal". The inferior alveolar canal is indicated by arrows. (From Abrahams JJ. CT assessment of dental implant planning. Oral Maxillofac Surg Clin North Am 1992;4:1–18.)

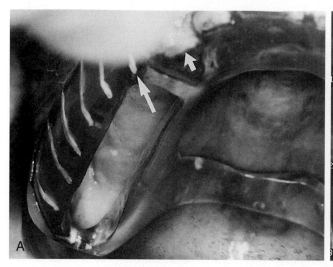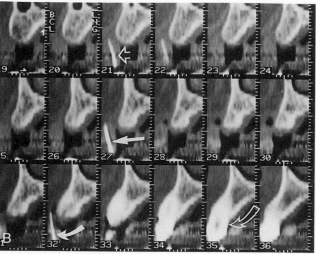

**FIGURE 15-6** Surgical implant procedure. **A,** A stent with six vertical markers has been placed over the alveolar ridge and residual teeth. The sixth marker (*long arrow*) is adjacent to the right canine (*short arrow*) and will be demonstrated on the CT images. This marker appears as a dot on the axial image and as a line on the cross-sectional image. **B,** Cross-sectional views demonstrating markers 4 (*open arrow*), 5 (*straight arrow*), and 6 (*curved arrow*) of the stent. Note that marker number 6 is adjacent to the right canine (*open curved arrow*). By placing the stent on the patient during surgery, the surgeon knows that the bone under marker 6 is as depicted by cross-sectional image 32. (From Abrahams JJ. The role of diagnostic imaging in dental implantology. Radiol Clin North Am 1993;31(1):163–180.)

mandibular joint, superior maxillary sinus, and floor of the mouth structures are visualized. These structures cannot be seen with intraoral radiography. With this technique, some soft-tissue structures attenuate the x-ray beam enough to be visualized and cause artifacts. The panoramic radiograph is limited, when compared with conventional intraoral radiography, by the necessity for careful technique, sensitivity to patient motion, and relatively poor spatial resolution.

Rotational panoramic radiographs are obtained by rotating a slender x-ray beam in a horizontal axis that is positioned extraorally. The principle is very similar to that of conventional x-ray tomography. With this technique, the focal spot of the x-ray tube anode acts as the dimension of the projection. To eliminate scatter and artifact, the x-ray beam is angled beneath the occipital condyles of the skull approximately – 4° to –7°. The patient remains stationary as the x-ray tube and film cassette holder both rotate around the patient's face during the exposure. The film is exposed though a narrow opening in the cassette that is usually flexible. These films are very technique sensitive. If the patient is improperly positioned, certain structures will be out of the focal trough (blurred). Even in properly positioned patients, the midline structures may be flattened and spread out or may be projected as a double image.

The normal anatomic structure seen in panoramic radiography are listed below and shown in Figures 15-7 and 15-8.

1. Mandibular condyles
2. Ramus of the mandible
3. Cervical spine
4. Maxillary sinus
5. Inferior turbinate
6. Inferior alveolar canal
7. Mental foramen
8. Nasal fossae
9. Dentition
10. Sigmoid notch
11. Mandibular coronoid process
12. Developing tooth bud
13. Hyoid bone

## INTRAORAL RADIOGRAPHY

An intraoral radiograph is obtained by placing a film packet in the mouth and projecting the x-ray beam at different angles from a position outside of the mouth toward the teeth. There are three types of intraoral radiographs, which are described as periapical, bitewing, and occlusal.

**FIGURE 15-7** Panoramic radiograph of jaws in an adult with extractions of mandibular third molars. This has caused supereruption (occlusal migration due to lack of contact by the opposing tooth) of teeth numbers 1 and 16. Hyoid bone (*white arrow*). Inferior alveolar canal (*arrowheads*). Dentition (mandibular left second molar) (*bold black arrow*). Right mental foramen (*thin black arrow*). Inferior nasal turbinate (*\**). Maxillary sinus (*M*).

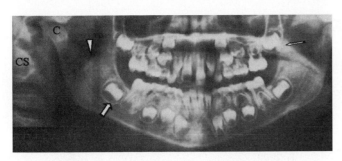

**FIGURE 15-8**    Panoramic radiograph of jaws in a child with mixed dentition (both primary and adult). Coronoid process (*thin white arrow*). Sigmoid notch of mandible (*arrowhead*). Mandibular condyle (*C*). Developing tooth bud of the permanent mandibular right first molar (*bold arrow*). Cervical spine (*CS*).

## Periapical Radiographs

The word *periapical* comes from *peri,* meaning "around," and *apical,* meaning "at the apex or end of the tooth root" (Fig. 15-9). This is the most common type of radiograph obtained in a dentist's office and has great spatial resolution, demonstrating exquisite detail compared with other techniques. Ideally, it is obtained by placing a film holder on the occlusal surface of the teeth and asking the patient to bite down to hold it in place. The film is attached to the end of the film holder within the patient's mouth on the lingual aspect, and an aiming guide is built into the other end of the film holder outside the patient's mouth. The aiming guide allows the dental x-ray tube to be aligned perpendicular to the film, thus preventing distortion. Periapical films allow the dentist to visualize the entire tooth, root, and surrounding structures, and to visualize the relationship of one tooth and its root to another. They allow the dentist to evaluate whether common entities such as caries and periodontal disease exist and, if so, their extent. This radiograph is also obtained during endodontal (root canal) procedures to measure tooth length and to determine whether the endodontal restoration (within the tooth root) is in the proper position. Periapical films have a vertical orientation, while the bitewing films have a horizontal orientation.

## Bitewing Radiographs

Bitewing radiographs (Fig. 15-10) demonstrate on a single film the position and extent of the crowns and coronal one-third of the interalveolar bone and portion of the roots of the maxillary and mandibular teeth. These radiographs, too, have excellent spatial resolution. A special bitewing holding device is placed on the occlusal surface of the tooth and the patient gently bites down to hold it in place. As with the periapical radiograph, an aiming device is ideally used to maintain a perpendicular relationship between the film and the x-ray beam. These films are commonly obtained to detect interproximal caries (between teeth), iatrogenically malplaced dental restorations, periodontal disease, and calculus (tartar) deposits; to evaluate pulp chamber shape and size; and to evaluate the occlusal relationship of teeth. They are not usually helpful for visualization of the root apices or periapical lesions such as a cysts or abscesses.

## Occlusal Radiographs

Occlusal radiographs are images of the incisal edges and occlusal surfaces of the teeth and a cross-section of the dental arches. The hard palate, upper lip, and base of the nose are seen in a maxillary occlusal radiograph. The mandibular occlusal radiograph records the floor of mouth, tongue, and lower lip. This type of radiograph is useful for determining the presence of foreign bodies, alveolar

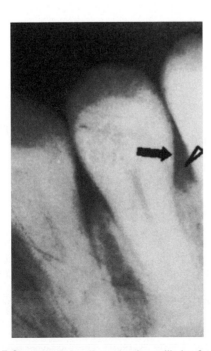

**FIGURE 15-9**    Periapical radiograph of mandibular first and second premolars. Cementoenamel junction (where enamel of tooth crown ends and cementum of root begins) (*black arrow*). The arrowhead points to the place where the alveolar crest of bone would normally be. Note that the bone is below this level secondary to loss from periodontal disease.

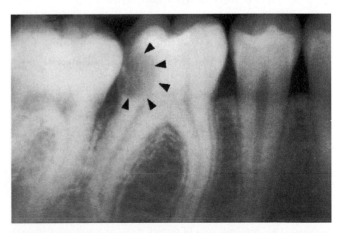

**FIGURE 15-10**    Bitewing radiograph of the mandibular second molar shows large interproximal carious lesion on the distal surface (*arrowheads*). Note that the root apices are not in the field of view on the bitewing radiograph.

fractures, and salivary duct calculi, as well as the position and relationship of impacted teeth.

## DENTAL PATHOLOGY SEEN ON RADIOGRAPHS

### Periodontal Disease

One of the most common abnormalities seen in dental radiographs is periodontal disease. This disease is a result of gingival inflammation (gingivitis), which leads to periodontitis (inflammation of the tooth socket) and then edentulism. Periodontal disease is very closely related to the patient's age and the amount of dental plaque accumulation. Accumulation of dental plaque at the free gingival margin causes the initial lesion of periodontal disease. Inflammatory exudates, gingival crevicular fluid, and leukocytes migrate into the gingival crevice. The collagen fibers within the gingiva near the free gingival margin become destroyed and replaced by inflammatory infiltrate and engorged vasculature. Subsequently, chemotactic substances from the maturing dental plaque cause a host response.

Initially, after about 4 days, early gingivitis develops, with associated swelling and erythema. Plaque then invades the periodontal ligament space, the gingival sulcus deepens through destruction of the junctional epithelium, and an inflammatory reaction against the plaque ensues at the free gingival margin. The periodontal membrane remains intact initially. After several weeks, inflammatory changes become more pronounced, and there is an increase in swelling and crevicular bleeding, with an associated increase in exudate. Predominantly plasma cells, along with T and B lymphocytes, are now found within the gingival sulcus. The lesion may exist for long periods, perhaps years, without progressing to the advanced lesion.[9]

As the lesion advances, plaque accumulates deep within the dental gingival junction, replacing the collagen fiber of the gingiva with inflamed connective tissue, ulceration of pocket epithelium, and increased crevicular fluid production. This results in destruction of the normal anatomy of the gingiva. Plaque and calculus then adhere to the root and tooth surface, attaching to irregularities in the cementum and absorbing bacterial endotoxin. Osteoclastic activity is then induced by factors from the dental plaque or inflammatory response. The supporting bone for the tooth is then lost.[10]

Some authors believe, however, that periodontal disease develops in response to infection by specific bacteria. Over 300 different microbial species have been identified that are associated with dental plaque and periodontal disease. Some, however, point to *Actinobacillus actinomycetemcomitans, Bacteroides indermedius,* and *Bacteroides gingivalis* as specific organisms that induce periodontal disease.

Most authors do agree that periodontal disease is a chronic disease that results in bone destruction (and supporting dental apparatus) at a rate of 0.2 mm per year. Some gingival plaque is thought of as inciting a host parasite response. This results in gingivitis followed by periodontal ligament attachment loss, increased gingival sulcus depth bone, and eventually tooth loss.

Normally, in the fully erupted dentition, the alveolar crest

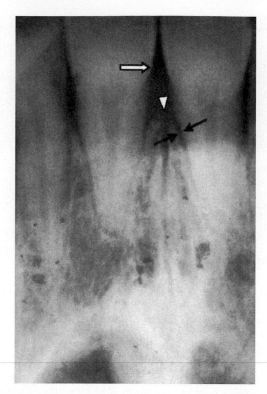

**FIGURE 15-11** Periapical radiograph of mandibular central incisors depicts mild loss of alveolar bone from periodontal disease. Alveolar crest (*arrowhead*) is eroded and is now located below the cementoenamel junction (*white arrow*). Concurrent minimal widening of the periodontal ligament space (*black arrows*) is noted.

of bone is located adjacent to the cementoenamel junction of the tooth (where the enamel of the crown meets the cementum of the root). In Figure 15-9, one can see that early periodontal disease has caused the alveolar crest to be slightly below where it should be. As the disease progresses, there is more loss of bone and widening of the periodontal ligament space, which appears radiographically as a widening lucency between the bone and root (Fig. 15-11). Eventually more bone is lost, resulting in a moderate degree of disease (Fig. 15-12), and finally advanced bone loss ensues (Fig. 15-12). In addition to being focal, periodontal disease may be generalized to involve the entire maxilla or mandible.

### Dental Caries

The next most common pathologic entity encountered on radiographs of the jaws is dental caries, an infectious disease associated with cavitation of the crown of an erupted tooth. Carious lesions are the result of mineral dissolution of the dental hard tissues by the acid metabolic products of carbohydrate fermenting bacteria. Since the enamel is composed primarily of inorganic salts, the process leads to formation of a cavity (carious lesion) due to demineralization from the altered pH. This is one of the most common diseases of humans and is more prevalent in societies that have a high percentage of processed, sugar-sweetened, sticky food. There is also a sex predilection, with a higher

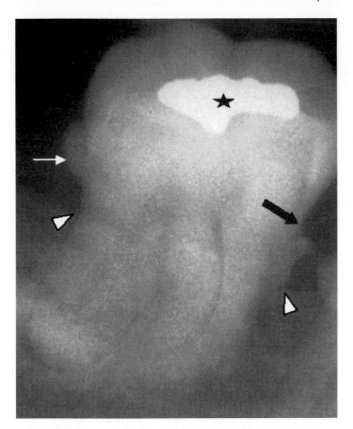

**FIGURE 15-12** Periapical radiograph depicts moderate loss of alveolar bone (*arrowheads*). Cementoenamel junction (*black arrow*). The star denotes the occlusal amalgum dental restoration. Adherent calculus (tartar), which is frequently seen with periodontal disease, surrounds the clasp of the removed partial denture (*white arrow*).

frequency in women. Dental caries are the largest cause of tooth loss in people below the age of 35.

All dental caries start at the tooth surface and can be divided into the following types: pit and fissure, smooth surface, root (cemental), and recurrent types. They may also be either acute or chronic.

*Pit and fissure* caries are the most common type, often appearing at an early age. *Pits and fissures* refer to the normal anatomic irregularities predominantly seen along occlusal surfaces of the posterior teeth. Fissures are also present along the buccal and lingual surfaces of the molars and, to a lesser degree, along the lingual surfaces of the anterior teeth. Pit and fissure caries typically occur on the occlusal surfaces (surface facing an opposing tooth) (Fig. 15-14) and, less commonly, on the buccal surface (facing the cheek) of the primary and secondary posterior dentition. Occasionally, the lingual surface (surface facing the tongue) may be affected.

*Smooth surface* caries occur on those surfaces of the teeth that are smooth, without pits and fissures. The smooth surfaces are not involved in mastication. Smooth surface caries most commonly occur in interproximal regions where contiguous teeth abut. They most frequently occur at the mesial (anterior) (Fig. 15-15) and distal (posterior) (Fig. 15-10) surfaces at the contact point with the adjacent tooth, but may also occur in the cervical region buccally or lingually. Nursing bottle caries is a type of smooth surface caries caused by leaving the feeding bottle containing milk or juice in the infant's mouth when sleeping. This is commonly seen on the labial surface of the dentition. Additionally, in adults, smooth surface carious lesions are usually secondary to alteration in the quantity or quality of saliva produced. This may also be seen with dry mouth secondary to radiation therapy.

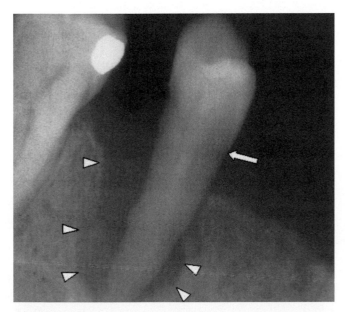

**FIGURE 15-13** Periapical radiograph of the maxillary second premolar demonstrates severe loss of alveolar bone from advanced periodontal disease (*arrowheads*). Note the location relative to the cementoenamel junction (*white arrow*).

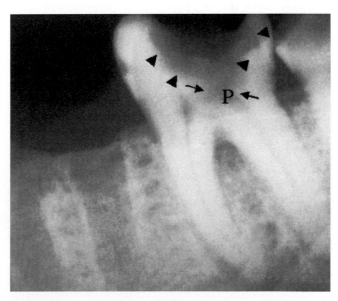

**FIGURE 15-14** Periapical radiograph depicts a large pit and fissure carious lesion (*arrowheads*) of the occlusal surface. The lesion has invaded the pulp chamber of the tooth (*P*), as outlined by black arrows.

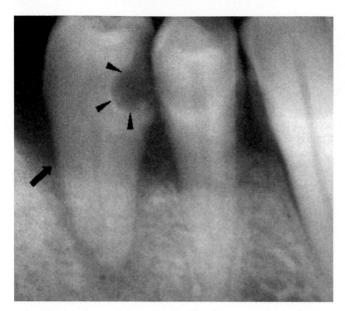

**FIGURE 15-15** Periapical radiograph depicts a large interproximal carious lesion of the mesial surface (*arrowheads*). Concurrent moderate loss of alveolar bone is noted (*black arrow*).

*Root (cemental)* caries occurs in older adults secondary to gingival recession. The exposed root surface is thin and soft, making the root vulnerable to the abrasive action of tooth brushing. Chemical erosion from bacterial acid production may also affect the root surface, causing erosion of the thin dentin layer. This may quickly invade the pulp cavity, resulting in a nonvital tooth.

*Recurrent* caries is a term used for caries that have formed around a dental restoration. These lesions may be due to weakness in the integrity of a restoration that results in marginal leakage. This allows food and bacteria to insinuate between the restoration and the remaining tooth structure, outside of the area that is cleaned. These lesions progress at variable speed, depending on the patient's diet, oral hygiene habits, and the degree of sclerosis of adjacent dentin.[11]

Rampant caries are often found in young patients. They occur because young teeth have large pulp chambers with short and wide dentinal tubules containing little sclerosis. When this condition is combined with a diet high in refined carbohydrates and sugars and poor oral hygiene, rapid extensive caries may develop.[12]

## REFERENCES

1. Laney WR, Tolman DE, Keller EE, et al. Dental implants: tissue-integrated prosthesis utilizing the osseointegrated concept. Mayo Clin Proc 1986;61:91–97.
2. Abrahams JJ. CT assessment of dental implant planning. Oral Maxillofac Surg Clin North Am 1992;4:1–18.
3. Abrahams JJ. The role of diagnostic imaging in dental implantology. Radiol Clin North Am 1993;31:(1):163–180.
4. Abrahams JJ, Levine B. Expanded applications of DentaScan: multiplanar CT of the mandible and maxilla. Int J Periodont Restor Dentistry 1990;10:464–467.
5. Abrahams JJ, Olivario P. Odontogenic cysts: improved imaging with a dental CT software program. AJNR 1993;14:367–374.
6. Delbalso AM, Greiner FG, Licata N. Role of diagnostic imaging in evaluation of the dental implant patient. Radiographics 1994;14: 699–719.
7. Fogelman D, Huang AB. Prospective evaluation of lesions of the mandible and maxilla: findings on multiplanar and three-dimentional CT. AJR 1994;163:693–698.
8. Yanagisawa K, Friedman C, Abrahams JJ. DentaScan imaging of the mandible and maxilla. Head Neck J 1993;15:1–7.
9. Ramfjord S, Ash M. Periodontology and Periodontics. Philadelphia: WB Saunders, 1979;Chaps 7, 10, 17, 23.
10. Regezi JA, Sciubba JJ. Oral Pathology. Philadelphia: WB Saunders, 1989;503–519.
11. Frank RM. Structural events in the caries process in enamel, cementum, and dentin. J Dent Res 1990;69:559–566.
12. Daculsi G, LeGeros RZ, Jean A, Kerebel B. Possible physico-chemical process in human dentin caries. J Dent Res 1987;66: 1356–1359.

## *16*

# Dental Implants and Related Pathology

*James J. Abrahams*

## DENTAL IMPLANTS

Dental implants are metal posts that are surgically implanted in the jaw to support a fixed dental prosthesis (Fig. 16-1). In the early development of implants, dentists attempted to imitate the natural anchorage system of the teeth, which are attached to the bony socket by the periodontal ligament. In addition to supporting the teeth, this ligament permits slight degrees of tooth motion within the socket. This ligament is visualized on plain radiographs as a thin radiolucent line situated between the lamina dura of the jaw and the tooth. The initial efforts to reproduce this ligament promoted growth of soft tissue between the oral implant and the bone.[1] These implants were often referred to as pseudoligaments or fibrous osseointegrated implants.[2, 3] However, the long-term results of these soft tissue–anchored implants were poor, and researchers redirected their efforts toward the possibility of anchoring the implants by direct contact with bone. Early long-term studies with these osseointegrated implants were optimistic, with success rates of 91% in the mandible and 81% in the maxilla.[4] Microscopic sections through bone-containing implants demonstrated the ability of osteoblasts to grow and integrate with the titanium posts, resulting in osseointegration.[5] The results of these early studies were corroborated by others, and this paved the road for the osseointegrated implants utilized today.[6]

There are three basic types of implants: root form (Fig. 16-1), blade (Fig. 16-2), and subperiosteal (Fig. 16-3). The osseointegrated, cylinder-shaped implants described previously are the root form because they simulate the shape of the root of a tooth. They are the ones most frequently used today and will be the type dealt with in this chapter. The blade implants are rectangular and are similar in shape to a razor blade. From the long side of the rectangle, one or more posts extend into the oral cavity to permit fixation of the prosthesis. The rectangular portion is implanted into the bone via a linear osteotomy, and the posts extend up above the gingiva. Lastly, the subperiosteal implants are metallic meshes that are custom built to fit over the alveolar process and under the periosteum. Several metallic posts extend from the mesh into the oral cavity (above the gingiva) to support the prosthesis. To customize these subperiosteal implants, the alveolar process must be surgically exposed so that a plaster impression can be obtained to manufacture the implant. After the implant is manufactured, the patient returns for a second surgical procedure that permits placement of the implant. The first surgical procedure can be eliminated if thin-slice axial CT is used to produce a 3D model of the jaw from which the prosthesis can be manufactured.

Osseointegrated root form implants are made up of several components (Fig. 16-4). The fixture is the portion of the implant that is surgically embedded in the osseous tissue of the jaw. It is made of titanium, a material that promotes osseointegration. The fixtures come in various sizes, typically ranging from 3.25 to 3.75 mm in diameter and 7 to 10 mm in length.[7] The size of the implant chosen is dependent upon the amount of available jaw bone. Dentists prefer the largest possible implant because it increases the surface area and thus provides stronger anchorage and more successful osseointegration. It is also preferable to have 1 to 1.5 mm of bone on either side of the implant and 1 to 2 mm of bone between the bottom of the implant and the adjacent structures (i.e., maxillary sinus, mandibular canal).[7] Fixtures can be threaded, unthreaded, or even coated with hydroxyapatite.[8]

The next component of the implant is the abutment (Figs. 16-1, 16-4), which is attached to the fixture to increase its

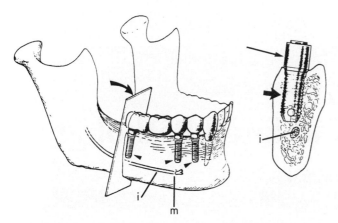

**FIGURE 16-1** View of the mandible illustrating the plane of orientation of the cross-sectional DentaScan images. The top of the plane (*curved arrow*) would correspond to one of the numbered perpendicular lines on the axial image in Figure 16-2A. Note how the height and width of the alveolar process and the location of the mandibular canal can be readily determined on the cross-sectional image. Three root form implants are seen (*arrowheads*) supporting a four-tooth prosthesis. The abutment (*thin arrow*) that is attached to the fixture (*broad arrow*) raises it above the surface of the bone and gingiva and into the oral cavity. Inferior alveolar canal (*i*), mental foramen (*m*). (From Langer B, Sullivan D. Osseointegration: its impact on the relationship of periodontics and restorative dentistry. Part 1. Int J Periodont Res 1989;9:86.)

(Fig. 16-4). The top of the abutment screw itself has a small screw hole, which allows the dental prosthesis to be attached by a screw that runs through the prosthesis and into the abutment screw. This screw is designed to be the weakest portion of the implant so that in the event of unforeseen stress, it, rather than the fixture, will break. Angled abutments are also available to correct for implants that are inserted at an angle rather than parallel to the residual teeth.

The prosthesis is composed of a strong metal framework (Fig. 16-4) that supports the prosthetic teeth. Because the implants actually support this framework, patients can have a full 14-tooth dental prosthesis supported by only six implants or a 3-tooth prosthesis supported by two implants, as shown in Figure 16-4.

## IMPLANT SURGICAL PROCEDURE

Dental implant surgery is a usually a two-stage procedure requiring a 4- to 6-month healing period between stages.[9] The healing period allows time for osseointegration to occur. In the first stage the fixture is installed; in the second stage the fixture is exposed, and the abutment is attached. The procedures are typically performed in the dentist's office, using local anesthetic.

### Fixture Placement

The first stage of surgery, fixture installation, is more extensive than the second stage and usually takes about 2

height to a level above the gingival surface. This occurs 3 to 6 months after the initial procedure, thus giving the fixture time to heal within the bone. The fixture is surgically exposed, and the abutment is attached with an abutment screw

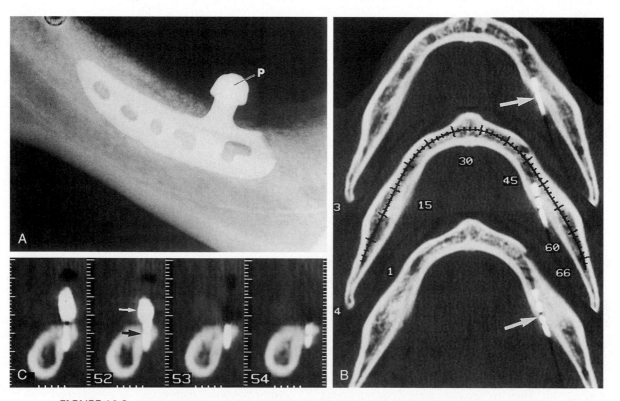

**FIGURE 16-2** Blade implant in mandible. **A,** Plain film illustrating a single post-blade implant. Note how the blade is inserted in the mandible after a linear osteotomy, while the post (*P*) extends above the level of the bone and gingiva. **B,** Axial views demonstrating the blade implant in mandible (*arrow*). **C,** Cross-sectional views illustrating the blade within the mandible (*black arrow*) and the post (*white arrow*) extending into the oral cavity above the level of the bone and gingiva.

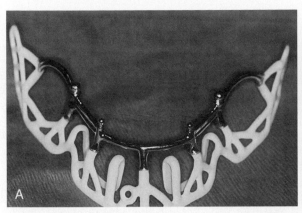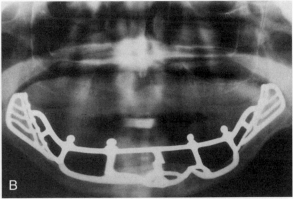

**FIGURE 16-3**   Subperiosteal implant. **A**, Photograph of a subperiosteal implant. The white portion fits under the periosteum and on top of the bone of the alveolar process, and the metallic-appearing portion extends above the gingiva to support the prosthesis. The subperiosteal portion (*white*) is often coated with hydroxyapatite to facilitate bone growth. **B**, Panoramic view demonstrating the subperiosteal implant on a severely atrophic mandible. The prosthesis has not been attached. (Courtesy of Dr. Wayne C. Jarvis, Williamsville, NY.)

hours, depending on the number of fixtures placed. Anesthesia is obtained by using local infiltration with lidocaine or a nerve block. A linear incision is then made along the buccal or lingual surface of the alveolar ridge, and a soft tissue flap, incorporating the periosteum, is reflected back (Fig. 16-5E). If the exposed bony ridge has a sharp or pointed surface secondary to buccolingual atrophy, an alveoloplasty may be performed to remove the sharp edge and provide a broad surface to install the fixtures. The anticipated implant site has been radiographically predetermined (Fig. 16-5A–D). Its position is then located on the patient either by measuring from an existing tooth or from another landmark that can be identified both on the films and on the patient or by using a stent with markers (Fig. 16-5B). Refer to the discussion of radiographic and surgical stents.

After the site has been identified on the patient, a series of graduated drill bits produce a hole in the bone. The hole is progressively widened to the appropriate size. A countersink widens the drill hole's entrance to accommodate the fixture head. The hole is then threaded with a titanium tap bur to accommodate the threaded fixture. Both drilling and threading are done at extremely low revolutions per minute (RPM), with copious irrigation to prevent heating and destruction of osteoblasts because osseointegration can only occur with viable cells. The top of the fixture has a threaded hole (Fig. 16-5G) to accommodate the abutment screw that is inserted during the second stage of the procedure. To prevent soft tissue and bone from growing into the hole while the patient is healing, a cover screw is used (Fig. 16-5E). The implant and cover screw are flush with the surface of the bone. To raise the height of the implant above the gingival surface, an abutment is later attached.

After the fixtures are placed, the tissue flap is sutured closed and the implants are allowed to heal for approximately 4 months in the mandible and 6 months in the maxilla (Fig. 16-5F). This promotes the process of osseointegration, thus forming a strong bond between the bone and the implant. Approximately 1 week after the initial surgery, the skin sutures are removed and the patient is fitted with an interim prosthesis, which typically is the one used before surgery. Because of the fixture, minor modifications of the old prosthesis may be necessary.

## Abutment Connection

The second stage of the procedure tends to be less traumatic for the patient and is typically carried out with only local infiltration of lidocaine. A pointed probe is used to locate the cover screws; after they are located, an incision is made to expose and remove them. Alternatively, a circular soft-tissue punch can be used to excise the tissue above the cover screw. The abutment is then attached to the fixture using the abutment screw. The top of the abutment screw has a screw hole that permits the prosthesis to be screwed into the fixture (Figs. 16-4 and 16-5H). Finally, a surgical pack is applied and retained for a short period by a healing cap.

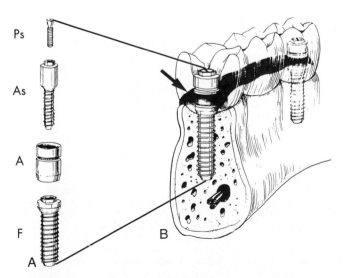

**FIGURE 16-4**   Illustration demonstrating the components of an implant (**A**) and two root form implants supporting a three-tooth prosthesis (**B**). For illustrative purposes, the black portion running through the prosthesis (*arrow*) represents the metal framework within the prosthesis. Prosthesis screw (*Ps*), abutment screw (*As*), abutment (*A*), and fixture (*F*).

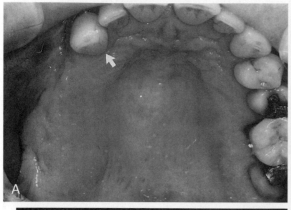

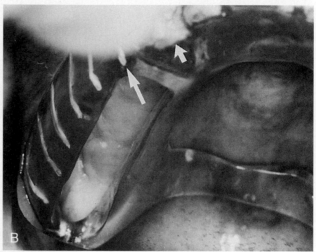

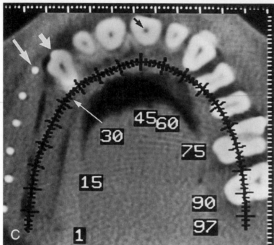

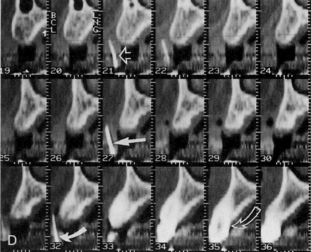

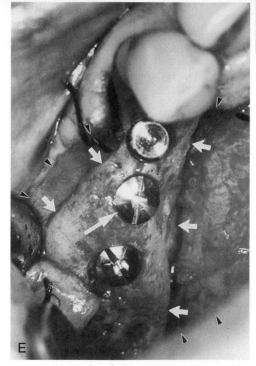

**FIGURE 16-5**  Surgical implant procedure. **A,** This patient, being evaluated for dental implants, is edentulous distal to the right maxillary canine (*arrow*). **B,** A stent with six vertical markers has been placed over the alveolar ridge and residual teeth. The sixth marker (*long arrow*) is adjacent to the right canine (*short arrow*) and will be demonstrated on the CT images. This marker appears as a dot on the axial image next to perpendicular line 32 (**C**) and as a line on cross-sectional image number 32 (**D**). **C,** Axial view demonstrating the sixth marker (*long thick arrow*) at perpendicular line 32 (*thin arrow*) and adjacent to the right canine (*short white arrow*). Note the radiolucent pulp in the center of the teeth (*black arrow*). **D,** Cross-sectional views demonstrating markers 4 (*open arrow*), 5 (*straight arrow*), and 6 (*curved arrow*) of the stent. Note that marker 6 is adjacent to the right canine (*open curved arrow*). By placing the stent on the patient during surgery, the surgeon knows that the bone under marker 6 is as depicted by cross-sectional image 32. **E,** An incision is made, and the gingival and periosteal flap (*arrowheads*) are held back with sutures. This exposes the bone of the alveolar process (*short thick arrows*). Holes are drilled, and three titanium implants are inserted into the bone. Note that the implants are flush with the bone, and their openings are covered with healing screw caps (*long arrow*).

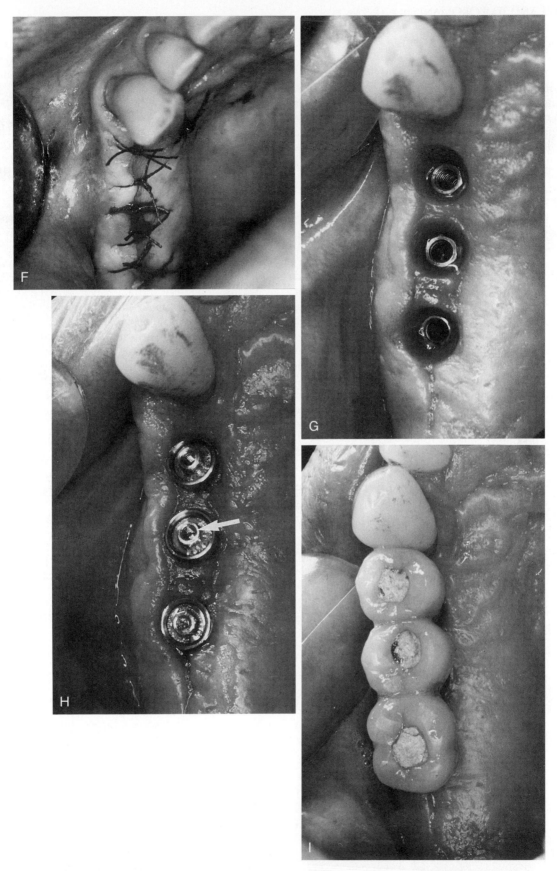

**FIGURE 16-5** *Continued.* **F,** The incision is sutured closed and permitted to heal for 4 months in the mandible and 6 months in the maxilla. **G,** Before this photograph was taken, a small incision was made to remove the healing caps. Healing abutments, which were attached to the implants, have been removed. The threaded opening of the implant is visualized. **H,** The permanent abutments, which raise the fixture above the gingival surface, have now been attached. The screw hole (*arrow*) in the center of the abutment will accommodate the screw that fixes the prosthesis. **I,** The prosthesis is now attached to the three implants. The screw heads are covered with a white compound. (From Abrahams JJ. The role of diagnostic imaging in dental implantology. Radiol Clin North Am 1993;31(1):163–180.)

## Prosthodontic Procedure

To make the prosthesis, an impression of the jaw with the abutments in place is made, using plaster or hydrocoloid. From this impression a cast of the mandible or maxilla is obtained. From this cast the prosthesis is made, aligning properly with the screw holes and properly aligning the prosthetic teeth with the occlusal plane. After the prosthesis is manufactured, it is fixed to the abutments with screws that typically come out the central fossa of the prosthetic teeth. A white compound is used to cover the screw holes (Fig. 16-5I).

## RADIOLOGY FOR ORAL IMPLANTS

To perform the implant procedure, the oral surgeon and dentist need to know the precise height, width, and contour of the alveolar process, as well as its relationship to the maxillary sinus and mandibular canal. Injury to the neurovascular bundle within the mandibular canal results in paresthesia or hypesthesia of the face, whereas perforation into the maxillary sinus increases the likelihood of implant failure and creates the potential for an oroantral fistula and antral infection. The precise dimensions of the alveolar process are important to determine preoperatively because atrophy of the alveolar ridge, which occurs in edentulous patients, may preclude the use of implants.

Before the development of CT dental reformatting programs, attempts were made to obtain this information with panoramic, intraoral, and cephalometric films. However, the panoramic film produced up to 25% distortion, making accurate measurements almost impossible. In addition, the width (thickness) of the alveolar process could not be determined by any of these techniques. Therefore the surgeon had to rely primarily on clinical assessment to determine if the alveolar process was thick enough to accommodate an implant. Unfortunately, it was common to find during surgery that there was insufficient bone for the implants. As a result, radiologists and dentists began to evaluate the efficacy of using CT to assess these patients.[10, 11] Axial and coronal images were only marginally helpful because of the streak degradation artifacts created by any dental restorations. However, reformatted images using thin-slice axial CT were found to be extremely useful because the streak artifact could be avoided, the anatomy could be displayed in multiple planes, the width of the alveolar process could be accurately assessed, and accurate, reproducible millimeter measurements could be made.

Reformatting software programs, which display multiple panoramic and cross-sectional images, soon became available (Figs. 15-2 and 15-3; Chapter 15).[12–15] The particular program used in this chapter is DentaScan. Although these programs were initially developed to assess implant patients, they have also gained popularity for evaluating all lesions of the jaw (Fig. 16-6).[16–19]

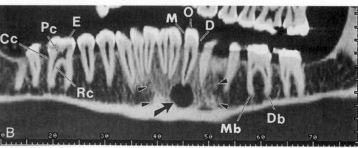

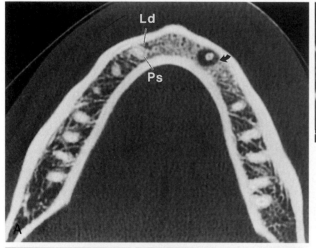

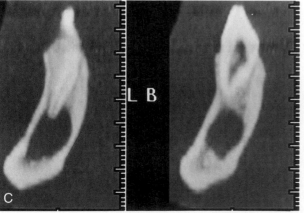

**FIGURE 16-6**   Mandibular DentaScan image demonstrating a radicular cyst surrounding the root apex of the left canine. **A,** Axial view demonstrating the radicular cyst (*black arrow*). The periodontal space (*Ps*), typically not seen on CT, can be visualized in this patient between the lamina dura (*Ld*) and the tooth. **B,** Panoramic view illustrating an area of sclerotic osteitis condensans (*arrowheads*) surrounding the radicular cyst (*black arrow*). The cervical constriction (*Cc*), pulp chamber (*Pc*), root canal (*Rc*), and dense enamel (*E*) are nicely demonstrated on the right first molar. The mesial (*M*), occlusal (*O*), and distal (*D*) surfaces of the left canine are demonstrated, as well as the mesiobuccal (*Mb*) and distobuccal (*Db*) roots of the left first molar. The lingual root of the left first molar is not seen in this plane. **C,** Cross-sectional views demonstrating the radicular cyst surrounding the root apex.

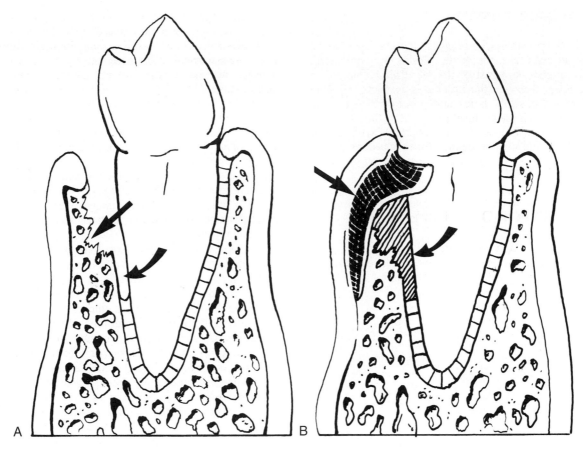

**FIGURE 16-7**    Illustration demonstrating a periodontal pocket and its repair. **A,** Bacterial overgrowth has attacked the periodontal ligament (*curved arrow*) and resorbed bone (*straight arrow*), creating this periodontal pocket. **B,** The periodontal pocket in **A** has now been packed with freeze-dried bone (*curved arrow*) and covered with a Gortex graft (*straight arrow*) to prevent ingrowth of soft tissue while the bone graft heals. The Gortex will be removed in approximately 6 weeks.

## RELATED PATHOLOGY

Most patients being scanned for dental implants have considerable oral pathology, often related to the inflammatory process that likely caused their edentulism. The inflammatory disease, which often starts as gingivitis (inflammation of the gums), can be divided into periodontal and endodontal disease. Periodontal disease refers to infection of the periodontal ligament along the sides of the root and the adjacent surrounding bone. Endodontal disease refers to infection and resorption of bone at the root apex.

## Periodontal Disease

Periodontal disease starts with gingivitis and the accumulation of bacteria-laden plaque around the teeth. This may harden into tartar or calculus, a tough, gritty material that is difficult to remove. The presence of this bacterial overgrowth produces inflammation of the gums, which presents clinically as swelling with frequent bleeding secondary to hyperemia from inflammation. If the infection is allowed to persist, the fibers that attach the gingiva to the tooth become involved, allowing bacteria to access the periodontal ligament (periodontitis). Once the periodontal ligament becomes involved, a periodontal pocket forms in which plaque accumulates adjacent to the root (Fig. 16-7A).

Routine dental hygiene at home does not adequately cleanse these infected regions, and the disease progresses. Eventually the periodontal ligament is destroyed, and the adjacent bone surrounding the root is resorbed.[20] Radiographically, periodontal disease is recognized by the associated bone loss that occurs. On CT, this bone loss appears as a radiolucency surrounding the root of the tooth (Fig. 16-8). The periodontal ligament, which appears as a radiolucency surrounding the root on radiographs (Fig. 16-9), is usually not resolved on CT because it is too thin. Therefore, radiolucency along the root of the tooth on CT usually implies periodontal disease. Because the resolution of radiographs exceeds that of CT, visualization of the periodontal ligament as a thin lucency between the root and lamina dura (surrounding cortical bone) (Fig. 16-9) is routinely seen. Widening of this periodontal space on radiographs implies periodontal disease (Fig. 15-10).

## Endodontal Disease

Another frequently encountered condition in this patient population is an inflammatory cyst surrounding the root

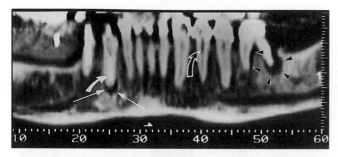

**FIGURE 16-8** Panoramic CT scan of mandible demonstrating periodontal disease. The radiolucency surrounding the root of the left first molar (*arrowheads*) is due to bone resorption from periodonitis. The periapical lucency around the root apex of the right canine (*long arrows*) is a radicular cyst secondary to a periapical abscess. Note the metal post in the pulp chamber secondary to a prior root canal procedure (*solid curved arrow*), and compare this with the normal radiolucent pulp chamber of the left first premolar (*open curved arrow*). A zone of relatively dense sclerotic bone (osteitis condensans) is identified surrounding both areas of disease. (From Abrahams JJ. The role of diagnostic imaging in dental implantology. Radiol Clin North Am 1993;31(1):163–180.)

apex called a radicular cyst.[21] Bacteria gains access to the pulp chamber through dental caries and travels down the root canal to the root apex, where either an acute abscess or a more chronic granuloma forms. Bone loss develops around the root apex, and this appears as a periapical radiolucency on CT (Fig. 16-6). When bacteria enters the pulp chamber through dental caries, it causes pulpitis with inflammation and edema. Because the tooth cannot expand, pressure builds within the pulp chamber and the diminished blood flow causes the tooth to die. Radicular cysts are therefore associated with nonvital teeth. The treatment is to drill through the pulp chamber and drain the abscess (root canal procedure). After this drainage is accomplished, the root canal is filled with a radiopaque material that also plugs the apical foramen. This is readily seen on CT as a radiodensity, rather than a radiolucency, in the region of the pulp chamber and root canal (Fig. 16-8, *curved arrow*).

## Osteitis Condensans

The chronic inflammatory changes of periodontal and endodontal disease can also cause reactive sclerosis in the adjacent bone, termed osteitis condensans. Radiographically, this appears as a relatively dense zone of bone surrounding an area of periodontal or endodontal disease (Fig. 16-8).[22] This condition is relatively benign, and treatment is directed at eradicating the underlying periodontal and endodontal disease.

## Maxillary Sinus Inflammation from Dental Disease

The close proximity of the root apexes to the maxillary sinus makes periodontal and endodontal disease potential sources of infection to cause maxillary sinus disease. It is not uncommon to find mounds of inflammatory tissue within the sinus adjacent to the root apices of diseased teeth. These

mounds frequently are misdiagnosed as mucous retention cysts or polyps on axial CT scans[23] (Fig. 16-10).

An oroantral fistula, which is an abnormal communication between the maxillary sinus and oral cavity, typically causes fluid and inflammatory changes in the maxillary sinus. These fistulas are often caused by tooth extractions but can also be caused by infection, trauma, tumors, etc.[24] Radiographically, the oroantral fistula presents as unilateral sinusitis with a bony defect in the floor of the maxillary sinus. This is best seen using dental CT reformatting programs (Fig. 16-11).

## Atrophy and Augmentation Procedures

Periodontal and endodontal disease eventually lead to edentulism. The resorption of bone, however, continues even after the teeth are lost. This is because the normal vertical stress applied to the bone from the teeth is no longer present and disuse atrophy occurs. It is believed that the use of dental implants retards this atrophic process. The disuse atrophy affects both the height of the alveolar process (Fig. 16-12A) and the width (Fig. 16-12B). When it is severe, the mandibular canal, which is normally covered by a considerable amount of bone, may lie just under the gingival surface.

Several augmentation procedures are now available for patients who have severe atrophy and have insufficient bone for implants. In the sinus lift procedure, the surgeon elevates

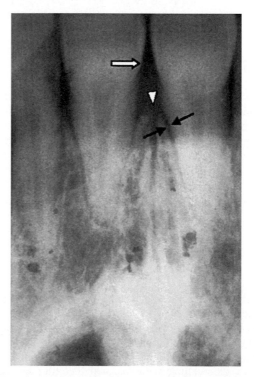

**FIGURE 16-9** Periapical radiograph of mandibular central incisors depicts mild loss of alveolar bone from periodontal disease. Alveolar crest (*arrowhead*) is eroded and is now located below the cemento-enamel junction (*white arrow*). Concurrent minimal widening of the periodontal ligament space (*black arrows*) is noted.

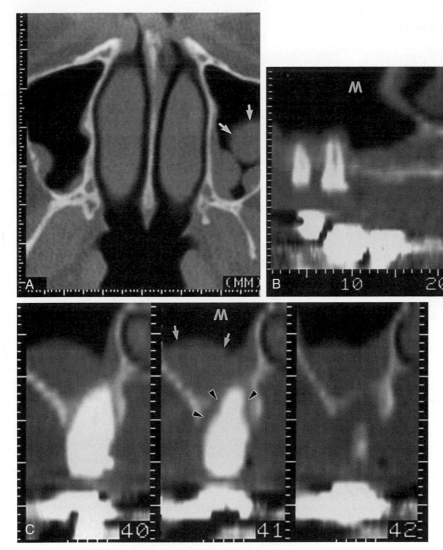

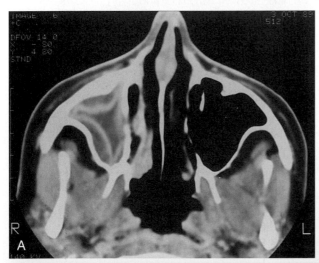

**FIGURE 16-10** Focal sinus disease adjacent to periodontal disease resembles a polyp or retention cyst. Axial (**A**), cross-sectional (**B**), and panoramic (**C**) DentaScan images of maxilla again show focal areas of maxillary sinus mucosal thickening (*white arrows*) centered over areas of periodontal disease (*arrowheads*). Mounds of focal mucosal thickening resemble polyps or retention cysts in the axial view (**A**, *white arrows*). Maxillary sinus (*M*), nasal septum (*N*). (From Abrahams JJ, Glassberg RM. Dental disease: a frequently unrecognized cause of maxillary sinus abnormalities. AJR 1996;166:1219–1223.)

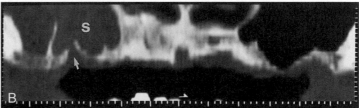

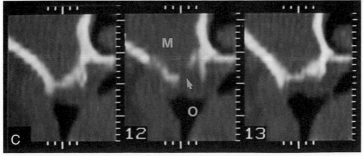

**FIGURE 16-11** A 45-year-old man with a left oroantral fistula. **A**, Standard axial CT scan at the level of the maxillary sinuses shows unilateral opacification of the ipsilateral sinus. **B**, Panoramic reconstructed CT scan from a dental reformatting program shows disruption of the bony floor of the maxillary sinus, with a fistula tract of soft-tissue density (*arrow*). Note the associated soft-tissue opacification of the ipsilateral maxillary sinus (*S*), whereas the contralateral sinus is aerated. **C**, Three cross-sectional CT scans are in true parallel planes to the alveolar ridge and show a fistula tract (*arrow*) and sinusitis. Oral cavity (*O*), maxillary sinus (*M*). (From Abrahams JJ, Berger SB. Oral-maxillary sinus fistula (oroantral fistula): clinical features and findings on multiplanar CT. AJR 1995;165:1273–1276.)

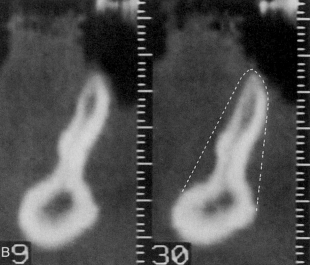

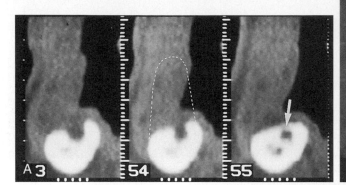

**FIGURE 16-12** Cross-sectional views of the mandible in two different patients demonstrating bone resorption and atrophy. **A,** Bone loss and atrophy of the height of the mandible in this patient cause the mandibular canal (*arrow*) to sit immediately under the gingival surface. The dotted line demonstrates how the bone contour might have appeared before atrophy. The patient has insufficient bone for implants. (From Abrahams JJ. The role of diagnostic imaging in dental implantology. Radiol Clin North Am 1993;31(1):163–180.) **B,** The width of the mandible in this patient has been considerably diminished due to atrophy. The dotted line again demonstrates how the bone might have appeared before atrophy. (From Abrahams JJ. CT assessment of dental implant planning. Oral Maxillofac Surg Clin North Am 1992;4:1–18.)

the periosteum in the floor of the maxillary sinus and packs a freeze-dried bone graft between the elevated periosteum and the bony floor. After this heals, it will increase the height of the alveolar bone available in the maxilla. In both the mandible and maxilla, various bone grafts alone, often from iliac crest, have been used to increase the height and width of the alveolar process. These grafts may be supplemented with freeze-dried bone.

Finally, if the implant is placed and either the buccal or lingual surface is exposed and uncovered by bone, a procedure known as guided tissue regeneration, which utilizes Gortex as a physical barrier, can be performed to regenerate the bone adjacent to the implant in the following manner. Bone graft is first packed around the exposed surface of the implant, and then a piece of Gortex fabric is placed between the bone graft and soft tissues. The Gortex acts as a barrier, preventing the soft tissues from growing into the bone graft, thus allowing time for the graft to take. Typically the Gortex remains in place for about 6 weeks and is then removed. This procedure can also be used when placing an implant in a fresh extraction socket and for filling a periodontal pocket with bone graft, as illustrated in Figure 16-7B.

## REFERENCES

1. Albrektsson T, Lekholm W. Osseo- integration: current state of the art. Dent Clin North Am 1989;33:537–544.
2. James R. The support system and perigingival defense mechanism of oral implants. J Oral Implant 1975;6:270–285.
3. Weiss C. Tissue integration of dental endosseous implants: description and comparative analysis of the fibro-osseous integration and osseous integration systems. J Oral Implant 1986;12:169–214.
4. Adell R, Lukholm U, Rockler B, et al. A 15-year study of osseointegrated implants in the treatment of the edentulous jaw. Int J Oral Maxillofac Surg 1981;10:387–416.
5. Branemark PI. Introduction to osseointegration. In: Branemark PI, Zarb G, Albrektsson T, eds. Tissue Integrated Protheses. Chicago and Berlin: Quintessence, 1985.
6. Albrektsson T. A multicenter report on osseointegrated oral implants. J Prosthet Dent 1988;60(1):75–84.
7. Delbalso AM, Greiner FG, Licata N. Role of diagnostic imaging in evaluation of the dental implant patient. Radiographics 1994;14:699–719.
8. Krauser JT. Hydroxyapatite-coated dental implants. Dent Clin North Am 1989;33:879–903.
9. Moy PK, Weinlaender M, Kenney EB, et al. Soft tissue modifications of surgical techniques for placement and uncovering of osseointegrated implants. Dental Clin North Am 1989;4:665–699.
10. McGivney GP, Haughton V, Strandt JA, et al. A comparison of computed-assisted tomography and data-gathering modalities in prostodontics. Int J Oral Maxillofac Surg 1986;1:55–68.
11. Wishan M, Bahat O, Krane M. Computed tomography as an adjunct in dental implant surgery. Int J Periodont Restor Dentistry 1988;8:31–47.
12. Rothman SLG, Chafetz N, Rhodes M, et al. CT in the pre-operative assessment of the mandible and maxilla for endosseous implant surgery. Radiology 1988;168:171–175.
13. Schwarz MS, Rothman SLGM, Chatetz N, et al. Computed tomography in dental implantation surgery. Dent Clin North Am 1989;33:555–597.
14. Schwarz MS, Rothman SLGM, Rhodes ML. Computed tomography. Part I. Pre-operative assessment of the mandible for endosseous implant surgery. Int J Oral Maxillofac Surg 1987;2:137–141.
15. Schwarz MS, Rothman SLGM, Rhodes ML, et al. Computed tomography. Part II. Pre-operative assessment of the mandible for endosseous implant surgery. Int J Oral Maxillofac Surg 1987;2:143–148.

16. Abrahams JJ. The role of diagnostic imaging in dental implantology. Radiol Clin North Am 1993;31(1):163–180.

17. Abrahams JJ, Olivario P. Odontogenic cysts: improved imaging with a dental CT software program. AJNR 1993;14:367–374.

18. Fogelman D, Huang AB. Prospective evaluation of lesions of the mandible and maxilla: findings on multiplanar and three-dimentional CT. AJR 1994;163:693–698.

19. Yanagisawa K, Friedman C, Abrahams JJ. DentaScan imaging of the mandible and maxilla. Head Neck J 1993;15:1–7.

20. Burgett F. Periodontal disease. In: Regezi JA, Sciubba JJ, eds. Oral Pathology: Clinical-Pathologic Correlations. Philadelphia: WB Saunders, 1989;503–519.

21. Regezi J, Sciubba J. Oral Pathology: Clinical-Pathological Correlation. Philadelphia: WB Saunders, 1989;301–336.

22. Regezi J, Sciubba J. Oral Pathology: Clinical-Pathological Correlation. Philadelphia: WB Saunders, 1989;390–404.

23. Abrahams JJ, Glassberg RM. Dental disease: a frequently unrecognized cause of maxillary sinus abnormalities? AJR 1995;166:1219–1223.

24. Abrahams JJ, Berger SB. Oral-maxillary sinus fistula (oro-antral fistula): clinical presentation and evaluation with multiplanar CT. AJR 1995;165:1273–1276.

*17*

# Jaw: Cysts, Tumors, and Nontumorous Lesions

## *Alfred L. Weber, Takashi Kaneda, Steven J. Scrivani, and Shahid Aziz*

**930**

# PATHOLOGIC STATES

## INTRODUCTION

Lesions developing within the jaws can arise from the dental elements, bone, nerves, or blood vessels. Classifications of these jaw lesions have varied considerably, with no universally accepted terminology. Some of these classifications have emphasized the presumed cell of origin of various tumors, while the cysts have been classified as being either developmental or inflammatory in etiology. However, as the theories of derivation evolve, classifications change. The World Health Organization (WHO) classification published in 1992 is widely accepted (Table 17-1).[1] In this classification, the tumors are separated into benign and malignant types and further subdivided based on the odontogenic tissue types involved in the generation of the lesion. This section does not precisely follow the WHO classification, and not all of the rare tumors mentioned in it are included in this chapter. Several excellent and more complete reference works are cited in the References (also see Chapters 6, 15, and 27 for further discussions of these lesions).[2, 3]

It should be noted that the groupings in this section are not precise. For instance, the various cemental lesions are grouped together under benign odontogenic tumors and tumor-like conditions. Clearly, many of these lesions could have just as easily been included in the fibroosseous category. It is hoped that the organization of this chapter will be helpful to those who are less familiar with maxillofacial lesions and allow this complex topic to be more readily understood. The cystic lesions are discussed first, followed by true tumors and tumor-like conditions. Finally, infections of the jaw are discussed.

## CYSTS

### Definition and Classification

A cyst is characterized pathologically as an epithelium-lined cavity that contains fluid or semisolid material.[4] In most cases, microscopic examination of the lining tissue, as well as the clinical and radiographic findings, is necessary to achieve a diagnosis.

Cysts frequently occur in the jaw and appear radiographically as either unilocular or multilocular lucent areas of varying size and definition. Cysts of the mandible can come to clinical attention by remodeling bone and thus weakening the mandible, causing functional disturbances, or by the effects of secondary cyst infection. Delayed tooth eruption and displacement and resorption of tooth roots are often seen on imaging, and the cyst's relationship to a tooth is an important differential diagnostic feature. On the basis of the cell of origin, cysts have been subdivided into odontogenic and nonodontogenic types.

Odontogenic cysts arise from tooth derivatives.[5] Frequently, odontogenic cysts are divided into inflammatory and developmental types, with the developmental variety not being directly associated with inflammation. In some lesions the pathogenesis is unclear. Histologic analysis of the epithelial layers, the presence of cyst calcification, and the clinical findings allow further subdivision of these cysts. The term *residual cyst* is frequently applied to any cyst (but specifically to a periodontal apical cyst) that remains or develops after surgical removal of a tooth.

Most odontogenic cysts are developmental in origin.[1] The fissural variety, as the name implies, arise along lines of fusion of the various bones and embryonic processes, and they are classified according to their anatomic location. Several cysts previously classified as fissural cysts have been moved into other categories, as their relationship to embryonic fusion or, alternatively, their worthiness of a separate category has been questioned. Developmental cysts

Table 17-1
## WHO HISTOLOGIC CLASSIFICATION OF JAW TUMORS AND CYSTS
The classification is provided for completeness. Classifications of jaw lesions vary,
and this chapter does not follow this classification exactly.

**Histologic Classification of Odontogenic Tumors**

**Neoplasms and Other\* Tumors Related to the Odontogenic Apparatus**
Benign
*Odontogenic epithelium without odontogenic ectomesenchyme\**
    Ameloblastoma
    Squamous odontogenic tumor
    Calcifying epithelial odontogenic tumor (Pindborg tumor)
    Clear cell odontogenic tumor

*Odontogenic epithelium with odontogenic ectomesenchyme, with or without dental hard-tissue formation\**
    Ameloblastic fibroma
    Ameloblastic fibrodentinoma (dentinoma) and ameloblastic fibroodontoma
    Odontoameloblastoma
    Adenomatoid odontogenic tumor
    Calcifying odontogenic cyst
    Complex odontoma
    Compound odontoma

*Odontogenic ectomesenchyme with or without included odontogenic epithelium\**
    Odontogenic fibroma
    Myxoma (odontogenic myxoma, myxofibroma)
    Benign cementoblastoma (cementoblastoma, true cementoma)

Malignant
*Odontogenic carcinomas*
    Malignant ameloblastoma
    Primary intraosseous carcinoma
    Malignant variants of other odontogenic epithelial tumors
    Malignant changes in odontogenic cysts

*Odontogenic sarcomas*
    Ameloblastic fibrosarcoma (ameloblastic sarcoma)
    Ameloblastic fibrodentinosarcoma and ameloblastic fibroodontosarcoma
    Odontogenic carcinosarcoma

**Neoplasms and Other Lesions Related to Bone**
Osteogenic neoplasms
    Cemento-ossifying fibroma (cementifying fibroma, ossifying fibroma)

Nonneoplastic bone lesions
    Fibrous dysplasia of the jaws

*Cementoosseous dysplasias*
    Periapical cemental dysplasia (periapical fibrous dysplasia)
    Florid cementoosseous dysplasia (gigantiform cementoma, familial multiple cementomas)
    Other cementoosseous dysplasias
    Cherubism (familial multiocular cystic disease of the jaws)
    Central giant cell granuloma
    Aneurysmal bone cyst
    Solitary bone cyst (traumatic, simple, haemorrhagic bone cyst)

Other Tumors
    Melanotic neuroectodermal tumor of infancy (melanotic progonoma)

**Epithelial Cysts**
Developmental
*Odontogenic*
    ''Gingival cysts'' of infants (Epstein pearls)
    Odontogenic keratocyst (primordial cyst)
    Dentigerous (follicular) cyst
    Eruption cyst
    Lateral periodontal cyst
    Gingival cyst of adults
    Glandular odontogenic cyst; sialoodontogenic cyst

*Nonodontogenic*
    Nasopalatine duct (incisive canal) cyst
    Nasolabial (nasoalveolar) cyst

Inflammatory
    Radicular cyst
    Apical and lateral
    Residual
    Paradental (inflammatory collateral, mandibular infected buccal) cyst

\*The enamel organ derives from the odontogenic epithelium developing from the ectoderm of the oral cavity. The dental papilla and follicle are considered ectomesenchymal, derived partly from the neural crest. Lesions that contain odontogenic ectomesenchyme, as well as the odontogenic epithelium, have the capability of producing dentin and enamel. Those without ectomesenchyme cannot. Some lesions arise primarily from the mesenchyme and appear to incidentally include ''odontogenic epithelium,'' but the odontogenic epithelium does not play a key role in producing the lesion.

From Kramer IRH, Pindborg JJ, Shear M. Histological Typing of Odontogenic Tumours, 2nd ed. Berlin and New York: Springer-Verlag, 1992;7–9.

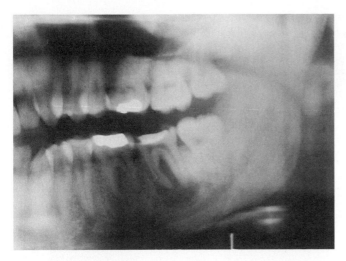

**FIGURE 17-1**   Radicular cyst of the left mandibular second molar tooth. Pantomogram of the mandible demonstrates a cystic, well-defined lesion around the apices of the lower left mandibular tooth. Note the sclerosis around the cyst and adjacent mandibular teeth, which is secondary to chronic osteitis.

include other cyst types derived from embryologic structures, such as dermoid cysts, and cysts arising from other causes, such as solitary bone cysts and aneurysmal bone cysts. Stafne's cyst is not a cyst at all but rather a variation in the development of the cortex of the bone.

## Odontogenic Cysts

### Periapical (Radicular) Cyst

Periapical (radicular) cyst is by far the most common odontogenic cyst.[1] It may form at any time during life, although the peak incidence is between 30 and 50 years of age. There is no sex predilection. This cyst is associated with carious teeth. Caries lead to infection of the pulp cavity and eventually pulp necrosis. Infection passes out of the apex of the root, resulting in apical periodontitis leading to an acute abscess or a more chronic granuloma. From these stages, the disease can quiesce and form the periapical (radicular) cyst. Most periapical cysts are discovered incidentally on radiography, but expansion of the cyst may cause a clinically noticeable displacement of teeth, and swelling and pain may occur when the cyst enlarges or becomes secondarily infected.

Radiographically, a radicular cyst is a well-circumscribed radiolucency arising from the apex of the tooth and bounded by a thin rim of cortical bone (Figs. 17-1 and 17-2). Large lesions may expand the cortical plates.[6] A radicular cyst can displace tooth structures and may cause slight root resorption. If the cyst occurs in the maxilla, extension into the maxillary sinus may be observed (Fig. 17-3). Radiographically, radicular cysts cannot be differentiated from periapical granulomas, which usually are less than 1.6 cm in diameter. On MR imaging, the lesions usually have high signal intensity on T2-weighted images and variable signal

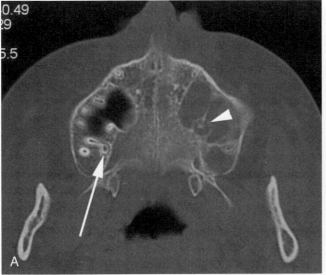

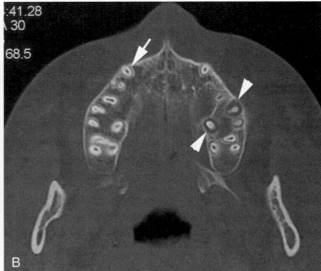

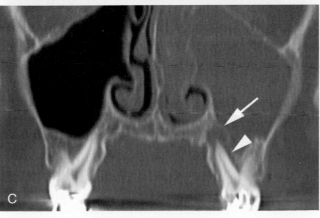

**FIGURE 17-2**   Periapical abscess and sinusitis. **A,** There is widening of the periodontal lucency separating the root tip from the lamina dura (*arrowhead*) of the affected tooth. Compare the relationship of the root tip/periodontal lucency and lamina dura on the opposite side (*arrow*). **B,** Slightly lower than **A.** The periodontal lucency is seen to affect multiple roots (*arrowheads*). Compare with the relationship of the canine tooth on the opposite side (*arrow*). **C,** Coronal image shows the opacification of the left maxillary sinus as well as the periapical abnormality (*arrow*). Note how the periodontal lucency (*arrowhead*) widens at the root tip, indicating the periapical abscess.

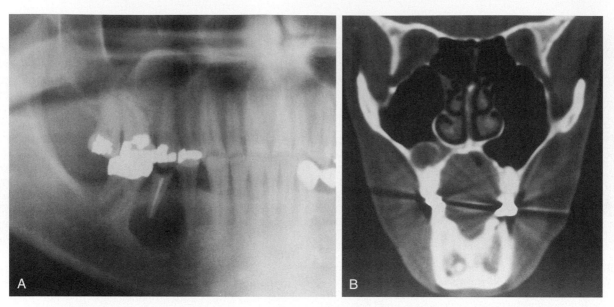

**FIGURE 17-3**  Radicular cyst. **A,** Pantomogram of the mandible and maxilla shows a radicular cyst around the apex of the right second premolar tooth within the mandible and around the apex of the upper right second premolar tooth. The upper radicular cyst bulges into the right antral cavity. **B,** Coronal CT of the paranasal sinuses shows the maxillary radicular cyst projecting into the floor of the right antrum.

intensity on T1-weighted images. On contrast-enhanced MR imaging, the cysts wall is usually thick and there is strong enhancement, probably representing inflammation.

### Dentigerous (Follicular) Cyst

The dentigerous cyst is the second most common odontogenic cyst after the inflammatory periapical cyst . The dentigerous cyst forms around the crown of an unerupted tooth (Figs. 17-4 and 17-5). This tooth will never erupt. Fluid collects between layers of epithelium or between the epithelium and the enamel. Most dentigerous cysts become evident during the third and fourth decades of life, and most (75%) are located in the mandible. In the usual case, the tooth crown projects into the lumen of the cystic cavity. The wall of the cyst tends to converge to the cementoenamel junction. With continued cyst growth, only a limited portion of the tooth may be attached to the cyst lining.

Dentigerous cysts vary greatly in size, ranging from less than 2 cm in diameter to those that cause massive expansion of the jaw. They may cause displacement of teeth, but apical resorption of tooth structures is uncommon. Fractures and superimposed infection may develop in the cyst. Dentigerous cysts do not demonstrate an extracystic soft-tissue mass, as seen in ameloblastomas, but ameloblastomas, mucoepidermoid tumors, and carcinomas may develop in the wall of the cyst.

On imaging, a mandibular dentigerous cyst appears as a well-circumscribed unilocular area of osteolysis that incorporates the crown of a tooth. The adjacent teeth are displaced and may be partly eroded. Dentigerous cysts in the maxilla often extend into the antrum, displacing and remodeling the bony sinus wall (Fig. 17-6). Large cysts may project into the nasal cavity or infratemporal fossa and may elevate the floor of the orbit. In the mandible, buccal or lingual cortical expansion and thinning are noted. On MR imaging, the contents of the cyst show high signal intensity on T2-weighted images and low to intermediate signal intensity on T1-weighted images. The tooth itself is an area of signal void (Fig. 17-7). The lining of the cyst is thin and regular in thickness and may show slight enhancement after contrast injection.

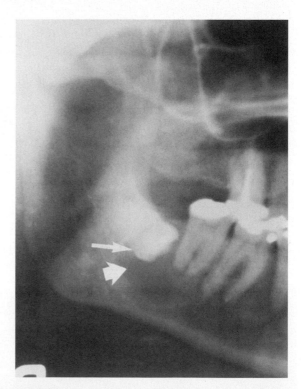

**FIGURE 17-4**  Dentigerous cyst. Pantomogram of the mandible shows a sharply marginated, oval-shaped cyst in the body of the right mandible (*short arrow*). The crown (*long arrow*) of the impacted third molar tooth is incorporated into the posterior portion of the cyst.

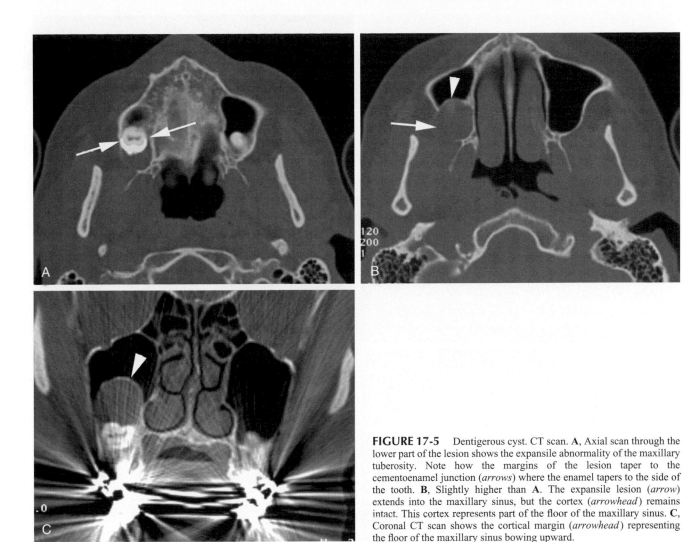

**FIGURE 17-5**    Dentigerous cyst. CT scan. **A**, Axial scan through the lower part of the lesion shows the expansile abnormality of the maxillary tuberosity. Note how the margins of the lesion taper to the cementoenamel junction (*arrows*) where the enamel tapers to the side of the tooth. **B**, Slightly higher than **A**. The expansile lesion (*arrow*) extends into the maxillary sinus, but the cortex (*arrowhead*) remains intact. This cortex represents part of the floor of the maxillary sinus. **C**, Coronal CT scan shows the cortical margin (*arrowhead*) representing the floor of the maxillary sinus bowing upward.

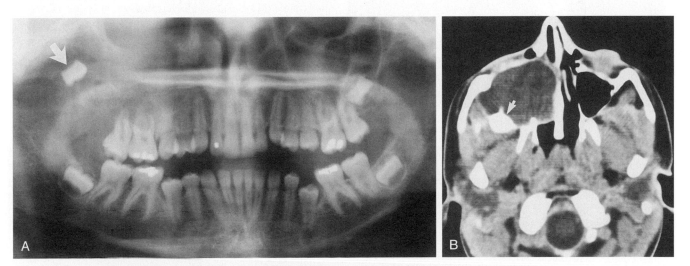

**FIGURE 17-6**    Dentigerous cyst. **A**, Pantomogram of the mandible and maxilla shows a displaced tooth in the upper lateral aspect of the right maxilla (*arrow*). There is a poorly defined expansile lesion in the same region. **B**, Axial CT demonstrates an expansile cystic lesion within the right antral cavity, with extension into the right nasal cavity and infratemporal fossa. Note the localized density at the posterior margin of this cyst representing a tooth that is incorporated into the cyst (*arrow*).

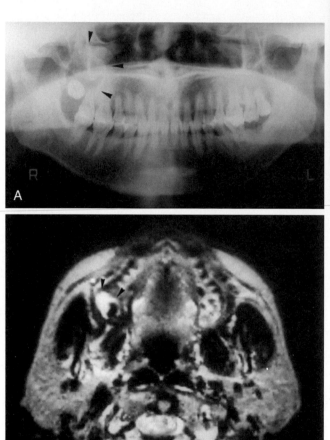

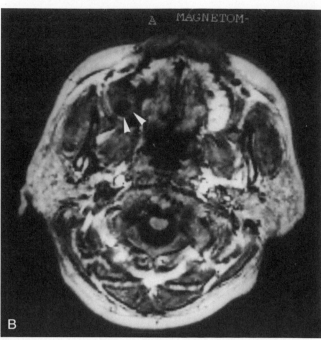

**FIGURE 17-7** Dentigerous cyst. **A**, Pantomogram shows a well-defined lesion with an unerupted tooth involving the right maxillary sinus (*arrowheads*). Dentigerous cyst is strongly suspected, but unilocular ameloblastoma and OKC cannot be ruled out. **B**, Axial T1-weighted image reveals an unerupted tooth as signal void (*arrowheads*) within a low-intensity lesion. **C**, Axial T2-weighted MR image reveals a pericoronal lesion of homogeneously high intensity (*arrowheads*). MR findings suggest a pericoronal cyst containing homogeneous fluids and an unerupted tooth, most likely a dentigerous cyst.

### Odontogenic Keratocyst

Odontogenic keratocysts (OKC) account for 3% to 11% of all jaw cysts and occur twice as often in the mandible as in the maxilla.[7–9] These cysts are found in patients of all ages, but the peak incidence is in the second and third decades of life. This cyst has been classified as a separate type of bone cyst because of its aggressive biologic behavior and histologic structure. Histologically, the cyst is lined by a stratified keratinizing squamous epithelium. The epithelium is characteristically thin, six to eight cell layers, and the keratinization is usually of the parakeratin type. Parakeratin has nuclei in the layer of keratin that borders the lining of the cyst. There is no keratogranular layer in the wall. Parakeratinization is a more disordered type of keratin

formation than orthokeratinization. With the formation of orthokeratin, there is a granular layer and nuclei are not sloughed into the keratin. Orthokeratinizing epithelium is considered to reflect the normal keratinization process, as seen in the epithelial layer of the skin.

In the keratocyst, the interface between the epithelium and the connective tissue is flat, without rete ridge formation. The basal layer is prominent, with palisading cells containing darkly staining and enlarged nuclei. Daughter (satellite) cysts or microcysts may be observed microscopically. The recurrence rate has been variously reported as being between 20% and 60%. This high recurrence rate is thought to be the result of the specific abnormal biology of these cysts. Various hypotheses have been proposed in an attempt to explain this rate and solve this problem.[10, 11]

The diagnosis depends on the cyst's microscopic features and is independent of its location and radiographic appearance. This cyst is a radiolucent lesion that may be multiloculated, with a smooth or scalloped border (Fig. 17-8). These cysts are characteristically located in the body and ramus of the mandible and may occur in conjunction with an impacted tooth (Figs. 17-9 and 17-10). The lesion usually grows along the length of the mandible and does not usually resorb teeth roots. CT shows a well-defined unilocular or multilocular cystic radiolucency with a bony sclerotic margin and bulging of the bony cortex (Fig. 17-11).

Sometimes the content of the cyst shows higher density than water due to keratinized material.[12] The MR imaging appearance is variable but typically shows a cystic pattern with a regularly thin wall, heterogeneous intensity of fluid contents, and weak contrast enhancement of the cyst wall (Fig. 17-12).[13] The signal intensity on T2-weighted sequences is usually high but is variable, depending on the protein concentration of the contents.

One variant of the OKC has a true orthokeratinizing epithelial lining (see above). Although truly a keratocyst, the lesion exhibits significantly less aggressive behavior than the parakeratinizing variant. Some prefer to categorize these lesions separately as an orthokeratinizing keratocyst rather

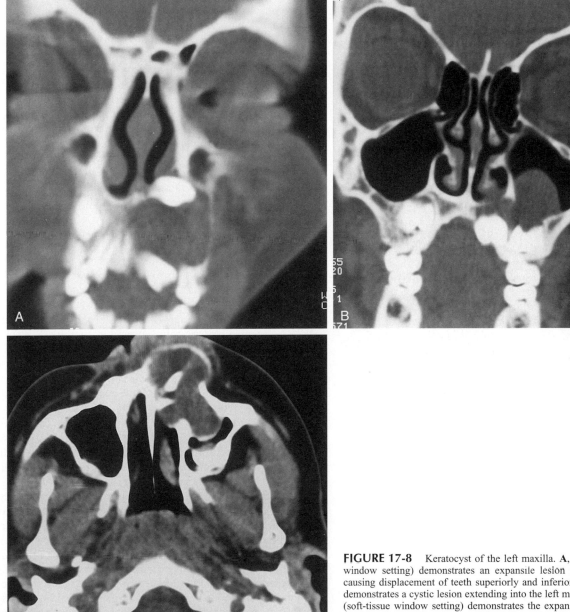

**FIGURE 17-8**   Keratocyst of the left maxilla. **A,** Coronal CT (bone window setting) demonstrates an expansile lesion in the left maxilla causing displacement of teeth superiorly and inferiorly. **B,** Coronal CT demonstrates a cystic lesion extending into the left maxilla. **C,** Axial CT (soft-tissue window setting) demonstrates the expansile cyst in the left maxilla, the anterior portion of the left nasal cavity, and the adjacent maxillary antrum. Note the low attenuation of the cyst and the tooth remnants at the medial aspect of the cyst.

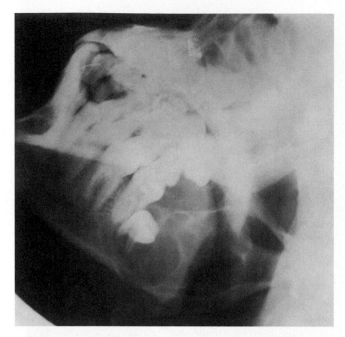

**FIGURE 17-9**   Keratocyst. Oblique view of the mandible shows a multiloculated cyst in the posterior body of the mandible, angle of the mandible, and ramus. The third molar tooth is incorporated into the anterior part of the cyst. There is encroachment on the posterior aspect of the second molar tooth. Note that there is also expansion, with thinning of the anterior wall of the ascending ramus.

than a variant of the typical keratocyst. At imaging, the two lesions cannot be distinguished unless studies over time show the aggressive growth more typical of the parakeratinizing OKC.

The surgical management of OKC demands special attention because of the aggressive biologic behavior of these benign lesions.[14] Surgical treatment over the years has included decompression and marsupialization, enucleation and curettage, and local and en bloc resection and reconstruction. Various adjuvant methods of treatment have been used to decrease the potential for recurrence or to deal with a recurrence. These include extraction of teeth in continuity with the cyst, excision of overlying mucosa, and treatment of the surrounding bone with peripheral ostectomy, chemical cautery, or cryosurgery. Many of these lesions, especially recurrences, are treated with some combination of these surgical techniques. Regardless of the management strategy employed or the surgical outcome, these patients must be closely followed for many years.

The term *primordial cyst* is now usually considered to be synonymous with OKC. However, some consider the term to be more appropriately applied only to the rare cysts that contain nonkeratinized squamous epithelium rather than the typical keratinized lining typical of the keratocyst.[2] Primordial cysts are considered to arise from a degenerated enamel organ and are therefore found in place of a missing tooth (Fig. 17-13).

## Basal Cell Nevus Syndrome (Gorlin's or Gorlin-Goltz Syndrome)

Basal cell nevus syndrome (nevoid basal cell carcinoma syndrome) is a genetic disorder inherited as an

autosomal dominant trait with variable penetrance and expressivity.[15, 16] The syndrome becomes apparent between 5 and 10 years of age. There is no sex predilection, and many patients with this syndrome have slight mental retardation. The syndrome comprises a number of features that are classically grouped into five categories: cutaneous, skeletal, ophthalmologic, neurologic, and sexual. Among the most common features are multiple cysts of the jaw, multiple basal cell carcinomas, skeletal abnomalities, and ectopic calcifications. At least two of these findings must be present to establish a diagnosis.

The multiple jaw cysts develop early in childhood[17]; they may be either unilocular or multilocular and often prove to be keratocysts varying in size from 1 mm to several centimeters (Fig. 17-14). Many investigators have suggested that the OKCs in basal cell nevus syndrome are histologically and biologically different from the solitary OKCs not associated with this syndrome. Those associated with the syndome occur earlier and are more likely to recur after excision. However, this concept is not universally agreed upon. Some investigators believe that the cysts associated with this syndrome are just larger, multilocular, and tend to have more frequent satellite microcysts that may account for their clinical behavior. Nevoid basal cell carcinomas tend to appear later than cysts, usually before 30 years of age, and are found especially on the face, trunk, neck, and arms. The most common skeletal abnormalities are bifid ribs, synostosis of ribs, kyphoscoliosis, vertebral fusion, mild ocular hypertelorism, prognathism, polydactyly, and frontal and temporoparietal bossing. The ectopic calcifications occur most frequently in the falx cerebri and other areas of the dura.

## Calcifying Odontogenic Cyst (Gorlin Cyst)

A calcifying odontogenic cyst is a rare developmental odontogenic lesion having features of both a cyst and a solid neoplasm. It was defined as a distinct entity by Gorlin et al. in 1962[18] and is listed by the WHO as an odontogenic epithelial cyst having odontogenic ectomesenchyme, with or without dental hard tissue formation. In the most recent WHO classification, the calcifying odontogenic cyst is also classified as a tumor.[1] The terms *calcifying odontogenic cyst* and *odontogenic ghost cell tumor* are used. The ghost cell tumor designation results from a characteristic cell found in the wall of the cyst. Ghost cells have eosinophilic cytoplasm and no nuclei. These cells can calcify.

The lesion occurs at many ages but is most commonly found in the second or third decade of life, with an almost equal sex distribution and a similar incidence in the mandible and the maxilla. Those in the maxilla are usually anterior. Radiographically, the cyst may present as a unilocular or multilocular radiolucency with discrete, well-defined margins containing scattered calcifications of irregular size (Figs. 17-15 and 17-16).[19–22] Such opacities may produce a "salt-and-pepper-like" appearance. Displacement of teeth or root resorption is occasionally seen. The lesion is sometimes associated with unerupted teeth. If it is seen along with a complex odontoma, those opaque components may be seen to merge (Fig. 17-15). The radiologic appearance may be similar to that of adenomatoid odontogenic tumor, ameloblastic fibro-odontoma, or calcifying epithelial odontogenic tumor (Pinborg).

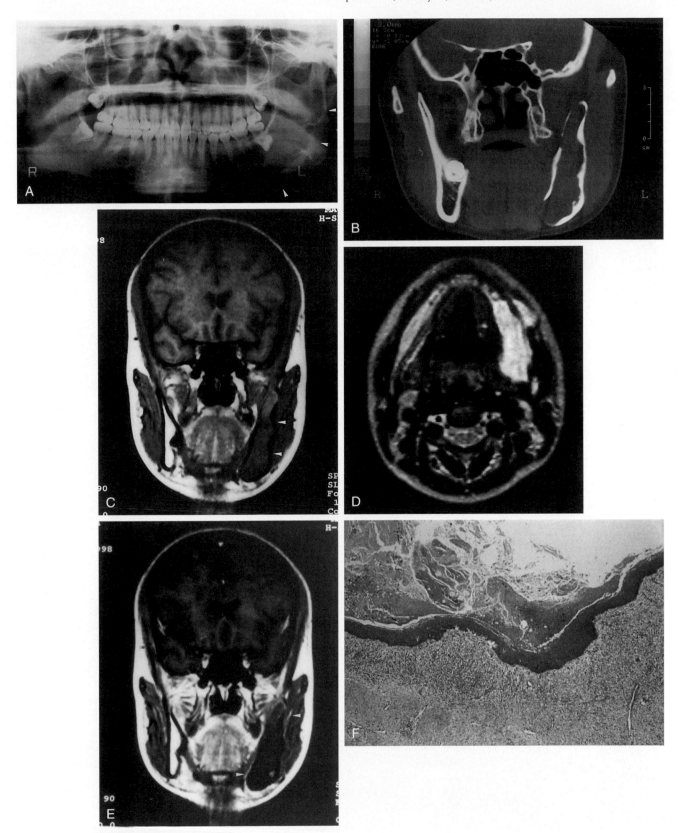

**FIGURE 17-10**   Unilocular odontogenic keratocyst in a 20-year-old woman. **A,** Panoramic radiograph shows a large, unilocular, expansile lesion (*arrowheads*) in the left side of the mandible. There is no root resorption of adjacent teeth. **B** Coronal CT shows an expansile unilocular lesion in the mandible. The bony sclerotic margin and bulging of the bony cortex can be seen. **C,** Axial T1-weighted MR image reveals a lesion of heterogeneously low to intermediate signal intensity in the mandible (*arrowheads*). **D,** On this axial T2-weighted MR image, the fluid contents of the cyst are heterogeneous in intensity. **E,** Gadolinium-enhanced MR image shows a thin cyst wall with weak enhancement. The cyst contents have heterogeneously low to intermediate signal intensity. The lack of solid tissue argues against the diagnosis of ameloblastoma, and OKC is suspected. **F,** Photomicrograph shows that the cyst has a uniformly thin wall with keratinization histopathologically (H & E. Original magnification ×100.)

### Other Odontogenic Cysts

As stated, there is overlap in the descriptions of several entities. Several terms or named cysts deserve mention for completeness.[2, 3]

The lateral periodontal cyst is considered to be a developmental cyst arising from epithelial remnants in the periodontal ligament along the lateral aspect of the tooth root. It is not inflammatory and should be distinguished from the occasional occurrence of an inflammatory lateral radicular cyst that can occur here as well. The botryoid odontogenic cyst may simply be a multicystic variant of the lateral periodontal cyst.

Several cysts are thought by some to be most likely of an inflammatory origin, arising from epithelial rests in the periodontal space. The lateral radicular cyst has been mentioned as analogous to the periapical radicular cyst but occurring along the lateral aspect of the root. The term *paradental cyst* also describes an inflammatory cyst along the sides of the root. Originally described along the lateral aspect of the third molar, the term has been applied to other teeth as well.

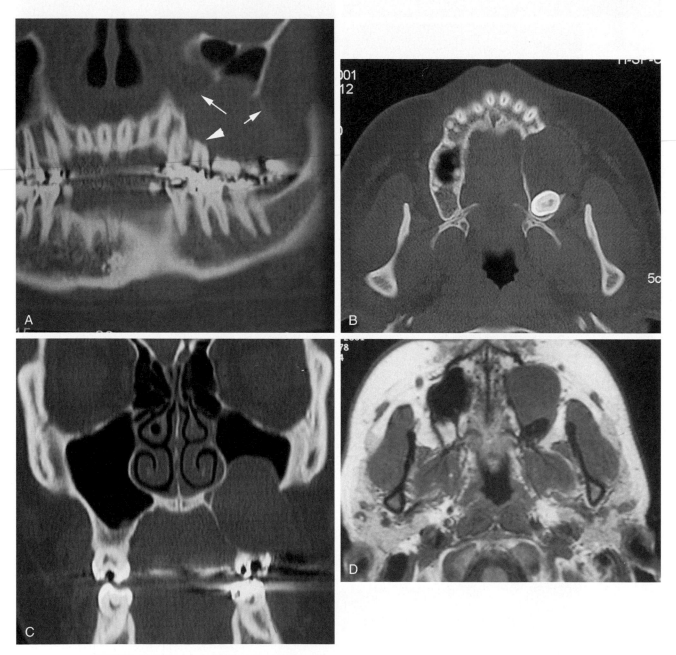

**FIGURE 17-11**   OKC. **A,** Panoramic reformat from multidetector spiral CT scan. The OKC is seen as an expansile abnormality in the left maxilla. Note the intact cortical line (*arrows*) as the lesion expands outward. Multiple root tips (*arrowhead*) are shortened and eroded. **B,** Axial bone algorithm CT shows the expansile abnormality in the lower maxilla. The lesion does have a relationship to the unerupted molar but does not show the typical configuration of a dentigerous cyst. **C,** Coronal CT shows the expanding abnormality enlarging the alveolar process and extending into the maxillary sinus. **D,** Axial T1-weighted MR image. The lesion shows low signal intensity.

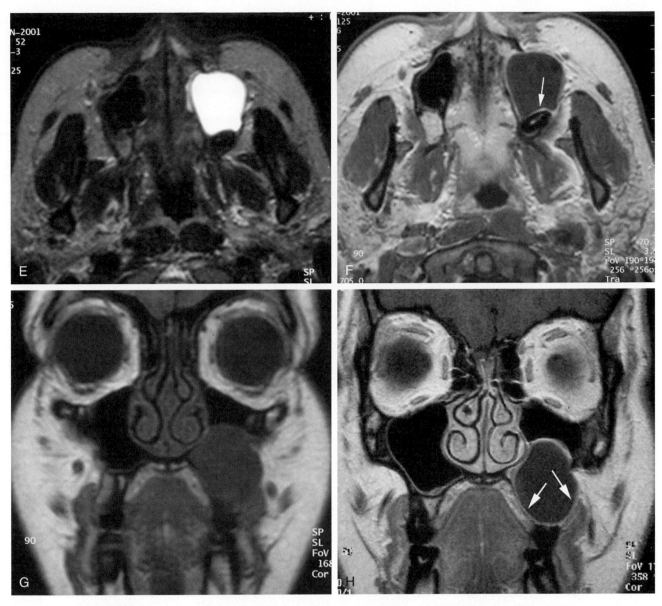

**FIGURE 17-11**   *Continued.* **E,** The lesion is homogeneously bright on this T2-weighted image. OKC can also be heterogeneous. **F,** Axial T1 postgadolinium image shows a thin, regular enhancing margin. Note that a thin soft-tissue enhancing margin (*arrow*) borders and "covers" the tooth. **G,** Coronal T1-weighted image. **H,** Coronal T1-weighted image after gadolinium enhancement shows the thin, regular enhancing wall (*arrows*) of the keratocyst.

The buccal bifurcation cyst arises from the periodontium at the bifurcation of the lateral (buccal) roots of the mandibular molars, usually the first. The roots tend to tip lingually. Although it is considered most likely related to inflammation, inflammation is not always present. The term *paradental cyst* (see above) has been applied to this lesion as well.[3]

## Nonodontogenic Cysts and Pseudocysts

### Incisive Canal Cyst (Nasopalatine Duct Cyst)

A nasopalatine duct cyst (incisive canal cyst) is a nonodontogenic developmental cyst or fissural cyst arising in the nasopalatine duct near the anterior palatine papilla.[23, 24] It is the most common nonodontogenic cyst. The cysts probably arise from epithelial remnants in the incisive canal. They can occur at any age but are most frequently found in the fourth and sixth decades of life, with no sex predilection. These cysts are usually asymptomatic, but some patients note swelling in the palate, especially when the cyst is primarily in the incisive papilla. Alternatively, the anterior maxilla can be remodeled forward, elevating the columella of the nose. Occasionally, patients notice a discharge of mucoid material and a salty taste through what are thought to be remnants of embryonic ductal structures on the palate.

Many of these cysts are small and are found on routine plain film radiographic surveys. It may be difficult on imaging to differentiate between an enlarged incisive fossa and an incisive canal cyst. The incisive canal cyst is always located at or close to the midline and usually is round or ovoid, although it may be heart-shaped (Fig. 17-17). A condensed rim of cortical bone is often seen along the periphery, and the lesion may displace the roots of the central incisor teeth.

The nasolabial or nasoalveolar cyst is considered most likely a fissural cyst arising adjacent to bone at the root apex of the incisors just beneath the lip. It may scallop the bone along the anterior cortex of the maxilla. This lesion is also discussed in Chapter 6.

Several terms are no longer used. The term *globulomaxillary cyst* referred to a cyst located between the lateral incisor and the canine tooth, at the site thought to correspond to a developmental fusion line between the lateral nasal and maxillary processes.[25, 26] Today there is evidence that these cysts do not arise from "trapped" epithelium but are probably simply cysts of odontogenic origin (Fig. 17-18). A cyst in this location is now thought to be either a radicular cyst or perhaps a keratocyst.

The median palatal cyst is now frequently grouped with nasopalatine cysts rather than considered a separate entity.

### Solitary, Simple, or Hemorrhagic Bone Cyst (Traumatic Bone Cyst)

Solitary, simple, or hemorrhagic bone cysts are seen more frequently in men than in women and are usually found in young people, with 70% occurring in the second decade of life.[27, 28] The etiologic factors are usually obscure. Yet, whether this cyst results from an injury not associated with a fracture that causes an intramedullary hematoma that disintegrates, producing the cyst within the bone, or is perhaps the result of aseptic necrosis or degeneration of an earlier benign tumor, the end result appears to be the same. A hemorrhagic bone cyst is a unilocular cavity that can be partly filled with a clear or sanguineous fluid. The cyst lining

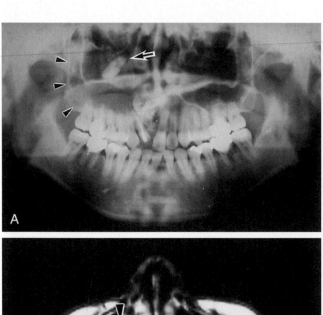

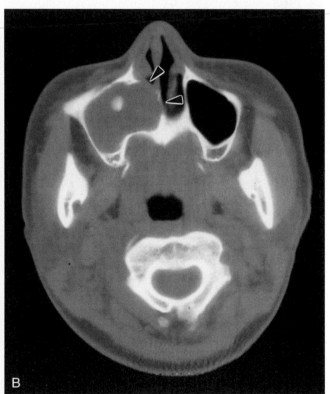

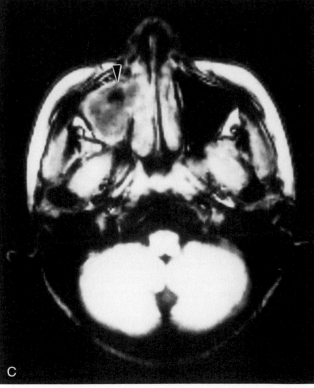

**FIGURE 17-12** OKC. **A,** Pantomogram shows a unilocular lesion (*arrowheads*) with an impacted tooth (*arrow*) in the right side of the maxilla. **B,** Axial CT shows an expansile unilocular lesion extending into the nasal cavity (*arrowheads*). **C,** Axial T1-weighted MR image reveals a cystic lesion of heterogeneously intermediate to low signal intensities with signal void (*arrowhead*) suggesting the impacted tooth in the maxilla.

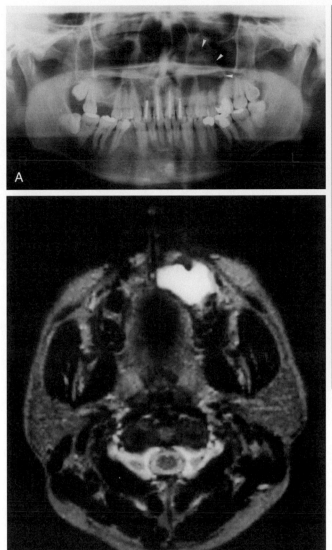

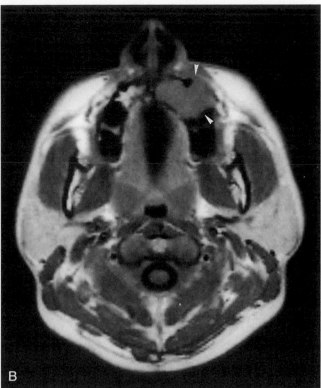

**FIGURE 17-13** Primordial cyst in a 35-year-old man. **A,** Pantomogram shows a well-defined unilocular radiolucent lesion extending from the left upper premolar region into the left maxillary sinus (*arrowheads*). Differentiation between ameloblastoma, OKC, and primodial cyst is difficult. **B,** Axial T1-weighted MR image reveals an expansible low-intensity lesion in the left maxilla (*arrowheads*). **C,** Axial T2-weighted MR image shows the well-defined lesion of homogeneously high intensity. MR findings suggest a cyst other than OKC, but further differentiation is difficult.

consists of a loose vascular connective tissue that may have areas of recent or old hemorrhage.[29, 30]

Because these solitary bone cysts often are asymptomatic, most are discovered incidentally during examination of the teeth, and it is believed that some of them regress spontaneously. These lesions are most commonly located in the mandibular marrow space that extends posteriorly from the premolar region. Less often, they may occur in the incisor area of the mandible. Radiographically, these cysts are slightly irregular in shape and size and have poorly defined borders, and the outline of the cyst between the roots of the teeth has a scalloped appearance (Fig. 17-19). Larger cysts may extend into the interdental space. The ramus and body of the mandible may be slightly expanded (Fig. 17-20). The radiographic features are not sufficiently specific to be diagnostic. On MR T1-weighted images, the cyst may show variable signal intensities ranging from low to high according to the age of the hematoma. CT may be helpful to evaluate the contents of the cyst, as a relatively high density is consistent with blood products, but the density can be variable.

These lesions are usually investigated surgically with a single diagnostic and therapeutic procedure. Using a minimally invasive technique, the surgeon can evaluate the lesion and sample tissue. Healing usually takes place with reossification.

### Aneurysmal Bone Cyst

These rare lesions are far more common in children than in adults, in females than in males, and in the mandible than in the maxilla or zygoma.[31–34] They usually present with a rapidly growing swelling that can be markedly disfiguring, and there is usually no pain or paresthesia. There can be spontaneous bleeding from around the teeth or from areas of mucosal trauma. Although there is often a history of prior trauma, these cysts can occur without this history, and they may be associated with a preexisting intraosseous pathologic process. Radiographically, these lesions are often multiloculated, with areas of bone destruction (Fig. 17-21). On CT or MR imaging, fluid-fluid levels may be present, a finding strongly suggestive of this entity. Histologically,

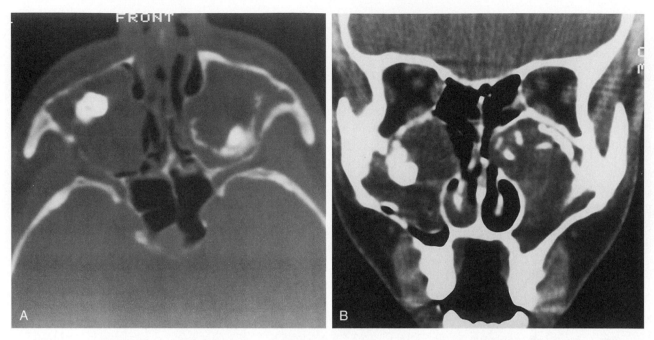

**FIGURE 17-14** Bilateral maxillary keratocysts in a patient with the basal cell nevus syndrome. **A,** Axial CT (bone window setting) through the maxillary antra shows slightly expansile lesions in both antral cavities reflected by a cystic bony rim in the left antral cavity and some lateral expansion and thinning of the wall of the right antrum. Note the displaced teeth on the left and right within the cystic lesions. **B,** Coronal CT (soft-tissue window setting) demonstrates bilateral cystic lesions in the maxillary antra, with part of a thin rim of surrounding bone seen in the left antrum. Note the displaced tooth in the upper part of the right antral cavity and the low attenuation of the cyst contents.

they are epithelium-lined, blood-filled cavities with accumulations of immature connective tissue, multinucleated giant cells, osteoid, and inflammatory cells. Numerous approaches have been used to treat these lesions, including interventional radiologic procedures, low-dose radiation therapy, and multiple types of surgical enucleation and resection. More recently, these and other types of giant cell lesions have been treated with calcitonin, interferon, and direct intralesional steroid injections.[35, 36]

### Static Bone Cavity (Stafne Cyst)

A Stafne cyst is a pseudocyst. The cortex of the mandible bows inward into the medullary space of the mandible. A

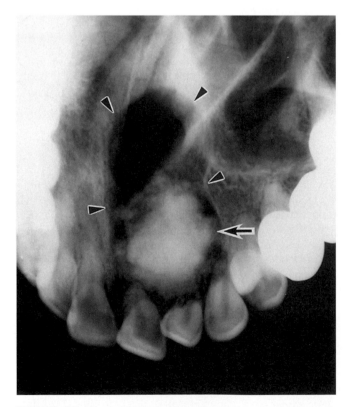

**FIGURE 17-15** Calcifying odontogenic cyst. Occlusal radiograph shows a unilocular lesion (*arrowheads*) with odontoma (*arrow*) in the right side of the maxilla. Calcified tissue can be observed adjacent to the odontoma.

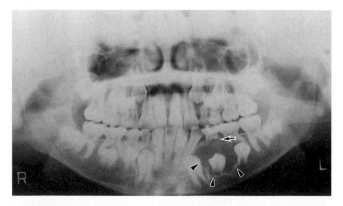

**FIGURE 17-16** Calcifying odontogenic cyst. Pantomogram shows a pericoronal calcifying odontogenic cyst (*arrowheads*) with tiny calcifications. Root resorption can be observed at the left side of the milk tooth (*arrow*).

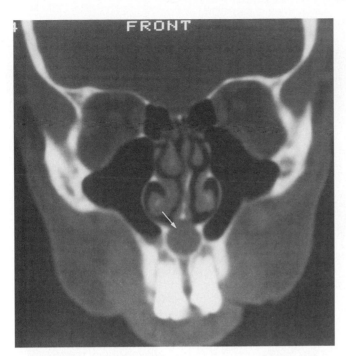

**FIGURE 17-17**    Nasopalatine cyst. Coronal CT (bone window setting) shows a cyst with bony expansion in the nasopalatine duct between the upper central incisor teeth (*arrow*). There is a slight bulge into the adjacent nasal cavity.

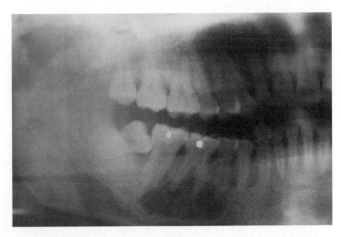

**FIGURE 17-19**    Hemorrhagic bone cyst in the body of the right mandible. Pantomogram of the mandible shows a sharply defined, oval-shaped cyst around the apices of the molar and premolar teeth of the right mandible.

Radiographically, the radiolucency has a well-defined border, often with a sclerotic margin, and varies in size from 1 to 2 cm (Figs. 17-22 and 17-23). The cortex follows along the lateral aspect of the abnormality, projecting into the bone. Diagnostic evaluation is usually needed to rule out lesions that are actually located within the bone.

### Medullary Pseudocyst

The number of trabeculae crossing the medullary cavity of the mandible is variable. An area with relatively few trabeculae can give the appearance of a lucency mimicking a cyst on a plain film or parorex. Usually there is no sharp or sclerotic margin. In the adult, most of the medullary space is filled with fat, so the diagnosis of pseudocyst is readily made by the characteristic density on CT or signal intensity on MR imaging.

Stafne cyst appears as an elliptical ovoid or round radiolucency usually located on the medial surface of the posterior mandible, often near the angle of the mandible below the mandibular canal and the mylohyoid line of the mandible (Fig. 17-22). Stafne cysts occur more frequently in men than in women and have been reported in patients from 20 to 70 years of age. Most are discovered by 50 years of age. These asymptomatic lesions are usually detected incidentally on routine radiographs of the mandible.[37] The bone "defect" usually contains submandibular salivary gland tissue or fat.[38] The cortex is intact, separating the medullary space of the mandible from the soft tissues in the submandibular space along the medial aspect of the bone (Fig. 17-23). Bilateral lesions have been described.

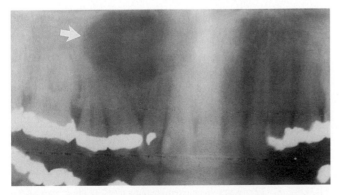

**FIGURE 17-18**    "Globulomaxillary cyst." Pantomogram shows a cystic structure (*arrow*) in the right maxilla causing divergence of the roots of the lateral incisor and canine tooth.

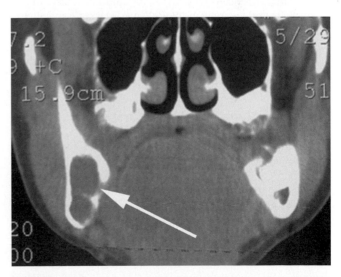

**FIGURE 17-20**    Traumatic simple (posttraumatic) bone cyst. The abnormality enlarges the body of the mandible, with some thinning of the bony wall (*arrow*).

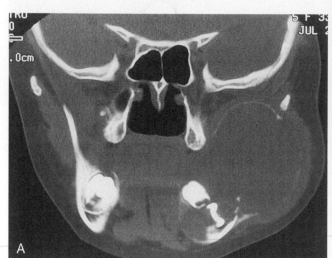

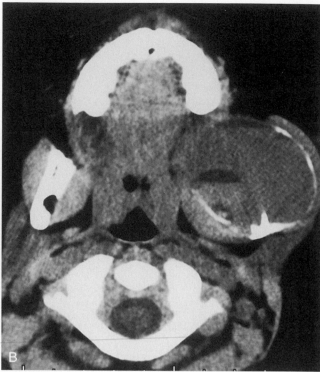

**FIGURE 17-21** Aneurysmal bone cyst of the left mandible. **A,** Coronal CT through the posterior portion of the mandible shows an expansile lesion in the left mandible. Note the thin, bony rim around the cyst and misplacement of teeth in the mandible at the lower aspect of the cyst. **B,** Axial CT through the ascending ramus of the mandible shows a cystic, expansile lesion with several fluid-fluid levels.

# BENIGN ODONTOGENIC TUMORS AND RELATED TUMOR-LIKE CONDITIONS

Odontogenic tumors result from an abnormal proliferation of the cells and tissues involved in odontogenesis.[39, 40] They represent a diverse group of lesions that are classified according to the origin of the various layers of tooth development. Based on the histologic findings, these tumors have been divided into epithelial, mesodermal, and mixed tissue tumors of odontogenic origin.[3] The radiographic appearance of odontogenic tumors varies, and many of them cannot be differentiated from the cysts previously described.

## Ameloblastoma (Epithelial Origin)

An ameloblastoma is a benign epithelial odontogenic tumor thought to arise from ameloblasts (enamel-forming cells).[41–43] It is found with about equal frequency in men and women and has a peak incidence in the third and fourth decades of life, with two thirds of cases occurring before 40 years of age. Ameloblastomas account for approximately 18% of odontogenic tumors; 81% are located in the mandible, and the remaining 19% are found in the maxilla. Half of the mandibular lesions are located in the molar regions. An ameloblastoma is a slow-growing, painless mass that may reach a considerable size; swelling is the most common presenting symptom. Ameloblastoma may mani-

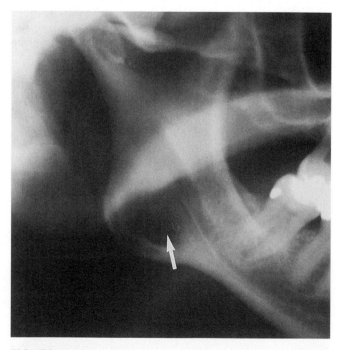

**FIGURE 17-22** Static bone cavity (Stafne cyst). Oblique view of the mandible shows an oval-shaped "cavity" in the angle of the mandible (*arrow*) below the mandibular canal. This lucency is simply a deformity of the medial cortex.

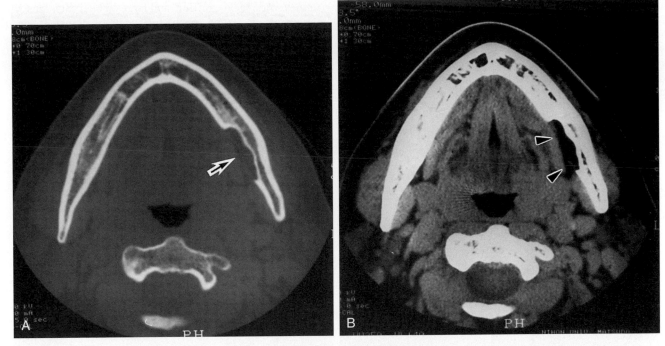

**FIGURE 17-23**   Static bone cavity (Stafne cyst). **A,** Axial CT (bone tissue window setting) shows a defect (*arrow*) with adjacent thinning of the lingual cortex. Note, however, that the cortex is complete along the lateral aspect of the abnormality. **B,** Axial CT (soft-tissue window setting) shows the static bone cavity containing adjacent fat (*arrowheads*).

fest in a number of histologic patterns, including the follicular, plexiform, acanthomatous, keratinizing, granular cell, basal cell, and clear cell types. In 1984 Eversole et al. described a desmoplastic variant of ameloblastoma.[44] This unusual variant was characterized histologically by an abundant densely collagenous stroma (desmoplasia) with small nests and strands of odontogenic epithelium.[3]

Radiographically, an ameloblastoma is radiolucent and either multilocular or unilocular (Figs. 17-24 and 17-25). The unilocular lesions occur most often in the maxilla (Fig. 17-26). The multilocular form often has been described as having a honeycombed or bubble-like appearance, and the loculi may be oval or spherical and vary in size. Ameloblastomas can vary in size from a small cyst confined to the alveolus to a large cyst that causes extensive destruction of the mandible or maxilla. The tumor has a tendency to break through the cortex of the bone, with subsequent tumor extension into the adjacent soft tissues (Figs. 17-27 and 17-28). There can be bony expansion of variable degree, sometimes with scalloped marginal sclerosis, and there is no periosteal new bone formation. Loss of the lamina dura, erosion of the tooth apex, and displacement of the teeth are also commonly seen. MR imaging findings in ameloblastomas include mixed patterns of solid and cystic components, irregularly thick walls, papillary projections, and marked enhancement of the walls and septa (Fig. 17-29). The demonstration of papillary projections and solid components on contrast-enhanced T1-weighted images is especially helpful in differentiating ameloblastomas from various other cysts (Fig. 17-30).[45] However, the desmoplastic variant of ameloblastoma shows unusual radiographic features such as a mixed radiolucent-radiopaque appearance with poorly defined borders. Because of its appearance, it

can be mistakenly diagnosed as a fibroosseous lesion (Fig. 17-31).[46, 47]

The biologic behavior of these lesions has been of great interest and debate. Numerous clinical and histopathologic studies have evaluated the several varieties of ameloblas-

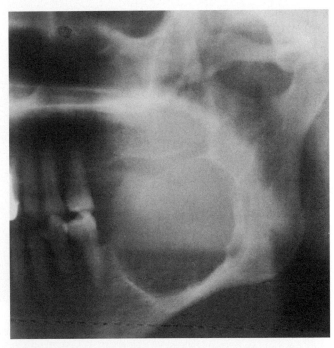

**FIGURE 17-24**   Ameloblastoma. Oblique view of the mandible shows a large cystic lesion in the body and ramus of the mandible, with attenuation and loss of bone superiorly. The lesion has broken through the upper part of the mandible.

toma in an attempt to relate the clinical picture, histologic pattern, and biologic behavior to provide more appropriate treatment. However, at this time, there does not seem to be any good correlation and the treatment strategies remain predominantly surgical. A variety of approaches have been advocated based on the individual patient. These include curettage and adjuvant treatment of the surrounding soft tissues, wide local excision, and large en bloc excisions with immediate or staged reconstruction. A malignant form of ameloblastoma accounts for 1% of the ameloblastomas. With recurrent tumors and delayed reconstructions, CT, MR imaging, and technetium bone scanning can be helpful in evaluating whether a soft-tissue mass is a recurrence or fibrous healing.

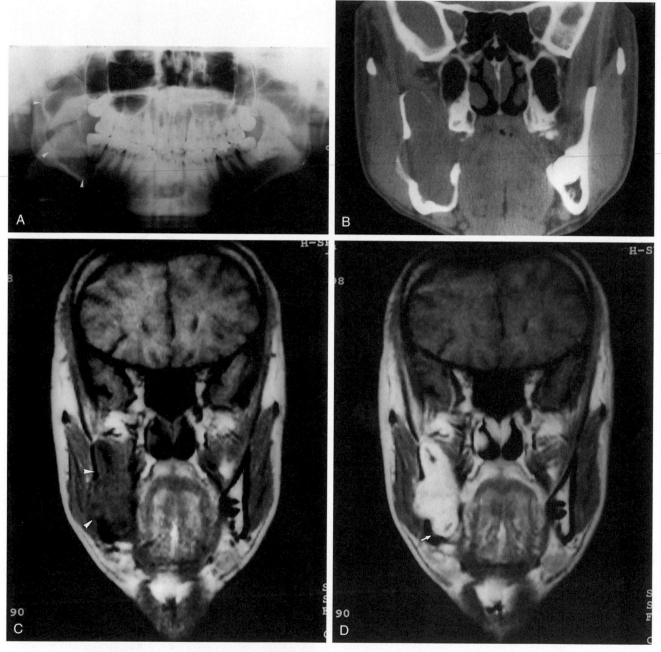

**FIGURE 17-25** Multilocular ameloblastoma in a 25-year-old man. **A**, Pantomogram shows a large, multilocular, expansile lesion in the right side of the mandible (*arrowheads*). There is no root resorption of adjacent teeth. A cystic lesion is suspected. **B**, Coronal CT shows the expansile multilocular lesion, with bulging of the bony cortex without perforation. **C**, Coronal T1-weighted MR image reveals a lesion of homogeneously low signal intensity in the mandible (*arrowheads*). **D**, Enhanced coronal MR image shows the markedly enhanced solid lesion in the mandible. The mandibular canal can be seen under the solid mass (*arrow*).

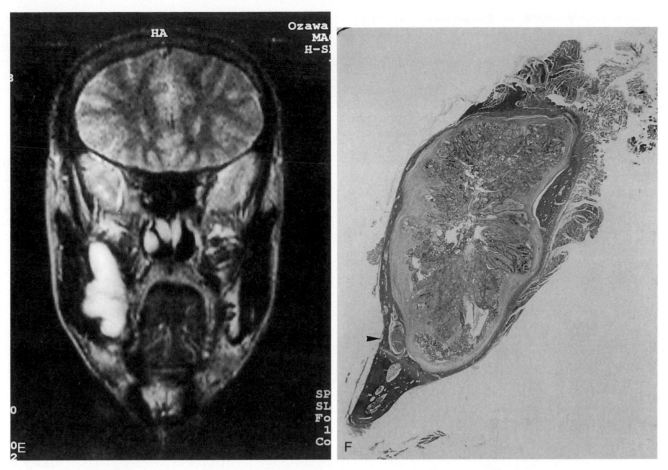

**FIGURE 17-25**   *Continued.* **E,** Coronal T2-weighted MR image reveals the tumor and fluid content to be of homogeneously high signal intensity. Solid ameloblastoma is suspected preoperatively, but other solid tumors cannot be ruled out. **F,** Photomicrograph shows complete solid tumor of ameloblastoma. (H&E. Original magnification ×100.) The mandibular canal is seen under the tumor (*arrowhead*).

## Calcifying Epithelial Odontogenic Tumor (Pindborg Tumor)

A calcifying epithelial odontogenic tumor is composed of polyhedral epithelial cells in a fibrous stroma that contains acidophilic homogeneous structures that commonly calcify.[48–50] At first diagnosis the average age of the patient is about 40 years, with an age range of 12 to 78 years. There is no sex predilection. Many of these tumors are located in the premolar-molar area of the mandible, and in half of the cases they are associated with the crown of an impacted tooth.

Radiographically, the lesion usually is a mixed radiolucent and radiopaque mass that may be unilocular but more often is multilocular and honeycombed. It has poorly defined, irregular borders that reflect its aggressive behavior, which is similar to that of the ameloblastoma. Radiopaque densities of varying degree may be located close to the crown of an impacted tooth (Fig. 17-32). Curettage is the preferred treatment, but recurrence or extensive tumor involvement should be treated by resection.

## Odontoma (Mixed Tumor)

An odontoma is a benign tumor made up of the various components of teeth (e.g., enamel, dentin, cementum, and pulp). It is also designated as a composite lesion because of the admixture of several types of tissue.[5, 51–54] During its maturation, an odontoma passes through the same stages as a developing tooth, but dentin and enamel are laid down in an abnormal pattern. In the initial stage of development, a radiolucent area develops because of bone resorption by the odontogenic tissues. In the intermediate and late stages, progressive calcification takes place, initially characterized by small, speckled calcific densities that eventually form radiopaque masses surrounded by a lucent ring. These tumors may be discovered in any location of the dental arches and are situated between the roots of teeth.

Both forms of odontoma (complex and compound) are frequently associated with unerupted teeth. It is noteworthy that compound odontomas occur most often in the anterior jaw, whereas complex odontomas tend to occur in the posterior jaw. A developing odontoma without calcification or with few calcifications is difficult to diagnose radiographically and usually cannot be differentiated from other similar-appearing lesions.

### Complex Odontoma

Complex odontomas (complex composite odontomas) account for 24% of all odontomas.[52, 53] These lesions are composed of dental tissues arranged in a disorderly pattern and bearing no morphologic similarity to normal or rudimentary teeth (Figs. 17-33 and 17-34). Complex odontomas most commonly occur in patients aged 10 to 25 years, and males and females are affected equally. The lesion usually is asymptomatic and most frequently is located in the premolar and molar regions in the mandible, although it is sometimes found in the maxilla. Most lesions are small, measuring only a few millimeters, but some may reach a considerable size.

Radiographically, these lesions are well-demarcated radiopaque masses, often with radiating structures. Occasionally, the tumor is surrounded by a narrow radiolucent zone, and there usually is a nearby unerupted tooth. The preferred therapeutic treatment is enucleation. Cancellous bone grafting may be appropriate, depending on the size and location of the surgical defect.

### Compound Odontoma

Compound odontoma (compound composite odontoma) consists of dental tissues that are similar to a normal tooth, having a more orderly pattern than that seen in complex odontoma.[54] The lesion is composed of many tooth-like structures, with enamel, dentin, cementum, and pulp arranged as in a normal tooth (Figs. 17-35 and 17-36). The

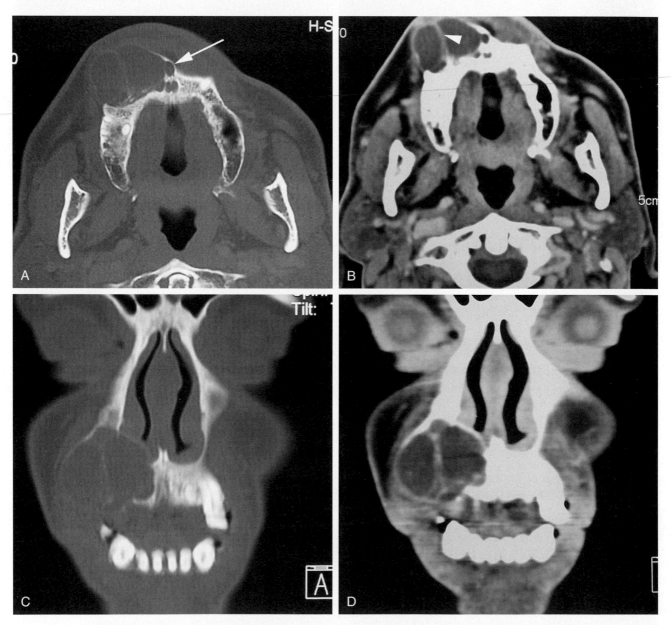

**FIGURE 17-26**  Ameloblastoma of the maxilla. **A,** Expansile abnormality with multiple loculations extends away from the alveolar process of the maxilla. Note the secondary cystic extension (*arrow*) to the midline. **B,** Soft-tissue algorithm (postcontrast) shows an enhancing septation (*arrowhead*) within the lesion. **C,** Coronal bone algorithm. The lesion elevates the floor of the nasal cavity. **D,** Coronal soft-tissue algorithm.

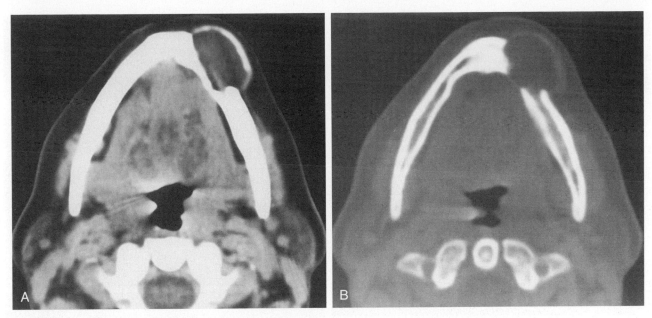

**FIGURE 17-27**   Ameloblastoma. **A,** Axial CT (soft-tissue window setting) shows an expansile lesion in the body of the left mandible and adjacent symphysis with marked lateral expansion. **B,** Axial CT (bone window setting) defines the boundary of this expansile lesion to better advantage. Also, note the erosion of the lingual surface of the mandible.

differentiation of teeth varies from case to case, and the number of teeth involved may be surprisingly high.

Most compound odontomas (60%) occur in the second and third decades of life, and there is no sex predilection. The tumor frequently is located in the incisor-canine region of the maxilla. It is usually small but may occasionally displace teeth or interfere with their eruption; the lesion is otherwise asymptomatic. Radiographically, several small, rather well-defined, malformed or rudimentary teeth are demonstrated, surrounded by a radiolucent zone that is caused by a fibrous capsule. The teeth contained in a

compound odontoma are dwarfed and usually distorted, with simple roots (Fig. 17-37). Most of these lesions are well encapsulated and easily enucleated, and recurrences are not encountered after enucleation.

### Ameloblastic Fibroodontoma

An ameloblastic fibroodontoma is a mixture of ameloblastic tissue and a composite odontoma. It is a rare lesion that can occur at any age but is more prevalent in children than in adults, being rare after the age of 13 years. This tumor is more common in the mandible (premolar-molar

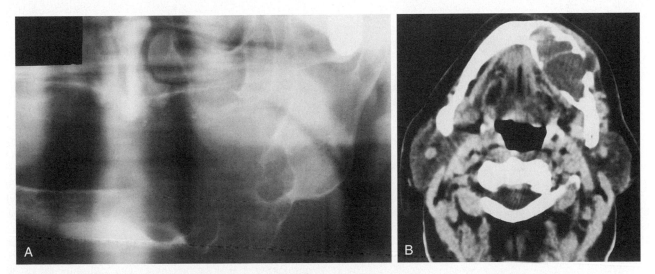

**FIGURE 17-28**   Ameloblastoma. **A,** Pantomogram of the mandible shows a multiloculated aggressive lesion in the body and ramus of the mandible with considerable loss of bone. **B,** Axial CT (soft-tissue window setting) shows the expansile lesion in the body and ramus. There is loss of bone medially and laterally. There is general low attenuation and slightly septated soft-tissue densities within the lesion. A small component of the tumor has penetrated through the lateral cortex into the adjacent soft tissues.

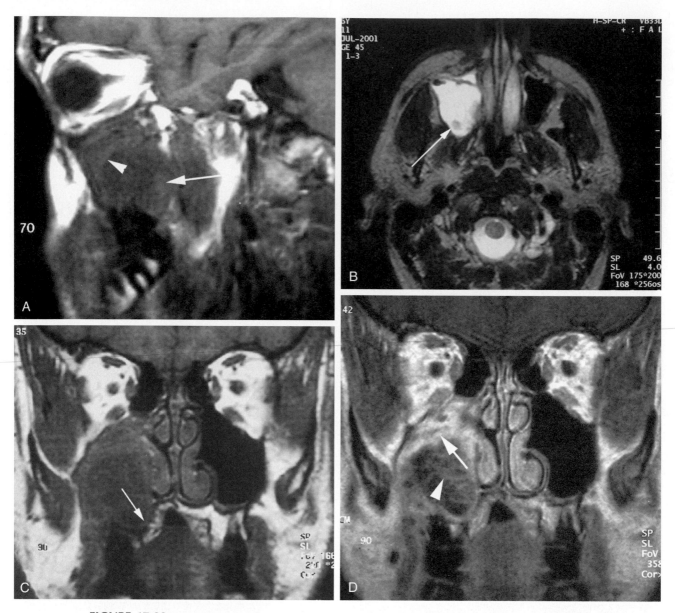

**FIGURE 17-29**   Ameloblastoma of the maxilla. **A**, Sagittal T1-weighted image shows an expansile lesion extending into the maxillary sinus. The superior margin of the lesion (*arrowhead*) extends into this sinus. An area of slightly higher signal (*arrow*) is a more nodular tissue extending into the primarily cystic abnormality. **B**, Axial T2-weighted image. The soft-tissue nodule (*arrow*) has lower signal than most of the cystic fluid. **C**, Coronal T1-weighted image. The lesion expands the palate and the alveolar process (*arrow*). **D**, Postcoronal T1-weighted image shows the nodular enhancement (*arrow*) along the margin. There is also an enhancing septation (*arrowhead*) within the lesion. Compare this to the pregadolinium image.

region) than in the maxilla, and it is always associated with developing teeth. Painless swelling or absence or displacement of teeth are the most common signs leading to its diagnosis.

Radiographically, the tumor has a lucent, well-defined margin with a solitary mass or several small radiopaque masses that may resemble miniature teeth (Fig. 17-38). Radiographic differentiation from other odontomas is not possible, and inadequate removal may be followed by a recurrence.

### Adenomatoid Odontogenic Tumor

An adenomatoid odontogenic tumor, formerly known as adenoameloblastoma, is a tumor of odontogenic epi-

thelium with duct-like structures and with varying degrees of inductive changes in the connective tissue.[3] It is relatively rare, accounting for approximately 3% of all odontogenic tumors.[55, 56] The tumor is seen more frequently in female patients. It usually occurs in the second decade of life and is present as a slow-growing, painless swelling. The maxilla is involved nearly twice as frequently as the mandible. Radiographically, the tumor is associated with the crown of an embedded tooth mimicking a dentigerous cyst. The radiolucency is well demarcated. Some tumors have a totally radiolucent center; others have punctate calcifications either sprinkled throughout (giving a cloud-like appearance) or in clusters (Fig. 17-39). The tumor can displace or prevent the eruption of teeth, especially the canine. Root resorption is rarely encountered. The radiologic appearance may be similar to that of calcifying odontogenic cyst, ameloblastic fibroodontoma, and calcifying epithelial odontogenic tumor.[57]

## Odontogenic Myxoma

An odontogenic myxoma appears to be a true odontogenic tumor, originating from the mesodermal portion of the odontogenic apparatus.[3] This tumor, which is not found in bones outside the jaw, accounts for about 3% to 6% of

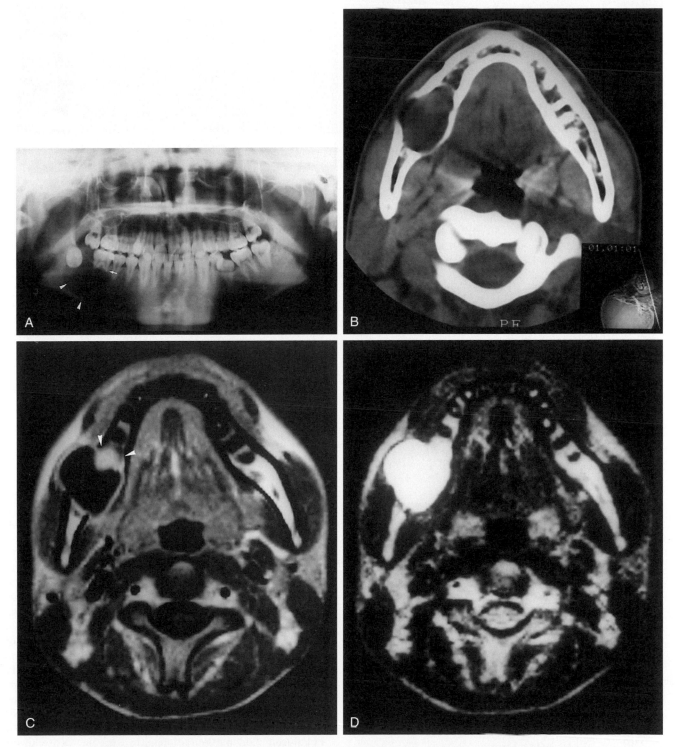

**FIGURE 17-30**    Unilocular ameloblastoma. **A,** Panoramic radiograph shows a large, unilocular, expansile lesion with an unerupted tooth in the right side of the mandible (*arrowheads*). There is root resorption of adjacent teeth (*arrow*). A cystic lesion is suspected. **B,** Axial CT shows an expansile unilocular lesion, with bulging of the bony cortex without perforation. **C,** Enhanced axial MR image shows a papillary projection (*arrowheads*) along the walls of the unilocular lesion. **D,** Axial T2-weighted MR image reveals the lesion to be of high signal intensity.

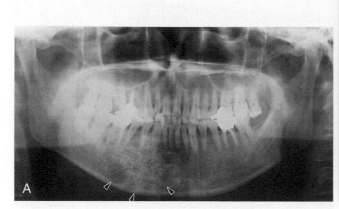
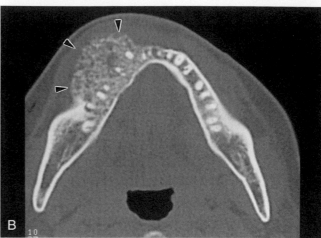

**FIGURE 17-31** Desmoplastic variant of ameloblastoma in the mandible. **A,** Panoramic radiograph shows a diffuse, mixed radiolucent-radiopaque lesion in the mandible (*arrowheads*). **B,** Axial CT shows a definite buccal expansile radiolucent-radiopaque lesion (*arrowheads*). (Courtesy of Dr. T. Kurabayashi, Dept. of Dental Radiology, Tokyo Medical and Dental University, Tokyo.)

odontogenic tumors.[58, 59] It occurs most often in the second and third decades of life, with no sex predilection. The tumor consists of rounded and angular cells lying in an abundant mucoid stroma; the lesion is painless, locally invasive, and slow-growing. If untreated, odontogenic myxomas eventually may cause extensive destruction of bone with marked cortical expansion. The mandible and maxilla are involved with about equal frequency; however, in the mandible, the body and ramus are most commonly affected.

Radiographically, several radiolucent areas of varying size are present, septated by straight or curved bony trabeculae that form triangular, quadrangular, or square-shaped compartments (Figs. 17-40 and 17-41).[60, 61] Unilocular cysts have also been described. The radiographic margins of the tumor may be well or poorly defined, and the lesion may simulate ameloblastoma, central giant cell granuloma, or

hemangioma. This tumor is benign but very aggressive and rapidly growing. It shows little encapsulation and often extends through bone, with a propensity to invade local soft tissues. It may appear to expand in thin layers into and through bone, as well as into the adjacent soft tissues.

Because of its histology and behavior, the treatment of choice has become wide en bloc resection rather than simple enucleation.[59] A tumor-free margin must be resected because of the tumor's local invasiveness and its tendency to recur. A recurrence rate of 25% after curettage has been reported.

## CEMENTAL LESIONS

### Periapical Cemental Dysplasia and Florid Cemental Dysplasia (Florid Cementoosseous Dysplasia)

Periapical cemental dysplasia is a rare lesion that occurs most often in the mandibular region, although in rare cases the lesion may develop in the maxilla.[62–65] It always occurs at the roots of teeth. This lesion is more common in women (average age at diagnosis is 40 years) and among Africans/African Americans. In almost half of the patients, pain is the initial symptom; in other patients, a hard swelling may develop that may cause facial asymmetry.

The initial lesion, which is caused by a proliferation of connective tissue from the periodontal membrane, appears as a well-defined radiolucency.[63] However, it subsequently may be transformed into a radiopaque calcified mass. These lesions can be divided radiographically into three stages: (1) a rather well-defined radiolucency at the apex of a tooth (osteolytic or early stage); (2) a lesion that is partly radiolucent and partly radiopaque, with the dense tissue initially central in the lesion (cementoblastic or mixed stage); and (3) a lesion that is transformed into a mineralized radiopaque mass surrounded by a narrow radiolucent zone (mature stage) (Figs. 17-42 and 17-43). The in-

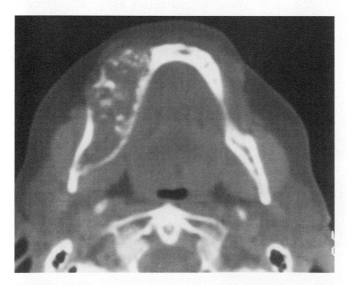

**FIGURE 17-32** Pindborg tumor. Axial CT (bone window setting) shows marked expansion of the right mandible with loss of bone in the lateral cortex. Multiple calcific densities are noted within the lesion.

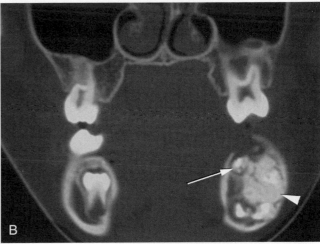

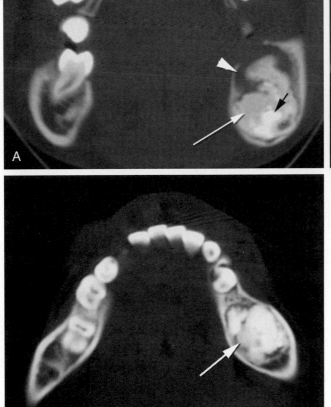

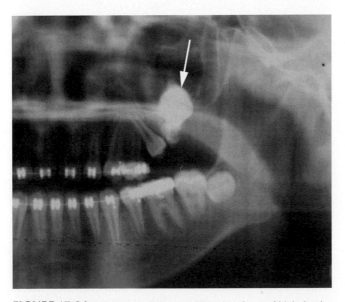

**FIGURE 17-33** Complex odontoma. This lesion has some characteristics of both complex and compound odontoma. CT scan. **A,** Coronal CT shows the expansile abnormality in the mandible. There is amorphous material (*white arrow*) without differentiation into individual teeth. There are, however, several small areas of apparent tooth formation, but they are incomplete (*black arrow*). Note the lucency between the mineralization and the cortex (*arrowhead*). **B,** Slightly more anteriorly, the amorphous material (*arrowhead*) is again noted. There does appear to be an attempt at small tooth formation (*arrow*). **C,** The lesion (*white arrow*) is seen expanding the lower ramus of the mandible.

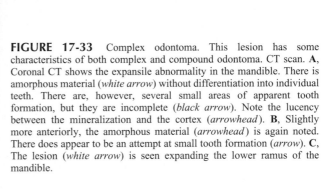

**FIGURE 17-34** Complex odontoma, There is a focus of high density (*arrow*) in the region of the maxillary alveolus. There is disordered organization of dental tissue but no obvious true tooth element.

volved tooth is normal in color and responds normally to tests of vitality.

Periapical cemental dysplasia does not require treatment unless the lesion becomes infected or other disturbing symptoms occur. The treatment of choice is enucleation, with or without extraction of the involved tooth. No recurrences have been reported.

Florid cemental dysplasia (florid cementoosseous dysplasia) is a diffuse form of periapical cemental dysplasia (Fig. 17-44). Pain has been described, but many patients are asymptomatic. There is no clearly defined distinction between multiple periapical cemental dysplasia lesions and florid cemental dysplasia.

The diagnosis is made with plain films or occasionally with CT. MR imaging is not considered helpful (Fig. 17-45).

## Benign Cementoblastoma

Also called a true cementoma, a benign cementoblastoma is a rare neoplasm of functional cementoblasts characterized by the formation of a cementum or cementum-like mass connected with a tooth root.[66, 67] The lesion occurs most

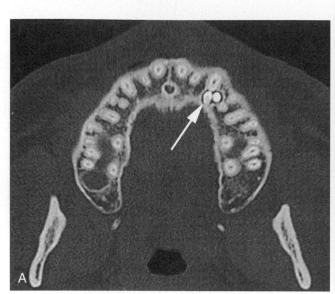

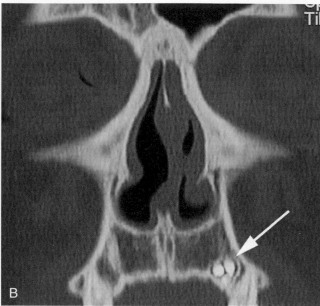

**FIGURE 17-35**   Compound odontoma. CT scan. **A**, Axial image shows small structures containing both enamel and dentine apparently forming small dental units (*arrow*). **B**, Coronal CT showing a small compound odontoma (*arrow*).

frequently in men under 25 years of age, is solitary, and usually is located in the molar or premolar region, with the mandibular first molar being most frequently involved. Benign cementoblastomas are most often associated with permanent teeth, but primary teeth may also be affected.

Radiographically, the tumor is well defined, with central dense radiopaque material being attached to the tooth root and a surrounding radiolucent zone of uniform width, which represents the peripheral nonmineralized tissues of the formative cellular layers.[68] These tumors have a tendency to expand the cortical bone of the jaws. The lesion is easily enucleated because it is benign and surrounded by a capsule.

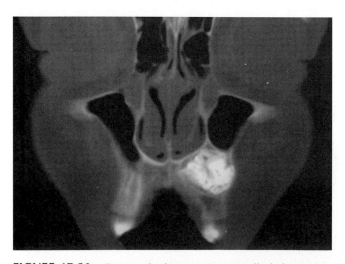

**FIGURE 17-36**   Compound odontoma. An expansile lesion with a well-defined cortical margin contains small, malformed dental structures similar to normal teeth.

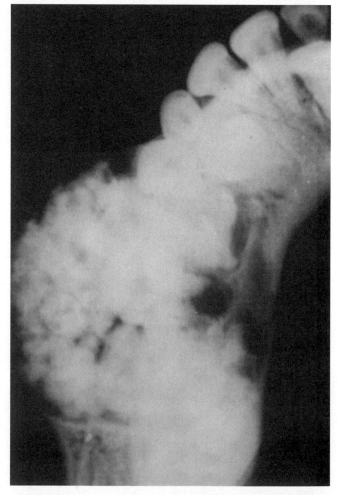

**FIGURE 17-37**   Compound odontoma. Semiaxial view of the mandible shows a calcified lesion expanding the outer cortex of the mandible. The lesion contains multiple malformed teeth. Note the surrounding lucent zone between the expanded cortex and the malformed teeth.

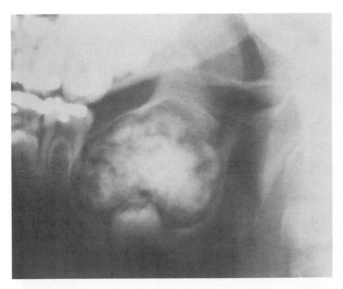

**FIGURE 17-38**   Ameloblastic fibroodontoma. Oblique view of the mandible shows an expansile lesion in the posterior body and ramus of the mandible. Amorphous calcific densities are noted within the lesion. There is a radiolucent zone between the calcified mass and the adjacent expanded cortex. Note the impacted third molar tooth, which is incorporated in the inferior part of the lesion.

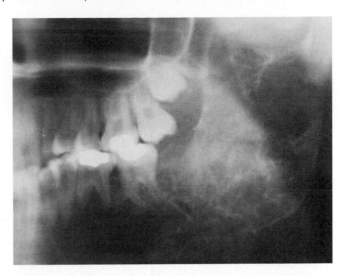

**FIGURE 17-40**   Myxoma of the mandible. Pantomogram of the mandible shows multiple small, irregular lucent areas within the mandible bounded by thickened trabeculae. The lesion more anteriorly demonstrates an ill-defined lucent area beneath the molar teeth. There is extension of this myxoma through the cortex of the mandible, best illustrated inferiorly near the angle of the mandible.

# BENIGN NONODONTOGENIC TUMORS

Benign nonodontogenic tumors are not unique to the jawbone, being found in other parts of the skeleton as well. Their radiographic appearance in the jaw does not differ significantly from their appearance in other bones if one takes into account any abnormalities the lesions may cause to adjacent tooth structures. The discussion of these lesions is based mainly on their tissue of origin.

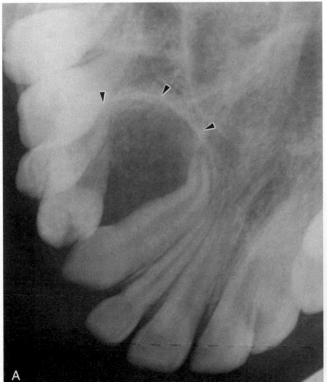

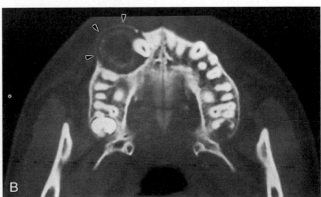

**FIGURE 17-39**   Adenomatoid odontogenic tumor. **A,** Occlusal view shows a well-defined radiolucent lesion with curved margins, tooth displacement, and small internal calcifications in the maxilla (*arrowheads*). **B,** Axial CT shows the well-defined rounded lesion with the incorporated canine and tiny calcifications (*arrowheads*).

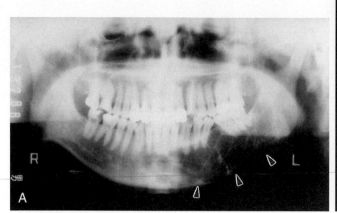

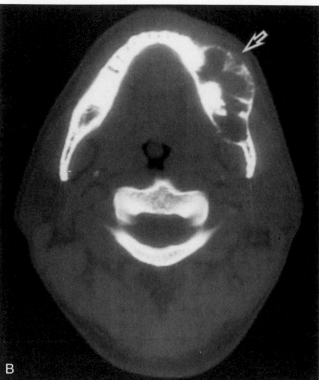

**FIGURE 17-41**   Myxoma of the mandible. **A,** Pantomogram shows an ill-defined lesion with straight septa and tooth displacement (*arrowheads*). **B,** Axial CT (bone window setting) shows buccal expansion of the lesion with straight septa (*arrow*).

## Exostosis

Exostoses are localized outgrowths of bone that vary in size and can be either flat, nodular, or slightly pedunculated protuberances on the surface of the mandible or maxilla.[69–71] The cause of these exostoses of the jaw is unknown. Three types of exostosis are identified according to their location: the torus mandibularis, the torus palatinus, and multiple (maxillary) exostoses. They resemble the compact form of osteoma. The exostoses are differentiated primarily by their typical location.

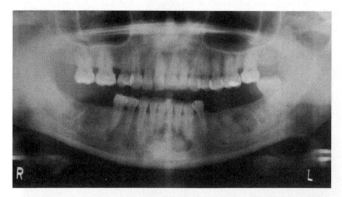

**FIGURE 17-42**   Periapical cemental dysplasia. Pantomogram of the mandible shows multiple sclerotic foci within the mandible, especially at the symphysis and body on the left. Some of these sclerotic areas merge imperceptibly with the mandible. Other densities are surrounded by a lucent ring. The radiographic appearance shows the evolution from lucent areas in the early stages, to mixed stages, and finally to the sclerotic stage.

Radiographically, exostoses are recognized as areas of increased bony density projecting from the mandible or maxilla. Exostoses composed of compact bone are of uniform radiopacity, whereas those that contain a marrow space have trabeculations. Some exostoses are difficult to demonstrate radiographically, particularly small ones and those that are superimposed on the teeth. An enostosis is a related lesion that originates from the inner cortex of the jaw as an area of osteosclerosis.

Torus mandibularis is an outgrowth of bone on the lingual surface of the mandible (Figs. 17-46 to 17-48). It usually is situated above the mylohyoid line, opposite the bicuspid teeth.[44] The size, shape, and number of exostoses vary. The mandibular tori are usually bilateral, but this condition has been found to be unilateral in 20% of cases. The reported incidence in the United States ranges between 6% and 8%, with no sex predilection.

Torus palatinus is a flat, spindle-shaped, nodular or lobular exostosis that arises in the middle of the hard palate (Figs. 17-49 and 17-50). The cause is unknown, but some theories suggest that it may be a hereditary condition.[63, 64] The incidence in the United States varies between 20% and 25%, with women being affected more often. Although torus palatinus may occur at any age, its peak incidence is before the age of 30 years. Radiographically, the torus palatinus is radiopaque, with distinct borders, and is composed of either dense compact bone or a shell of compact bone with a center of cancellous bone. Often a midline suture can be identified through the lesion. Surgical removal is indicated if the torus interferes with swallowing or if a denture must be constructed for prosthetic tooth replacement.

Multiple exostoses of the maxilla (Fig. 50) arise from the buccal or lingual surfaces of the maxilla, primarily in the molar region.[71] They appear as small, nodular, bony masses.

## Osteoma

An osteoma is a benign neoplasm composed of compact or cancellous bone, usually in an endosteal or periosteal location.[72–74] These tumors vary greatly in size and, if large, can cause disfigurement. The average age at occurrence is 50 to 60 years, and twice as many women as men are affected. These lesions occur most often in the paranasal sinuses, especially in the frontal and ethmoid sinuses. The next most common site is the jaw, and the mandible is affected more often than the maxilla.

Osteomas have a characteristic radiographic appearance. They are well-circumscribed, sclerotic bony masses attached by a broad base or pedicle to the surface of the mandible. Root absorption may occur when the osteoma is located in the vicinity of a tooth. The need for surgical removal is determined clinically because osteomas have not been found to become malignant.

Gardner's syndrome, which is inherited as an autosomal dominant trait, consists of multiple osteomas, multiple colonic polyps, epidermoid and sebaceous cysts, desmoid tumors of the skin, and impacted supernumerary and permanent teeth (Fig. 17-51). The multiple osteomas often precede the onset of the colonic polyps, and these polyps almost always eventually become malignant.[75–78] Osteomas have a predilection for the frontal bone, maxilla, and mandible, although they may be observed in any of the bones of the cranium or facial skeleton. Osteomas of the jaw usually appear early in life, most often in the second decade.

## Osteochondroma

An osteochondroma is a benign lesion thought to arise from overgrowth of cartilage at a growth site. These lesions have been reported most frequently in the coronoid and condylar processes.[79, 80] Radiographically, they usually appear as radiopaque extraosseous projections. Although it has been suggested that these tumors are very slow-growing and may have malignant potential, this is not universally agreed upon. Complete surgical removal is the treatment of choice, and recurrence is rare.

## Chondroma

Chondromas are slow-growing lesions that presumably arise from cartilaginous remnants in bone.[81] They produce destruction of normal bone and appear as lytic lesions in the body of the mandible and occasionally in the condyle. Full delineation of condylar lesions often requires CT or MR imaging. Histologically, they are neoplasms of hyaline cartilage that are usually homogeneous in appearance. Therefore, these lesions have high signal intensities on T2-weighted MR images, while T1-weighted MR images often shows low signal intensities similar to those of water. It may be difficult to distinguish between benign and malignant lesions when unusual mitotic activity is identified. Surgical removal with wide margins is the preferred treatment.

## Synovial Chondromatosis

Synovial chondromatosis is a proliferation of synovial tissues with the formation of cartilaginous particles in the

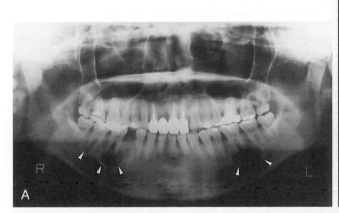
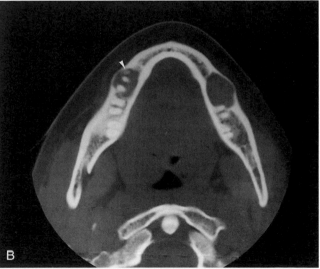

**FIGURE 17-43**   Cemental dysplasia in the mandible. **A,** Pantomogram shows multiple periapical radiolucent lesions with radiopaque areas in the mandible (*arrowheads*). This appearance may be indistinguishable from that of radicular cyst. **B,** Axial CT shows one expansile low-density lesion with tiny calcifications (*arrowhead*) and another expansile lesion without calcification. These are the early stages of cemental dysplasia.

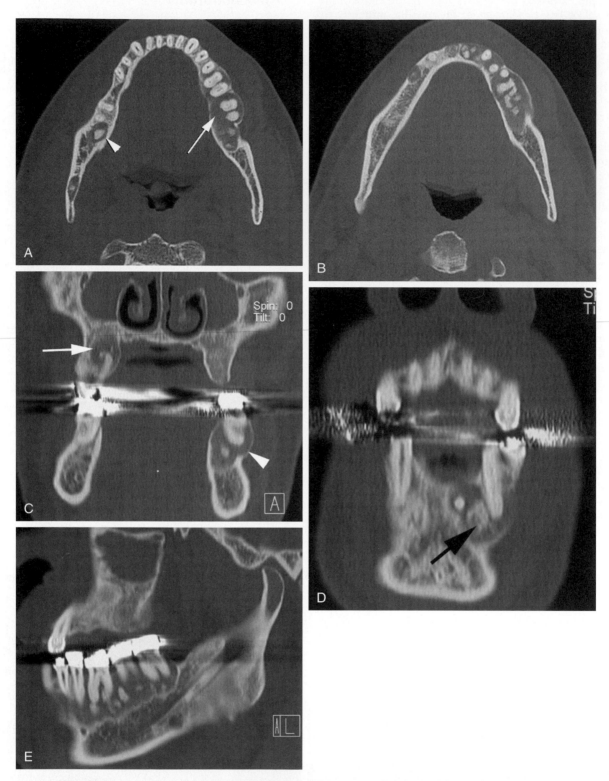

**FIGURE 17-44**    Florid cementoosseous dysplasia. **A,** Axial scan shows the expansile abnormality involving the mandible. The lesion is well corticated and has abnormal density (*arrow*) between the tooth roots and the margin of the lesion. An abnormality is also seen on the opposite side (*arrowhead*). **B,** Slightly caudad image shows that the lesion follows the mandible to the midline. Isolated root tips are involved on the opposite side. **C,** Coronal image shows the lesion in the mandible (*arrowhead*) as well as in the maxilla (*arrow*). There is expansion of bone. The abnormal bone is closely applied to the root tips. **D,** There is mineralization within the lesion (*black arrow*). This reflects the beginning of maturity of the lesion. **E,** Sagittal image shows the lesion involving multiple tooth roots. There are areas of mineralization within the lesion.

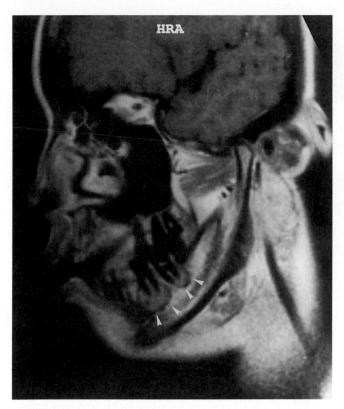

**FIGURE 17-45**   Cemental dysplasia of the mandible in a 38-year-old woman. Oblique sagittal T1-weighted MR image reveals multiple low signal intensities with tiny signal voids in the periapical region (*arrowheads*). Preoperative diagnosis of cemental dysplasia is made by radiography, and MR imaging is not useful for differentiation.

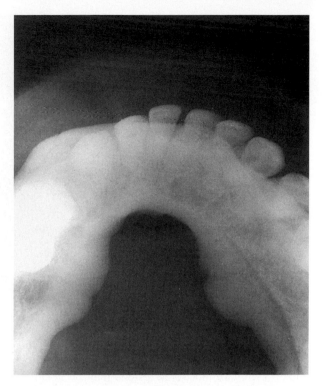

**FIGURE 17-46**   Torus mandibularis. Dental view demonstrates bony exostoses along the lingual surface of the mandible bilaterally.

synovium that can ossify and migrate into the TMJ space. Symptoms vary widely, but patients often complain of intermittent periarticular swelling, pain, and limitation of motion. Radiographic findings depend on the extent of the proliferative process and include joint effusion, anatomic derangement of the normal joint structures with widening of the joint space, irregularity of the joint's articular surfaces, and evidence of calcified or ossified particles within the joint space. Surgical removal of the lesion and synovectomy is the usual treatment, and in most cases the articular disk does not need to be reconstructed. In cases where reconstruction is deemed necessary, the most common procedure is a vascularized, pedicled temporalis muscle flap interposed between the condyle and the articular fossa of the temporal bone (see Chapter 18).

## Giant Cell Lesions

Giant cell lesions of the maxillofacial skeleton make up a continuum of clinically distinct yet histologically very similar pathologic conditions.[82-89] Giant cell granuloma, giant cell tumor, brown tumor of hyperparathyroidism, and cherubism are clinically separate entities that fall into this category. Whether or not the ''true'' giant cell tumor of long bones exists in the maxillofacial skeleton continues to be controversial. Most authors now believe that there is an analogy between the two lesions and that they may represent

a spectrum of a similar pathologic process. Several groups have carried out histomorphometric studies to examine the biologic behavior of these lesions to classify them more correctly, with the aim of correlating histologic and clinical behavior. Based on the clinical, radiologic, and histologic findings, the designation of giant cell lesions of the jaws as either aggressive or nonaggressive may be of more help to the clinician than designation of all of these lesions as belonging to one group.

Giant cell granulomas occur most frequently in the second and third decades of life, and they occur twice as frequently in women as in men. Painless swelling is the most

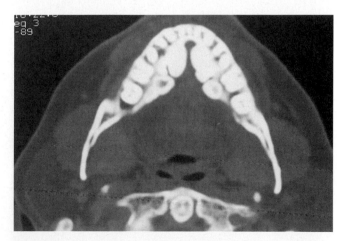

**FIGURE 17-47**   Torus mandibularis. Axial CT (bone window setting) through the mandible demonstrates bilateral bony exostosis of the lingual surface of the mandible.

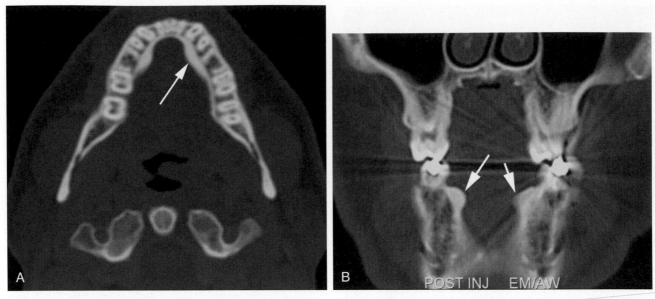

**FIGURE 17-48**   Torus mandibularis. **A,** Axial image shows the thickening of the cortex (*arrow*) along the inner (lingual) margin of the mandible. **B,** Coronal image shows the torus (exostosis) in cross section (*arrows*).

common symptom, but some lesions may be noted as an incidental finding during routine radiographic screening. The mandible is affected in about two thirds of the reported cases, with most tumors being located in the anterior mandible between the second premolar and the second molar, often with extension across the midline. On occasion, these lesions may exhibit a more aggressive clinical and radiographic appearance.

Radiographically, the lesion most often has a radiolucent, multilocular, honeycombed appearance, with tiny bony septae traversing the involved area (Fig. 17-52). When present, the various loculi are irregular in shape and vary in size; however, unilocular tumors without trabeculation do occur.

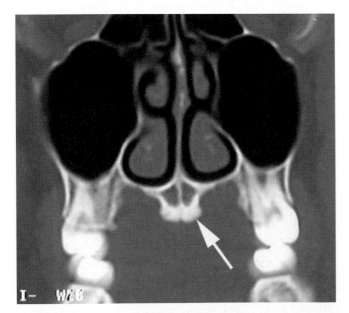

**FIGURE 17-49**   A torus palatinus (*arrow*) extends from the midline of the palate.

Often there is rather marked expansion, with thinning of the cortical plates, and perforation may occur in large lesions. If the mass is adjacent to teeth, displacement and root resorption are seen. Lesions, especially those in the antral region, produce "ground-glass" radiopacities and occasional calcifications (Figs. 17-53 and 17-54). Treatment modalities include enucleation and curettage with local osteotomy, chemical cautery, electrocautery, cryotherapy, and en bloc resection.[82, 83] Calcitonin, interferon alpha, and intralesional steroids are newer modalities that have been somewhat successful in treating more aggressive and recurrent lesions.

## LANGERHANS' HISTIOCYTOSIS (HISTIOCYTOSIS X)

Histiocytosis X is a spectrum of diseases with a proliferation of lipid-laden Langerhans' cells (histiocytes) accompanied by a significant inflammatory response.[90-99] This process can be focal or widely disseminated, acute or chronic, and benign or malignant. The cause of this disease remains unknown, although genetic factors, infectious agents, and immunologic abnormalities have been suggested. In 1987, the Writing Group of the Histiocyte Society proposed that the term *Langerhans' cell histiocytosis* replace *histiocytosis X* because Langerhans'-type histiocytes are a unique identifier for this disease.[98] Based on the clinical presentation, three variants have been described: Letterer-Siwe disease (disseminated acute histiocytosis), Hand-Schuller-Christian disease (disseminated chronic histiocytosis), and eosinophilic granuloma (localized histiocytosis).

### Letterer-Siwe Disease

Letterer-Siwe disease is the acute, widely disseminated form of histiocytosis X.[95] It is generally fatal and usually

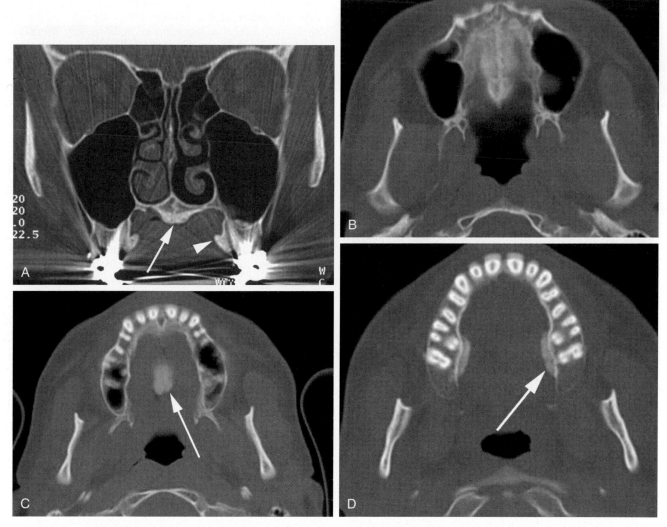

**FIGURE 17-50**   Torus palatinus and exostosis. CT scan. **A**, Coronal CT shows the torus palatinus (*arrow*) in the midline and the small bilateral maxillary exostosis (*arrowhead*) extending from the medial aspect of the alveolar process. **B**, Axial CT through the palate. **C**, Slightly inferiorly, the torus palatinus (*arrow*) is visualized. **D**, Slightly inferior to **C**. The maxillary exostosis (*arrow*) is identified. The lesion is bilateral.

occurs in infants under 1 year of age. Lesions are usually present in several bones and may appear as multiple small, rounded radiolucencies with well-defined borders. If teeth are present in the affected regions, they are frequently mobile, and there is associated gingival bleeding.

## Hand-Schuller-Christian Disease

Hand-Schuller-Christian disease is the disseminated chronic skeletal and extraskeletal form of histiocytosis X.[96] It is the intermediate stage between eosinophilic granuloma and Letterer-Siwe disease. It occurs mostly in children (twice as often in boys as in girls) from the first to the tenth year of life. The three classic signs of the disease (single or multiple sharply defined calvarial defects, unilateral or bilateral exophthalmos, and diabetes insipidus) are noted in about 10% of patients. Other organs such as the lymph

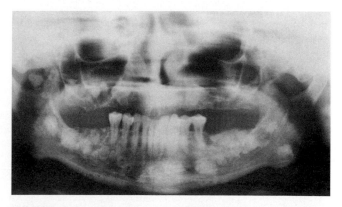

**FIGURE 17-51**   Gardner's syndrome. Pantomogram of the mandible and maxilla demonstrates multiple osteomas within the mandible and the alveolar portion of the maxilla. There is some conglomeration of the osteomas, especially in the body of the right mandible.

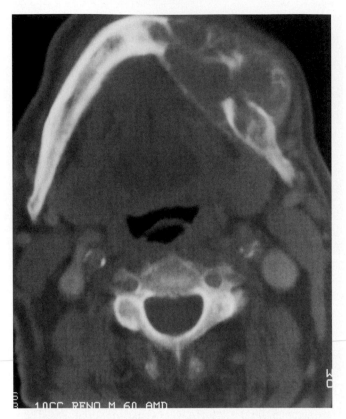

**FIGURE 17-52**   Giant cell granuloma of the left mandible. Axial CT (bone window setting) demonstrates a loculated, expansile lesion involving the ramus, body, and symphysis of the mandible.

nodes, liver, spleen, lungs, and skin may be involved. The first indication of the disease often appears in the oral structures, either in the form of red, spongy gingiva or premature loss of teeth. The typical radiographic appearance is one of irregular, lucent defects in the mandible and maxilla. The affected teeth appear to be "floating in space" as a result of marked destruction of the alveolar bone. The disease is slowly progressive, and the mortality rate may be as high as 60%.

## Eosinophilic Granuloma

Eosinophilic granuloma is the mildest and most favorable form of histiocytosis X.[97] There is a male predilection, with a peak frequency in the third decade of life. The average age of patients with eosinophilic granuloma of the jaw is higher than that of patients with lesions in other parts of the body, and frequent sites are the skull and the tooth-bearing areas of the mandible. The lesion may be an incidental radiographic finding and may manifest as local pain, swelling, tenderness, or fever and general malaise. Eosinophilic granuloma of the mandible causes well-demarcated areas of osteolysis that may appear "punched out." Maxillary lesions usually are not as well demarcated as those in the mandible.

The area of bone involvement is characterized by irregular lucent patches having no reactive sclerosis but often showing cortical destruction (Fig. 17-55). These patches may appear as single or multiple areas of rarefaction simulating jaw cysts, periapical granulomas, or periodontal disease (Fig. 17-56). Early radiographic findings include

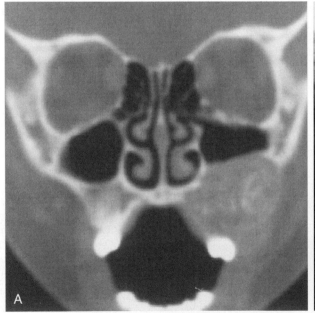

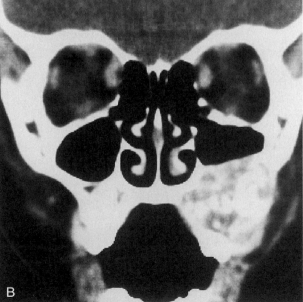

**FIGURE 17-53**   Giant cell granuloma of the left maxilla. **A,** Coronal CT (bone window setting) shows an expansile lesion in the left maxilla bulging into the left lower antrum and adjacent oral cavity. Note the calcific densities within the lesion. **B,** Coronal CT (soft-tissue window setting) demonstrates to better advantage the calcific and bony densities within the expansile lesion.

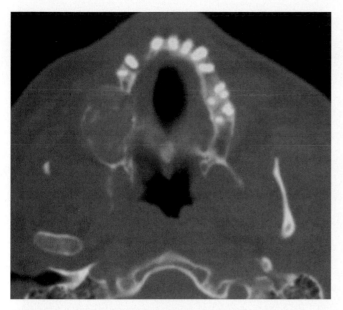

**FIGURE 17-54**   Giant cell lesion of the mandible. Axial CT scan. There is expansion of the alveolar process, and foci of mineralization are seen. The appearance of this lesion mimics that of fibrous dysplasia.

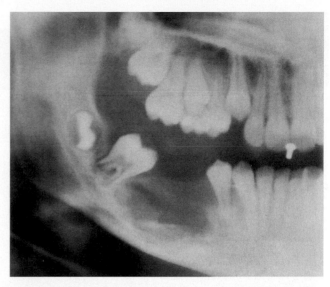

**FIGURE 17-55**   Eosinophilic granuloma in the right mandible. Pantomogram of the mandible shows a lucent, irregular, fairly well defined area in the body of the mandible between the second molar tooth and the first premolar tooth. There is some loss of the lamina dura of the lower second molar tooth.

destruction of the alveolar bone crest and interdental septum and loss of the cortical outline of a tooth follicle or the lamina dura. The teeth in the involved regions become loose, float in space, and are exfoliated.

Unifocal lesions may be curetted and packed with cancellous bone.[99] With several recurrences or persistent residual granulomas, low-dose irradiation and cortisone treatment may be beneficial. Cytostatic agents (vinblastine, cyclophosphamide, and etoposide) also have been used successfully. Other treatment modalities include immunotherapy (suppressin A, cyclosporin), hormonal therapy, intralesional steroids, and bone marrow transplantation.

# FIBROOSSEOUS LESIONS

## Fibrous Dysplasia

Fibrous dysplasia is a lesion of unknown cause, diverse histopathology, and uncertain pathogenesis that is most commonly seen in the first three decades of life.[100–106] It occurs more frequently in the maxilla than in the mandible, where it usually arises in the posterior regions of the bone. There are considerable microscopic variations in the different lesions, as evidenced by fibrous tissue alternating with trabeculae of coarse woven bone and less organized lamellar bone. The three forms of fibrous dysplasia are monostotic fibrous dysplasia, polyostotic fibrous dysplasia (in which multiple bony lesions, often unilateral, occur), and Albright's syndrome.

Monostotic fibrous dysplasia occurs equally often in males and females and is encountered frequently in children and young adults, with a mean age of 27 years.[102] The clinical symptom usually is painless swelling of the involved bone; however, neurovascular compromise may cause symptoms. Typically, there is involvement of the jaw, as

noted by bulging of the labial or buccal plates, malalignment and displacement of teeth, protuberance of the maxilla, or enlargement of the maxilla or zygoma with proptosis. There also can be skull base disease.

Polyostotic fibrous dysplasia manifests early in life, often with an insidious onset. The disease is characterized by bone deformities, and in some cases there is associated bone pain. In this form of fibrous dysplasia, the skull and face are frequently involved, often with obvious asymmetry secondary to bone expansion. Jaw involvement develops slowly and usually presents with facial deformity, overgrowth of the alveolar bone, and displacement of teeth. There can be marked enlargement of the maxilla, with involvement of the maxillary sinuses, nasal cavities, orbit, and base of the skull. Craniofacial fibrous dysplasia is generally not a functionally devastating disease unless the lesion involves the orbit and skull base; when this happens, blindness, pituitary dysfunction, and vital neurovascular compromise may occur.

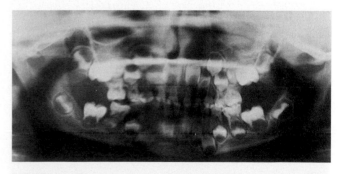

**FIGURE 17-56**   Diffuse eosinophilic granuloma in the mandible. Pantomogram of the mandible shows loss of the lamina dura of erupted and partially erupted tooth follicles. This is especially evident at the second lower right molar tooth.

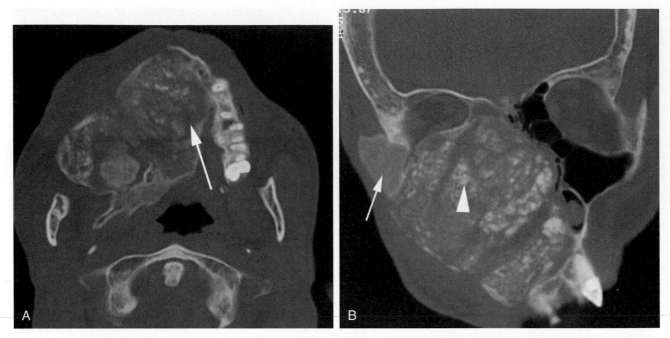

**FIGURE 17-57** Fibrous dysplasia of the maxilla. There is gross expansion of the maxilla. The lesion contains multiple consistencies including soft tissue, bone, and perhaps cartilage. **A**, Axial image with multiple punctate areas of mineralization (*arrow*). The low density may represent fibrous tissue or a cystic component. **B**, Coronal image shows small foci of calcifications (*arrowhead*) that may represent chondroid matrix. This makes differentiation from chondrosarcoma difficult. The lateral part of the abnormality (*arrow*) has a typical "ground glass" appearance.

Albright's syndrome is a developmental defect of unknown cause. It consists of cutaneous pigmentation, precocious puberty, and multiple skeletal lesions. Young girls are affected most often.

The radiologic appearance of fibrous dysplasia can vary considerably, usually depending on the degree of bone present within the lesion (Figs. 17-57 to 17-60). One appearance is that of a unilocular or multilocular, primarily radiolucent lesion with a well-defined border. Interspersed bony trabeculae are often present within the lucent area, rendering the lesion partially radiopaque (Fig. 17-61). Another appearance is that of a marked homogeneous increase in bone density associated with bone expansion, which reflects the predominant histologic finding of bony

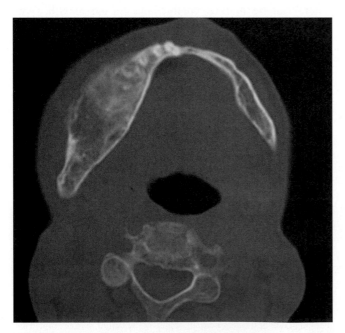

**FIGURE 17-58** Fibrous dysplasia. There is an expansile abnormality of the mandible. The mineralization suggests osteoid as well as lucencies representing fibrous tissue.

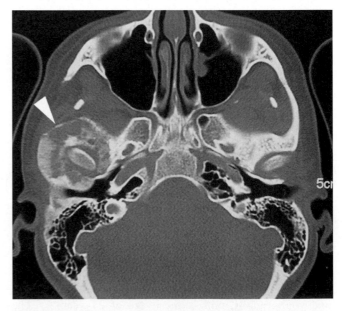

**FIGURE 17-59** Fibrous dysplasia of the glenoid. There is expansion of the bone of the glenoid. This abnormality contains "ground glass" as well as soft-tissue density presumably representing fibrous tissue. Note that the cortex (*arrowhead*) is intact. The lesion does not involve the condylar head.

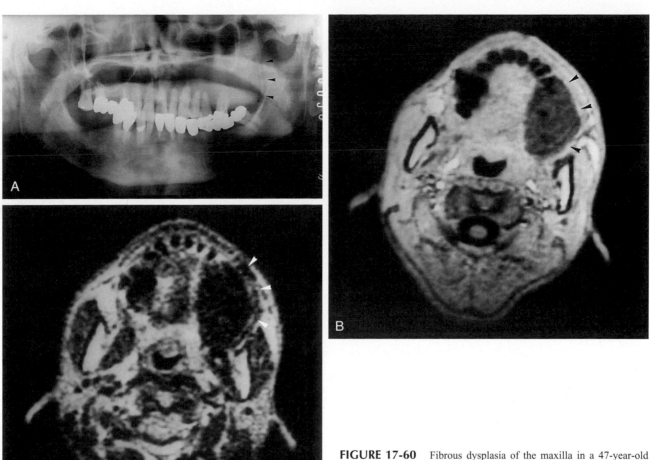

**FIGURE 17-60**   Fibrous dysplasia of the maxilla in a 47-year-old man. **A**, Pantomogram shows a diffuse radiopaque lesion in the maxilla (*arrowheads*). Fibrous dysplasia is most likely; osteomyelitis is not considered because of the lack of clinical symptoms and signs. **B**, Enhanced axial T1-weighted image reveals a low-intensity mass in the left side of the maxilla (*arrowheads*). **C**, Axial T2-weighted image demonstrates a low-intensity mass (*arrowheads*). MR findings suggest an expansible fibrous lesion, and fibrous dysplasia is suspected.

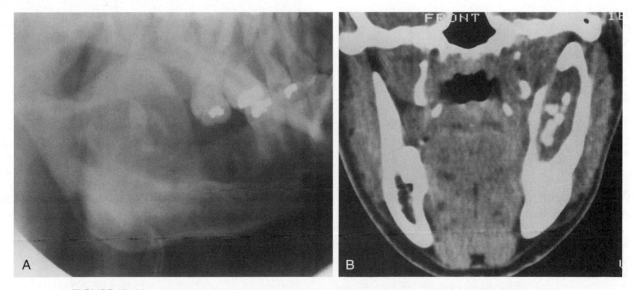

**FIGURE 17-61**   Monostotic fibrous dysplasia in the left mandible. **A**, Oblique view of the left mandible shows a sclerotic expansile lesion in the ramus of the mandible, with extension into the coronoid process. There are some calcific densities within the central anterior part of this lesion. **B**, Coronal CT (soft-tissue window setting) shows the expansile nature of the lesion in the ramus. Calcified densities are noted within the lesion.

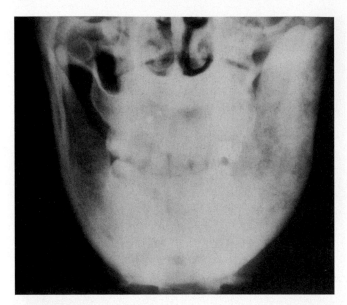

**FIGURE 17-62**   Monostotic fibrous dysplasia. Posteroanterior view of the mandible shows an expansile sclerotic lesion involving the left ramus of the mandible, with extension into the angle and body of the left mandible.

trabeculae with only a few scattered areas of fibrous tissue (Fig. 17-62). This is sometimes referred to as a ground-glass appearance, which is more evident on CT. Cystic lesions of appreciable size cause thinning and remodeling of the cortex, but they rarely perforate the cortex or produce new periosteal bone. Although the lesion may cause resorption of the roots of erupted teeth, this is rare. MR imaging findings also depend on the variety of components of the disease, especially on T2-weighted images. The fibrous components often shows enhancement after contrast administration. If the lesion has rich cartilaginous components or cystic changes, its signal intensities can be brighter: the former show gradual enhancement, while the latter show no enhancement.

The disease is usually self-limiting, often not progressing after the third decade of life. Surgical treatment usually is limited to a cosmetic debulking and recontouring of the bone. However, an accelerated progression of the disease has been noted with early and aggressive surgical manipulation, sometimes mandating additional surgery. Only small lesions can be removed by enucleation. Because there is a low incidence of malignant transformation of fibrous dysplasia, regular and careful follow-up should be maintained.

## Ossifying Fibromas (Cemento-Ossifying Fibromas, Cementifying Fibromas)

The ossifying fibroma is an encapsulated, benign neoplasm consisting of fibrous tissue that contains various amounts of irregular bony trabeculae.[107, 108] As the lesion matures, the areas of ossification increase in number and coalesce, accounting for the lesion's progressively increasing radiodensity. These lesions may be difficult to distinguish from fibrous dysplasia histologically, but they are

sharply demarcated and not uncommonly encapsulated masses that behave as benign neoplasms. In the recent WHO classification,[3] cemento-ossifying lesions (both neoplastic and dysplastic) are listed in the category of neoplasms and other lesions related to bone, although benign cementoblastoma, generally accepted as being essentially cementogenic, has been included in the neoplasms and other tumors related to the odontogenic apparatus category. Ossifying (cemento-ossifying) fibroma is found more often in females and may occur at any age, but it is most common in the third and fourth decades of life. The lesion develops predominantly in the mandible and is usually situated at the roots of the teeth or in the periapical region. It generally is asymptomatic, but a progressive increase in size may eventually cause swelling of the jaw.

Radiographically, the lesion usually has a distinct boundary, unlike fibrous dysplasia, and in the early stages it presents as a lucent area. As the lesion matures, bone densities appear, transforming the lesion into a radiopaque mass surrounded by a "halo" of less ossified tissue (Fig. 17-63). One aggressive variety of ossifying fibroma is referred to as juvenile ossifying fibroma. This term designates a very actively growing destructive lesion that is histologically identical to the routine ossifying fibroma. This lesion affects individuals younger than 15 years of age and occurs exclusively in the maxilla.

The treatment of ossifying fibroma is usually surgical enucleation. However, for some forms of this lesion, especially the juvenile form that is prone to recur, broader surgical resection should be considered.

## Paget's Disease (Osteitis Deformans)

Paget's disease of bone is a chronic disease characterized by abnormal functioning of osteoblasts and osteoclasts resulting in poorly mineralized and deformed bones.[109, 110] There is a slightly higher male predominance, and the incidence increases with age. There are also reports of an occasional familial pattern. Although the exact cause remains unknown, numerous theories have been proposed regarding its development, including a slow viral infection, hormonal abnormalities, a vascular anomaly, an autoimmune-type connective tissue disorder, and a true neoplasia. Malignant transformation, although not a common occurrence, has been reported in the jaws and is a constant concern. This is of particular concern if the region has been previously irradiated.

In the craniofacial skeleton, involvement of the skull, maxilla, and mandible is common. Headache, dizziness, hearing loss, and other cranial nerve abnormalities may result from the skull base involvement. The maxilla is involved more commonly than the mandible. The jaw lesions cause bone enlargement, separation of teeth with generalized widening of the interdental spaces, ill-fitting dentures, and frequently neuralgia-type pain.

Radiographically, the jaw lesions have a variable appearance, depending on the stage of disease progression. There can be "punched-out" radiolucent areas, mixed areas giving a "cotton wool-like" appearance, and more densely sclerotic areas. The jaw lesions frequently show evidence of rarefaction and sclerotic change in the alveolar bone, with loss of the lamina dura surrounding the teeth and hypercementosis of the roots of teeth. Radionuclide scanning can identify the presence of disease based on the presence of areas of biologic activity. Laboratory findings typically include elevations in serum alkaline phosphatase and urinary hydroxyproline. Serum calcium and phosphorus levels are usually normal.

Clinical management may consist of no more than closely following the patient. When more severe disease exists or when the bone lesions in the craniofacial skeleton cause symptoms, therapeutic intervention is usually indicated. Nonsurgical treatment can include steroids and the use of calcitonins and diphosphonates. Surgical procedures must be carried out with great care because the abnormal bone is often very vascular, and significant bleeding can occur.

## VASCULAR LESIONS

Vascular lesions of the head and neck are a perplexing group of problems that have generated significant debate and confusion regarding terminology and classification.[111–117] Descriptive, anatomic-pathologic, and embryologic classification schemes have been devised and debated and generally have not offered clinicians significant treatment guidance. The classification developed by Mulliken and Glowacki in 1982 is based on the cellular kinetics of the anomalous vessels and provides a diagnostic and therapeutic approach based on the biologic behavior of the lesion.[114] In this classification, two entities exist: hemangiomas and vascular malformations.

## Hemangioma

Hemangiomas are usually not identified at birth, but they appear soon thereafter. They are present in 12% of all children by 1 year of age. They go through a rapid proliferation phase during the first year of life followed by a much slower involution phase, which usually reaches partial or complete resolution by 5 to 7 years of age.

Hemangiomas are 2 to 2½ times more common in females than in males, and there is no racial predilection. Hemangiomas are found most often in the skull and vertebrae, and although common in the head and neck, they are rarely located in the jaw. They are benign tumors with vessels that have marked endothelial turnover, and there are increased numbers of mast cells that are thought to play a role in the pathophysiology of these lesions.

Although most hemangiomas can be diagnosed by the history and physical findings, some are difficult to fully evaluate clinically and warrant imaging studies. Radiographically, hemangiomas of the mandible appear as ill-defined radiolucent lesions usually involving the inferior alveolar canal (Fig. 17-64). Some lesions may have a cystic or occasionally a multilocular shape. CT and MR imaging are particularly helpful for deeper lesions and those thought to involve bone. Doppler ultrasound and angiography may also be employed. Angiography of hemangiomas shows a well-circumscribed mass, usually with prolonged parenchymal staining and tissue blush.

Treatment is based on correctly identifying the lesion and distinguishing it from a vascular malformation. Kaban and Mulliken pointed out, in their review of vascular anomalies of the maxillofacial region, that many reported hemangiomas were in fact vascular malformations.[113] Management of maxillofacial hemangiomas often consists of counseling and

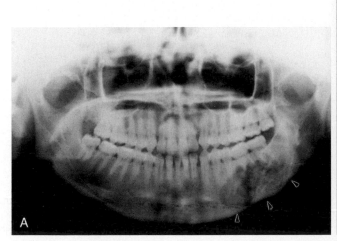
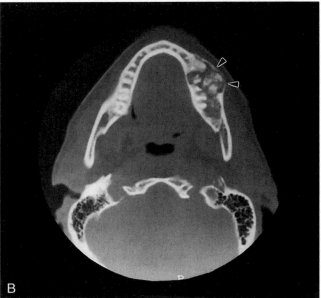

**FIGURE 17-63**   Cemento-ossifying fibroma in the mandible. **A,** Pantomogram shows a well-defined mixed radiolucent-radiopaque lesion (*arrowheads*). **B,** Axial CT (bone window setting) demonstrates a buccal expansile lesion with some calcifications in the mandible. The surrounding buccal bony cortex is barely preserved (*arrowheads*).

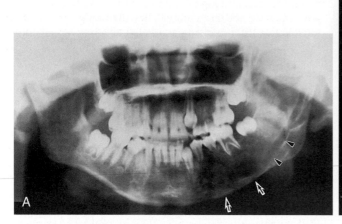

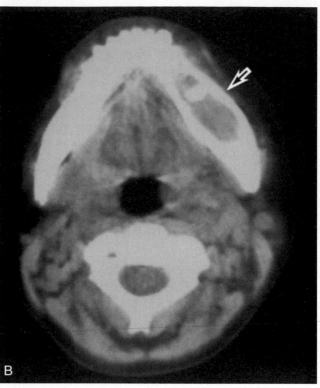

**FIG. 17-64** Central hemangioma in the mandible. **A,** Pantomogram shows a large radiolucent lesion in the mandible (*arrows*). The inferior alveolar nerve canal has been widened, and its course has been altered (*arrowheads*). **B,** Axial CT (soft-tissue window setting) shows a well-defined, slightly expansile lesion (*arrow*). Note the increased density within the lesion suggesting blood rather than cystic fluid. (Courtesy of Dr. T. Kurabayashi, Dept. of Dental Radiology, Tokyo Medical and Dental University, Tokyo.)

parental support along with observation. If significant functional problems ensue, treatment consists of steroid therapy, compression therapy, radiotherapy, embolization, and treatment with interferon alpha.[116, 117] Surgery is reserved for small lesions and as a secondary procedure to correct cosmetic deformities.

## Vascular Malformation

Vascular malformations are usually present at birth, but they may not be clinically evident until some inciting event occurs.[114] Their growth parallels normal body growth and is influenced by numerous additional factors. There is no sex predilection. Vascular malformations can be composed solely of capillary, venous, arterial, or lymphatic tissues or can be a combination of these tissues. They are subdivided into high-flow and low-flow lesions based on their clinical and angiographic patterns. In the maxillofacial region they frequently involve bone.

Radiographically, the lesion appears as a radiolucent area, often traversed by delicate bony trabeculae forming variously sized small cavities. In large vascular malformations the cortex may be thinned, remodeled, or eroded.[108] If the trabeculae are arranged in a radiating pattern, a sunburst or spoke wheel appearance results. In some cases, there may be a single radiolucent lesion with a sclerotic or ill-defined border that simulates a cyst. Root absorption, loss of the lamina dura, and exfoliation of teeth have also been

reported, and a bruit may be heard or a thrill palpated over the lesion. Spontaneous bleeding around the involved teeth is a problem in the jaws.

Management of vascular malformations mandates a thorough knowledge of the pathologic process and the relevant anatomy. Small lesions may be treated with sclerosing agents, radiotherapy, cryotherapy, laser treatment, or conventional surgical techniques. Larger lesions, particularly high-flow and arteriovenous malformations, are best treated with embolization techniques, with or without surgical resection.

## NEUROGENIC TUMORS

Benign neurogenic tumors, which include schwannomas (neurilemommas), neurofibromas, and traumatic neuromas, occasionally are found centrally within the jaw.[118–121] They may occur at any age, and there is little or no sex predilection. Most of these slow-growing lesions arise in the mandible and cause pain or paresthesia.

A schwannoma is usually encapsulated and composed of two distinct histologic components: Antoni type A tissue and Antoni type B tissue.[119] A neurofibroma arises from the connective tissue sheath of nerve fibers and has axons traversing the unencapsulated tumor.[118, 119] It may occur as a solitary lesion or as multiple lesions associated with neurofibromatosis. Solitary neurofibromas may originate in the oral mucosa or may occur within the jaws.

Radiographically, these lesions may present as solitary radiolucencies associated with the inferior alveolar canal or as multilocular radiolucencies that produce extensive bone damage, with cortical remodeling and even perforation. On occasion, the intraosseous tumor may perforate the cortex of the jaw and extend into the overlying soft tissues. A schwannoma, arising from the nerve within the inferior alveolar canal, may cause bulbous, elongated enlargement of the canal, and a neurofibroma adjacent to bone may produce a saucer-shaped erosive defect on the surface of the bone.

Treatment is surgical but depends on the size and location of the lesion. Smaller lesions can often be removed without significant damage to the nerve or surrounding tissues and without the need for major reconstructive surgery. Larger lesions, especially those with significant bone involvement, usually require larger surgical exposure with enucleation or en bloc surgical resection, often with additional treatment modalities such as cautery or cryotherapy of the bone. When these techniques are needed, surgical reconstruction is mandatory, often with a microsurgical nerve repair.

# MALIGNANT TUMORS

Malignant tumors can be grouped into three categories: (1) lesions that invade the mandible and maxilla secondarily from adjacent soft-tissue structures of the oral cavity and sinuses, (2) tumors that arise primarily within the mandible and maxilla, and (3) metastatic tumors from distant sites. The radiographic appearance of malignant lesions often allows differentiation from benign tumors and cysts; however, a biopsy is necessary to establish the final diagnosis. For proper treatment planning, it is important to assess the extent of the malignant tumor radiographically before surgery or radiation therapy. CT and MR imaging have proven valuable in assessing the extent of tumors outside the mandible and maxilla, as well as in assessing disease extension within the bone or metastases to the neck.

## Carcinoma

Most carcinomas encountered in the jaw originate in the oral cavity (lip, tongue, buccal mucosa, gingiva, floor of the mouth, and palate) and maxillary sinuses, and they secondarily invade the mandible and maxilla.[122–125]

Radiographically, the osseous involvement manifests early at the alveolar ridge with a saucer-shaped erosive defect. This defect may be shallow and well defined, but in time an irregular cavity can be formed. There is usually no evidence of bony sclerotic or periosteal reaction. Therefore, superficial erosion of the alveolar crest in the tooth-bearing regions may initially mimic periodontal disease. Radiographically, carcinoma usually appears as a radiolucency with irregular margins (Fig. 17-65). Permeative disease extension may create a "moth-eaten" appearance. The radiographic findings are nonspecific, and the tumor cannot be differentiated from other malignant lesions. Pathologic fractures are common complications in advanced cases.

Odontogenic carcinoma is a carcinoma arising within the bone without a lesion of the mucosa.[1] These rare malignancies arise from epithelial remnants left behind by the process of tooth formation, hence the use of the term *odontogenic*. Odontogenic carcinoma can be subcategorized according to its apparent origin. Malignant ameloblastoma represents transformation from a benign ameloblastoma. Primary intraosseous carcinoma arises without preexisting ameloblastoma. Some carcinomas may arise in preexisting odontogenic cysts.

Primary intraosseous carcinoma may develop from epithelial components that participate in the development of the teeth or from epithelial cells that become enclosed within the deeper structures of the jaw during embryonic development. About 90% of these lesions are found in the mandible; they occur more frequently in men than in women, and their peak incidence is in the sixth and seventh decades of life. Although uncommon, this lesion is now recognized as a distinct entity. The lesion typically has an irregular margin. No mucosal abnormality is seen.

Carcinomatous transformation of the epithelium in an odontogenic cyst is a rare event, although it has been reported in dentigerous cysts, radicular cysts, residual cysts, and keratocysts. None of the reported cases affected individuals over 40 years of age. Radiographically, the lesion resembles a cyst with a circumscribed margin. In the area of malignant degeneration the margin may become ill-defined, irregular, or moth-eaten.

Ameloblastoma is rarely malignant.[1–3] The WHO classification of 1992, however, does include malignant ameloblastoma[1] as a category. It defines malignant ameloblastoma as "a neoplasm in which the pattern of an ameloblastoma and cytological features of malignancy are shown by the primary growth in the jaws and/or by any metastatic growth." There is controversy regarding exact terminology.[2, 126–128] Some advocate restriction of the term *malignant ameloblastoma* to an ameloblastoma that, although histologically benign, shows a malignant nature by metastasizing. The metastasis shows the histologic pattern of the original tumor, again without cytologic indicators of malignancy. There are tumors that do have typical cytologic findings of malignancy including increased and abnormal mitoses, nuclear pleomorphism, and so on. The term *ameloblastic carcinoma* has been advocated for these rare lesions. They may metastasize as well. Neither term should be applied to a histologically benign tumor that simply shows aggressive local extension even though involvement of key contiguous structures may be life-threatening. The radiologist should simply realize that the controversy related to terminology exists and that clarification of terms is appropriate in the individual case or in reports in the literature.

Malignant variants of ameloblastoma may arise de novo or in relation to a preexisting ameloblastoma. The lesions are most commonly found in the jaw. The imaging findings may be inseparable from those of benign ameloblastoma, but locally aggressive tumors can have a more irregular margin.

Other rare malignant epithelial lesions include clear cell odontogenic carcinoma and malignant odontogenic ghost cell tumor. The clear cell lesion must be distinguished from metastatic renal cell carcinoma. Immunohistochemical markers help make this differentiation. The term *malignant ghost cell tumor* (odontogenic ghost cell carcinoma) has been applied to a histologically malignant solid tumor related to calcifying odontogenic cyst.

## Mucoepidermoid Carcinoma

Mucoepidermoid carcinoma can also arise within the jaw.[129–132] Women are affected twice as often as men, and the average age at diagnosis is 46 years. The radiographic changes consist of ill-defined lytic or multilocular cystic areas that are often indistinguishable from squamous cell carcinoma (Fig. 17-66). CT and MR imaging are extremely helpful in delineating the extent of disease in the mandible and the surrounding soft tissues, as well as in identifying cervical lymph node involvement. An accurate tissue diagnosis is also mandatory to plan appropriate therapy, which usually consists of combined radiation therapy, chemotherapy, and surgery. A pretreatment oral examination and dental evaluation is necessary to diag-

nose any tooth and gum pathology that needs to be eliminated before initiating radiotherapy or chemotherapy. Also, when surgical resection is planned, appropriate prosthetic reconstruction strategies can be planned before surgery, allowing better functional results and greater patient satisfaction.

## Metastatic Jaw Tumor

Metastatic tumors to the mandible or maxilla may be the first indication of an occult malignancy or the first evidence of dissemination of a known primary tumor. Patients with metastatic lesions may be asymptomatic or may complain of symptoms similar to those found with other primary malignant tumors. Metastases to the mandible are four times more frequent than those to the maxilla, and the most common primary tumors are in the breast, lung, kidney (hypernephroma), thyroid, prostate, and stomach.

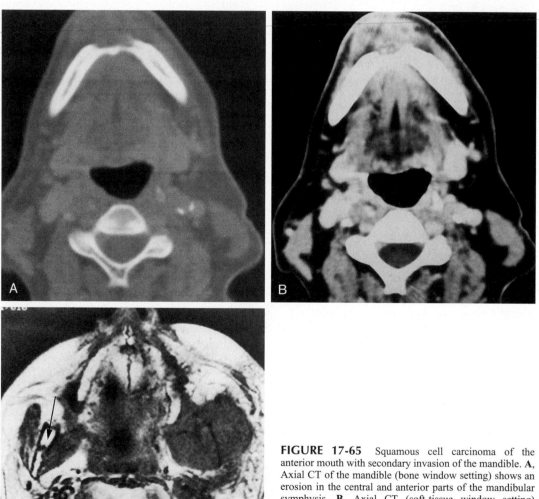

**FIGURE 17-65** Squamous cell carcinoma of the anterior mouth with secondary invasion of the mandible. **A,** Axial CT of the mandible (bone window setting) shows an erosion in the central and anterior parts of the mandibular symphysis. **B,** Axial CT (soft-tissue window setting) demonstrates a lesion in the anterior mouth, with extension into the mandible. Again, note the erosion in the anterior cortex and adjacent medullary portion of the mandible. **C,** Another patient. Axial T1-weighted MR image shows a large squamous cell carcinoma in the left cheek and retromolar trigone that has infiltrated the ramus of the mandible. The normal high signal intensity of marrow (*arrow*) is seen on the right side.

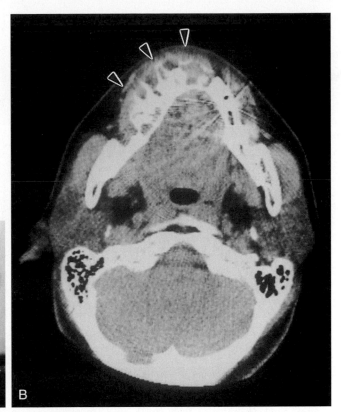

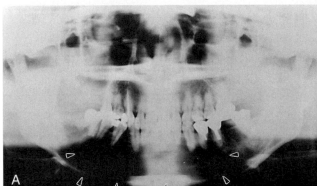

**FIGURE 17-66** Mucoepidermoid tumor in the mandible. **A,** Pantomogram shows an ill-defined radiolucent lesion in the anterior part of the mandible (*arrowheads*). **B,** Axial CT of the mandible (soft-tissue window setting) demonstrates the ill-defined soft-tissue density lesion with multiple bony trabeculae. The surrounding buccal bony cortex is destroyed (*arrowheads*). (Courtesy of Dr. T. Kurabayashi, Dept. of Dental Radiology, Tokyo Medical and Dental University, Tokyo.)

In most instances, the bone destruction caused by a metastatic lesion is radiographically similar to that caused by a primary tumor, and the area of destruction within the mandible may be localized, bilateral, or diffuse (Fig. 17-67). On occasion a mixed lesion of lytic and blastic areas may be encountered, usually from a carcinoma of the breast. In rare cases, metastasis from a carcinoma of the prostate may cause diffuse osteoblastic change.

When metastatic disease is suspected, a thorough search for the primary site and other sites of metastatic involvement should be immediately initiated, and a biopsy for definitive tissue diagnosis should be performed. A team approach with coordination among the internist, radiologist, oncologist, surgeon, and other health care providers involved in the care of the cancer patient is the optimal approach to an often difficult problem.[133–140]

## Sarcoma

### Osteogenic Sarcoma

Osteogenic sarcoma is a malignant tumor of the bone in which neoplastic cells produce a variable amount of osteoid.[141–147] According to the predominant tissue observed microscopically, these lesions are classified as osteoblastic, chondroblastic, or fibroblastic. About 6.5% of osteogenic sarcomas arise in the jaw.

Primary osteogenic sarcoma usually affects children and young adults, with a peak incidence in the second decade of life. However, osteogenic sarcomas of the mandible and maxilla have their peak incidence a decade later. The mandible is affected more often than the maxilla, and there is no sex predominance. The main symptoms are swelling

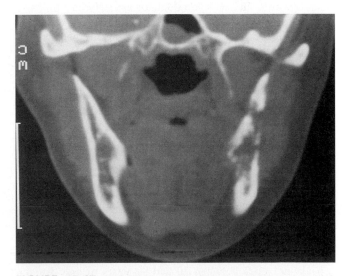

**FIGURE 17-67** Carcinoma of the breast metastatic to the left mandible. Coronal CT through the mandible (bone window setting) shows a lytic destructive lesion in the ramus of the left mandible. There is no new bone formation.

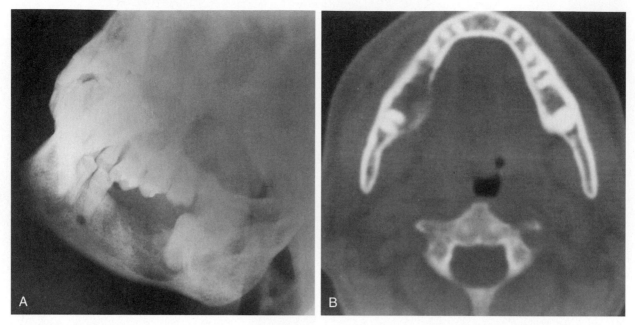

**FIGURE 17-68**    Osteogenic sarcoma of the mandible. **A,** Oblique view of the mandible shows an ill-defined lucent area in the body of the right mandible. There is loss of the lamina dura of the remaining third molar tooth. There is also invasion of the mandibular canal. **B,** Axial CT (bone window setting) shows ill-defined destruction, with expansion of the body of the right mandible.

and pain, but paresthesias, loose teeth, and bleeding have been reported.

Radiographically, osteogenic sarcoma can cause lytic bone destruction with indefinite margins (osteolytic type) (Fig. 17-68), an area of sclerosis (osteoblastic type) (Figs. 17-69 and 17-70), or a mixed pattern. The osteoblastic type is the most common one in the jaw. Some osteosarcomas show a sunburst effect caused by radiating mineralized tumor spicules (Fig. 17-71). Cortical breakthrough, with tumor outside the jaw, is a common finding in advanced cases. Because a symmetrically widened periodontal membrane may be the earliest radiographic finding of osteogenic sarcoma of the jaw, this tumor must be differentiated from other diseases such as sclerodoma or acrosclerosis that also cause widening of the periodontal membrane.

Osteosarcomas can be easily assessed by CT because this modality identifies lesions that contain calcium, osteoid, or both. However, the extent of tumor spread within the marrow space or outside of the jaw may be seen better with MR imaging. Patients with mandibular osteosarcomas have a better prognosis than those with maxillary tumors; however, patients with mandibular or maxillary osteosarcomas are prone to develop either a recurrence or distant metastases, especially to the lungs. Treatment is surgical excision, usually followed by radiation therapy and possibly chemotherapy.

### Fibrosarcoma

Fibrosarcoma of the jaw is a rare lesion that occurs predominantly in the mandible.[148, 149] Onset can occur at any age but is most common before the age of 50 years, with a peak incidence between 20 and 40 years of age. Among these tumors, peripheral and central fibrosarcomas have been differentiated. The rare central form most frequently develops in the mandibular canal and causes central bone

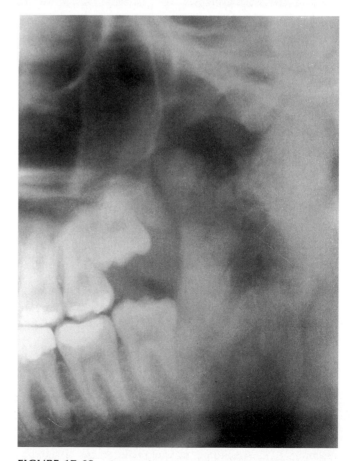

**FIGURE 17-69**    Osteogenic sarcoma of the left mandible. Pantomogram of the mandible shows a sclerotic lesion in the ascending ramus of the mandible and coronoid process. The boundaries of the mandible are poorly defined posteriorly. There is extension of this sclerotic tumor into the upper left mandibular canal.

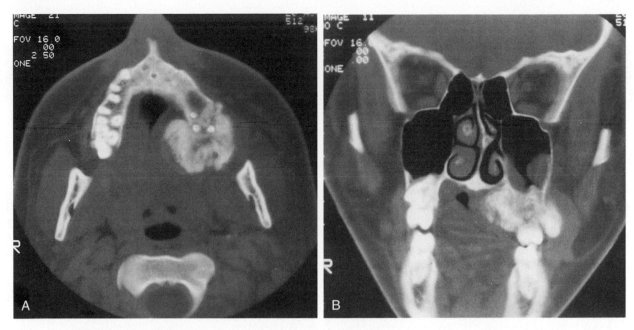

**FIGURE 17-70**   Chondroblastic osteosarcoma of the left maxilla. **A,** Axial CT through the maxilla demonstrates a sclerotic, destructive lesion in the left maxilla, with extension into the lower portion of the left antrum. **B,** Coronal CT demonstrates the sclerotic, destructive, expansile lesion in the left maxilla and in the lower left maxillary antrum.

destruction, with gradual expansion leading to cortical erosion in larger lesions. The more prevalent peripheral type originates from the periostium or the periodontal membrane, frequently in the body and angle of the mandible. Radiographically, erosive changes are encountered at the alveolar ridge or at the inferior border of the mandible; the depth of the defect varies, depending on the stage of tumor development. Usually an extramandibular soft-tissue mass of variable size is palpated.

An ameloblastic fibrosarcoma has been described as a mixed epithelial/mesenchymal lesion.[2] Only the mesenchymal component is malignant. The epithelial component most

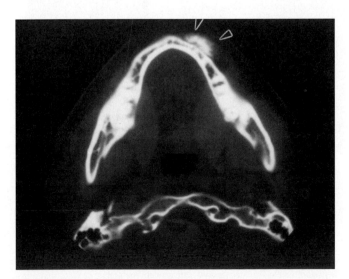

**FIGURE 17-71**   Osteogenic sarcoma in the anterior part of the mandible. Axial CT demonstrates a mass with periosteal reaction suggesting the typical "sun-ray" appearance in the mandible (*arrowheads*).

closely resembles an ameloblastic fibroma. This lesion is extremely rare. The terms *odontogenic sarcoma* and *ameloblastic fibro-odontosarcoma* have been used to refer to similar lesions.[150]

The term *carcinosarcoma* has been applied to a rare lesion in which both the epithelial and mesenchymal components are malignant.

### Ewing's Sarcoma

Ewing's sarcoma occurs predominantly in children and young adults between 5 and 25 years of age, and males are affected twice as frequently as females.[151–154] In one series of studies, jaw involvement occurred in 13% of cases, and this lesion occurs 10 times more frequently in the mandible than in the maxilla. Radiographically, the lesion has a mottled, irregular, lucent appearance, with sclerosis interspersed in a small percentage of tumors. Perpendicular bony spicules and extensive bone destruction may be found at the cortices. The characteristic onion-peel (onion skin) layering of new subperiosteal bone is often absent in the jaw. This tumor tends to metastasize early, often to multiple bony sites, making treatment difficult and the prognosis poor. Treatment usually involves a combination of radiotherapy and chemotherapy.

## Malignant Lymphoma

Malignant lymphoma is derived from lymphocytes and reticulum (histiocytic) cells that are in different stages of development, and the disease can have either a regional or a systemic distribution.[155–157] Lymphomas in the head and neck occur predominantly in the neck nodes, oral cavity, nasopharynx, and occasionally in the sinuses. However, primary lymphoma of bone may occur in the mandible and maxilla. Such bone lymphomas are predominantly histio-cytic (large cell) lymphomas; they occur more frequently in the mandible than in the maxilla, and there is a male predominance. Radiographically, there are no pathogno-monic findings. In the mandible, most often there are ill-defined lytic destructive areas of variable size (Fig. 17-72). Radiation therapy and chemotherapy are the primary treatment modalities.

## Multiple Myeloma

Although single lesions may occasionally occur, multiple myeloma is characterized by multiple or diffuse bone involvement.[158–161] Myeloma occurs most frequently in patients 40 to 70 years of age, with males being affected twice as frequently as females. In patients with multiple myeloma of the jaw, mandibular lesions are far more common, and there is a predilection for the angle, ramus, and molar tooth regions. The typical radiographic appear-ance is that of "punched-out," regular, circular, or ovoid radiolucencies with no circumferential bone reaction, especially when the skull is involved (Fig. 17-73). The cortex of the mandible may be perforated, but expansion of bone is not demonstrated. If the lesion is extensive, the entire bone may be destroyed, and bone destruction frequently is associated with hypercalcemia.

Treatment of multiple myeloma is primarily medical. Chemotherapy is the primary modality, often along with anabolic steroids, fluoride, calcium, and vitamin D. Solitary bone lesions most often are treated with radiation therapy. When surgery of jaw lesions is planned, consideration of the

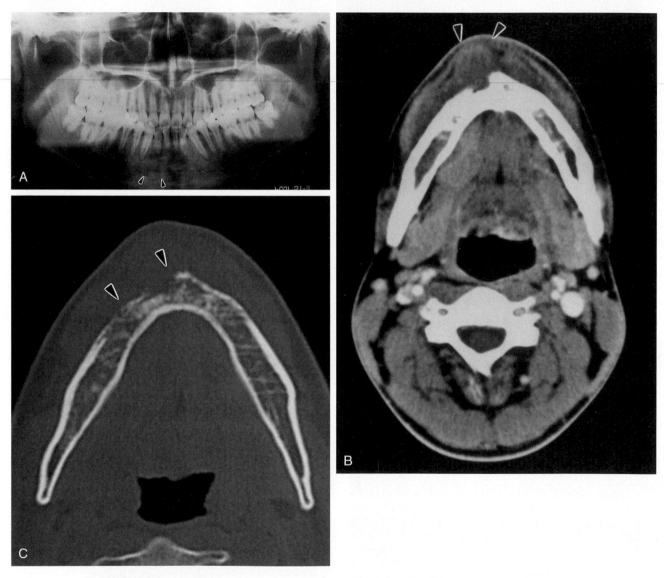

**FIGURE 17-72** Lymphoma in the mandible. **A,** Pantomogram shows an ill-defined radiolucent lesion in the anterior part of the mandible (*arrowheads*). **B,** Axial CT of the mandible (soft-tissue window setting) demonstrates the soft-tissue density lesion in the anterior part of the mandible involving the surrounding soft tissue (*arrowheads*). **C,** Axial CT (bone window setting) demonstrates the ill-defined lesion (*arrowheads*), with permeative destruction of the buccal bony cortex (*arrowheads*). (Courtesy of Dr. T. Kurabayashi, Dept. of Dental Radiology, Tokyo Medical and Dental University, Tokyo.)

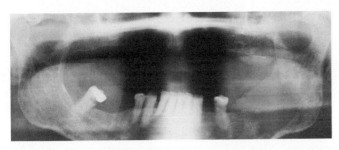

**FIGURE 17-73**   Multiple myeloma of the mandible. Pantomogram of the mandible shows a large, destructive lesion in the body and ramus of the left mandible, with extramandibular extension at the alveolus. There is the suggestion of a pathologic fracture at the anterior aspect of this lytic defect. Also, note the multiple "punched-out" lucent areas throughout the mandible, especially in the left ramus, consistent with foci of multiple myeloma.

patient's hematologic status is necessary to avoid untoward complications.

## Leukemia

Leukemia may involve the jaw bones; in one series of patients with acute leukemia, 63% of cases had disease in the jaw.[162-164] An early radiographic finding is loss of the lamina dura with loosening of the teeth. This is often followed by varying degrees of lytic bone destruction (Fig. 17-74). Treatment is primarily medical management, and special attention should be paid to reducing the chance of oral infection and bleeding.

# INFLAMMATORY CONDITION OF THE MANDIBLE

## Osteomyelitis

Osteomyelitis, an inflammation of bone and bone marrow, may develop in the jaw as a result of odontogenic infection or the sequelae of various other conditions including underlying systemic diseases (immunocompromise) and focal injuries such as trauma, complicated fractures, and large doses of radiation therapy.[165-167] Development of osteomyelitis is rare in normal healthy people because of early administration of antibiotic therapy but can be associated with tuberculosis, diabetes, agranulocytosis, neutropenias, leukemia, uremia, sickle cell anemia, severe anemia, and febrile diseases such as typhoid.[165] The mandible is made up of a well-developed periosteum, a solid cortex, and a liberal spongiosa in the subapical region of the body of the mandible. The spongiosa also extends into the ascending ramus and the mental protuberance. The thick cortex is not easily penetrated by suppurative processes, and the infection can easily involve the whole mandible. Therefore, osteomyelitis of the mandible is more frequently and severely widespread than that of the maxilla.

Osteomyelitis may present radiographically as (1) suppurative osteomyelitis, (2) sclerosing osteomyelitis, (3) osteomyelitis with periositis, (4) tuberculous osteomyelitis, and (5) osteoradionecrosis.[160, 163] The disease may be either acute or chronic and may involve different clinical courses, depending on its nature.[166]

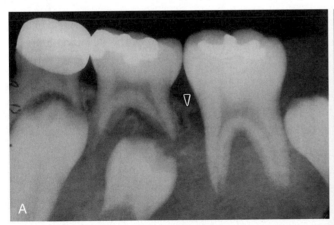

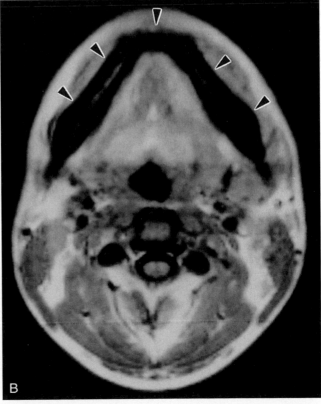

**FIGURE 17-74**   Leukemia of the mandible. **A**, Periapical film demonstrates general rarefaction and loss of the lamina dura (*arrowhead*). **B**, Axial T1-weighted MR image shows diffuse low signal intensity in the entire mandible (*arrowheads*). Normal fatty marrow has been completely replaced by leukemic infiltration.

## Suppurative Osteomyelitis

Acute suppurative osteomyelitis is sudden in onset and runs a very acute course. Such cases are associated with a severe constitutional reaction: high fever, rapid pulse, vomiting, delirium, and prostration.[165] In some instances, the disease may run a chronic course with slow onset, slight fever, and moderate pain. Radiologic findings can differ, depending on the course of the disease. On conventional radiographs, the bone usually has a normal appearance in the early stage (the first 8 to 10 days) of the disease. Later radiographs can show single or multiple irregular radiolucencies with poorly defined margins.[167] Chronic osteomyelitis shows a variety of bone reactions including completely radiolucent areas, mixed radiolucent and radiopaque areas, and completely radiopaque areas.

Bone scintigraphy and MR imaging can detect the early stage of the diseases.[168–170] Bone scintigraphy is useful in examining patients with suspected osteomyelitis. Radionuclide studies may signify the possibility of early-stage osteomyelitis before osseous changes are apparent on plain radiographs. Technetium-99m methylene diphosphonate ($^{99m}$Tc-MDP) bone scans are sensitive indicators of altered osteoblastic activity, but local disturbances in vascular perfusion, clearance rate, permeability, and chemical binding also affect imaging.[168] On standard $^{99m}$Tc-MDP bone scans, however, it is sometimes difficult to differentiate soft-tissue uptake from bone uptake in patients with known cellulitis and possible underlying osteomyelitis. MR imaging has been reported to be useful in the initial diagnosis of osteomyelitis. Its MR imaging appearance depends on a variety of factors, including the patient's age, the type and virulence of the offending organism, and the presence of an underlying medical conditions.[170] In a normal population of patients over 30 years old, the entire medulla of the mandible usually shows high signal intensities suggesting fatty marrow when spin echo images are used.[171] On MR imaging, bone marrow lesions of osteomyelitis show low signal intensity on T1-weighted images and high signal intensity on T2-weighted images. Sequestrum reveals low signal intensity on both T1- and T2-weighted images. Soft-tissue abnormalities are also evaluated on MR images, showing signal intensity patterns similar to those of marrow lesions, soft-tissue edema, blurring fat planes, and sometimes an abnormal fluid collection (Fig. 17-75).[169]

Contrast enhancement may improve the accuracy of the evaluation of osteomyelitis. Patients with active osteomyelitis show enhancement in medullary bony lesions. Infected areas are usually hypervascular, and the contrast moves into the extracellular fluid compartment because of altered vascular permeability.[172] This enhancement can be seen in soft-tissue components outside the infected areas of the mandible.

## Osteomyelitis with Periostitis

Osteomyelitis with periostitis was erroneously described in the past as Garre osteomyelitis. It is simply a variant of osteomyelitis in which a periosteal reaction predominates, leading to subperiosteal deposition of new bone.[173, 174] This condition is characterized by the formation of new bone on the surface of the cortex over infected areas of spongiosa. The new bone formation is a response of the inner surface of the periosteum to stimulation by a low-grade infection that

has spread through the bone and penetrated the cortex. The disease is seen almost exclusively in children and rarely occurs in persons over 30 years of age.[173] The mean age varies from 12 to 13.3 years, with a 1.4:1 male predominance. Patients have facial asymmetry resulting from a bony, hard swelling of the mandible.

Radiographs of this disease show laminar periosteal new bone (the so-called onion peel appearance), which is most evident on the inferior, buccal, or lingual aspect of the mandible (Fig. 17-76). In some cases, there may be accompanying radiolucent or osteosclerotic osteomyelitic changes, and small sequestra can often be seen. The differential diagnosis for a condition that resembles osteomyelitis with periositis includes Ewing's sarcoma, fibrous dysplasia, osteogenic sarcoma, infantile cortical hyperostosis, and peripheral osteomas.

## Tuberculous Osteomyelitis

Tuberculous osteomyelitis is a specific infection caused by the acid-fast bacillus *Mycobacterium tuberculosis*. The oral tissue is involved by this organism via three routes: direct inoculation, extension from adjacent sites of infection, or hematogenous seeding.[175, 176] Radiographs of this disease show rarefaction with ill-defined borders and formation of sequestra, but sometimes there may be accompanying periosteal new bone formation (Fig. 17-77). The differential diagnosis includes nonspecific osteomyelitis, malignant tumors, and eosinophilic granuloma.

## Sclerosing Osteomyelitis

Sclerosing osteomyelitis of the mandible is a predominantly proliferative reaction of bone representing resistance of the host to low-grade infection.[166] In patients with chronic sclerosing osteomyelitis, bone is deposited along the osseous cortex and existing trabeculae, resulting in thickening of the cortex and trabeculae and reduction or obliteration of the marrow spaces.[177]

Sclerosing osteomyelitis of the mandible has been divided into focal and diffuse types. The focal type, also known as periapical osteitis, is a common condition with a pathognomonic appearance. The radiographs show a well-circumscribed periapical radiopaque area of sclerotic bone (Fig. 17-78). The patient is easily cured by endodontic treatment or extraction of the affected tooth. The diffuse type is an uncommon disease that creates diagnostic and therapeutic problems.[177–179] Clinically, recurrent pain and swelling are typical symptoms. In the early stages of diffuse sclerosing osteomyelitis and in younger patients, the mandibular volume increases due to periosteal deposition of new bone. However, diffuse osteolytic changes are a more prominent feature than sclerosis. In the established chronic stages and in older patients with less prominent periosteal reactivity, the mandibular volume is reduced and sclerosis is more obvious, with smaller and fewer osteolytic zones. A distinctive radiographic and CT scan pattern is that of diffuse endosteal sclerosis with simultaneous involvement of the alveolar and basal bones and extension to the angle, ramus, or condyle, with indistinct borders. In the chronic stages, diffuse sclerosing osteomyelitis must be differentiated from other radiopaque lesions such as diffuse cemento-

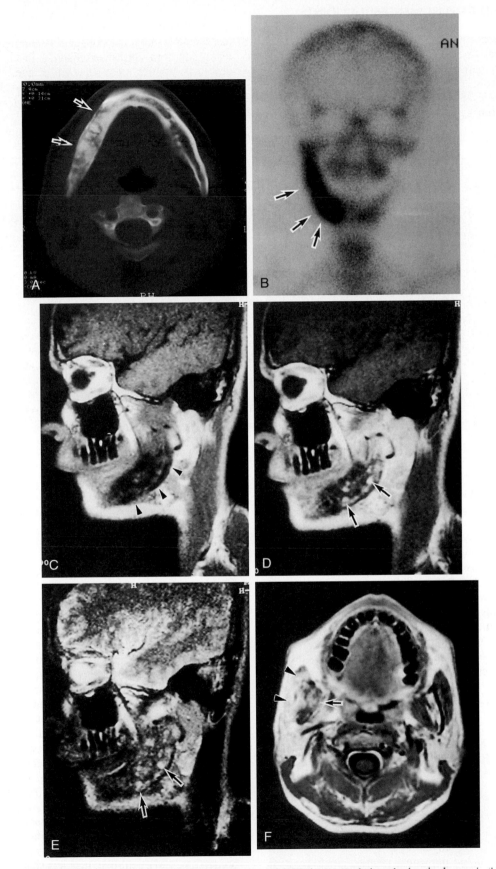

**FIGURE 17-75** Chronic suppurative osteomyelitis. **A,** Axial CT shows osteolytic and sclerotic changes in the right side of the mandible. Cortex has been destroyed (*arrows*). **B,** Anterior view of bone scintigraphy shows increased activity in the right side of the mandible (*arrows*). **C,** Sagittal T1-weighted MR image shows low-intensity areas from the molar to the ramus region (*arrowheads*). **D,** Enhanced sagittal T1-weighted MR image demonstrates areas of patchy enhancement (*arrows*), which is consistent with residues of infected bone marrow. **E,** Sagittal T2-weighted MR image shows heterogeneous low to high signal intensities. Residues of inflammatory bone marrow show high-intensity foci (*arrows*). **F,** Enhanced axial T1-weighted MR image demonstrates enhancement in the ramus region (*arrow*). The right masseter muscle shows swelling and enhancement (*arrowheads*).

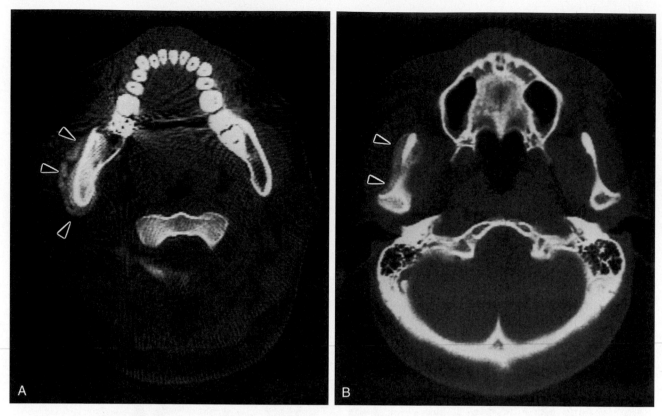

**FIGURE 17-76** **A** and **B**, Osteomyelitis with periositis. Axial CT (bony window setting) shows multilayered periosteal reaction of irregular thickness in the right side of the mandible (*arrowheads*).

sis, sclerosing cemental masses of the jaw, and florid osseous dysplasia in radiographic examinations.[176]

MR imaging shows abnormally thickened cortex with a signal void. There may be defects in the cortex and decreased signal intensity of bone marrow on T1-weighted images. The medullary cavity has increased signal intensity on T2-weighted images. Diffuse enhancement with gadolinium can be seen outside of the mandible when soft tissue is involved. In management, some authors report that an early diagnosis is of the utmost importance, and the patient should be kept under observation for several years.[177–179] However, similarities to other radiopaque lesions such as diffuse cementosis, sclerosing cemental masses of the jaw, florid osseous dysplasia, Ewing's sarcoma, osteosarcoma, and metastasis, as well as the lack of pathognomonic features,

signify that the diagnosis of this disease should be established by a combination of clinical, radiographic, and histologic findings.

## Osteoradionecrosis

Osteoradionecrosis is a pathologic process that sometimes follows heavy irradiation of bone and is characterized by a chronic, painful necrosis accompanied by late sequestration and sometimes permanent deformity.[180, 181] The radiation effects are endothelial cell death, hyalinization resulting from amyloid degeneration, and thrombosis of vessels. The periosteum undergoes fibrosis, and bone osteocytes and osteoblasts become necrotic, with fibrosis of the marrow spaces. Bone trabeculae are reduced in width and number, so that there is an increase in the size of the marrow spaces, which contain necrotic debris. These changes are progressive and lead to necrosis of bone and sequestration, although there is no clear line of demarcation between vital and nonvital bones. Radiologically, the bone can be normal in the early stages. The progression of the bone change is slow and slight. In advanced cases, there are multiple radiolucent areas with poorly defined borders and enlarged, irregular trabecular spaces (with the typical moth-eaten appearance) containing areas of sequestra (Fig. 17-79).

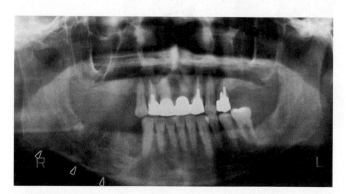

**FIGURE 17-77** Tuberculosis osteomyelitis. Pantomogram shows ill-defined borders and formation of sequestra (*arrowheads*).

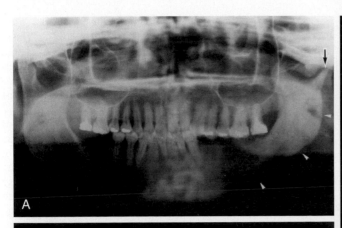

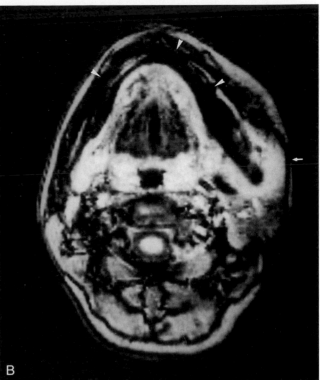

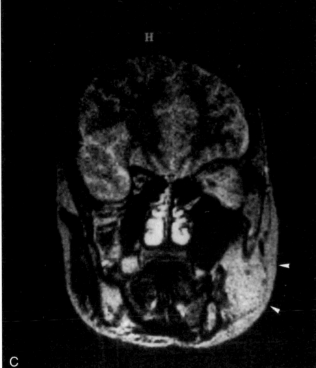

**FIGURE 17-78**   Sclerosing osteomyelitis. **A,** Pantomogram shows a radiopaque lesion in the left side of the mandible (*arrowheads*). The left head of the condyle is deformed (*arrow*). **B,** The entire mandible reveals low signal intensity in this axial T1-weighted MR image (*arrowheads*). Soft tissues around the left side of the mandible show high intensity and hemorrhage or fatty degeneration of the masseter muscle (*arrow*). **C,** Coronal T2-weighted MR image demonstrates expansile change of high intensity in the left side of the mandible (*arrowheads*). MR imaging reveals a larger extent of the lesion than does a pantomogram, and extensive inflammation was suspected.

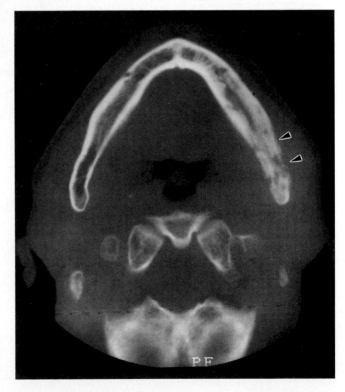

**FIGURE 17-79**   Osteoradionecrosis. Axial CT shows osteolytic and sclerotic changes in the left side of the mandible in a patient previously treated by radiation therapy. Destruction of the mandibular cortex can be seen (*arrowheads*).

SECTION TWO

# SYSTEMATIC APPROACH TO IMAGING DIAGNOSIS OF JAW LESIONS

*Takashi Kaneda, Manabu Minami, Hugh D. Curtin, Mitsuaki Yamashiro, Yoshiaki Akimoto, Kuni Ohtomo, Hiroyuki Okada, and Hirotsugu Yamamoto*

The objective of this section is to present a systematic approach to the diagnosis of jaw lesions using various imaging findings.

Odontogenic tumors comprise about 10% of all tumors of the oral cavity and about 2.4% of all lesions biopsied by dentists in the United States.[3, 182] After clinical examination, the patient with a suspected jaw lesion is first referred for plain radiography, pantomogram, or sometimes CT. The radiologic examination is part of the overall diagnostic process. Oral surgeons need a differential diagnosis of the disease as well as an exact assessment of the topography and extent of the lesion. Infiltration into surrounding tissues must also be evaluated.

Radiologic diagnosis of jawbone lesions has used conventional radiography including dental and occlusal films, pantomography, conventional tomography, and CT.[183–185] More recently, MR imaging has allowed excellent soft-tissue differentiation, and its increasing application is beginning to have an impact on the diagnosis of dento-maxillofacial lesions.[186–190]

As discussed in the previous section, few radiographic or imaging appearances are pathognomonic for a specific lesion. Based on all imaging modalities, the disease pattern may indicate several different diseases of either odontogenic or nonodontogenic origin. The question is, "How do we use the imaging modalities to differentiate these jawbone lesions?" What is needed is an effective, systematic approach to solve this problem.

Conventional radiography and pantomography provide screening imaging in various pathologic conditions of the maxilla and mandible and may suggest the need for further radiologic examinations such as CT or MR imaging. Imaging in at least two planes is necessary to analyze the lesion and adjacent tissues properly. Currently, multidetector CT provides images in multiple planes from a single spiral scan acquisition. Dental reformatting software also provides cross-sectional as well as panoramic sectional imaging.

When a jaw lesion is first identified, inflammation related to a tooth is usually considered first because of the high incidence of caries and related periapical disease. Inflammation can progress and lead to several different pathologic

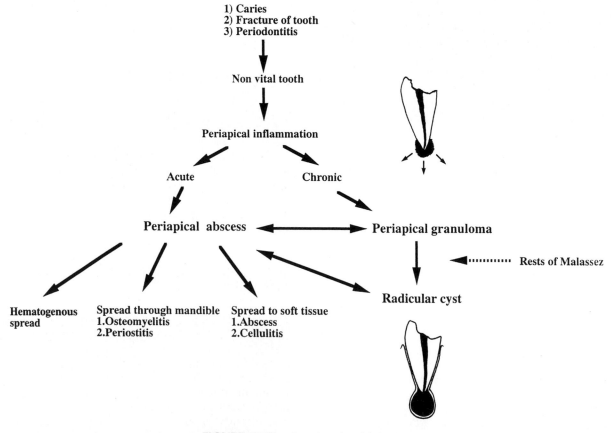

**FIGURE 17-80** Sequelae of tooth infection.

# Jawbone lesions

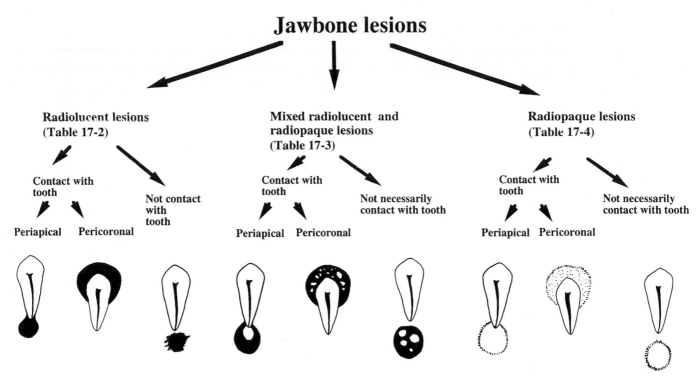

**FIGURE 17-81**   Systematic approach using radiologic examination of jawbone lesions.

conditions including periapical inflammation, periapical granuloma, periapical abscess, and radicular cyst (Fig. 17-80). Specifically, periapical inflammation or periapical granuloma is initiated and maintained by degeneration products of necrotic pulp tissue of a nonvital tooth. Stimulation of the resident epithelial rests of Malassez occurs in response to the products of inflammation. When the infection reaches the periapical tissue, many different tissue reactions may occur, depending on the nature of the infection and the resistance of the host.

If an inflammatory pathology can be excluded as a potential diagnosis, then the various tumors and cysts must be considered.

As previously discussed, the radiologic analysis for differential diagnosis primarily depends on changes in density, character of the margin, location, relationship to the teeth (including root resorption), and other radiologic findings (Fig. 17-81). The lesion may have a radiolucent, radiopaque, or mixed appearance. The margin may be sharp or indistinct, sclerotic or well corticated. Other useful radiologic findings are (1) the degree of extension, (2) the internal architecture of the lesion, (3) changes in the cortex of the mandible, and (4) periosteal reactions and soft-tissue changes. The relationship to a particular part of a tooth is extremely useful in the diagnosis of jaw lesions.[1, 191, 192]

## RADIOLUCENT LESIONS

### Well-Defined Radiolucent Lesions

Maxillomandibular lesions most frequently show a unilocular pattern or a multilocular pattern with internal septa.[1, 191, 192] A number of odontogenic and nonodontoge-

nic lesions including periapical lesions, cyst of the globullomaxillary region, dentigerous cyst, primodial cyst, OKC, and ameloblastoma can present as well-defined radiolucent lesions (Table 17-2). When the lesion is equal or less than 2 cm in diameter, most of the lesions can be well evaluated by radiography alone. When radiolucent lesions are more than 2 cm in diameter, addition of MR imaging can be useful, especially for the evaluation of internal structures and the nature of the content, as stated below.[193]

### Ill-Defined Radiolucent Lesions

Ill-defined radiolucent lesions are produced by inflammation and by malignancies of the jaw including carcinoma and osteosarcoma. Most carcinomas involving the jaws are invading from the lesions of the oral mucosa. Some may be metastatic deposits from primary tumors in distant sites.[185, 191, 192]

## MIXED RADIOLUCENT-RADIOPAQUE LESIONS

A mixed radiolucent-radiopaque appearance (Table 17-3) can result from the presence of two or more tissues with different radiographic densities, varying degrees of maturation of the inflammatory soft tissue within the lesion, and localized resorption and apposition of new bone within or around the lesion. This appearance may indicate osteomyelitis, an immature fibroosseous lesion, or tumor.[185, 191, 192] The location of the lesion sometimes gives the clue for differentiation, but is not always a definite differential point.

**Table 17-2**
**RADIOLUCENT LESIONS OF THE JAWS**

| | Periapical | Pericoronal | No Contact with Tooth |
|---|---|---|---|
| **Cysts** | | | |
| **Common** | | | |
| Radicular cyst (radicular granuloma) | O | | |
| Residual cyst | | | O |
| Dentigerous cyst | △ | O | |
| Primordial cyst | | | O |
| Odontogenic keratocyst | | O | △ |
| Globulomaxillary cyst | | | O |
| Nasopalatine duct cyst | | | O |
| Incisive canal cyst | | | O |
| Lateral periodontal cyst | O | △ | |
| Static bone cavity | | | O |
| | | | |
| **Uncommon** | | | |
| Traumatic bone cyst | | | O |
| Aneurysmal bone cyst | | | O |
| Calcifying odontogenic cyst (early stage) | | O | |
| | | | |
| **Tumors** | | | |
| **Common** | | | |
| Ameloblastoma (multilocular or unilocular) | △ | O | O |
| Cemento-ossifying fibroma | O | | △ |
| Cementoblastoma (early stage) | O | | |
| Periapical cemental dysplasia (early stage) | O | | |
| Odontogenic fibloma | | △ | O |
| Giant cell granuloma | △ | O | |
| Malignant neoplasm | △ | △ | O |
| | | | |
| **Uncommon** | | | |
| Ameloblastic fibroma and myxoma | | O | |
| Calcifying epithelial odontogenic tumor (early stage) | | O | |
| Odontogenic myxoma | | △ | O |
| Odontogenic fibloma | | △ | O |
| Odontoma (premineralized stage) | | | O |
| Cementifying and ossifying fibroma (early stage) | O | | △ |
| Histiocytosis X | | | O |
| Metastatic carcinoma | | | O |
| | | | |
| **Others** | | | |
| Osteomyelitis | O | O | ∧ |

O, Common; △, uncommon.

# RADIOPAQUE LESIONS

Radiopacity in the jawbones is produced mainly by osteosclerosis, thickening of the cortex, cemental masses, or impacted teeth. Radiopaque lesions in the maxillomandibular region are usually fibroosseous lesions, inflammation, or tumors.[185, 191, 192] These lesions are considered to be best differentiated by a combination of plain radiography and high-resolution CT (Table 17-4).

# MR IMAGING

MR imaging (Fig. 17-82) has an advantage over plain films and CT in that it directly visualizes bone marrow characteristics, is more sensitive to contrast enhancement, better evaluates soft-tissue involvement, and provides multiple planes of imaging without radiation. MR imaging is said to be less useful in examining cortical bone because of the lack of signal generated by compact bone. However, invading tumors involving the cortex can be identified, as the intermediate signal of the tumor replaces the signal void usually seen in the cortex. MR imaging is less frequently affected than CT by artifacts related to dental materials, but the images can be seriously distorted by dental materials with high ferrous content. Artifacts related to dental materials on MR imaging are mainly dependent on the strength of the magnetic field, the specific pulse sequence and scan direction, and the nature of the dental materials. In addition, some injury to the gingiva is unavoidable at dental treatment and subsequent implantation of dental bur

**Table 17-3**
**MIXED RADIOLUCENT-RADIOPAQUE LESIONS OF THE JAWS**

| | Periapical | Pericoronal | Not Necessarily in Contact with Tooth |
|---|---|---|---|
| **Common** | | | |
| Cementoma (intermediate stage) (periapical cemental dysplasia) | ○ | | |
| Calcifying odontogenic cyst | △ | ○ | |
| Cemento-ossifying fibroma | ○ | | △ |
| Adenomatoid odontogenic tumor | | ○ | |
| Calcifying epithelial odontogenic tumor | | ○ | △ |
| Odontoma (intermediate stage) | △ | ○ | |
| Fibrous dysplasia, cherubism | | | ○ |
| Paget's disease | | | ○ |
| Osteitis | ○ | △ | |
| **Uncommon** | | | |
| Cementoblastoma | ○ | | |
| Ameloblastic fibroodonotoma | | ○ | △ |
| Odontogenic fibroma | | | ○ |
| Ameloblastic fibrodentinoma | | ○ | △ |
| Osteoblastoma | | | ○ |
| Hemangioma | | | ○ |
| Chondroma, chonodrosarcoma | | | ○ |
| Ewing's sarcoma | | | ○ |
| Lymphoma | | | ○ |
| Osteoblastic metastasis | | | ○ |
| Osteosarcoma | | | ○ |
| Histocytosis X | | | ○ |
| Osteomyelitis (chronic stage) | | | ○ |
| Osteoradionecrosis | | | ○ |
| Ossifying subperiosteal hematoma | | | ○ |
| Cemental mass | ○ | | |

○, Common; △, uncommon.

fragments into the gingiva may occur, resulting in local image distortion.[194]

MR imaging has been reported to be superior to CT in the evaluation of certain characteristics of apparently cystic lesions, giving better information about the inner consistency of the lesion with demonstration of cystic or solid components, thickness of cyst walls, and heterogeneity of fluid content. For example, an OKC frequently shows heterogeneous intensity of fluid contents on MR imaging, while other types of cysts usually show more homogeneous fluid intensity. Some cysts, especially inflammatory cysts, can be misdiagnosed as having a mixed or solid pattern on noncontrast studies and require contrast-enhanced examinations for accurate diagnosis.[190] These findings can be most easily evaluated in lesions larger than 2 cm in diameter.

MR imaging is also useful in differentiating ameloblastoma from larger cysts by demonstrating thick walls and papillary projections, especially on contrast examinations.[188] Other types of maxillomandibular benign tumors show well-defined solid components and some enhancement on contrast-enhanced T1-weighted images, but these findings are usually less helpful in separating various diagnoses. Maxillomandibular malignant tumors show ill-defined inhomogeneous enhancement on gadolinium-enhanced T1-weighted images. The findings are nonspecific but are useful in the evaluation of tumor extension for preoperative planning.

With osseous lesions in the maxillomandibular region, conventional tomography and CT are superior to MR imaging because of their better detection of calcification and cortical abnormality.

## Acknowledgment

We thank Manabu Minami, M.D., Department of Radiology, the University of Tokyo, Japan, and Hugh D. Curtin, M.D., Department of Radiology, Massachusetts Eye and Ear Infirmary, and Harvard Medical School for their advice and editorial comments in helping us prepare this section.

Table 17-4
### RADIOPAQUE LESIONS OF THE JAWS

| | Periapical | Pericoronal | Not Necessarily in Contact with Tooth |
|---|:---:|:---:|:---:|
| **Common** | | | |
| Odontoma (complex, compound) | | ○ | △ |
| Cementoma (mature), periapical cemental dysplasia | ○ | | |
| Fibrous dysplasia | | | ○ |
| Condensing osteitis, focal sclerosing osteitis | ○ | ○ | |
| Paget's disease | | | ○ |
| Sclerosing osteomyelitis | ○ | | △ |
| Unerupted or impacted tooth | ○ | | △ |
| Sclerotic cemental masses | ○ | | |
| Unerupted or impacted tooth | ○ | | △ |
| **Uncommon** | | | |
| Cemento-ossifying fibroma | ○ | | △ |
| Chrondroma, chondrosarcoma | | | ○ |
| Exostosis, osteochondroma | | | ○ |
| Idiopathic osteosclerosis | | | ○ |
| Osteoblastoma, osteoid osteoma | | | ○ |
| Torus mandibularis or palatinus | | | ○ |
| Osteoblastic metastasis | | | ○ |
| Osteosarcoma | | | ○ |

○, Common; △, uncommon.

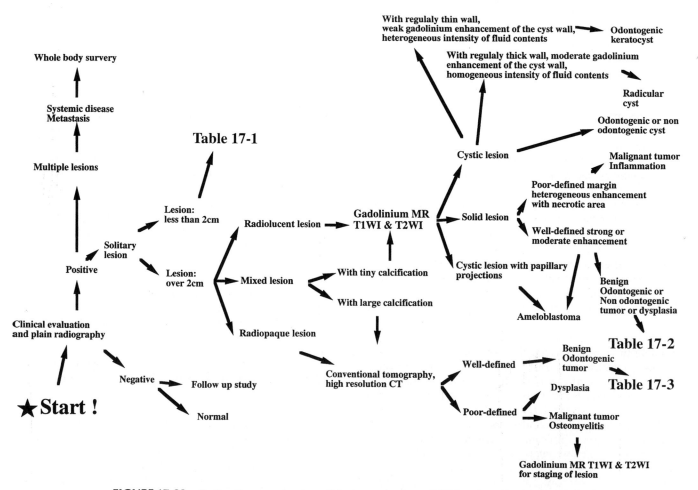

**FIGURE 17-82**    Systematic approach using radiologic examination and MR imaging of jawbone lesions.

# DENTAL ANOMALIES AND SYSTEMIC DISEASE

## *Jorge Bianchi and Hugh D. Curtin*

The purpose of this section is not to provide a complete description of every dental anomaly with a correlating imaging appearance or to discuss extensively the various manifestations of systemic disease. Rather, its purpose is to describe those conditions that may be seen incidentally during imaging of the head and neck and that may be questioned during interpretation of an examination done for an unrelated reason. It is hoped that some of the terminology will prove useful to the reader. A systemic disease will usually be obvious by the time the patient comes to imaging. Almost all of the dental anomalies described here are best shown by plain dental radiographs.

## DENTAL ANOMALIES

Dental anomalies include variations in the shape, size, number, and morphology of the teeth. These types of abnormalities are relatively frequent and are usually diagnosed by the general dentist with plain radiographic films. Although most anomalies occur as isolated entities, some are associated with extraoral abnormalities. The various tooth structures (enamel, dentin, cementum, and periodontal ligament) have different embryologic origins, and abnormalities affecting a particular tooth structure may be associated with disorders of extradental tissues that have a similar embryologic origin.

## Supernumerary Teeth

Supernumerary teeth are simply extra teeth (Fig. 17-83). They occur mainly in the anterior region of the maxilla. A supernumerary tooth in the anterior maxilla is called a mesiodens.[195] An extra tooth seen posterior to the molar area is called a distomolar or distodent. The term *paramolar* has been used to describe a supernumerary tooth in the region of the molars. It can be lingual (medial), buccal (lateral), or occur between the normal molars. The term has been used to describe a distomolar as well. Supernumerary teeth are usually smaller than normal teeth and are more common in the permanent dentition. They are present in 1% to 4% of the population.[196] Syndromes associated with supernumerary teeth include Gardner's syndrome and cleidocranial dysplasia, but a supernumerary tooth is most commonly seen as an isolated phenomenon.[197]

The presence of supernumerary teeth may affect the normal eruption of teeth and therefore future appropriate positioning of the teeth. Thus, the dentist may want to know the position and orientation of the mesiodens in the maxilla or jaw, as the position, orientation, and inclination of the mesiodens can be significant in potential treatment.

Palatal orientation refers to the position of the tooth facing the hard palate. Buccal orientation refers to the position of the tooth facing the cheek and the buccal mucosa of the alveolar process. The dentist can plan extractions or orthodontic treatment (teeth alignment) knowing the posi-

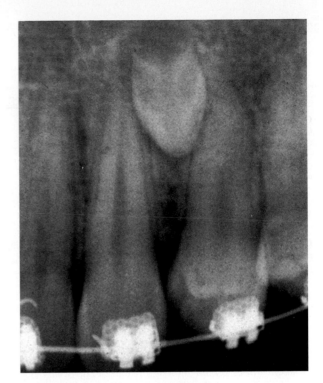

**FIGURE 17-83** Supernumerary tooth. Periapical view of the anterior maxilla shows a supernumerary tooth between the left canine and first premolar.

tion and orientation of the mesiodens. Distomolars or paramolars may also have different inclinations and positions that can affect normal occlusion.

## Hypodontia

Hypodontia is the absence of one or more teeth.[198] This condition occurs in permanent dentition in 5% to 10% of the population. The most common missing teeth excluding the third molars are the mandibular second premolars and maxillary lateral incisors, respectively.[198, 199] Disorders associated with missing teeth include ectodermal dysplasia, epidermolysis bullosa, and a variety of other disorders.[200]

Ectodermal dysplasia is an X-linked recessive disorder characterized by the absence or deficient development of at least two derivatives of the ectoderm such as the teeth, hair, and nails (Fig. 17-84). Charles Darwin identified the first case in the 1860s.

Epidermolysis bullosa is a rare genetic disorder characterized by blister formation on the mucosa or skin that develops in response to minor trauma.

Radiation treatment can affect the normal development of the teeth, and missing teeth is a common consequence of radiation therapy in children.

## Macrodontia and Microdontia

Macrodontia and microdontia refer to correlations between the size of a tooth and its correspondent on the opposite side of the arch.[199–201] Teeth may be bigger or smaller (Fig. 17-85) in a normal healthy individual. However, macrodontia and microdontia can affect the space available in the jaws for the teeth and therefore can affect normal occlusion. This may lead to misalignment of the teeth in the arch.

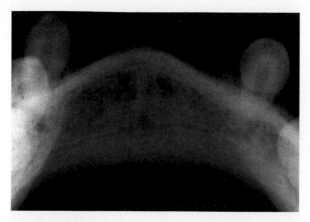

FIGURE 17-84   Ectodermal dysplasia. Occlusal view. Abnormal teeth with absence of central incisors.

## Dens in Dente (Dens Invaginatus)

Dens in dente results from an invagination of the outer surface of the tooth into the inner part of the tooth (Figs. 17-86 and 17-87).[202, 203] It occurs most frequently in permanent upper lateral incisors. It can occur in any region of the tooth but usually affects the crown of the tooth, with the enamel folding inward. The vitality of the tooth may be compromised. When the abnormality involves the root of the tooth, the defect is lined by cementum.[202, 203]

## Pulp Stones

Pulp stones are calcifications in the pulp chamber of the tooth (Figs. 17-88 and 17-89). The etiology is unclear, but there may be a direct relationship with increased age. The molar teeth are most commonly affected, but pulp stones can affect any tooth. At clinical inspection, a tooth with a pulp stone looks like any other tooth. A pulp stone may make root canal treatment difficult or impossible. Pulp calcifications have been found in association with tumoral calcinosis, dentin dysplasia, and Ehlers-Danlos syndrome.[204]

## Enamel Pearls

Enamel pearls are small spherical enamel masses located at the root of the molars and are found in 2% of the

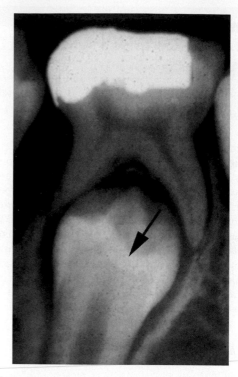

FIGURE 17-86   Dens in dente. Periapical view shows an unerupted bicuspid with an invaginated cusp (*arrow*) consistent with dens in dente.

population (Figs. 17-90 and 17-91).[205] There can be a small pulp chamber extending from the parent tooth. Enamel pearls can distort the periodontal space and may predispose the patient to periodontal disease, but usually they are not considered to have clinical significance. Occurring beneath the gingiva, they are not usually clinically obvious.

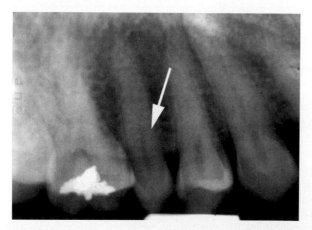

FIGURE 17-85   Microdontia. A periapical view of the right posterior maxilla shows a small second premolar (*arrow*).

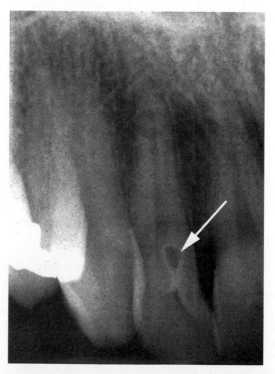

FIGURE 17-87   Dens in dente. Periapical view of the right maxilla shows a dens in dente in the lateral incisor. Invagination of the enamel (*arrow*) and pulp chamber is noted.

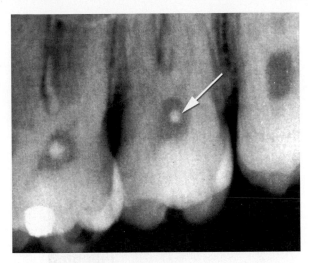

FIGURE 17-88 Periapical view of the right posterior maxilla. The first and second permanent molars show pulp stones in the pulp chamber (*arrow*).

## Amelogenesis Imperfecta

Normal enamel is the densest material in the human body. Enamel covers the outer surface of the teeth and is almost 100% inorganic, composed mainly of hydroxyapatite crystals. Its attenuation value at CT is 3000 HU. Amelogenesis imperfecta is a developmental disorder that involves generalized abnormal enamel formation.[3] Strong autosomal and recessive X-linked associations have been documented.[206] The enamel is very thin (Fig. 17-92). The dentin can be seen through the enamel, giving the tooth a darker or, in some cases, a yellow-brown color. Frequently the enamel will fracture easily and the teeth wear down quickly. In some

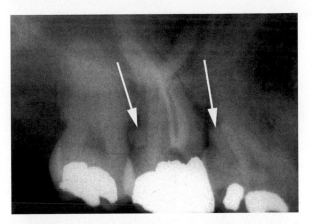

FIGURE 17-90 Enamel pearls. Periapical view of the right posterior maxilla. Enamel pearls are seen in the cervical portion of the first and second permanent molars (*arrows*).

variants the teeth readily absorb stains, adding a darkened component to the already abnormal appearance.[207]

The radiographic appearance varies with the subtype.[3, 207, 208] The enamel may be of normal density but very thin (hypoplastic form). The thickness initially may be relatively normal but the density is low, at times even lower than the radiographic appearance of dentin (hypomaturation or hypocalcified form). All forms erode or wear easily and the enamel may be worn down, giving a squared-off appearance to the crown.

## Dentinogenesis Imperfecta

Dentinogenesis imperfecta (DI) is an autosomal dominant developmental disturbance of dentin formation.[209] Dentin is the inner layer of the tooth structure and has a more organic matrix than the enamel. DI can affect both primary

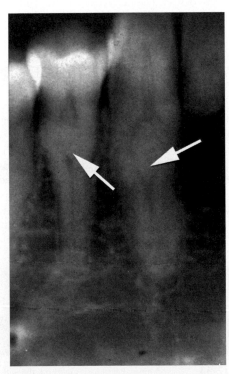

FIGURE 17-89 Periapical view of the right posterior mandible. The right permanent canine and first bicuspid show pulp stones in the pulp chamber (*arrows*).

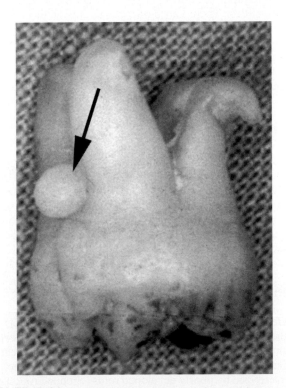

FIGURE 17-91 Enamel pearl. An enamel pearl (*arrow*) is seen on the cervical portion of the tooth.

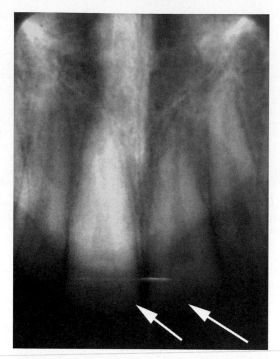

**FIGURE 17-92** Amelogenesis imperfecta. Periapical view of the anterior maxilla. Dentin, pulp chamber, and cementum are present, but there is no or very thin enamel (*arrows*).

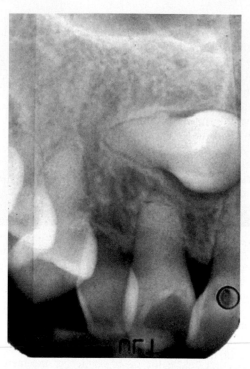

**FIGURE 17-93** DI. Periapical view of the right maxilla shows pulp chamber obliteration and short teeth consistent with DI. An impacted canine is also seen.

and secondary dentitions and has no sex predilection. It may be associated with osteogenesis imperfecta but can occur in isolation, without associated skeletal abnormalities.[210] The term *hereditary opalescent dentin* has been applied to the isolated defect variant. The teeth may be translucent and vary in color from yellow to gray. The enamel fractures easily, and the teeth wear readily.[210]

Radiographic features of DI can include a variety of abnormalities. There can be a constriction of the cervical portion of the tooth (junction between enamel and cementum). The roots can be narrowed or short. There can be partial or complete obliteration of the pulp chamber (Fig. 17-93). The lucency is replaced by an opacity that is more characteristic of dentin.

## Taurodontia

Taurodontia or taurodontism is an inherited anomaly characterized by enlarged pulp chambers of the teeth (Fig. 17-94). The pulp chamber's size is increased. Clinically, teeth with taurodontia appear no different than normal teeth. The radiographic identification of taurodonia is important because of the risk of exposing the pulp chamber during dental procedures.

## Dentin Dysplasias

Dentin dysplasia is a rare dental anomaly. It is an autosomal dominant condition characterized by abnormal tooth and root formation.[211] Dentin dysplasias have two variants. Dentin dysplasia type 1 (radicular type) is characterized by poorly developed roots (chopped roots) and

obliterated pulp chambers. The crown of the tooth may have normal color or may be slightly darker than normal. Radiologically, obliteration of the pulp cavity is present at birth. In dentin dysplasia type 2 (coronal type), the tooth has the same appearance as in DI. Clinically, the tooth is translucent. Radiography shows narrowing or obliteration of the pulp chamber occurs. Obliteration of the pulp chamber occurs later in dentin dysplasia than in DI. Dentin dysplasia is an uncommon condition.[211]

## DENTAL MANIFESTATION OF METABOLIC AND SYSTEMIC CONDITIONS

A number of metabolic diseases that affect bone biology can also affect the teeth and surrounding structures including the bone, the lamina dura, and the periodontal ligament. Conditions such as hyperparathyroidism, osteoporosis, renal osteodystrophy, and rickets may lead to altered trabeculation of bone, loss or thinning of lamina dura, and a "ground glass" appearance of bone. The dentist may identify this radiographic sign during a regular plain film examination.

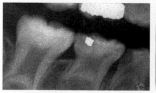
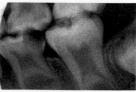

**FIGURE 17-94** Taurodontia. Periapical views of the left and right posterior mandibles. Enlarged pulp chambers are noted.

Systemic conditions such as scleroderma (progressive systemic sclerosis) can present with generalized enlargement of the periodontal ligament (PDL) space.[212–214] The precise explanation of the finding is not known, but the abnormality has been attributed to an obliterative microvascuopathy and a thickened periodontal membrane.[212] The reduction in vascularity of the PDL space may predispose the patient to superimposed periodontal disease as well. This finding is not universal in patients with scleroderma. The differential diagnosis of enlarged PDL space includes occlusal trauma, orthodontic braces (alignment device), and malignancies. Orthodontic appliances pulling on the tooth will usually enlarge one aspect of the PDL space at the expense of the opposite side. The PDL space is narrowed on the side to which the tooth is being "pulled." Malignancies in the jaws such as leukemia, lymphomas, sarcomas, primary lesions, or metastasis may present with teeth "floating in space," localized alveolar bone destruction, and enlarged PDL spaces. "Floating teeth" are also seen in histiocytosis.

Patients with scleroderma can have bone changes as well, and there can be pronounced erosions at points of muscle attachment. Erosions or scalloping of the bone can be seen in the area of the angle of the mandible or more anteriorly where the anterior belly of the digastric attaches to the mandible. There can also be involvement of the coronoid process or condyle.

# REFERENCES

1. Kramer IRH, Pindborg JJ, Shar M. Histological Typing of Odontogenic Tumours: World Health Organization: International Histological Classification of Tumours, 2nd ed. Berlin: Spring-Verlag;1992:1–42.
2. Sciubba JJ, Fantasia JE, Kahn LB. Tumors and cysts of the jaw. In: Rosai J, ed. Atlas of Tumor Pathology. Washington, DC: Armed Forces Institute of Pathology, 2001.
3. White SC, Pharoah MJ. Oral Radiology: Principles and Interpretation, 4th ed. St. Louis: CV Mosby, 2000.
4. Weber AL, Easter KM. Cysts and odontogenic tumors of the mandible and maxilla. I. Contemp Diagn Radiol 1982;5(25):1.
5. Borg G, Persson G, Thilander H. A study of odontogenic cysts with special reference to comparisons between keratinizing and non-keratinizing cysts. Swed Dent J 1974;67:311–325.
6. Shrout MK, Hall MJ, Hildebolt CE. Differentiation of periapical granulomas and radicular cysts by digital radiometric analysis. Oral Surg 1993;76:356–361.
7. Donoff RB, Guralnick WC, Clayman L. Keratocysts of the jaw. J Oral Surg 1972;30:800–884.
8. Brannon RB. The odontogenic keratocyst: a clinicopathologic study of 312 cases. I. Clinical features. Oral Surg 1962;42:54–72.
9. Brennon RB. The odontogenic keratocyst: a clinicopathologic study of 312 cases. II. Histologic features. Oral Surg 1977;43:233–255.
10. Shear M. Developmental odontogenic cysts: an update. J Oral Pathol Med 1994;23:1–11.
11. Forssell K, Forssell H, Kahnberg KE. Recurrences of keratocysts: a long-term follow up study. Int J Oral Maxillofac Surg 1988;17:25–28.
12. Yonetsu K, Bianchi JG, Troulis MJ, Curtin HD. Unusual CT appearance in an odontogenic keratocyst of the mandible: case report. AJNR 2001;22(10):1887–1889.
13. Minami M, Kaneda T, Ozawa K, et al. Cystic lesions of the maxillomandibular region: MR imaging distinction of odontogenic keratocysts and ameloblastomas from other cysts. AJR 1996;166:943–949.
14. Williams TP, Connor FA. Surgical management of the odontogenic keratocyst: aggressive approach. J Oral Maxillofac Surg 1994;52:964–966.
15. Koutnik AW, Kolodny SC, Hooker SP, et al. Multiple nevoid basal cell epithelioma, cysts, of the jaws, and bifid ribs syndrome: report of a case. J Oral Surg 1975;33:686–689.
16. Gorlin RJ, Goltz RW. Multiple nevoid basal cell epithelioma, jaw cysts, I and bifid ribs. N Engl J Med 1960;262:908–912.
17. Woolgar JA, Rippin JW, Browne RM. The odontogenic keratocyst and its occurrence in the nevoid basal cell carcinoma syndrome. Oral Surg Oral Med Oral Pathol 1987;64:727–730.
18. Gorlin RJ, Pindborg JJ, Clausen FP, Vickers RA. The calcifying odontogenic cyst: a possible analogue of the cutaneous calcifying epithelioma of Malherbe: an analysis of 15 cases. Oral Surg 1962;15:1235–1243.
19. Lello GE, Makek M. Calcifying odontogenic cyst. Int J Oral Maxillofac Surg 1986;15:637–644.
20. Tanimoto K, Tomita S, Aoyama M, et al. Radiographic characteristics of the calcifying odontogenic cyst. Int J Oral Maxillofac Surg 1988;17:29–32.
21. Buchner A. The central (intraosseous) calcifying odontogenic cyst: an analysis of 215 cases. J Oral Maxillofac Surg 1991;49:330–339.
22. Devlin H, Horner K. The radiological features of calcifying odontogenic cyst. Br J Radiol 1993;66:403–407.
23. Abrams A, Howell FV, Bullock WK. Nasopalatine cysts. Oral Surg 1963;16:306–332.
24. Campbell JJ, Baden E, Williams AC. Nasopalatine cyst of unusual size: report of case. J Oral Surg 1973;31:776–779.
25. Christ TF. The globulomaxillary cyst: an embryologic misconception. Oral Surg 1970;30:515–526.
26. Little JW, Jakobsen J. Origin of the globulomaxillary cyst. J Oral Surg 1978;31:188.
27. Huebner GR, Turlington EG. So-called traumatic (hemorrhagic) bone cysts of the jaw. Oral Surg 1971;31:254–265.
28. Saito Y, Hoshina Y, Nagamine T. Simple bone cyst: a clinical and histopathological study of fifteen cases. Oral Surg Oral Med Oral Pathol 1992;74:487–491.
29. Suei Y, Tanimoto K, Wada T. Simple bone cyst: evaluation of contents with conventional radiography and computed tomography. Oral Surg Oral Med Oral Pathol 1994;77:296–301.
30. Biewald HF. A variation in the management of hemorrhagic, traumatic or simple bone cyst. J Oral Surg 1987;25:627.
31. Ellis DJ, Walters PJ. Aneurysmal bone cyst of the mandible. J Oral Surg 1972;34:26–32.
32. Gruskin SE, Dablin DC. Aneurysmal bone cyst of the mandible. J Oral Surg 1968;26:523–528.
33. Steidler NE, Cook RM, Reade PC. Aneurysmal bone cysts of the jaws: a case report and review of the literature. Br J Oral Surg 1970;16:254–261.
34. Reyneke JP. Aneurysmal bone cyst of the maxilla. Oral Surg 1978;45:441–447.
35. Karabouta I, Tsodoulos S, Trigonidis G. Extensive aneurysmal bone cyst of the mandible: surgical resection and immediate reconstruction. Oral Surg Oral Med Oral Pathol 1991;71:148–150.
36. Robinson PD. Aneurysmal bone cyst: a hybrid lesion? Br J Oral Maxillofac Surg 1985;23:220–226.
37. Stafne EC. Bone cavities situated near the angle of the jaw. J Am Dent Assoc 1942;29:19–69.
38. Buchner A, Carpenter WM, Merrell PW, Leider AS. Anterior lingual mandibular salivary gland defect. Oral Surg Oral Med Oral Pathol 1991;71:131–136.
39. Regezi JA, Kerr DA, Courtney RM. Odontogenic tumors: analysis of 706 cases. J Oral Surg 1978;36:771–778.
40. Weber AL, Easter KM. Cysts and odontogenic tumors of the mandible and maxilla. II. Contemp Diagn Radiol 1982;5(36):1.
41. Small IA, Waldron CA. Ameloblastoma of the jaw. Oral Surg Oral Med Oral Pathol 1955;8(3):281–297.
42. Hylton RP, McKean TW, Albright JE. Simple ameloblastoma: report of case. J Oral Surg 1972;30:59.
43. Mehlish DR, Dahlin DC, Masson JK. Ameloblastoma: a clinicopathologic report. J Oral Surg 1972;30:9–22.
44. Eversole LR, Leider AS, Hansen LS. Ameloblastomas with pronounced desmoplasia. J Oral Maxillofac Surg 1984;42:735–740.
45. Minami M, Kaneda T, Yamamoto H, et al. Ameloblastoma in the maxillomandibular region: MR imaging. Radiology 1992;184:389–393.

46. Kaffe I, Buchner A, Taicher S. Radiographic features of desmoplastic variant of ameloblastoma. Oral Surg 1993;76:525–529.

47. Ng KH, Siar CH. Desmoplastic variant of ameloblastomas in Malaysians. Br J Oral Maxillofac Surg 1993;31:299–303.

48. Franklin CD, Hindle MO. The calcifying epithelial odontogenic tumor: report of four cases, two with long-term follow-up. Br J Oral Surg 1976;13:230–238.

49. Franklin CD, Pindborg JJ. The calcifying epithelial odontogenic tumor. Oral Surg 1976;42:753–765.

50. Pindborg JJ. A calcifying epithelial odontogenic tumor. Cancer 1958;11:838–843.

51. Tratman EK. Classification of odontomes. Br Dent J 1951;91:167–173.

52. Curreri RC, Masser JE, Abramson AL. Complex odontoma of the maxillary sinus: report of a case. J Oral Surg 1975;33:45–48.

53. Caton RB, Marble HB Jr, Topazian RG. Complex odontoma in the maxillary sinus. J Oral Surg 1973;36(5):658–662.

54. Thompson RD, Hale ML, McLeran JH. Multiple compound composite odontomas of maxilla and mandible: report of case. J Oral Surg 1968;26:478–480.

55. Regezi JA, Kerr DA, Courtney RM. Odontogenic tumors: analysis of 760 cases. J Oral Surg 1978;36:771–778.

56. Daley TD, Wysocki GP, Pringle GA. Relative incidence of odontogenic tumors and oral and jaw cysts in a Canadian population. Oral Surg 1994;77:276–280.

57. Philipsen HP, Reichart PA, Zhang KH, et al. Adenomatoid odontogenic tumor: biologic profile based on 499 cases. J Oral Pathol Med 1991;20:149–158.

58. Gundlach KK, Schulz A. Odontogenic myxoma: clinical concept and morphological studies. J Oral Pathol 1977;6(6):343–358.

59. Hendler BH, Abaza NA, Quinn P. Odontogenic myxoma, surgical management and an ultrastructural study. Oral Surg 1979;47:203–217.

60. Davis RB, Baker RD, Alling CC. Odontogenic myxoma: clinical pathologic conference, case 24. J Oral Surg 1978;36:534–538.

61. Peltola J, Magnusson B, Happonen R-P, Borrman H. Odontogenic myxoma: a radiographic study of 21 tumours. Br J Oral Maxillofac Surg 1994;32:298–302.

62. Zegarelli EV, Kutscher AH, Napoli N, et al. The cementoma: a study of 235 patients with 435 cementomas. Oral Surg 1964;17:219–224.

63. Vegh T. Multiple cementomas (periapical cemental dysplasia). Oral Surg 1976;42:402–406.

64. Chaudhry AP, Spink JH, Gorlin RJ. Periapical fibrous dysplasia (cementoma). J Oral Surg 1958;16:483.

65. Waldron CA. Fibro-osseous lesions of the jaws. J Oral Maxillofac Surg 1993;51:828–835.

66. Hamner JE III, Scofield HH, Cornyn J. Benign fibro-osseous jaw lesions of periodontal membrane origin: analysis of 249 cases. Cancer 1968;22:861–878.

67. Cherrick HM, King OH Jr, Lucatorto FM, et al. Benign cementoblastoma: a clinicopathologic evaluation. Oral Surg 1974;37:54–63.

68. Eversole LR, Sabes WR, Dauchess VG. Benign cementoblastoma. J Oral Surg 1973;36:824–830.

69. Suzuki M, Sakai T. A familial study of torus palatinus and torus mandibularis. Am J Phys Anthropol 1960;18:263.

70. King DR, Moore GE. An analysis of torus palatinus in a transatlantic study. J Oral Med 1976;31:44–46.

71. Bhaskar SN, Cutright DE. Multiple enostosis: report of cases. J Oral Surg 1968;26:321–326.

72. Weinberg S. Osteoma of the mandibular condyle: report of case. J Oral Surg 1977;35:929–932.

73. Noren GD, Roche WC. Huge osteoma of the mandible: report of a case. J Oral Surg 1978;36:375–379.

74. Alling CC, Martinez MG, Ballard JB, et al. Osteoma cutis: clinical pathologic conference, case 5 II. J Oral Surg 1974;32:195–197.

75. Halse A, Roed-Petersen B, Lund K. Gardner's syndrome. J Oral Surg 1975;33:673–675.

76. McFarland PH, Scheetz WL, Knisley RE. Gardner's syndrome: report of two families. J Oral Surg 1968;26:632–638.

77. Neal CG. Multiple osteomas of the mandible associated with polyposis of the colon (Gardner's syndrome). Oral Surg 1969;28:628–631.

78. Witkop CJ. Gardner's syndrome and other osteognathodermal disorders with defects in parathyroid functions. J Oral Surg

79. Ramon Y, Horowitz I, Oberman M, et al. Osteochondroma of the coronoid process of the mandible. Oral Surg 1977;43:696–697.

80. Allan JH, Scott H. Osteochondroma of the mandible. Oral Surg 1974;37:556–565.

81. Chaudry AP, Robinovitch MR, Mitchell DF, et al. Chondrogenic tumors of the jaws. Am J Surg 1961;102:403–411.

82. Waldron CA, Shafer WG. Central giant cell reparative granuloma of the jaws. Am J Clin Pathol 1966;45:437–647.

83. Wesley RK, Horan M, Helfrick JF, et al. Central giant cell granuloma of the mandible: clinical pathologic conference, case 25 I. Oral Surg 1978;36:713.

84. Smith GA, Ward PH. Giant-cell lesions of the facial skeleton. Arch Otolaryngol 1978;104:186–190.

85. Curtis ML, Hatfield CG, Pierce JM. A destructive giant cell lesion of the mandible: report of a case. J Oral Surg 1979;37:432–436.

86. Chuong R, Kaban LB, Kozakewich H, et al. Central giant cell lesions of the jaws: a clinicopathologic study. J Oral Maxillofac Surg 1986;44:708–713.

87. Whitaker SB, Waldron CA. Central giant cell lesions of the jaws: a clinical, radiologic, and histopathologic study. Oral Surg Oral Med Oral Pathol 1993;75:199–208.

88. Pogrel MA. The use of liquid nitrogen cryotherapy in the management of locally aggressive bone lesions. J Oral Maxillofac Surg 1993;51:269–273.

89. MacIntosh RB. Surgical management of benign nonodontogenic lesions of the jaws. In: Peterson LJ et al, eds. Principles of Oral and Maxillo-Facial Surgery, Vol. 2. Philadelphia: Lippincott, 1992;713–753.

90. Lichtenstein L. Histiocytosis X: integration of eosinophilic granuloma of bone: Letterer-Siwe disease and Schuler-Christian disease as related manifestation of a single nosologic entity. Arch Pathol 1953;56:84–102.

91. Rapidis AD, Langdon JD, Harvey PW, et al. Histiocytosis X. Int J Oral Surg 1978;7:76–84.

92. Scott J, Finch LD. Histiocytosis X with oral lesions: report of case. J Oral Surg 1972;30:748–753.

93. Soskolne WA, Lustmann J, Azaz B. Histiocytosis X: report of six cases initially in the jaws. J Oral Surg 1977;35:30–33.

94. Sigala JL, Silverman S Jr, Brody HA, et al. Dental involvement of histiocytosis. Oral Surg 1972;33:42–48.

95. Lieberman PH et al. A reappraisal of eosinophilic granuloma of bone, Hand-Schuller-Christian disease and Letterer-Siwe syndrome. Medicine 1969;48:375–400.

96. Maw RB, McKean TW. Hand-Schuller-Christian disease: report of case. J Am Dent Assoc 1972;85:1353–1357.

97. Ragab RR, Rake O. Eosinophilic granuloma with bilateral involvement of both jaws. Int J Oral Surg 1975;4:73–79.

98. Chu T, D'Angio GJD, Favara B. Histiocytosis syndromes in children. Lancet 1987;1:208–209.

99. David R, Oria RA, Kumar R, et al. Radiologic feature of eosinophilic granuloma of bone. AJR 1989;153:1021–1026.

100. Waldron CA, Giansanti JS. Benign fibro-osseous lesions of the jaws: a clinical-radiologic-histologic review of sixty-five cases. II. Benign fibro-osseous lesions of periodontal ligament origin. Oral Surg 1973;35:340–350.

101. Cangiano R, Stratigos GE, Williams FA. Clinical and radiographic manifestations of fibro-osseous lesions of the jaws: report of five cases. J Oral Surg 1971;29:872–881.

102. Hayward JR, Melarkey DW, Megquier J. Monostotic fibrous dysplasia of the maxilla: report of cases. J Oral Surg 1973;31:625–627.

103. Eversole LR, Sabes WR, Rovin S. Fibrous dysplasia: a nosologic problem in the diagnosis of fibro-osseous lesions of the jaws. J Oral Pathol 1972;1:189–220.

104. Waldron CA, Giansanti JS. Benign fibro-osseous lesions of the jaws: a clinical-radiologic-histologic review of sixty-five cases. I. Fibrous dysplasia of the jaws. Oral Surg 1973;35:190–201.

105. Waldron CA, Giansanti JS. Benign fibro-osseous lesions of the jaws: a clinical-radiologic-histologic review of sixty-five cases. II. Benign fibro-osseous lesions of periodontal ligament origin. Oral Surg Oral Med Oral Pathol 1973;35:340–350.

106. Schlumberger HG. Fibrous dysplasia (ossifying fibroma) of maxilla and mandible. Am J Orthod 1946;32:579–587.

107. Sherman RS, Sternbergh WCA. Roentgen appearance of ossifying fibroma of bone. Radiology 1948;50:595–609.

108. Waldron CA. Ossifying fibroma of mandible: report of 2 cases. Oral Surg Oral Med Oral Pathol 1953;6:467–473.

109. Anderson JT, Dehner LP. Osteolytic form of Paget's disease. J Bone Joint Surg (Am) 1976;58:994–1000.

110. Gee JK, Zambito RF, Argentieri GW, et al. Paget's disease (osteitis deformans) of the mandible. J Oral Surg 1972;30:223–227.

111. Lund BA. Hemangioma of the mandible and maxilla. J Oral Surg 1972;22:234.

112. Macansh JD, Owen MD. Central cavernous hemangioma of the mandible: report of two cases. J Oral Surg 1972;30:293–296.

113. Kaban LB, Mulliken JB. Vascular anomalies of the maxillofacial region. J Oral Maxillofac Surg 1986;44:203–213.

114. Mulliken JB, Glowacki J. Hemangiomas and vascular malformations in infants and children: a classification based on endothelial characteristics. Plast Reconstr Surg 1982;69:412–422.

115. Boyd JB, Mulliken JB, Kaban LB, et al. Skeletal changes associated with vascular malformations. Plast Reconstr Surg 1984;74:789–795.

116. Ezekowitz RAB, Mulliken JB, Folkman J. Interferon alpha-2a for life threatening hemangiomas of infancy. N Engl J Med 1992;326:1456–1463.

117. Ricketts RR, Hatly RM, Corden BJ, et al. Interferon alpha-2a for the treatment of complex hemangiomas of infancy and childhood. Ann Surg 1994;219:605–612.

118. Shklar G, Meyer I. Neurogenic tumors of the mouth and jaws. Oral Surg 1963;16:1075–1093.

119. Shimura K, Allen EL, Kinoshita Y, et al. Central neurilemmoma of the mandible: report of a case and review of the literature. J Oral Surg 1973;31:363–367.

120. Prescott GH, White RF. Solitary, central neurofibroma of the mandible: report of case and review of the literature. J Oral Surg 1978;28:305.

121. Singer CF, Gienger GL, Kulborn TL. Solitary intraosseous neurofibroma involving the mandibular canal: report of case. J Oral Surg 1973;31:127–129.

122. Nolan R, Wood NK. Central squamous cell carcinoma of the mandible: report of a case. J Oral Surg 1976;34:260–264.

123. Coonar HS. Primary intraosseous carcinoma of maxilla. Br Dent J 1979;147:47–48.

124. Lapin R, Garfinkel AW, Catania AF, et al. Squamous cell carcinoma arising in a dentigerous cyst. J Oral Surg 1973;31:354–358.

125. Sigal R, Zagdanski AM, Schwaab G, et al. CT and MR imaging of squamous cell carcinoma of the tongue and floor of the mouth. RadioGraphics 1996;16:787–810.

126. Eversole LR. Malignant epithelial odontogenic tumors. Semin Diagn Pathol 1999;16(4):317–324.

127. Slootweg PJ, Muller H. Malignant ameloblastoma or ameloblastic carcinoma. Oral Surg Oral Med Oral Pathol 1984;57(2):168–176.

128. Nagai N, Takeshita N, Nagatsuka H, et al. Ameloblastic carcinoma: case report and review. J Oral Pathol Med 1991;20(9):460–463.

129. Shear M. Primary intra-alveolar epidermoid carcinoma of the jaw. J Pathol 1997;97:645–651.

130. Sirsat MV, Sampat MB, Shrikhande SE. Primary intra-alveolar squamous cell carcinoma of the mandible. Oral Surg 1973;35:366–371.

131. Fredrickson C, Cherrick HM. Central mucoepidermoid carcinoma of the jaws. J Oral Med 1978;30:80–85.

132. Schultz W, Whitten JB. Mucoepidermoid carcinoma in the mandible: report of case. J Oral Surg 1969;27:337–340.

133. Adler CI, Sotereanos GC, Valdivieso JG. Metastatic bronchogenic carcinoma of the maxilla: report of case. J Oral Surg 1973;31:543–546.

134. Al-Ani S. Metastatic tumors to the mouth: report of two cases. J Oral Surg 1973;31:120–122.

135. Appenzeller J, Weitzner S, Long GW. Hepatocellular carcinoma metastatic to the mandible: report of case and review of literature. J Oral Surg 1971;29:668–671.

136. Carter DG, Anderson EE, Currie DP. Renal cell carcinoma metastatic to the mandible. J Oral Surg 1977;35:992–993.

137. Cherrick HM, Demkee D. Metastatic carcinoma of the jaws. J Am Dent Assoc 1973;87:180–181.

138. Moss M, Shapiro DN. Mandibular metastasis of breast cancer. J Am Dent Assoc 1969;78:756–757.

139. Aniceto GS, Penin AG, de la Mata Pages R, Moreno JJM. Tumors metastatic to the mandible: analysis of nine cases and review of the literature. J Oral Maxillofac Surg 1990;48:246–251.

140. Hishberg A, Leibovich P, Buchner A. Metastatic tumors to the jawbones: an analysis of 390 cases. J Oral Pathol Med 1994;23:337–341.

141. Garrington GE, Scofield HH, Cornyn J, et al. Osteosarcoma of the jaws: analysis of 56 cases. Cancer 1967;20:377–391.

142. Caron AS, Hajdu SI, Strong EW. Osteogenic sarcoma of the facial and cranial bones: review of 43 cases. Am J Surg 1971;122:719–725.

143. Wilcox JW, Dukart RC, Kolodny SC, et al. Osteogenic sarcoma of the mandible. Review of the literature and report of case. J Oral Surg 1973;31:49–52.

144. Clark JL, Unni KK, Dahlin DC, et al. Osteosarcoma of the jaw. Cancer 1983;51:2311–2316.

145. Wannfors K, Hammarstrom L. Periapical lesions of mandibular bone: difficulties in early diagnostics. Oral Surg 1990;70:483–489.

146. Lindquist C, Teppo L, Sane J, et al. Osteosarcoma of the mandible: analysis of nine cases. J Oral Maxillofac Surg 1986;44:759–764.

147. Yagan R, Radivoyevitch M, Beillon EM. Involvement of the mandibular canal: early sign of osteogenic sarcoma of the mandible. Oral Surg 1985;60:56–60.

148. Taconis WK, van Rijssel TG. Fibrosarcoma of the jaws. Skeletal Radiol 1986;15:10–13.

149. Wright JA, Kuehn PG. Fibrosarcoma of the mandible. Oral Surg 1973;36:16–20.

150. Slater LJ. Odontogenic sarcoma and carcinosarcoma. Seminars Diagn Pathol 1999;16:325–332.

151. Borhgelli RF, Barros RE, Zampieri J. Ewing sarcoma of the mandible: report of case. J Oral Surg 1978;36:473–475.

152. Carl W, Schaaf NG, Gaeta J, et al. Ewing's sarcoma. J Oral Surg 1971;31:472–478.

153. Wood RE, Nortje CJ, Hesseling P, Grotepas F. Ewing's tumor of the jaw. Oral Surg 1990;69:120–127.

154. Yalcin S, Turoglu HT, Ozdamar S, et al. Ewing's tumor of the mandible. Oral Surg 1993;76:362–367.

155. Steg RF, Dahlin DC, Gores RJ. Malignant lymphoma of the manible and maxillary region. Oral Surg Oral Med Oral Pathol 1959;12:128.

156. Keyes GC, Balaban FS, Lattanzi DA. Periradicular lymphoma: differentiation from inflammation. Oral Surg 1988;66:230–235.

157. Cohen MA, Bender S, Struthers PJ. Hodgkin's disease of the jaws. Oral Surg Oral Med Oral Pathol 1984;57:413–417.

158. Miller CD, Goltry RR, Shenasky JH. Multiple myeloma involving the jaws and oral soft tissue. Oral Surg 1969;28:603–609.

159. Tabachnick TT, Levine B. Multiple myeloma involving the jaws and oral soft tissue. J Oral Surg 1976;34:931–933.

160. Tamir R, Pick AI, Calderon S. Plasmacytoma of the mandible: a primary presentation of multiple myeloma. J Oral Maxillofac Surg 1992;50:408–413.

161. Furutani M, Ohnishi M, Tanaka Y. Mandibular involvement in patients with multiple myeloma. J Oral Maxillofac Surg 1994;52:23–25.

162. Curtis AB. Childhood leukemias: osseous change in jaws on panoramic dental radiographs. J Am Dent Assoc 1971;88:844–847.

163. Michaud M, Baehner RL, Bixler D, et al. Oral manifestations of acute leukemia in children. J Am Dent Assoc 1977;95:1145–1150.

164. Sela MN, Pisanti S. Early diagnosis and treatment of patients with leukemia: a dental problem. J Oral Med 1977;32:46–50.

165. Shafer WG, Hine MK, Levy BM. A Textbook of Oral Pathology, 4th ed. Philadelphia: WB Saunders, 1983;479–510.

166. Parker ME. Infection of the teeth and jaws. In: Farman AG, Nortje CJ, Wood RE, eds. Oral and Maxillofacial Diagnostic Imaging. St. Louis: Mosby Year Book, 1993;181–209.

167. Hudson JW. Osteomyelitis of the jaws: a 50-year perspective. J Oral Maxillofac Surg 1993;51:1294–1301.

168. Rohlin M. Diagnostic value of bone scintigraphy in osteomyelitis of the mandible. Oral Surg Oral Med Oral Pathol 1993;75:650–657.

169. Kaneda T, Minami M, Ozawa K, et al. Magnetic resonance imaging of osteomyelitis in the mandible: comparative study with other radiological modalities. Oral Surg Oral Med Oral Pathol 1995;79:634–640.

170. Unger E, Moldofsky P, Gatenby R, Hartz W, Broder G. Diagnosis of osteomyelitis by MR imaging. AJR 1988;150:605–610.
171. Kaneda T, Minami M, Ozawa K, et al. Magnetic resonance appearance of bone marrow in the mandible at different ages. Oral Surg Oral Med Oral Pathol 1996;82:229–233.
172. Morrison WB, Schweitzer ME, Block GW, et al. Diagnosis of osteomyelitis: utility of fat-suppressed contrast-enhanced MR imaging. Radiology 1993;189:251–257.
173. Wood RE, Nortje CH, Grotepass F, et al. Periostitis ossificans versus Garre's osteomyelitis. 1. What did Garre's really say? Oral Surg 1988;65:773–777.
174. Nortje CH, Wood RE, Grotepass F, et al. Periostitis ossificans versus Garre's osteomyelitis. 2. Radiologic analysis of 93 cases in the jaws. Oral Surg 1988;66:249–260.
175. Sephariadou-Mavropoulo T, Yannoulopolous A. Tuberculosis of the jaws. Oral Maxillofac Surg 1986;44:158–162.
176. Wood RE, Housego T, Nortje CJ, Padayachee A. Tuberculous osteomyelitis in the mandible of a child. Pediatr Dent 1987;9:317–320.
177. Van Merkesteyn JPR, Groot RH, Bras J, McCarrol RS, Bakker DJ. Diffuse sclerosing osteomyelitis of the mandible: a new concept of its etiology. Oral Surg Oral Med Oral Pathol 1990;70:414–419.
178. Jacobsson S. Diffuse sclerosing osteomyelitis of the mandible. Int J Oral Surg 1984;13:363–385.
179. Marx RE, Carlson ER, Smith BR, Toraya N. Isolation of *Actinomyces* species and *Eikenella corrodens* from patients with chronic diffuse sclerosing osteomyelitis. J Oral Maxillofac Surg 1994;52:26–33.
180. Marx RE. Osteoradionecrosis: a new concept in its pathology. J Oral Surg 1983;1:283–288.
181. Marx RE, Johson RD. Studies in the radiobiology of osteoradionecrosis and their clinical significance. Oral Surg Oral Med Oral Pathol 1987;64:379–390.
182. MacClatchey KD. Odontogenic lesions: tumors and cysts. In Batsakis JG, ed. Tumors of the Head and Neck: Clinical and Pathological Considerations, 2nd ed. Baltimore: Williams & Wilkins, 1979;210–238.
183. Eversole LR, Rovin S. Differential radiographic diagnosis of lesions of the jaw bones. Radiology 1972;105:277–284.
184. Hertzanu Y, Mendelsohn DB, Cohn M. Computed tomography of mandibular ameloblastoma. J Comput Assist Tomogr 1984;8:220–223.
185. Wood NK, Goaz PW. Differential Diagnosis of Oral and Maxillofacial Lesions, 5th ed. St. Louis: Mosby Year Book, 1997;238–518.
186. Belkin BA, Papageorage MB, Fakitsas J, Bankoff MS. A comparative study of magnetic resonance imaging versus computed tomography for the evaluation of maxillary and mandibular tumors. J Oral Maxillofac Surg 1988;46:1039–1047.
187. Cohn MA, Mendelsohn DB. CT and MR imaging of myxofibroma of the jaws. J Comput Assist Tomogr 1990;14:281–285.
188. Minami M, Kaneda T, Yamamoto H, et al. Ameloblastoma in the maxillomandibular region: MR imaging. Radiology 1992;184:389–393.
189. Kaneda T, Minami M, Ozawa K, et al. Magnetic resonance imaging of osteomyelitis in the mandible: comparative study with other radiological modalities. Oral Surg Oral Med Oral Pathol 1995;79:634–640.
190. Minami M, Kaneda T, Ozawa K, et al. Cystic lesions of the maxillomandibular region: MR imaging distinction of odontogenic keratocysts and ameloblastomas from other cysts. AJR 1996;166:943–949.
191. Langlaris RP. Radiology of the jaws. In: Delbalso AM, ed. Maxillofacial Imaging. Philadelphia: WB Saunders, 1990;313–373.
192. Reeder MM, Bradley WG Jr. Gamuts in Radiology, 3rd ed. New York: Springer-Verlag, 1993;104–110.
193. Kaneda T, Minami M, Curtin HD, et al. Maxillomandibular lesions: assessment of gadolinium-enhanced MR images. Radiology 1998;209(P):613–614.
194. Kaneda T, Minami M, Curtin HD, et al. Dental bur fragments causing metal artifacts on MR images. AJNR 1998;19:317–319.
195. Grahnen H, Lindahl B. Supernumerary teeth in the permanent dentition: a frequency study. Odont Rev 1961;12:290.
196. Grimanis GA, Kyriakides AT, Spyropoulos ND. A survey on supernumerary molars. Quintess Int 1991;22:989.
197. Yusolf WZ. Non-syndrome multiple supernumerary teeth: literature review. J Can Dent Assoc 1990;56:147.
198. Al Emran S. Prevalence of hypodontia and developmental malformation of permanent teeth in Saudi Arabian school children. Br J Orthod 1990;17:115.
199. Thorburn DN, Ferguson MM. Familial ogee roots, mobility, oligodontia and microdontia. Oral Surg Oral Med Oral Pathol 1992;74:576–581.
200. O'Dowling IB, McNamara TG. Congenital absence of permanent teeth among Irish school-children. J Ir Dent Assoc 1990;36:136–138.
201. Garn SM, Lewis AB, Kerewsky BS. The magnitude and implications of the relationship between tooth size and body size. Arch Oral Biol 1968;13:129.
202. Soames JV, Kuyebi TA. A radicular dens invaginatus. Br Dent J 1982;152:308.
203. Yip WW. The prevalence of dens invaginatus. Oral Surg 1974;38:80.
204. Pope FM et al. Ehlers-Danlos syndrome type 1 with novel dental features. J Oral Pathol Med 1992;21:418–421.
205. Moskow BS, Canut PM. Studies on root enamel. II. Enamel pearls: a review of their morphology, localization, nomenclature, occurrence, classification. J Clin Periodontol 1990;17:275–281.
206. Witkop CJ Jr, Saulk JJ. Heritable defects of enamel. In: Stewart RE, Prescott GA, eds. Oral Facial Genetics. St. Louis: CV Mosby, 1976;151–226.
207. Crawford PJ, Aldred MJ. X-linked amelogenesis imperfecta: presentation of two kindreds and a review of the literature. Oral Surg 1992;73:449.
208. Via WF Jr. Enamel defects induced by trauma during tooth formation. Oral Surg 1968;25:49.
209. Witkop CJ Jr. Amelogencsis imperfecta, dentinogenesis imperfecta and dentin dysplasia revisited: problems in classification. J Oral Pathol 1988;17:547.
210. Schwartz S, Tsipouras P. Oral findings in osteogenesis imperfecta. Oral Surg 1984;57:161.
211. Ciola B, Bahn SL, Goviea GL. Radiographic manifestations of an unusual combination of type 1 and type 2 dentin dysplasia. Oral Surg Oral Med Oral Pathol 1978;45:317–322.
212. Wood RE, Lee P. Analysis of the oral manifestations of systemic sclerosis (scleroderma). Oral Surg Oral Med Oral Pathol 1988;65(2):172–178.
213. White SC, Frey NW, Blaschke DD, et al. Oral radiographic changes in patients with progressive systemic sclerosis (scleroderma). J Am Dent Assoc 1977;94(6):1178–1182.
214. Alexandridis C, White SC. Periodontal ligament changes in patients with progressive systemic sclerosis. Oral Surg Oral Med Oral Pathol 1984;58(1):113–118.

# 18

# Temporomandibular Joint

*P.L. Westesson, Mika Yamamoto,*
*Tsukasa Sano, and Tomohiro Okano*

The purpose of an imaging assessment of the temporomandibular joint (TMJ) is to graphically depict clinically suspected disorders of the joint. For many years, plain film radiography done mainly in a transcranial projection was the most commonly used method of making this assessment. This modality has major limitations because it is sensitive only to changes in the osseous components and depicts just the lateral aspect of the joint. With the evolution of newer imaging modalities such as arthrography, computed tomography (CT), and, most importantly, magnetic resonance (MR) imaging, the soft tissues of the joint could be appreciated. This allowed a better understanding of the anatomy and pathophysiology of internal derangements related to disk displacement.[1]

This chapter begins with descriptions of the anatomy and function of the TMJ and then provides an overview of the various imaging modalities available for evaluating the TMJ. Because most TMJ imaging is directed toward assessment of internal derangements or related degenerative joint changes, the sections addressing imaging methods emphasize the key findings in these important disorders. A variety of miscellaneous diseases that affect the TMJ are then covered, and an algorithm for imaging patients with TMJ problems is given.

## ANATOMY OF THE TMJ

Interpreting TMJ imaging studies requires an understanding of the pathophysiology of the joint and a knowledge of both normal and pathologic anatomy of the joint and surrounding structures. Therefore, a description of joint anatomy, joint pathology, function, and dysfunction is presented in some detail.

The mandible and the temporal bone comprise the osseous components of the TMJ. The head of the mandibular condyle comprises the inferior component of the joint, and the temporal bone contributes the glenoid fossa and articular tubercle, forming the superior osseous (or skull base) part of the joint (Fig. 18-1). Unlike most other joints of the body, which have cartilaginous coverings, the articulating surfaces

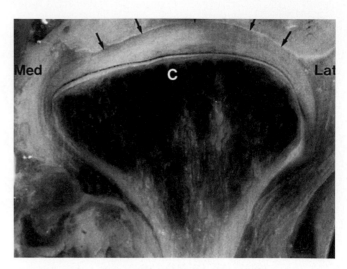

**FIGURE 18-2**   Normal TMJ in coronal section. The disk (*arrows*) is crescent-shaped and located over the condyle. Medially and laterally, the disk is attached to the condyle and capsule. The condyle (*C*) is indicated.

of the TMJ are covered by a thin layer of dense fibrous tissue.

The TMJ disk is a biconcave fibrous structure located between the mandibular condyle and the temporal component of the joint. The disk is round to oval, with a thick periphery and a thin central part. The mediolateral dimension of the disk is approximately 20 mm. In a sagittal section the normal disk appears biconcave, with the anterior and posterior thicker parts of the disk, respectively, referred to as the anterior and posterior bands.[2] In the normal joint the posterior band is located over the condyle, and the central thin zone is located between the condyle and the posterior part of the articular tubercle (Fig. 18-1). The anterior band is located under the articular tubercle. In the coronal plane, a section through the disk is crescent-shaped (Fig. 18-2). A joint capsule surrounds the joint, emerging from the temporal bone and extending like a funnel inferiorly to attach to the neck of the condyle. The medial and lateral edges of the disk attach to the capsule and then to the mandible at the inferior edge of the medial and lateral poles of the condyle (Fig. 18-2). Posteriorly, the disk is attached to the temporal bone and to the condyle by the posterior disk attachment. This attachment is extremely important in internal derangements of the TMJ. This region has also been referred to as the bilaminar zone or the retrodiskal tissue. The structure consists of loose fibrous connective and elastic tissue components. The posterior disk attachment has traditionally been called the bilaminar zone because initial histologic studies indicated that the upper part was elastic tissue and the lower part consisted of more connective tissue. However, more recent histologic studies have failed to confirm the bilaminar nature of the posterior disk attachment. Despite this, the term *bilaminar zone* continues to be used in both clinical and scientific work. The bilaminar zone also contains many small blood vessels. Anteriorly, the disk is attached to the joint capsule, and in the anteromedial portion of the joint the disk also merges with the upper head of the lateral pterygoid muscle.

There are two joint spaces, or compartments. The superior space separates the glenoid and articular eminence

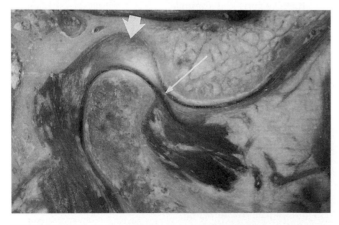

**FIGURE 18-1**   Normal TMJ in sagittal section. Biconcave disk in the normal superior position. The posterior band of the disk (*thick arrow*) is lying over the condyle. The central thin zone of the disk (*thin arrow*) is between the anterior prominence of the condyle and the articular eminence.

of the temporal bone from the disk and its attachments. The inferior joint space separates the disk and its attachments from the condyle of the mandible. The anterior recess is a small space in the inferior joint compartment anterior to the condyle. The posterior recess is the part of the inferior joint space posterior to the condyle. The lower part of the bilaminar zone (posterior disk attachment) curves downward to attach to the condylar neck and thus forms the posterior boundary of the posterior recess of the inferior joint compartment.

## FUNCTION OF THE TMJ

The function of the TMJ is complex because the upper and lower joint compartments principally act as two small joints within this same joint capsule. This allows for proportionally greater movement of the TMJ in relation to the actual size of the joint. The principal function of the disk is to permit relatively large movements within a small joint while maintaining stability. Rotation and translation occur in both the upper and lower joint spaces. However, translation occurs predominantly in the upper space, and rotation is more evident in the lower joint space. In the initial phase of jaw opening, the condyle rotates in the lower joint compartment. After this initial rotation, translation occurs in the upper and subsequently in the lower joint space. During translation, the condyle and the disk translate (slide) together under the articular tubercle. During all mandibular movements, the central thin part of the disk is located

between the condyle and the articular tubercle. This suggests that the thick periphery of the disk and the thick posterior and anterior bands act as functional guides for the joint. This normal joint function can be identified in anatomic specimens of the TMJ (Fig. 18-3).

## INTERNAL DERANGEMENT RELATED TO DISPLACEMENT OF THE DISK

*Internal derangement* is a general orthopedic term implying a mechanical fault that interferes with the smooth action of a joint.[3] Internal derangement is thus a functional diagnosis, and for the TMJ the most common internal derangement is displacement of the disk.[4-9] Most often the disk displaces in an anterior, anterolateral, or anteromedial direction. Thus the posterior band of the disk prolapses anteriorly, relative to the superior surface of the condyle (Figs. 18-4 and 18-5), instead of remaining in position between the condyle and glenoid fossa. As a consequence, the condyle is positioned under the posterior disk attachment rather than under the disk, and the condyle closes on the posterior attachment (bilaminar zone or retrodiskal tissues) rather than on the disk itself. The central thin part of the disk lies inferior to the articular tubercle.

Studies have shown that the disk frequently is also displaced in a medial (Fig. 18-6) or lateral direction.[10-13] Posterior disk displacement (Fig. 18-7) does occur, but it is rare. When present, it is frequently seen in combination with

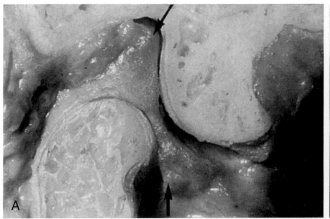

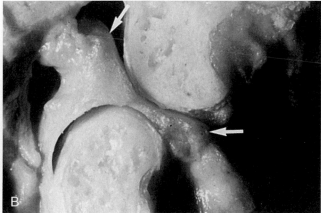

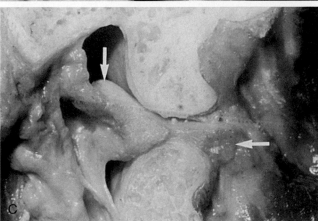

FIGURE 18-3  Normal TMJ function. **A,** Normal TMJ in the closed-mouth position. The anterior and posterior bands of the disk are indicated by arrows. **B,** Normal TMJ in the half-open mouth position. Anterior and posterior bands of the disk are indicated by arrows. **C,** Normal TMJ in the open-mouth position. Anterior and posterior bands of the disk are indicated by arrows.

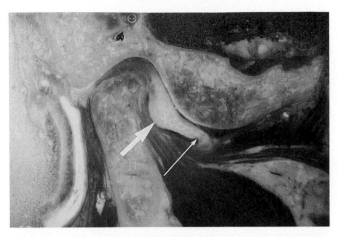

**FIGURE 18-4** Anterior disk displacement. The disk is anteriorly displaced, with its posterior band (*thick arrow*) located forward of the condyle. Note that the central thin zone of the disk (*thin arrow*) is separated from the anterior prominence of the condyle.

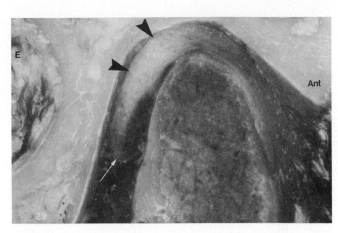

**FIGURE 18-7** Posterior disk displacement. The disk (*arrowheads*) is posterior to the condyle. The external auditory canal (*E*) and anterior (*Ant*) are indicated for orientation. Inferiorly and posteriorly there is folding of the disk (*thin arrow*) similar to what is seen with anterior disk displacement.

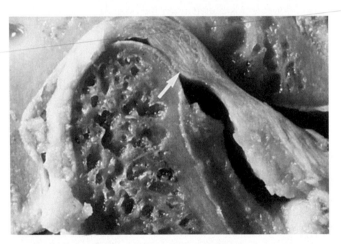

**FIGURE 18-5** Anterior disk displacement. The disk is anteriorly displaced, with its posterior band (*arrow*) located slightly forward of the condyle.

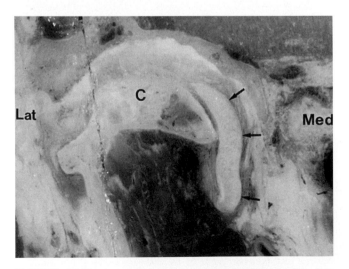

**FIGURE 18-6** Coronal section of TMJ showing medial disk displacement. The disk is indicated by arrows. The condyle (*C*) is sclerotic.

medial disk displacement. A general classification of the different types of disk displacement of the TMJ is shown in Box 18-1. Pure lateral and pure medial sideways displacements of the disk also occur, but not as commonly as in combination with anterior displacement.[11–13] The combination of anterior and lateral or medial displacement is called rotational displacement, whereas pure lateral or pure medial displacement is called sideways displacement.[11]

The functional aspects of disk displacement include displacement with or without reduction. The functional categories of internal derangement are illustrated in Figure 18-8. In disk displacement with reduction (Fig. 18-8B) the disk is anteriorly displaced in the closed-mouth position but reverts to a normal superior position during opening. In disk displacement without reduction (Fig. 18-8C) the disk lies anterior to the condyle during all mandibular movements, and the normal condyle–disk relationship is not reestablished.

## Disk Displacement with Reduction

When a displaced disk reduces to a normal position, a click is usually heard. When the jaw closes, the disk again

---

**BOX 18-1**

**TERMINOLOGY FOR DESCRIBING THE POSTION OF THE DISK**

| | |
|---|---|
| Normal | Superior |
| Abnormal | Anterior, partial or complete |
| | Anteromedial rotation |
| | Anterolateral rotation |
| | Medial sideways |
| | Lateral sideways |
| | Posterior |

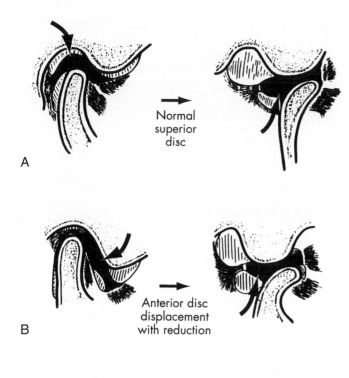

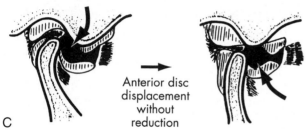

Normal
superior
disc

A

Anterior disc
displacement
with reduction

B

Anterior disc
displacement
without
reduction

C

**FIGURE 18-8** Schematic drawing of a normal TMJ and different categories of internal derangement. The disk is black and is indicated by the curved arrows. **A,** Normal. **B,** Anterior displacement with reduction. **C,** Anterior displacement without reduction.

displaces anteriorly, usually during the last phase of the closing movement of the jaw, and again a click is commonly heard. The closing click usually is less prominent than the opening click. The cyclic nature of disk displacement was described by Ireland in 1951.[14] The clicking sound has been shown to be caused by the impact of the condyle hitting the temporal bone component of the articulation after the condyle has passed under the posterior band of the disk.[15, 16]

## Disk Displacement without Reduction

In disk displacement without reduction (Fig. 18-8C) the disk remains displaced relative to the condylar head, regardless of the jaw position. In the initial stages of this condition, jaw opening is typically limited and the jaw deviates to the side of the affected joint. However, this clinical characteristic is typical only during the initial (early) phase; with time, the opening capacity of the TMJ increases and the jaw no longer deviates to the affected side. This is the result of stretching or progressive elongation of the posterior disk attachment and, to a lesser extent, deformation

of the disk itself. In the early stage, disk displacement without reduction is usually not associated with joint sounds.

## Disk Deformity

The normal disk is biconcave when viewed in the sagittal plane (Fig. 18-3). In the early stages of internal derangement the disk remains normal in shape. However, the displaced disk begins to deform, as noted by thickening of the posterior band and shortening of the entire anteroposterior length of the disk (Fig. 18-9).[4, 9, 17–19] Additionally, both the central thin part and the anterior band decrease in size. The end result is a biconvex disk configuration and a stretched, elongated, and thinned posterior disk attachment. The gross changes of the disk are associated with histologic alterations within the disk that lead to metaplastic hyaline cartilage, hyalinization, and accumulation of foci of calcium deposits and abnormal collagen patterns.[20, 21] Changes also occur in the posterior disk attachment itself, leading to fibrosis and narrowing of vessels.[22, 23] Histologic studies of the posterior disk attachment in joints with disk displacement have shown narrowing of the arterial lumen, increased density of fibroblasts, and hyalinization of loose connective tissue.[24]

## Late-Stage Changes Following Disk Displacement

In the late or chronic stages of disk displacement without reduction, the disk is deformed and has a stretched, torn, or detached posterior attachment; communications between the upper and lower joint spaces (perforation) are often seen.[8, 9, 19, 25] Most commonly the perforations are found in the posterior disk attachment, at its junction with the disk itself (Fig. 18-10). Infrequently, perforations are found in the disk per se.[19] Thus, although traditionally this condition has been designated *perforation of the disk*, this is not anatomically correct, as the perforations are usually found in the posterior disk attachment rather than in the disk proper.

Osseous changes involving the condyle and temporal

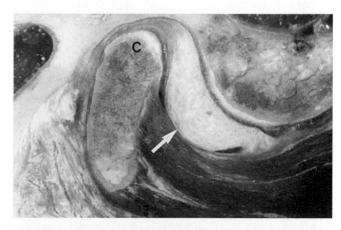

**FIGURE 18-9** Anterior displacement and deformation of the disk. The disk (*arrow*) is biconvex. The condyle (*C*) articulates with the posterior disk attachment.

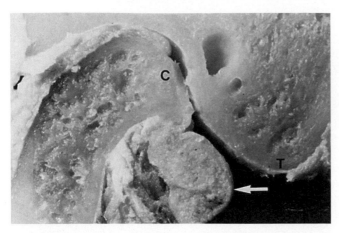

**FIGURE 18-10**    Anterior displacement and extensive deformation of the disk (*arrow*), with perforation of the posterior disk attachment. The condyle (*C*) is flattened, with an anterior osteophyte and surface irregularities.

bone often occur as sequelae of disk displacement.[7-9, 18, 26] Osseous changes consist of flattening and osteophytosis of the mandibular condyle and flattening of the temporal component of the articulation. These changes are more commonly observed in the lateral part of the joint and can be detected on plain film imaging. It should be noted that osseous changes are relatively late findings in the disease process, and it is often difficult to differentiate radiographically between advanced remodeling and degenerative joint disease.

## Clinical Aspects of Internal Derangement

The preceding classification of disk position and function is based only on anatomic and functional aspects. In the clinical setting the patient's history, signs, and symptoms must be incorporated into the staging of the disease. Patients may complain of pain or of clicks when opening and closing the mouth. Physical examination may show tenderness on palpation of the joint or associated muscles. Palpable clicks or crepitus on movement of the jaw may be clinically evident, and abnormalities of occlusion or deviation of the jaw on opening may also suggest TMJ abnormality.

However, the clinical assessment of the TMJ has definite limitations. Multiple studies have shown that the accuracy of the physical examination in predicting the status of the joint is about 70%.[27-33] The intensity and location of pain in a study of more than 200 patients did not distinguish patients with internal derangement from those without internal derangement, and there was no consistent relationship between occlusion and the status of the joint. These studies indicate that physical examination alone is not reliable in determining the status of the joint.[28-34]

The situation is further complicated by the fact that clinical signs of TMJ internal derangement are relatively common in the general population. An epidemiologic study of more than 400 individuals ranging in age from 28 to 73 years showed clinical evidence of internal derangement in 39%. Most of these individuals had functional symptoms with clicking or limitation of opening, but the majority did not have any pain associated with the dysfunction. Studies of

asymptomatic volunteers using both arthrography and MR imaging have shown disk displacement in approximately 20% to 25% of this population.[35-37] The finding of anatomic abnormalities in the joints of asymptomatic individuals is not unique to the TMJ. Similar observations have been shown in MR studies of the knee, cervical spine, and lumbar spine.[38-42]

The prevalence of disk displacement in symptomatic individuals is much higher than in a normal population.[43] In view of the high incidence of displacement in asymptomatic patients, the precise relationship of symptoms to the displacement is difficult to define. Disk displacement has been found in approximately 80% of patients with symptoms of TMD referred for MR imaging.[44] Several forms of disk displacement have been demonstrated in up to one third of asymptomatic volunteers.[44-46] One study analyzing the type of disk displacement in patients and asymptomatic volunteers showed that most of the volunteers have early stage disk displacement, and more severe displacements are seen in symptomatic patients.[47] However, complete disk dislocations are found incidentally in patients without complaints referable to the TMJ. Perhaps further investigation of these apparently asymptomatic patients could determine some degree of joint dysfunction, but clearly more work is necessary before the precise relationship between disk position and pain can be confidently defined.

Among patients presenting with TMJ symptoms, there is a significant prevalence of young females, and in the clinical population the female/male ratio has been between 5:1 and 10:1. The reason for the female dominance among TMJ patients is not fully understood. Cadaver studies have found that approximately 50% of elderly individuals have an internal derangement, with no significant difference between the sexes.[48]

Because of the difficulty in the clinical evaluation of a potential disk displacement, imaging must be done to define the anatomy of the joint and to determine the relationship of the disk to the condyle. The purpose of an imaging study is to identify and characterize the anatomy in a patient who presents with symptoms. Because of the overlap of morphologic abnormalities in symptomatic and asymptomatic individuals, imaging findings should always be interpreted in light of clinical findings. Similarly, the choice of imaging studies must depend on the clinical evaluation, and an algorithm for TMJ imaging can be made based upon prior clinical and imaging experience.

An appropriate patient evaluation integrates the imaging and clinical findings. A workable classification of TMJ disorders, related to internal derangement, is also necessary for communication among clinicians and radiologists. The classification developed by Wilkes[9] encompasses clinical, radiographic, and morphologic observations and categorizes internal derangement into early, intermediate, and late stages. This classification is presented in Box 18-2.

## IMAGING

### Transcranial and Transmaxillary Projections

The most common and most well-established plain film technique for examination of the TMJ is the transcranial

## BOX 18-2

### CLASSIFICATION OF INTERNAL DERANGEMENT

**Early Stage**

Clinical — No significant mechanical symptoms other than reciprocal clicking (early in opening movement, late in closing movement, and soft in intensity); no pain or limitation in opening motion

Radiologic — Slight forward displacement; good anatomic contour of disk; normal tomograms

Surgical — Normal anatomic form; slight anterior displacement; passive incoordination (clicking) demonstrable

**Early-Intermediate Stage**

Clinical — First few episodes of pain; occasional joint tenderness and related temporal headaches; beginning of major mechanical problems; increase in intensity of clicking sounds; joint sounds later in opening movement; and beginning transient subluxations or joint catching and locking

Radiologic — Slight forward displacement; slight thickening of posterior edge or beginning of anatomic deformity of disk; normal tomograms

Surgical — Anterior displacement; early anatomic deformity (slight to mild thickening of posterior edge); well-defined central articulating area

**Intermediate Stage**

Clinical — Multiple episodes of pain, joint tenderness, temporal headaches, major mechanical symptoms: transient catching, locking, and sustained locking (closed locks); restriction of motion; difficulty (pain) with function

Radiologic — Anterior displacement with significant anatomic deformity or prolapse of disk (moderate to marked thickening of posterior edge); normal tomograms

Surgical — Marked anatomic deformity with displacement; variable adhesions (anterior, lateral, and posterior recesses); no hard-tissue changes

**Intermediate-Late Stage**

Clinical — Characterized by chronicity with variable and episodic pain, headaches, variable restriction of motion; undulating course

Radiologic — Increase in severity over intermediate stage; abnormal tomograms; early to moderate degenerative remodeling; hard-tissue changes

Surgical — Increase in severity over intermediate stage; hard-tissue degenerative remodeling changes of both bearing surfaces; osteophytic projections; multiple adhesions (lateral, anterior, and posterior recesses); no perforation of disk or attachment

**Late Stage**

Clinical — Characterized by crepitus on examination; scraping, grating, grinding; variable and episodic pain; chronic restriction of motion; and difficulty with function

Radiologic — Anterior displacement; perforation with simultaneous filling of upper and lower compartments; filling defects; gross anatomic deformity of disk and hard tissues; abnormal tomograms; essentially degenerative arthritic changes

Surgical — Gross degenerative changes of disk and hard tissues; perforation of posterior attachments; erosions of bearing surfaces; multiple adhesions equivalent to degenerative arthritis (sclerosis, flattening, and anvil-shaped condyle, osteophytic projections, and subcortical cystic formation).

From Wilkes CH. Internal derangement of the TMJ. Pathologic variations. Arch Otolaryngol Head Neck Surg 1989;115:469-477.

projection (Fig. 18-11). The lateral aspect of the joint is well visualized, but the central and medial parts of the joint are not clearly seen because the x-ray beam is not tangent to these articular surfaces. This disadvantage is partly compensated for by the fact that most of the early osseous changes occur laterally in the joint.[49]

It has been recommended that, in addition to the transcranial projection, an anteroposterior projection should be used to depict the central and medial parts of the condyle. A transmaxillary projection (Fig. 18-12) or a transorbital projection also is suggested.[50]

## Tomography

Complex motion tomography has been recommended for detection of early osseous changes (Fig. 18-13). Studies have demonstrated that a clearer depiction of the osseous anatomy can be gained from tomography than can be gained from transcranial radiography.[51] Tomography may also be performed in the coronal plane, providing information about the medial and lateral poles of the condyle, which are usually not adequately depicted on the sagittal tomograms. The disadvantage of tomography is the rather large radiation dose delivered to the lens of the eye. To a large extent, tomography has been replaced by CT, which probably represents the most effective modality for demonstrating osseous abnormalities.

## Arthrography

### Development of TMJ Arthrography

Early attempts at TMJ arthrography were undertaken by Nørgaard in the 1940s.[52, 53] However, this procedure was not adopted by many clinicians. It was considered technically difficult and painful for the patient, and the information gathered was not considered of great value for treatment planning and evaluation of prognosis. Only a few descriptions of TMJ arthrography appeared in the literature over the ensuing 25 years.

Toward the end of the 1970s several articles appeared, describing the clinical and arthrographic characteristics of internal derangement related to displacement of the disk.[7, 8, 54–56] These arthrographic studies were actually the first to depict displacement of the disk, a pathologic entity that had been suspected earlier.[14, 57-61] During the following years, considerable enthusiasm developed for TMJ arthrography, and a large number of publications describing the usefulness of the technique appeared. The changed attitude toward TMJ arthrography can be traced to the following factors: (1) use of an image intensifier to facilitate joint puncture and to study and document joint dynamics, (2) identification of disk displacement as a common cause of TMJ pain and dysfunction, and, probably most important, (3) introduction of new, conservative surgical methods for treating disk displacement.[7, 8, 54, 55, 62–66] These newer treatment methods required accurate information about the status and function of the joint. The use of a nonionic contrast

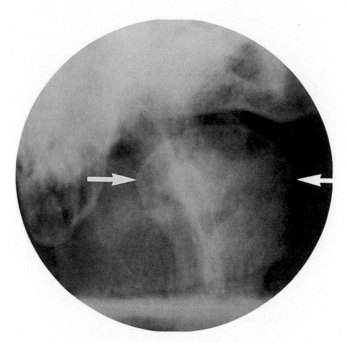

**FIGURE 18-12** Transmaxillary radiograph of TMJ. The lateral and medial poles of the condyles are indicated by arrows.

medium, which made the examination less painful, and the combination of arthrography and tomography, also influenced the increased use of arthrography.[6, 25]

### Single- and Double-Contrast Arthrography

Injection of contrast medium into only the lower space (Fig. 18-14) is a simplification of the original arthrographic technique, in which contrast medium was injected into both upper and lower joint spaces.[5, 54, 55] This simplification

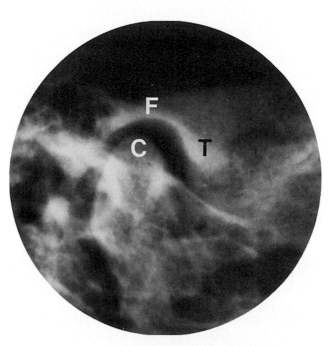

**FIGURE 18-11** Transcranial radiograph of TMJ. The condyle (C), fossa (F), and tubercle (T) are indicated.

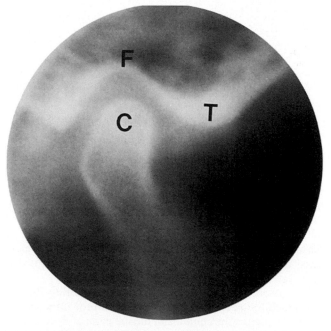

**FIGURE 18-13** Sagittal tomogram of TMJ. The condyle (C), fossa (F), and tubercle (T) are indicated.

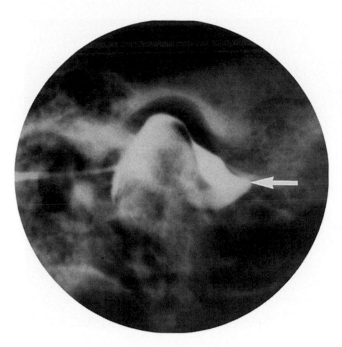

**FIGURE 18-14**   Lower compartment arthrogram of TMJ showing anterior disk displacement. The prominent anterior recess (*arrow*) of the lower joint space is a sign of disk displacement.

further popularized the use of arthrography; currently, single-contrast lower-compartment arthrography is the most commonly used arthrographic technique.[5, 54]

Double-contrast arthrography (Fig. 18-15) is a variant of arthrography in which injection of iodine contrast medium is combined with injection of air.[6, 17, 25, 56, 67, 68] The double-contrast study is superior to the single-contrast study in its demonstration of the configuration of the disk and the posterior disk attachment (Figs. 18-15 and 18-16). However, the double-contrast technique is technically more difficult to perform, because it requires cannulation of both the upper and lower joint spaces and the injection of both contrast medium and air.

### Indications and Contraindications

MR imaging has almost completely replaced arthrography for establishing the position of the disk relative to the condyle, and many institutions have eliminated arthrography as a diagnostic procedure. Arthrography can still be done to assess the position and function of the disk in patients with pain and dysfunction suggesting internal derangement. Perforations of the disk or retrodiskal attachments can be identified as contrast injected into the inferior compartment passes freely into the superior compartment of the joint. Arthrography can be used in patients with TMJ disk displacement with reduction to determine the mandibular position that reestablishes a normal condyle–disk relationship.[54, 69] The purpose of this would be to establish the optimum position for initiating protrusive splint therapy (conservative therapy).[54, 69] Infrequently, arthrography is performed to delineate loose bodies within the joint spaces, for diagnostic aspiration of joint fluid, for intraarticular injection of cortisone, or for evaluation of the TMJ after trauma.

There are indications that arthrography occasionally relieves patients' symptoms.[70] Manipulation and lavage of the joint was shown to improve mobility and decrease pain in a small clinical study.[70] The mechanism is not fully understood, and the precise indications for therapeutic arthrography must await further studies.

An infrequent contraindication for TMJ arthrography is infection in the preauricular area, which could potentially result in contamination of the joint during the arthrographic procedure. In patients with previous reactions to contrast medium, other modalities such as MR imaging should be considered. However, arthrography has been performed on such patients without any premedication, and there was no untoward reaction. Bleeding disorders and anticoagulation medication also are relative contraindications to arthrography.

### Radiologic Equipment and Procedure

A fluoroscopic table or a C-arm unit with an image intensifier is necessary equipment for this study. Because of the small size of the TMJ, it is also useful to be able to magnify the image to about three times its normal size. The capability for spot filming and videotape recording is valuable for documentation and the evaluation of joint dynamics. For double-contrast arthrography, tomography is also needed.

The examination is explained to the patient. The patient is placed on the tabletop in a laterally recumbent position, and the head is oriented so that the side to be injected faces up. The head is slightly tilted, and the transcranial projection is optimized with fluoroscopy. Opening and closing movements of the jaw, with attention to the condyle and fossa, are recorded on videotape before contrast medium is injected.

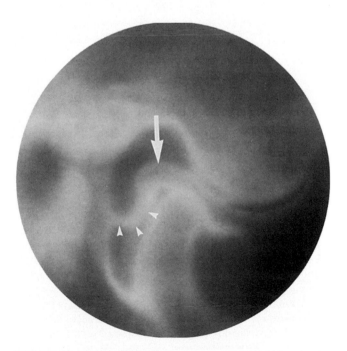

**FIGURE 18-15**   Dual space double-contrast arthrotomogram showing the disk (*arrow*) in a superior position. The mouth was half open, and the redundant posterior disk attachment (*arrowheads*) is seen between the disk and the posterior capsule. The upper and lower joint spaces are radiolucent due to the intraarticular injection of air.

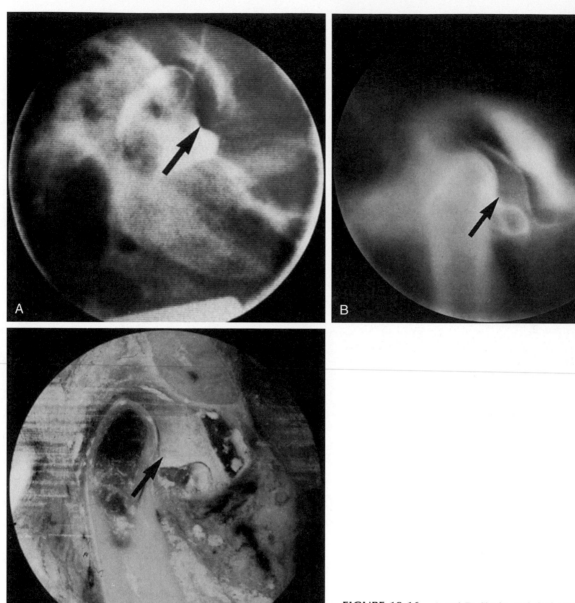

**FIGURE 18-16** **A** and **B**, Single- and dual-space double-contrast arthrotomography. **C**, Corresponding cryosection of TMJ with anterior disk displacement. The location of the posterior band is indicated by arrows.

### Technique for Single-Contrast Arthrography

The superoposterior aspect of the condyle is clinically and fluoroscopically identified and indicated on the skin by a metal marker.[71] The area is marked with a pen, and a local anesthetic (1% to 2% lidocaine) is injected. The joint is punctured with a 23-gauge, 3/4 to 1 inch scalp vein needle introduced perpendicular to the skin surface, and contrast medium (nonionic iodine, 300 mg/ml) is injected into the lower joint space (Fig. 18-17A). Contrast medium is injected until optimum visualization of the joint space has been achieved, as determined by fluoroscopic observation of the joint space. Usually between 0.2 and 0.4 ml of contrast medium is injected. The needle is then withdrawn from the joint space, but the tip of the needle is left in the soft tissue lateral to the joint. The patient is asked to open and close the mouth several times while the image is recorded on

videotape. The free flow of contrast medium around the top of the condyle and into the anterior recess of the inferior space indicates a successful injection. Simultaneous filling of the upper joint space indicates a perforation of the disk or retrodiskal attachments. In joints with perforation, additional contrast medium usually needs to be injected for optimum image quality. Spot films are obtained in at least the closed- and open-mouth positions and at additional positions where abnormalities are clearly seen.

If the diagnosis is not clear from these images, it may be helpful to also inject contrast medium into the upper joint space (Fig. 18-17B). This can be done either by withdrawing the needle slightly and then directing it superiorly into the upper joint space (if the needle was left in place after the initial injection) or by reinserting it while the patient is holding the mouth half open. Injection of the upper joint

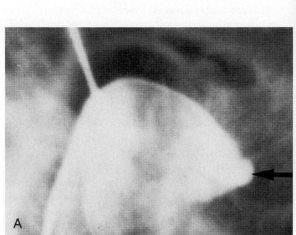
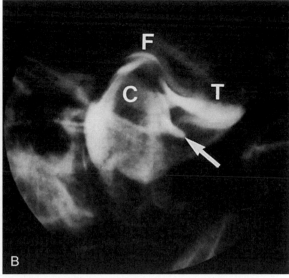

**FIGURE 18-17**  **A**, Single-contrast arthrogram of a normal TMJ with contrast injection into the lower joint compartment only. The small anterior recess of the lower joint compartment (*arrow*) suggests a normal superior disk position. **B**, Normal TMJ demonstrated by a single-contrast arthrogram with contrast injection into both the upper and lower joint spaces. The condyle (*C*), fossa (*F*), and tubercle (*T*) are indicated. The arrow indicates the anterior recess of the lower joint space.

space allows clearer delineation of the disk because both its inferior and superior surfaces are now coated by contrast medium.

### Technique for Double-Contrast Arthrography

If double-contrast arthrography is to be performed, the joint spaces are punctured with catheters (Angiocath 0.8 mm in diameter and 25 mm in length) instead of needles.[17, 25] Contrast medium is injected via extension tubes and aspirated after the dynamic phase of the study. Room air is then injected via new extension tubes, and images are obtained on an upright tomographic unit such as the Phillips

polytome. A complete description of the double-contrast technique is given elsewhere.[72]

### Arthrographic Findings of the Normal TMJ

In a normal TMJ, the posterior band of the disk is located superior to the condyle in the so-called 12 o'clock position relative to the mandibular condyle (Fig. 18-18). The lower joint space has a relatively small anterior recess. However, studies of normal individuals without symptoms have shown great variation in the size of this recess despite the location of the disk in the superior position.[73] At maximum opening the disk is located inferior to the articular tubercle, and the

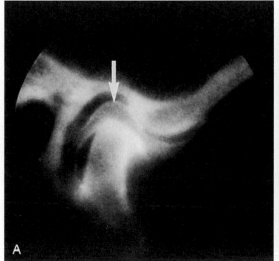
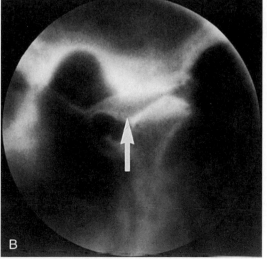

**FIGURE 18-18**  **A**, Normal TMJ with dual-space double-contrast arthrotomography in the closed-mouth position. The posterior band (*arrow*) of the disk is located over the condyle. **B**, Normal TMJ dual-space double-contrast arthrotomography in the open-mouth position. The posterior band (*arrow*) of the disk is located posterior to the condyle.

condyle articulates with the central thin zone and the posterior part of the disk (Fig. 18-18).

### Abnormal Findings

Displacement of the disk with reduction (Fig. 18-19) and without reduction (Fig. 18-20) are the most frequent pathologic findings in TMJ arthrography. Principally this means that the posterior thick part (posterior band) of the disk is located anterior to the condyle in the closed-mouth position, and the condyle closes on the posterior disk attachment (bilaminar zone). An arthrographic sign of disk displacement in single-contrast lower compartment arthrography is enlargement of the anterior recess of the lower joint space (Fig. 18-19).

In disk displacement with reduction the disk is usually biconcave, although there may be some minor enlargement of the posterior band. This corresponds to the early-intermediate stage in the classification scheme described by Wilkes[9] (Box 18-2). In disk displacement without reduction a more extensive deformity of the disk is frequently encountered, and this corresponds to the late stage in the same classification scheme.[9] This is consistent with the deformities observed in pathologic specimens, which include thickening and shortening of the anteroposterior dimension of the disk. Perforation of the posterior disk attachment is another sign of late-stage internal derangement. Perforation is indicated by passage of contrast medium from the lower to the upper joint space (Fig. 18-21) when only the inferior space is injected.

Demonstration of pathology other than internal derangement is distinctly uncommon at TMJ arthrography. Patients with symptoms such as clicking and locking may occasionally have one or more loose bodies within the joint space.[74]

Synovial chondromatosis, osteoarthrosis, or osteochondritis dissecans are the three principal causes of loose bodies in a joint.

Inflammatory joint disease such as rheumatoid arthritis is another pathologic entity that may affect the TMJ. However, this is usually diagnosed clinically, and patients with these diseases are rarely seen for TMJ arthrography. Osseous changes associated with rheumatoid arthritis can be clearly demonstrated with tomography or CT.

### Complications Following Arthrography

Serious complications after arthrography are rare; no cases of infection following arthrography have been reported in the literature. Transient facial nerve palsy may result from extensive injection of a local anesthetic agent around the condyle and condylar neck, and the patient may have mild to moderate local discomfort for 1 to 2 days after the procedure. The use of nonionic or low-osmolality contrast media has been helpful in reducing the patient's discomfort.

## Computed Tomography

CT scanning gives excellent definition of the bony contours of the mandibular head and the glenoid fossa. Axial imaging gives good definition of the head of the condyle, but sagittal and coronal planes are needed for evaluation of the actual joint surfaces. Though direct sagittal scanning of the TMJ (Figs. 18-22 and 18-23) has been done in the past, most institutions use axial scanning with sagittal reconstructions.[75-77] Both techniques have been reported to be successful in demonstrating internal derangement and

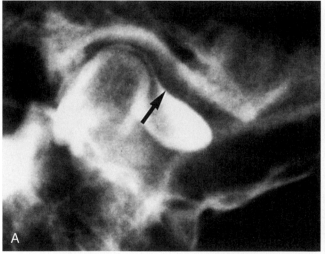
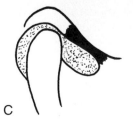
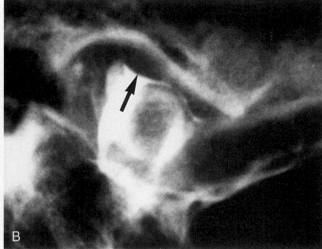
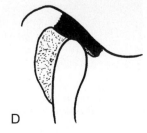

**FIGURE 18-19** **A** and **C**, Anterior disk displacement demonstrated with single-contrast lower compartment arthrography. The posterior band (*arrow*) of the disk is located anterior to the condyle. **B** and **D**, After reduction the disk is in a normal superior position with the posterior band (*arrow*) posterior to the condyle.

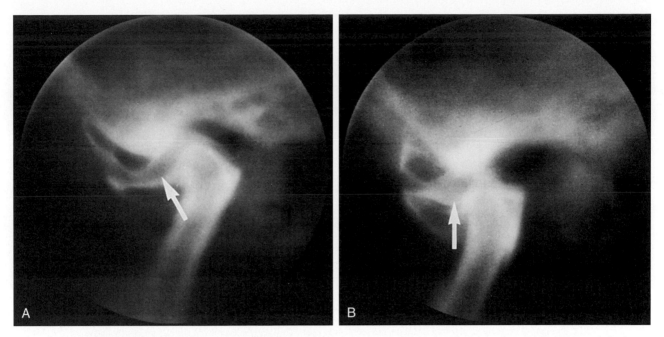

**FIGURE 18-20**   Anterior disk displacement without reduction, double-contrast arthrogram. **A** and **B**, With closed mouth and maximum mouth opening, the disk is located anterior to the condyle. The position of the posterior band is indicated by arrows.

osseous disease.[78–80] Currently, multidetector CT scan technology using very thin collimation allows coronal and sagittal reformatted images that rival direct scan images (Fig. 18-24). The use of CT for diagnosis of disk position has decreased rapidly during the past decade because of the superiority of MR imaging with surface coils (Fig. 18-25).[81] Although CT is not used for visualization of the disk, it is still the best means of examining the osseous structures of the joint.

The two main reasons to use CT in evaluation of the TMJ today are for evaluation of fractures and postsurgical changes involving the osseous components of the joint. Thus, CT can clearly demonstrate the integrity of the glenoid fossa and note the presence of extensive erosions. Perforation into the middle cranial fossa after alloplastic implants also is shown best on CT.

CT is also frequently used for evaluation of potential pathology in the contiguous tissues. Although MR imaging has certain advantages in evaluation of soft tissues, CT gives excellent information regarding the soft tissues and has the benefit of providing detailed images of the contiguous temporal bone and skull base. Calcifications are more easily appreciated on CT. This information can be gathered with the same single scan acquisition done to provide the images of osseous components of the joint.

### Technique for CT Scanning

Sagittal images are preferable to axial or coronal images for disk visualization. Coronal and sagittal images are equally good when evaluating the integrity of the roof of the glenoid fossa, a common indication for CT in patients who have received alloplastic TMJ implants. Axial scanning is

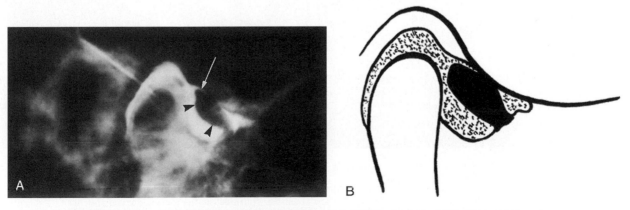

**FIGURE 18-21**   Perforation. **A**, Contrast material was injected into the lower joint space, and there is an overflow (*arrow*) to the upper joint space indicating perforation. The disk (*arrowheads*) is anteriorly displaced and deformed. **B**, Schematic drawing of **A**.

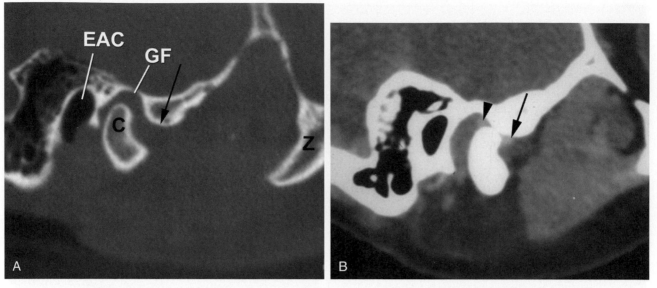

**FIGURE 18-22** Direct sagittal CT of the TMJ. **A,** Bone algorithm shows the position of the condyle (*C*) in the glenoid fossa (*GF*) in the closed-mouth position. *EAC,* External auditory canal; *arrow,* articular eminence; *Z,* zygoma. **B,** Soft-tissue algorithm with the mouth slightly open. The condyle has moved slightly anteriorly and is not completely seated in the glenoid. There is good visualization of the disk. Anterior thick band (*arrow*), posterior thick band (*arrowhead*).

performed with 1 mm (or less) collimation, and sagittal and coronal images are reformatted from the original axial data. Three-dimensional reformatted images can be generated from the same data set (Fig. 18-26).

Before the advent of spiral CT machines, direct sagittal imaging required patients to be placed in uncomfortable positions, with the neck bent sharply to one side. In some cases, an additional stretcher was used to position the patient in the direct sagittal CT imaging plane.[75, 76] The stretcher was placed laterally at an angle with respect to the scanner table and the scanner gantry. Once the patient was in the correct position, scans were performed at 1 to 2 mm intervals from the medial to the lateral poles of the condyle. Additional images were obtained at maximum mouth opening. To minimize radiation, open-mouth images were taken in only a single plane through the center of the

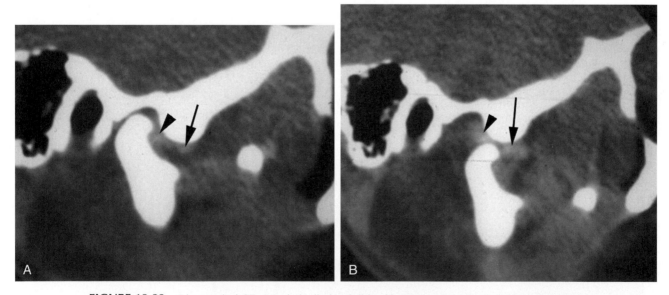

**FIGURE 18-23** Direct sagittal CT. Anteriorly displaced disk with recapture (reciprocal click). **A,** Soft-tissue setting shows the condyle positioned posteriorly in the glenoid fossa. The posterior thick band (*arrowhead*) is demonstrated anterior to the condyle. The anterior thick band (*arrow*) is seen just inferior to the articular eminence. Normally, the condyle should articulate with the thin part of the disk visualized between the anterior and posterior thicker bands. **B,** Open-mouth position. The condyle now has a normal relationship to the disk articulating with the thin area between the posterior thick band (*arrowhead*) and the anterior thick band (*arrow*). The disk has been recaptured.

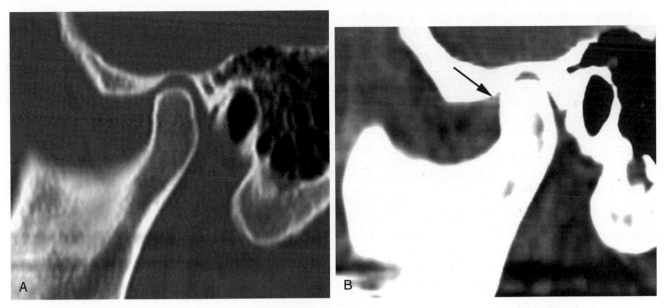

**FIGURE 18-24** Multidetector CT with sagittal reformats. Normal TMJ. **A,** Sagittal reformatted image; the bone algorithm shows the normal relationship of the condyle to the glenoid and the articular eminence. **B,** Soft-tissue sagittal reformat shows a small focus of high density (*arrow*) just anterior to the condylar head. This represents the anterior thick band. This position is considered to be normal.

condyle. CT scans are reconstructed for both bone detail and soft-tissue detail, eliminating the need for conventional radiography or tomography.

### CT Findings

When the disk is normal and thus positioned superior to the condyle, it is usually relatively difficult to visualize (Fig. 18-24). Indeed, the inability to see the disk anterior to the condyle and inferior to the tubercle has been interpreted as a diagnosis of normal disk position (Fig. 18-25). The lateral pterygoid fat pad is the fat around the lateral pterygoid muscle. Some fat is also seen between the two bellies of the lateral pterygoid muscle. If the disk is dislocated, it will distort this fat (Fig. 18-27). Scans with a wide mouth opening usually produce optimum images of the disk but are seldom performed, as MR imaging has become the preferred modality for identifying the disk and its position.

When the disk is anteriorly displaced, it appears as a high-attenuation small mass anterior to the condyle, inferior to the tubercle, and within the low-attenuation lateral pterygoid fat pad (Fig. 18-27). The configuration of the disk typically cannot be determined by CT because the soft-tissue separation is not sufficient for this purpose. The depiction of the disk on CT depends on the disk's density and size. Thus, if the disk is thin and small, it usually is not identified on CT, leading to a higher incidence of false-negative diagnoses. On the other hand, if the disk is large, it can be demonstrated by CT.

## Magnetic Resonance Imaging

MR imaging has been used to image the TMJ since 1984, and imaging quality has continuously improved since that time.[1, 10, 82-89] A major advantage of MR imaging over all other radiographic imaging techniques is the absence of radiation to the patient. This is especially pertinent for TMJ imaging, because a significant number of the patients are young females.[64] The soft-tissue differentiation of MR imaging is also superior to that of all other imaging modalities that have been applied to this joint, and at this time MR imaging is the primary imaging technique for most clinical presentations.

The objective of MR imaging of the TMJ is to document soft- and hard-tissue abnormalities of the joint and its surrounding structures. The ability of MR imaging to visualize the soft-tissue structures around the joint is another advantage of this modality over arthrography, and a comparison of these two imaging modalities on the same joint shows this fact (Fig. 18-28).

### Magnetic Field Strength and Comparison with CT

Scanners with magnetic field strengths ranging from 0.05 to 2 Tesla are currently in clinical use; however, studies that compare the image quality of these scanners with different magnetic field strengths are scarce. One study compared images from two different scanners obtained with equal acquisition time and demonstrated significantly better image quality with the high-field system (Fig. 18-29).[90] Although the lower image quality of the 0.3 Tesla scanner could be somewhat compensated for by increasing the acquisition time (the number of excitations) by a factor of about 4, in clinical work this increases the risk of motion artifact.[90]

Some principal advantages and disadvantages of MR imaging compared with CT are outlined in Box 18-3. Contraindications for MR imaging are outlined in Box 18-4.

### Surface Coil and Scanning Technique

The oblique sagittal and oblique coronal planes are standard for MR imaging of the TMJ (Fig. 18-30). A standard imaging protocol is shown in Table 18-1. The use of the dual surface coil technique for imaging of the left and right TMJs at the same time has been of great value because the time on the scanner can be significantly shortened for bilateral TMJ imaging.[91, 92] Bilateral abnormalities are seen in up to 60% of patients with pain and dysfunction who initially present with unilateral symptoms.[93, 94]

MR imaging is performed using the body coil as the transmitter and the two surface coils as the receivers. Surface coils are essential for good image quality, and a diameter between 6 and 12 cm provides an optimal signal-to-noise ratio in most patients. The standard imaging protocol obtains oblique sagittal and oblique coronal images perpendicular and parallel to the long axis of the mandibular condylar head (Fig.18-30).[95] Sagittal images should be obtained in both closed- and open-mouth positions to determine the function of the disk. Coronal images are usually obtained only in the closed-mouth position. The

protocol shown in Table 18-1 may need to be adjusted, depending on the performance of the scanner and the type of surface coils used.

Proton density images are preferable to T1-weighted images for outlining morphology because of the ''greater latitude'' and better visualization of disk tissue relative to the surrounding joint capsule and cortical bone. T2-weighted images are obtained routinely to document the presence of joint effusion and inflammatory changes in the joint capsule. Because of the arthrographic effect created by the high signal intensity of the joint effusion on T2-weighted images, these images also may be useful for outlining perforations. T2-weighted images obtained in both sagittal and coronal planes frequently help outline the joint effusion.

Fast spin-echo T2-weighted images provide a better signal-to-noise ratio than standard T2-weighted images.

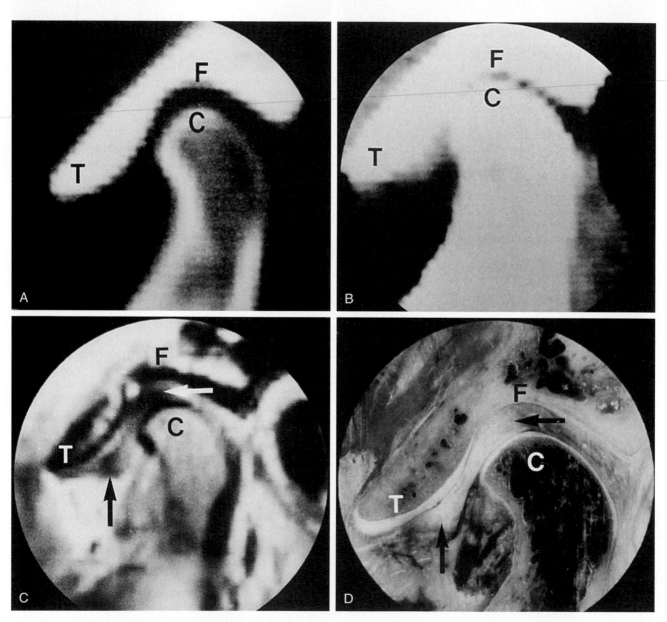

**FIGURE 18-25** CT in hard-tissue (**A**) and soft-tissue (**B**) settings, MR imaging (**C**), and corresponding cryosection (**D**) of a TMJ with the normal superior disk position. The tubercle (*T*), fossa (*F*), and condyle (*C*) are indicated. The anterior and posterior bands of the disk are indicated by arrows.

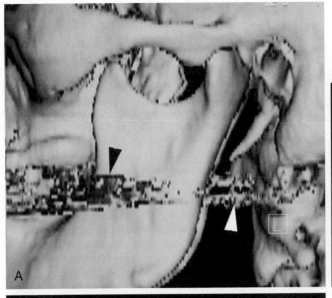

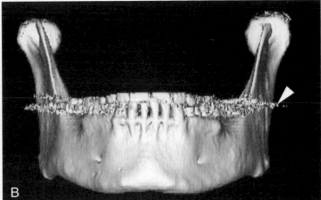

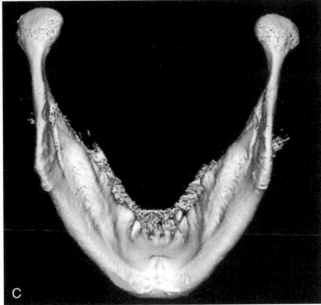

**FIGURE 18-26** Three-dimensional reformatted images. **A,** Lateral view. Note the "spray artifact" (*arrowheads*) due to dental restorations. **B,** Anterior view of the electronically disarticulated mandible. Again, note the artifacts from dental restorations (*arrowhead*). **C,** View from posterior and inferior of the disarticulated mandible.

However, the standard proton density images provide superior soft-tissue separation, and many imagers prefer standard spin-echo images because they are sharper than fast spin-echo images. Open-mouth images are obtained to determine the function of the disk. Syringes of various sizes or commercially available bite block devices are used to stabilize the patient's jaw in the open-mouth position (Fig. 18-31). Slice thickness should be 3 mm or less. The gap or interval between slices should be 0.5 to 1.5 mm for the sagittal images; for the coronal images it should be reduced to about 0.3 mm to obtain at least one good image through the center of the condyle. The anteroposterior dimension of the condyle is usually about 8 to 10 mm, and volume averaging is a greater problem for coronal images than for sagittal images. By angling the coronal images along the horizontal long axis of the condyle, images of both left and right joints can be obtained simultaneously. In the rare instance in which the slices of the left and right joints

interfere with each other, separate scans of the left and right joints should be obtained.

The coronal images are valuable in identifying medial and lateral displacements of the disk. Additionally, the osseous anatomy of the condyle can sometimes be better appreciated in the coronal plane.

If the patient's oral splint is to be assessed, additional oblique sagittal images are obtained with the splint in place. The same scanning parameters are used for the closed-mouth sagittal images.

### MR Imaging Findings of the Normal TMJ

MR imaging nicely shows the normal TMJ anatomy in the sagittal and coronal planes (Figs. 18-32 and 18-33). In the sagittal plane the disk is biconcave, with the posterior band (posterior thick part) lying over the condyle. The central thin zone articulates against the anterior prominence of the condyle. Because the fibrous connective tissue of the

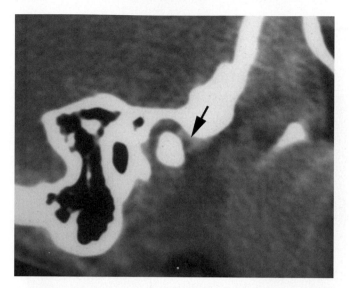

**FIGURE 18-27** Direct sagittal CT scan with a soft-tissue setting depicting an anteriorly displaced disk. The image of the disk has a relatively high CT attenuation contrasted against the fat close to the lateral pterygoid muscle. The arrow points to the thin portion of the disk.

the muscles reach their attachments to the disk and condyle. This fibrous band is seen as a linear low-signal structure just inferior to the position of the disk, and it should not be mistaken for the disk. This is a particular problem when the disk is medially or laterally displaced and the fibrous band of the lateral pterygoid muscle is the only low-signal structure anterior to the condylar head.

In MR imaging scans obtained at maximum mouth opening, the central thin zone of the disk is visualized between the condyle and the tubercle (Fig. 18-33B). The posterior band of the disk articulates against the posterior surface of the condyle, as has been demonstrated in anatomic specimens (Fig. 18-3).

In the coronal plane (Fig. 18-33C), the normal disk has a crescent shape. The medial aspect of the disk attaches just inferior to the medial pole of the condyle and to the medial capsule. Similarly, the lateral part of the disk attaches just inferior to the lateral pole of the condyle and to the lateral capsule (Fig. 18-2). Normally, the lateral and medial capsules are visualized and do not bulge outward.

### Disk Displacement

Displacements of the disk in the anterior (Fig. 18-34), anteromedial, or anterolateral direction are the most common findings observed when interpreting MR images of patients with clinical signs and symptoms of internal derangement.[43] In the sagittal plane the disk is noted to be displaced when its posterior band is anterior to the condyle (Fig. 18-34).

disk has low signal intensity, the disk usually can be distinguished from the surrounding tissues, which have higher signal intensity. The cortices of both the condylar and temporal bone components of the joint have low signal intensity, but the articular coverings of the joint have higher signal intensity. This makes the outline of the osseous components easily visible. The posterior disk attachment has relatively high signal intensity compared with the posterior portion of the disk itself because of the fatty tissue in the posterior disk attachment. MR imaging is the only modality that consistently allows the disk to be distinguished from its posterior attachment.

The upper and lower heads (or bellies) of the lateral pterygoid muscle are seen extending anteriorly from the TMJ. The upper belly can be followed into the anterior margin of the disk. The lower belly attaches to the anterior surface of the condylar neck. There is a thin, fibrous band at the junction of the upper and lower heads at the point where

Disk displacement may be complete or partial. In complete disk displacement, the entire mediolateral dimension of the disk is displaced anterior to the condyle. In partial disk displacement, only the medial or lateral part of the disk is displaced anterior to the condyle. Most frequently, the lateral part is displaced anteriorly and the more medial part of the disk is still in a normal superior position. Partial disk displacement is frequently seen in joints with disk displacement with reduction (Fig. 18-35); the disk is displaced anteriorly in the lateral part of the joint (Fig. 18-35A) and is in a normal position in the medial part of the joint (Fig. 18-35B). This is probably because the displaced part of the disk, being anchored by the normally positioned medial

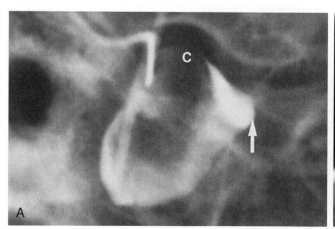
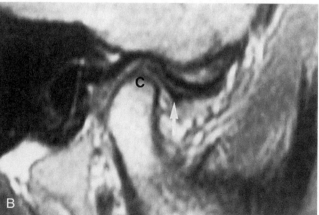

**FIGURE 18-28** **A**, Arthrogram. **B**, MR image of the same TMJ showing the normal superior disk position. The anterior recess of the lower joint compartment is indicated by an arrow in the arthrogram. In the MR image the disk is located superior to the condyle. The condyle (*C*) is noted in both studies.

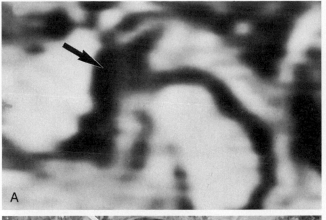

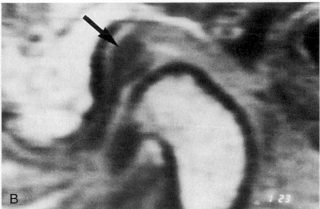

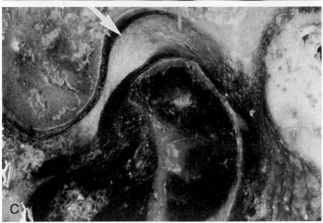

**FIGURE 18-29**   **A** and **B**, MR images with 0.3 Tesla and 1.5 Tesla. **C**, Corresponding cryosection showing the normal superior disk position (*arrow*). The image quality of the 1.5 Tesla scanner is superior to that of the 0.3 Tesla scanner when comparable imaging times are used.

portion of the disk, is allowed to revert to its normal position on opening without being squeezed between the two joint components as much as in cases with a complete anterior disk displacement.

Frequently, the anterior disk displacement is combined with either medial or lateral displacement. Initially, when MR imaging was done in the true coronal plane, medial displacements were considered more prevalent than lateral displacements. This was probably the result of the scanning technique rather than pathologic changes because, with oblique coronal images parallel to the horizontal long axis of the condylar head, medial and lateral displacements are seen with approximately the same frequency. In most cases, the sagittal images show the anterior component of the displacement, and the coronal images show the medial or lateral component. In approximately 10% of patients

---

### BOX 18-3

### ADVANTAGES AND DISADVANTAGES OF MR IMAGING COMPARED WITH CT

| Advantages | No ionizing radiation |
| | Fewer artifacts from dense bone and metal clips |
| | Imaging possible in several planes without moving the patient |
| | Superior anatomic detail of soft tissues |
| Disadvantages | High initial cost of the scanner Special site planning and shielding |
| | Patient claustrophobia in magnet |
| | Inferior images of bone |

---

### BOX 18-4

### CONTRAINDICATIONS TO MR IMAGING

| Absolute | Patients with cerebral aneurysm clips |
| | Patients with cardiac pacemakers |
| Relative | Ferromagnetic foreign bodies in critical locations (e.g., eyes) |
| | Metallic prosthetic heart valves |
| | Claustrophobic or uncooperative patients |
| | Implanted stimulator wires for pain control |
| Not contra-indications | Metallic prostheses |
| | Orthodontic fixed appliances |

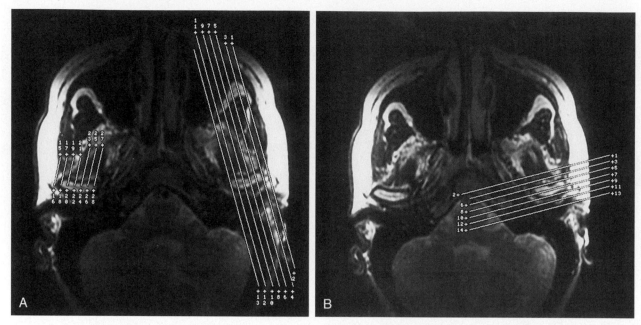

**FIGURE 18-30**   Axial scout images for sagittal (**A**) and coronal (**B**) MR images. The orientations of the sagittal and coronal images are outlined. It is important to cover the area of the lateral and medial poles of the condyle with the sagittal images. For the coronal images, one image should be through the center of the condyle.

presenting with TMJ pain and dysfunction, there is a pure lateral or pure medial disk displacement that is not detected on sagittal images (Fig. 18-36).[10] The displacement can be dramatic in both the lateral (Fig. 18-36) and medial (Fig. 18-37) directions. When the disk is displaced medially or laterally in combination with anterior displacement, it is called rotational disk displacement (Box 18-1).

The empty fossa sign seen in the sagittal images (Fig. 18-38) is an indication of a medial or lateral disk displacement. When the disk displaces in a medial direction, the lateral capsular tissue is pulled between the condyle and glenoid fossa and gives the appearance of an "empty" fossa. Thus, when the disk is not clearly seen in the glenoid fossa in the closed-mouth position (Fig. 18-38), medial or lateral disk displacement should be suspected. The coronal images are examined for verification. Medial and lateral disk displacement may or may not (Fig. 18-38) reduce on

### Table 18-1
### SCANNING PARAMETERS FOR MR IMAGING

| Image | Scanning Time |
|---|---|
| **Axial Localizer**<br>TR/TE = 300 ms; 16 ms<br>NEX = 0.5<br>FOV = 18 cm<br>Slice thickness = 3 mm<br>Matrix = 256 × 128 | 25 sec |
| **Sagittal, Closed Mouth**<br>TR/TE = 2000 ms; 19/80 ms<br>NEX = 0.5–0.75<br>FOV = 10–12 cm<br>Slice thickness = 3 mm<br>Matrix = 256 × 192 | 3 min, 52 sec |
| **Sagittal, Open Mouth**<br>TR/TE = 1500 ms; 19/80 ms<br>NEX = 0.75<br>FOV = 10–12 cm<br>Slice thickness = 3 mm<br>Matrix = 256 × 128 | 2 min, 42 sec |
| **Coronal, Closed Mouth**<br>TR/TE = 2000 ms; 19/80 ms<br>NEX = 0.5–0.75<br>FOV = 10–12 cm<br>Slice thickness = 3 mm<br>Matrix = 256 × 192 | 3 min, 52 sec |

*FOV*, field of view; *NEX*, number of excitations.

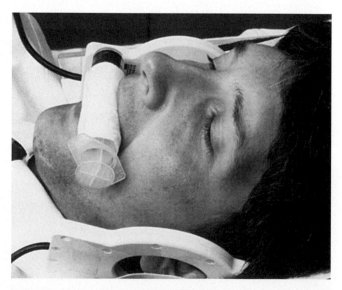

**FIGURE 18-31**   Clinical positioning with dual surface coils and a syringe between upper and lower teeth used as a bite block.

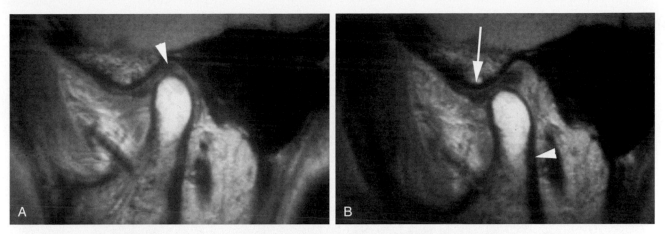

**FIGURE 18-32** Normal MR imaging, Normal TMJ. **A,** The posterior thick band (*arrowhead*) is located immediately superior to the condylar head. Just anterior to this band is the central thin region. The low signal just anterior to the condylar head is the anterior thick band. The disk gives a ''bowtie'' appearance due to the anterior and posterior thick bands. **B,** Open-mouth position. The mouth is slightly open. The disk has translated down anteriorly so that the anterior thick band of the disk is immediately inferior to the articular eminence (*arrow*). The condylar head has rotated with respect to the disk. Note how the posterior edge of the mandible has rotated posteriorly (*arrowhead*) compared to **A.**

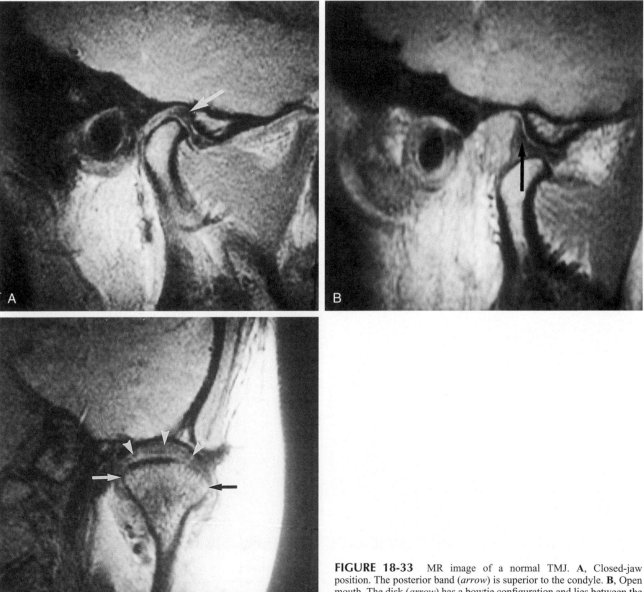

**FIGURE 18-33** MR image of a normal TMJ. **A,** Closed-jaw position. The posterior band (*arrow*) is superior to the condyle. **B,** Open mouth. The disk (*arrow*) has a bowtie configuration and lies between the condyle and the articular tubercle. **C,** Coronal image. The medial and lateral poles of the condyle (*arrows*) are clearly visualized. The disk (*arrowheads*) is crescent-shaped and is seen superior to the condyle.

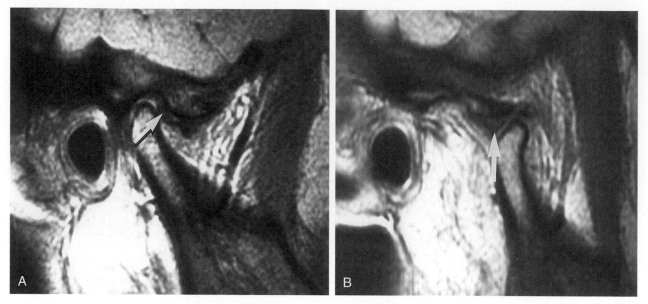

**FIGURE 18-34** Disk displacement with reduction. **A,** A posterior band of the displaced disk (*arrow*) is anterior to the condyle. **B,** Open-mouth image shows the posterior band (*arrow*) in a normal relationship posterior to the condyle. This indicates reduction on opening.

opening. The function of the disk with sideways displacement is more difficult to evaluate than with anterior displacement because the location of the disk is best seen in the coronal plane in the closed position and the sagittal plane in the open position.

MR images obtained at maximum mouth opening determine whether the disk displacement reduces. In displacement with reduction (Fig. 18-34) the disk position normalizes during jaw opening. In disk displacement without reduction (Fig. 18-39) the disk remains anterior to the condyle in all mandibular positions. Disk displacement with reduction practically always precedes late-stage disk displacement without reduction.

### Disk Deformity

Deformity of the disk (Fig. 18-9) resulting from chronic displacement can usually be demonstrated by MR imaging (Fig. 18-40). Initial deformity includes thickening of the

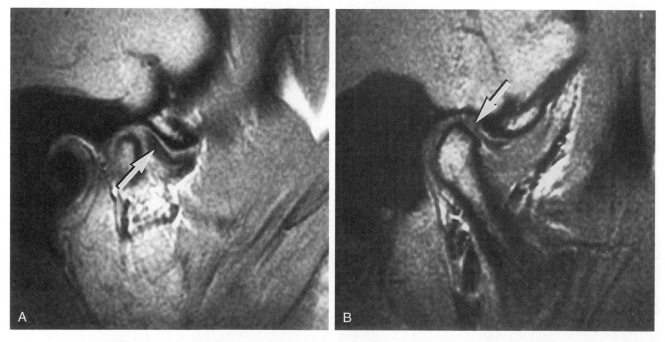

**FIGURE 18-35** Partial anterior disk displacement. **A,** In the lateral part of the joint, the disk (*arrow*) is anteriorly displaced. **B,** In the medial part of the joint, the disk (*arrow*) is located in a normal superior position. This indicates partial anterior disk displacement.

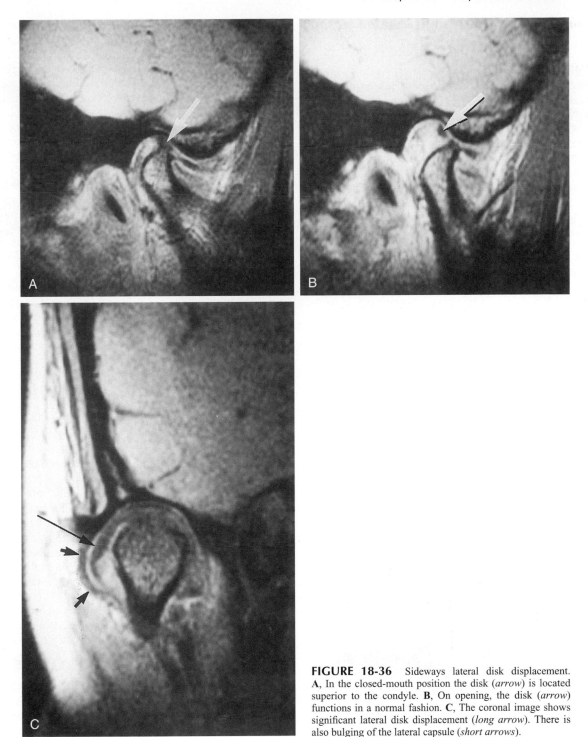

**FIGURE 18-36**   Sideways lateral disk displacement. **A,** In the closed-mouth position the disk (*arrow*) is located superior to the condyle. **B,** On opening, the disk (*arrow*) functions in a normal fashion. **C,** The coronal image shows significant lateral disk displacement (*long arrow*). There is also bulging of the lateral capsule (*short arrows*).

posterior band. Late-stage deformity may include a rounder, biconvex disk or a severely diminished amount of disk tissue. Disk deformation is significant in the clinical management of patients because a deformed disk usually cannot be repositioned surgically, and more aggressive surgical treatment with diskectomy may be necessary. It is therefore important to evaluate the degree of disk deformity and communicate this information to the referring clinician.

Another form of tissue alteration secondary to disk displacement is the formation of the so-called pseudodisk

(Fig. 18-41). A pseudodisk appears as a band-like structure of low signal intensity replacing the normally bright signal from the posterior disk attachment. Histologically, it is thought to represent the fibrotic change that occurs in the posterior disk attachment in response to pressure from the condyle against the loose tissue of the posterior disk attachment (bilaminar zone). It has been suggested that this fibrotic change in the posterior disk attachment is associated with decreasing pain, but this has not been confirmed in systematic studies.[96, 97]

# Other Findings and Conditions Related to Internal Derangement

### Joint Effusion

An assessment of the amount of joint fluid is essential because small amounts of fluid are seen outlining the articular surfaces in both normal and abnormal individuals (Fig. 18-42).[98] Large accumulations of joint fluid (Fig. 18-43) are seen only in symptomatic patients. Such effusions are best seen in T2-weighted MR imaging.

Joint fluid is significantly more prevalent in painful joints than in nonpainful joints.[98] Not all individuals with pain have joint effusion, but a significant accumulation of joint effusion is likely to be associated with pain and the status of the disk.[99-101] Joint effusion may also have some diagnostic value, as the fluid outlines the morphology of the disk and may outline a perforation in the posterior disk attachment (Fig. 18-44).

### Osteoarthritis

Osteoarthritis is frequently seen in joints with long-standing disk displacement without reduction.[18, 26] Disk displacement seems to be a precursor of osteoarthritis. Osteoarthritis is infrequently seen in joints with a normal superior disk position, occasionally in disk displacement with reduction, and more frequently when disk displacement without reduction has been present for some time. Imaging evidence of osteoarthritis can be seen in teenagers with disk displacement without reduction. Disk displacement and internal derangement are, however, only one cause of osteoarthritis, the common final pathway for a multitude of primary joint lesions.

Osteoarthritis is characterized radiographically by flattening and irregularities of the articular surfaces, osteophy-

tosis, and erosion (Figs. 18-45 and 18-46). There may be irregularity of the glenoid fossa, particularly when there is bone-to-bone contact because of a tear in the disk or retrodiskal tissues. The distinction between early arthritis and advanced remodeling on MR imaging, as well as on other imaging modalities, is difficult to define, and overlap will exist.

Osteoarthritis has been suggested as a source of pain. However, osteoarthritis is present in a large proportion of older individuals and is usually completely asymptomatic. It is well recognized that symptoms related to TMJ dysfunction decrease with age, and are often remitting and self-limited.[102-105] The discrepancy between imaging findings and patient symptoms indicates the need for a good clinical examination to determine which imaging findings are significant.

### Marrow Abnormalities of the Mandibular Condyle

Claims have been made, based on comparison with other joints, that areas within the bone marrow of the condyle having low signal intensity on T1-weighted images (variable signal on T2-weighted images) represent osteonecrosis (avascular or aseptic necrosis) (Figs. 18-47 to 18-50).[89, 106] However, based on this MR imaging appearance, other etiologies such as sclerosis or fibrosis of the bone marrow cannot be ruled out.

Multiple MR imaging studies have described abnormalities of the mandibular condyle similar to the appearance of osteonecrosis (aseptic necrosis) in the femoral head.[107-111] One study used core biopsy to document that edema and osteonecrosis may occur in the marrow of the mandibular condyle.[112] Histologic evidence of bone marrow edema was also found without evidence of osteonecrosis, suggesting that edema may be a precursor to osteonecrosis, as is known from investigation of other joints.[112] MR findings suggesting bone marrow edema include intermediate signal intensity on T1-weighted and proton density images and increased signal intensity on T2-weighted image (Fig. 18-48).

Osteoarthritis may develop secondary to osteonecrosis in the TMJ (Fig. 18-50).[112, 113] However, edema and osteonecrosis are separate entities from osteoarthritis and do occur without osteoarthritis.[113]

Avascular necrosis is best characterized in the hip. Predisposing factors include sickle cell disease, alcoholism, and steroid therapy. Avascular necrosis in the mandibular condyle probably has a different etiology and has not been associated with the same systemic factors but rather with local trauma from internal derangement.[89] Disk displacement may be one factor that leads to bone marrow changes.[109-111, 113, 114]

Abnormal bone marrow of the mandibular condyle may be seen in less than 10% of joints with TMJ disease.[113, 115] A study has shown markedly greater pain in joints that have bone marrow alterations in the mandibular condyle compared to joints with normal bone marrow.[116] Increased intraarticular pressure in conditions such as synovitis and hemophilia has also been suggested as an etiology of osteonecrosis.[117] A relationship between osteonecrosis and larger amounts of joint fluid has also been described.[111, 112]

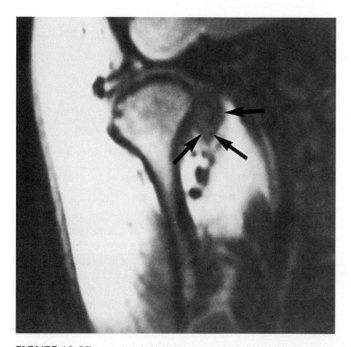

**FIGURE 18-37**   Medial disk displacement. Coronal MR image shows the disk (*arrows*) displaced medial to the condyle.

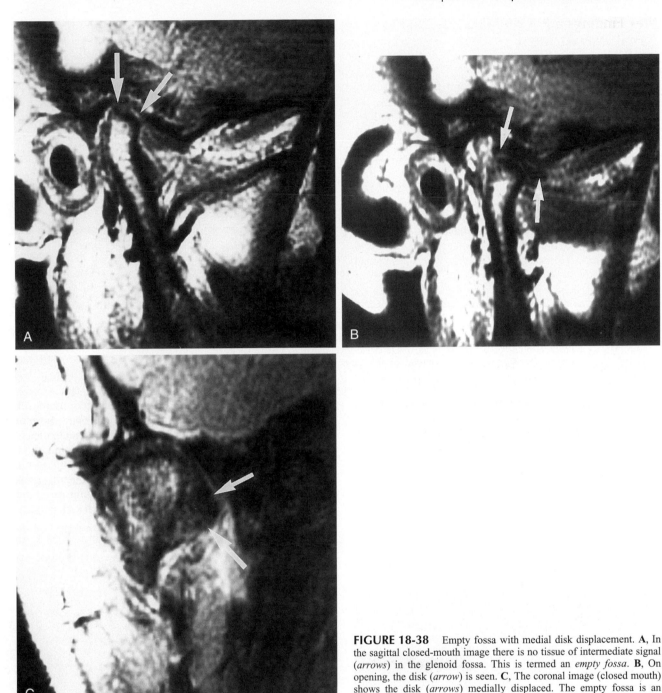

**FIGURE 18-38**   Empty fossa with medial disk displacement. **A,** In the sagittal closed-mouth image there is no tissue of intermediate signal (*arrows*) in the glenoid fossa. This is termed an *empty fossa.* **B,** On opening, the disk (*arrow*) is seen. **C,** The coronal image (closed mouth) shows the disk (*arrows*) medially displaced. The empty fossa is an indication of medial or lateral disk displacement.

## Osteochondritis Dissecans

Loose bodies are seldom found in the TMJ. One loose body in the joint space associated with a defect in the condyle of the same size can be characterized as osteochondritis dissecans.[89] In this condition, a small part of the condyle is dislodged into the joint space and acts as a small, loose body (Fig. 18-51). The condition has been described as being associated with avascular necrosis, although the relationship between the two conditions is not fully understood.[89] Osteochondritis dissecans has been demonstrated in a cadaver joint (Fig. 18-52). Multiple loose bodies are discussed in the section on Synovial Chondromatosis.

## Stuck Disk

In the normal opening sequence, the disk moves relative to both the condyle and the temporal bone component of the joint. Most of the movement in the upper joint compartment represents translation. The disk slides or translates relative to the glenoid. In the lower joint compartment the predominant motion is rotation. The condyle rotates within the concavity of the disk. Translation or sliding of the condyle relative to the disk is normally minimal. It has been suggested in the arthroscopic literature that inability of the disk to move, relative to the glenoid fossa, is a significant cause of pain and dysfunction.[28] This observation has not been extensively and systematically documented, but there

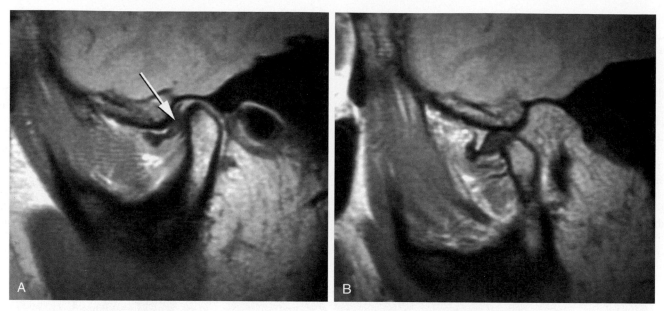

**FIGURE 18-39** Anterior displacement without reduction (closed lock). **A,** The head of the condyle is posteriorly positioned in the glenoid fossa. The posterior thick band of the disk (*arrow*) is completely anterior to the condylar head. **B,** Upon opening of the mouth, the condyle moves to a point just inferior to the articular eminence. Rather than recapturing the disk, it pushes the disk anteriorly and does not regain the normal relationship.

are indications that MR definition of a stuck disk (Figs. 18-53 and 18-54) may be associated with pain and dysfunction.[118] As the patient opens the mouth, the disk maintains a constant relationship to the glenoid while the condyle rotates and may translate relative to the disk.

### Lock

The most frequent situation with locking of the TMJ is the inability of the patient to open the mouth completely. This is most frequently caused by anterior disk displacement without reduction.

The open lock condition is encountered more infrequently. In this condition, the patient can open the mouth widely but is temporarily or permanently unable to close the mouth. This condition sometimes requires manipulation of the jaw by the patient or a health care professional to move the mandible into place. These patients frequently present in the emergency room but rarely for imaging assessment.

There are two different causes of the open lock condition.

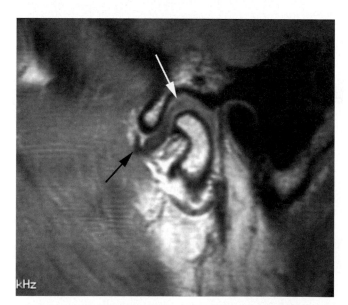

**FIGURE 18-40** Disk deformation. The disk is anteriorly displaced. There is thickening of the posterior band (*black arrow*) and folding of the disk. The lack of signal from the retrodiskal attachments (*white arrow*) suggests fibrosis secondary to the chronic trauma of the dislocation.

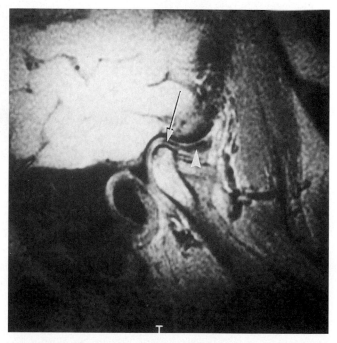

**FIGURE 18-41** Fibrosis of the posterior disk attachment. The disk (*arrowhead*) is anteriorly displaced. There is an area of low signal in the posterior disk attachment (*long arrows*), which indicates fibrosis.

In the classic situation, the condyle is luxated (subluxed or dislocated) in front of the articular eminence, and the articular eminence prevents the condyle from retruding back into the glenoid fossa. In the other situation, the condyle translates anteriorly to the anterior band of the disk, and the disk prevents the condyle from retruding back into the glenoid fossa (Fig. 18-55). Characteristically, in this situation the disk is folded behind the condyle (Fig. 18-55). It is usually not possible to differentiate between the two causes on physical examination. Although acute management with reduction of the subluxation is similar in both situations, if definitive surgery is necessary, it differs depending on the cause of the subluxation. If the disk is blocking the reversion of the condyle, surgery has to be directed to the disk. If the articular eminence is the cause of the patient's inability to close the mouth, surgery must focus on the bone.

## Accuracy of TMJ Imaging

Knowing the diagnostic accuracy of an imaging modality is essential for its clinical use. The accuracy of tomography, arthrography, CT, and MR imaging has been investigated in several studies on fresh autopsy material (Tables 18-2 and 18-3 on p. 1029).[81, 119–122] All techniques have demonstrated relatively high accuracy in determining osseous conditions and disk position; however, MR imaging has the highest accuracy and demonstrates both joint structures and the soft tissues surrounding the joint.

The accuracies noted in Tables 18-2 and 18-3 are from investigations performed without the biases of clinical work. The figures are relevant for the comparison between the different techniques because the studies were performed under the same conditions. In a clinical situation, however, additional information about the patient is available that

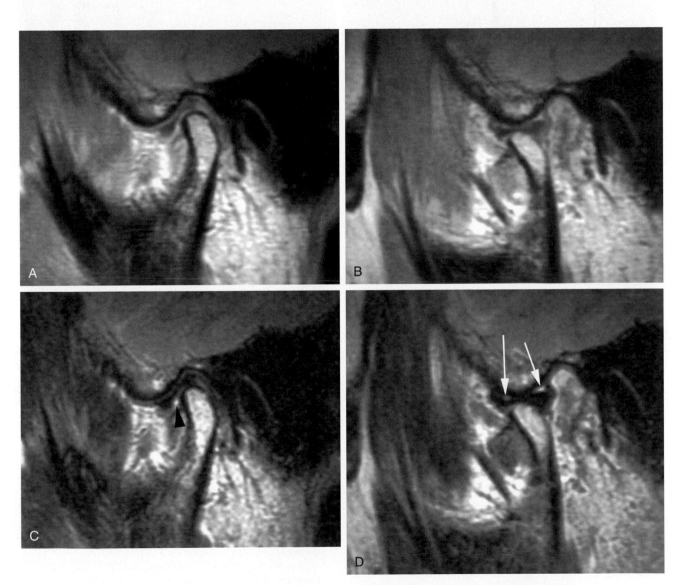

**FIGURE 18-42**   Normal TMJ with minimal joint fluid. **A,** Proton density image, closed-mouth position. The disk is seen in the normal location. The condyle is in the normal position relative to the glenoid fossa. **B,** Open-mouth position. The disk and condyle have translated downward beneath the articular eminence. **C,** T2-weighted image, closed-mouth position. A very small amount of high signal (*arrowhead*), which may represent a small amount of fluid in the anterior recess of the inferior joint space. **D,** T2-weighted image, open-mouth position, shows a small amount of fluid (*arrows*) in the superior joint space.

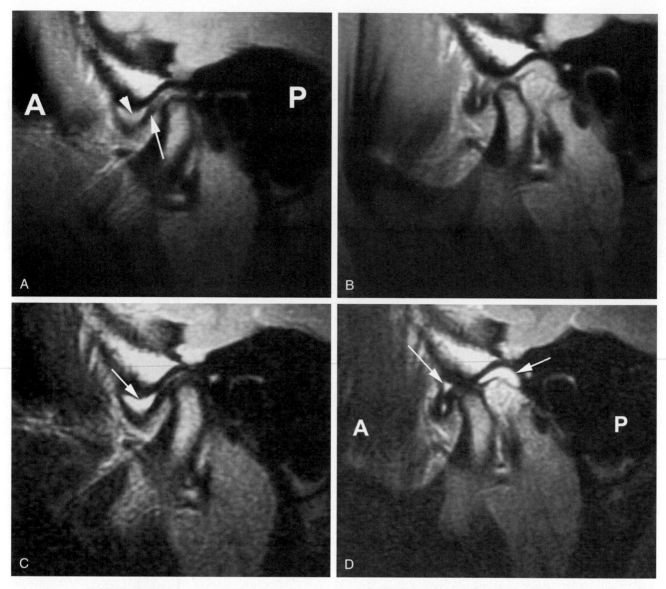

**FIGURE 18-43** Large amount of joint fluid (effusion) in a painful joint. Closed lock (anterior displacement without recapture). **A,** Proton density image. The disk is completely dislocated anteriorly in the closed-mouth position. The fluid (*arrowhead*) in the upper joint compartment can be appreciated even on the proton density image. Posterior thick band (*arrow*). **B,** Open-mouth position, proton density image. The condyle pushes the disk anteriorly but does not recapture. The disk is deformed. **C,** T2-weighted image, closed-mouth position. The bright fluid (*arrow*) in the upper compartment of the joint is easily appreciated. **D,** Open-mouth position. The fluid in the joint (*arrows*) is more clearly seen on the T2-weighted image. Anteriorly, the fluid outlines the upper contour of the disk. Posteriorly, the fluid outlines the superior surface of the bilaminar folds (retrodiskal tissues). *A,* anterior; *P,* posterior.

might help further improve interpretation of the image. In addition, by detecting medially or laterally displaced disks, the multiplanar imaging capability of MR imaging may provide even greater accuracy (Fig. 18-56). A recent study demonstrated the accuracy of MR imaging in determining disk position and configuration to be more than 90%.[123]

## Imaging After Treatment

Imaging after surgical treatment is indicated in patients who continue to have symptoms that might be related to intraarticular pathology such as recurrence of disk displacement, intraarticular adhesions, or inflammatory changes. Although surgery is performed for a variety of pathologies of the jaw and TMJ, most surgery is done for patients with internal derangements. For this reason, imaging of the postoperative joint is discussed in this section.

The primary goal of treatment of TMJ disorders is to eliminate pain and dysfunction. Secondary goals are restoration of normal anatomy and prevention of disease progression. If a patient continues to have symptoms after treatment, imaging is frequently helpful in determining the etiology of the problem.

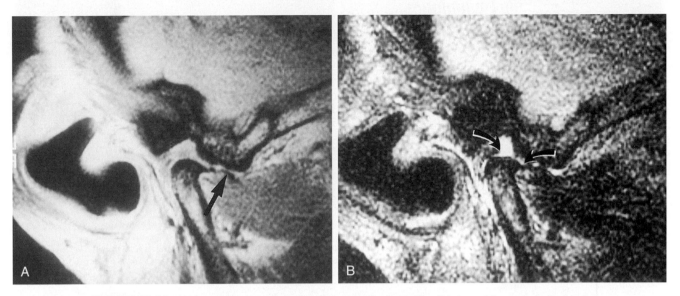

**FIGURE 18-44**   Disk perforation demonstrated with proton density. **A,** The disk (*arrow*) is anteriorly displaced and extensively deformed. There is an anterior osteophyte of the condyle indicating degenerative changes. Also, the component is flattened. **B,** In the T2-weighted image the defect in the posterior disk attachment (*arrows*) is well outlined by the joint effusion.

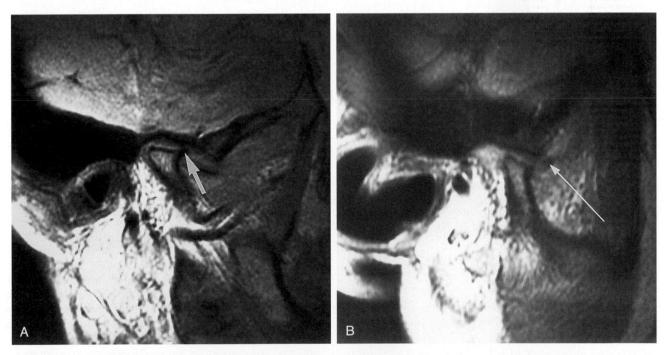

**FIGURE 18-45**   Osteoarthritis. **A,** Proton density closed-mouth image shows an anterior osteophyte of the condyle (*arrow*) and superior flattening. The glenoid fossa is widened, and the articular tubercle is flattened. These changes are consistent with degenerative joint disease. **B,** On opening, the two flat articular surfaces slide against each other and a small part of the disk remains anterior (*arrow*).

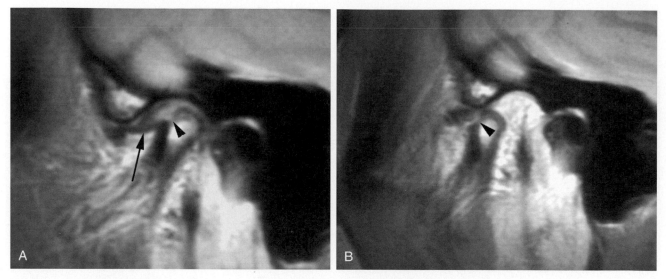

**FIGURE 18-46**   Osteoarthritis with erosion of the condylar head. **A,** Proton density MR image shows a defect (*arrowhead*) in the head of the condyle. The disk is completely dislocated anteriorly, with the posterior thick band (*arrow*) completely anterior to the condylar head. **B,** Open-mouth position. The condyle pushes the disk anteriorly but does not recapture. Note how the posterior thick band fits into the cortical defect (*arrowhead*) and the head of the condyle.

## Treatment Modalities for TMJ Internal Derangement

Conservative treatment of TMJ internal derangement includes reassurance, observation, occlusal adjustment, bite splints, nonsteroidal antiinflammatory medications, muscle relaxants, and physical therapy. Arthroscopic surgery includes lysis and lavage of adhesions and disk repositioning. Open joint surgery includes disk repositioning, diskectomy without replacement, diskectomy with autologous implant, and joint reconstruction with rib grafts. The use of alloplastic disk replacement implants has been discontinued.

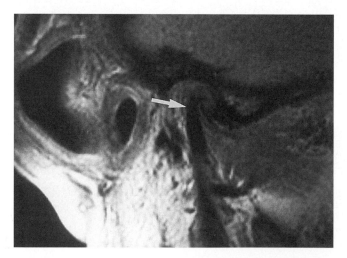

**FIGURE 18-47**   Sclerosis of the condyle and condyle neck. A proton density image shows decreased signal from the entire condyle head and condyle neck (*arrow*). This may indicate sclerosis, fibrosis, or possibly avascular necrosis. No histologic proof was available in this case.

## Imaging Techniques after Surgical Treatment

Before the availability of MR imaging, plain films (Fig. 18-57), tomography, and arthrography were used to evaluate patients after surgery. Plain films and tomography show only the osseous structures, and there is often a need for soft-tissue evaluation as well. Arthrography can be difficult to perform once surgery has been done because the anatomy is altered and the joint spaces are narrowed as a result of peripheral and intraarticular adhesions (Fig. 18-58). For this reason, MR imaging is a preferable method of examination in most postoperative patients.[1, 82, 83]

Postoperative MR imaging is helpful in confirming whether surgical treatment has corrected the position of the displaced disk. Frequently, however, the disk remains anteriorly displaced after disk-repositioning surgery. This is seen in both symptomatic and asymptomatic individuals, and less emphasis should be placed on the position of the disk after surgery because symptoms may be associated more with peripheral adhesions than with disk position per se.

In patients who have undergone diskectomy, there is a soft-tissue interface between the condyle and the glenoid fossa (Fig. 18-59), which is a natural replacement for the extirpated disk.[124] This is a normal postsurgical development. On MR imaging this soft tissue has intermediate to high signal intensity compared to fibrous adhesions, which have low signal intensity (Fig. 18-60). The most important imaging assessment in these patients is to evaluate for peripheral or intraarticular adhesions following diskectomy, because such adhesions (Fig. 18-60) frequently are the cause of the patient's limited opening and pain. Thickening of the lateral joint capsule is also frequently seen after surgery (Fig. 18-61) in both symptomatic and asymptomatic individuals and is probably of limited clinical significance as long as the scar tissue does not extend into the joint space. The amount of scar tissue in the lateral capsule wall varies

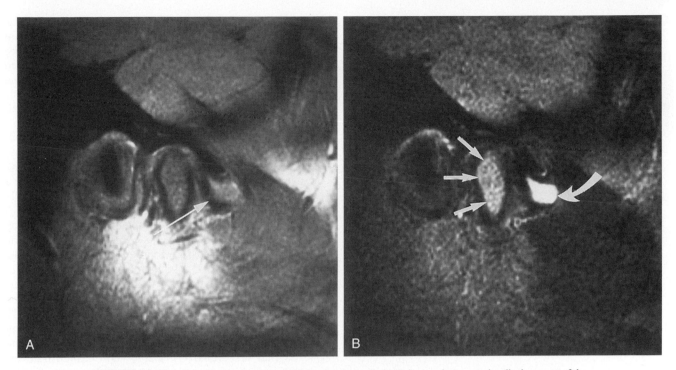

**FIGURE 18-48**   Bone marrow edema. **A**, Proton density sagittal MR image shows anterior displacement of the disk (*arrow*). **B**, T2-weighted image shows increased signal in the bone marrow of the condyle (*arrows*). There is also a large effusion (*curved arrow*) in the upper joint space. The increased signal in the bone marrow indicates bone marrow edema.

significantly among patients; some scar tissue in asymptomatic patients is quite large but does not extend into the joint space (Fig. 18-61).

Complete fibrous (Fig. 18-60) or bony ankylosis may occur after surgery in a few instances. Jaw motion is severely restricted, but opening can be up to about 10 mm, even with a heavy fibrous ankylosis. In bony ankylosis there is no motion. CT or tomography is preferred over MR imaging for demonstration of these bony changes.

## Alloplastic Implants

During the 1980s and early 1990s, alloplastic implants were used to replace the disk. Two types of implants, Proplast Teflon (Figs. 18-62 and 18-63) and silicone rubber material (Silastic) were mainly used. The Proplast implants were intended to be permanent, whereas the silicon implants were used either on a temporary or a permanent basis. The initial results were favorable and these surgical techniques

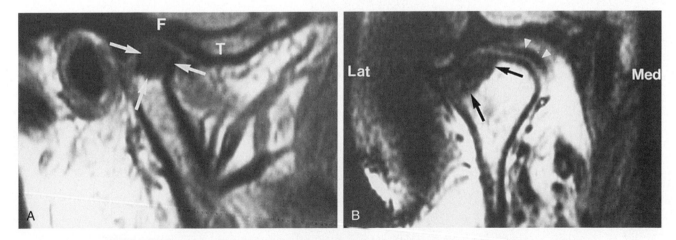

**FIGURE 18-49**   Probable aseptic necrosis. **A**, Sagittal MR image showing decreased signal from the bone marrow in the upper part of the mandibular condyle (*arrows*). The fossa (*F*) and tubercle (*T*) are indicated. **B**, Coronal MR image of the same joint as in **A** showing the low signal intensity area (*arrows*) in the lateral part of the joint. In the medial part of the condyle, the disk is seen superior to the condyle (*arrowheads*) and laterally the disk is absent, suggesting perforation.

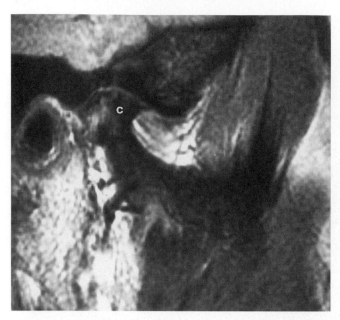

**FIGURE 18-50** Sagittal proton density MR image showing degenerative changes of the mandibular condyle (*C*). A core biopsy of this condyle showed avascular necrosis.

quickly gained popularity, although clinical studies to support long-term success were lacking. After about 2 to 4 years, patients frequently developed gradually increasing pain. This was later shown to be due to fragmentation of the implant material and a foreign body giant cell reaction to this material. Although the reaction to the particulated material was similar with both Silastic and Proplast, it seemed more aggressive with Proplast. Clinically, the patient presented with pain, and radiographically erosive changes of the bone have been observed (Fig. 18-64). The long-term prognosis for TMJ alloplastic implants is poor, and probably all implants eventually have to be removed.

While the implants are still in place, imaging evaluation is frequently necessary. The principal findings relate to the extent of erosive change of the glenoid fossa and the mandibular condyle. The integrity of the glenoid fossa is critical since erosions can extend into the middle cranial fossa (Fig. 18-63). For the initial evaluation of a patient with a TMJ alloplastic implant, both MR imaging (Fig. 18-62) and CT (Figs. 18-63 and 18-65) may be necessary. MR imaging shows the extent of the soft-tissue alteration (Fig. 18-62), fragmentation of the implant material, and expansion of the joint capsule. CT is valuable for assessment of bones, especially the integrity of the glenoid fossa (Fig. 18-63B). For follow-up examination, CT with coronal or sagittal images is the optimal imaging modality. Irregularity of the implant is best appreciated on CT. Sagittal or coronal CT images best demonstrate the implant and show erosive changes of the condyle most clearly. The status of the condyle following the temporary use of Silastic is best appreciated on CT, as is the bony ankylosis that may occur between the condyle and the glenoid fossa (Fig. 18-64).

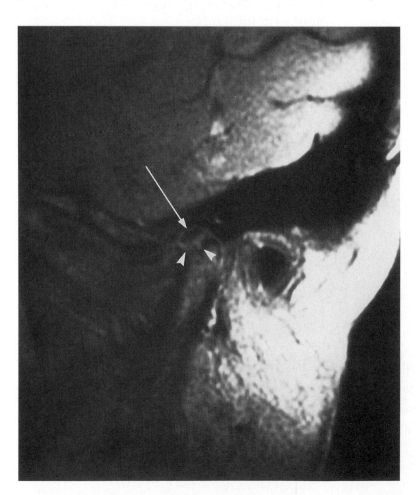

**FIGURE 18-51** Osteochondritis dissecans. Sagittal MR image shows a defect in the upper part of the condyle (*arrowheads*) and a corresponding structure in the glenoid fossa, which was interpreted as a loose body (*long arrow*). This condition is consistent with osteochondritis dissecans.

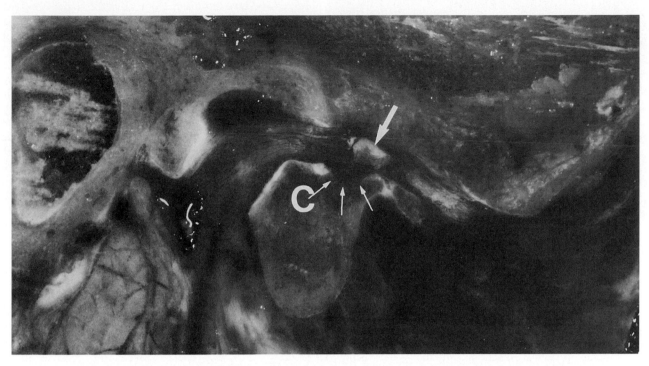

**FIGURE 18-52**   Osteochondritis dissecans. Cadaver specimen with advanced degenerative changes and a loose body (*thick arrow*) in the joint space with a corresponding defect in the mandibular condyle (*thin arrows*). Condyle (*C*).

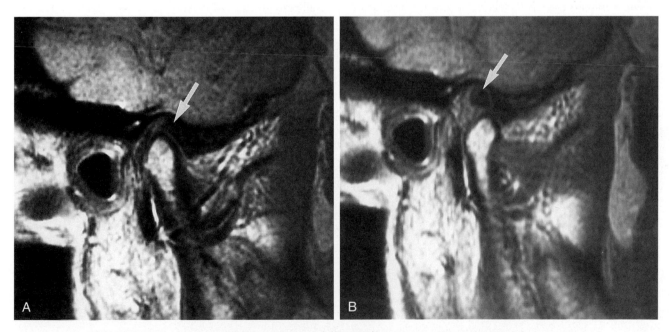

**FIGURE 18-53**   Stuck disk. Sagittal proton density MR images with a closed mouth (**A**) and maximal mouth opening (**B**) in a patient with limitation of mouth opening. The disk (*arrow*) is located in the normal superior position with a closed mouth. On opening, the disk does not move out of the glenoid fossa and the condyle does not translate all the way down to the articular eminence. This is consistent with a stuck disk condition.

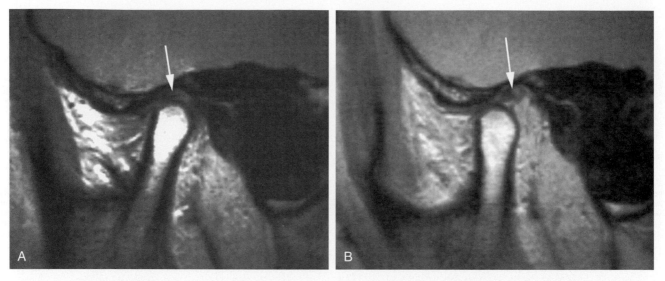

**FIGURE 18-54** Stuck disk. **A,** In the closed-mouth position, the condyle has a normal relationship to the disk. The posterior edge of the posterior thick band (*arrow*) is located immediately superior to the condylar head. **B,** In the open-mouth position, the condyle has translated anteriorly and now is seated on the thick anterior portion of the disk. The disk has not moved relative to the glenoid and the articular eminence. Note that the posterior edge of the disk (*arrow*) remains at the same point as in the closed-mouth image.

## Total Joint Replacement

Total replacement of the TMJ has been attempted for many years.[125, 126] There continue to be problems with stabilization of both the glenoid and condyle parts of the prosthesis, and these patients frequently present for imaging evaluation. In a situation where there are large metallic implants, neither CT nor MR imaging is feasible because of degradation artifacts. Plain films and tomography are the only imaging modalities available (Fig. 18-66). The assessment should concentrate on motion between the implant and the underlying bone, osteolytic changes of the bone, and evidence of loosening of the implant.

## Costochondral Grafts

Costochondral grafts were formerly used for reconstruction of the TMJ and have recently regained popularity since the alloplastic joint prostheses have essentially been abandoned.[127] Imaging of costochondral grafts can be done with plain films, tomography, CT, and MR imaging. MR imaging gives good images of the cartilaginous part of the graft. CT shows the osseous part of the graft but does not show the cartilaginous segment as well (Figs. 18-67 and 18-68). The size and orientation of the cartilaginous segment are represented by the apparent gap between the osseous part of the graft and the skull base, and the cartilage itself can

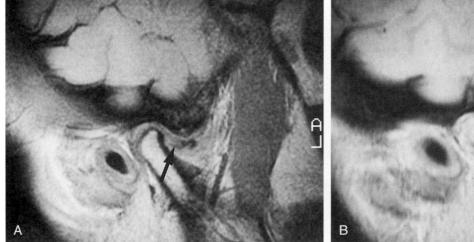
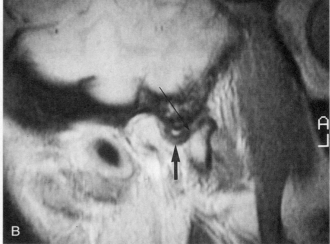

**FIGURE 18-55** Subluxation in front of the disk. **A,** Proton density sagittal MR image shows the disk (*arrow*) anterior to the condyle. The disk is deformed. **B,** On maximal mouth opening the condyle is in front of the disk (*arrow*), and the disk is preventing the condyle from reverting back into the glenoid fossa. The long arrow indicates the anterior edge of the disk.

**Table 18-2**
**ACCURACY OF TMJ IMAGING OSSEOUS CHANGES**

| Imaging | Accuracy (%) | Sensitivity | Specificity |
|---|---|---|---|
| Tomography | 63–85 | 0.47 | 0.94 |
| CT | 66–87 | 0.28–0.75 | 0.91–1.0 |
| MR imaging | 60–100 | 0.50–0.87 | 0.71–1.0 |

Modified from Lindvall AM, et al. Radiographic examination of the temporomandibular joint. Dentomaxillofac Radiology 1976;5:24–32; Bean LR, et al. Comparison between radiologic observations and macroscopic tissue changes in temporomandibular joint. Dentomaxillofac Radiol 1977;6:90–106; Rohlin M, et al. Tomography as an aid to detect microscopic changes of the temporomandibular joint. Acta Odontol Scand 1986;44:131–140; Tanimoto K et al. Comparison of computed tomography with conventional tomography in the evaluation of temporomandibular joint disease: a study of autopsy specimens. Dentomaxillofac Radiol 1990;19:21–27; Westesson P-L, et al. CT and MRI of the temporomandibular joint: comparison using autopsy specimens. AJR 1987;148:1165–1171; Westesson P-L et al. Temporomandibular joint: comparison of MR images with cryosectional anatomy. Radiology 1987;164:59–64; Hansson L-G et al. MR imaging of the temporomandibular joint: comparisons of images of specimens made at 0.3T and 1.5T with cryosections. AJR 1989;152:1241–1244; and Tasaki MM, Westesson P-L. Temporomandibular joint: diagnostic accuracy with sagittal and coronal MR imaging. Radiology 1993;186:723–729.

**Table 18-3**
**ACCURACY OF TMJ IMAGING FOR DISK POSITION**

| Imaging | Accuracy (%) | Sensitivity | Specificity |
|---|---|---|---|
| Lower space, single-contrast arthrography | 84–100 | 0.95 | 0.76 |
| CT | 40–67 | 0.45–0.85 | 0.50–0.87 |
| MR imaging | 73–95 | 0.86–0.90 | 0.63–1.0 |

Modified from Westesson P-L et al. Temporomandibular joint: Correlation between single-contrast videoarthrography and post mortem morphology. Radiology 1986;160:767–771; Schellhas KP et al. The diagnosis of temporomandibular joint disease: two-compartment arthrography and MR. AJNR 1988;51:341–350; Tanimoto K et al. Computed tomography versus single-contrast arthrotomography in evaluation of the temporomandibular joint disc. A study of autopsy specimens. Int J Oral Maxillofac Surg 1989;18:354–358; Westesson P-L et al. Temporomandibular joint: Comparison of MR images with cryosectional anatomy. Radiology 1987;164:59–64; Hansson L-G et al. MR imaging of the temporomandibular joint: comparisons of images of specimens made at 0.3T and 1.5T with cryosections. AJR 1989;152:1241–1244; Westesson P-L et al. CT and MRI of the temporomandibular joint: comparison using autopsy specimens. AJR 1987;148:1165–1171; and Tasaki MM, Westesson P-L. Temporomandibular joint: diagnostic accuracy with sagittal and coronal MR imaging. Radiology 1993;186:723–729.

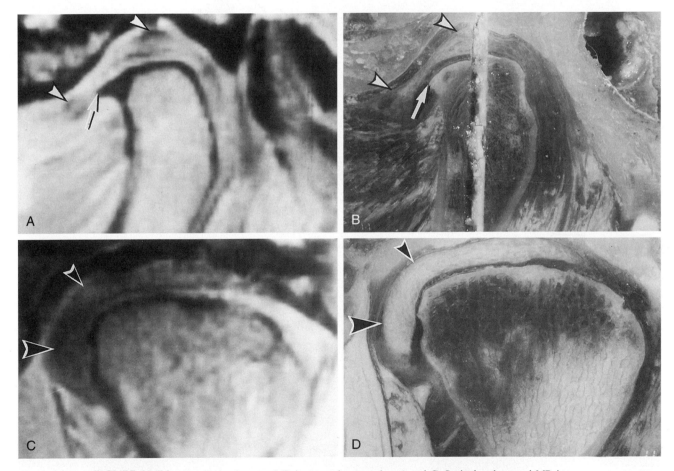

**FIGURE 18-56**   Correlation between MR image and cryosection. **A** and **C**, Sagittal and coronal MR images show the disk (*arrowheads*) superior to the condyle in the sagittal view (**A**) but medially displaced in the coronal view (**C**). **B** and **D**, The corresponding cryosections confirm the MR images. The condyle also demonstrates an anterior osteophyte (*arrow* in **A**).

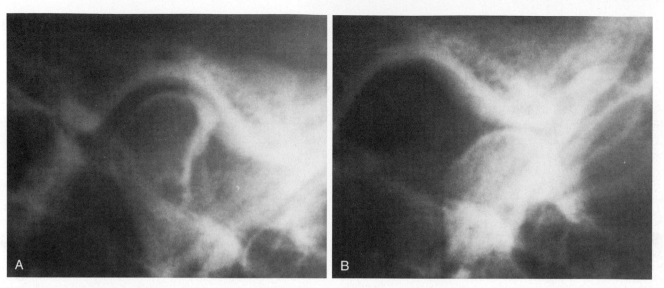

**FIGURE 18-57**    Transcranial plain film in the closed-mouth (**A**) and open-mouth (**B**) positions 29 years after diskectomy. The osseous structures are relatively normal, with only a decreased joint space. The outline of the condyle and temporal joint components is smooth, without evidence of degenerative joint disease.

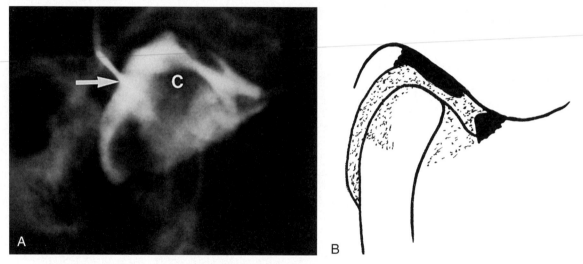

**FIGURE 18-58**    **A** and **B**, Postsurgical arthrogram and schematic drawing. Contrast medium was injected into the lower joint space (*arrow*), and there is a perforation to the upper joint space. Peripheral adhesions make the joint space smaller than normal. A disk plication had been performed 2 years before this arthrogram was obtained.

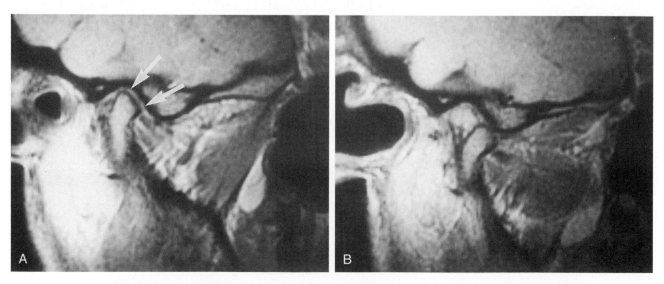

**FIGURE 18-59**    Successful diskectomy. **A**, Closed-mouth MR image shows an area of intermediate to high signal (*arrows*) in the joint space. This is the normal appearance after a successful diskectomy. **B**, On opening, the condyle translates anteriorly and inferiorly, and there is no evidence of fibrous ankylosis.

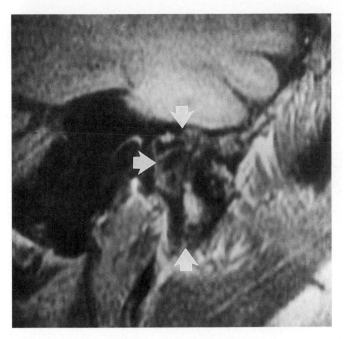

**FIGURE 18-60**   Intraarticular adhesions following diskectomy. Sagittal MR image 2 years after diskectomy. There is an irregular area of low signal intensity in the entire joint region (*arrows*). This is indicative of extensive fibrous adhesions.

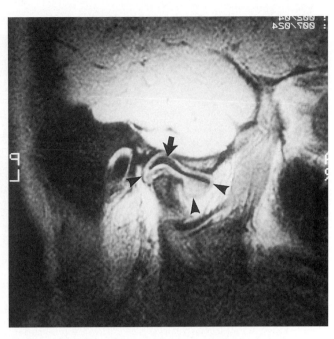

**FIGURE 18-62**   Alloplastic TMJ implant. Sagittal proton density MR image shows an alloplastic TMJ implant (*arrow*). The implant has been in place for 3 years, and there is an expanded capsule (*arrowheads*) surrounding it. Degenerative changes of the condyle with an anterior osteophyte are seen.

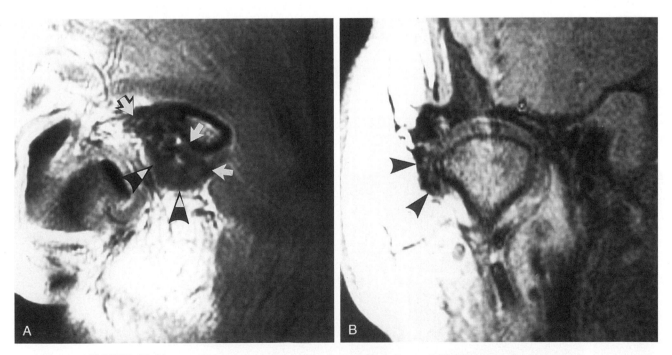

**FIGURE 18-61**   Scar tissue in the lateral capsule. Sagittal (**A**) and coronal (**B**) MR images after diskectomy. There is an irregular area of decreased signal in the lateral capsule wall (*arrows*) indicative of scar tissue. Coronal image (**B**) shows the area confined to the capsule wall. This fibrous tissue (*arrowheads*) does not extend into the joint space.

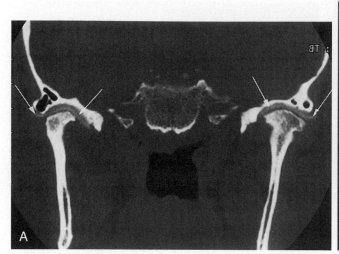

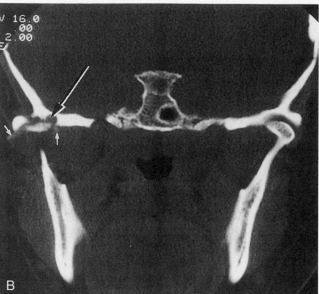

**FIGURE 18-63**   **A,** Coronal CT scan of a patient with bilateral Proplast Teflon implants (*arrows*) in good condition. There is no evidence of erosions into the middle cranial fossa, and the implants appear intact and with a good relationship to the condyle and glenoid fossa. **B,** Erosions of the glenoid fossa secondary to an alloplastic implant. Coronal CT scan of another patient with a Proplast Teflon implant (*short arrows*) and erosions of the glenoid fossa (*long arrow*). Also note that the implant is difficult to outline due to partial fragmentation.

sometimes be demonstrated. Points of contact between the osseous part of the graft and the skull base can be demonstrated, and sclerosis of the bone may be present. Fusion can occur, causing progressive limitation of opening. CT imaging with 3D reconstructions allows for a more graphic demonstration of the relationship between the joint components; however, portions of the cartilaginous graft are still not visualized (Fig. 18-69).

## Metallic Artifacts

Metallic artifacts are frequently seen in MR imaging of postoperative osseous structures. The metallic artifact

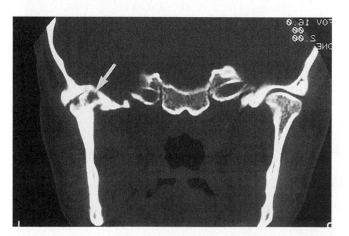

**FIGURE 18-64**   Erosions and bony ankylosis following temporary Silastic implant. Coronal CT scans through the TMJ show extensive erosive changes of the right condyle. There is bony ankylosis between the condyle and the glenoid fossa and the medial part of the joint. The patient used a temporary Silastic implant for a few months. These extensive radiographic changes are the sequelae from the use of the implant.

appears as an area of signal void bordered by areas of high signal intensity (Fig. 18-70). Even very small metallic particles can cause significant areas of loss of signal, and thus minuscule pieces shredded from metallic instruments used to scrape the bone could be sufficient to create a significant artifact. These small artifacts are seen in both symptomatic and asymptomatic patients after surgery, and they are probably of no clinical significance.[124] The most important aspect of the metallic artifact is that it may prevent further MR imaging.

## MISCELLANEOUS CONDITIONS INVOLVING THE TMJ

Though most imaging evaluations are done for possible internal derangements and their sequelae, many other types of pathology occasionally affect the TMJ. Tumors, systemic arthritides, and congenital anomalies may be found during an evaluation of the TMJ or during assessment for suspected pathology in the adjacent head and neck region.

### Tumors and Tumor-Like Conditions of the TMJ

#### Synovial Chondromatosis

The TMJ is infrequently affected by tumors. The most common neoplastic lesion affecting the TMJ is probably synovial chondromatosis.[128, 129] This tumor can be locally aggressive, and cases with intracranial extension have been described.[130, 131] It is a benign lesion characterized by formation of multiple small "pearls" of cartilage, usually within the joint space. MR imaging can show synovial chondromatosis primarily affecting the upper joint space

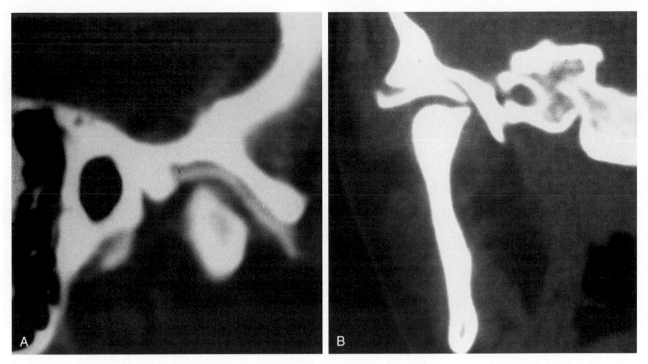

**FIGURE 18-65**   CT scan in the sagittal (**A**) and coronal (**B**) planes showing an implant in a good position.

(Fig. 18-71) or both the upper and lower joint spaces (Fig. 18-72). There is often significant joint expansion, and there may be multiple areas of low signal intensity that represent the pearls (Fig. 18-72). The clinical presentation of patients with synovial chondromatosis is similar to the general presentation of TMJ pain and dysfunction, and the findings are usually detected with imaging studies or at surgery. Evaluation can be done with both MR imaging and CT.[132–134]

### Pigmented Villonodular Synovitis

Pigmented villonodular synovitis is a benign proliferative disease or tumor affecting the synovial lining of joints as well as tendons. There is nodular synovial proliferation and hemarthrosis. Pathology shows a mixture of histiocytes, giant cells, and spindle cells. There is evidence of hemorrhage with intracellular hemosiderin. The condition rarely involves the TMJ.[135–141] An enlarging mass is centered in the TMJ or the lesion may seem to extend away from the joint. The lesion tends to be dense on CT.

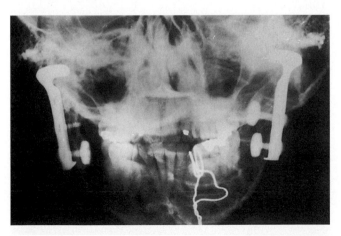

**FIGURE 18-66**   Bilateral total joints. Anterior posterior plain film shows bilateral total replacement. The condyle fragments are attached to the ramus of the mandible. Proplast Teflon fossa implants are attached to the articular eminence and the zygomatic arch with screws. Also note the osteosynthesis in the left symphysis region from an old mandibular fracture.

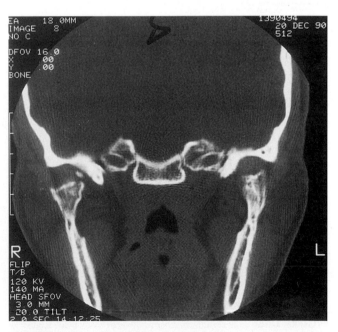

**FIGURE 18-67**   Bilateral costochondral grafts. Coronal CT scan of an asymptomatic patient with bilateral costochondral grafts. Note how the grafts are integrated into the ramus of the mandible. The most superior cartilaginous parts of the grafts are not well visualized on CT.

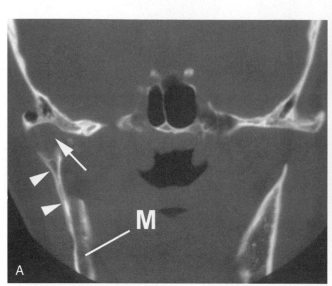

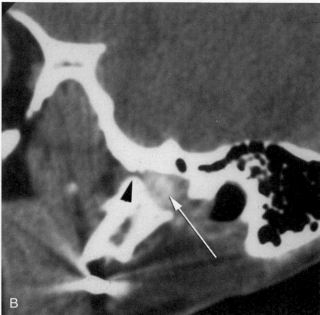

**FIGURE 18-68**   Costochondral graft CT. **A,** Coronal CT scan shows the osseous portion of the costochondral graft (*arrowheads*) attached to the lateral aspect of the native mandible (*M*). The chondral part of the graft (*arrow*) is seen as a lucency separating the osseous part of the graft from the glenoid. **B,** The cartilage portion of the graft (*arrow*) is seen more clearly on the sagittal reformatted image. Note that the edge of the osseous portion of the graft (*arrowhead*) is very close to the articular eminence.

The head of the condyle is usually eroded, and in more extensive cases the skull base may also be involved. The hemorrhage by-products give the lesion low signal on both T1- and T2- weighted images (Fig. 18-73). Indeed, the extensive iron deposition can give a pronounced susceptibility artifact, particularly on T2-weighted MR images.

### Osteochondroma

Osteochondroma is probably the second most common neoplastic lesion affecting the TMJ. Osteochondroma (Fig. 18-74), osteoma, and condyle hyperplasia are difficult to differentiate clinically and on imaging studies. MR imaging can define these conditions in both the sagittal and coronal planes, but CT may delineate more precisely the extension of the tumor and its relationship to anatomic structures medial to the TMJ region.

**FIGURE 18-69**   Three-dimensional right-sided costochondral graft in an asymptomatic patient. Note that the graft is integrated into the mandible. The superior cartilaginous portion of the graft is not well visualized on the CT scan. The image was obtained in a partial mouth-open position.

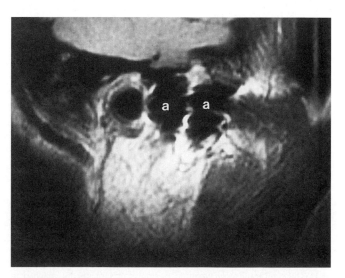

**FIGURE 18-70**   Metal artifact. MR proton density image of a joint with metallic wires. These artifacts (*a*) are characterized by irregular areas of signal void bordered by areas of high signal.

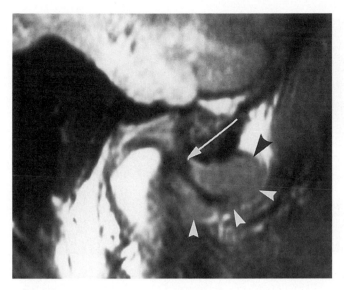

**FIGURE 18-71**   Synovial chondromatosis. Sagittal MR image showing expansion of the upper and lower joint spaces (*arrowheads*). The disk (*arrow*) is anteriorly displaced.

## Calcium Pyrophosphate Arthropathy (Pseudogout)

Calcium pyrophosphate dihydrate (CPPD) deposition disease, or pseudogout, infrequently affects the TMJ. Involvement can be mild or quite severe. Mild cases of this condition have been described with subtle calcifications in the disk and in the joint space (Fig. 18-75).[142–144] Clinically, the patient presents with pain and dysfunction similar to the symptoms of other TMJ patients. There can be associated swelling and degenerative changes in the joint. CT is the best imaging modality for demonstration of the minute intraarticular calcifications. More extensive cases present with enlarging masses.[143, 145–147] Calcification can be demonstrated on a CT scan. There can be significant erosion of the contiguous skull base as well as the condyle. Malignancy may be suspected because of the apparent aggressiveness and bone "destruction" shown at imaging (Fig. 18-76). The pathology can also suggest sarcoma, and thus the importance of considering this benign diagnosis so that aggressive therapy inappropriate for this benign disease can be avoided.[145, 146, 148, 149]

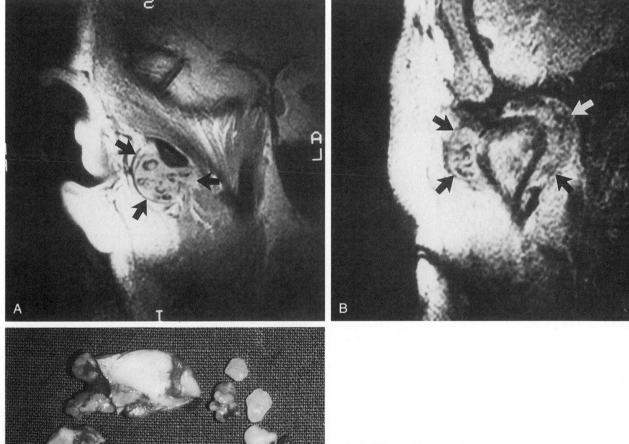

**FIGURE 18-72**   Synovial chondromatosis. **A,** Sagittal proton density MR image from the lateral aspect of the TMJ. There is expansion of the joint capsule (*arrows*), with multiple areas of low signal. **B,** Coronal proton density MR image. In the coronal image there is expansion of both the lateral and medial capsule walls (*arrows*). This indicates a neoplastic intraarticular process. The finding of multiple areas of low signal within the expanded joint capsule is consistent with synovial chondromatosis. **C,** Small bodies of cartilaginous material removed from a joint (another patient) with synovial chondromatosis.

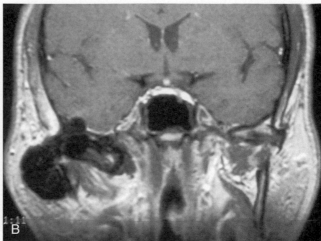

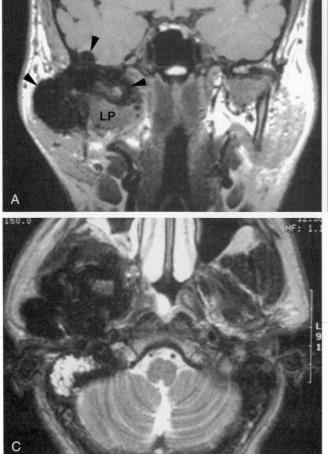

**FIGURE 18-73** Pigmented villonodular synovitis. **A,** Coronal T1-weighted precontrast image shows a mass (*arrowheads*) of very low signal in the region of the head of the condyle. The lesion "squeezes" above the lateral pterygoid muscle (*LP*). The configuration is typical of lesions arising in the joint compartment. **B,** T1-weighted postcontrast image. No significant enhancement is seen within the lesion. **C,** T2-weighted images shows extremely low signal due to the blood by-products characteristic of this lesion. Fluid is seen in the mastoid because this lesion interferes with eustachian tube function. (Courtesy of Dr. Tim Larson.)

### Synovial Cysts and Simple Bone Cysts

Synovial cysts of the TMJ have been reported but are rare (Fig. 18-77).[150, 151] They present with unilateral pain and possible enlargement of the condyle head, and there can be associated swelling.

Simple bone cysts are most frequently located in the body of the mandible. However, they may occur in the condyle head (Fig. 18-78), and often the remaining joint components are normal.

### Rare Lesions and Tumors

Eosinophilic granuloma may also present as a lytic lesion involving the mandibular condyle and ramus (Fig. 18-79). Rarely, tumoral calcinosis has been described involving the joint and contiguous muscles.[152] The calcified lesions are best defined on CT scan.

Chondrosarcoma and synovial cell sarcoma, as well as other sarcomas, can occasionally involve the TMJ. Meningiomas, chondroblastomas, and a variety of other tumors may extend into the joint from the contiguous bone, as can malignancies of the external ear and parotid gland.

### Metastatic Disease in the TMJ Region

Fewer than 1% of all tumors metastasize to the maxillofacial area.[153-155] Adenocarcinoma is the most common of all metastatic tumors in the jaw, accounting for 70% of the cases. A review of 115 cases of mandibular metastasis found that 30% were metastases from breast carcinoma, 16% from kidney, 15% from lung, 8% from colon and rectum, 7% from prostate, 6% from thyroid, 5% from stomach, 4% from skin, 3% from testes, and other sites represented less than 1% each. Most metastases are found in the molar and premolar regions of the mandible, and only a few cases of metastasis to the mandibular condyle have been reported. Most cases with metastasis to the TMJ region have presented with TMJ-related symptoms.[154] Lymphoma can also rarely involve the TMJ (Fig. 18-80), and bone regeneration may occur after chemotherapy (Fig. 18-80B).[156]

## Arthritides

The TMJ is involved in approximately 50% of patients with rheumatoid diseases such as rheumatoid arthritis, ankylosing spondylitis, and psoriatic arthritis. Imaging is an important adjunct to the clinical diagnosis and is particularly valuable for follow-up of patients with these diseases. Plain films and panoramic images are standard, but MR imaging may be indicated to evaluate the soft-tissue involvement of these diseases.[157] Morphologically, inflammatory arthritis is characterized by synovial proliferation and secondary erosive changes of the bone (Fig. 18-81). Studies with MR imaging have shown potential for accurate evaluation of the soft-tissue components of the joint (Fig. 18-82).[85, 86] A study indicated the additional value of contrast-enhanced images for defining the area of inflammatory change within the joint and in the periarticular soft tissue (Fig. 18-82B).[157] Only limited experience is available with MR imaging of other inflammatory arthritides such as psoriatic arthritis and ankylosing spondylitis. Gout rarely involves the TMJ.[158] There can be erosion of the condyle and swelling of the tissues contiguous to an acutely painful joint. Rarely, the skull base can be eroded.

## Acute Trauma

Plain films, panoramic examinations, or CT may be done for acute trauma to the mandible. Most patients do not come to imaging specifically for the TMJ, but in many patients with condylar neck and mandibular fractures there is also injury to the TMJ. Such TMJ trauma is frequently not recognized until after the acute clinical course. MR imaging may occasionally show fractures and effusions not seen on other imaging studies (Fig. 18-83), and thus MR imaging could be helpful in evaluating patients with acute pain following trauma to the face and jaw despite other negative examinations. The external auditory canal should also be closely examined when a jaw fracture is suspected.

Both CT and MR imaging may be helpful in cases with intracapsular fractures (Fig. 18-84). Although CT may show the positional relationship of the osseous fragments, MR imaging (Fig. 18-84) shows any associated disk abnormality. In a situation where reconstructive surgery is contemplated, 3D reconstructions (Fig. 18-84D) may be helpful to evaluate the positional relationships between the joint components.

Penetrating trauma to the TMJ is relatively rare, but it warrants imaging evaluation. It can cause fracture, hematoma, and dislocations. CT is the preferred method of examination, and it is important to obtain both axial and coronal images (Fig. 18-85).

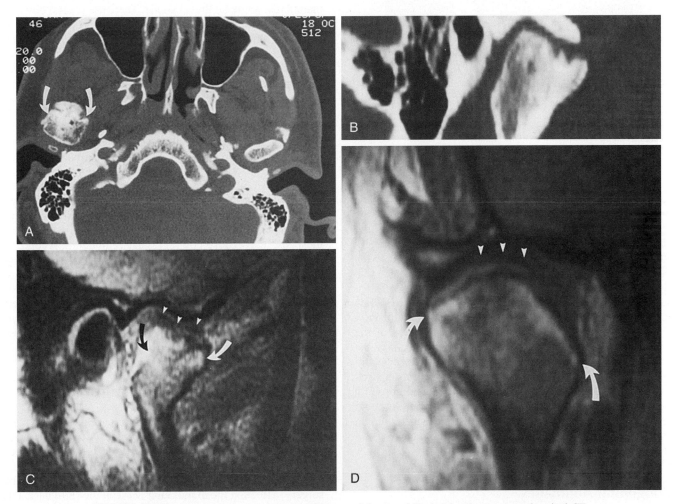

**FIGURE 18-74**   Osteochondroma of the mandibular condyle. **A** and **B**, Axial and reconstructed sagittal CT scans show the right condyle (*arrows*) to be two to three times larger than the left condyle. There is also irregular mineralization in this condyle. **C** and **D**, Sagittal and coronal MR images of the same joints show mixed low and high signal from the enlarged parts of the condyle (*curved arrows*). The temporal component is normal. The disk (*arrowheads*) is biconcave and located in a normal superior position. (Courtesy of Dr. Donald Macher, Rochester, New York.)

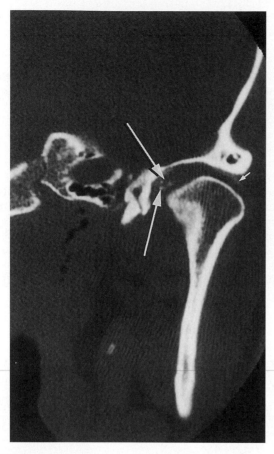

**FIGURE 18-75** Pseudogout. Coronal CT scan of a patient with chronic TMJ pain and normal disk position on an MR image (not shown). There are subtle calcifications in the joint space (*arrows*). Aspiration showed pyrophosphate crystals.

## Coronoid Hyperplasia

Hyperplasia or elongation of the coronoid process of the mandible can mimic symptoms of TMJ internal derangement with limitation of jaw opening. This condition has been extensively described, and a study has indicated that elongation of the coronoid process may occur in up to 5% of patients with TMJ symptoms and limitation of jaw opening.[159–161] If the coronoid process is significantly elongated, it can impact on the zygomatic process of the maxilla, causing limitation of jaw opening. CT scans in the axial or sagittal plane, performed in the closed- and open-mouth positions, are valuable in the imaging assessment of patients with a clinical suspicion of coronoid hyperplasia because they can demonstrate the coronoid impaction on the maxilla (Fig. 18-86). Surgical treatment with removal of the coronoid process usually yields good results.

## Congenital Anomalies

### Bifid Condyle

Congenital anomalies of the TMJ are relatively rare. The most common congenital anomaly is probably the so-called bifid condyle. This implies a partial or complete separation of the condyle into a lateral and a medial half (Fig. 18-87). This is usually of no clinical significance other than in the rare situation in which surgery should be performed and preoperative knowledge of the morphology is important. The picture of a bifid condyle is characteristic on coronal imaging and should be distinguished from acquired pathologic conditions with remodeling and degenerative joint disease.

### Hemifacial Microsomia

The TMJ is affected in other conditions such as hemifacial microsomia with underdevelopment of the TMJ. Frequently, there is a flat articular eminence and a small mandibular condyle (Fig. 18-88). The mastoid typically is underdeveloped, with no aeration. The disk is usually in a normal location in hemifacial microsomia. In advanced cases the entire ramus, condyle, and coronoid process of the mandible are not developed (Fig. 18-89).

### Asymmetry of the Mandible

Asymmetry of the mandible is a frequent clinical presentation. The most prominent facial features include a shift of the chin to the short side and prominence of the mandibular angle on the long side. There are several obvious causes of mandibular asymmetry such as trauma with fractures, tumors, and congenital anomalies. In many cases, however, the cause of mandibular asymmetry leading to facial deformities is unclear on physical examination, and imaging assessment may be warranted.[162, 163]

Mandibular asymmetry can result principally from enlargement of the condylar head (condylar hyperplasia) on the long side (Fig. 18-90) or from decreased condyle growth (condylar hypolasia) (Fig. 18-91) or degenerative joint disease on the short side (Fig. 18-92).[163–165] Imaging studies are done to determine the cause of mandibular asymmetry and for treatment planning. The imaging evaluation of mandibular asymmetry is outlined in Box 18-5 on page 1049. Soft-tissue imaging is important, and MR imaging may be performed as well as CT. Condylar hypoplasia is most frequently caused by regressive remodeling secondary to long-standing internal derangement; however, the condyle may have a relatively normal appearance, without evidence of degenerative joint disease. The joint appears to be more sensitive to regressive remodeling if the internal derangement occurs during the growth and development phase. However, mandibular asymmetry and change in occlusion have also been described in adults.

## Atrophy of the Muscles of Mastication

Atrophy of the muscles of mastication is occasionally seen in patients who are unable to open their mouths. These atrophic changes in the muscles are most frequently secondary to trauma or orthognathic surgery.[88, 166] Less often, they may occur secondary to a tumor (or tumor surgery) affecting the mandibular nerve at the skull base. On MR imaging the atrophic changes of the muscles of mastication are usually reflected as fatty replacement.

Following orthognathic surgery, there is frequently asymptomatic muscle atrophy.[166] Occasionally, this is associated with chewing difficulties and fatigue in the jaw

*Text continued on page 1046*

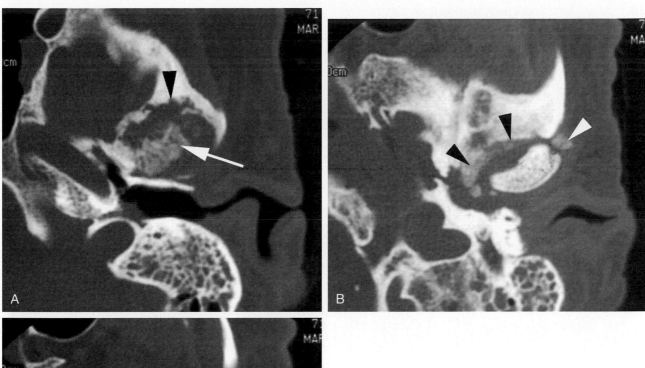

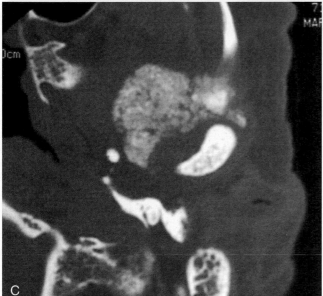

**FIGURE 18-76** Calcium pyrophosphate arthropathy, axial CT scan. At the initial histopathologic examination, the lesion was thought to be malignant. **A**, There is erosive expansion of the glenoid including erosion of the articular eminence (*arrowhead*). Amorphous calcific material is seen in the joint space (*arrow*). **B**, The calcific material (*arrowheads*) wraps around the anterior surface of the condylar head. **C**, Scan slightly caudad to **A** and **B** shows the amorphous calcific material anterior to the condylar head. The small rings suggest a chondroid matrix, as in synovial chondromatosis, but histopathologic examination showed calcium pyrophosphate dihydrate crystals.

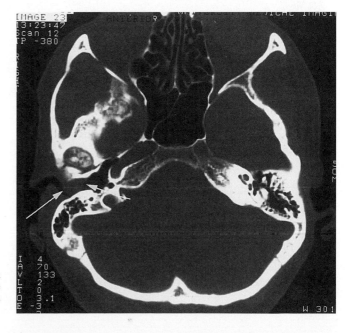

**FIGURE 18-77** Synovial cyst. Axial CT scan of a patient with a 1 cm synovial cyst (*arrows*) extending into the external auditory canal. There are extensive degenerative changes of the condyle head. At surgery the cyst was found to extend into the joint through the bony fissure.

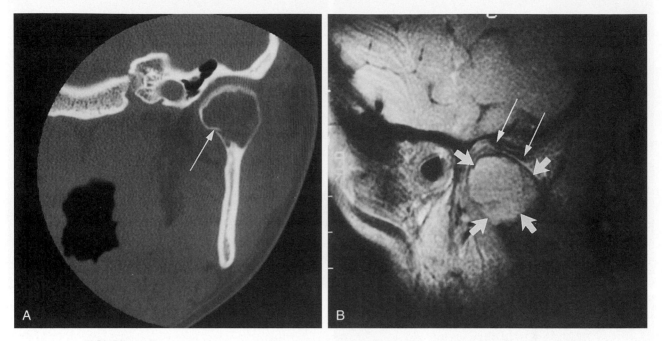

**FIGURE 18-78** Simple bone cyst. **A,** Coronal CT scan shows a large cystic lesion involving the entire condyle head. There is expansion and enlargement of the condyle and thinning of the cortex. Medially and inferiorly (*arrow*) there is a small pathologic fracture. **B,** Sagittal proton density MR image shows intermediate signal of the expanded bone marrow of the condyle (*thick arrows*). The disk (*long arrows*) is in the normal location.

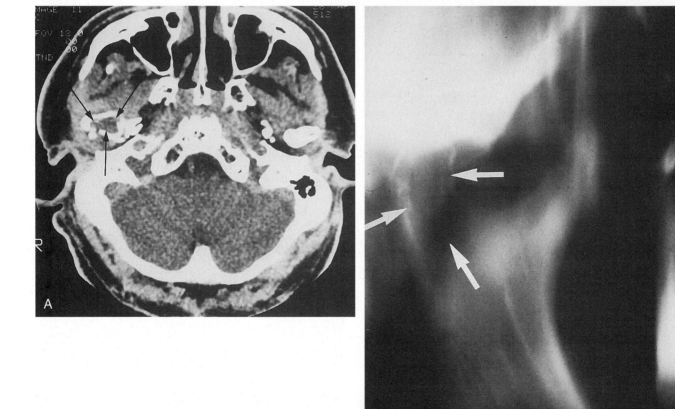

**FIGURE 18-79** Eosinophilic granuloma. **A,** Axial CT scan through the TMJ shows expansion and lytic changes of the right condyle (*arrows*). **B,** Sagittal tomogram shows the lesion to extend down into the neck of the condyle. (Courtesy of Dr. Susan White, Gainesville, Florida.)

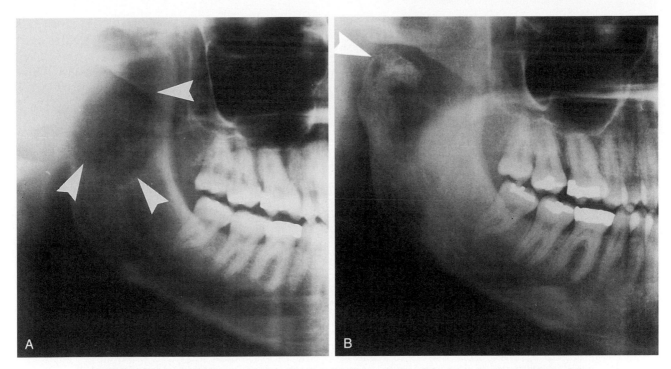

**FIGURE 18-80**   Metastatic lymphoma to the TMJ. **A**, Large osteolytic defect involving the condyle, condyle neck, coronoid process, and upper half of the ascending ramus (*arrowheads*). **B**, Following chemotherapy, there was regeneration of the condyle neck and condyle (*arrowhead*). The patient died 1 year later from intracranial and generalized metastasis.

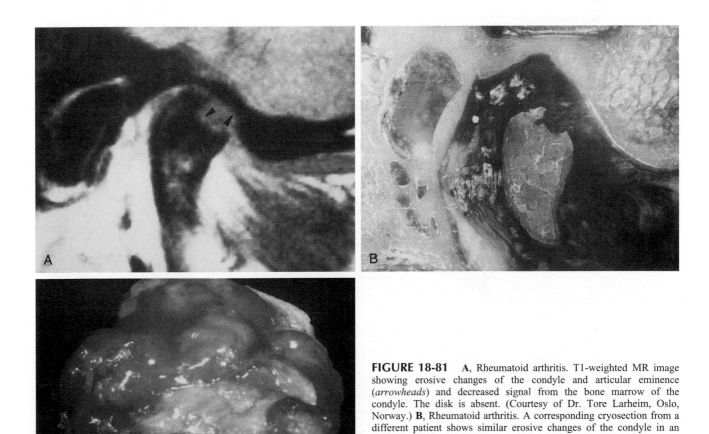

**FIGURE 18-81**   **A**, Rheumatoid arthritis. T1-weighted MR image showing erosive changes of the condyle and articular eminence (*arrowheads*) and decreased signal from the bone marrow of the condyle. The disk is absent. (Courtesy of Dr. Tore Larheim, Oslo, Norway.) **B**, Rheumatoid arthritis. A corresponding cryosection from a different patient shows similar erosive changes of the condyle in an individual with a long history of rheumatoid arthritis. There is extensive granulation tissue in the joint and periarticular area. **C**, Rheumatoid arthritis. Anterior aspect of the condyle from another individual with a long history of rheumatoid arthritis shows extensive synovial proliferation overlying the entire condyle head.

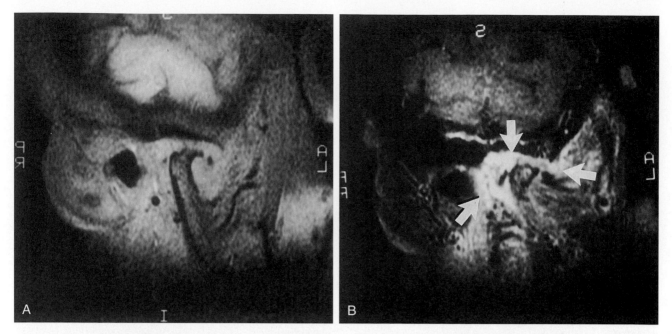

**FIGURE 18-82** Rheumatoid arthritis with contrast enhancement. **A,** Sagittal proton density image shows advanced degenerative disease of both the condyle and the temporal joint component. **B,** With contrast enhancement there is significant enhancement in the joint and the periarticular area (*arrows*). This indicates the area of synovial proliferation. There is also a small area of meningeal enhancement of unclear clinical significance.

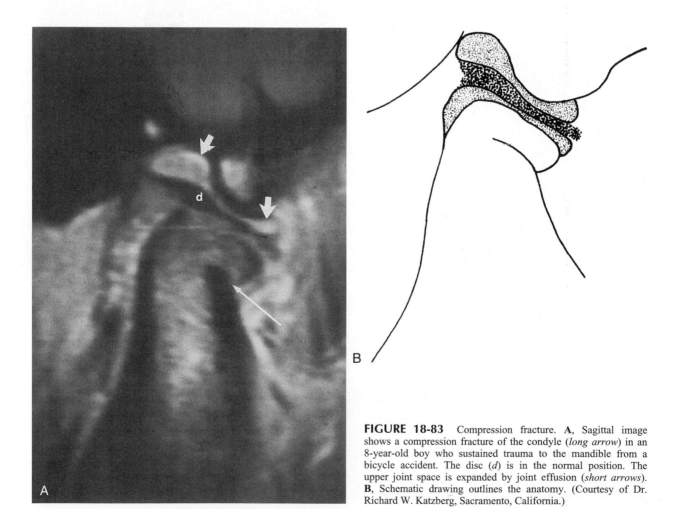

**FIGURE 18-83** Compression fracture. **A,** Sagittal image shows a compression fracture of the condyle (*long arrow*) in an 8-year-old boy who sustained trauma to the mandible from a bicycle accident. The disc (*d*) is in the normal position. The upper joint space is expanded by joint effusion (*short arrows*). **B,** Schematic drawing outlines the anatomy. (Courtesy of Dr. Richard W. Katzberg, Sacramento, California.)

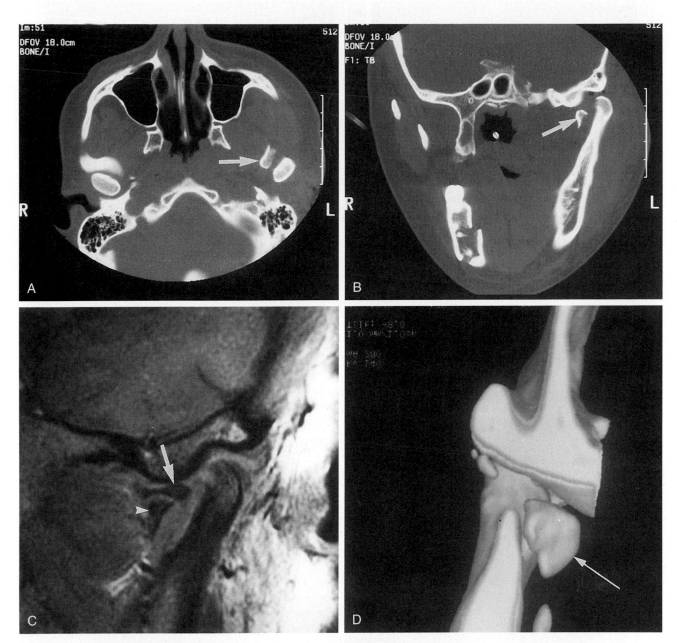

**FIGURE 18-84**   Intracapsular fracture with displacement of a condyle fragment and disk. **A,** Axial CT scan shows fracture of the medial part of the condyle (*arrow*) with anterior and medial displacement. **B,** Coronal CT scan confirms the inferior medial displacement of the condyle fragment (*arrow*) and shows small intraarticular air collections. Note the contralateral mandibular body fracture. **C,** Sagittal proton density MR image shows the condyle fragment (*arrowhead*) anteriorly and inferiorly displaced. The disk (*arrow*) is located superior to the fragment but is anteriorly and inferiorly displaced relative to the remaining condyle. **D,** Coronal three-dimensional reconstruction of CT image demonstrates the inferior medial location of the displaced fragment (*arrow*).

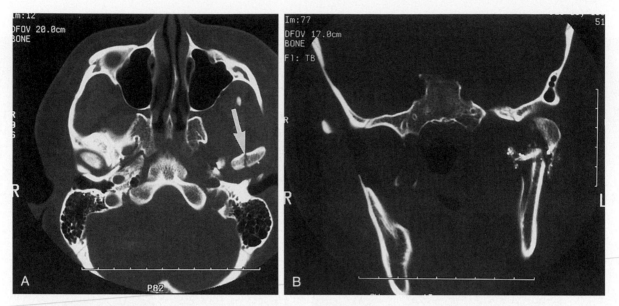

**FIGURE 18-85**   Penetrating trauma to the TMJ. **A,** Axial CT scan through the condyle shows a sagittal fracture in the center of the condyle head. **B,** Coronal image through the joint shows comminuted fractures with displacement of the medial fragment. Axial and coronal views are supplementary because the displacement was not well appreciated on the axial image.

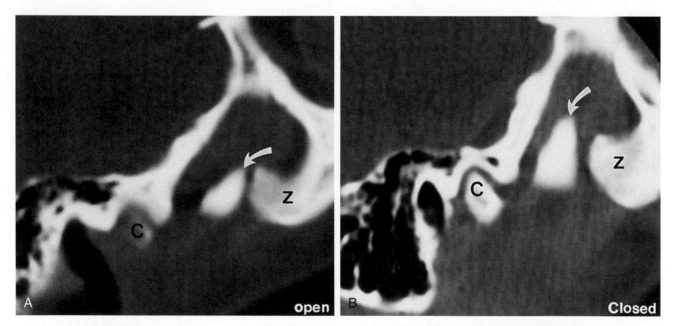

**FIGURE 18-86**   Coronoid hyperplasia restricting mouth opening. **A** and **B,** Direct sagittal CT scans in the open-mouth and closed-mouth positions showing the elongated coronoid process (*arrows*) interfering with the zygomatic process (*z*) of the maxilla at the open-mouth position. The condyle (*C*) is in the glenoid fossa.

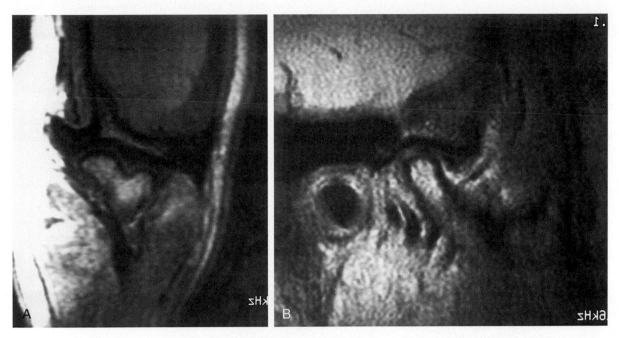

**FIGURE 18-87** Bifid condyle. **A,** Coronal MR image shows the characteristic appearance of a bifid condyle. **B,** Sagittal MR image shows a normal appearance of the condyle and disk.

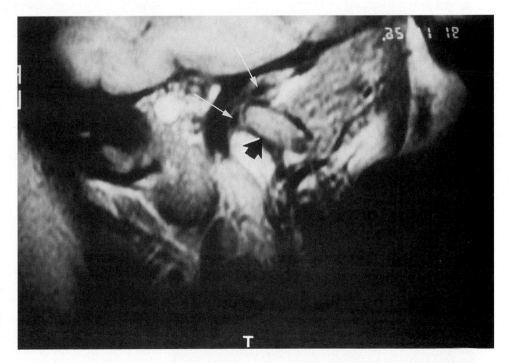

**FIGURE 18-88** Hemifacial micro-somia. Sagittal MR image of a young patient with hemifacial microsomia. The temporal bone is underdeveloped. The mastoid is not aerated; instead, there is fat filling the mastoid air cells. The mandibular condyle (*thick arrow*) is underdeveloped, with a curvature poste-riorly. The disk (*thin arrows*) is in a normal relationship with the condyle. The articular eminence is absent, and the condyle is essentially articulating against the flat skull base. The lateral pterygoid muscle appears normal.

muscles; in these cases, MR imaging is the best imaging modality. Electromyography may be of some value when asymmetric recordings of the left and right sides can be documented.

## MISCELLANEOUS IMAGING

### Radionuclide Imaging

Studies have suggested that radionuclide imaging of the TMJ (Fig. 18-93), using conventional skeletal imaging techniques, may be a valuable screening test for osseous disease.[167, 168] The technique can be performed easily, and the radiation dose to the patient is low.[1] An advantage of the technique is that conditions outside the joint also may be easily detected. Radionuclide imaging has not gained popularity for TMJ imaging. This is probably because it is nonspecific, and frequently a second imaging modality is needed to determine the nature of the problem and to form a treatment plan.

### Thin-Section MR Imaging

There is continuous ongoing development in MR imaging technology. The signal-to-noise ratio and soft-tissue and spatial resolution are improved each time MR scanners are upgraded. This means that the image quality can be expected to continue to improve, and experimental MR images with improved spatial and soft-tissue resolution (Fig. 18-94) may soon be available commercially. Figure 18-94 was obtained on an autopsy TMJ specimen. It shows significantly improved spatial and soft-tissue resolution because of thinner slice thickness and a smaller field of view. In this image the trabecular pattern of the condyle can be clearly identified, and the perforation of the disk and the osteophyte of the condyle, protruding into the perforation, can be seen with exquisite detail.

### Dynamic MR Imaging

The time needed to acquire an image is also rapidly decreasing, and within the next few years, one may be able

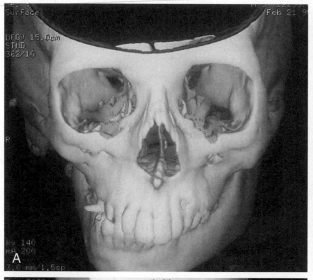

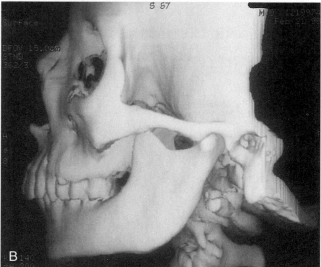

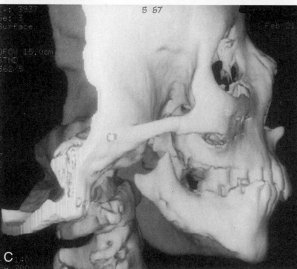

**FIGURE 18-89** Hemifacial microsomia. Three-dimensional CT scan shows asymmetry of the maxillofacial and mandibular regions. **A,** The right side of the face is underdeveloped. **B,** The left side of the face has a normal configuration and size. **C,** The right side of the face shows the diminished size of the body and ramus of the mandible. The midface structures are also underdeveloped in this 9-year-old female with hemifacial microsomia. Note in the frontal view (**A**) that there is a crossbite on the right side, with the mandibular teeth occluding on the buccal side of the maxillary teeth.

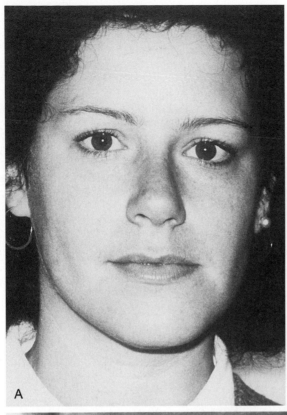

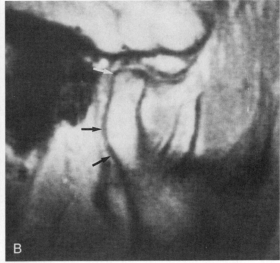

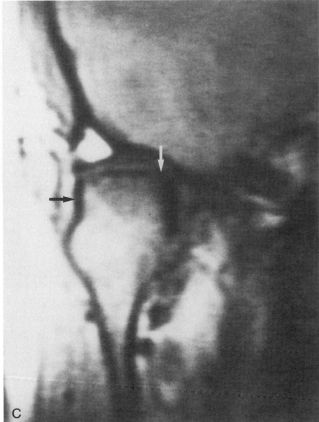

**FIGURE 18-90**   Mandibular asymmetry caused by condyle hyperplasia. **A,** Photograph. **B** and **C,** Sagittal and coronal MR images of the right condyle of a patient with deviation of the chin to the left. The MR images show elongation of the condyle and condyle neck (*arrows*) as the cause of mandibular asymmetry.

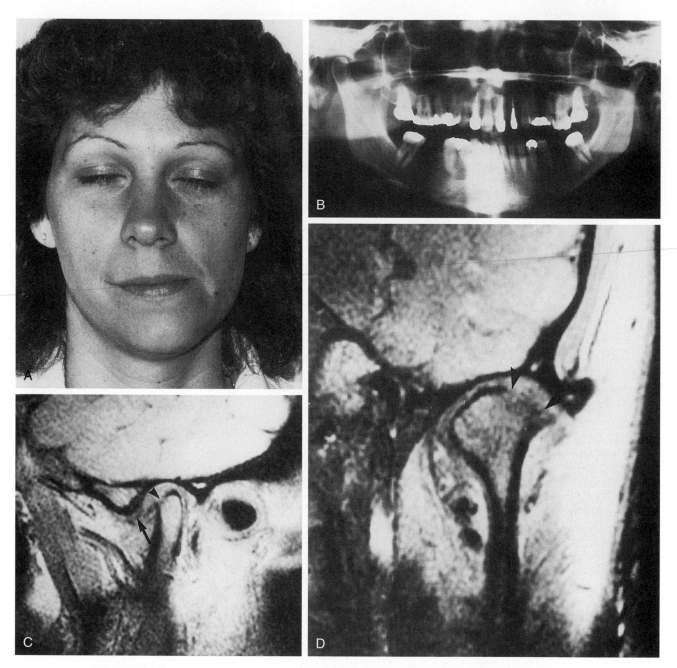

**FIGURE 18-91**    Mandibular asymmetry secondary to condyle hypoplasia. **A**, Photograph. **B**, Panoramic image. **C**, Sagittal MR image. **D**, Coronal MR image. There is deviation of the chin to the left. Panoramic view (**B**) shows a normal configuration on the right side of the mandible. The left side shows shortening of the ramus and regressive remodeling of the left condyle. MR images (**C** and **D**) show erosive changes of the condyle (*arrowheads*) and anterior disk displacement (*arrow*). The diminished size of the left condyle was the cause of the asymmetry in this patient.

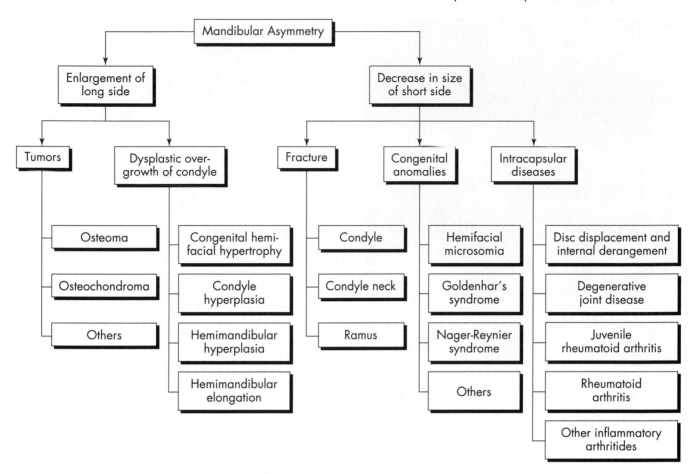

**FIGURE 18-92**    Etiologies of mandibular asymmetry.

to obtain real-time dynamic MR images. This will make possible the study of joint dynamics without injection of contrast medium or a local anesthetic. Pseudodynamic imaging with magnetic resonance is possible today, but its value for diagnostic work is not fully understood.[169] Multiple images are collected with the mouth opened to different widths, and the images are rapidly viewed on a *cine loop*. This creates the illusion of a real-time examination even though the images were acquired at separate points in time. However, the position of the disk can be followed, and the snapping of the condyle over the back of the disk can be appreciated.

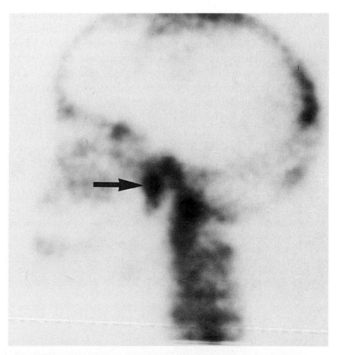

**FIGURE 18-93**    Radionuclide imaging of a patient with condylar hyperplasia of the left TMJ (*arrow*).

---

**BOX 18-5**

**IMAGING STRATEGY FOR PATIENTS WITH MANDIBULAR ASYMMETRY**

1. Lateral and anterior posterior cephalograms
2. Lateral tomograms of TMJs, including entire mandibular ramus
3. MR imaging or arthrography of both left and right TMJs

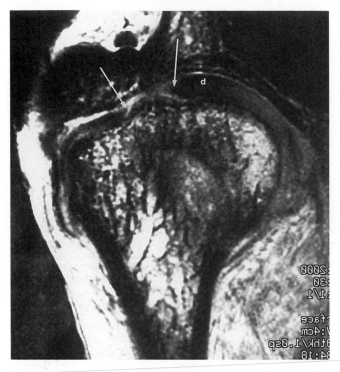

**FIGURE 18-94** High-resolution MR image. This experimental MR image was obtained with a slice thickness of 1.5 mm and a field of view of 4 cm. The perforation of the disk (between the *long arrows*) and the osteophyte of the condyle filling the perforation are well visualized. The disk (*d*) is indicated for orientation.

## MR Spectroscopy

The third area that will probably develop into a more useful clinical tool is MR spectroscopy. This may be helpful in evaluating metabolic and biochemical changes in the joints and muscles. Previous reports have suggested abnormalities of lactate accumulation in the intervertebral peridiskal tissues of the spine in the presence of degeneration and herniation.[170] MR spectroscopy has also been applied to experimental situations and appears capable of showing changes in areas of inflammation.[171]

## REFERENCES

1. Katzberg RW. Temporomandibular joint imaging. Radiology 1989; 170:297–307.
2. Rees LA. The structure and function of the mandibular joint. Br Dent J 1954;96:125–133.
3. Adams JC, Hamblen DL. Outline of Orthopedics, 13th ed., London: Churchill Livingstone, 2001;135.
4. Eriksson L, Westesson PL. Clinical and radiological study of patients with anterior disc displacement of the temporomandibular joint. Swed Dent J 1983;7:55–64.
5. Katzberg RW, Dolwick MF, Helms CA, et al. Arthrotomography of the temporomandibular joint. AJR 1980;134:995–1003.
6. Westesson PL. Double-contrast arthrography and internal derangement of the temporomandibular joint. Swed Dent J Suppl 1982;13:1–57.
7. Wilkes CH. Arthrography of the temporomandibular joint in patients with the TMJ pain-dysfunction syndrome. Minn Med 1978;61:645–652.
8. Wilkes CH. Structural and functional alterations of the temporomandibular joint. Northwest Dent 1978;57:287–294.
9. Wilkes CH. Internal derangements of the temporomandibular joint. Arch Otolaryngol 1989;115:469–477.
10. Brooks SL, Westesson PL. Temporomandibular joint: value of coronal MR images. Radiology 1993;188:317–321.
11. Katzberg RW, Westesson PL, Tallents RH, et al. Temporomandibular joint: magnetic resonance assessment of rotational and sideways disc displacements. Radiology 1988;169:741–748.
12. Liedberg J, Westesson PL. Sideways position of the temporomandibular joint disk: coronal cryosectioning of fresh autopsy specimens. Oral Surg Oral Med Oral Pathol 1988;66:644–649.
13. Liedberg J, Westesson PL, Kurita K. Sideways and rotational displacement of the temporomandibular joint disk: diagnosis by arthrography and correlation to cryosectional morphology. Oral Surg Oral Med Oral Pathol 1990;69:757–763.
14. Ireland VE. The problem of the "clicking jaw." Proc R Soc Med 1951;44:363–372.
15. Isberg-Holm AM, Westesson PL. Movement of disc and condyle in temporomandibular joints with clicking: an arthrographic and cineradiographic study on autopsy specimens. Acta Odontol Scand 1982;40:151–164.
16. Isberg-Holm AM, Westesson PL. Movement of disc and condyle in temporomandibular joints with and without clicking: a high speed cinematographic and dissection study on autopsy specimens. Acta Odontol Scand 1982;40:165–177.
17. Westesson PL. Arthrography of the temporomandibular joint. J Prosthet Dent 1984;51:534–543.
18. Westesson PL, Rohlin M. Internal derangement related to osteoarthritis in temporomandibular joint autopsy specimens. Oral Surg Oral Med Oral Pathol 1984;57:17–22.
19. Westesson PL, Bronstein SL, Liedberg J. Internal derangement of the temporomandibular joint: morphologic description with correlation to function. Oral Surg Oral Med Oral Pathol 1985;59: 323–331.
20. Bessette RW, Katzberg RW, Natiella JR, et al. Diagnosis and reconstruction of the human temporomandibular joint after trauma or internal derangement. Plast Reconstr Surg 1985;75:192–205.
21. Kurita K, Westesson PL, Sternby NH, et al. Histologic features of the temporomandibular joint disk and posterior disk attachment: comparison of symptom-free persons with normally positioned disks and patients with internal derangement. Oral Surg Oral Med Oral Pathol 1989;67:635–643.
22. Blaustein DI, Scapino RP. Remodelling of the temporomandibular joint disk and posterior attachment in disk displacement specimens in relation to glycosaminoglycan content. Oral Surg Oral Med Oral Pathol 1986;78:756–764.
23. Isberg AM, Isacsson G. Tissue reactions associated with internal derangement of the temporomandibular joint: a radiographic, cryomorphologic, and histologic study. Acta Odontol Scand 1986;44:160–164.
24. Pereira FJ Jr, Lundh H, Eriksson L, et al. Histologic characterization of the TMJ in patients and asymptomatic persons. Manuscript in preparation.
25. Westesson PL. Double-contrast arthrotomography of the temporomandibular joint: introduction of an arthrographic technique for visualization of the disc and articular surfaces. J Oral Maxillofac Surg 1983;41:163–172.
26. Westesson PL. Structural hard-tissue changes in temporomandibular joints with internal derangement. Oral Surg Oral Med Oral Pathol 1985;59:220–224.
27. Paesani D, Westesson PL, Hatala MP, et al. Accuracy of clinical diagnosis for TMJ internal derangement and arthrosis. Oral Surg Oral Med Oral Pathol 1992;73:360–363.
28. Roberts D, Schenck J, Joseph P, et al. Temporomandibular joint: magnetic resonance imaging. Radiology 1985;155:829–830.
29. Roberts CA, Tallents RH, Espeland MA, et al. Mandibular range of motion versus arthrographic diagnosis of the temporomandibular joint. Oral Surg Oral Med Oral Pathol 1985;60:244–251.
30. Roberts CA, Tallents RH, Katzberg RW, et al. Clinical and arthrographic evaluation of temporomandibular joint sounds. Oral Surg Oral Med Oral Pathol 1986;62:373–376.
31. Roberts CA, Tallents RH, Katzberg RW, et al. Comparison of internal derangements of the TMJ to occlusal findings. Oral Surg Oral Med Oral Pathol 1987;63:645–650.

32. Roberts CA, Tallents RH, Katzberg RW, et al. Clinical and arthrographic evaluation of the location of TMJ pain. Oral Surg Oral Med Oral Pathol 1987;64:6–8.

33. Roberts CA, Tallents RH, Katzberg RW, et al. Comparison of arthrographic findings of the temporomandibular joint with palpation of the muscles of mastication. Oral Surg Oral Med Oral Pathol 1987;64:275–277.

34. Anderson GC, Schiffman EL, Schellhas KP, et al. Clinical vs. arthrographic diagnosis of TMJ internal derangement. J Dent Res 1989;68:826–829.

35. Drace JE, Enzmann DR. Defining the normal temporomandibular joint: closed-, partially open-, and open-mouth MR imaging of asymptomatic subjects. Radiology 1990;177:67–71.

36. Kircos LT, Ortendahl DA, Mark AS, et al. Magnetic resonance imaging of the TMJ disk in asymptomatic volunteers. J Oral Maxillofac Surg 1987;45:852–854.

37. Westesson PL, Eriksson L, Kurita K. Temporomandibular joint: variation of normal arthrographic anatomy. Oral Surg Oral Med Oral Pathol 1990;69(4):514–519.

38. Boden SD, Davis DO, Dina TS, et al. Abnormal magnetic resonance scans of the lumbar spine in asymptomatic subjects. A prospective investigation. J Bone Joint Surg (Am) 1990;72:403–408.

39. Boden SD, Davis DO, Dina TS, et al. A prospective and blinded investigation of magnetic resonance imaging of the knee. Abnormal findings in asymptomatic subjects. Clin Orthop 1992;282:177–185.

40. Kornick J, Trefelner NE, McCarty S, et al. Meniscal abnormalities in the asymptomatic population in MR imaging. Radiology 1990;177:463–465.

41. Nagendak WG, Fernandez FR, Halbrun LK, et al. Magnetic resonance imaging of meniscal degeneration in asymptomatic knees. J Orthop Res 1990;8:311–320.

42. Shellock FG, Morris E, Deutsch AL, et al. Hematopoietic bone marrow hyperplasia: high prevalence on MR images of the knee in asymptomatic marathon runners. AJR 1992;158:335–338.

43. Paesani D, Westesson PL, Hatala M, et al. Prevalence of internal derangement in patients with craniomandibular disorders. Am J Orthod Dentofacial Orthop 1992;101:41–47.

44. Tasaki MM, Westesson PL, Isberg AM, Tallents RH, Ren YF. Classification and prevalence of temporomandibular joint disk displacement in patients and asymptomatic volunteers. Am J Orthod Dentofac Orthop 1996;109:249–262.

45. Katzberg RW, Westesson PL, Tallents RH, Drake CM. Orthodontics and temporomandibular joint internal derangement. Am J Orthod Dentofac Orthop 1996;109:515–520.

46. Katzberg RW, Westesson PL, Tallents RH, Drake CM. Anatomic disorders of the temporomandibular joint disc in asymptomatic subjects. J Oral Maxillofac Surg 1996;54:147–153.

47. Larheim TA, Westesson P, Sano T. Temporomandibular joint disk displacement: comparison in asymptomatic volunteers and patients. Radiology 2001;218:428–432.

48. Widmalm S-E, Westesson PL, Kim I-K, et al. Temporomandibular joint pathosis related to sex, age, and dentition in autopsy material. Oral Surg Oral Med Oral Pathol 1994;78:416–425.

49. Oberg T, Carlsson GE, Fajers CM. The temporomandibular joint: a morphologic study of human autopsy material. Acta Odontal Scand 1971;29:349–384.

50. McCabe JB, Keller SE, Moffet BC. A new radiographic technique for diagnosing temporomandibular joint disorders. J Dent Res 1959;38:663.

51. Omnell K-A, Peterson A. Radiography of the temporomandibular joint utilizing oblique lateral transcranial projections: comparison of information obtained with standardized technique and individualized technique. Odontol Rev 1976;26:77–92.

52. Nørgaard F. Artografi av kaebeleddet. Preliminary report. Acta Radiol 1944;25:679–685.

53. Nørgaard F. Temporomandibular Arthrography. Thesis. Copenhagen: Munksgaard, 1947.

54. Farrar WB, McCurty WL Jr. Inferior joint space arthrography and characteristics of condylar paths in internal derangements of the TMJ. J Prosthet Dent 1979;41:548–555.

55. Katzberg RW, Dolwick MF, Bales DJ, et al. Arthrotomography of the temporomandibular joint: new technique and preliminary observations. AJR 1979;132:949–955.

56. Westesson PL, Omnell K-Å, Rohlin M. Double-contrast tomography of the temporomandibular joint. A new technique based on autopsy examinations. Acta Radiol (Diagn) (Stockh) 1980;21:777–784.

57. Annadale T. Displacement of the inter-articular cartilage of the lower jaw and its treatment by operation. Lancet 1987;1:411.

58. Burman M, Sinberg SE. Condylar movement in the study of internal derangement of the temporomandibular joint. J Bone Joint Surg (Br) 1946;28:351–373.

59. Farrar WB. Diagnosis and treatment of anterior dislocation of the articular disc. NY J Dent 1971;41:348–351.

60. Pringle JH. Displacement of the mandibular meniscus and its treatment. Br J Surg 1918;6:385–389.

61. Silver CM, Simon SD, Savastano AA. Meniscus injuries of the temporomandibular joint. J Bone Joint Surg (Am) 1956;38A:541–552.

62. Bell KA, Walters PJ. Videofluoroscopy during arthrography of the temporomandibular joint. Radiology 1983;147:879.

63. Dolwick MF, Riggs RR. Diagnosis and treatment of internal derangements of the temporomandibular joint. Dent Clin North Am 1983;27:561–572.

64. Lundh H, Westesson PL, Kopp S, et al. Anterior repositioning splint in the treatment of temporomandibular joints with reciprocal clicking: comparison with a flat occlusal splint and an untreated control group. Oral Surg Oral Med Oral Pathol 1985;60:131–136.

65. McCarty WL, Farrar WB. Surgery for internal derangements of the temporomandibular joint. J Prosthet Dent 1979;42:191–196.

66. McCarty WL. Surgery. In: Farrar WB, McCarthy WL, eds. A Clinical Outline of Temporomandibular Joint Diagnosis and Treatment, 7th ed. Montgomery, Ala: Normandie Publications, 1982.

67. Arnaudow M, Haage H, Pflaum I. Die Doppelkontrastarthrographie des Kiefergelenkes. Dtsch Zahnarztl Z 1968;23:390–393.

68. Arnaudow M, Pflaum I. Neue Erkenntnisse in der beurteilung bei der Kiefergelenktomographie. Dtsch Zahnarztl Z 1974;29:554–556.

69. Tallents RH, Katzberg RW, Macher DJ, et al. Arthrographically assisted splint therapy: 6-month follow-up. J Prosthet Dent 1986;56:224–226.

70. Ross JB. The intracapsular therapeutic modalities in conjunction with arthrography: case reports. J Craniomandib Disord 1989;3:35–43.

71. Katzberg RW, Westesson PL. Temporomandibular Joint Arthrography, Section I. Single Contrast Arthrography. In: Diagnosis of the temporomandibular joint. Philadelphia: WB Saunders, 1993;101–142.

72. Katzberg RW, Westesson PL. Double Contrast Arthrography. In: Diagnosis of the Temporomandibular Joint. Philadelphia: WB Saunders, 1993;143–165.

73. Westesson PL, Eriksson L, Kurita K. Reliability of a negative clinical temporomandibular joint examination: prevalence of disk displacement in asymptomatic temporomandibular joints. Oral Surg Oral Med Oral Pathol 1989;68:551–554.

74. Anderson QN, Katzberg RW. Loose bodies of the temporomandibular joint: arthrographic diagnosis. Skeletal Radiol 1984;11:42–46.

75. Manzione JV, Seltzer SE, Katzberg RW, et al. Direct sagittal computed tomography of the temporomandibular joint. AJNR 1982;3:677–679.

76. Manzione JV, Katzberg RW, Brodsky GI, et al. Internal derangement of the temporomandibular joint: diagnosis by direct sagittal computed tomography. Radiology 1984;150:111–115.

77. Helms CA, Morrish RB Jr, Kircos LT, et al. Computed tomography of the meniscus of the temporomandibular joint: preliminary observations. Radiology 1982;145:719–722.

78. Manco LG, Messing SG, Busino LJ, et al. Internal derangements of the temporomandibular joint evaluated with direct sagittal CT: a prospective study. Radiology 1985;157:407–412.

79. Sartoris DJ, Neumann CH, Riley RW. The temporomandibular joint: true sagittal computed tomography with meniscus visualization. Radiology 1984;150:250–254.

80. Thompson JR, Christiansen EL, Hasso AN, et al. The temporomandibular joint: high resolution computed tomographic evaluation. Radiology 1984;150:105–110.

81. Westesson PL, Katzberg RW, Tallents RH, et al. CT and MRI of the temporomandibular joint: comparison with autopsy specimens. AJR 1987;148:1165–1171.

82. Harms SE, Wilk RM, Wolford LM, et al. The temporomandibular joint: magnetic resonance imaging using surface coils. Radiology 1985;157:133–136.

83. Katzberg RW, Schenck J, Roberts D, et al. Magnetic resonance imaging of the temporomandibular joint meniscus. Oral Surg Oral Med Oral Pathol 1985;59:332–335.

84. Katzberg RW, Besettte RW, et al. Normal and abnormal temporomandibular joint: MR imaging with surface coil. Radiology 1986;158:183–189.

85. Larheim TA. Imaging of the temporomandibular joint in rheumatic disease. In: Westesson PL, Katzberg RW, eds. Imaging of the Temporomandibular Joint, Vol. 1. Cranio Clinics International. Baltimore: Williams & Wilkins, 1991;133–153.

86. Larheim TA. Imaging of the temporomandibular joint in juvenile rheumatoid arthritis. In: Westesson PL, Katzberg RW, eds. Imaging of the Temporomandibular Joint, Vol. 1. Cranio Clinics International. Baltimore: Williams & Wilkins, 1991;155–172.

87. Manzione JV, Katzberg RW, Tallents RH, et al. Magnetic resonance imaging of the temporomandibular joint. J Am Dent Assoc 1986;113:398–402.

88. Schellhas KP. MR imaging of muscles of mastication. AJR 1989;153:847–855.

89. Schellhas KP, Wilkes CH, Fritts HM, et al. MR of osteochondritis dissecans and avascular necrosis of the mandibular condyle. AJNR 1989;10:3–12.

90. Hansson L-G, Westesson PL, Katzberg RW, et al. MR imaging of the temporomandibular joint: comparison of images of autopsy specimens made at 0.3 T and 1.5 T with anatomic cryosections. AJR 1989;152:1241–1244.

91. Hardy CJ, Katzberg RW, Frey RL, et al. Switched surface coil system for bilateral MR imaging. Radiology 1988;167:835–838.

92. Shellock FG, Pressman BD. Dual-surface-coil MR imaging of bilateral temporomandibular joints: improvements in imaging protocol. AJNR 1989;10:595–598.

93. Isberg A, Stenstrom B, Isacsson G. Frequency of bilateral temporomandibular joint disc displacement in patients with unilateral symptoms: a 5-year follow-up of the asymptomatic joint. A clinical and arthrotomographic study. Dentomaxillofac Radiol 1991;20:73-76.

94. Sanchez-Woodworth RE, Tallents RH, Katzberg RW, et al. Bilateral internal derangements of temporomandibular joint: evaluation by magnetic resonance imaging. Oral Surg Oral Med Oral Pathol 1988;65:281–285.

95. Musgrave MT, Westesson PL, Tallents RH, et al. Improved magnetic resonance imaging of the temporomandibular joint by oblique scanning planes. Oral Surg Oral Med Oral Pathol 1991;71:525–528.

96. Manzione JV, Tallents RH. "Pseudomeniscus" sign: potential indicator of repair or remodeling in temporomandibular joints with internal derangements. Presented at Radiologic Society of North America. Radiology 1992;185(suppl):175.

97. Paesani D, Westesson PL. MR imaging of the TMJ: decreased signal from the retrodiscal tissue. Oral Surg Oral Med Oral Pathol 1993;76:631–635.

98. Westesson PL, Brooks SL. Temporomandibular joint: relation between MR evidence of effusion and the presence of pain and disk displacement. AJR 1992;159:559–563.

99. Larheim TA, Westesson PL, Sano T. MR grading of temporomandibular joint fluid: association with disk displacement categories, condyle marrow abnormalities and pain. Int J Oral Maxillofac Surg 2001;30:104–112.

100. Rudisch A, Innerhofer K, Bertram S, Emshoff R. Magnetic resonance imaging findings of internal derangement and effusion in patients with unilateral temporomandibular joint pain. Oral Surg Oral Med Oral Pathol Oral Radiol Endod 2001;92:566–571.

101. Larheim TA, Katzberg RW, Westesson PL, Tallents RH, Moss ME. MR evidence of temporomandibular joint fluid and condyle marrow alterations: occurence in asymptomatic volunteers and symptomatic patients. Int J Oral Maxillofac Surg 2001;30:113–117.

102. Pereira FJ Jr, Lundh H, Westesson PL, Carlsson LE. Clinical findings related to morphologic changes in TMJ autopsy specimens. Oral Surg Oral Med Oral Pathol 1994;78:288–295.

103. Lundh H, Westesson PL, Kopp S. A three year follow-up of patients with reciprocal temporomandibular joint clicking. Oral Surg Oral Med Oral Pathol 1987;63:530–533.

104. Rasmussen OC. Description of population and progress of symptoms in a longitudinal study of temporomandibular arthropathy. Scand J Dent Res 1981;89:196–203.

105. Randolph CS, Greene CS, Moretti R, Forbes D, Perry HT. Conservative management of temporomandibular disorders: a posttreatment comparison between patients from a university clinic and from private practice. Am J Orthod Dentofacial Orthop 1990;98:77–82.

106. Schellhas KP, Wilkes CH. Temporomandibular joint inflammation: comparison of MR fast scanning with T1-and T2-weighted imaging techniques. AJR 1989;153:93–98.

107. Schellhas KP, Wilkes CH, Omlie MR, Peterson CM, Johnson SD, Keck RJ, Block JC, Fritts HM, Heithoff KB. The diagnosis of temporomandibular joint disease: two-compartment arthrography and MR. AJR 1988;151:341–350.

108. Schellhas KP. Internal derangement of the temporomandibular joint: radiologic staging with clinical, surgical, and pathologic correlation. Magn Reson Imaging 1989;7:495–515.

109. Schellhas KP, Wilkes CH. Temporomandibular joint inflammation: comparison of MR fast scanning with T1- and T2-weighted imaging techniques. AJR 1989;153:93–98.

110. Schellhas KP, Wilkes CH, Fritts HM, Omlie MR, Lagrotteria LB. MR of osteochondritis dissecans and avascular necrosis of the mandibular condyle. AJR 1989;152:551–560.

111. Schellhas KP. Temporomandibular joint injuries. Radiology 1989; 173:211–216.

112. Larheim TA, Westesson PL, Hicks DG, Eriksson L, Brown D. Osteonecrosis of the temporomandibular joint: correlation of magnetic resonance imaging and histology. J Oral Maxillofac Surg 1999;57:888–898.

113. Sano T, Westesson PL, Larheim TA, Rubin SJ, Tallents RH. Osteoarthritis and abnormal bone marrow of the mandibular condyle. Oral Surg Oral Med Oral Pathol Oral Radiol Endod 1999;87:243–252.

114. Reiskin AB. Aseptic necrosis of the mandibular condyle: a common problem? Quintessence Int 1979;2:85–89.

115. Lieberman JM, Gardner CL, Motta AO, Schwartz RD. Prevalence of bone marrow signal abnormalities observed in the temporomandibular joint using magnetic resonance imaging. J Oral Maxillofac Surg 1996;54:434–439.

116. Sano T, Westesson PL, Larheim TA, Takagi R. The association of temporomandibular joint pain with abnormal bone marrow of the mandibular condyle. J Oral Maxillofac Surg 2000;58: 254–257.

117. Resnick D, Sweet DE, Madewell JE. Osteonecrosis and osteochondrosis. In: Resnick D, ed. Bone and Joint Imaging, 2nd ed. Philadelphia: WB Saunders, 1996;941–959.

118. Rao VM, Lliem MD, Farole A, et al. Elusive "stuck" disk in the temporomandibular joint: diagnosis with MR imaging. Radiology 1993;189:823–827.

119. Westesson PL, Rohlin M. Diagnostic accuracy of double-contrast arthrotomography of the temporomandibular joint: correlation with postmortem morphology. AJR 1984;143:655–660.

120. Westesson PL, Bronstein SL, Liedberg J. Temporomandibular joint: correlation between single-contrast videoarthrography and postmortem morphology. Radiology 1986;160:767–771.

121. Westesson PL, Katzberg RW, Tallents RH, et al. Temporomandibular joint: comparison of MR images with cryosectional anatomy. Radiology 1987;164:59–64.

122. Westesson PL, Bronstein SL. Temporomandibular joint: comparison of single- and double-contrast arthrography. Radiology 1987; 164:65–70.

123. Tasaki M, Westesson PL. Temporomandibular joint: diagnostic accuracy with sagittal and coronal MR imaging. Radiology 1993;186:723–729.

124. Hansson L-G, Eriksson L, Westesson PL. Temporomandibular joint: magnetic resonance evaluation after diskectomy. Oral Surg Med Oral Pathol 1992;74:801–810.

125. Kent JN, Misiek DJ, Akin RK, et al. Temporomandibular joint condylar prosthesis: a ten-year report. J Oral Maxillofac Surg 1983;41:245–254.

126. Kent JN, Block MS, Homsey CA, et al. Experience with a polymer glenoid fossa prosthesis for partial or total temporomandibular joint reconstruction. J Oral Maxillofac Surg 1986;44: 520–533.

127. Lindqvist C, Jokinen J, Paukku P, et al. Adaptation of autogenous costochondral grafts used for temporomandibular joint reconstruction: a long-term clinical and radiologic follow-up. J Oral Maxillofac Surg 1988;46(6):465–470.

128. Heffez LB. Imaging of internal derangements and synovial chondromatosis of the temporomandibular joint. Radiol Clin North Am 1993;31:149–162.

129. Nomoto M, Nagao K, Numata T, et al. Synovial osteochondromatosis of the temporomandibular joint. J Laryngol Otol 1993;107:742–745.

130. Quinn PD, Stanton DC, Foote JW. Synovial chondromatosis with cranial extension. Oral Surg Oral Med Oral Pathol 1992;73;398–402.

131. Sun S, Helmy E, Bays R. Synovial chondromatosis with intracranial extension: a case report. Oral Surg Oral Med Oral Pathol 1990;70:5–9.

132. Boccardi A. CT evaluation of chondromatosis of the temporomandibular joint. J Comput Assist Tomogr 1991;15:826–828.

133. Herzog S, Mafee M. Synovial chondromatosis of the TMJ: MR and CT findings. Am J Neuroradiol 1990;11:742–745.

134. van Ingen JM, de Man K, Bakri I. CT diagnosis of synovial chondromatosis of the temporomandibular joint. Br J Oral Maxillofac Surg 1990;28:164–167.

135. Rickert RR, Shapiro MJ. Pigmented villonodular synovitis of the temporomandibular joint. Otolaryngol Head Neck Surg 1982;90(5):668–670.

136. Lapayowker MS, Miller WT, Levy WM, Harwick RD. Pigmented villonodular synovitis of the temperomandibular joint. Radiology 1973;108(2):313–316.

137. Curtin HD, Williams R, Gallia L, Meyers EN. Pigmented villonodular synovitis of the temporomandibular joint. Comput Radiol 1983;7(4):257–260.

138. O'Sullivan TJ, Alport EC, Whiston HG. Pigmented villonodular synovitis of the temporomandibular joint. J Otolaryngol 1984;13(2):123–126.

139. Song MY, Heo MS, Lee SS, et al. Diagnostic imaging of pigmented villonodular synovitis of the temporomandibular joint associated with condylar expansion. Dentomaxillofac Radiol 1999;28(6):386–390.

140. Bemporad JA, Chaloupka JC, Putman CM, et al. Pigmented villonodular synovitis of the temporomandibular joint: diagnostic imaging and endovascular therapeutic embolization of a rare head and neck tumor. AJNR 1999;20(1):159–162.

141. Klenoff JR, Lowlicht RA, Lesnik T, Sasaki CT. Mandibular and temporomandibular joint arthropathy in the differential diagnosis of the parotid mass. Laryngoscope 2001;111(12):2162–2165.

142. Dijkgraaf LC, Liem RS, de Bont LG. Temporomandibular joint osteoarthritis and crystal deposition diseases: a study of crystals in synovial fluid lavages in osteoarthritic temporomandibular joints. Int J Oral Maxillofac Surg 1998;27(4):268–273.

143. Goudot P, Jaquinet A, Gilles R, Richter M. A destructive calcium pyrophosphate dihydrate deposition disease of the temporomandibular joint. J Craniofac Surg 1999;10(5):385–388.

144. Jibiki M, Shimoda S, Nakagawa Y, Kawasaki K, Asada K, Ishibashi K. Calcifications of the disc of the temporomandibular joint. J Oral Pathol Med 1999;28(9):413–419.

145. Olin HB, Pedersen K, Francis D, Hansen H, Poulsen FW. A very rare benign tumour in the parotid region: calcium pyrophosphate dihydrate crystal deposition disease. J Laryngol Otol 2001;115(6):504–506.

146. Jordan JA, Roland P, Lindberg G, Mendelsohn D. Calcium pyrophosphate deposition disease of the temporal bone. Ann Otol Rhinol Laryngol 1998;107(11 Pt 1):912–916.

147. Vargas A, Teruel J, Trull J, Lopez E, Pont J, Velayos A. Calcium pyrophosphate dihydrate crystal deposition disease presenting as a pseudotumor of the temporomandibular joint. Eur Radiol 1997;7(9):1452–1453.

148. Kurihara K, Mizuseki K, Saiki T, Wakisaka H, Maruyama S, Sonobe J. Tophaceous pseudogout of the temporomandibular joint: report of a case. Pathol Int 1997;47(8):578–580.

149. Slater LJ. Distinguishing calcium pyrophosphate dihydrate deposition disease from synovial chondrosarcoma. J Oral Maxillofac Surg 1998;56(5):693–694.

150. Lopes V, Jones JAH, Sloan P, et al. Temporomandibular ganglion or synovial cyst? Oral Surg Oral Med Oral Pathol 1994;77:627–630.

151. McGuirt WF, Myers EN. Ganglion of the temporomandibular joint. Presentation as a parotid mass. Otolaryngol Head Neck Surg 1993;109:950–953.

152. Noffke C, Raubenheimer E, Fischer E. Tumoral calcinosis of the temporomandibular joint region. Dentomaxillofac Radiol 2000;29(2):128–130.

153. Bhaskar SN. Synopsis of Oral Pathology. St. Louis: CV Mosby, 1977;304–324.

154. Ruben MM, Jui B, Cozzi GM. Metastatic carcinoma of the mandibular condyle presenting as temporomandibular joint syndrome. J Oral Maxillofac Surg 1989;47:511–513.

155. Zachariades N. Neoplasms metastatic to the mouth, jaws and surrounding tissues. J Craniomaxillofac Surg 1989;17:283–291.

156. Ruggiero SL, Donoff RB. Bone regeneration after mandibular resection: report of two cases. J Oral Maxillofac Surg 1991;49:647–651.

157. Smith HJ, Larheim TA, Aspestrand F. Rheumatic and nonrheumatic disease in the temporomandibular joint: gadolinium-enhanced MR imaging. Radiology 1992;185:229–234.

158. Barthelemy I, Karanas Y, Sannajust JP, Emering C, Mondie JM. Gout of the temporomandibular joint: pitfalls in diagnosis. J Craniomaxillofac Surg 2001;29(5):307–310.

159. Isberg A, Isacsson G, Nah KS. Mandibular coronoid process locking: a prospective study of frequency and association with internal derangement of the temporomandibular joint. Oral Surg Oral Med Oral Pathol 1987;63:275–279.

160. Langenbeck B. Augeborene kleinheit des unterkiefers; kiefersperre verbunden, geheilt durch resection der processus coronoidei. Archiv Klin Chir 1860;1:30.

161. Munk PL, Helms CA. Coronoid process hyperplasia: CT studies. Radiology 1989;171:783–784.

162. Markey RJ, Potter BE, Moffett BC. Condylar trauma and facial asymmetry: an experimental study. J Maxillofac Surg 1980;8:38–51.

163. Wang-Norderud R, Ragab RR. Unilateral condylar hyperplasia and the associated deformity of facial asymmetry. Scand J Plast Reconstr Surg Hand Surg 1977;11:91–96.

164. Lineaweaver W, Vargervik K, Tomer BS, et al. Posttraumatic condylar hyperplasia. Ann Plast Surg 1989;22:163–171.

165. Katzberg RW, Tallents RH, Hayakawa K, et al. Internal derangements of the temporomandibular joint: findings in the pediatric age group. Radiology 1985;154:125–127.

166. Westesson PL, Dahlberg G, Hansson L-G, et al. Osseous and muscular changes after vertical ramus osteotomy. An MRI study. Oral Surg Oral Med Oral Pathol 1991;72:139–145.

167. Collier DB, Carrera GF, Messer EJ, et al. Internal derangement of the temporomandibular joint: detection by single-photon emission computed tomography. Radiology 1983;149:557–561.

168. Katzberg RW, O'Mara RE, Tallents RH, et al. Radionuclide skeletal imaging and single photon emission computed tomography in suspected internal derangements of the temporomandibular joint. J Oral Maxillofac Surg 1984;42:782–787.

169. Bell KA, Jones JP, Miller KD, et al. The added gradient echo pulse sequence technique: application to imaging of fluid in the temporomandibular joint. AJNR 1993;14:375–381.

170. Diamant B, Karlsson J, Nachemson A. Correlation between lactate levels and pH in disks in patients with lumbar rhizopathies. Experientia 1969;24:1195–1196.

171. Alder ME, Dove SB, Murrah VA, et al. Magnetic resonance spectroscopy of inflammation associated with the temporomandibular joint. Oral Surg Oral Med Oral Pathol 1992;74:515–523.

# Index

Note: Page numbers followed by f indicate figures; those followed by t indicate tables.

## A

AAO-HNS nodal classification system, 1872, 1874t–1875t
ABCs. *See* Aneurysmal bone cysts (ABCs).
Abducens nerve, 542
  branchial arches and, 1759
Aberrant fusion proteins, chromosome translocation to generate, oncogene activation by, 2277–2278
Abscesses
  Bezold, 1178f
  cerebellar, 1179f
  cerebral, nasal dermal sinus resection for, 34–35
  epidural
    in sinusitis, 582f
    with mastoiditis, 1182, 1182f
  epiglottic, 1569f
  in submandibular gland space, 1821f
  in toxoplasmosis, 778f
  intracranial, 250
  laryngeal, 1672f
  of masticator space, 1822f, 1990f
  of oral cavity, 1400, 1401f–1403f, 1402
  of pinna, 2108f
  of sphenoid sinuses, 582f
  orbital, 575, 578f
  parotid, 2027, 2027f, 2028f, 2042f, 2047f
  peritonsillar, 1504–1505, 1506f, 1565f, 1566f
  postoperative, following craniofacial resection, 435f
  retropharyngeal, 1565f, 1817f, 1820f
  septal, 380
  subperiosteal, 580f–582f, 580–581
ACCs. *See* Acinic cell carcinomas (ACCs); Adenoid cystic carcinomas (ACCs; AdCCs).
Achalasia, 2211f

Achondroplasia, 1110t, 1165f
  of skull base, 857
Acinic cell carcinomas (ACCs), 2096
Acoustic nerve, hamartomas of, 1303, 1311f
Acoustic schwannomas, 1276–1285
  bilateral, 1277–1278, 1278f
  clinical evaluation with, 1278–1279, 1279f
  imaging appearance of, 1280–1285
    on computed tomography, 1280, 1281f, 1282f, 1283
    on magnetic resonance imaging, 1280f–1284f, 1283–1284
    secondary changes and, 1284–1285, 1285f
    size, location, and configuration and, 1280, 1280f–1283f
  incidence and terms for, 1276–1277, 1277t
  intracanalicular, 1303
  pathology of, 1277
  treatment of, 1279–1280
Acquired immunodeficiency syndrome (AIDS). *See also* Human immuno-deficiency virus (HIV) infections.
  coccidioidomycosis in, 1896
  neoplasia in, 2289–2290
  pharynx and, 1509, 1510f, 1511f, 1511–1512
  sinusitis in, 255
Acrocephalosyndactyly. *See* Apert's syndrome; Craniofacial dysostosis; Pfeiffer syndrome; Saethre-Chotzen syndrome.
Acromegaly, sinus enlargement in, 250f
Actinomycosis
  salivary glands and, 2037–2038
  sinonasal, 232–234

AdCCs. *See* Adenoid cystic carcinomas (ACCs; AdCCs).
Adductor paralysis, 1682, 1683f
Adelaide craniosynostosis. *See* Muenke syndrome.
Adenitis
  lacrimal, orbital pseudotumors and, 587, 590f
  retropharyngeal, 1505f
Adenoameloblastomas, 952–953, 957f
Adenocarcinomas
  basal cell, of salivary glands, 2084–2086, 2085f
  buccal, 1994f
  laryngeal, 1645
  low-grade, of salivary glands, 2096–2097, 2097f
  metastatic, lymph nodes in, 1927f, 1928f
  not otherwise specified, of salivary glands, 2104–2105, 2105f, 2106f
  ocular, 513
  of hard palate, 1444f
  of lacrimal gland, 644f
  of oral cavity, 1440, 1444f
  of parotid gland, with perineural tumor spread, 879f
  recurrent, following craniofacial resection, 435f
  sinonasal, 272, 274, 276–277, 282f
    intestinal-type, 274, 276–277
Adenoid(s)
  hypertrophic, 1509, 1510f, 1578, 1578f, 1579f
  retention cysts of, 1579f
Adenoid cystic carcinomas (ACCs; AdCCs)
  of facial nerve, 1327f
  of lacrimal gland, 645f
  of oral cavity, 1433, 1438, 1440f–1442f
  of parapharyngeal space, 1972, 1977f